PRACTICAL OBSTETRIC PROBLEMS

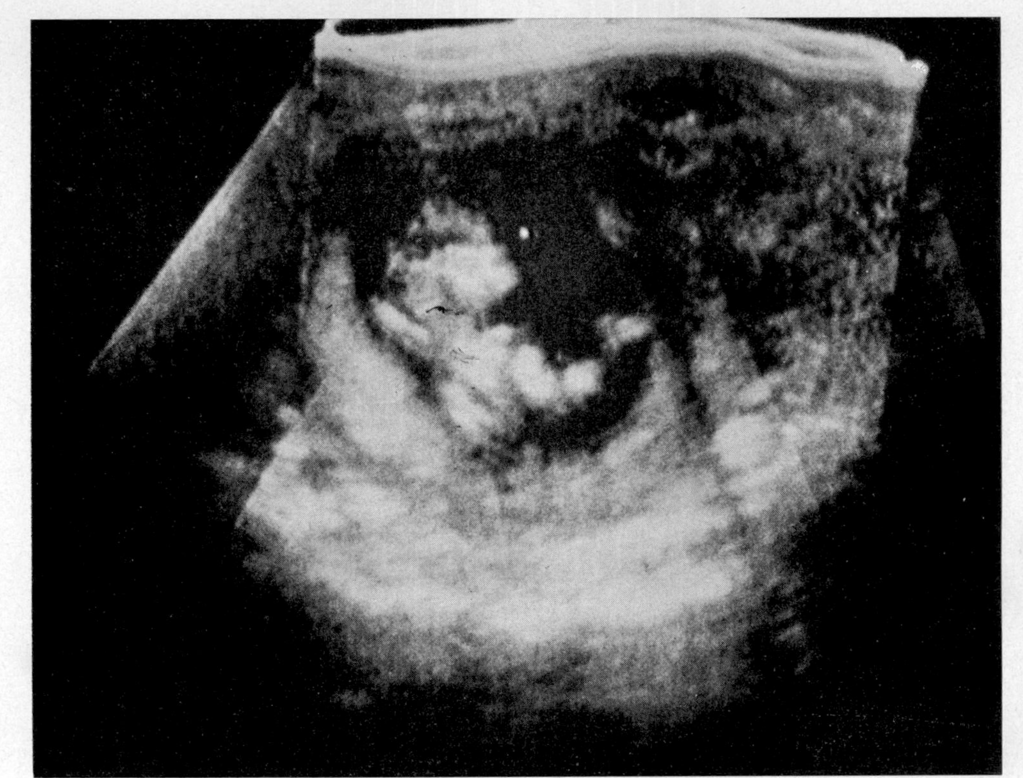

Diasonograph ultrasonogram (Nuclear Enterprises Ltd) of normal fetus of twelve-and-a-half weeks gestation (menstrual age).

(By courtesy of Editor, *British Journal of Radiology*.)

Practical Obstetric Problems

IAN DONALD

C.B.E., M.D., B.S. (Lond.), B.A. (Cape Town), F.R.C.S. (Glasg.), F.R.C.O.G., F.C.O.&G.(S.A.) Hon.F.A.C.O.G.

Emeritus Regius Professor of Midwifery, University of Glasgow; Honorary Research Consultant, National Maternity Hospital, Dublin; Formerly Reader, University of London, Institute of Obstetrics and Gynaecology, Hammersmith Hospital; One time Reader in Obstetrics and Gynaecology St. Thomas's Hospital Medical School, London; Eardley Holland Gold Medallist, Royal College of Obstetricians and Gynaecologists; Blair Bell Gold Medallist, Royal Society of Medicine; McKenzie Davidson Bronze Medallist, Royal College of Radiologists; Victor Bonney Prize, Royal College of Surgeons of England

Fifth edition

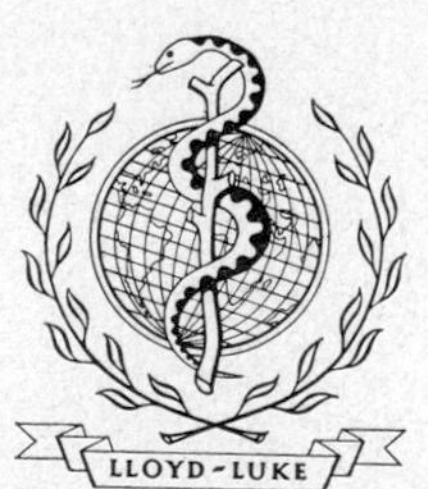

LLOYD-LUKE (MEDICAL BOOKS) LTD
49 NEWMAN STREET
LONDON
1979

FIRST EDITION . .	1955
Reprinted . .	1956
SECOND EDITION .	1959
Reprinted . .	1960
Reprinted . .	1961
THIRD EDITION . .	1964
Reprinted . .	1966
FOURTH EDITION .	1969
Reprinted . .	1972
Reprinted . .	1974
FIFTH EDITION . .	1979

PRINTED AND BOUND IN ENGLAND BY
THE PITMAN PRESS
BATH

ISBN 0 85324 132 5

To all who have known doubt, perplexity and fear as I have known them,
To all who have made mistakes as I have,
To all whose humility increases with their knowledge of this most fascinating subject,

THIS BOOK IS DEDICATED

PREFACE TO FIFTH EDITION

TWENTY-FOUR years ago, when I wrote the preface to the first edition, I wondered what it was that drove a man to write a textbook. My friend, Professor Philip Rhodes, now of Newcastle upon Tyne, has since supplied the cynical answer that it was in the hope of learning something about the subject. I now know that he was right and after all these years it is still true. There has been much to learn since the last edition and in order to keep the book within manageable size every possible scrap of dead wood has had to be cut away, without, I trust, spoiling the anecdotal flavour.

A large new section has been inserted on the prenatal diagnosis of fetal handicap. This is an emotive subject since there is, as yet, little constructive therapy to offer except in cases of Rh haemolytic disease. The growing importance of genetics has been fully outlined by my colleague Professor Ferguson-Smith. It is an issue which has to be squarely faced, especially when the ever-growing multiplicity of antenatal screening tests comes under review by the media.

Another colleague, Dr Robert Logan, has supplied a new section on biochemistry, including an account of the methods involved. It may instruct the obstetrician on what to expect from the biochemist, and vice versa. With yet another conversion, this time to SI units, we seem to have gone to ground now with moles and millimoles!

More is written and less is known about the subject of toxaemia of pregnancy than any other. I am delighted therefore to welcome the contribution of Dr Ronald Weir, formerly of the M.R.C. Blood Pressure Unit in Glasgow, with whom we have co-operated at the Queen Mother's Hospital for many years.

It was with great sadness that, because of the untimely death of my friend Gordon Garland, I had to take on the revision of his chapters myself.

Recent developments in neonatal paediatrics have been far-reaching, and I have been lucky to have had so much help and advice from Dr John McLaurin, who has disabused my mind of much that I had hitherto taken for granted.

Medically speaking, the most fascinating and eventful period of a child's life is that part of it spent *in utero*; the book is increasingly orientated towards that aspect, and matters like lecithin:sphingomyelin ratios and intra-uterine growth retardation are bandied about with conversational familiarity. It is when we come to labour itself, however, that the greatest change in outlook has occurred, thanks largely to the active and modern management which has been so outstandingly successful at Holles Street, Dublin, and this without recourse to difficult forceps delivery or an increase in the incidence of Caesarean section.

Needless to say, the section on sonar (ultrasonics) has had to be completely re-written, and I am grateful to the editors of the Silver Jubilee number of the *Indian Journal of Obstetrics and Gynaecology* for permitting me to include much of what I published in that journal.

To my secretary, Miss Adèle Ure, I am as grateful as ever for her help, and for delaying her well-earned retirement until after my own.

This edition, which has had to cover so much new ground, has taken me over four years to complete. I have, of course, been busy at other things too, to say nothing of a couple of operations to replace my mitral valve and an increasing tempo of research—and publication. The patience, therefore, of my friend and publisher Douglas Luke is beyond all praise. He certainly deserved better.

Looking back over a long clinical lifetime, one tends to forget, or take for granted, one's successes; it is the failures which stand out like keloid scars, never to be forgotten and, hopefully, a warning to others. I have to recognise that if there is any classic mistake which I have not myself made it is simply because of the lack of time in which to commit it. It makes one wondrously sympathetic towards others in trouble. No apology is therefore made for the highly personal emphasis in this book.

A teacher's greatest contribution has been achieved when his pupils finally know more than he does himself. With this tribute to those whom I have had the privilege of instructing I conclude this, my last Obstetrical Will and Testament.

Glasgow
1978

IAN DONALD

PREFACE TO FIRST EDITION

THE art of teaching is the art of sharing enthusiasm. The teacher must, therefore, love what he teaches if he is not to become "as a tinkling cymbal". If, then, exuberance occasionally bubbles through the pages of this book, I know that my past students will understand, and I ask no forgiveness.

I have often wondered what drives men to write a textbook. In my case it was the persuasiveness of my publisher. He felt, and of course he is right, that there was a place for a book of a practical sort which would appeal to the clinician who lives in the rough and tumble of it all, as well as to aspirants for additional diplomas in the subject.

We agreed upon a strategic size, and therefore, we hope, upon a palatable price, but apart from that I was given a completely free hand. I gladly accepted the excuse to omit the inevitable dreary irrelevance of such matters as ovulation, menstruation, conception, infertility, diagnosis of pregnancy and the early development of the ovum, which can be found in most textbooks of midwifery, making them heavy upon the knee as well as upon the mental digestion of the reader. Having got bid of this burden, I found myself free to get down to the real business of midwifery. In doing so I may or may not have pleased my public (if any) but I certainly pleased myself. The would-be pianist does not struggle through his Beethoven because of the imagined needs of a hypothetical audience. His efforts are owed to the Master. It is in this spirit that I have written, and I can only hope that some will find it infectious.

The task of nearly two years has been made pleasurable by all the willing and at times argumentative help I have had from colleagues and friends, above all, Gordon Garland, who has scrutinised every sentence I have written and at times supplied sobering criticism. I owe much to his encouragement, though it would not be fair to hold him in any way responsible for my statements. In addition to writing two chapters on the malpresentations he has read the proofs and has provided many of the illustrations. The toxaemias of pregnancy are not easy to deal with in a modern way without becoming "woolly", and I am therefore very glad of Harvey Carey's chapter thereon with his uncompromising clarity. Hilda Roberts, besides giving most of my anaesthetics in the last two years, has devoted years of practical research to the relief of pain in labour and has very fittingly written this chapter.

My views upon the misuse of the antibiotics are so strong that I thought it a good plan to seek the help of one whose views are even stronger and certainly more expert. I therefore asked William Hayes for a chapter on these lines before his recent visit to the U.S.A. The book is worth while if only for this authoritative piece of work, the like of which is not to be found in most other volumes.

Illustrations are often more of a problem to the author than the text itself, unless he happens to be a collector from lifelong habit. A great many are the work of the photographic and X-ray departments of the Postgraduate Medical School and Hammersmith Hospital, whose help is gratefully acknowledged. In other instances acknowledgements are made in the appropriate places. The line drawings are by Miss Pat Burrows who, besides her rapid skill, has the convenient property of being able to rise to the occasion demanded, regardless of the Sabbath.

One could not write a book, even of this modest size, in the midst of ordinary professional activity, without the help of a good secretary, and I have been fortunate in Miss Joan Bush. She worked fast and well, and her cheerful composure helped to prevent things from getting out of hand when time appeared to be running short.

The Postgraduate Medical School library is a remarkable place, the more so because of the efficiency of the Librarian, Miss Atkins, for whose help I am much indebted.

I started this preface by alluding to the persuasiveness of my publisher, but Mr. Douglas Luke is more than that. He is a delightful slave driver, but he is also patient and meticulous, for all his enthusiasm. Our association has been a very happy one, although I will try to discourage him, for the present, from making me write another book.

It would not be fair, in all these acknowledgements, to omit mention of my long-suffering wife and family, who have put up with me and my book for so many months. Most of the time that I gave to the task was really their time and their contribution has been the calm with which they have managed to surround my domestic life and without which I would surely have failed.

In retrospect it has been worth while and if, in the pages that follow, I have at times provoked, instructed and amused, then I am content.

September 1954 IAN DONALD

CONTENTS

CHAPTER I

THE SCOPE OF ANTENATAL CARE

As the hazards to the mother of pregnancy and labour continue to recede, so too have those to the fetus come to be recognised more acutely during its intra-uterine existence. The first 38 weeks of human life spent in the allegedly protected environment of the amniotic sac are medically more eventful and more fraught with danger and accident than the next 38 years in the lifespan of most human individuals. The scope therefore of antenatal care is widening rapidly in this direction.

We are only on the threshold of a new and far more important type of antenatal care than hitherto, and, inasmuch as prevention is always better than cure, it is the function of antenatal care to reduce the need for desperate measures at the time of delivery. Unfortunately the present situation leaves little room for more than "divine discontent", since we cannot yet match the recent improvement in labour room tactics with those of antenatal care itself. Nevertheless, gone are the days, I hope, of the hospital "cram clinic" which treated its patients like machine parts on an assembly line, being mainly concerned with the prevention of eclampsia, the correction of malpresentation and recognising disproportion, if it could. The ability to see 60 patients in 65 minutes is a type of pre-war insult—according to the patient little more recognition than the status of an appendage of her gravid uterus and its contents. To a woman who may have waited an hour or more in an unattractive waiting space in even less attractive company, the rapid exposure of her bulging abdominal surface and the overhearing of a few muttered remarks to some assistant writing notes, followed by a hurried dismissal, must have seemed a travesty of medical care as indeed it was. Yet such tactics have not entirely died out.

If the survey of the present position is disquieting, at least a brief look back into history gives comfort for what has been done in a relatively short period of time.

History

Antenatal care began as a social service in Paris in 1788 for women who had committed the double inconvenience of being both pregnant and destitute (femmes abandonnées). These pitiable creatures were housed, sometimes two or three to a bed, in the Hôtel Dieu and Hôpital Salpetrière from the thirty-sixth week of pregnancy onwards.

For over a hundred more years the problem of disposal seems to have been a more pressing objective than treatment or preventive care. To some extent this was due to a failure to recognise the importance of emergencies peculiar to the gravid state and illnesses occurring in pregnancy found their way to an unwelcome reception in general wards whose staff feared, with good reason, that the patient might do something awkward like going into labour and generally making a nuisance of herself in unsuitable surroundings.

It was in Edinburgh at the very end of the last century that the first effective medical and scientific interest was shown in the antenatal patient. In 1902 the first antenatal bed (all of one bed in fact) was endowed for the purpose. Admittedly Ballantyne's original concern was fetal deformity and stillbirth but this soon came to embrace a wider interest in maternal well-being which, on more general adoption by the end of the 1914–18 war, had swamped concern for the unborn child. In fact until the period following the last war it was thoughtlessly assumed that antenatal care which was good enough for the mother was good enough to cover the needs of the baby as well.

A few heretics talked about "antenatal paediatrics" but they were not taken very seriously. This complacency has been shaken first by the recognition of the possible effects of certain viruses upon the baby following Gregg's observations in 1941, in Australia,[6] on the association between maternal rubella in early pregnancy and cataract, secondly by Dr Alice Stewart's enquiry into the harmful effects of X-rays upon the fetus, increasing the hazard of leukaemia in later childhood[21] and, finally at the end of 1961, came the terrible tragedy of thalidomide-deformed babies, so promptly spotted, reported and acted upon[9, 10, 18, 20] after the association between this drug and limb and intestinal deformities was first suspected in Western Germany. The firm supplying thalidomide very rightly withdrew the drug from sale at the first suggestion of responsibility, but even so it was reckoned that not less than 800 babies in this country alone were likely to have been damaged. If such a catastrophe could follow the taking, in early pregnancy, of so apparently harmless a sedative and anti-emetic as thalidomide then what of the possible effects of all sorts of other agencies—drugs, poisons, radiations, metabolic diseases, even psychosomatic and stress disorders? The intra-uterine vulnerability of the baby is now in all our minds and congential abnormalities can no longer be accepted with fatalism. And so the wheel has turned full circle and Ballantyne's original teratological interest is revived.

Perinatal Mortality

Obstetrical units throughout the country have been stimulated to a sort of self examination by the ever-increasing practice of studying perinatal mortality statistics, which reached its most intensive peak in the nation-wide Perinatal Mortality Survey instituted by the National Birthday Trust.[14] Perinatal mortality is defined as the sum of stillbirths and deaths within the first week of life, because there is a good deal of overlap in the aetiology of both types of disaster. As people like Sir Dugald Baird have repeatedly pointed out, this rate depends a good deal upon the social standards of different areas and there is danger of comparing like with unlike. For example, in a poor industrial area like Glasgow the rate is considerably worse than in the country as a whole and the rate improves in the more prosperous Southern parts of England. Provisional figures from the quarterly return of the Registrar-General, Scotland, are 28 per 1000 births for Glasgow in 1972, but 22 per 1000 for Great Britain as a whole (Office of Population Censuses and Surveys, General Register Office, Scotland). Even the best obstetrical care can to some extent be offset by bad social conditions, at least as far as perinatal and mortality statistics go.

Five social classes are conveniently recognised as follows:—

I. Professional workers, directors and departmental managers.
II. So-called "white collared workers", small farmers, small shopkeepers, sales representatives and teachers.
III. Skilled artisans, foremen and clerical workers without administrative responsibility.
IV. Semi-skilled workers, but in reasonably regular employment.
V. Labourers—both employed and unemployed, the Epsilons of Aldous Huxley's *Brave New World*.

So much for our democratic society.

Adverse influences on fetal development.—It is now clear that agents lightly tolerated by the mother can damage the rapidly growing tissues of her child. Here is fresh scope for antenatal care not only in a negative sense but positively as well to improve a child's endowment at birth.

Perinatal mortality is too loosely accepted these days as an index of the standard of obstetrical care, and one might go much further and ask, "What about the survivors?" After all, our interest is with the living and not the dead and the casual phrase, "Alive and Well" gives little indication how well in fact the baby has survived its antenatal hazards and those attending its birth.[3, 4] It would be suprising if influences, either chemical or physical, which reached the baby during the critical stages of its intra-uterine development did not have possible far-reaching effects upon its intellectual and physical capacity, quite apart from the more obvious forms of handicap. Here lies one of the biggest gaps in obstetrical knowledge. Even so-called intra-uterine asphyxia can only be explained in a minority of cases, yet macerated stillbirth is simply the end-product of intra-uterine subnutrition and suboxygenation. The damaging effects of X-rays[21] and rubella virus[6] are among the few that are well known.

The tragedy of fresh stillbirth is becoming relatively uncommon in obstetrical units. Apart from unexplained macerated stillbirths, the large components of perinatal loss are represented by fetal abnormalities, abruptio placentae, pre-eclamptic toxaemia, while fresh obstetrical stillbirths commonly associated with cord accidents and post-maturity only come fifth down the list. In all this the association of prematurity stands out prominently in between two-thirds and three-quarters of the total, sometimes as cause and sometimes as effect.

Drugs

In spite of an intensive witch-hunt for possibly teratogenic drugs, in addition to thalidomide, remarkably little has so far been substantiated. There are two reasons for this—firstly, the natural incidence of fetal abnormality (namely 2–3 per cent of all babies, alive or dead) for which no explanation can be found, and, secondly, the matter of species difference which to some extent invalidates the observations made on experimental animals, such as rodents, which do not apply in the case of the human fetus. Nevertheless there is every need for a large corporate effort to be made by all practitioners, as encouraged by the Royal College of General Practitioners, to report possible associations between fetal abnormality and drugs given in early pregnancy. Any suspected association, even though remote, should be forwarded promptly in writing to the Medical Assessor, Committee on Safety of Medicines, 33 Finsbury Square, London, E.C.2.

So far it is recognised that androgenic steroids may masculinise a female fetus if used within the first trimester and there is a general belief that some of the synthetic progestational agents may likewise produce androgenic effects. A most interesting and disastrous complication has come to light in the case of giving large doses of diethylstilboestrol in early pregnancy, sometimes as a means of endeavouring to encourage abortion. A surviving female fetus may, twenty years later, develop a primary carcinoma of the vagina. This sort of phenomenon provides fresh food for cautious thought about possible "morning-after" pills to reduce the risk of pregnancy from unprotected sexual intercourse.

The corticosteroids have from time to time been blamed for causing cleft palate, as is known to occur experimentally in mice and possibly other fusion failures as well, but the risk is not a large one and may certainly be less than that of withholding such drugs from a mother who very genuinely needs them. Nevertheless the matter deserves caution.

Because most hormones given therapeutically can cross the placenta their effect on the fetal endocrine system should be anticipated. Antithyroid drugs may so depress the activity of an otherwise normal fetal thyroid gland that the fetal pituitary may endeavour to overcome the defect by increasing its output of thyroid-stimulating hormone, the fetus as a consequence developing a goitre. Fortunately the effect is reversible. Even the indiscriminate ingestion of iodides, often available without prescription across the counter for self-medication for bronchitis and asthma, can produce congenital goitre in a baby and hypothyroidism sometimes associated with mental retardation.[2]

Oral hypoglycaemic agents used in the treatment of diabetics may have an undesirable effect on the fetus inasmuch as they may cross the placenta and affect the baby who is by no means diabetic, and is vulnerable to prolonged hypoglycaemia.

Many drugs, including quinine, and of course lead and ergot poisoning, may cause fetal death, but the pregnant patient of today does not encounter such hazards.

If anticoagulants have to be given during pregnancy, heparin, which does not affect the fetus, is far safer than the "Coumadin" class of drugs, which may cause fetal bleeding from coagulation defects. It is prudent to stop the use of drugs such as warfarin and phenindione at least a fortnight, preferably more, before anticipated delivery, during which period the use of heparin, which does not cross the placenta, is far safer.

Quite apart from teratogenic effects many drugs which readily cross the placenta can adversely affect the child, such as, for example, hexamethonium bromide, once used to reduce blood pressure in pre-eclamptic toxaemia as a ganglionic blocking agent, which had the disastrous effect of producing paralytic ileus in the baby.

It is generally thought that molecules with a molecular weight of less than 1000 diffuse across the placenta easily, but larger molecules may require some more active process of transportation. Surprisingly the known effects on the fetus are much less in evidence than the known incidence of transplacental migration. The most serious teratogenic agents in addition to thalidomide include the antineoplastic and suppressive drugs, which hardly concern us, but of serious import today is the now recognised danger of chromosomal damage and stunted growth in offspring of lysergic acid diethylamide (LSD) drug-takers.[11]

Increasing numbers of manic-depressive patients are now being fairly effectively controlled by lithium salts, the teratogenic effects of which are known to exist in rats and mice. A register of lithium babies has been started on a Scandinavian scale.[17] There is an even greater need to control this medication during pregnancy because it is known that the renal lithium clearance rates rise at this time. The risk of teratogenesis would appear to be less in the human fetus than in rodents but the matter is still *sub judice*.

The use of anticonvulsive drugs for the control of epilepsy in the pregnant mother is always likely to raise doubts as to safety. Naturally the control of epilepsy must be the primary concern though the minimum medication necessary to achieve it is clearly desirable. Phenobarbitone and the barbiturates generally are more dangerous during labour or just before delivery because they may accumulate within the fetus whose liver in the neonatal period is less competent at detoxicating them, particularly if premature. Most sophisticated anticonvulsants such as phenytoin, primidone and sulphathiazine have been associated with a doubling in the incidence of major congenital malformations such as congenital heart disease, cleft palate, microcephaly and mental subnormality, but it is suggested that these malformations probably have a multifactorial aetiology in epilepsy such as heredity and environmental factors, and it is even suggested that any teratogenic action may be mediated by interference with folic acid metabolism.[13, 19] The risk to the individual case is not a large one but it is a general safe principle to prescribe the minimum amount of any medication, particularly drugs operating on the nervous system, in the first trimester of pregnancy at the very least.

Maternal addiction to narcotic drugs such as heroin can appear as a neonatal addiction too, with serious withdrawal symptoms after birth, of which there have been some sad instances recorded recently with this growing abuse in our society. Another addiction, though in this case less socially objectionable, namely cigarette smoking, has been shown in Aberdeen[23] to produce mild intra-uterine growth retardation and babies with significantly lower birth weights than in control cases. Even the vitamins are not without their potential harmful effects, particularly vitamin D, which if given in massive doses may produce hypercalcaemia and possibly adverse mental effects on the child. A maternal dose not exceeding 400 units a day, however, is safe. Large doses of vitamin K in the mother can produce hyperbilirubinaemia and kernicterus in the baby.

Of the antibiotics, prolonged administration of streptomycin can be potentially ototoxic to the fetus, but perhaps most striking of all is the danger of giving tetracyclines to the mother in pregnancy. The tetracycline molecule chelates very readily with metallic ions such as calcium so that it is deposited in bones and teeth. In the case of bones the drug is gradually eliminated in the course of the natural turnover of the chemical constituents, but not so with teeth which may be hideously discoloured. Fortunately it is the deciduous teeth which suffer more than the permanent teeth since it is they which undergo mineralisation *in utero* whereas the permanent front teeth do not start the process until a few months after birth. The discoloration of a young child's teeth so produced, besides being psychologically harmful because of the disfigurement, may, by this very fact, make the child less attractive to relatives whose affection might otherwise be lavished more generously upon it. This process in the deciduous teeth extends from the fourteenth week of gestation until after term and there is therefore good reason for not giving tetracyclines unless the mother is suffering from some infection for which no other antibiotic is suitable, a most unlikely state of affairs. Tetracyclines have the further disadvantage that the blood levels may rise very high because of diminished excretion by diseased kidneys, for example, when treating pyelonephritis and the liver may consequently suffer toxic effects.

Another antibiotic not favoured in pregnancy is Cycloserine which is said to be damaging to the early embryo and might cause microcephaly. It is a useful drug in gynaecology but I have no experience of it in obstetrics. Chloramphenicol is also an undesirable antibiotic in pregnancy because it inhibits protein synthesis.

Ototoxicity applies not only to streptomycin but to the other aminoglycoside antibiotics, for example, kanamycin, gentamicin and vancomycin and these should therefore only be used when specifically essential.

Tranquillisers are almost a feature of modern daily life. Because of their usefulness they tend to be overprescribed and it is suprising that they have not been more directly incriminated as yet in producing fetal handicap. Nevertheless two of the most commonly used, namely diazepam and chlordiazepoxide cross the placenta readily and can depress neurological activity in the fetus at birth if given incautiously right up to that time.

All live viral vaccines, and these include rubella, smallpox, measles, poliomyelitis and yellow fever are potentially dangerous to the fetus in pregnancy.[22]

The suggestion has been made that thalidomide acted as a teratogen not by producing such abnormalities as phocomelia directly but by acting as an immunosuppressive drug which prevented the alleged homograft rejection by the mother of a fetus that was spontaneously deformed; in other words that it prevented the natural riddance through abortion of such biologically unacceptable offspring, but experimental work on the survival of skin homografts in rabbits has shown that thalidomide did not in any way prevent or postpone their rejection[1] and for the time being this ingenious explanation of the action of thalidomide cannot be accepted as a more likely alternative to the theory of direct teratogenicity.

Maternal Mortality

Midwifery has largely ceased to be the blood-and-thunder subject which it was less than thirty years ago. In terms of maternal mortality alone the improvement has been staggering. Since 1970 the rate has been less than 2 per 10,000 births and each succeeding year shows a slight further drop, whereas in 1928 just under three thousand women in England and Wales died as a result of pregnancy or associated complications, an incidence of one in 226. The figure is now getting very near to the irreducible minimum and has to include coincident accidents and diseases.

According to Ministry of Health figures in the report covering the three-year period 1967–69 for England and Wales[12] avoidable factors were deemed to be present in no less than 56 per cent of cases. Poor antenatal care and injudicious delegation of responsibility, particularly in cases ill-prepared for anaesthesia, were frequently involved.

The following is a list of the major complications causing maternal death during this period.

Abortion		117
Pulmonary Embolism		75
Toxaemia		53
Haemorrhage		
abruptio placentae	16	
placenta praevia	9	
postpartum	16	
	—	
		41
Anaesthesia		34
Sepsis (not abortion)		33
Ectopic pregnancy		31
Amniotic fluid embolism		27

It is interesting to reflect that in the early 1930's natural death from haemorrhages occurred in more than double the above figures of 41 in one Glasgow hospital alone in a year.

The biggest drop has been shown in an analysis by Douglas (1955) to have occurred between 1942 and 1952.[5] This period witnessed three very important events: firstly, the universal availability of banked blood throughout the country, introduced earlier under the stimulus of war; secondly, the introduction of antibiotics, starting with penicillin, to reinforce the control of sepsis already begun by the sulphonamides and, thirdly, the establishment of the National Health Service.

The full impact of this last-mentioned social reform will only be truly evaluated in years to come, but one of the more obvious benefits is the growth, in numbers and quality, of the hospital registrar class of practitioners who form the backbone of hospital midwifery today. This result may not have been intentional but the standards demanded by the Royal College of Obstetricians and Gynaecologists have seen to it that a good obstetric registrar is worth his weight in consultant gold.

The slow but steady improvement in anaesthetic services in maternity units is also a major contribution to maternal safety, although far too often emergency anaesthetics have still to be given by the inexperienced and the unskilled. The provision of antenatal beds in maternity units, although often abused inasmuch as many women have to spend needlessly long periods thus incarcerated because of the present inability to assess all risks accurately, has come hand-in-hand with the general recognition of the classes in whom booking for delivery in key obstetrical hospital units is positively indicated.

Domiciliary Delivery

Whatever the merits of this, and they are considerable, there is no doubt that domiciliary midwifery is dying in the more highly developed populations of the world socially, such as the white population of the United States, Sweden and Australia, much in the same way as traditional tonsillectomy on the kitchen table is more or less gone for good. It is also the avowed policy in Great Britain to provide maternity beds for every pregnant woman in the land, if she so wishes it, and most do. This trend would have more to be said for it if many hospitals were not rather grisly, out-of-date places with out-of-date thinking, especially on matters like visiting and patient freedom, and occasionally run by a human species of dragon, and if only food in all hospitals could be treated with the dignity and intelligent artistry which cooking deserves and if private nursing homes were not often so ruinously expensive. Discipline in hospital which varies from the irksome to the terrifying can almost be reminiscent of one's days at boarding school in childhood. It is essential in all new hospital planning that these objections be vigorously and consciously overcome as they have been in our new Queen Mother's Hospital, where open visiting is allowed and where children are allowed to visit their mothers and "see the new baby". Irregular dismissals, against medical advice, are therefore rare indeed and we keep no such register; nor is any notice, other than a direction notice, allowed to be displayed for the instruction of patients, including futile restrictions on smoking; the latter only encourages secret smoking in lavatories and bathrooms to the detriment of the drains and the general hygiene of the place.

In opening the Queen Mother's Hospital we gave serious thought to this question of open visiting with children coming into hospital and decided, as has been proved to be the case, that the advantages in patient morale far outweighed the risks, particularly in long-stay cases. A woman's chief reason for dismissing herself from hospital against advice is that she is worried about what is going on at home and nothing can more readily reassure her than the right of her other children to visit her. Apart from an occasional drunken husband late at night and the theft of a few ashtrays, we have had absolutely no trouble and working class women are just as capable of behaving like duchesses, if given a chance, as anybody else. We feared that swarms of children might turn the place into a sort of Red Indian camp on a Sunday afternoon, but their behaviour has been overawed and demure. Husband attendance has been noticeably at peak levels when there is a television broadcast in the day rooms of a celebrated prize fight. The one hazard which has worried us is not so much some exotic infection introduced from outside, because, after all, the mother and her baby are returning to home and shopping in crowded departmental stores, but the possibility that one woman's child incubating whooping cough may infect the baby of another patient. Children are, therefore, not allowed to see the babies of other patients and, of course, the Paediatric Department with its vulnerable premature babies has to be out of bounds to the general public. This experiment in human kindness towards patients has paid enormous dividends in producing a really happy hospital, in which patients feel free to walk away into the main corridors of the hospital, furnished with tables and chairs, where family groups can sit and watch the world, at least within the hospital, go by, and are no longer under the eye of the Ward Sister. This policy has made it possible to combine high standards of medical care with simultaneous removal of so-called advantages of being at home within the bosom of the family, which, to a parous woman, simply means bondage to the sink and the kitchen stove from which she deserves a proper rest in the immediate postnatal period.

The case for hospitals, lies in their ability to provide everything from expert anaesthesia to massive blood transfusion and all the facilities which modern medical science can offer. The dangers of cross-infection are proportional to the overcrowding of the unit and the degree to which it is overworked. Recognising that hospitals have much to provide in safety and in coping with emergencies, there has been a natural attempt to extend the practice of 24 or 48 hour admissions just to cover labour. In other words to turn the hospital into a sort of public convenience, or sausage machine, where simply the mechanics of labour and its potential hazards are coped with. This doleful expedient can produce a good showing as far as the percentage of institutional deliveries and gives the bureaucrats in charge of taxpayers' money the very excuse they need for not building any new maternity units. In Bradford, however, be it remembered, the institution of this principle was done in order to provide antenatal beds which were badly needed and which could only be got at the expense of a longer lying-in period, and the object was not simply to stuff more patients through the labour wards per unit period of time. The argument uses a parous woman's home-sickness and anxiety about her other children as an excuse for dumping her at 48 hours notice back into the midst of all her domestic cares and responsibilities and can be squashed simply by providing the type of hospital which treats her and her family as human beings. The idea that the patient's family doctor can have much control over what she gets up to the minute he has turned his back is, of course, absurd. The parous woman who is most harassed and worried about getting home to resume her domestic responsibilities is the one who is most in need of TLC (tender, loving care). As for the idea of simply using institutions as places where the patient, already in established labour, can be hurried into, there to complete her second and third stages before being wrapped up and sent home a few hours later, is a travesty in human management; nor is the back seat of a taxi a suitable alternative to a Labour Ward bed.

The effect upon midwives and hospital staff, and their recruitment into obstetrics of this sordid, mechanistic approach to labour, hardly needs mentioning, although there is so much present talk of improving human relations in hospital. The country can't eat its cake and have it. Admittedly with slick organisation there may be few maternal disasters and only a few babies will escape the recognition of acute neonatal emergencies within the first few days of life, ranging from jaundice to attacks of sudden hypoglycaemia, to say nothing of some more obscure congenital handicaps, as has been pointed out in a hospital in a very poor Brooklyn district where I had the privilege of working for a month as Guest Professor.[7] It is agreed that a lying-in period of fourteen days is absurdly extravagant and even ten days, although desirable, is longer than absolutely necessary and we have compromised in Glasgow in the normal case at six days. A woman who says she will only come into hospital for 48 hours and that those are her conditions is the case that requires urgent investigation by the Medical Social Service Department to estimate and eliminate the reasons; this form of blackmail, in fact, need not be a problem.

Full-blown, key obstetric units are, of course, expensive, both in equipment and staffing. Selection, screening and filtration should be, therefore, at a very high level, since the need for a flying squad simply condemns domiciliary and small unit obstetrical practice in retrospect.

Indications for Specialist Hospital Delivery

Bad social conditions alone due to overcrowding, lack of sanitation, or the presence of disease in the family are all too often indications enough, but many could be adequately dealt with in satellite obstetric units. The young girl with the illegitimate pregnancy, however, comes into a special category and often needs rather more than medical care because of her background problems. The illegitimacy rate in cities like Glasgow and Dundee, and curiously enough, in country districts like Wigtownshire in the extreme South West of Scotland, are much worse than for the country as a whole and the rate would appear to be rising in cities. Nevertheless while it has been obvious for generations to all the less youthful of our citizens that the country is steadily going to the dogs, it should be remembered that exactly 100 years ago the illegitimacy rate in the country was over 10 per cent and that our glorious island history furnishes instances of far worse periods of social and moral degradation than we face at present. The illegitimacy rate is no better in spite of wholesale "legalised" abortion.

Under the modern National Health Service the Medical Social Services are reaching a high degree of efficiency, especially in aftercare. The following, however, are the chief medical and obstetrical indications for delivering in specialised hospital units which are, to our way of thinking, absolute.

1. *Grand multipara*
   Chief hazards:
   - Uterine rupture
   - Cervix and vault rupture
   - Postpartum haemorrhage
   - Shock and anaemia
   - Antepartum haemorrhage (all varieties)
   - Malpresentation
   - Prematurity
   - Hypertensive disease
   - Precipitate labour

2. *Previous third-stage abnormality*
   especially haemorrhage, retained placenta or previous manual removal.

   Hazard—repetition common even after an intervening normal third stage.

3. *All major medical disorders*
   e.g. Cardiac disease, diabetes, tubercle, thyrotoxicosis, cardiovascular disorders, unresponding anaemia, etc.

4. *Twins or triplets*
   Chief hazards:
   - Postpartum haemorrhage
   - Antepartum haemorrhage

Malpresentation
Anaemia
Difficulties or delay in delivering second twin
Prematurity
Pre-eclampsia and eclampsia
Hydramnios.

5. All *malpresentations* including multiparous breech
   Hazards:
   High operative delivery rate
   Higher fetal risks.

6. *B.O.H.* (bad obstetric history)
   especially in the "recurrent" group of calamity (see Chapter IV):
   e.g. Postmature stillbirth
   Intra-uterine death (IUD)
   Fetal abnormality (FA).

7. *Disproportion* actual or suspect
   Hazards: obvious
   All European women with height of less than five feet (1·5m) should be included.

8. *Previous Caesarean section, myomectomy or hysterotomy*
   Hazard: ruptured uterus
   Increased incidence of unsatisfactory labour necessitating further Caesarean section.

9. *All hypertensive states*
   Hazards:
   IUD
   Eclampsia
   Cerebral vascular accident
   Abruptio placentae.

10. *Prematurity and history of repeated premature labour*
    Best incubator for transport to hospital is mother's uterus.

11. *Rh-negative women with antibodies* and hitherto non-immunised patients with Rh-postive husbands who are ABO compatible (see Rh Chapter)
    Hazard: Fetal or neonatal death from haemolytic disease.

12. *Gynaecological abnormality*, including history of operation on cervix, or repair of prolapse, stress incontinence or fistula, or third-degree perineal tear.
    Hazard: Cervix or vaginal vault may split suddenly. Pelvic tumours may complicate pregnancy, labour and/or puerperium.

13. *Primiparae*
    Age over 30 or where fetal head is high at term
    Hazards: Inertia and unforeseen dystocia—this may well be a "premium pregnancy".

14. *History of infertility.*

15. *Gross obesity* (see Chapter IV)

16. *Age alone.* Regardless of parity, i.e. over 35 years, or under 18 years. The latter are often in particular need of attention both medical and social.[16]

The above list is given in order of priority yet it has taken a paediatrician to point out our shortcomings even today in applying this standard of selection. Neville Butler, director of the National Birthday Trust Fund Survey of Perinatal Mortality[14] dispelled any complacency at a meeting at the Royal College of Obstetricians and Gynaecologists on October 18th, 1961, with figures that remind us that all was far from well, even in G.P. units where the same selection should apply as for domiciliary booking. He pointed out that some of these units were booking the same sort of cases as consultant units (*Lancet* 1961, **2,** p. 976) and that high-risk mothers such as primiparae over the age of 30, women over 35 and grand multiparae formed 15 per cent of all cases booked in G.P. units. From these 15 per cent came a quarter of the 480 perinatal deaths in G.P. cases booked and delivered in these units in the period reviewed. This might have been partly "bad luck" (if such a thing exists in midwifery), but Butler criticised the standard of antenatal care in many instances; for example, the haemoglobin was not estimated in 46 per cent of cases nor the rhesus group in 5 per cent, nor was the blood pressure taken at every visit in 16 per cent. Compared with these distressing intimations the organisation of the G.P. units in the Oxford region, as described by Stallworthy at the same meeting, shows what can be achieved by a high standard of selection and liaison with parent or key hospitals, namely a halving of perinatal mortality in 5000 deliveries to the striking figure of 13 per thousand.

The progressive integration of general practitioners in the practice of hospital-based obstetrics should help to iron out existing disparities in the standard of obstetric care.

Not least among the many benefits to womankind of this generation and the children of the next as a result of the ever-widening scope of modern antenatal care, is the fact that to many of the population it represents the first comprehensive health check-up since leaving school, and its implications go far beyond immediate obstetrical considerations.

If a woman can reach delivery as fit as she was at the start of her pregnancy, then why not fitter? Notable examples are cases of nutritional anaemia diagnosed early in pregnancy and many cases of cardiac disability which are thoroughly supervised and treated throughout pregnancy.

It lies within the power of antenatal care to stamp out congenital syphilis utterly; the incidence of eclampsia can be lowered to an irreducible minimum; premature labour can to some extent be prevented; and many of the more dramatic disasters of labour itself forestalled by the early recognition of their causes. Above all, the patient's emotional reactions to her pregnancy and forthcoming labour are paramount and, by one means or another, it is one of the important functions of this work to engender confidence and to eliminate fear.

Antenatal Classes

These vary widely in their scope and efficiency, but all have the primary objective of fighting ignorance and fear based on ignorance. As far as hospital clinics go they provide a splendid opportunity for the patient to get to know more about the place where she is going to face her coming ordeal and about the perople who are going to help her through it and what they do for her. The confidence and trust engendered and the personal contacts established make a great difference to morale. These classes, like so many booklets, devote the greater part of their effort to baby management thereby focusing the patient's mind less on labour and its difficulties and more on the goal to be achieved, namely a healthy baby. Our own hospital now offers to every pregnant woman enrolling 8 classes in mothercraft, 8 in physiotherapy, including lessons in muscular relaxation in a gymnasium and talks on the physiology of pregnancy and labour. Between two and three times a month a film show is organised for patients, and husbands too, showing what is known to us as the "Barnet Sound film".* always to very full houses in our main lecture theatre. There is also a course of what are called "adoptive" classes, numbering 3, which were pioneered by our midwifery staff for the benefit of women who, though not patients, are planning to adopt babies and require instruction and, above all, reassurance. A special Sister is appointed to look after those patients who have expressed a desire to breast-feed. This wish is deliberately ascertained antenatally and without moral pressure and for those so choosing much can be done in the antenatal preparation of the breasts to ensure subsequent

* Film produced by Professor Ingelman-Sundberg and Dr Miriam Furjehelm, obtainable from Educational Foundation Audio Visual Aids Library, Paxton Place, London, S.E. 27.

success. Questions and discussion are an important part of antenatal instruction in all its aspects and they help to make the patient feel that she is not on her own and unique in her problems but one of a helpful and interested community. Tours of the hospital are undertaken and the patients are given an opportunity to practise on self-administered anaesthetic machines.

All the above dedicated work is making a tremendous difference to the whole spirit of the hospital and the attitude of the patients and their friends and relatives, and could well be copied by units with a so-called stricter outlook. That this sort of attitude only works in a well-developed social community is not true because we have established an explant in Nairobi at the Kenyatta National Hospital, where a similar philosophy prevails.

Routine Procedures

The following is a brief summary:

History-taking

This is quite an art and should not be left to members of the nursing staff, nor should it take the nature of form-filling. It should be dealt with under three headings—medical history, obstetrical, and family history. Details of previous hospitalisation should be entered, and specific enquiry should be made into a history of rheumatism, chorea, fits, nervous breakdowns, pleurisy and urinary infections. The usual dreary negative list with which one is presented includes mumps, scarlet fever, a distant family history of twins and, oddly enough, diphtheria, and is obstetrically irrelevant.

The obstetric history should note the menstrual rhythm and any irregularities. This information may help later to settle a doubt about the maturity of the fetus. Any period of antecedent involuntary sterility is also worth recording. Fully summarised details should be obtained of all previous deliveries and abortions; in each instance the complications of pregnancy, if any, should be listed; whether the labour was premature or overran the patient's dates, whether it was induced, and if so why; the nature and duration of the labour, the birth weight of the child, details of its survival or fate, puerperal complications and the duration of successful breast feeding.

The family history should take account of hypertension, diabetes, pulmonary tuberculosis and rheumatic heart disease, all of which may be of some relevance.

The present symptoms, if any are volunteered, are recorded, but it is doubtful if leading questions do not prove misleading. Most women reply in the affirmative if asked about headaches, backache or discharge, and almost half of them admit to constipation if questioned directly. There is not much point in making an impressive list of symptoms too irrelevant for the patient to bother to mention.

Booking Examination

The earlier the better. The patient should be weighed and a specimen of urine examined for protein and sugar and, if vomiting has not yet ceased, for acetone. The examination of the urine simultaneously for protein and glucose has been enormously simplified by the introduction of reagent strips which will handle both tests at the same time, such as, for example Bili-Labstix, supplied by Ames Co. Ltd.

We now screen the urine of every patient at the first attendance at the antenatal clinic by the clean-catch Uricult dipslide technique (see Chapter XI). Symptomless bacteriuria is not uncommon and, if of a significant amount, should be treated before rather than after upper urinary tract infection gets a hold.

General medical examination should include the teeth and gums, and a search is made for signs of oral and nasopharyngeal sepsis. The thyroid is palpated and the triangles of the neck are examined for the presence of enlarged glands. While the patient is sitting up for this, the vertebral column should be looked at for any signs of deformity. There now follows an examination of the heart and chest and a detailed inspection of the nipples. Now, and not before, the blood pressure is taken, the patient having settled down so that a reliable reading can be obtained. The abdomen is next examined, particular attention being paid to the size of the uterus, if palpable. The hand and nails are examined for evidence of tremor, oedema, nail biting, koilonychia and pallor of the nail beds. The legs are looked at for the presence of varicose veins and oedema, and the feet for serious degrees of deformity. The size of shoe is worth noting as an index of bony stature.

Routine blood testing is now undertaken for an increasing variety of purposes and at present we require at least 20 ml taken by venepuncture to be disposed of in a variety of receptacles for:

1. Wassermann, Kahn and VDRL reactions;
2. Another specimen for blood grouping including Rh grouping and the estimation of antibody titres if any are present. The results of Rh-negative antibody tests are entered on the antenatal clinic sheet in red ink;
3. A small unclotted specimen is necessary for haemoglobin testing and for full blood values if below 12 g per 100 ml;
4. Drops of blood are placed on blotting paper slides for Guthrie testing. This is in order to pick up the rare cases which would otherwise be missed of maternal phenylketonuria. These women

have abnormally high levels of phenylalanine in their blood which adversely affects the mental development of the fetus and may also be associated with other varieties of growth retardaation. Such babies may thus inherit imbecility from their mothers without the latter suffering from the disease themselves, but the proper dietetic management of the patient could prevent this dreadful effect. In spite of carrying out this routine test for some years now we have yet to pick up a case of undiagnosed maternal phenylketonuria, to the best of my recollection, but this does not provide the excuse for overlooking the possibility. Any women known to suffer from this disorder should be discouraged from embarking upon a pregnancy until her serum levels can be maintained at a safe level (certainly below 15 mg per 100 ml) since fetal damage may be inflicted at a very early stage even before the diagnosis of pregnancy is established;[24]

5. A further blood-screening test which we have now adopted is the estimation of alphafetoprotein levels by radioimmunoassay. The hope is to obtain warning thereby of neural-tube developmental defects, since clearly it is not possible to employ amniocentesis for all pregnant women whose history does not indicate it. This test requires a further 10 ml of unclotted blood;
6. Units undertaking assays of serum oestrogens and other steroids have to obtain a further 20 ml of clotted blood. It can be seen therefore that the usual requirement of 20 ml of blood will soon be short of requirement unless, or until, more subtle micromethods are introduced.

Provided there has been no recent bleeding, a vaginal examination is now made. Any discharge present is cultured, the position and size of the uterus is noted and pelvic tumours excluded. It is not often worth while attempting an assessment of the pelvic size or shape at this stage of pregnancy. This is better deferred until the softening and relaxation of the soft parts facilitate a more accurate assessment.

The Radiological Advisory Panel of the Department of Health and Social Security has recommended that it is not advisable to X-ray pregnant women except in special circumstances. This includes chest radiography which should only be carried out by full size films with strictly limited field size. Nevertheless it is important not to miss undiagnosed pulmonary tuberculosis in pregnancy. In healthy communities this risk is small enough to make routine chest radiography unnecessary in pregnancy provided the patients have a record of a normal chest X-ray within the last five years or are known to have had a successful BCG vaccination; but chest X-rays are usually desirable in immigrants from underdeveloped countries, in diabetics, in those with a history, family or personal, of tuberculosis and in those who are socially deprived. Chest radiography should not be denied to a woman whose state of ill health or clinical signs indicate the need for it.

By now one should have a very fair estimate of the patient and her reactions. If pregnancy is normal, there should be no hesitation in telling her so and questions should be both encouraged and answered. Their very nature may indicate an important though unspoken fear that there may be something wrong with the baby.

Subsequent Visits

Provided pregnancy continues without complications, the patient should be seen at least every month until the 28th week, thereafter every fortnight until the 36th week, and then weekly until delivery. At each of these subsequent visits she is weighed, since any excessive gain often signifies undue water retention and the pre-eclamptic diathesis. The weight gain should not exceed 2½ kilograms in any one month or 0·9 kg in a week. At each visit, of course, the urine is tested for protein and the blood pressure is recorded.

The maximum permissible weight gain throughout the whole of pregnancy is about 10 kg although up to 12½ kg does not call for more than vigilance. One-third of this weight increase is put on in the first twenty weeks, another third in the next ten weeks from the 20th to the 30th week, and the remaining third between the 30th week and term. Every encouragement should be given to the patient in the view that there is no need to put on weight permanently just because of having babies although this is often a very handy excuse.

The value of antenatal cervical cytology is far more debatable than that of postnatal cytology which should never be omitted. The chance of getting false positive results antenatally is not inconsiderable and it would be as well to repeat the smear test before rushing into cervical biopsy which may give the patient very real cause for alarm. While, of course, it is important never to miss a case of invasive cancer of the cervix in pregnancy, the results of antenatal cytology are not entirely an unmixed blessing and far more people suffer from the fear of cancer as a result than the disease itself. I cannot recall a single case of invasive cervical cancer in pregnancy that owed its detection to routine antenatal cervical smearing. The practice of routine cytological screening however is to be commended when dealing with the class of patient liable to default from postnatal attendance.

It is our practice to estimate the haemoglobin at every antenatal visit and to record the result on the patient's notes before the doctor even sees the patient. This is a counsel of perfection and is paying enormous dividends in stamping out anaemia long before labour, in reducing the need for parenteral iron therapy by the detection of iron deficiencies early on, by spotting folic acid deficiencies earlier than they otherwise would be and in calling for a much earlier investigation of a patient's anaemia when it fails to respond to treatment. Failing this at least four readings should be obtained in pregnancy, namely at booking, at somewhere around 20–24 weeks gestation, at 32–34 weeks gestation and near term. Of all antenatal services the detection and correction of anaemia in good time is probably more important than all others.

Abdominal palpation of the uterus becomes increasingly important as pregnancy advances, but even in the early stages it should not be omitted, as, by this time, an assessment of the period of gestation in relation to uterine size is easier; also the sooner twins are diagnosed the kinder for the patient, who will have thereby more time for additional preparations. The patient should be instructed to note the first fetal movements felt, as this, too, will help to pinpoint the period of gestation. An experienced multipara can recognise them at the sixteenth week but a primigravida will not be aware of them before the eighteenth and often the twentieth week.

At the 34th week, estimation of the haemoglobin should be made in all cases, since iron deficiency anaemia can creep on very surreptitiously, but rapidly, in pregnancy and, if the patient happens to be Rh-negative, a further test for antibodies is worth doing, although it is very unusual for iso-immunisation to occur during the first pregnancy without some placental accident. If, however, antibodies are detected in the booking blood specimen the test should be repeated at least monthly, since any rise in antibody titre may call for earlier investigation by amniocentesis and possibly elective treatment.

At the 36th week in primigravidae, a full digital assessment of the pelvis is undertaken, as described in the chapter on disproportion. The information so obtained is of immense value. It is better not to leave this examination any later, because any vaginal interference during the last four weeks of pregnancy should be undertaken with full aseptic and antiseptic ritual. It is true that pathogenic microorganisms introduced by such an examination do not usually survive very long in the vagina, but one cannot be certain that labour may not supervene while the organisms still retain their potency if the examination is too long deferred.

The relationship of the fetal head to the pelvic brim becomes more important as term approaches. The deeply engaged head can easily be mistaken for the engaged breech with extended legs and vice versa. A rectal examination often helps to settle the point, and at the same time the ripeness of the cervix can be assessed.

Diet

It is not so much what a woman eats that matters as what she fails to eat, and the deficiencies are more important than the excesses. One thing is certain, the baby will be the last to suffer in cases of malnutrition, for it is the complete parasite.

Although malnutrition in England and America is uncommon, the same cannot be said for subnutrition, and the subject still retains its importance. Since the baby will take the best of what is going, its size and development are only reduced materially in advanced malnutrition, but there is no doubt that the incidence of prematurity is influenced by the mother's diet and her social circumstances. The growth and development of the fetus are more related to the social background in the patient's own childhood and to genetic factors than to the variations in maternal diet ordinarily encountered in the present pregnancy and, as a corollary, it is no longer reckoned that a woman can procure an easier delivery with a small baby by dietary restriction[23].

The first requisite is an adequate supply of fluid, and the patient should be advised to take two pints or a litre of fluid over and above her usual intake. It is the best and most natural defence against constipation and helps to tread down stasis in the urinary tract with its resultant liability to infection.

Constipation is very largely a neurosis, and its evils are much exaggerated, but nothing is to be gained by the passage of hard, abrasive stools, and one's first attack on such a problem should be to ensure an adequate fluid intake, and secondly, to see that the diet contains enough cellulose-containing foods, commonly referred to as "roughage". Of these, fruits, vegetables and especially prunes are among the most important. The use of purgative drugs is often ill-advised and even more often unnecessary. Of all of them, paraffin is perhaps one of the most vicious because of its apparent and alleged harmlessness. By coating the villous crypts in the small intestine it must, to some extent, interfere with absorption from the gut. What the patient therefore gains in having loose, oily stools she loses in vitamin and mineral intake.

A dietitian reviews the diet of all our patients on booking and issues advice. The normal quantitative requirements of a woman in pregnancy need not exceed, 2500 calories a day. A hundred grammes of animal protein and 100 g of fat per day are desirable levels of intake, but it is not much use telling a woman to eat 100 g of protein a day if she does not know where it comes from nor how to measure it, and it is important, therefore, to give her only the plainest and most simple advice. The majority of patients are not very much interested in the subject of diet, and those that are have usually least reason to be so and often present a neurotic predisposition. Most well-to-do people eat a reasonably well-balanced diet, but it is among the poorer classes that mistakes are made. In the latter, carbohydrates, because of their cheapness, are relied upon largely to fill up the gaps. Unfortunately, they cannot replace the value of high-class protein from animal sources.

Even the apparently well-nourished, however, are liable to a deficient intake of iron and vitamin D, and iron deficiency anaemia is still much too common. The daily requirements of iron are about 20 mg, and during the last three months of pregnancy the baby makes its greatest demands upon the available store. Liver, green vegetables and meat are natural sources of iron, but any case exhibiting a haemoglobin less than 85 per cent (12·6 g) should receive a supplementary supply for which the ferrous salts are eminently suitable. As discussed later in the chapter on Anaemia, we have found that the dietary intake of both iron and folic acid is deficient in an industrial population such as we are dealing with in Glasgow and it is our present practice to prescribe, in addition to iron, a very small supplement of folic acid of 300 micrograms a day such as Ferrograd Folic, one tablet daily on an empty stomach.

Two pints of milk a day would go very far towards meeting all the dietary demands of the pregnancy, but few women can bring themselves to drink that much. One pint a day at least should be insisted upon. The essential calcium requirements are thereby met, although other natural sources are fruits and vegetables.

Phosphorus, also necessary for skeletal growth, is supplied by eggs, cheese, milk, meat, liver and oatmeal. A diet deficient in either calcium or phosphorus predisposes the baby to the development of rickets or a latent tendency to this disease and the subsequent liability to dental caries. These propensities, engendered during intrauterine life, persist into infancy and childhood, even though the diet after birth may be sound. Extreme cases of deficiency can provoke osteomalacia in the mother, but this disease is limited mainly to famine-stricken areas.

The role of vitamin D in the prevention of rickets is now universally appreciated. In areas where sunshine is short and eggs too expensive to buy and fresh milk taken in insufficient quantity, vitamin D deficiency is a very real danger.

The stress laid upon vitamin D should not detract from the importance of all the other vitamins, but the deficiency effects of these in pregnancy are less obvious. So far as we can tell at present a normal middle-class diet reinforced as above, and with orange juice and at least a pint of milk, will meet the nutritional demands of normal pregnancy.

The issue of free milk to all expectant mothers is now being stopped and is reserved for the less privileged who are receiving supplementary benefits or are in special need, for mothers who already have two children under school age regardless of the income of the family and for the children as well after the first two. The conditions are outlined in leaflet W.11 issued by the Health Department of the United Kingdom which is about as difficult for a working class woman to fill up as an Income Tax Return; in other words daunting in the extreme. Vitamin tablets too are included in the bureaucratic largesse or can be bought cheaply with less form-filling at Maternity and Child Welfare Clinics.

The enlightened policy of recent years officially adopted in regard to the nutrition of the poorer classes has practically stamped indigenous rickets out of existence, and dental health among the new generation of children would have been even better had it not been for the sinister increase in juvenile addiction to sweet eating. The recent flood of immigrants particularly from Pakistan, has however, re-introduced this problem in the U.K.

Smoking, an expensive, useless and dirty habit at the best of times and one often betraying a neurotic predisposition, has even less to be said in its favour in pregnancy. To forbid it, of course, would set up more conflicts in the psychologically handicapped addict than she or her family would be likely to endure, but an Aberdeen enquiry[8] showed that the mean birth weight of the babies of mothers who smoke is lower and the prematurity rate higher than in non-smokers and that the difference cannot be attributed to the fact that smoking is commoner amongst the lower social grades and higher degrees of parity.

Rest

This is even more important than exercise. A minimum of nine hours in bed at night, preferably ten, is recommended, and during the afternoon the expectant mother should be encouraged to lie down or at least put her feet up for one hour. This is often very difficult, especially for the parous patient who is most in need of it. A system of home helps is available, but the scope is still too limited.

Exercise

The mental effect of exercise upon the patient is perhaps even more important than the nature of the exercise itself and the muscles which it is designed to train. Speaking as a mere male, it can be admitted confidentially that housework is the most exhausting of all forms of exercise and easily the most distasteful, while the mental effect which it can produce is little short of deplorable. As a form of exercise, therefore, for the pregnant woman, it cannot be recommended on this count. Exercise, then, to be of much value, should provide a mental break from routine humdrum activity. This means getting out of the house into the open air. It might be added that shopping does not count as exercise—in fact, it is even more harassing than housework.

Of all types of exercise, walking, short of fatigue, is the most natural and suitable. Golf and bathing are admirable, although diving is obviously contra-indicated. Sports as energetic as tennis are not suitable after the first two months, and horse riding is positively foolhardy. The only objection to cycling is the danger of falling off. It is far better to allow an experienced cyclist to continue her activities for as long as she wishes than to encourage in her any idea of invalidism.

Exercises in pregnancy designed to promote relaxation in labour in the hope of expediting it and making it less painful are popular. Physiotherapists, as a whole, are keen to co-operate in this type of antenatal treatment, and many hospitals hold classes in relaxation. The least that can be said for them is that they can do no harm and may indirectly benefit the patient by encouraging her in the view that she is thereby insuring herself against an unsatisfactory labour. Apart from these incidental and psychological effects, their value is by no means proven. A noteworthy contrast is the patient who spends the last few weeks of her pregnancy in hospital because of cardiac disease, and it is notorious how seldom inertia complicates labour in these cases. Relaxation classes provide good opportunities for instructing patients in the physiology of childbearing and in the hygiene of pregnancy and are of particular value in eliminating ignorance, which often lies at the root of many of the patient's unspoken fears. More than this, however, cannot be claimed for antenatal education and exercises, although an enlightened view would be that this is justification enough.

An interesting analysis[15] divided 2700 primigravidae into three groups, all matched in age. The first group consisted of 1000 patients trained fully in relaxation exercises and techniques in addition to all the other incidental instruction on diet, hygiene and physiology. The second group received the instruction but not relaxation training, and the third, control group, had neither exercises nor lectures. The differences in the ensuing labours in respect of duration, need for forceps, analgesia and the incidence of postpartum haemorrhage were negligible, while the perineal laceration rate in the exercise group was highest of all.

Travel

For the patient who has a known tendency to abort, travel is contra-indicated during the early months of pregnancy, especially at what would have been periods of menstruation. In other respects, the chief thing against travel during pregnancy is the fatigue which it may involve and, towards the end of pregnancy, the possibility of labour supervening in inconvenient circumstances. Long car journeys should be interrupted about every two hours in order to allow a change of position and the re-establishment of healthy circulation. Travel by air has no risks peculiar to pregnancy and is particularly suitable for long journeys because of its alleged freedom from fatigue.

However, as an air traveller now of almost world-wide experience I am often forced to a contrary point of view and am reminded of the old saying, "Time to spare, go by Air."

Air travel, however, has made absolute the need for yellow-fever inoculation which, astonishingly, has not yet reached India from Africa since the necessary mosquitoes are available in both countries under the most unfavourable circumstances. Even in pregnancy it may therefore be mandatory.

Coitus

People vary very widely in their inclinations in this respect, and it is a good rule not to offer unsolicited advice unless there are very strong reasons for doing so, for example in cases of recurrent abortion. To the patient, however, who asks for advice on such a private matter, it should be stated that, ideally speaking, there should be abstinence between the 8th and 14th weeks of pregnancy and in the last four weeks as well. This advice should be given very gently, because one can never be wholly certain of the patient's marital background.

The use of the lateral position in coitus certainly prevents deeper penetration and possible hazard to the pregnancy and this is well worth remembering when counselling married women with mitral cardiac disease, where the combination of tachycardia and the supine position may cause acute pulmonary distress.

Dental Hygiene

Dental treatment is available free of charge throughout pregnancy and for one year after confinement but far too many women are more afraid of the dentist than they are of having a baby! It is commonly believed that dental caries is liable to progress rapidly because of the calcium demands of the fetus, although this is not fully proven. The view, however, is too widely held to be erroneous and, quite apart from the question of progressive caries, oral sepsis may menace the safety of labour. Reparative dental work can safely be carried out at any stage of pregnancy, but dental extractions under a general anaesthetic are best undertaken in mid-pregnancy. The danger lies not so much in the extraction as in the anaesthetic, the risks being mainly those of asphyxia, which is particularly liable to occur in these cases when nitrous oxide is administered none too expertly. A fluoride-containing preparation such as Zymafluor can be taken orally in the hope of discouraging caries but is no substitute for oral hygiene.

Breasts

Much can be done in pregnancy to prepare the breasts for successful lactation. The nipples can be trained in protraction by manipulation, and the wearing of Waller shells in the later weeks of pregnancy will often overcome apparently stubborn degrees of retraction.

The skin of the nipples requires no preparation other than ordinary washing with soap and water and careful drying. During the last few weeks of pregnancy the patient may, with advantage, be taught the art of manual expression of the breasts to encourage the early flow of colostrum and clearance of the ducts; the baby would otherwise have to perform the same task in the face of a possibly engorged and unyielding breast.

Notification of Birth

Under the Notification of Birth Acts of 1907, 1915 and 1965 notification has to be made of all births, alive or still, to the local Medical Officer of Health by whom notification forms are supplied. This responsibility lies upon the doctor or the midwife attending the patient at delivery and must be complied with within 21 days. At the same time the Registration Advice Card is given to the husband or next of kin of the mother advising him of where and how to register the birth, also within the period of 21 days. Neonatal deaths are registered on the usual type of Death Certificate. In the case of stillbirth no death grant is payable (normally £9) but the mother is entitled to her maternity allowance for six weeks after birth, as if the baby had lived.

Booklets

Patients often ask for some advice on suitable literature to study during pregnancy. The choice will largely depend upon the patient's educational background. There are too many excellent publications to specify, and one would hesitate to proclaim an exclusive choice. An excellent booklet entitled *The Health of Mother and Child* is produced as a result of joint efforts on the part of the Department of

Health for Scotland and the City of Glasgow Corporation and has been made available at special rates to all local authorities. The book gives advice on hygiene in pregnancy, is well illustrated, and gives an excellent outline of the care, clothing and feeding of the baby.

The National Baby Welfare Council issues *Baby Book* which is full of useful information about pregnancy, labour and baby management and the British Medical Association publishes a similar excellent booklet *You and Your Baby* composed of a number of short articles by eminent contributors, some of which have already appeared in *Family Doctor*. It is distributed through Maternity and Child Welfare Centres.

Many hospitals, including our own, issue their own booklet which is a mine of information about how to get an ambulance, whom to ring when labour supervenes and what to do if various complications occur, what to wear, what to eat, what to do and what not to do, what to bring into hospital and what the visiting arrangements are. A specimen is included at the end of this book as an appendix.

Monetary Benefits Available

All pregnant women in the United Kingdom, regardless of their social position, are entitled to maternity benefits, provided at least 26 current health insurance contributions have been paid by the patient or her husband, or have been credited. The Maternity Grant payable is £25 for which application should be made on Form BM4 obtainable from the Local Social Security Office or from the patient's clinic. This form should be accompanied by a certificate of expected confinement on Form FW8 or if the baby is already born at the time of application, the baby's Birth Certificate. There is an additional grant of £25 for each twin surviving more than 12 hours after birth. The present weekly Maternity Allowance is now (1977) £14.70 beginning 11 weeks before the baby is due and continuing until the baby is seven weeks old. Late claims are correspondingly reduced if paid employment is undertaken during the period for which the patient would otherwise be eligible for an allowance. Prematurity is no disqualification provided the pregnancy has lasted at least 28 weeks. Full details of the benefits allowable are given on leaflet W.11 already referred to.

It is important that a claim should be made before delivery as otherwise payments may be restricted to the seven postnatal weeks. Unmarried patients receive not only the Maternity Allowance but also a dependent's allowance for the baby and an allowance for other dependent children during the six weeks following delivery.

The maternity allowance is still payable to an unmarried mother even though the child is placed for adoption and the amount in any case continues to be payable even in the event of stillbirth or neonatal death. Total disqualification for allowances follows resumption of employment, emigration, death or, sad to relate, imprisonment.

REFERENCES

1. BORE, P. J. and SCOTHORNE, R. J. (1966). *Lancet*, **1,** 1240.
2. CARSWELL, F., KERR, M. M. and HUTCHISON, J. H. (1970). *Lancet*, **1,** 1241.
3. DONALD, I. (1966). *J. Coll. gen. Practit.*, **13,** No. 60, Suppl. **1,** 40.
4. DONALD, I. (1966). *Proc. roy. Soc. Med.*, **59,** 184.
5. DOUGLAS, C. A. (1955). *J. Obstet. Gynaec. Brit. Emp.*, **62,** 216.
6. GREGG, H. M. (1941). *Trans. ophthal. Soc. Aust.*, **3,** 35.
7. HELLMAN, L. M., KOHL, S. G. and PALMER, J. (1962). *Lancet*, **1,** 288.
8. HERRIOT, A., BILLEWICZ, W. Z. and HYTTON, F. F. (1962). *Lancet*, **1,** 771.
9. LENZ, W. (1962). *Lancet*, **1,** 45.
10. MCBRIDE, W. G. (1961). *Lancet*, **2,** 1358.
11. MARTIN, E. W. (1971). *Hazards of Medication*, pp. 274–280 and 345. Philadelphia: Lippincott.
12. Ministry of Health. *Report on Confidential Enquiries into Maternal Deaths in England & Wales*, 1967/69. London: H.M. Stationery Office.
13. MONSON, R. R., ROSENBERG, L., HARTZ, S. C., SHAPIRO, S., HEINONEN, O. P. and SLONE, D. (1973). *New Engl. J. Med.*, **289,** 1049.
14. *Perinatal Mortality Survey* (1958). National Birthday Trust Fund, by N. R. BUTLER, and D. G. BONHAM. Edinburgh: Livingstone.
15. RODWAY, H. E. (1957). *J. Obstet. Gynaec. Brit. Emp.*, **64,** 545.
16. RUSSELL, J. K. (1970). *Practitioner*, **204,** 401.
17. SCHOU, M., GOLDFIELD, M. D., WEINSTEIN, M. R. and VILLENEUVE, A. (1973). *Brit. med. J.*, **2,** 135.
18. SMITHELLS, R. W. (1962). *Lancet*, **1,** 1270.
19. SPEIDEL, B. D. and MEADOW, S. R. (1972). *Lancet*, **2,** 839.
20. SPEIRS, A. L. (1962). *Lancet*, **1,** 303.
21. STEWART, ALICE (1956). *Lancet*, **2,** 477.
22. STIRRAT, C. M. and BEARD, R. W. (1973). *Prescribers' J.*, **13,** 135.
23. THOMSON, A. M. (1951). *Brit. J. Nutr.*, **5,** 158.
24. YU, J. S. and O'HALLOVAN, M. T. (1970). *Lancet*, **1,** 210.

CHAPTER II

ABORTION AND INTRA-UTERINE DEATH

THE abortion scene has altered drastically in both the United Kingdom and the United States since virtually an abortion on demand principle, at least for those who can pay for it, has been legalised in both countries. This may not have been the intention of most of our legislators but is nevertheless a matter of fact.

An attempt to provide safeguards against wanton and indiscriminate abortion was made in the British Abortion Act of 1967 but these were doomed to failure because of the breadth of interpretation which could be applied to the working of the Act. In the briefest possible terms British law does not now regard it as unlawful to abort a woman if two Practitioners of more than a few years standing "in good faith" consider such is necessary for the following reasons:

1. in the interests of the woman's life;
2. in the interests of her health, mental as well as physical;
3. in the interests of the health, mental and physical, of other existing children, and
4. if there is a risk of serious fetal handicap.

The operative phrase here is "in good faith". This is at some times less evident than at others.

One good point was the control of premises where legalised abortions could be carried out and another was the insistence on notification. In so far as this last condition is fulfilled some useful statistical information might emerge as in other countries. In the United Kingdom the annual legalised abortion rate continued to rise steadily every year reaching approximately 156,000 for England and Wales in 1973, although about one-third of these were private patients from abroad—a form of invisible export which does the British medical profession little credit. It is difficult to see at what point this rising curve will level out but my guess, to judge from other countries with similar cultural standards, would be at about one-third of the rate for all births. In other words, a quarter of a million annually. This sort of thing is not medicine; it is sociological scavenging and will not be discussed further in this book, nor will its social implications. Volumes of ink and rhetoric have been spilt already.

Criminal abortion, including self-afflicted abortion, still continues in our midst as does illegitimacy.

Spontaneous abortion is beyond the patient's control and its incidence can only roughly be guessed since the rate is bound to include cases of deliberate interference with a pregnancy which the patient is unwilling to disclose. An approximate figure, for example from Sweden and Czechoslovakia, is about ten per cent, and is fairly constant. It is almost certainly higher than the natural abortion rate.

It is interesting to observe that whereas in supposed spontaneous abortion the aborted material examined shows a chromosome abnormality in about 22 per cent,[10] no chromosomal abnormalities were found in the series of induced abortions, ectopic pregnancies and stillbirths at the same time. Further, the more ill the aborting patient on admission to hospital, the more likely is criminal interference to be suspected.

The incidence of abortion in cases attending an antenatal clinic is bound to be lower than other quoted rates because the patient who takes the trouble to book early at an antenatal clinic is presumably interested in the pregnancy, and it is from this group of patients that the incidence of abortion as a natural phenomenon should be calculated. The figure then would be found to be less than 5 per cent, after about the first ten weeks. Earlier cases are often not recognised as such.

Mortality and Causes of Death

One of the chief causes of death, even nowadays, is sepsis, although antibiotics have made a great difference. The effects of sepsis are very often magnified by haemorrhage, which ranks as the second factor in causing the patient's death. Thirdly, shock may kill the patient, but in these cases the shock is nearly always due to the method employed in interfering with the pregnancy. Lastly, anuria and uraemia may carry the patient off some days later following severe shock and haemorrhage.

In recent years the actual number of women who die as the result of an abortion is measurable in dozens rather than hundreds (in 1972 the number for England and Wales was twenty-three). According to the Registrar-General, even in 1966, before the passage of the Abortion Act, the number of women dying from abortion was fifty-three, whereas in 1912 it had been three hundred and thirteen. The dramatic drop came in 1944 onwards presumably due to penicillin and improved blood transfusion facilities.

In strictly medical terms nearly all abortion deaths should be regarded as unnecessary. It is not medicine which stands condemned but our Society and the present state of our culture, which lies at the root of the problem.

The safety of any method of abortion is inversely related to the stage of gestation at which it is undertaken. Standard surgical methods of procuring abortion by dilatation and curettage or dilatation and vacuum aspiration become increasingly hazardous from the tenth week of pregnancy onwards and by the twelfth week of pregnancy the size of the fetal head makes such dilatation of the cervix necessary as to endanger not only the patient's immediate health but her subsequent reproductive capacity. These methods are positively contra-indicated from this time onwards. Abdominal hysterotomy, surely about the easiest operation in the whole of abdominal gynaecological surgery, carries even greater risks mainly from pulmonary embolism. It is for this reason that deliberate killing of the fetus *in situ* within the uterus with hypertonic saline injections and such-like are much in vogue, with occasional fearful neurological consequences if injection is inadvertently made into the maternal blood stream. The use of the prostaglandins applied extra-amniotically is to be preferred in mid-trimester abortion and is discussed more fully in the next chapter.

Symptoms and Signs of Abortion

The first symptom is that of bleeding, which precedes the onset of pain. Any case, therefore, who presents with the symptom of pain before bleeding should be suspect of suffering from some other condition, for example ectopic pregnancy. Where there has been interference, pain may also come first.

At this stage there should be no fever, and the aborting patient who has a temperature, while the cervical os is yet closed, is likely to be either a case of criminal interference or one suffering from some other febrile illness, for example poliomyelitis, pyelitis, an acute infectious fever or some such general disturbance which demands recognition and of which the threat to abort is an incidental result. Bearing these possibilities in mind, one should be ready to spot mischief farther afield before it is too late, and I can recall a sad instance of the recognition of poliomyelitis being put off, simply because septic abortion was diagnosed.

Following the onset of bleeding, intermittent uterine contractions occur which are painful and, after a variable interval, something more than blood clot is passed. If the patient's general condition is worse than can be accounted for by the estimate of the quantity of blood lost, other possibilities must be considered, particularly that of haemoperitoneum. The diagnosis of abortion is not difficult, provided it is thought of. I know a colleague who, for example, divides all patients in the childbearing period of life into four categories: the married and pregnant, the married and not pregnant, the unmarried and not pregnant, and the unmarried and pregnant, and in all cases in this age group the evidence of pregnancy, recent or present, should be sought if one is to avoid being caught out.

The appearance of the blood lost *per vaginam* should also be noted, being, as a rule, brighter and more copious than in cases of ectopic gestation, though this is by no means invariable. In assessing the patient's general condition, the pulse, pallor and blood pressure are vital observations, but there is one sign of the utmost gravity which must here be noted and, if encountered in any case of genital haemorrhage, provides a desperate warning of the patient's nearness to death. The sign is that of ballooning of the vagina, due to extreme atony of the vaginal musculature, so that on vaginal examination one gets the impression of a huge cavern filled with clots, whose walls seem to be almost out of reach and in which it is often quite difficult to reach the cervix. Such a case is in urgent need of resuscitation before any attempt is made to move her.

To decide whether an abortion is threatened or inevitable is often difficult, in the absence of sophisticated sonar techniques. Many "threatened" abortions are, in fact, inevitable due to the death of the fetus, and it is often impossible before the process of cervical dilatation starts to decide whether the case is worth striving to save from aborting. Where products of conception are passed and recognised, or where they can be felt projecting through the cervix and when the cervix itself is dilated, the inevitability of the abortion is obvious, and it only remains to be decided whether the ovum has been passed wholly, partly or not at all; in other words, whether the inevitable abortion is complete, incomplete or missed. It is in such matters that sonar is particularly useful. As a general rule, the more severe the bleeding and the more definite the intermittent pains of uterine contraction, the more likely is the case to abort inevitably, although the accepted signs of inevitable abortion have yet to appear.

Any patient in whom early pregnancy is suspected, who is bleeding more than slightly or who has a temperature or in whom pain is a prominent feature, should be examined *per vaginam* on admission to hospital, not only to exclude other differential diagnoses, but also to decide what measures if any should be undertaken forthwith to expedite the abortion process and control the bleeding.

On vaginal examination in cases of inevitable abortion two types of findings are likely to be encountered. In the first, the uterine body is bulky and the cervix is open; and one may be aware of retained products and clot within the cavity of the uterus but not easily within reach. This situation is more dangerous from the probability of further haemorrhage than the second group, in which a uterine fundus, only slightly enlarged, appears to be sitting on top of a widely dilated lower segment and cervical canal from which products of conception can be easily picked out. In this latter instance the

PLATE I

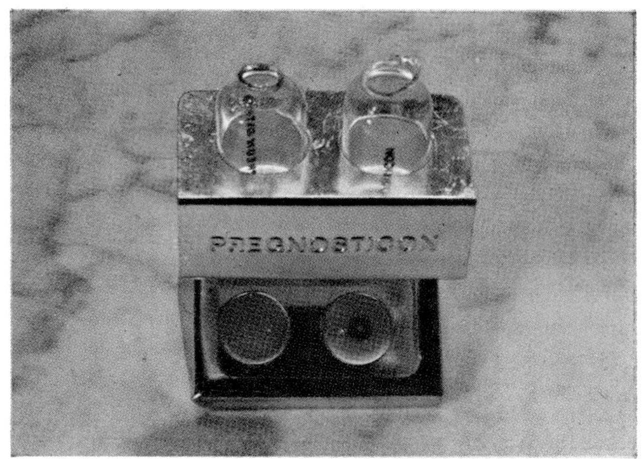

The Pregnosticon 2-Test Rack

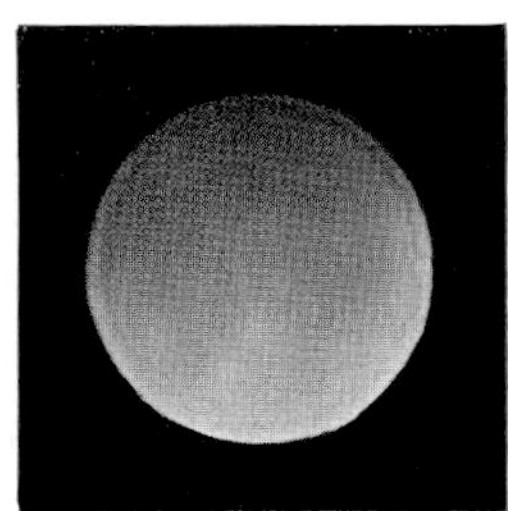

(a) Negative Result

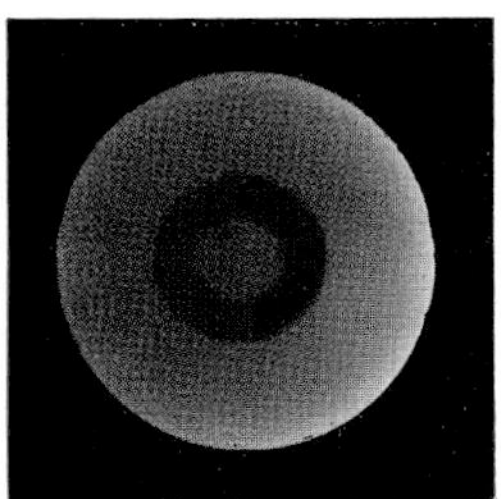

(b) Positive Result

The Pregnosticon Test

(By courtesy of Organon Laboratories, Ltd.)

abortion process is far more nearly complete and if the products of conception can be withdrawn easily by means of a sponge forceps, further bleeding may cease and it is even possible that little other than decidual remnants may be found on subsequent curettage. Vaginal examination is therefore very useful in distinguishing the two types of case and their urgency. These examinations should be carried out with at least some regard to asepsis and limiting the introduction of infection and it is our practice to cleanse the vulva with an antiseptic cream and to make the examination with dry, sterile gloves and wearing a mask but we do not usually regard a full scrub-up as necessary.

It is in the cases of mild bleeding that a conservative attitude is indicated. A vaginal examination may turn a threatened abortion into an inevitable one, or so it is said, although I think that an examination of this vigour is neither indicated nor necessary. The more honest reason for deferring vaginal examination in these cases is that any severe bleeding which might presently arise cannot then be attributed to it. The case, then, is regarded as one of threatened abortion until the signs of abortion are manifest, even though in a number of cases optimism is not rewarded. Any cases, however, who continue to bleed, even though slightly, for more than four or five days must be examined vaginally and by speculum, as otherwise, from time to time, other pelvic pathological lesions will be missed, for example carcinoma of the cervix, cervical erosion and polyp.

Immunological Tests for Pregnancy

These are absolutely invaluable because of the quick answers given and they are of particular help in deciding whether or not the patient may have a continuing pregnancy and one for which it is worth adopting a conservative attitude. The immunological tests can be carried out as ward side-room procedure and fall into two groups: the single urine drop method, or the small test tube. The first is very rapid (e.g. Gravindex) and may give an answer within a few minutes; the second, (e.g. Pregnosticon or Prepuerin) take about two hours, and in our experience at least are a little more accurate, mainly because observer error is associated with naked eye observation of precipitation in the case of the drop test. This, however, can be overcome by using a microscope under low power.

The principle is the same in all of them. One of the ingredients is an anti-human chorionic gonadotrophic serum which, when added to a pregnant patient's urine, is neutralised by the chorionic gonadotrophins in it. The other reagent is a suspension or erythrocytes or latex particles which are coated or primed with human chorionic gonadotrophin. Normally these erythrocytes or latex particles inter-react with the anti-HCG serum and are precipitated either as visible granules in the case of the slide test or as a diffuse yellow-brown sediment in the test tube. This is a negative result but if the patient's urine contains free chorionic gonadotrophin because of the existence of pregnancy, this substance reacts first with the anti-HCG serum and provided sufficient HCG is present the primed erythrocytes or latex particles are not sedimented by the neutralised anti-HCG and settle in the test tube as a characteristic brown ring at the bottom. This indicates a positive result. In the case of the Pregnosticon test (Organon) which we chiefly use, a fresh suspension of erythrocytes primed with human chorionic gonadotrophin is made up with the suspension fluid provided. Meanwhile 0·1 ml of urine, if necessary diluted to whatsoever titre is being estimated, is added to an ampoule of anti-HCG serum. The urine is best filtered first and the likelihood of false positives, particularly in women over 40 and who may be approaching the menopause, is reduced by diluting with an equal quantity of water. To the mixture of urine which has now had an opportunity to react with the anti-HCG serum, if any HCG is, in fact, present, is now added 0·4 ml of the primed cell suspension. The triple mixture should then be shaken for about a minute and left to settle in a special rack for 2 hours without disturbance. A clear brown ring indicates a positive result (Plate 1). This test can be undertaken at room temperature and does not even require centrifugation and, as can be seen, the minimum of apparatus is needed. It is as well to set up a control tube at the same time to eliminate inaccuracies in reading and to check the activity of the reagents which have a limited shelf life of not more than twelve months when stored at between 0° C and 4° C. A made-up suspension of primed erythrocytes and suspension fluid is not reliable after more than a week of storage.

These tests are extremely sensitive and false negatives are rare, but false positives are by no means infrequent especially if proper precautions are not taken. As Sharman reported,[56] proteinuria may itself provide a false positive and he recommended separating it from the urine when present in more than trivial amount, by precipitation with an equal volume of saturated solution of ammonium sulphate followed by filtration. Alternatively, the urine may be acidified, drop by drop, with 33 per cent acetic acid until slightly acid to litmus, heated to about 70° C and then filtered. Fortunately, boiling the urine does not affect the human chorionic gonadotrophin as far as this test is concerned. Any blood present in the urine, as may indeed occur in cases of abortion, should be filtered off or a catheter specimen used, because haemoglobin itself is a protein and may tend to give false positives. Urine, also, which is excessively alkaline may give a false positive even in the absence of protein. False results can also be due to cleaning pipettes with detergents or soaps which should not be used, and for cleansing purposes a bichromate solution or plentiful distilled water is recommended.

These immunological tests by their accuracy and speed, commonly able to detect pregnancy within the first ten days after the first missed period, are much to be preferred to tablets combining progestational and oestrogenic hormones administered to the patient in the hope of inducing withdrawal bleeding and thereby satisfying her that she is not pregnant. Furthermore, the tablet test has the objection that the result is not known

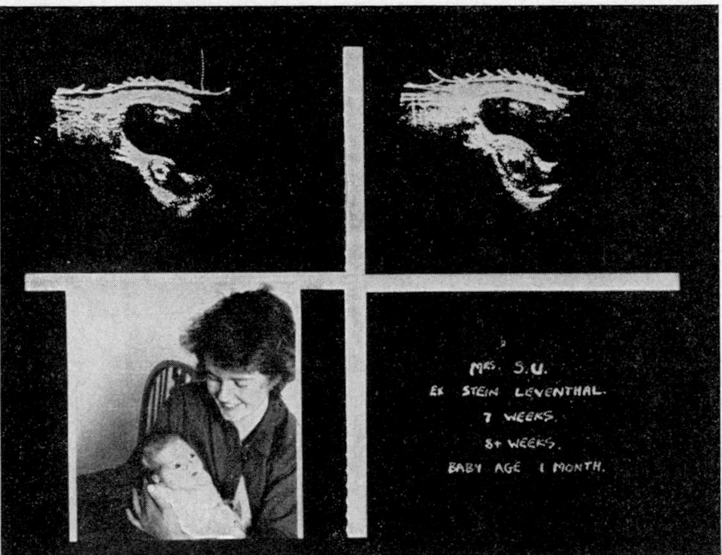

2/FIG. 1.—An ultrasonogram in an early and unexpected pregnancy in a patient previously operated on for Stein-Leventhal syndrome. Top left picture shows a longitudinal section, cranialwards to the left with the level of the symphysis pubis marked by a vertical line. Behind a distended bladder (black) there is seen a normal sized anteverted uterus containing a small, white ring representing a gestation sac of seven weeks. The ultrasonogram, top right, shows the same patient ten days later. Note how both the uterus and the gestation sac have grown. The bottom picture shows the same baby a few months old.

for a few days and is not reliable in women with abnormal bleeding patterns in whom a pregnancy diagnosis test is most urgently wanted. In the case of a continuing pregnancy a woman might be encouraged to blame the tablets for any abnormality of the fetus which might subsequently appear, however unfounded her suspicions. Since in any busy gynaecological unit the immunological tests are being done every day, often in considerable numbers, there would appear to be no point in using the hormone tablet test, although it might be useful in general practice.

Sonar (ultrasonography).—Even quicker and more useful is ultrasonography since we have the apparatus to hand and in daily use, and the first signs of an early gestation sac show up as a white ring within the uterus as early as five-and-a-half weeks after the first day of the last period and with even more clarity by the sixth week;[23, 25] after which time the progressive growth of the gestation sac can be observed and the maturity estimated (Fig. 1). Even twin gestation sacs at seven-and-a-half weeks have been revealed (Fig. 2) indicating the earliest known diagnosis of multiple pregnancy. The feat achieved with sonar at Queen Charlotte's Hospital in London of confidently diagnosing quintuplets

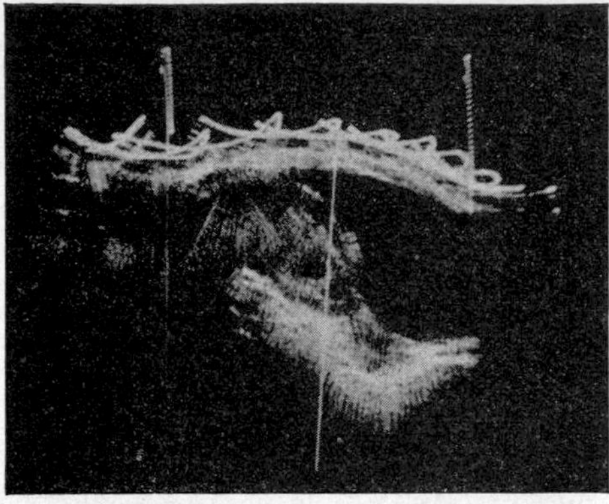

2/FIG. 2.—Twin gestation sacs (indicated by white intermediate vertical line) found at eight weeks' gestation although urine tests for pregnancy negative. L.S. behind moderately full bladder to the right.

(By courtesy of the Editor, *Brit. J. Radiol.*)

at the ninth week was indeed remarkable.[9] Furthermore, the level of gestation whether in the upper or lower uterine segment can also be seen and we have a strong suspicion, at present being followed up, that the likelihood of abortion is related in some measure to the level of implantation of the sac (Fig. 3). Finally in cases of blighted ovum, failure of development of a normal-looking sac has been observed many weeks before abortion has ultimately taken place (Fig. 4 *a–d*).

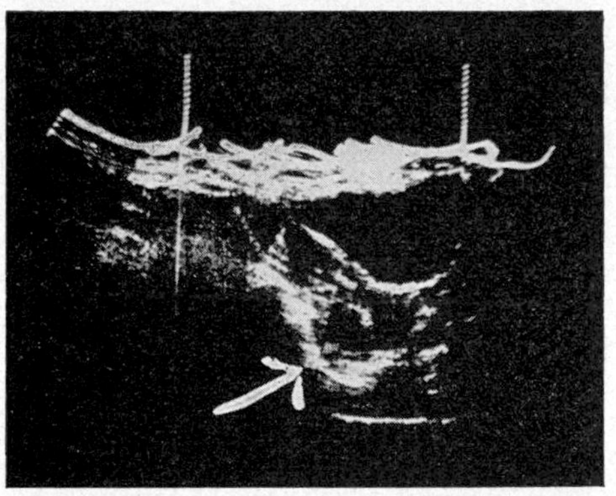

2/FIG. 3.—Low implantation of gestation sac in a case of recurrent abortion. An abnormally shaped uterus is visible behind a partially filled bladder in longitudinal section. The sac can be made out in the lower segment. The patient again aborted four weeks later.

(By courtesy of the Editor, *Brit. J. Radiol.*)

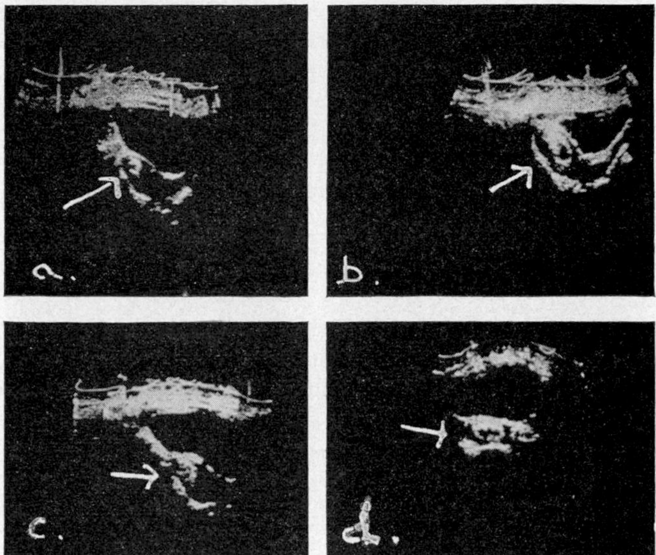

2/Fig. 4.—Blighted ovum in a case of recurrent abortion due to genetic defect *viz.* translocation on chromosome III in husband.

(*a*) Shows apparently normal gestation sac at six weeks in upper segment of uterus behind full bladder. L.S.

(*b*) At eight weeks, growth of gestation sac has clearly occurred. L.S.

(*c*) At nine and a half weeks. No further growth, in fact shrinkage although urine tests still positive. L.S.

(*d*) 10½ weeks—no further sign of growth, just a crenated sac. T.S. behind full bladder.

Patient aborted for the fifth time ten days later. No fetus.

(By courtesy of the Editor, *Brit. J. Radiol.*)

With good ultrasonic apparatus it is usually possible, using the full bladder technique,[21] to pick out what we call the fetal pole, quite often during the sixth week of amenorrhoea and with reasonable certainty by the seventh. If this cannot be identified by the eight week and the gestation sac on careful searching appears to be empty, we begin to question the existence of an active and continuing pregnancy regardless of the urinary gonadatrophin test results. The technique has been elaborated further in this Unit by Robinson who measures the crown-rump length in millimetres and adduces the gestation period to within a matter of days.[53]

Blighted Ovum

This term is used to describe the fertilised ovum whose development becomes arrested early in pregnancy before the end of the first trimester. It differs from missed abortion largely in degree but particularly because of the absence of properly developed and recognisable fetal parts. The phenomenon of blighting has been recognised for over a quarter of a century but it is only with the advent of sonar that it is possible to diagnose it while still *in utero* and to confirm the long existing suspicion that it is a common type of reproductive failure. We are not in a position to give an accurate estimate of the incidence since, although we often find several cases a week, the population studied is selected in the sense that the patient either has a bad history of recurrent abortion or has been threatening to abort already, and for this reason ultrasonic examination is requested, but the figure must be somewhere around a quarter of all conceptuses. It is Nature's method, after all, of rejecting the failed pregnancy. Fetal abnormalities which go through to term are simply the tip of the iceberg. The following then are the ultrasonic features of a blighted ovum[26]

1. Loss of definition of the gestation sac. This may be seen to be poorly formed and often actually fragmented. Sometimes the ring is incomplete with a break in its contour.
2. Absent fetal echoes. We have frequently observed an enlarging gestation sac in which it is impossible to find any fetal pole.
3. A gestation sac which is consistently small for dates and fails to enlarge.
4. Absence of fetal heart.

Using Robinson's technique[51] we would expect to be able to detect the fetal heart after seven weeks amenorrhoea and certainly by eight weeks, by which time failure to demonstrate fetal cardiac activity is almost pathognomonic of blighted ovum, regardless of urinary gonadotrophic tests. The ultimate fate of these cases is spontaneous abortion of a minor type when, to the accompaniment of bleeding—sometimes not much more than a period, tissue which is frequently not recognised or not recognisable is passed. If we can obtain the material fresh enough we endeavour by tissue culture to establish whether there was some genetic abnormality. As far back as 1969 it was reckoned that 12 per cent of clinically recognised pregnancies were intrinsically defective and that chromosone abnormalities were about forty times more frequent in early spontaneous abortions than in babies reaching term.[11] It is particularly tragic that this condition of ovum blighting tends to be recurrent in the same patient, but at least the ability to determine that the pregnancy is doomed at an early stage before later disappointment and, even better, to demonstrate reassuringly the presence of a fetal heart in an active and continuing pregnancy, has made a great deal of difference to the management of these cases.

Differential Diagnosis

The most important differential diagnosis is that of ectopic gestation, in which the clinical findings are by no means always characteristic. In this instance, however, the onset of pain tends to precede that of bleeding, a history of fainting attacks is characteristic, the patient's symptoms and general condition may be out of proportion to the amount of blood lost, vaginal tenderness and pain on moving the cervix gently are usually marked, a boggy indefinite mass may be felt either behind the uterus or to one side of it, and the vaginal loss often has a dark "prune-juice" appearance. Abdominal rigidity is very rare.

A prolonged clinical lifetime has not, however, reduced the number of mistakes which I (and incidentally my colleagues) from time to time make, resulting either in a missed diagnosis or occasionally in an unnecessary laparotomy. Cases frequently present in altogether atypical fashion. Commonly, a persistently positive immunological urine test leads one to treat a case of continuing mild vaginal bleeding as one of threatened abortion, with only vague clinical signs within the pelvis. Ultimate curettage in such a case shows only decidua and no villi, which should immediately alert one to the diagnosis of a pregnancy elsewhere. Even a negative urine test does not eliminate the possibility of a tubal mole with continuing invasive properties. Such a mistake once resulted in a massive haemoperitoneum some days after I had discharged the patient from hospital. This incident was brought to our notice by the inevitable "chortle" letter which one receives from time to time from rival hospitals, advising one of errors committed and how the patient was snatched from the jaws of death by their own superior clinical acumen. Perhaps the most dangerous pitfall of all is to rely upon examination under anaesthesia. A tubal pregnancy on the point of rupture can be so provoked the minute the examining fingers approach it, with the result that nothing is now felt and the patient may be returned to the ward where, if she is not very closely watched, her collapse from haemoperitoneum may not be observed until too late. I know of two fatal instances of this sort in other hospitals. Once when visiting one of the London Teaching Hospitals I noticed two cases who appeared to have been to the operating theatre twice in the one day and to have had massive transfusions, and my inquiries prompted the confession that both had been examined under anaesthesia to exclude ectopic pregnancy and had been brought back to the theatre in a hurry later the same day. The dangers of examining the patient with an ectopic pregnancy in the anaesthetised and non-protesting state have led many clinicians to preach that if there is a suspicion from history or signs of ectopic pregnancy, laparotomy should be undertaken forthwith and that it is better to look inside unnecessarily than to miss the diagnosis. This was indeed my teaching until the new fibre optic peritoneoscopes came on the market.

Laparoscopy

This now features very prominently in our gynaecological practice and we may undertake as many as ten cases in a week. Among the indications for this simple and useful investigation are possible ectopic pregnancy. For the process we anaesthetise and catheterise the patient in the dorsal position, and then tilt her into the Trendelenburg position and induce a pneumoperitoneum with helium or carbon dioxide or both through a needle introduced a few centimetres below the umbilicus. A fibre optic laparoscope is then introduced, as described by Steptoe[57] at the lower border of the umbilicus and an immediate view of the pelvic viscera from above is obtained often superior to that provided at laparotomy by some surgeons. If tubes and ovaries are normal and the pouch of Douglas clear of inflammatory disease or endometriosis, we take the opportunity of inspecting the appendix as well. We take a good deal of trouble at the end of the operation to evacuate as much gas as possible from the pneumoperitoneum and the patient suffers so little disturbance that she can be dismissed safely the next day. If, on the other hand, an ectopic pregnancy is seen it is a simple matter to proceed with the patient under the same anaesthetic to laparotomy. A considerable personal experience of posterior culdoscopy has now been discarded because of the inferior view obtained and all the palaver of having to turn the patient round into the Trendelenburg position from the genu-pectoral in order to proceed to operation in the positive case. Armed with facilities for laparoscopy it is now inexcusable to miss the diagnosis of ectopic pregnancy in either direction and, in fact, since adopting the technique in my department this mistake has been made only once, by a junior who happened to be on duty and who had not confidently mastered laparoscopic technique.

All types of functional uterine haemorrhage may simulate abortion, particularly cases of metropathia haemorrhagica, in which a period of amenorrhoea may have preceded the onset of the loss, but pain is never a feature of such bleeding apart from that due entirely to the passage of large clots.

Fibroids, likewise, may produce bleeding, together with signs of uterine enlargement, and occasionally there is associated pain due either to the attempt on the part of the uterus to extrude a fibroid polyp, or, occasionally, due to acute degeneration in the fibroid, but fibroids never, repeat never, produce amenorrhoea. Other pelvic lesions which may present as cases of apparent abortion include new growths of the cervix and polyps.

Hydatidiform mole comes into the differential diagnosis of abortion and this is dealt with more fully later in the chapter.

Now and then the bleeding comes neither from uterus nor cervix, but from a torn vessel in a ruptured hymen from which, occasionally, haemorrhage can be very profuse, to the point of exsanguination and vaginal ballooning as already described. Such a possiblity was very sharply brought home to me on a Service Outstation during the war. The girl was pulseless, the vagina was ballooned with atony and full of a bewildering mass of clots, so that I had difficulty in identifying the cervix at first. There was so much blood and clot about that I did not at once recognise the source of the haemorrhage, which was from a large hymenal tear, and I assumed that she was aborting.

Lastly, a patient who has recently, secretly, delivered herself of a baby at term can easily be mistaken for a case of abortion if not very carefully examined, for the uterus is bulky and bleeding, and only careful examination of the cervix and perineum for tell-tale signs of laceration may prevent one from making a humiliating mistake. I have been caught out by just such a case seen for the first time, and it was the police who later dealt with the matter of a newborn strangled infant found within a cupboard in the patient's room. The placenta, incidentally, was never found!

Treatment of Threatened Abortion

Rest in bed with sedation is the keystone of treatment, and hormone therapy is of no more than very questionable value once the threat to abort is manifest. Morphine is not recommended. It often induces vomiting and even more often appears to expediate abortion. Sodium amytal, 0·2 g (3 gr) four-hourly, is far more effective. At this stage, the use of progesterone often appears to act more as an abortifacient than as a remedy. Occasionally isoxsuprine (Duvadilan) may appear to damp down uterine activity but we are not enthusiastic, especially when one bears in mind that with a normally implanted ovum or one known by sonar to be alive and growing and in which there is no cervical incompetence, the chances of pregnancy continuing successfully on its own are very high.

There is certainly nothing to commend the exhibition of progestational agents without evidence of deficiency and this is hard to come by because even normal cases show wide variations in pregnanediol excretion. Although present-day methods of assay are in themselves becoming more accurate[15, 32] it has been suggested[54] that 24-hour outputs below 4 mg are more likely to be associated with abortion, but these may well include cases of missed abortion. It is our experience that ultrasonography gives a far more reliable and ready answer to whether or not pregnancy is continuing. After the eleventh week it should be possible to pick up the fetal heart by the ultrasonic Doppler effect[31]. Any pulsating structure and particularly, of course, the fetal heart or cord, will modify the frequency of an echo to an ultrasonic beam reflected from it. It will thus give a signal which, even in early pregnancy, has a recognisable rate of around 140 beats per minute and is readily identified as fetal in origin. This proof of continuing intra-uterine life is as reassuring to the patient who can hear it on the loud-speaker, as to the clinician who may be in doubt that pregnancy is continuing and whether to regard a case of continued bleeding as salvable.

Patients should be kept in bed until all signs of fresh bleeding have ceased for at least forty-eight hours, and the bowels should be left strictly alone. At the end of five days a vaginal examination is made to ensure that all is well, a urinary pregnancy test is performed, and the patient advised before discharge to avoid heavy lifting, sexual intercourse and powerful purgation, at least until safely past the 16th week.

A study of the changes in cervical mucus is often helpful. It is very simple to carry out and involves the removal of a small quantity of mucus from the cervical canal with a throat swab, after first mopping the surface of the cervix. The specimen so obtained is spread fairly thickly on a dry slide, without coverslip, and examined under low-power microscopy about twenty minutes later, after it has had time to dry.

It has long been known that the quantity and appearance of this mucus is related to oestrogen and progesterone activity and in 1946 Papanicolaou observed fern-like crystallisation in the first half of the menstrual cycle which tended to disappear in the second half. Furthermore, these crystals were absent in pregnancy and after the menopause.

Typical fern-like crystals are seen in Fig. 5 and they are believed to consist of sodium and potassium chloride bound with a small amount of organic material. Their presence is an indication of oestrogen activity, whereas their appearance can be modified or inhibited by progesterone (Fig. 6). This latter picture is characteristic of the premenstrual part of the cycle, indicating that ovulation has occurred. If there are endocervical cells only and no crystals after an expected period has been missed, this appearance suggests pregnancy, the phenomenon being believed due to oestrogen activity now balanced by progesterone.

By contrast the picture of ovarian inactivity, e.g. after the menopause, is shown in Fig. 7, which is lacking in both crystals and cells.

The presence of blood spoils the test so that it cannot be employed until bleeding has settled down, but in cases of repeated abortion, before a threat develops, complete absence of crystals and the presence of endocervical cells indicates a good prognosis. As a test

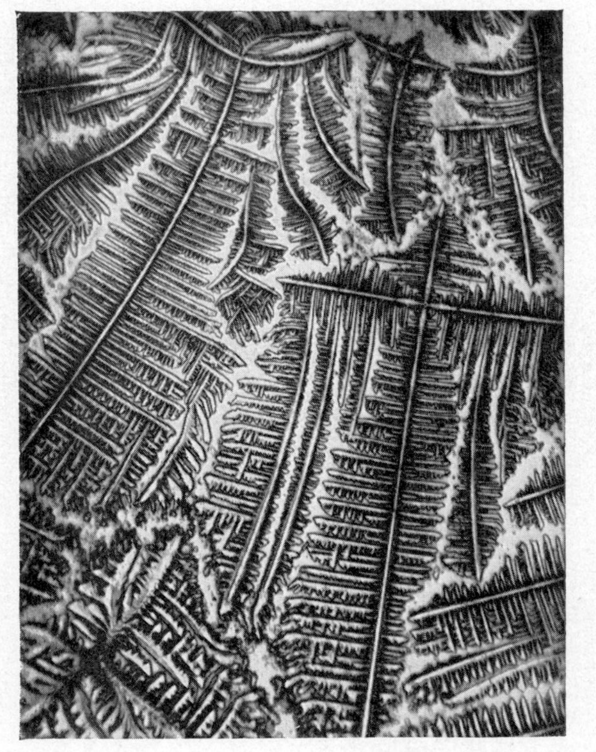

2/FIG. 5.—Cervical mucus salt crystals (indicating unbalanced oestrogen activity and incompatible with pregnancy).

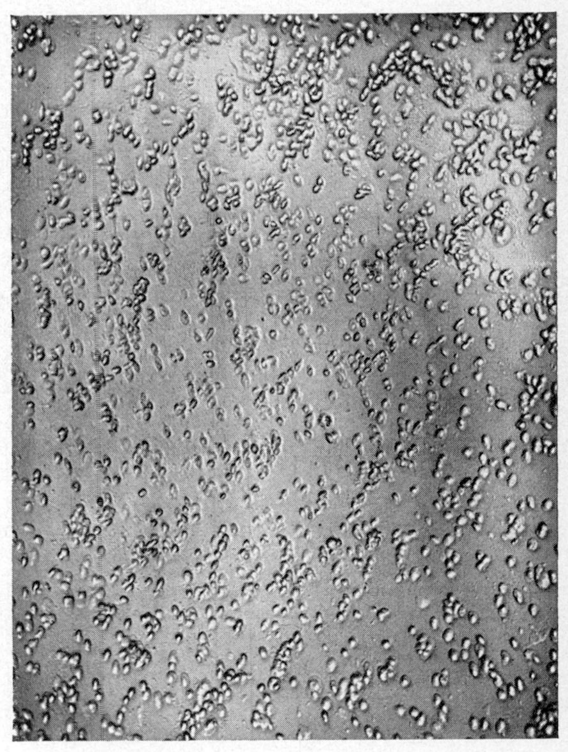

2/FIG. 6.—Cervical mucus. Premenstrual and normal pregnancy. (Progesterone effect.)

for pregnancy it is only reliable in a negative sense, fern-like crystals excluding the diagnosis, whereas their absence might be due either to the premenstrual or the early gravid state. However, if an intramuscular injection of oestradiol, 10 mg, fails to produce the crystals four days later, pregnancy can be fairly reliably assumed. This test is not now used by us because of our ultrasonic and urine-testing facilities. We also regard it as unsafe.

Often, however, one gets an equivocal result with atypical ferning (Fig. 8). This appearance commonly indicates that all is not well with the pregnancy and precedes early abortion some days later. The injection of medroxyprogesterone (Depo-Provera, Upjohn) (125–250 mg) can reverse this picture and abolish the ferns, but the pregnancy may already be past salvage and disappointments are common.

This simple test, therefore, can clearly exclude the diagnosis of pregnancy, e.g. at the menopause or in metropathia haemorrhagica, can help to confirm that active pregnancy is continuing, or can give warning to expect a threat to abort in the near future.

Incidentally crystals have been reported in the cervical mucus of cases of hydatidiform mole.[36]

We seldom use Depo-Provera injections nowadays without biochemical proof of the need for it. Norethisterone preparations are not favoured because of the risk of masculinising a female fetus *in utero*.

The efficacy of all treatments, whether bizarre or rational, must be viewed against the natural recovery rate.

Even though threatened abortion may be successfully treated, the pregnancy continues at greater risk than normal, premature labour, intra-uterine fetal death and antepartum haemorrhage of both main varieties being about three times as common as usual. The evidence that threatened abortion increases the incidence of subsequent fetal abnormality is less clear.[59, 61] Fetal abnormality is far less likely to be the result of threatened abortion than the cause of abortion itself.

The use of radioimmunossay of human placental lactogen (HPL) levels has been found helpful in predicting the outcome in cases of threatened abortion,[28] levels being very low in cases becoming inevitable.

Treatment of Complete Abortion

In the case of an abortion which is adjudged complete by inspection of the ovum which has been passed no local treatment is indicated, but any patient who bleeds more than enough to stain a pad every few hours should be suspected of still retaining products of conception. There is a general tendency in hospital practice to explore and

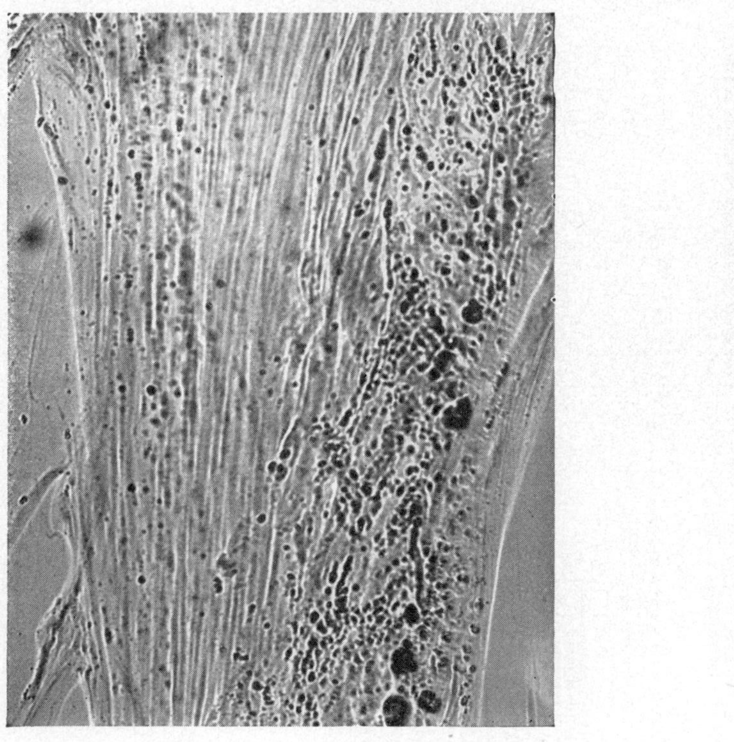

2/FIG. 7.—Postmenopausal cervical mucus. (Ovarian inactivity.)

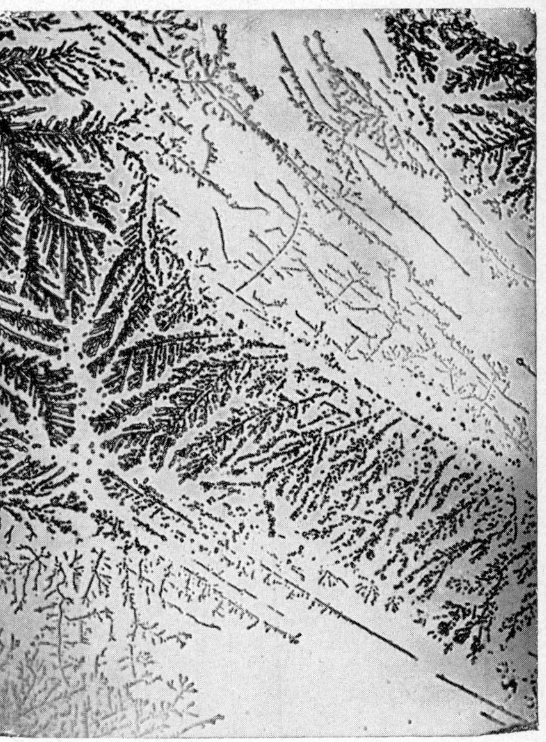

2/FIG. 8.—Atypical crystals in cervical mucus.

(FIGS. 5–8 by courtesy of Dr R. R. Macdonald[37] and the Editor *J. Obstet. Gynaec. Brit. Cwlth.*)

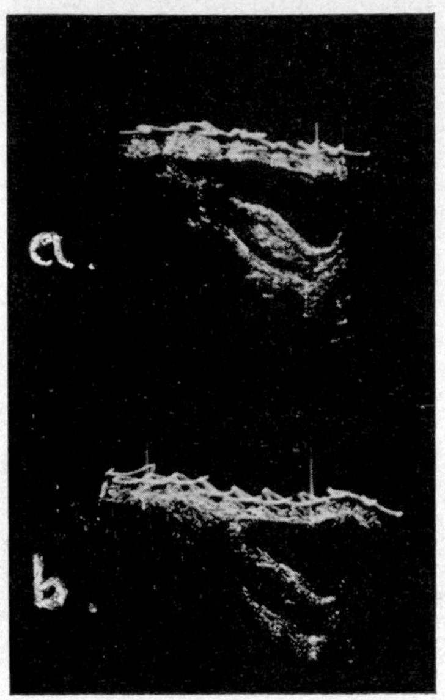

2/Fig. 9.—Retained products of conception. Bleeding eight weeks after delivery though uterus well involuted. (*a*) and (*b*) Before and after evacuation of uterus at which a piece of placental tissue was removed.

(By courtesy of the Editor, *Brit. J. Radiol.*)

curette the uterus in every case of abortion occurring in the first three months of pregnancy however completely the products of conception may appear to have been passed and however little post-abortum bleeding there may be, on the ground that in about a quarter of these cases readmission would otherwise be necessary for persistent or recurring bleeding. This may be sound hospital economics but is not sufficient reason for unthinkingly subjecting a large number of women unnecessarily to an operation which yields only shreds of decidua.

Our present practice of sparing patients an unnecessary operation who already have an empty uterus and in whom bleeding has practically ceased has made an appreciable difference to clinical management and duration of hospital stay.[52]

Ultrasonic examination of the post-abortum uterus[25] can reveal whether the uterine cavity contains a sufficient quantity of retained products to justify curettage (Fig. 9*a* and *b*). This operation after a recent abortion is not totally harmless, quite apart from the immediate risks of perforation or of disseminating infection. If, in a subsequent pregnancy, the placenta happens to be sited over an area of uterine damage caused by the curette there is great danger of uterine rupture. One of the most dramatic cases of haemoperitoneum that I can recall concerned a young woman in her twenty-eighth week of pregnancy who was admitted on a Saturday afternoon so ill that the differential diagnosis ranged from abruptio placentae to most other conceivable intra-abdominal surgical catastrophes. A diagnosis of acute haemoperitoneum was established by needle aspiration and at laparotomy the placenta was found bulging through the uterine fundus, presumably at the site of an undiagnosed perforation some years earlier at the time of curettage, following a sixteen weeks abortion. She lost her uterus, her baby and very nearly her life, being saved only by very rapidly induced hypothermia on the operating table and the usual gamut of resuscitative measures. Another such instance is demonstrated in Plate II.

The motto, "Is your curettage really necessary?" could well be applied to many aspects of gynaecology besides this one and I take great satisfaction in discharging a patient without routine curettage when neither her bleeding nor uterine size, nor ultrasonic findings indicate the need for it.

The administration of ergot may assist involution, and retention of urine should be watched for. The patient, provided her general condition is good, can be allowed up as soon as she feels like it, and a sterile vaginal examination is made. If the cervix is by now closed and the uterus involuting well, the patient may be discharged home in a few days. A retroversion of the uterus, if present, is worth correcting and maintaining in correction with a Hodge pessary after the first post-abortum week because it is always possible that it may have been an aetiological factor in the abortion, and the chances of cure are better now than subsequently, after full involution of the uterus and its supports has taken place.

Treatment of Incomplete Abortion

In these cases, the placenta or chorion is wholly or partly retained within the uterus, and as long as this is so the patient is liable to bleed. One's objective, therefore, is to encourage the uterus to complete the process and turn an incomplete abortion into a complete one. To this end, ergometrine 0·5 mg intramuscularly is given and repeated, if necessary, in four hours. As an alternative, oxytocin in doses of 5 to 10 units may be given, coupled with morphine 15 mg (gr $\frac{1}{4}$). A great favourite is what is called the "triple mixture" of an injection of all three as above simultaneously. Very often this will prevent further serious bleeding and will allow adequate time for restoring the patient's blood volume where necessary and preparing her properly for the operating theatre, including the passage of some hours since food was last taken. Under this scheme it is seldom that the patient has to be taken to the operating theatre in the middle of the night and she can await a safer operation and anaesthetic deliberately undertaken next morning. Only in the unlikely event of uncontrollable haemorrhage or in cases of suspected uterine rupture is emergency operation immediately indicated, but such cases are often better treated by preliminary resuscitation. Rapid deterioration of the patient's condition meanwhile should alert one to some hideous associated catastrophe, such as a case I recall in which an abortionist had avulsed the whole of the patient's sigmoid colon through a rent in the uterus and, for a time, unbeknown to those in attendance on the patient, the torn end of the descending colon was discharging faeces copiously into the peritoneal cavity. Her life was eventually saved by total hysterectomy and terminal colostomy and the doctors were promptly threatened with legal proceedings for carrying out such an operation without the patient's written consent. The abortionist, whose identity was known, escaped prosecution.

The delivery of the placenta usually occurs within a few hours, but occasionally it is retained for longer. If it is not delivered within 12 hours, its spontaneous and complete expulsion becomes less likely, especially with the progressive tendency of the cervix to close, so that the patient continues at some risk of bleeding, and the placental mass may become infected *in utero*. One can usually wait safely up to 12 hours for the placenta in cases of abortion, but further delay is without profit, and it should then be removed by exploration of the uterine cavity under an anaesthetic. If the patient bleeds meanwhile, however, the situation is altogether different, and haemorrhage demands intervention in its own right. Ergometrine should be given in the first instance and will, in the majority of cases, control bleeding at least for the time being. The necessary preparations for blood transfusion are made and a vaginal examination with full antiseptic precautions is undertaken. This can be done in the ward, but should be deferred preferably until the ergometrine has been given and taken effect. Often a mass of placental tissue will be found lying within the cervical canal, from which it can be quite simply picked out with the finger or sponge forceps without an anaesthetic, but if this fails or bleeding is provoked, the patient should be taken to the theatre forthwith, anaesthetised and the abortion completed by evacuation of the uterus.

Under no circumstances should operative intervention be undertaken without ensuring that the patient's general condition permits it. Some cases are already so exsanguinated and shocked that immediate attention must first be given to their resuscitation. Blood transfusion is the most important single measure, but very great care must be taken in cross-matching, not only because of the dangers of transfusion reactions immediately but also because of the great risk of subsequent anuria to which this particular type of patient is exposed. It is much safer to have a blood drip running before anaesthesia is induced so that any reaction can be noticed at once. Dextran infusions may provoke clotting defects and we never

PLATE II

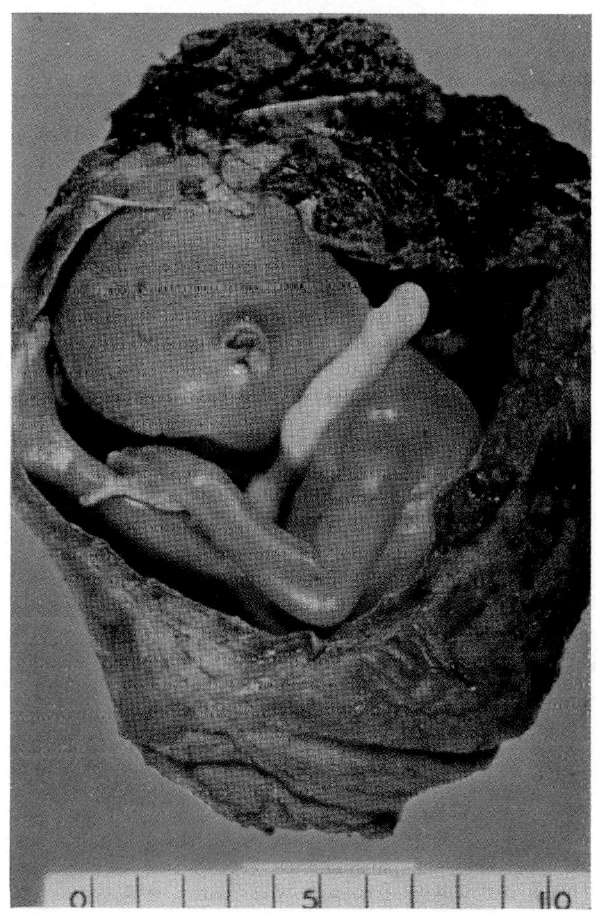

A case of spontaneous uterine rupture at twenty-three weeks due to placenta percreta involving the entire fundus and posterolateral aspect of the uterus in a patient who had previously been curetted twice because of haemorrhage following a twin abortion complicated by coliform sepsis. The patient had no living children.

(By courtesy of Dr A. Lobo, Nairobi)

use them now. The intravenous injection of methedrine 20 mg is often useful in desperate cases to produce an immediate rise in blood pressure, and the continuous administration of oxygen by mask is helpful in addition to other general measures, such as judicious warmth and the raising of the foot of the bed. Hydrocortisone added to the drip infusion or transfusion is of inestimable value in the really shocked case and has the additional advantage that it is very hard to produce overdosage. 500 mg can be added to the half litre and up to a total of 2 g may have to be given in desperate cases. In less serious cases 100 mg may be added to the half litre. Treatment with hydrocortisone should thereafter be tapered over the course of the next few days.

As soon as the patient's systolic blood pressure begins to approach 100 mm of mercury, the operation may be started under thiopentone anaesthesia. The vulva is shaved and painted with antiseptic and a catheter is passed. These measures are often better deferred until the patient is already on the operating table. The vagina is emptied of blood cot and, if bleeding threatens to start again, more ergometrine can be added to the intravenous drip. The cervix is usually already dilated sufficiently to admit a finger, but if not, it should be gently and slowly dilated to size 16 Hegar, in order to allow the passage of a finger. A half-hand should be pushed into the vagina and either the index or middle finger, whichever is more convenient, is passed into the uterus. The internal finger cannot, as a rule, be inserted farther into the uterus than the proximal interphalangeal joint unless the cervix is well dilated and it is, therefore, difficult to obtain access to the whole of the internal uterine surface. It is now that the other hand, working through the abdominal wall, performs the most important function by pressing the uterus down over the internal finger, so that the whole of the uterine interior can be properly explored. This requires a good anaesthetic with adequate muscular relaxation. The gloved finger thus loosens up all the retained placental tissue and is the only really safe instrument for the purpose. Having loosened the tissue, the sponge forceps may now be used, and their function is simply to pick out the fragments from the uterine cavity. This is far preferable to plunging about wildly inside the uterine cavity with sponge forceps, tearing out the placenta piecemeal. The best forceps to use are those having no ratchet, as one thereby retains a sense of feel of what is being grasped. The instrument should be inserted very gently until the top of the uterus is lightly felt, the blades are then opened, rotated through a right angle and closed on the material to be removed. The uterus can be perforated with the greatest ease, but the preliminary exploration of its cavity with the finger will reduce the risk by appraising one of its dimensions, and the prior injection of ergometrine will harden its musculature and provide additional protection. Brisk bleeding demands further digital exploration rather than the blind use of metallic instruments. If the uterus is perforated in the course of this operation—and the first warning thereof may be the prolapse of omentum or bowel into the birth canal—the only safe measure is immediate laparotomy and repair of the rent. It will, therefore, be appreciated that the evacuation of the pregnant uterus demands the availability of proper theatre facilities.

Properly done, the whole placenta may be delivered in one piece. After its delivery, the uterus should be finally explored with the finger to make sure that no portion remains. If the uterus has been properly evacuated, there should be little more bleeding than follows dilatation and curettage in the non-gravid patient. Continued haemorrhage almost certainly indicates incomplete removal of placenta and the need for further exploration. A breathing space for the surgeon can be obtained, in cases of profuse haemorrhage requiring hastened blood transfusion, by digital compression of the uterus. For this at least two fingers are pressed up into the vaginal vault on either side of the cervix and the uterine body compressed through the abdominal wall against them. By this means also, the uterus can be rubbed up to contract after evacuation is completed in order to reduce the collection of clot within its cavity which, by its presence, may provoke yet more bleeding.

In less recent cases of incomplete abortion, curettage of the uterine wall may be necessary, and for this purpose there is no instrument more suitable than the spoon type of curette. The same precautions, as before, against perforating the uterus must, of course, be taken. The flushing curette is popular with many surgeons, but is seldom necessary. It often appears to start up unnecessary bleeding, it breaks down the natural defence barriers which are forming against infection, and injudicious use may force liquid up the Fallopian tubes. In any case, it makes a great mess.

The use of intra-uterine packing is debatable. Certainly plugging will effectively stop haemorrhage, but the most efficient way of arresting bleeding is to empty the uterus properly, in which case the plug is not necessary and serves to increase the risk of uterine sepsis.

The use of chemotherapy and antibiotics is clearly indicated as cover in cases known to be septic, but it is a mistake to use these substances simply as a protective umbrella under which to operate, for they may mask the true bacteriology of infection when it later reveals itself.

Transplacental Haemorrhage and Rh Sensitisation in Abortion

Using the Kleihauer technique it has been found that the incidence of transplacental haemorrhage in genuinely spontaneous abortion is small, at around 6 per cent with no significant haemorrhages of over five fetal cells per hundred low power fields. However, where termination of pregnancy has been deliberately undertaken the picture is altogether different and approximately a quarter of the cases are found to have suffered transplacental bleeding which in some was sufficiently severe to be capable of iso-immunising the patient.[43] These findings are amply confirmed by other workers in Newcastle[44, 45] and it is routine practice throughout the country to give the contents of a small-dose vial of anti-D gamma globulin for all abortions which are inevitable or therapeutic where the patient is Rh negative. The Rh grouping of the male partner could neither be known nor trusted. This dose of prophylactic anti-D is of 50 μg. The injection should be given within 36 hours of abortion, since Rhesus antigens have been found on fetal red cells as early as the 38th day of pregnancy.[5]

Treatment of Septic Abortion

So far, the two indications given for surgical evacuation of the uterus are, firstly, haemorrhage, and secondly, unduly long retention of placental tissue *in utero*. Nothing has yet been said of the place of evacuation in established sepsis, and here opinions vary.

As a general rule our preference is not to intervene surgically in the presence of uncontrolled uterine sepsis because of the danger of converting a local infection into a general one, which is infinitely more dangerous. When necrotic tissue is readily accessible and can be picked out, this, of course, should be done as before. Cultures, both aerobic and anaerobic should be obtained before any antiseptics are introduced into the genital tract and, pending the return of sensitivity reports from the bacteriologists, broad-spectrum antibiotics should be exhibited in serious cases in massive dosage. This therapy should become more specific as soon as the bacteriologist's report is available. A continuing tachycardia indicates the need for blood culture, as do rigors. Failure to respond within 48 hours suggests either the development of a pelvic abscess or some hitherto undiagnosed complication, such as uterine perforation or rupture in criminally induced cases, for which curettage would do nothing but harm.

The hazards of surgical evacuation of the uterus are greatly increased in septic abortion because the uterus is even more easily perforated and infected material can be readily disseminated. The need to perform laparotomy in such a case might well indicate hysterectomy as the safest course, a tragedy which might never have occurred if steps had been taken first to master the infection. If meanwhile, however, there is no response to treatment, an unlikely event, it may be necessary to explore the uterus after 36 hours.

In cases developing septicaemia the responsible organism is most often the *Staphylococcus aureus*, the anaerobic *Streptococcus* or *Clostridium welchii*. Haemolytic streptococci usually yield very readily to antibiotics and are less often fatal today. *Escherichia coli* infections are commonly responsible and may be associated with bacteraemic shock.

Clostridium welchii is often cultured on routine examination of patients in whom there is no clinical evidence of gas infection; nevertheless, when this organism gains a foothold the case comes into a class of its own. The presence of damaged or devitalised tissue is essential for its growth and, therefore, this type of sepsis is particularly favoured by criminal methods of interference, including the use of the syringe. The patient has a subnormal temperature, a rapid, thready pulse, a very low blood pressure and oliguria. Consciousness is retained to the last, and X-rays may show the presence of gas. Anti-gas gangrene serum in doses of 100,000 units should be injected four-hourly at first, penicillin should be massively prescribed, ileus is treated by gastric or duodenal suction and intravenous glucose saline, and very carefully matched blood should be given with judicious care. The patient undoubtedly needs the last, but the presence of oliguria allows of no more than a limited fluid intake (see section on anuria).

In summary, the presence of retained products in septic abortion is not in itself generally accepted by most of us as a primary reason for routine evacuation. The patient, if she is going to die, will do so because of a generalised infection rather than the local condition, and every effort must be made to attend to this first. In the wide choice of antibiotics now available, we can defy the basic principles of surgery with less penalty, but, even so, penicillin affords no justification for routine and ill-considered interference.

Endotoxic Shock

This is also sometimes referred to as "bacteraemic shock" and is chiefly associated with infection by Gram-negative organisms, particularly *E. coli*. Whereas Gram-positive organisms produce exotoxins which can inflict their damage at a distance, the originating bacteria meanwhile multiplying, in the case of Gram-negative organisms endotoxins may be released from the cell wall of the bacteria in the course of their death. The endotoxin so produced is not specific to any particular organism, although most commonly originating from the coliforms, and consists of a phospholipopolysaccharide which is closely linked to a protein and acts as a pyrogen and also destroys other living cells, particularly leucocytes, by increasing the permeability of the lysosomes within them. This accounts for the leucopenia so commonly associated with endotoxic shock. Hydrocortisone, apart from its other effects upon the vasomotor system, acts directly by countering this abnormal permeability.

Endotoxic shock differs very significantly from the other two types, namely the oligaemic or hypovolaemic and the cardiac type following infarction. The action of endotoxin is mainly peripheral and its chief effect is one of vasoconstriction so that there is a reduced venous return to the heart. Pyrexia may be a notable feature.

Metabolic effects are profound with mounting acidosis due to tissue hypoxia and an initial hyperglycaemia giving place to hypoglycaemia. Hypovolaemia is not normally a feature of the condition and therefore fluid-replacement therapy, especially in the presence of oliguria, may be dangerous.

There are three main stages in the production of endotoxic shock. The first is one of vasoconstriction with ischaemic hypoxia and the release of catecholamines. The second is the stage of stagnant hypoxia with apparent oligaemia. In the third stage, acidosis becomes profound and cardiac failure supervenes. The mortality of the condition varies with the efficacy of treatment, but may be between 50 and 70 per cent.

Cases of septic abortion sometimes demonstrate the Schwartzmann reaction. This involves diffuse intravascular coagulation which exhausts all the available clotting factors, to which is added the state of severe circulatory shock. As a result there is prolonged bleeding time, thrombocytopenia and diminished clot stability but the process is not primarily fibrinolytic. The intravascular coagulation is preceded by a phase of hypercoagulability which might call for the use of heparin to prevent the consumption of fibrinogen and all the other clotting factors involved. Ecchymoses, further haemorrhages and renal damage from fibrin thrombi simply indicate how far the condition has gone. Increasing thought is being given these days to the exhibition of heparin but for this to be rationally undertaken the assistance of a high-grade haematological department at hand is essential.

The clinical features of endotoxic shock are sudden and often unexpected collapse with rigors and pyrexia. The condition is not confined by any means to septic abortion and sometimes follows bladder instrumentation in males. Because of vasoconstriction there is marked peripheral cyanosis. The association of hypotension and rigors helps to distinguish endotoxic shock from the other two main types, namely, cardiac and oligaemic in which there is usually no such association. The systolic blood pressure is often 60 mm Hg or less and the patient is cold and clammy, becomes easily delirious and lapses into coma. Respiratory hyperventilation due to acidosis may be observed and, as already mentioned, there is initial leucopenia. Further examination of the blood shows a low Po_2 and a base deficit.

The haematocrit reading will only be raised if there has been associated fluid loss; otherwise it is likely to be normal. Measurement of the central venous pressure will, with most certainty however, indicate oligaemia if present, in which case it will be reduced, unlike myocardial or pulmonary infarction in which the CVP is raised.

The treatment has to be prompt and courageous. Fluid loss must be replaced, preferably under direct monitoring of the central venous pressure, which will not only give guidance as to the adequacy of replacement but will give warning of overhydration and congestion. The fluid used may be blood in cases associated with haemorrhage, 5 per cent intravenous glucose or a plasma volume expander such as Rheomacrodex. A poor urine flow may indicate intravenous mannitol, as in the treatment of anuria. The need for hydrocortisone is urgent and in a severe case 1 g should be given immediately intravenously, followed by doses ranging up to 500 mg per half litre of intravenous fluid in the worst cases. Overdosage with hydrocortisone is not to be feared and up to 3·5 g can be administered in 24 hours. It produces peripheral vasodilatation which may call for more fluid replacement already being monitored. Vasopressor drugs are normally dangerous and should be given only if there is obvious cardiac failure. Metaraminol (Aramine) is favoured by some because it increases renal blood flow and a dosage of up to 200 mg in the hour in 5 per cent dextrose has been recommended, though I have no personal experience of doses exceeding half that amount.[13] In any case this drug is overshadowed in importance by hydrocortisone which may be life-saving. Acidosis is corrected by sodium bicarbonate, starting with 100 mEq and correcting according to blood examination. Meantime the infection must be vigorously countered and pending a bacteriologist's report, including blood culture, a wide-spectrum but non-toxic antibiotic should be given in maximum dosage and for this purpose cephaloridine is the best yet available. It is non-toxic and avoids the great disadvantage of the tetracyclines of an uncontrollable build-up if there is any renal shut-down. In using artificial plasma volume expanders a watch must be kept against the development of hypofibrinogenaemia. The value of isoprenaline as a dilator of peripheral vessels is somewhat debatable because of its associated hypotensive effect which must be watched for. The use of hyperbaric oxygen is much disputed because of the already existing vasoconstriction which is part of the pathology of the condition. However, one of our cases near to death with this condition revived so quickly in a hyperbaric pressure chamber that it was tempting not to regard her dramatic recovery as a coincidence; but it has to be admitted she was receiving the rest of the gamut of treatment at the same time, although our use of hydrocortisone in this case was timid by modern standards.

Oliguria in spite of all the above indicates a very bad prognosis, but once the infection is mastered and urine secretion is adequate, recovery is unbelievably fast and apparently complete. These cases can be amongst the most terrifying in clinical practice and a matter of a few hours only may determine the issue of life or death.

Treatment of Missed Abortion

The greatest pitfall in this case is to diagnose missed abortion when, in fact, active pregnancy is continuing. To eliminate this mistake there is only one safe rule, namely, to wait and see, for there is no immediate need to intervene. Proof should be fully afforded before taking active steps; the urine pregnancy tests should be negative, the uterus after adequate observation should be seen not to enlarge, and all the signs of continuing pregnancy should have abated. Ultrasonic examination may clearly indicate the cessation of further growth, but of particular use is the ultrasonic Doppler effect, which is capable of picking up the fetal heart from the eleventh week onwards in many cases, and certainly by the twelfth or thirteenth week and thus immediately dispel the diagnosis of intra-uterine death[31]. After the sixteenth week X-rays may help (Fig. 10*a* and *b*). The patient will nearly always safely and spontaneously discharge the contents of her uterus in due course, certainly within the next nine months, though she may be irked by the delay and inconvenienced by a persistent dark vaginal loss. Our own record is a case which failed to deliver in spite of repeated attempts with oxytocin over the course of two years. There is however, a very real danger of a clotting defect, usually due to hypofibrinogenaemia, developing if a dead fetus is retained *in utero* for more than a month.[3] Most of us nowadays therefore will intervene in the absence of spontaneous abortion by the end of a month. One should proceed to an oxytocin drip in escalating dosage.[35] There is, of course, in such a case, no danger of uterine rupture and one can start straight off with 10 units of oxytocin in half a litre of intravenous dextrose or saline running at 25 drops a minute and increasing the concentration according to effect, if necessary up to 100 units of oxytocin to the half litre. Usually much less is effective, but the drip therapy may have to be repeated more than once with a day or two's rest in between. If hypofibrinogenaemia has developed before delivery, this must be corrected by fibrinogen replacement, but most instances of this ugly complication, however, are concerned with retained hydropic fetuses due to Rh haemolytic disease.

Surgical interference is to be avoided because of the appalling risks of sepsis, particularly from anaerobic organisms like *Cl. welchii*. Such attempts at uterine evacuation are often unpleasantly haemorrhagic and the cervix may prove very unyielding. I have used laminaria

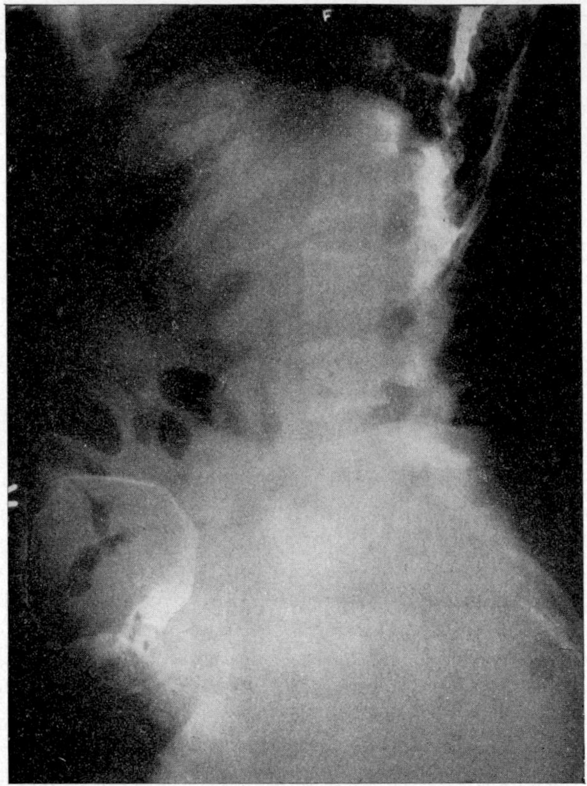

2/FIG. 10(*a*).—Intra-uterine death. X-ray showing appearance of a skull in intra-uterine death of the fetus. Note overlap of the bones of the vault (Spalding's sign).

tents in the past but only good luck, rather than good management, prevented catastrophe. A dead fetus *in utero* provides an anaerobe with the most perfect culture medium it could ever hope to encounter and the folly of surgical interference is likely to turn what is no more than a nuisance to the patient into a rapidly fatal infection.

In the unlikely event of really determined oxytocin drip therapy failing, recourse may be had to the addition of prostaglandin E2 infusions[50] up to a maximum of 4 μg/minute.

Injections of hypertonic solutions into the amniotic cavity are regarded by us as neither necessary nor safe.

CAUSES OF ABORTION, AND PROPHYLAXIS

The question of criminal interference and the degree to which it is practised have already been discussed. The majority of cases of septic

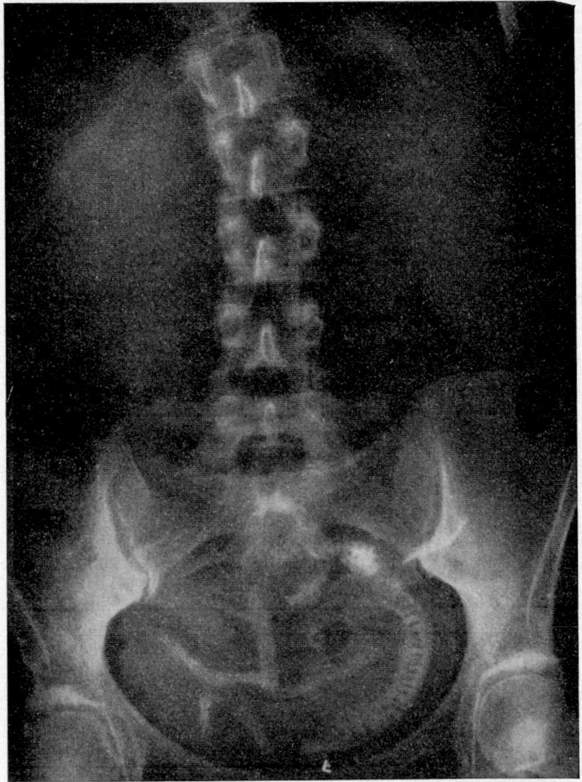

2/FIG. 10 (*b*).—Intra-uterine death. Note gross distortion of fetal spinal column.

(FIG. 10 *a* and *b* by courtesy of Dr J. W. McLaren.)

abortion are so caused, likewise cases of severe uterine haemorrhage early in pregnancy with a tightly closed cervix. The most horrifying method I have yet encountered was in Baghdad where I saw a young multipara who had dipped a feather into sewage and pushed it into her cervix. She died on the fifth day of septicaemia in spite of heroic attempts to save her. I gathered that the "method" was far from unusual.

So far, no medicinal method is reliably effective in a patient not naturally disposed to abort. Of the local methods employed, crochet hooks and sticks of slippery elm have tended to give place to the nowadays more common practice of violent syringing with Dettol or soap-and-water solutions, and I remember a case who managed to fill her peritoneal cavity, to the degree of shifting dullness, with a large quantity of soap suds. It nearly killed her, and when, after her recovery, we commented upon her recklessness, she answered firmly that the advertisements guaranteed the purity of the soap flakes! The modern fat-solvent detergent soaps are even more dangerous and we have had a case in whom it is believed a considerable quantity of the substance got into her central nervous system, which, besides nearly killing her, produced practically a complete quadriplegia, and to this

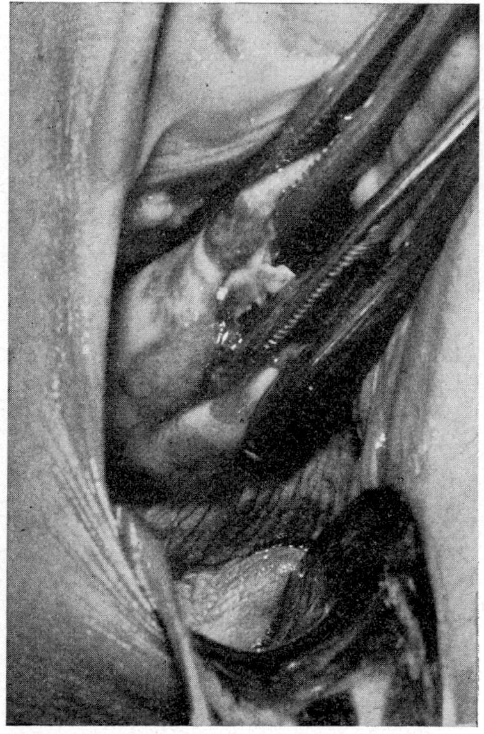

2/FIG. 11.—Potassium permanganate ulceration of cervix and fornices causing repeated and profuse haemorrhage.

(By courtesy of the late Dr G. W. Garland.)

day she can only move one arm slightly and continues a vegetable existence. Potassium permanganate crystals have also come into vogue. Besides being ineffective they ulcerate the fornices and cervix, and may cause profuse bleeding (Fig. 11).

Of spontaneous abortions, no cause either local or general can be found in more than half. Many cases are due to faulty development of the ovum, for which genetic factors may be to blame, and more attention is now being paid to the minute examination of these aborted fetuses for evidences of early abnormality.[30]

The present view is that bleeding in early pregnancy is not a cause of fetal abnormality but rather that the abnormality is a primary cause of the abortion. The extent to which this is recognised naturally depends upon the zeal with which many early specimens are obtained and without the help of sonar these would naturally be missed. However, even so, Carr reckoned that the prevalance of chromosomes anomalies in spontaneous abortions is about 36 per cent.[12] Bearing the above factors in mind even this striking figure is likely to be an understatement. These estimates have been further confirmed since at Guy's hospital in London a simultaneous series of therapeutic abortions were found to be chromosomally normal.[17] Nearly half of the abortuses which were chromosomally abnormal were autosomal trisomics, approximately 30 per cent chromosome monosomics, approximately 13 per cent triploids, and the remainder were made up of mosaics, double trisomic and tetraploid abortuses. Three had translocations.

The possible role of oral contraceptives in causing an increased incidence of abortion with a chromosomal anomaly, mainly polyploidy, is being investigated in the case of women conceiving within six months of abandoning this medication. These defects are incompatible with continuing fetal life and merit a more detailed investigation.[11]

The more carefully spontaneously aborted material is examined the more often will there be found some chromosomal abnormality. This involves immediate tissue culture of the material as soon as it is passed and this is only possible if it is fresh enough to culture. The material should be put in a sterile jar and taken immediately to the cytogenetic laboratory. We are fortunate in having such facilities and at the end of this chapter Professor Malcolm Ferguson-Smith gives an account of chromosome anomalies as a prominent cause of spontaneous abortion.

Of particular interest to us is the study by sonar (Fig. 12), of the process of ovum blighting. We have thus been able to foretell an inevitable abortion often weeks before it occurred.[25]

If, for any reason, the fetus dies *in utero*, abortion becomes inevitable, but this is only begging the question. General maternal diseases such as syphilis, nephritis, diabetes and infections associated with hyperpyrexia have long been accepted as causes, though nowadays they operate less commonly. Lead poisoning is now rare in England and is seldom a cause.

Profound anaemia, malnutrition and hypothyroidism are all significant aetiological factors, and it will be seen that a search (if worth while) for the cause of abortion demands an examination of the patient in a wide sense, including Wassermann reaction, thyroid and renal function and haematological investigation.

Rh iso-immunisation is not now regarded as a significant cause, for the abortion rate is no higher in Rh-negative patients. Perhaps one of the most important single factors is the trauma of sexual intercourse which may easily provoke abortion in the early weeks of pregnancy in a woman whose hold on pregnancy is none too secure.

Emotional factors such as severe shock and great fatigue may also result in the interruption of pregnancy.

Examination of the pelvic organs may reveal local conditions which might reasonably be inculpated. The significance of retroversion, for example, in this respect is debated, as about 10 per cent of all

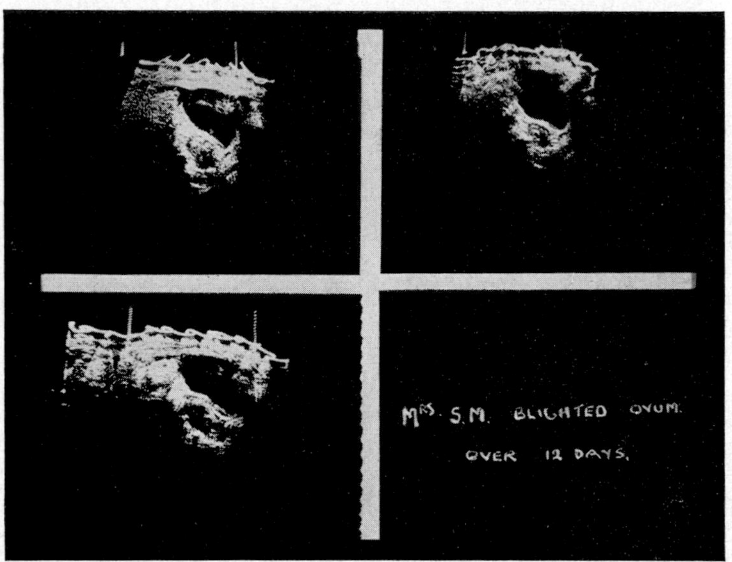

2/Fig. 12.—A case of blighted ovum. Ultrasonograms taken in longitudinal section (cranialwards to the left) over a period of twelve days. The distended bladder (large black area) permits a view of the uterus behind, which is not appreciably enlarged and contains only a speckled and non-growing mass. The patient was a recurrent aborter and again passed a blighted ovum.

(By courtesy of Year Book Medical Publishers, Inc.)

women have a retroverted uterus which is without pathological significance. Nevertheless, such a uterus does in fact abort rather more easily than one in normal position, and when abortion is recurrent there is much to be said for correcting the retroversion between pregnancies. When a patient with a history of abortion is found to be pregnant again with a retroverted uterus, she should be warned of the dangers of intercourse in the early months of pregnancy and before the retroversion has corrected itself. The use of the lateral position in coitus is certainly safer than the dorsal because it prevents deeper penetration. The prognostic value of hormone estimations is dubious and low output levels may be the result of abortion rather than indicating a cause in cases where a pregnancy is already beyond salvage.[33] Consequently such measurements of oestriol and pregnanediol excretion are of little help in determining the management of recurrent abortion,[39] although they are thoroughly worth while obtaining in order to provide a useful yardstick much later in pregnancy when the problem of dysmaturity comes on the horizon.

If a retroverted uterus is found early in pregnancy, the patient should be advised to encourage its spontaneous correction by lying on her front as often and for as long as she can and by seeing to it that her bladder is never allowed to become overfilled.

Fibroids are frequently associated with infertility and are often blamed for abortion, though their role in this respect is by no means general. Myomectomy between pregnancies, however, often increases a patient's chances of conception and carrying her pregnancy to term.

Deep lacerations of the cervix and high cervical amputation undoubtedly favour abortion, and cases of cervical incompetence, with membranes bulging through a partially dilated os, commonly abort in the second trimester. Dilatation of the cervix, as a treatment for spasmodic dysmenorrhoea, may also render the cervix incompetent, especially when the operation has resulted in splitting of the internal os rather than a careful overall stretching. Therapeutic abortion by the vaginal route undoubtedly increases the chances of abortion or premature labour in subsequent pregnancy.[66] In a country like Hungary where therapeutic abortions are considerably more common than deliveries the rise in prematurity to over 14 per cent has given cause for great disquiet. We now recognise that the cervix may be functionally incompetent even though the structural defect may not be obvious.

The question of genital hypoplasia as a factor is worth discussing, and patients with maldevelopment of the uterus are particularly less likely to conceive or, having done so, to retain their pregnancies. The diagnosis of hypoplasia is often made on evidence which is too slender and should be based upon more than a clinical impression of uterine size. Measurement of the cavity by a sound and hysterography are frequently necessary to justify the diagnosis. This is an important matter, because patients are often treated with oestrogens in the hope of increasing genital development; but a woman who has passed puberty cannot, by taking thought, or stilboestrol either, for that matter, add one cubit to her uterine stature. Vitamin deficiency, particularly of alphatocopherol (vitamin E), has long been known to produce abortion in rats, but the evidence that this occurs in humans is too slender to justify further comment.

Certain prophylactic measures are well worth enjoining. The avoidance of undue fatigue, especially at period times, and the lifting of heavy weights, continence during the first 14 weeks, and a quiet existence will greatly reduce the likelihood of abortion. Very hot baths are said to be harmful, and spirituous liquor and other such dissipations should be eschewed. To a patient who has aborted before, or in whom the threat to abort has already developed and subsided, advice in these respects is essential.

Prophylactic progesterone injections are given far more often than evidence of progesterone deficiency, if any, is discovered to justify their use.

The indulgence in very active forms of sport, including horse-riding, is of course asking for trouble.

Advice is often sought on the question of travel. Journeys by air are not contra-indicated, especially in these days of pressurised cabins at high altitudes. Lengthy journeys by car should be punctuated by halts at frequent intervals to allow the patient to move about and change her position.

Another common query is the advisability of anaesthesia for minor operations, such as dental extraction. The main risk here is that of asphyxia due to some anaesthetic accident. For this reason, the use of nitrous oxide is somewhat undesirable. Most dentists prefer to postpone, if possible, such an operation until the second trimester, because there is always the possibility that the patient might abort anyway and be encouraged to blame the operation for it.

Habitual Abortion

In defining habitual abortion most of us would accept an abortion sequence of not less than three, though patients are naturally anxious about their prospects after a sequence of two, in which case a recurrent factor can be less accurately inferred. Malpas[41] found that there was a recurrent factor in 1 per cent of women, whereas 17 per cent of women abort from random and accidental causes which are not recurrent. All the possible causes, both local and general, which have already been mentioned will have to be reviewed and excluded by examination. Nevertheless, causative factors in recurrent abortion are discernible in less than half the cases. Faulty early development of the embryo is an important recurrent factor, and ovum blighting as already described may be repeated in subsequent pregnancies.

There have been rumblings that women anaesthetists are more prone to spontaneous abortion (as well as involuntary infertility) and have an increased incidence of congenital fetal abnormality. This has been looked into in our own Department, with confirmatory results but with the comforting reflection that those who had given up work did better than those who are still in active anaesthetic practice.[34] A possible explanation is the teratogenic effect of volatile anaesthetic agents which may be absorbed by staff in operating theatres. If these findings are confirmed all such toxic atmospheric pollutants in operating theatres will have to be eliminated by elaborate exhaust systems which do not at present exist.

Listeria monocytogenes, an organism little noticed hitherto because of its resemblance to diphtheroids, is known to be a cause of abortion in certain animals and evidence is accumulating in Western Germany that in humans too such an infection may be a cause of habitual abortion as well as perinatal mortality.[55]

Listeria can be found in the seminal fluid of husbands and in the cervical mucus of some women who habitually abort[48] but so far there has been little reported of the infection in this country and our own pathologists strongly deny any suggestion from me that they have been missing the characteristic granulomata over the last few years. Nevertheless, we may hear more of this matter and its importance lies in its easy curability with antibiotics, particularly demeclocycline hydrochloride (Ledermycin).

The majority of cases are unexplained, and treatment, therefore, becomes empirical. It might be pointed out here that any treatment has to be seen against the background of the spontaneous cure rate. Malpas found that following one previous abortion the spontaneous cure rate was between 50 and 78 per cent with the chances propressively diminishing with each successive abortion until, after a sequence of four, they had reached very slender proportions.

In patients who habitually abort during the second trimester it is occasionally found that the cervix is already partially dilated, allowing the membranes to bulge, often some weeks before abortion starts Presently liquor starts to leak away, followed in a few days by abortion, or in some cases there is no such additional warning. It would appear that in these cases the mechanical factor of cervical incompetence might be responsible and a variety of operations have been designed, mainly modifications or simplifications of the Shirodkar type of operation. The membranes must first be reduced within the uterus and then, by one means or another, the cervical canal is reformed and practically closed by unabsorbable sutures.

The modification of this operation which we now use is that devised by Gavin Boyd in Belfast and is simplicity itself. The cervix is gently drawn down with two sponge forceps applied to anterior and posterior lips of the cervix (preferable to vulsella which often tear the softened cervix) and a simple braided tantalum wire suture is inserted as a purse string round the outside of the cervix taking four "bites" at the level of the internal os and without displacing the bladder by dissection. The knot is carefully tightened, just enough to provide a slight resistance to the passage of a No. 6 Hegar dilator and not tight enough to endanger the blood supply of the cervix. A commonly employed alternative is nylon tape, but it does not tie so well as tantalum wire. The latter is nowadays hard to get and braided nylon has to suffice.

This operation probably works by interfering with uterine polarity by discouraging the internal os and neighbouring lower segment from "taking up". If this is indeed the case it would be logical to extend the indications for the operation and not to await the gross signs of incompetence itself. The purpose after all is not to make the cervix apparently competent but to discourage uterine contractions which will dilate the cervix and so achieve abortion. On this basis it is our practice to use the operation in cases with a history of two previous abortions without apparent cause occurring after the first ten weeks and in whom there is no evidence of blood clotting defect nor of cervical mucus fern-like crystals indicating oestrogen/progesterone imbalance. There is always a disheartening risk that one may be trying by such a stitch to "lock up" a pregnancy already doomed and it is now our invariable practice to observe continuing intra-uterine growth over a period of some days by sonar before operating.

Such criteria may dilute some of the worst cases with others that might have been normal anyway. One of our cases started to abort some time after the operation and, on the wire suture being hurriedly removed, bleeding and contractions ceased and the pregnancy continued uninterrupted.

A suitable time to operate is at the fourteenth week although we have no hesitation in doing so earlier, even the tenth week, where the history indicates it. If labour supervenes, the stitch, of course, should be removed. Sometimes the patient aborts in spite of the presence of the stitch and nearly always it will be found that the encircling stitch has cut out of the posterior lip of the cervix and the products of conception have been passed through the cervix behind what is left of the stitch. A deep bite posteriorly is therefore essential when inserting it. I usually take a second bite here.

The suture is removed at the onset of labour or at the 38th week, whichever is the sooner. The procedure is so simple and harmless that it has every right to take its place among all the more picturesque attacks upon the problem, none of which can be scientifically evaluated for want of suitable untreated controls. These patients are usually desperate women who would not take kindly to being an "untreated control".

We do not recommend operation between pregnancies. The non-pregnant cervix does not heal predictably after trachelorrhaphy and it is impossible to gauge the desired degree of closure until pregnancy is well established.

An extreme instance of this type of deformity as a cause of recurrent abortion was shown in a case of mine who, at her first labour elsewhere delivered the baby through the back of the lower uterine segment and through the posterior fornix, by-passing the cervix entirely. The injury cannot have been noticed at the time, or repair there and then might have succeeded, but she was now left with a hole in the posterior fornix through which a finger could be poked into the uterus. Surprisingly she conceived, to her great distress, with monotonous regularity and had a series of abortions, each bloodier than the last. A diaphragm contraceptive was of course useless and her husband unco-operative. I tried to persuade her to accept an attempt at repair (offered without noticeable conviction) and finally yielded to her request for hysterectomy to prevent yet a fifth haemorrhagic disaster. Today I would have offered her sterilisation by bilateral tubal diathermy through a laparoscope.

Sequelae of Abortion

Many women suffer years of ill health following a serious abortion, and follow-up supervision is therefore important. The patient may have very great difficulty in restoring a normal haemoglobin level; post-abortum anaemia may reduce her health and efficiency for years to come and may easily prejudice the outlook in a further pregnancy. The detection and correction of anaemia are, therefore, the most important items of aftercare.

Infection contracted at the time of abortion may persist in a chronic form, giving rise to continued ill health, pain, dysmenorrhoea, menorrhagia and dyspareunia, while tubal occlusion puts an end to the patient's reproductive career.

A uterus which was not previously retroverted may now be found so, and the malposition may become permanent. It is often associated with subinvolution and the more chronic form of pelvic sepsis, and chronic cervicitis, with its associated symptom of vaginal discharge, may persist for years. A history of abortion in the first pregnancy is associated with a much higher incidence of threatened abortion and premature labour in the next.[38] A report from Queen Charlotte's Hospital in London[66] showed that there was a ten-fold increase in the incidence of second trimester abortion following vaginal termination of pregnancy. The perinatal death rate is appreciably higher due to prematurity, fetal abnormality or both.

It is likely that a common aetiological factor operates in this class of recurrent misfortune. Very occasionally hysterosalpingography undertaken in the investigation of cases of recurrent abortion or infertility may indicate some abnormality of the Müllerian system, most commonly a septate uterus. As a general rule the more complete the Müllerian duplication the less obstetrical trouble is the patient likely to encounter but on taking age, fertility and history into account a decision to operate and correct the anatomical defect is justified. Any pregnancies successfully ensuing call for elective delivery by Caesarean section.

HYDATIDIFORM MOLE

The cause of this strange condition is unknown, but it must be due to a defect of the ovum, because it can co-exist with a healthy twin. Hydatidiform degeneration can also be partial without belonging to a separate twin and I have had a case in which normal villi were interspersed with gross hydatidiform change and a developing fetus. So far we have thrice demonstrated by sonar the co-existence of hydatidiform mole and normal fetus, and have had the courage to make the pre-operative diagnosis. The problem of what to do next was solved in all instances by either acute pre-eclampsia or haemorrhage so that therapeutic abortion became not a matter of opinion but of necessity (Fig. 13). A change, partly degenerative and partly hyperplastic, occurs in the chorionic villi, causing them to take the form of

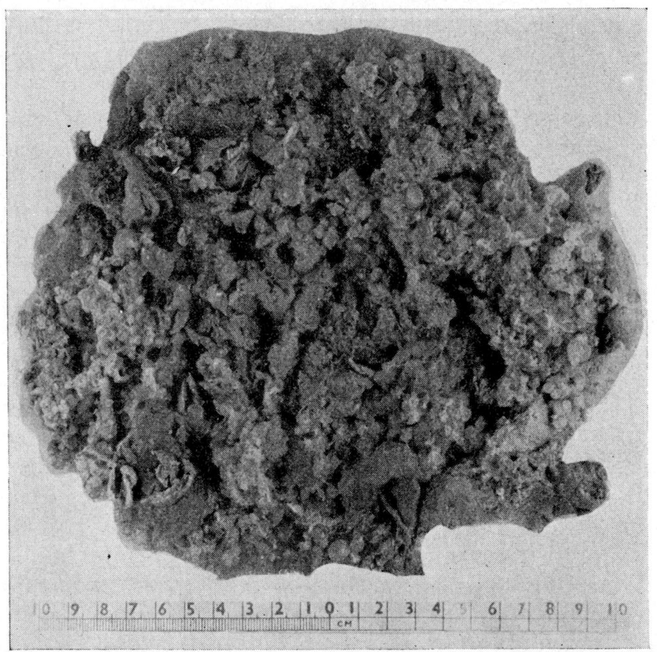

2/Fig. 13.—A case of hydatidiform degeneration interspersed with normal villi and an actively growing fetus within the sac. Fulminating pre-eclampsia necessitated therapeutic abortion.

cysts which vary in size from a grape seed to a cherry. Most commonly the entire villous system undergoes vesicular change and no fetus or normal placenta can be found within the uterus, but occasionally these changes may only partially affect an otherwise normal placenta. Both trophoblastic layers, namely syncytium and Langhan's layer, persist, but the mesodermal core of the villus undergoes a myxomatous change and its blood vessels disappear (Fig. 14). The vesicles, of course, draw their nourishment from the maternal blood supply. Because of the persistence of the trophoblastic elements, the power to invade the decidua persists, and may even cause penetration of the uterine wall. Maternal blood vessels encountered are easily entered, so that small trophoblastic elements may be swept into the general maternal circulation. The syncytium shows a marked tendency to budding, and the Langhan's layer shows proliferative activity, but it is difficult from histological examination to judge whether or not a particular hydatidiform mole is benign or malignant the latter being much less common. Commonly there is enlargement of both ovaries due to multiple theca-lutein cysts. They are the result of the stimulus of high circulating chorionic gonadotrophin levels in the blood and after riddance of the mole they regress spontaneously.

The disease, though uncommon, is by no means rare, since many cases are not reported. A rough estimate of the incidence would be about 1 in 2000 pregnancies. In China, and Malaysia where there is a large Chinese population, the disease is about four times as common.

Symptoms

The cardinal symptom is bleeding, though its presence is by no means invariable. It may be preceded by a sanious, watery discharge, most commonly between the 3rd and 4th month of pregnancy. It is usually unremittent and occasionally very profuse. All the usual symptoms of pregnancy are present in full measure, and vomiting, for example, may be exaggerated to the degree of hyperemesis. The patient is likely to become progressively more anaemic and nearly always looks far from well. Pain is not usually present, unless concealed bleeding within the uterus occurs to an appreciable degree or the mole becomes infected. Pre-eclamptic toxaemia is often superadded, and eclampsia may develop at an early stage of pregnancy.

Diagnosis

Examination of the patient reveals all the usual signs of early pregnancy, but the uterus is, more often than not, larger than the period of gestation would suggest. Occasionally the size of the uterus is normal, and uncommonly it may actually be smaller than normal.

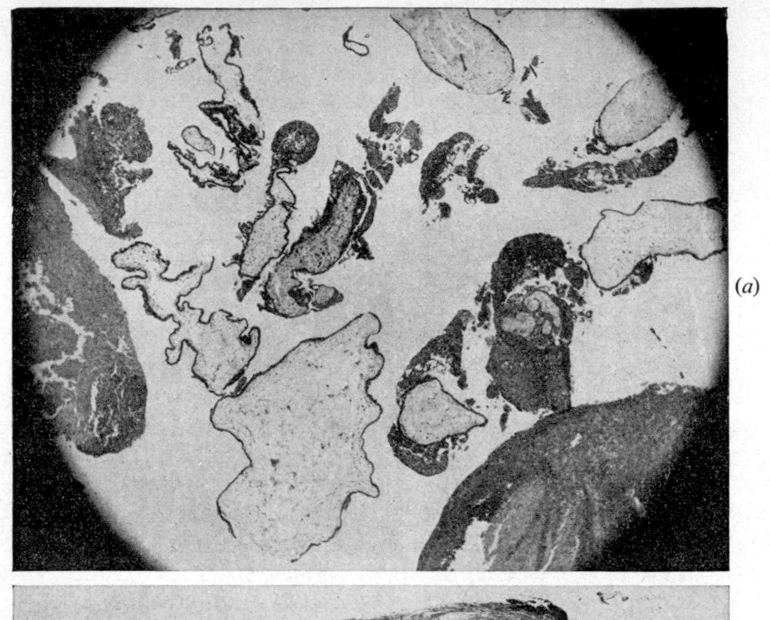

(*a*)

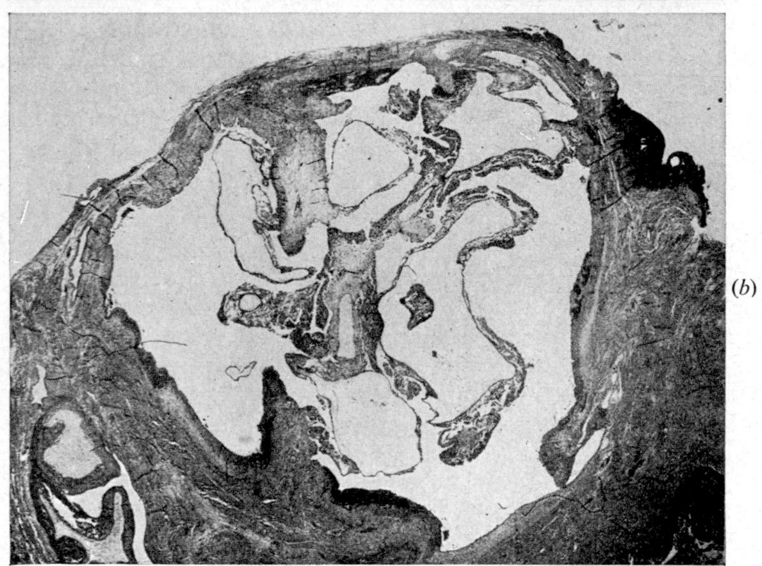

(*b*)

2/FIG. 14 (*a*).—Hydatidiform mole. Chorionic villi are enlarged by oedema, are devoid of blood vessels and some of them have hyperplastic trophoblast.

2/FIG. 14 (*b*).—"Malignant" hydatidiform mole. Mole removed 8 weeks previously. Friedman test became positive again. Hysterectomy specimen. Low-power magnification showing hydatidiform mole embedded in myometrium and deeper invasion by some hyperplastic trophoblast (bottom left corner). Patient recovered.

(By courtesy of Prof. C. V. Harrison.)

Brews found that the uterus was unduly enlarged five times as frequently as diminished.[6] Palpation of the uterus gives an impression which is hard to describe but is not quite normal, and its consistency appears to the touch to be more doughy than cystic. On bimanual examination ballottement cannot be elicited, since the whole cavity of the uterus is filled with vesicles instead of fetus and liquor amnii. A straight X-ray of the lower abdomen is often helpful in one sense, inasmuch as the radiographic evidences of fetal parts rule out all major degrees of hydatidiform mole. As one is usually in doubt, however, long before the 16th week, the usefulness of radiological examination is somewhat limited, since fetal parts cannot be seen earlier than this.

Signs of pre-eclamptic toxaemia are occasionally present, being rare in early pregnancy except in cases of hydatidiform mole. The urine contains large quantities of chorionic gonadotrophin, so that a pregnancy test may be positive in one-in-a-hundred dilution; but this is not conclusive, because even normal pregnancies may give positive results in these dilutions within the first 100 days. I have even had cases where the pregnancy test on the urine was only positive undiluted and in one case the test was even negative, so too much reliance cannot be placed on gonadotrophin levels in the urine.

Occasionally ovarian theca-lutein cysts may be detected on careful vaginal examination. These cysts are often as large as tennis balls, although the size is variable.

It is very difficult to be certain of the diagnosis of hydatidiform mole before the spontaneous discharge of vesicles *per vaginam*, which may not be observed for some weeks. The most important and common differential diagnosis is that of threatened abortion in a pregnancy otherwise normal; therefore, an expectant line of treatment often has to be adopted for a long time. Serious mistakes in intervention are commonly made in the belief that a hydatidiform mole is present because of a positive pregnancy test in high dilution and because of errors in the patient's dates. My own researches in the diagnostic uses of ultrasonic echo sounding (sonar) have naturally extended to this problem and our apparatus[18, 19] can distinguish between early fetal parts *in utero* and a mass of vesicles, by displaying the echoes from these structures on the face of a cathode ray tube, which is photographed. The dot-like echoes from clusters of vesicles (Fig. 15*a*) can be almost suppressed by reducing the amplification or "gain" of the apparatus (Fig. 15*b*) whereas fetal echoes are not only demonstrable, strong and clear from the tenth week onwards, but cannot be suppressed by the same reduction in gain settings (Fig. 15*c*). Our positive identification of hydatidiform mole by this means now extends to many dozens of cases, while the method has proved equally valuable in excluding the diagnosis of hydatidiform

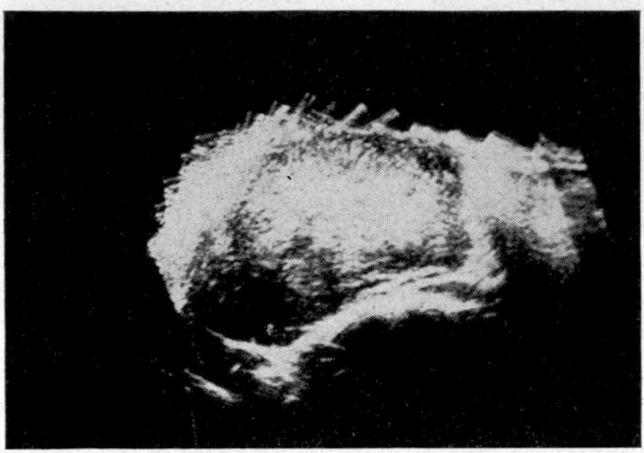

2/Fig. 15 (*a*).—Ultrasonogram in longitudinal section of uterus containing hydatidiform mole. High-gain amplification.

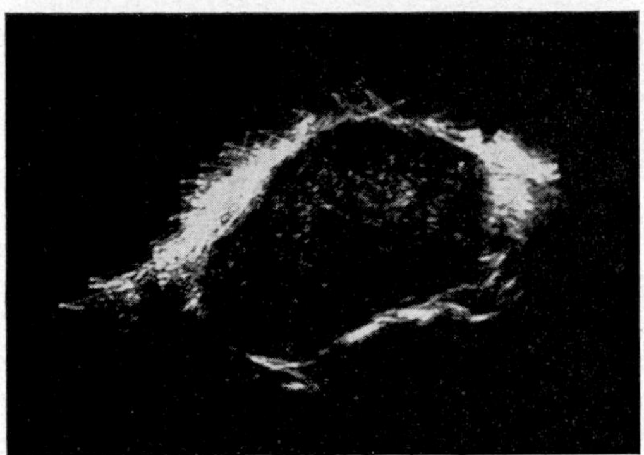

2/Fig. 15 (*b*).—Ultrasonogram. Same case as Fig. 15*a*. Reduced gain practically extinguishes echoes of hydatidiform mole, unlike fetal echoes.

(Fig. 15 *a* and *b* by courtesy of the Editor *Brit. J. Radiol.*)

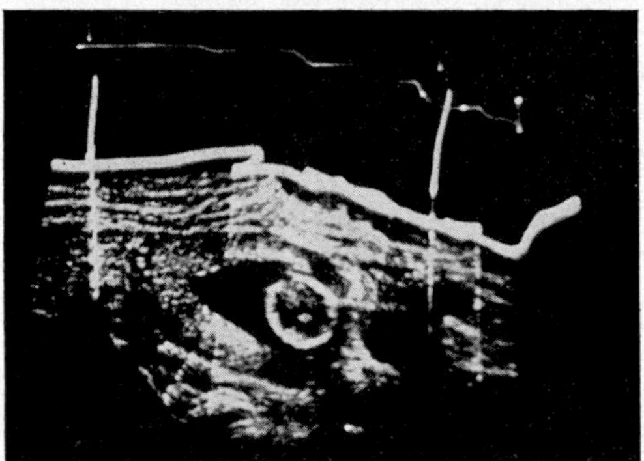

2/Fig. 15 (*c*).—Ultrasonogram. Normal pregnancy of 15-week gestation, showing fetal echoes. Note fetal head.

mole by demonstrating fetal echoes long before standard radiology would be of any help.

A carneous mole or missed abortion may be confused with hydatidiform mole, but here the uterus ceases to enlarge, the symptoms of pregnancy regress, and the urine test usually becomes negative within about a fortnight. It was suggested as long ago as 1949[29] that a hydatidiform mole may in fact arise in the placental remnants of a missed abortion which has not died and we have from time to time demonstrated what would appear to be a small sac in the midst of the molar mass by sonar before abortion.[22, 23] The possibility is therefore suggested that one of the hazards of a retained missed abortion is the subsequent development of hydatidiform change, particularly if the chorionic gonadotrophin tests remain positive.

A retroverted gravid uterus incarcerated within the pelvis and causing retention of urine is another diagnostic possibility, but vaginal examination should rule this out.

Fibroids in association with pregnancy may be accompanied by a threat to abort, and the uterine enlargement due to their presence may contribute to error. A fibroid undergoing myxomatous degeneration can give ultrasonic appearances in pregnancy deceptively like those of hydatidiform mole—a serious mistake which can best be prevented by confirming the diagnosis at the higher ultrasonic frequency of 5MHz which is now our rule.[24]

Sometimes the uterus containing a hydatidiform mole may be so large that it reaches almost to the xiphisternum and hydramnios may be diagnosed, although there is no fluid thrill, no ballottement, and bleeding is the predominant symptom.

Needless to say, everything that is passed and all pads should be very carefully inspected, as otherwise the passage of a few tell-tale vesicles may be missed and the true diagnosis consequently put off, the patient meanwhile becoming steadily more anaemic and requiring treatment on that account. Often the first indication of the presence of hydatidiform mole is the onset of its spontaneous expulsion, which is frequently incomplete at first and accompanied by profuse haemorrhage (Fig. 16).

Treatment

As soon as the condition is definitely diagnosed, steps should be taken to empty the uterus or to encourage it to empty itself, because further delay will only increase the risks of haemorrhage. In women in the younger age groups, spontaneous evacuation, encouraged, if necessary, by a full medical induction, including the use of a brisk oxytocin drip, is the most satisfactory outcome, but the risks of malignancy increase with the patient's age, so that over the age of 40 hysterectomy is undoubtedly the safest course. Recently we had a case of hydatidiform mole in a widow aged 53. The diagnosis was not made until after hysterectomy (no preliminary curettage) and to my even greater fury the specimen was not photographed! We recall this as the case of the merry widow who had the correct treatment for the wrong reason.

An escalating oxytocin drip starting with 10 units to the half litre and rising, if necessary, to ten times that concentration is nowadays

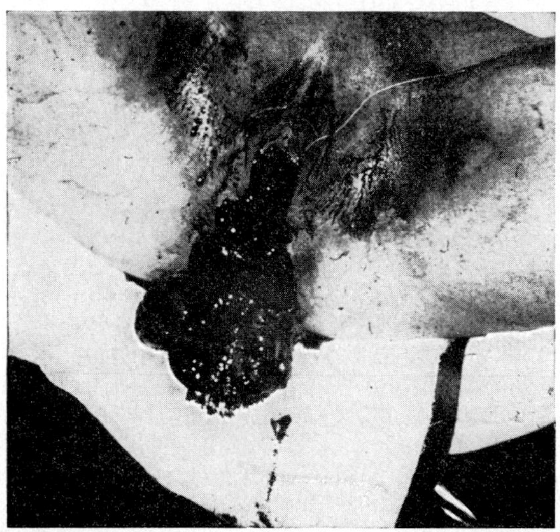

2/FIG. 16.—Hydatidiform mole in process of being aborted.

the most commonly used method of getting the patient to abort the mole. It is most likely to work if the abortion process has already started as demonstrated by the preliminary passage of some vesicles. The attempt can be repeated. Often, however, this meets with no success, and one is left with the alternatives of some type of surgical induction and evacuation or resorting to abdominal hysterotomy. When the mole is expelled, either spontaneously or as the result of drug induction, the uterus should always be explored with the gloved finger because expulsion is frequently incomplete. In other cases, the patient makes no attempt to get rid of her mole and the cervix remains tightly closed. Laminaria tents to dilate the cervix have been advocated in the past and I have used them (which dates me), but even these can fail to bring on abortion, and the dangers of infection are considerable, dangers which are enhanced by a state of anaemia and the presence of quantities of suitable culture material within the uterus. A single tent inserted within the cervix is seldom adequate, and, if possible, two or three should be inserted side by side. The resulting amount of dilatation of the cervix is then usually sufficient after 24 hours to allow the passage of a finger into the uterine cavity.

The alternative of dilating the cervix with metal dilators, although less likely to provoke sepsis, may result in considerable tearing of the cervix and lower segment, because sufficient dilatation must be achieved to allow a finger to be passed with ease. Digital exploration of the uterine cavity must not only be thorough but reasonably brisk, as great haemorrhage can attend the manoeuvre. One should always use a slow intravenous oxytocin drip, 10 units in 500 ml, during the operation to harden up the soft, atonic uterine wall. No instrument other than the gloved finger is safe for the purpose because of the exceptional ease with which the uterine wall can be perforated, especially if its integrity has been undermined by direct invasion by trophoblast. A blood transfusion already set up as a precautionary measure may be life-saving. Ergometrine, likewise, should be at hand for intravenous use for the immediate control of any undue haemorrhage. The size of the uterine cavity may be such as to make it impossible to explore more than a fraction of its volume forthwith, and the procedure is to pass the half-hand into the vagina and to loosen up as much of the mole as can be reached and to pick out the loosened fragments with ovum forceps, the other hand, meanwhile, being kept upon the body of the uterus through the abdominal wall, steering it towards the internal finger. As the uterus shuts down with the successive removal of each mass of tissue, more and more of the uterine cavity comes within digital reach until, by judicious bimanual manipulation, the entire internal surface can be thoroughly explored. More recently a colleague, Maung, from Burma, has introduced me to a splendid method of evacuating a large hydatidiform mole employing the vacuum aspiration abortion curette, which I have found most useful. While an oxytocin drip is running the cervix is dilated no more than necessary to admit one of the larger sizes of vacuum curette without loss of suction, if necessary clamping the cervix. This is introduced no more than to the half-way level of the uterine contents. Suction is then applied up to 200–250 millimetres of mercury, the curette being rotated slowly at this level. It therefore sucks out the hydatidiform mole from within its centre, the uterus meanwhile reducing its size as the contents are sucked out and with the help of the oxytocin. This manoeuvre costs the patient far less blood than previous methods and the mole is practically entirely eliminated before the decidual surface of the uterus is disturbed.

Having emptied the uterus, more ergometrine is given to control bleeding, and it may be necessary for a couple of minutes to resort to bimanual compression. This can be a very messy and bloody operation, and it is necessary to get a move on if an undue quantity of blood is not to be lost. Curettage should be repeated 5 to 7 days later after delivery of the mole, whether spontaneous or assisted, in order to remove residual fragments.

For these reasons, there is much to be said for abdominal hysterotomy when the cervix is tightly closed, and when two or more escalating oxytocin drips have failed. I have never yet regretted "chickening-out" and performing abdominal hysterectomy if vaginal abortion threatens to be difficult or dangerous. The lower segment approach can usually be made. It has, moreover, the advantage that the uterus can be inspected for the presence of the penetrating variety of mole which may justify proceeding to hysterectomy. Certainly less blood will be lost in evacuating the uterus by the abdominal route, and the situation is much more easily kept under control. At laparotomy, the presence of quite large lutein cysts may be observed, usually bilateral, and their sheer size may encourage one to resect them, but they should be left strictly alone, as they always absorb and disappear within the next few weeks.

In a more elderly patient in whom hysterectomy is indicated, it is a good plan to suture the cervix before proceeding, to prevent the dissemination of trophoblastic tissues.

As may be gathered, this is a dangerous condition. The immediate risks are those of haemorrhage, shock and sepsis, yet in spite of these, mortality is not as high as one would expect. Further curettage, one to two weeks after the mole is aborted, is recommended as part of the routine follow-up in all cases delivered *per vaginam.*

Since the beginning of 1973 a Register has been established by the Department of Health and Social Security and the Royal College of Obstetricians and Gynaecologists for purposes of follow-up over a two-year period with a service laid on of serial estimations of urinary gonadotrophin levels. It is reckoned that there are about 800 or more cases of hydatidiform mole in the United Kingdom annually but because of the very real risk that a small percentage of them may suffer a more invasive type of mole or even go on to choriocarcinoma it is a matter of great importance to identify those in need of special treatment such as chemotherapy at the earliest possible moment. Frequent estimations of human chorionic gonadotrophin levels provide a good early-warning system. The most sensitive methods of testing are by radioimmunoassay but because of the expense it is agreed that this testing should be centralised. The Centres supplying this service through the R.C.O.G. at present are Charing Cross Hospital in London, The Jessop Hospital in Sheffield, and the University of Dundee. Frequent chest X-ray examinations are recommended as long as the gonadotrophic levels remain abnormal. Bagshawe and his colleagues in London have shown that when treatment is instituted within two to six months of the previous hydatidiform mole chemotherapeutic drugs are more effective, better tolerated, and have a better chance of prolonged remission. The reverse is the case with delays in treatment.[1, 2]

There remains the tricky question of how long a patient who has had a hydatidiform mole should wait before embarking upon another pregnancy and whether oral contraceptives are meanwhile safe. The usual advice to wait for a period of two years is to prevent the confusion in diagnosis which may arise when the gonadotrophin levels reappear because of a pregnancy rather than as indications of choriocarcinomatous change. This kind of doubt can be at once resolved at a very early stage in units equipped with suitable sonar apparatus and my own practice would be to permit pregnancy if

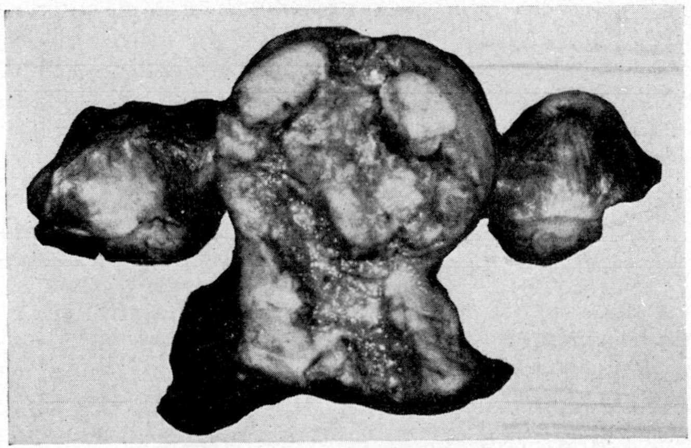

2/Fig. 17.—Hysterectomy specimen of choriocarcinoma. Presented as incomplete septic abortion. Satisfactory recovery.

gonadotrophic tests had been normal for a period of 12 months. Oral contraceptives are without known danger in this interim period.

Choriocarcinoma (chorion epithelioma).—Apart from the immediate risks, the remote danger of choriocarcinoma is a serious matter, and estimates of its likelihood vary around 10 per cent, although European figures are generally lower. This highly malignant condition may follow normal pregnancy, abortion or tubal pregnancy, but the risk is immeasurably greater after hydatidiform mole. If choriocarcinoma is going to develop, it will almost certainly do so within two years, and seldom in under two months, although Fig. 17 shows a uterus originally evacuated for septic abortion, not once but twice within a fortnight because of continued bleeding and discharge and in which the curettings showed choriocarcinoma on the second occasion. The patient has remained well since. Usually tests become negative within a few weeks of expulsion of a hydatidiform mole although I once had a case in which they remained positive in undiluted urine for just over a year. She subsequently had a normal pregnancy. What is particularly significant is a test which becomes positive after a period of being negative, and it may be very difficult to tell at first whether a patient has developed a choriocarcinoma or has started a fresh pregnancy. Ultrasonography may help, as already indicated. Positive results in dilutions of 500 or over are almost pathognomonic of choriocarcinoma and indicate the need for immediate panhysterectomy or chemotherapy. A diagnostic curettage may settle the point by yielding the necessary histological evidence, but it is by no means a certain method of excluding this dreadful complication, because the growth may be embedded within the uterine wall and may not be accessible to the exploring curette (Figs. 18 and 19).

A discussion of the varying grades of malignancy of choriocarcinoma would be out of place in this book, but the very serious prognosis is due to its rapid and widespread dissemination by the blood stream, even before warning signs of irregular vaginal bleeding occur, and the patient may present with haemoptysis as the first sign. Other signs of developing choriocarcinoma are the appearance of metastatic deposits in the lower vagina and vulva, and uterine enlargement.

The serious outlook for these cases has been transformed by the use of amethopterin (methotrexate-Lederle). This substance (4-amino-N^{10}-methylpteroylglutamic acid) acts as a folic acid antagonist. Folic acid (pteroylglutamic acid) is prevented by methotrexate from conversion into folinic acid (citrovorum factor) which is essential for the synthesis of nucleic acid and hence the mitotic process. It would appear to be particularly applicable to this virulent type of tumour.[42] It has been suggested[14] that it should be given even before hysterectomy, especially where metastases are already evident, in the belief that surgical manipulation increases spread of the disease. This chemotherapy or nothing approach to treatment, however, has been more recently queried from Singapore by Tow and Cheng,[60] who have shown that timely hysterectomy in cases where the tumour is localised to the uterus is well worth carrying out and that chemotherapy has its major role in the management of metastatic choriocarcinoma. We ourselves have treated cases by chemotherapy using the dosage scheme of Bagshawe and McDonald.[1] This takes the form of combined treatment using methotrexate and 6-mercaptopurine. Methotrexate is administered by mouth in divided doses totalling 25 mg a day, usually for a five-day course provided the patient's general condition can stand it. More recently the intravenous route has been used. Likewise 6-mercaptopurine in divided doses totalling 600 mg a

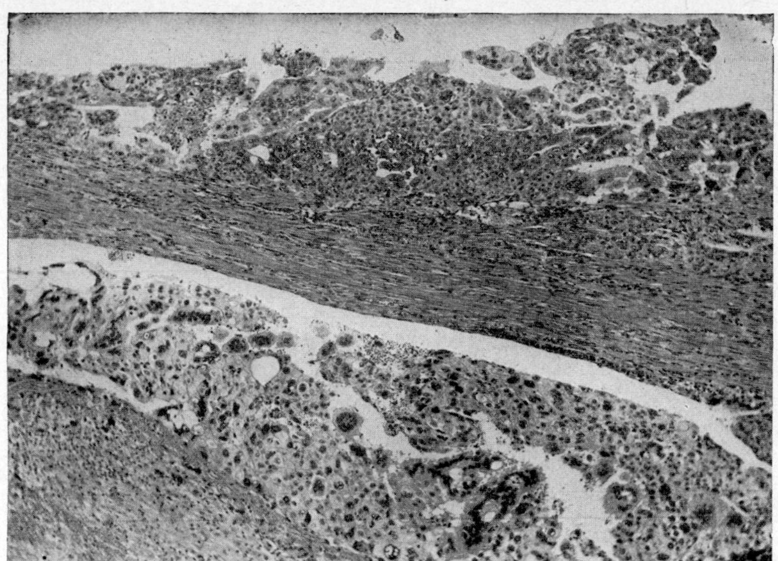

2/Fig. 18 (*a*).—Choriocarcinoma invading myometrium. In the upper parts of the field the Langhans cells and syncytium are present together; in the lower part, the tumour consists largely of syncytium. The myometrium is also infiltrated with neutrophils.

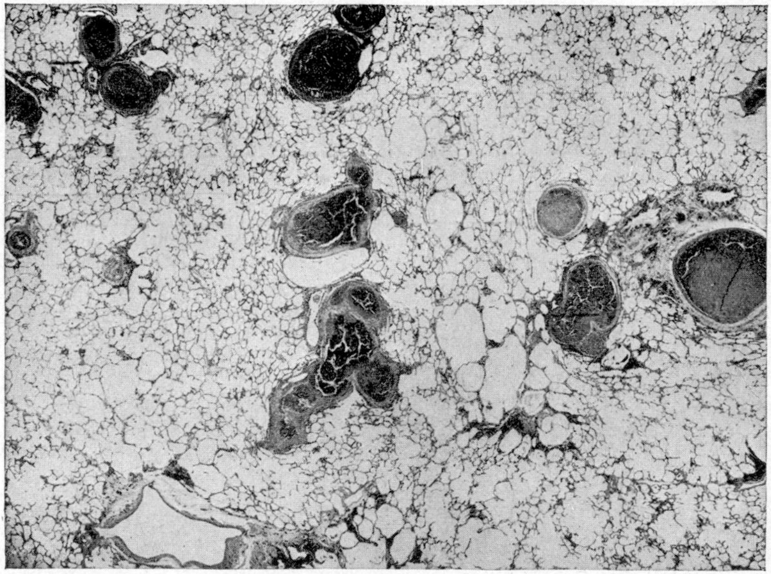

2/Fig. 18 (*b*).—Choriocarcinomatous metastases. Low-power view of lung showing pulmonary arteries distended by masses of tumour and thrombosis.

(By courtesy of Prof. C. V. Harrison.)

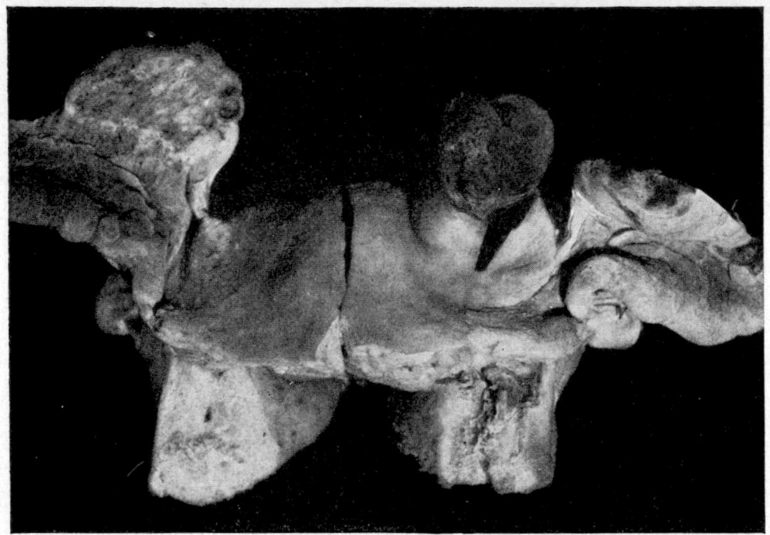

2/FIG. 19 (*a*).—Perforating choriocarcinoma. Patient continued bleeding after abortion at three months. Curetted twice—sections not conclusive. Admitted subsequently with acute haemoperitoneum. Recovered.

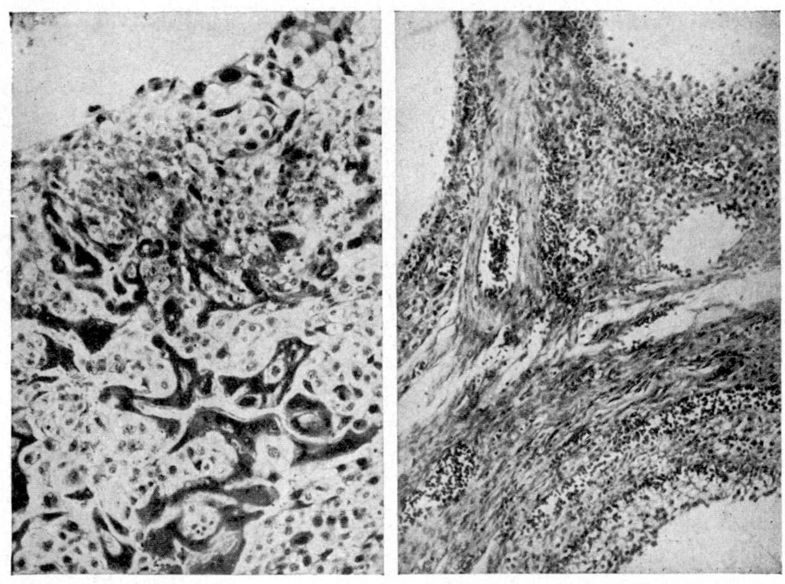

2/FIG. 19 (*b*).—Same case. Curettings. Choriocarcinoma.

2/FIG. 19 (*c*).—Same case. Theca-lutein cysts.

(By courtesy of the late Dr G. W. Garland.)

day are given at the same time. This latter drug is toxic to fetal tissues and is an antagonist to hypoxanthine and adenine. As soon as the white cell count starts to fall antibiotic cover is instituted. The patient must be nursed in isolation in an infection-free environment. The courses may have to be repeated especially if the gonadotrophin pregnancy tests become positive again suggesting recrudescence of the disease. Side-effects are severe but usually come at the end of, or after, a 5-day course, so that the damage is already done by then. They consist of stomatitis going on to ulceration, intense dysphagia, vomiting, diarrhoea, occasionally jaundice, great susceptibility to infections, skin pigmentation and loss of hair. Some of these are due to profound leucopenia and thrombocytopenia which result from the treatment. There may be proteinuria as well. Fortunately these signs are usually reversible after the cessation of treatment, even the hair growing again.

It has been suggested that the effect of this treatment may be mitigated by prior aspiration of bone marrow, its storage under powerful refrigeration and reinjection after the end of treatment, but we have no personal experience of this.

To some extent methotrexate has an antidote in the form of folinic acid (citrovorum factor).

In the first of our own cases there was no antecedent pregnancy, the origin being teratomatous, and antibodies to her husband's leucocytes could not be demonstrated as might have been expected if the growth had originated from a pregnancy for which her husband was responsible.[27] There was no response and she died rapidly.

Another of our cases had had a hydatidiform mole some months earlier and had recently undergone total hysterectomy elsewhere for histologically proven choriocarcinoma.[20] She was now referred to us within a few weeks with metastatic deposits in the vaginal vault and vulva (Plate III, *a*) the latter being excruciatingly tender. She had pulmonary metastases and a haemoglobin level of 35 per cent. Her response to methotrexate was dramatic, so I rashly put her on as a case for the Glasgow Fellowship in which I was examining. To the candidate's horror he was greeted with torrential haemorrhage due to separation and sloughing of the vaginal and vulval deposits. The examination was halted while my co-examiner and I dealt hurriedly with the situation. Ultimately packing under anaesthesia was of no avail (obviously arterial bleeding) and I had to ligate the anterior division of the left internal iliac artery with strong silk before peace was restored. (The candidate passed!) Following two courses there are no signs of the original metastases (Plate III, *b*) and her urine pregnancy tests remain negative (over 7 years and now lost sight of) but at the time, as is usual with such treatment, she was reduced to a very wretched state with leucopenia, ulcerative stomatitis and dysphagia. Her hair, which threatened to fall out (Fig. 20), has since grown again and she has returned to running her farm and her husband as before.

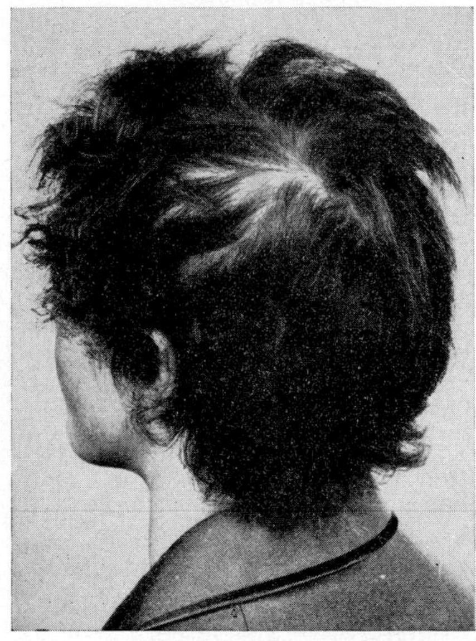

2/Fig. 20.—Loss of hair due to methotrexate.

Instances of recurrent hydatidiform mole are rare, much more so in fact than the development of choriocarcinoma. In my experience I have only once met a patient with a history of two such moles. Needless to say she presented with a request for an ultrasonic examination and we were able to demonstrate a normal pregnancy on this occasion.

INTRA-UTERINE FETAL DEATH

The term IUD (preferably used thus in the patient's hearing) embraces cases before the 28th week of pregnancy (missed abortion) and those occurring later which result in macerated stillbirth.

A very slovenly practice has grown up of referring to the intra-uterine contraceptive device as an IUD instead of an IUCD leaving out the "C". I well recall a case referred to me by an exasperated general practitioner, who had had one of his patients X-rayed for fetal parts since he suspected a pregnancy in spite of the previous insertion (elsewhere) of an intra-uterine contraceptive device. The radiologist reported not only the fetal parts, but that that "IUD" was present. The patient thus came to my clinic thoroughly alarmed

PLATE III

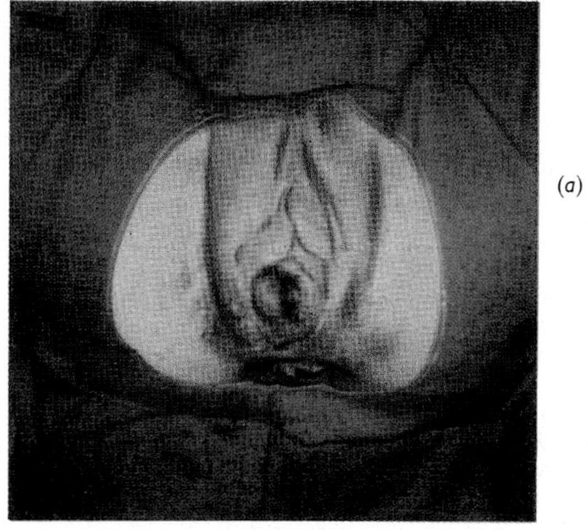

(a)

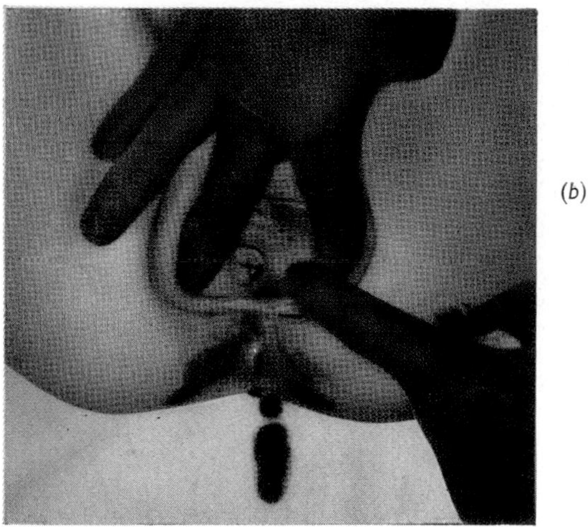

(b)

(*a*) Choriocarcinomatous deposit at vulva before treatment with methotrexate.

(*b*) Same case after treatment with methotrexate. Healed.

(By courtesy of Lederle Laboratories and John Wright and Sons, Ltd., Bristol.)

that her baby had "died *in utero*." Fortunately I was able to demonstrate to her an active fetal heart beat.

Maceration is a destructive aseptic process which first reveals itself by blistering and peeling of the fetal skin (Fig. 21). This appears between 12 and 24 hours after fetal death and in a case of stillbirth

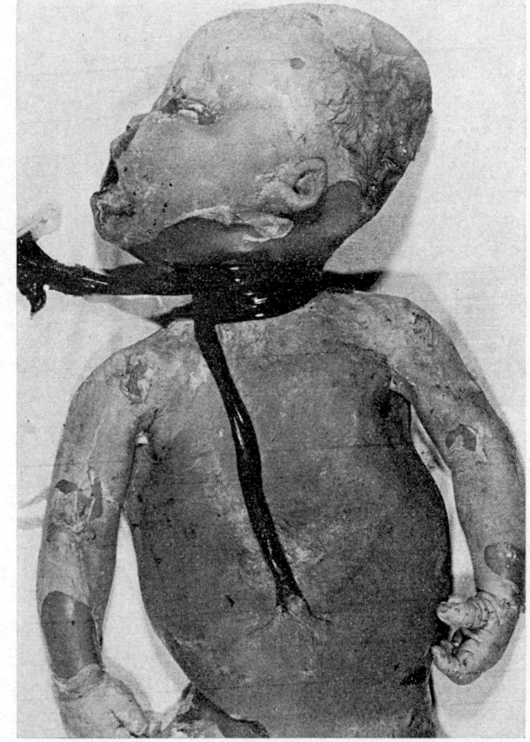

2/FIG. 21.—Fetal maceration. From *Diagnostic Ultrasound*, 1974. Ed. D. L. King, by courtesy of C. V. Mosby Co.

exculpates causes operating during labour except when labour is seriously prolonged.

The process, however, involves the whole body, giving rise to the characteristic radiological signs. The ligaments are softened and the vertebral column is liable to sag or collapse, especially with the patient in the erect posture. The ribs may concertina together and the skull bones, already loosened in their mutual attachments, overlap each other at the sutures because of the shrinkage of the brain (Spalding's sign, Fig. 10*a*).

It takes several days for Spalding's sign to appear after intra-uterine death, usually a week or more. Of all the radiological signs it is the most definite but is disqualified if the membranes are already ruptured or if labour is in progress. Spalding's sign may be present in an extra-uterine pregnancy which is still alive. Two X-rays taken within several hours with identical positioning may show total absence of fetal movement if the pictures are viewed superimposed. This is highly suggestive of fetal death.

Gas bubbles appear in the heart, aorta, vena cava, liver, cord and abdominal cavity[49] quite apart from infective putrefaction (Fig. 22*a* and *b*). These signs are very reliable in the diagnosis of intra-uterine death and, appearing within the first few days, provide the first conclusive evidence.[58]

Macerated stillbirth nearly always indicates fetal death in pregnancy and not in labour, and in most cases is caused by anoxia. By contrast, fresh stillbirth, i.e. non-macerated, usually indicates either death due to anoxia or trauma or both. The distinction is an important one in compiling a patient's past obstetric history or in attempting to pinpoint a cause for stillbirth. Unfortunately necropsy studies in macerated stillbirths are often unrewarding and, except in cases of haemolytic disease, syphilis and congenital malformation, may show nothing more than signs of asphyxia and even more often the tissues may be too softened and necrotic to be examined properly.

Causes of Macerated Stillbirth

One of the commonest is pre-eclamptic toxaemia. Because of the hypertensive spasm of the vessels supplying the maternal placental site the blood flow is seriously reduced and likewise therefore the oxygen supply rate to the baby. The difference in blood flow rates through the maternal placenta was first illustrated by Browne and Veall's isotope technique (1953) of measuring clearance rates of radiosodium from the choriodecidual space.[7] It is the small baby who, by its unsatisfactory growth, proclaims the inadequacy of its own placenta and who is most likely to die *in utero* before labour. Infarction of the placenta makes the fetal suboxygenation progressive and irreversible so that intra-uterine death is not far off. It would clearly be of the greatest importance to be able to foresee this disaster and to secure the baby's delivery before its unfavourable intra-uterine environment killed it. In this respect 24-hour oestriol excretion levels are of more use than pregnanediol and our practice is to average three consecutive days' collections. Even so, mistakes are liable to be made and the whole specimen may not be forwarded to the laboratory. We therefore do a creatinine excretion rate as well. The latter is fairly constant and any discrepancy quickly indicates that the 24-hour specimen is not complete. There is unfortunately quite a wide variation in what may be regarded as normal oestriol excretion, but the chart in the next chapter shows the normally accepted ranges at different stages of pregnancy. Of even greater usefulness, if the apparatus is available, is the study of intra-uterine growth by fetal biparietal cephalometry.[19, 64] The growth rate here is maximal between the 20th and 30th weeks, after which it tends to level off, but where growth apparently ceases death can be anticipated within a matter of ten days, especially if the evidence is reinforced by low oestriol levels. It is therefore our practice to carry out these sonar measurements at least once a week and sometimes twice a week in the cases obviously at risk.

Chronic hypertension operates in like fashion but the fetal prognosis on the whole is somewhat better, provided pre-eclamptic toxaemia does not supervene.

Chronic nephritis, fortunately an uncommon complication of pregnancy nowadays, has a very bad prognosis for the baby who frequently dies from placental infarction and anoxia before even the stage of viability is reached.

Hyperpyrexia, i.e. a body temperature over 39·4° C, can kill the fetus directly.

Diabetic pregnancy as a cause of IUD is dealt with in Chapter VI and haemolytic disease in Chapter XXVIII.

Fetal malformations may cause death before, during or after labour, according to their nature and extent.

Postmaturity, as a cause, is a disappointing matter since in such cases one is dealing with no particular disease in either mother or baby and one feels that had only labour been successfully induced a few days earlier the tragedy might have been prevented.

Syphilis, a traditional cause, has been practically eradicated from obstetric practice.

Placental insufficiency is commonly diagnosed in order to explain so-called idiopathic cases of intra-uterine death but this is begging the question. In about a fifth of cases of IUD no more definite reason can be given.

It will be seen, therefore, that any hope of effectively reducing the incidence of macerated stillbirth will depend upon the early detection and treatment of pre-eclamptic toxaemia and hypertension, the careful management of diabetes, including opportune termination of pregnancy, the judicious use of induction of labour in cases of Rh iso-immunisation and in established postmaturity, and the elimination of syphilis.

Clearly then, sound antenatal care has much to offer but cannot prevent all cases of intra-uterine death.

Management

The diagnosis having been established beyond all shadow of doubt from the clinical evidences of absent fetal heart sounds, absent movements, cessation of uterine growth and recession of all the other signs

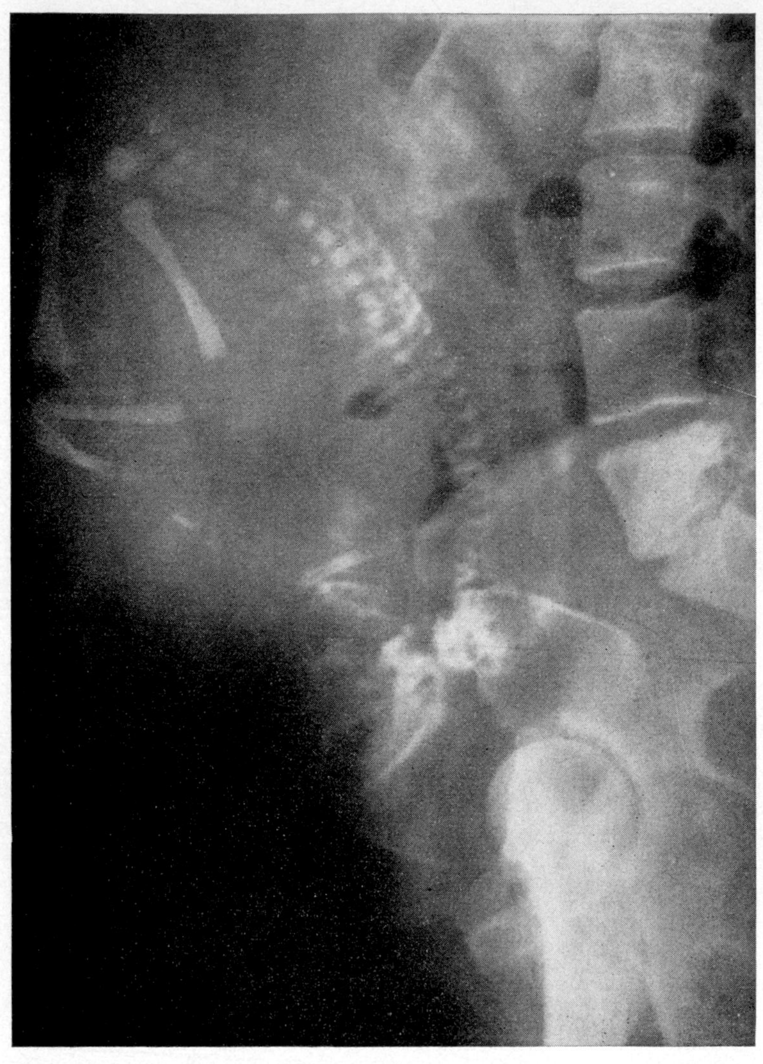

2/FIG. 22 (*a*).—Intra-uterine death. Gas present in cardiac chambers, abdominal aorta and superior mesenteric artery. This early sign is diagnostic of intra-uterine death. Spalding's sign is not yet visible.

(By courtesy of Dr Ellis Barnett.)

of continuing pregnancy and confirmed by the radiological signs mentioned above, one is faced with the choice of the following alternatives.

Firstly, a conservative attitude may be taken and spontaneous labour awaited. Secondly, attempts may be made to induce labour

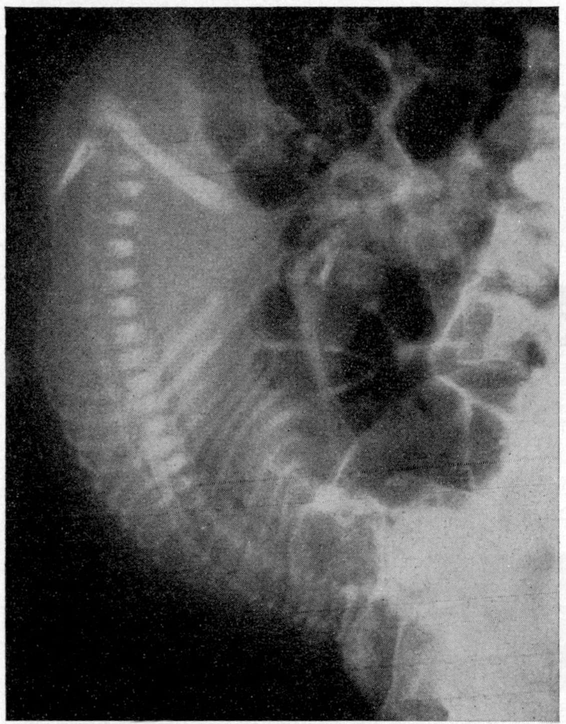

2/FIG. 22 (*b*).—Intra-uterine death during labour at 41½ weeks gestation. The first stage was prolonged and the fetus died slightly less than 24 hours before this picture was taken. Note the gas shadows in the thoracic and abdominal aorta and both common iliac vessels.

(By courtesy of Dr E. Sweet.)

medically. Thirdly, surgical methods of interfering with the pregnancy may be employed. The third choice is thoroughly dangerous and usually unnecessary. No one, of course, would dream of evacuation of the uterus by the abdominal route, the fetus is too large to remove from below and surgical induction of labour would be all that is left to choose from.

Surgical induction by any of the traditional methods, usually artificial rupture of the membranes, may not only reap the fearful penalty of an intra-uterine infection with gas-forming anaerobes but may fail to bring on labour, leaving one with a thoroughly nasty problem on hand.

If the patient is left strictly alone, labour will start usually within a month although occasionally the case may hang fire until term would have been reached. Very exceptionally the delay may be even longer. There are very few women who could face such an unhappy wait with equanimity and such therapeutic purism would hardly be humane. It is now recognised, moreover, that the prolonged retention of a dead fetus *in utero* may interfere with the coagulation mechanism in the blood. The defect is usually one of hypofibrinogenaemia. This was first noticed in the case of fetal death due to Rh iso-immunisation of the mother but it can occur in other varieties of intra-uterine death as well.[3]

Fortunately the disorder does not develop in less than four weeks after the death of the fetus, during which time the onset of labour, whether spontaneous or medically induced, is to be hoped for.

The modern technique of inducing labour or abortion in cases of intra-uterine death is to employ an escalating dosage of intravenous synthetic oxytocin, working within a few hours up to solution strengths occasionally of even 100 units per half-litre and increasing the drip rate up to 60 drops per minute, though this is seldom necessary.

An alternative is to use prostaglandins, F2α or E2. The former requires higher concentration (about five times) to be equally effective and does not appear to have any advantage over prostaglandin E2 (Prostin E2, dinoprostone). Toxic side-effects consist mainly of nausea, vomiting, diarrhoea, headache, vasovagal symptoms and locally a sore area in the neighbourhood of the receiving vein.

The intravenous route of medication is necessary since the genital tract is "out of bounds" because of the hazard of infection. Prostin E2 is made up in ethanol in strengths of 1 mg/ml in 0·75 ml or 5 ml ampoules. This strength, made up in 200 ml of saline solution, provides a dose of 5 micrograms/ml. By microinfusion pump 0·5–1 ml, i.e. 2·5–5 micrograms, can be infused per minute, not exceeding the upper dose for at least 4 hours.

If progress is not thereafter evident we favour giving intravenous oxytocin as well since the effect is apparently synergistic, prostaglandins reputedly sensitising the uterus to oxytocin and encouraging oxytocin release.

Intra-amniotic injection of hypertonic solutions.—One is faced with a hard core of cases, especially in the middle trimester of pregnancy, who will not go into labour as a result of oxytocin drip induction, and the method of injecting hypertonic solutions into the amniotic cavity may have to be considered. This was originally devised some 30 years ago but not really exploited until the present decade.[4, 16, 65] The technique was developed primarily as an alternative to abdominal hysterotomy in so-called "therapeutic" abortion and has been widely used in Sweden, in certain centres in the United Kingdom and in the United States. The use of hypertonic glucose[65] has proved too dangerous and at least two cases in these islands have been reported of fatal *Cl. welchii* infection following such an injection.[47] In one of them the gas pressure within the uterus was so great as to cause an amniotic embolus.[46] Therefore 20 per cent sodium chloride is preferable. The operation should not be performed on any uterus smaller than would apply to a 16-week gestation. After a preliminary infiltration of the area of the abdominal wall with local anaesthesic about midway between the umbilicus and the symphysis pubis in the midline, the patient is catheterised and then placed in a moderate Trendelenburg position to discourage bowel puncture. A spinal needle about 5 inches long may be used, or a fine trocar and cannula capable of carrying a polythene catheter is introduced into the amniotic cavity, which should be identified by the free withdrawal of liquor amnii and, above all, no blood. Sometimes with a dead fetus this fluid cannot be withdrawn, in which case about 100 ml of normal saline can be injected and then recovered. The attempt should be abandoned if there is any doubt about being in the amniotic cavity, because most of the fatalities and disasters are attributed to the intravascular injection of hypertonic saline. Having satisfied oneself that the end of the needle or the catheter is safely in the amniotic cavity, an additional precaution is to measure the intra-uterine pressure at the same time. In 50 millilitre steps liquor amnii is withdrawn and replaced by 20 per cent sodium chloride up to a maximum of 200 millilitres, observing throughout that the normal resting pressure of the uterus is maintained. Any sudden appearance of thirst should be immediately treated by dilute saline (0·2 per cent) infusion. Before removing the needle or cannula it should be rinsed with a little physiological saline.

The method, though fairly simple, is not without danger as may be expected and patients with cardiac or renal disease, also pre-eclampsia, are particularly at risk because, following this injection, the maternal serum shows an increased sodium concentration up to 160 mEq/l, increased volume and osmolality and on top of this an antidiuretic effect, so that cardiac patients may be precipitated into pulmonary oedema and the patients with renal disease may become anuric.[62] Three fatal cases of severe brain damage from intra-amniotic, hypertonic saline have been reported from the London Hospital,[8] and an impressive series of fatalities reported from Japan[63] has been sufficient to discourage a wider adoption of the method. The reported disasters have all concerned the deliberate termination of pregnancy, which makes them all the more tragic. When dealing with an intra-uterine death, the situation might well be worse, especially because of the difficulty sometimes of identifying the cavity. It is far preferable therefore to deal with the problem of intra-uterine death by medical means.

REFERENCES

1. BAGSHAWE, K. D. and MCDONALD, J. M. (1960). *Brit. med. J.*, **2,** 426.
2. BAGSHAWE, K. D., GOLDING, P. R. and ORR, A. H. (1969). *Brit. med. J.*, **3,** 733.
3. BARRY, A. P., GEOGHEGAN, F. and SHEA, S. M. (1955). *Brit. med. J.*, **2,** 287.
4. BENGSTSSON, L. and STORMBY, N. (1962). *Acta. obstet. gynec. scand.*, **41,** 115.
5. BERGSTROM, H., NILSSON, L., NILSSON, L. A. and RYTTINGER, L. (1967). *Amer. J. Obstet. Gynec.*, **99,** 130.
6. BREWS, A. (1939). *J. Obstet. Gynaec. Brit. Emp.*, **46,** 813.
7. BROWNE, J. C. M. and VEALL, N. (1953). *J. Obstet. Gynaec. Brit. Emp.*, **60,** 141.
8. CAMERON, J. M. and DAYAN, A. D. (1966). *Brit. med. J.*, **1,** 1010.
9. CAMPBELL, S. and DEWHURST, C. J., (1970). *Lancet*, **1,** 101.
10. CARR, D. H., (1967). *Amer. J. Obstet. Gynec.*, **97,** 283.
11. CARR, D. H. (1970). *Canad. med. Ass. J.*, **103,** 343.
12. CARR, D. H. (1970). In *Human Population Genetics*, ed. P. A. Jacobs and W. H. Price. (Pfizer Medical Monographs 5) p. 116.
13. CAVANAGH, D. and MCLEOD, A. G. W. (1966). *Amer. J. Obstet. Gynec.*, **96,** 913.
14. CHAN, D. P. C. (1962). *Brit. med. J.*, **2,** 957.
15. COYLE, M. G., GREIG, M. and WALKER, J. (1962). *Lancet*, **2,** 275.
16. CSAPO, A. (1966). In *Year Book of Obstetrics and Gynecology*, ed. J. P. Greenhill. Chicago: Year Book Med. Publishers.
17. DHADIAL, R. K., MACHIN, A. M. and TAIT, S. M. (1970). *Lancet*, **2,** 20.
18. DONALD, I., MACVICAR, J. and BROWN, T. G. (1958). *Lancet*, **1,** 1188.
19. DONALD, I. and BROWN, T. G. (1961). *Brit. J. Radiol.*, **34,** 539.
20. DONALD, I. (1962). In: *Methotrexate in the Treatment of Cancer*. Bristol: John Wright & Sons.
21. DONALD, I. (1962). *Brit. med. J.*, **2,** 1154.
22. DONALD, I. (1964). *Med. and Biol. Ill.*, **14,** 216.
23. DONALD, I. (1965). *Amer. J. Obstet. Gynec.*, **93,** 935.
24. DONALD, I. (1965). *J. Obstet. Gynaec. Brit. Cwlth*, **72,** 907.
25. DONALD, I. and ABDULLA, U. (1967). *Brit. J. Radiol.*, **40,** 604.
26. DONALD, I., MORLEY, P. and BARNETT, E. (1972). *J. Obstet. Gynaec. Brit. Cwlth*, **79,** 304.
27. DONIACH, I., CROOKSTON, J. H. and COPE, T. I. (1958). *J. Obstet. Gynaec. Brit. Emp.*, **65,** 553.
28. GENAZZARI, A. R., AUBERT, M. L., CASALI, M., FIONETTI, D. and FELBER, J. P. (1969). *Lancet*, **2,** 1385.
29. HERTIG, A. T. and EDMUNDS, H. W. (1940). *Arch. Path.*, **30,** 260.

30. Hertig, A. T. and Rock, J. (1949). *Amer. J. Obstet. Gynec.*, **38,** 968.
31. Johnson, W. L., Stegall, H. F., Lein, J. N. and Rushmer, R. F. (1965). *Obstet. and Gynec.*, **26,** 305.
32. Klopper, A., Michie, E. A. and Brown, J. B. (1955). *J. Endocr.*, **12,** 209.
33. Klopper, A. and MacNaughton, M. (1965). *J. Obst. Gynaec. Brit. Cwlth*, **72,** 1022.
34. Knill-Jones, R. P., Rodriguez, L. V., Mair, D. D. and Spence, A. A. (1972). *Lancet*, **1,** 1326.
35. Loudon, J. D. O. (1959). *J. Obstet. Gynaec. Brit. Emp.*, **66,** 277.
36. Macdonald, R. R. (1960). M.D. Thesis, Univ. of Glasgow.
37. Macdonald, R. R. (1963). *J. Obstet. Gynaec. Brit. Cwlth*, **70,** 580.
38. MacNaughton, M. C. (1961). *J. Obstet. Gynaec. Brit. Cwlth*, **68,** 789.
39. MacNaughton, M. (1966). *J. Obstet. Gynaec. Brit. Cwlth*, **73,** 290.
40. MacVicar, J. and Donald, I. (1963). *J. Obstet. Gynaec. Brit. Cwlth*, **70,** 387.
41. Malpas, P. (1938). *J. Obstet. Gynaec. Brit. Emp.*, **45,** 932.
42. Manly, G. A. (1961). *J. Obstet. Gynaec. Brit. Cwlth*, **68,** 277.
43. Matthews, C. D. and Matthews, A. E. B. (1969). *Lancet*, **2,** 694.
44. Murray, S., Barron, S. L. and McNay, N. A. (1970). *Lancet*, **1,** 632.
45. Murray, S. and Barron, S. L. (1971). *Brit. med. J.*, **3,** 90.
46. O'Driscoll, K. and Geoghegan, F. (1964). *Brit. med. J.*, **1,** 1113.
47. Pinkerton, J. H. M. (1966). *Brit. med. J.*, **1,** 1049.
48. Rappaport, F., Rabinovitz, M., Toaff, R. and Krochik, N. (1960). *Lancet*, **1,** 1273.
49. Roberts, J. R. (1944). *Amer. J. Roentgenol.*, **51,** 631.
50. Naismith, W. C. M. K. and Barr, W. (1974). *J. Obstet. Gynaec. Brit. Cwlth*, **81,** 146.
51. Robinson, H. R. (1972). *Brit. med. J.*, **4,** 466.
52. Robinson, H. R. (1972). *J. Obstet. Gynaec. Brit. Cwlth*, **79,** 90.
53. Robinson, H. R. (1973). *Brit. med. J.*, **4,** 28.
54. Russell, C. S., Paine, C. G., Coyle, M. G. and Dewhurst, C. J. (1957). *J. Obstet. Gynaec. Brit. Emp.*, **64,** 649.
55. Seeliger, H. P. R. (1961). *Listeriosis*. Basel: S. Karger.
56. Sharman, A. and Pearston, T. (1964). *J. med. Lab. Technol.*, **21,** 271.
57. Steptoe, P. C. (1967). *Laparoscopy in Gynaecology*, Chap. XVI. Edinburgh: Livingstone.
58. Stewart, A. M. (1957). *J. Obstet. Gynaec. Brit. Emp.*, **64,** 915.
59. Thompson, J. F. and Lein, J. N. (1961). *Obstet. and Gynec.*, **18,** 40.
60. Tow, W. S. H. and Cheng, W. C. (1967). *Brit. med. J.*, **1,** 521.
61. Turnbull, E. P. N. and Walker, J. (1956). *J. Obstet. Gynaec. Brit. Emp.*, **63,** 553.
62. Turnbull, A. C. and Anderson, A. B. M. (1966). *Brit. med. J.*, **1,** 672.
63. Wagatsuma, T. (1965). *Amer. J. Obstet. Gynec.*, **93,** 743.
64. Willocks, J., Donald, I., Duggan, T. C. and Day, N. (1964). *J. Obstet. Gynaec. Brit. Cwlth*, **71,** 11.
65. Wood, C., Booth, R. T. and Pinkerton, J. H. M. (1962). *Brit. med. J.*, **2,** 706.
66. Wright, C. S. W., Campbell, S. and Beazley, J. (1972). *Lancet*, **2,** 1278.

CHAPTER III

PRENATAL DIAGNOSIS OF FETAL HANDICAP

THE appalling problem of fetal handicap has, up to the present, been understated. It concerns not only the obstetrician but the paediatrician and in fact the whole of society, the family and the community. A congenital fetal abnormality often results in spontaneous abortion or perinatal death, commonly associated with prematurity, unforeseen stillbirth and, perhaps most harrowing of all, survival with disability or major handicap including mental retardation.

In the case of those fetuses reaching viability I have always used an oversimplified mnemonic, and as a rough guide the following approximation: about three in every hundred babies have a fetal abnormality, in a third of whom the disability is so great that they die shortly before, during or after birth; another third have a serious abnormality which nevertheless may be compatible with continued existence with or without major surgery and the remaining third have defects which still permit a life of fulfilment.

Major fetal abnormalities are indeed an important cause of perinatal death, in fact about 20 per cent.[7] The central nervous system and the heart and great vessels form the largest proportion which includes ventricular septal defects, aortic valves with only two cusps, atrial septal defects, patent ductus arteriosus, coarctation of the aorta, pulmonary stenosis, aortic stenosis, Fallot's tetralogy and transposition of the great vessels, the last-mentioned having a particularly high mortality. Of the central nervous system disorders, mercifully cases of anencephaly do not survive, but hydrocephalus and open spina bifida exposing the spinal cord are to some extent amenable to surgery, which nevertheless has to be very prompt to have much hope of functional success.

Intestinal malformations and genito-urinary defects are less tragic, but inborn errors of metabolism and enzyme deficiencies are usually associated with a high incidence of mental defect.

The genetic significance of much of the above is still unknown. Once the patient has had one such catastrophe her chances of having another as compared with the normal woman are multiplied about sixfold and after two fetal abnormalities, the risk rises to about seventy per cent.

Reviewing the prevalence of all chronic disabilities causing handicap in childhood, defined as a condition interfering with the ability to lead a normal life, Ross Mitchell[16] reckoned that about one child in six is affected. This is a staggering load which bears particularly heavily on the family.

It is now becoming increasingly the concern of obstetricians and paediatricians either to prevent or at least mitigate the problem. Methods of prenatal diagnosis are at last beginning to multiply.

Clinical examination of the mother in pregnancy is so imprecise in this respect as to be little better than soothsaying and the baby's normality or wellbeing defies accurate assessment. I myself can easily be a kilogram adrift in either direction in estimating a baby's weight, a figure far higher than that of any of my good midwifery sisters. Maturity assessment either clinically or radiologically has an error of plus or minus three weeks, although sonar has greatly narrowed the error. There is no reliable antenatal method yet of predicting a baby's endurance and capacity to withstand a difficult labour.

Certain maternal complications like pre-eclamptic toxaemia, diabetes, renal disorders and above all a bad obstetric history are well known to be associated with greater fetal hazard but these are no more than warning pointers, not to be neglected none the less.

A child's subsequent well-being may be influenced firstly by its genetic endowment, secondly by placental subnutrition and environmental factors and lastly by the accidents of the birth process itself.

There is a growing feeling that at least as far as intellectual endowment is concerned the last-mentioned category is the least important of the three. What is certain, however, is that nothing from conception onwards can improve matters; it can only prevent them from getting worse—and that a silk purse cannot be made out of a sow's ear.

Only Rhesus haemolytic disease provides any scope for treatment before birth. Otherwise induction of labour or more likely elective abortion in the more severely handicapped is all that can be offered, combined with genetic counselling which may modify the parents' attitude towards embarking upon another pregnancy in the future—hardly a happy subject. No method exists of improving genetic endowment.

In the previous chapter some time was spent on the subject of blighted ovum and its recognition, i.e. the fetus doomed to fail in its development during the first trimester.[11] An increasing percentage of these is identified as being due to genetic defect. This form of natural selection at best spares the mother greater unhappiness later on but the fear of giving birth to a handicapped child, especially one that is destined to be mentally retarded is almost universal in pregnant women today and reaches nightmare proportions in those who have had one such tragedy already and who face the possibility of another. As one of my patients, now nearly 40 years old, who had avoided a second pregnancy for nearly twenty years after her mongol son was born, remarked, "I've brought up one—I could not face another." Another patient at the same clinic, struggling with an increasingly heavy, paralysed and incontinent child with spina bifida, confessed that she did not see how she could physically, let alone mentally cope with a second. Genetic counsellors might tell her that the risk of a second child being thus affected was one in twenty, but who among us could face such odds? To be able to reassure the ninety-five per cent whose fears can be put at rest and to offer therapeutic abortion to the other five per cent facing a recurrent disaster is very much in line with current obstetrical thinking. The sanctity of human life has less meaning to many conscientious obstetricians when applied to a baby whose chances of fulfilment, particularly mental fulfilment, are denied to it from the first.

What can never be agreed amongst doctors or lay people is the degree of acceptable handicap and to the unfortunate parents the quandary is personal and greater still and often the responsibility of choice is too great for them to bear. No sympathetic doctor can escape involvement in their problem. Nevertheless in so far as the risk can be ascertained in a given case, modern obstetrics demands that the attempt be made.

Most important is the patient's obstetric history and where relevant that of the families of both partners. Apart from estimating the size of the pregnant uterus and the early recognition of hydramnios, clinical examination is of little help.

Radiology is both impracticable and positively contra-indicated before sixteen to eighteen weeks gestation and even then may be misleading.

Biochemical analysis, except in a few specific instances, only provides help after the halfway point in pregnancy.

Sonar, especially with gray scale developments in the future, may assist to a certain extent in recognising fetal abnormality. At the moment anencephaly is easy enough to recognise in the second trimester and the growth rate from the earliest stages of pregnancy, i.e. from six weeks amenorrhoea onwards, may help to provide a reassuring index of normality but no more than that. Details of cardiac activity and placental development are clearly feasible studies but are nowhere near fruition.

Antenatal screening for congenital defects is only possible where the mother's own condition might be responsible, for example in the case of Rh antibodies, or where she suffers a damaging condition such as rubella, which it is the function of antenatal care to recognise. The possibility of diagnosing fetal abnormality such as spina bifida however by estimating alphafetoprotein, as a screening procedure in the maternal serum of all patients in early pregnancy, opens up new horizons in perhaps one day helping to prevent a first tragedy rather than having to await the chance to prevent a second. This is more fully discussed later in the chapter.

Direct access to the fetus and its tissues however are only possible by amniocentesis. Fetoscopy, that is to say direct inspection with an optical instrument, however refined, inserted into the amniotic sac, can only be regarded as a research technique with hazards which are prohibitively high, for example, haemorrhage, abortion, infection and fetal death and the information yielded is hardly likely to be worthwhile.

This comment on fetoscopy would now be regarded by some as too pessimistic. Currently used for fetal blood sampling in cases of β-thalassaemia etc., the abortion rate is less than 10 per cent for a 25 per cent risk of severe abnormality.

Liquor amnii however is fairly easily and safely obtained from the 14th week of pregnancy onwards and provides living fetal cells in sufficient number, especially at sixteen weeks, for tissue culture and enzyme and the biochemical analysis of fetal metabolic products, so that it is becoming increasingly possible to diagnose or exclude an ever-growing selection of congenital disorders. This subject is dealt with fully in the section which follows by my colleague, Ferguson-Smith.

Genetic considerations are not the only ones that apply. At the moment speculation exceeds factual evidence about the environmental influences which may affect the child *in utero*. For instance it has always been a source of constant wonderment that the incidence of anencephaly and neural-tube defects should be so high in Ireland and the West of Scotland. A natural tendency of course is to blame our dismal climate. Even potato blight has been blamed, but Glasgow women do not eat blighted potatoes. By contrast mongolism is higher in New York than it is in Glasgow.

Sometimes risks can be calculated, foreseen and therefore prevented. This is most precise in the case of ionising radiations. Stewart and her colleagues, since their original publication in 1953 in the *Lancet*, have extended their observations[20, 21] by recognising that 6 per cent of all childhood malignancies are associated with exposure of the fetus *in utero* to X-rays. Furthermore whereas the general incidence of leukaemia is one in 12,000 children, after X-rays *in utero* the incidence is multiplied twentyfold to 1 in 600. This shows how vulnerable fetal tissues are to adverse environmental factors. Because of this risk, for example, radiographers who are not pregnant are allowed only to receive up to 3 rads over 13 weeks, but if they are pregnant, only one rad is permissible for the whole of pregnancy.

Diagnostic radiology of the pelvic regions in a potentially pregnant female can involve a dose to the fetus ranging from quarter of a rad up to about 5 rads, or even more, and even a dose as small as 1·4 rads doubles the natural incidence of childhood neoplasia and leukaemia.[9] By comparison background natural radiation runs between 1/8 and 1/10 of a rad per year.

Apart from drug teratogenesis which was mentioned in Chapter I, there are no other substantiated environmental hazards whose magnitude has been so precisely estimated. Any hope therefore of preventive action in reducing environmental fetal hazards must await a much wider knowledge.

General Antenatal Screening

There is an old English saying that a bird must first be caught before salt can be put on its tail. The great problem here is to recognise cases at risk by mass methods of screening which can be applied to all women in pregnancy. History alone may help to limit the selection but as yet there are no direct methods of diagnosing fetal abnormality by any non-invasive technique, except possibly by the use of sonar. Even however if all women were examined by sonar in early pregnancy the present limitations of the technique to two-dimensional scanning and lack of resolution would make it impossible to exclude any but the grossest abnormalities, for example, anencephaly, hydrocephaly and microcephaly. Spinal deformities can be demonstrated if very carefully and specifically sought,[6] likewise the capacity of the kidneys to secrete urine. Nevertheless these lesions are more often identified by hindsight than by foresight.

Ever since Brock and Sutcliffe in 1972[4] observed the association between severe fetal neural tube defects and raised alphafetoprotein levels in amniotic fluid, events have moved fast. Obviously it would be impracticable to subject every pregnant woman to amniocentesis and certainly more problems and complications would be caused thereby than one could even hope to prevent. The usefulness of the procedure depends on the care with which appropriate cases are selected for it. Often the indication is the history of a previously affected child in which case one can hope no more than to prevent a repeated tragedy. A mass screening technique might help to recognise the first affected child while still in early pregnancy. In our own series of the first 150 samples of amniotic fluid studies, spina bifida was detected by amniocentesis at 16 weeks gestation in two out of twenty pregnancies recognised to be at risk because of at least one previous tragedy and in both of these ultrasonography although undertaken for placental localisation had failed to recognise the neural tube defect, which is hardly surprising.[1] (Figs 1 and 2.)

Within less than two years of Brock and Sutcliffe's original paper, an anencephalic pregnancy was first diagnosed from recognising a raised alphafetoprotein level in maternal serum at 16 weeks which was then confirmed by amniocentesis.[5] This work was quickly confirmed in the months that followed, and was reviewed in a comprehensive leading article in *The Lancet*, 1974.[13] The success of this screening technique, which, be it remembered, merely helps to select cases for confirmatory amniocentesis, depends upon very precise and sensitive radioimmunoassay methods which can detect levels less than 100 nanograms per ml in the serum since the concentrations are likely to be about 500 times lower than in the amniotic fluid.

There is one very important proviso, however, in taking raised serum alphafetoprotein levels seriously and that is to bear in mind the possibility of multiple pregnancy. We have already been caught out in one instance in which the patient had a significantly raised level and in whom the diagnosis of twins was unfortunately not made in the course of a routine sonar localisation of the placenta before amniocentesis. The case in question aborted twin fetuses within the next two days following the amniocentesis, but the prognosis was further complicated because she had already threatened to abort spontaneously, so it is difficult to be sure which was the more relevant factor. Nevertheless the only method of making a diagnosis of twin pregnancy at the time when amniocentesis is normally carried out is by very thorough and careful sonar examination.

Serum alphafetoprotein screening programmes of course only apply to neural tube defects of open and more severe varieties. Other screening programmes involving amniocentesis are mainly restricted to classes known from age, family or past history to be particularly at risk. Down's syndrome or mongolism is now recognised as the predominant single cause of severe mental subnormality and although there is a growing tendency for fewer women above the age of 35 to embark on pregnancy, the prevalence of Down's syndrome is increasing, because more of these babies survive, according to the latest available figures from the New York State Department of Mental Hygiene and the Division of Epidemiology.[19]

Amniocentesis

The main indication for undertaking amniocentesis in later pregnancy is the study of Rh haemolytic disease but in early pregnancy the chief reasons are for the antenatal diagnosis of X-linked disorders such as haemophilia and Duchenne muscular dystrophy, for karyotyping and recognising cytogenetic abnormalities such as trisomy 21 (Down's syndrome) and for an ever-increasing number of recognisable inborn errors of metabolism associated with enzyme defects. Neural tube defects have already been discussed.

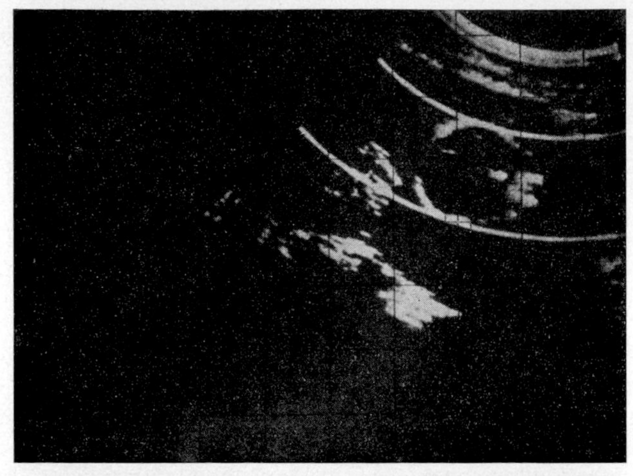

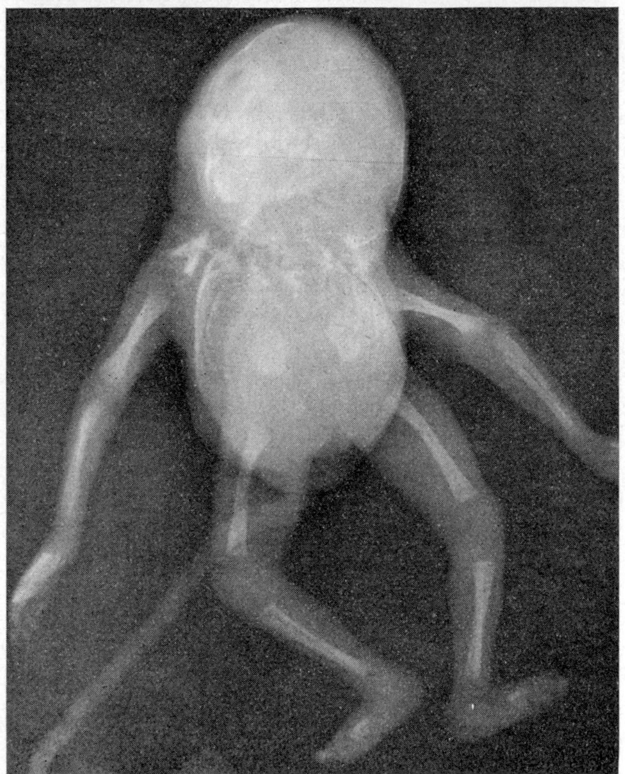

3/FIG. 1 (*see opposite*)

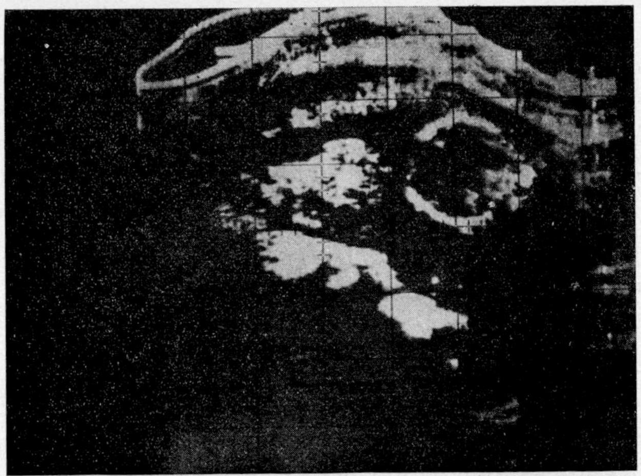

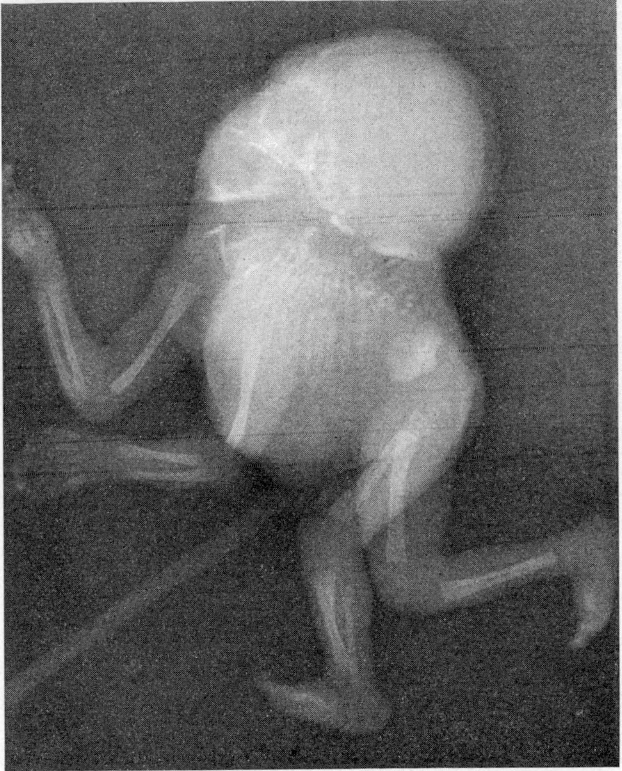

3/FIG. 1.—Iniencephaly. Too early for intra-uterine X-ray. Recognised by amniotic alphafetoprotein level raised to 5 times normal. Sonar failed to diagnose because of mistaken biparietal diameter as shown. The X-rays were taken after abortion by prostaglandins.

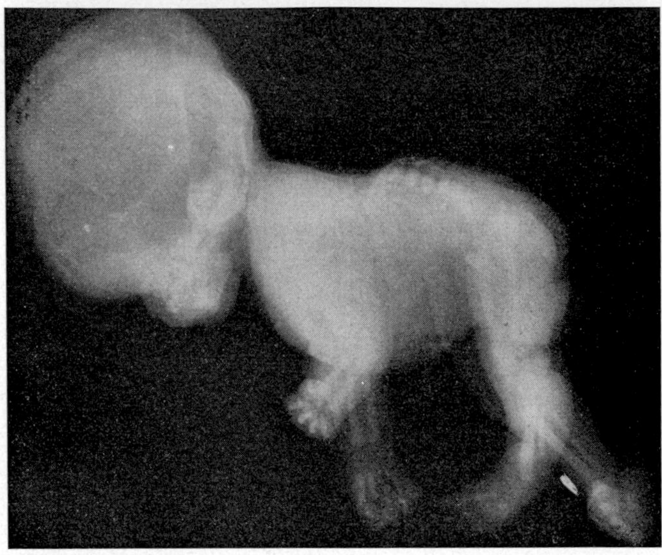

3/FIG. 2.—Gross spina bifida. X-ray after delivery. The acute lumbar kyphosis is always associated with irreversible paraplegia. (By courtesy of Dr E. M. Sweet.)

Technique

It is unthinkable to use the vaginal route because of the likelihood of infection and abortion. When making the puncture *per abdomen* the best time is undoubtedly at the sixteenth week, although the operation is possible at the fourteenth week, especially if an assistant pushes the uterus further up into the abdomen from below. Unfortunately amniocentesis carried out as early as fourteen weeks may fail to yield a sufficient amount of liquor amnii. At this stage the total available volume is only about 100 ml and it is as well not to aspirate much more than 5 ml. The cell yield for amniotic fluid cell culture may be insufficient and the operation may have to be repeated, so that in fact time is actually lost rather than saved. At sixteen weeks the operation is undoubtedly easier but even so can be most frustrating in the case of a "dry tap" and positively to be regretted in the case of a "bloody tap." In our view amniocentesis should not be undertaken without a proper sonar examination, not only to exclude twins but to localise the placenta exactly and to indicate the point and depth at which a pool of liquor amnii can be most safely tapped. For this reason we undertake the operation in the ultrasonics department and carry out the procedure immediately on the spot and before fetal movement can spoil the findings of the sonar examination.

The maturity must be known without doubt and this can be established by sonar at the same time, since the level of alphafetoprotein alters according to the state of maturity and any doubt on this point may invalidate the results. In Copenhagen[3] a hollow ultrasonic transducer is used through which the amniocentesis needle is passed under direct vision. The technique is certainly slick to watch but we have not adopted it ourselves since we are using our transducers for so many other purposes and dislike the idea of boiling them. Samples of maternal blood must be taken before and immediately after amniocentesis for Kleihauer testing since it is most important to recognise even minor fetomaternal transfusions of only a ml or two, as can be calculated from the number of fetal red cells thus identified. In the case of a rhesus negative woman even a small fetomaternal transfusion may sensitise her and it is now general practice to give a standard 100 μg dose of anti-D gamma globulin to all rhesus negative women whether the Kleihauer test is positive or not and whatever the group of the baby's alleged father. In spite of this precaution we have already had one case of rhesus iso-immunisation in a primigravid patient who had a standard amniocentesis with only a few fetal cells reported on the second Kleihauer test and in whom amniocentesis had been undertaken to exclude a neural tube defect because of the finding of a high serum alphafetoprotein. Rhesus antibodies appeared for the first time towards the end of pregnancy and the baby required an exchange transfusion.

The operation itself is deceptively simple. The point of entry and direction of the aspirating needle having been ascertained just before by sonar and marked with carbol fuchsin stain, the patient remains in the dorsal position on the original couch and full aseptic and antiseptic ritual is carried out. The selected point is infiltrated at skin level with 1 to 2 ml of 1 per cent lignocaine and the likely needle track further infiltrated with up to 6 to 7 ml in all, taking care to aspirate before injecting any more and particularly avoiding pumping any lignocaine into the liquor amnii itself.

My own practice is then to make a tiny nick in the skin with the point of a fine fistula knife which makes it easier to insert the needle without pressure and to appreciate the various layers penetrated. A spinal needle and stilette of gauge 20–22 is now inserted, confidently rather than tentatively, according to the angles of the predetermined track. This is more difficult than it sounds. Where the placenta has been found to be anterior the chances of a "bloody tap" are obviously greater and we consider it most important to avoid this. In any case if it occurs the blood must be sent for identification, whether fetal or maternal, because many of the "bloody taps" are due to maternal sources and are therefore less serious. Occasionally and to my annoyance one gets what I call a "dry tap," i.e. about as much fluid as one would expect to get out of a fibroid. The usual reason for this is that the needle is not travelling in the right axis and has either gone too far, or is blunt or is running tangentially inside the myometrium. It is therefore worth having an alternative site indicated in advance.

As soon as the amniocentesis needle enters the amniotic sac, removal of the stilette should be followed by a few drops of liquor amnii welling up. The first few drops are discarded in any case but the presence of any blood disqualifies the specimen and a fresh syringe must be used. Fifteen ml of clear amniotic fluid are a suitable size of specimen at 16 weeks and more than 20 ml is a dangerous amount and more likely to provoke abortion.

The patient's bladder, of course, should be empty but because of nervousness this is not always the case and occasionally one's genetic colleagues are irritated at receiving samples of elegantly pure urine. If there is any doubt about this on the part of the operator it is worth allowing a drop to dry on a slide and to examine under low-power microscopy for ferning crystals which indicate liquor amnii and not urine.

As soon as the sample has been obtained and despatched immediately to the genetics laboratory for culture etc., the needle is briskly removed and a little Nobecutane spray applied.

The procedure is perfectly painless for the patient and she should be warned at the time that it might be necessary to repeat the test in the course of the next fortnight. This precaution tends to minimise disappointment.

In later pregnancy amniocentesis involves some slight differences in approach. As usual the placenta is located beyond question and avoided. If possible the most fruitful area of fluid, which is sometimes disappointingly scanty, is sought either between the fetal limbs provided the placenta is not anteriorly situated and in this area, or alternatively behind the fetal neck and occiput.

In the regrettable absence of ultrasonic equipment in cases in which amniocentesis has nevertheless to be undertaken, one has to take a chance on harpooning an anterior placenta, preferably with the minimum possible movement and trauma. For this a site is commonly selected in early pregnancy about one-third of the way up the uterus from the top of the symphysis pubis or where the fetus can be clearly felt and avoided as above mentioned. Occasionally more satisfactory access can be obtained in later pregnancy by pulling the child by abdominal palpation in a ventral direction or even lifting up the presenting part above the pelvic brim to carry out the puncture in the midline suprapubically. This latter approach may decrease the chances of a "bloody tap" especially with anterior placentae which are reckoned not to be in the praevia position.

Hazards of Amniocentesis

As already hinted, damage to the placenta, particularly if it involves fetomaternal transfusion, has certainly to be reckoned with, and routine protection in Rh negative women with 100 μg of anti-D gamma globulin may not invariably protect them, yet larger amounts may be bad for the fetus itself.

The risks of abortion or premature labour have always to be faced although amniocentesis may be unjustly blamed. Serious bleeding may be associated with placental abruption and fetal haemorrhage is very readily lethal to the baby. I have had one case in which maternal bleeding progressed to haemoperitoneum necessitating laparotomy. This occurred in a woman who suddenly started vomiting before I was quick enough to remove the needle and a large maternal vein was torn open.

The danger of skewering the baby with the needle is ever in mind but seems to occur far less often than one would expect and anyway the fetus may react with palpable movements of protest.

The question of infection is a serious matter and yet again in our experience, and with the precautions taken, has not yet proved a cause of trouble, rather to my surprise. Intra-uterine fetal death should only be attributed to amniocentesis if it occurs within the first day or two and the indications for which the operation was done should be reviewed since they may be more relevant.

From the above it will be seen therefore that amniocentesis is not to be lightly or ill-advisedly undertaken.

Mid-Trimester Termination of Pregnancy

It goes without saying that if one subjects the patient to amniocentesis in order to determine the presence of a fetal abnormality a readiness to terminate the pregnancy in this unhappy event is automatically implied; otherwise matters would be better left unknown since the patient herself is not at risk. Normally most patients gladly accept the offer of such a diagnosis in the assurance that major fetal abnormality will be dealt with by selective abortion and the reassurance that all is well may save much maternal mental distress. However I have on occasion had a patient who for religious reasons stated that in any case she would take what was coming to her whatever the findings and for this reason felt that amniocentesis would be inappropriate.

Our own personal hostility to abortion on so-called "social grounds" as a method of long-stop contraception is modified when confronted with scientific evidence of serious disability which may threaten the intra-uterine baby's chance of a fulfilled life, particularly mental and spiritual fulfilment in so far as these can be foreseen. This raises an ethical issue on which the opinions of doctors can never be uniformly agreed. In the face of such incontrovertible evidence as a rising rubella antibody titre or a cast-iron genetic diagnosis of major disability reached by amniocentesis, I think the patient has a right to know the facts and to make some personal choice in the matter. This is altogether different from abortion on demand, whatever politicians or governments in their ill-informed ignorance may attempt to dictate.

Unfortunately in the majority of cases of congenital fetal handicap the need for termination of pregnancy is only established in the second trimester of pregnancy which, surgically speaking, is a much more serious matter than a simple vacuum aspiration within the first three months. Nevertheless it is such cases as these in my department which represent the majority of interruptions of pregnancy which, from the maternal point of view, are otherwise safe. We are very closely associated with a large Department of Medical Genetics but the number of terminations generally so indicated is not large and furthermore confirmatory justification for the termination is always sought from the Department of Pathology.

Mid-trimester Techniques of Termination

Of all methods of terminating a mid-trimester pregnancy, abdominal hysterotomy must be one of the easiest operations in the whole field of gynaecology and one in which control of blood loss is almost total, but its use is unjustified when operating because of fetal abnormality. One is left therefore with a choice of inducing abortion *per vaginam* by one of a number of techniques. Dilatation and curettage are out of the question since the fetal head is already too large to be safely delivered through the cervix without excessive dilatation, and haemorrhage can be very profuse.

The use of intra-amniotic hypertonic saline is very widely practised in some quarters but has never been popular in our part of the world. It involves amniocentesis under local anaesthesia through the abdominal wall using a Tuohy needle and the insertion of a polythene catheter. Following withdrawal of about 200 to 250 ml of liquor a similar amount of hypertonic saline is injected. This kills the fetus *in utero* and the patient is thereafter left to abort a dead fetus. Accidents have from time to time occurred in which the hypertonic saline is injected accidentally into the patient's own venous system with disastrous effects upon the central nervous system and sometimes death. Warning may be given by the subjective sensation of a raging thirst and this highly dangerous situation may be countered by the immediate intravenous injection of very dilute saline, such as 0·2 per cent. The use of hypertonic glucose for a short time enjoyed a brief vogue until accidents were reported due to the accumulation of gas under pressure because of gas-forming putrefaction by anaerobic bacilli in the presence of dead fetal material. The resulting intra-uterine pressure has even produced death from amniotic fluid embolism in a case in Dublin in whom abortion was being induced by this method because of known intra-uterine fetal death. Urea would appear to be safer, about 80 g dissolved in normal saline being instilled in place of the liquor amnii already removed.

Attempts to induce abortion by even massive doses of oxytocin given intravenously are almost doomed to failure in the absence of prior intra-uterine death of the fetus.

There the situation rested until prostaglandins came on the scene. Used intravenously prostaglandins are useless and produce vicious side-effects such as nausea, vomiting, headache, a very sore arm from chemical phlebitis, and intense diarrhoea, nor are they any more effective in inducing abortion by this route although they may sensitise the uterus to the action of oxytocin.

Attempts to limit the unpleasant side-effects of prostaglandins by intra-uterine administration have been very ineffectual in pregnancy of less than twelve weeks gestation[17] but when dealing with mid-trimester termination there is much more to be said for their use. There are two main prostaglandins available at present for this type of purpose, namely PGF2 alpha and PGE2. The E2 preparation (dinoprostone) is at least five times as powerful as the F2 alpha and appears to have fewer side-effects. Unfortunately it does not keep so well in hot climates.

The modern preferred method is to instil dinoprostone directly into the uterus where it exerts its effect with less absorption into the maternal circulation and undesirable side-effects and one has the choice of either the intra-amniotic or the extra-amniotic route. Our own preferred method is to use the extra-amniotic technique.[15]

The operation requires no general anaesthesia but in the case of a really anxious patient (and this is often so because of the general psychological upset of facing termination after four months amenorrhoea) intravenous Valium (diazepam) may do much to make the procedure more tolerable. Working under full theatre aseptic conditions a Foley catheter of French gauge 12–14 is introduced through the cervix under direct vision. It should have a 15 ml balloon which is introduced well past the internal os and then inflated with sterile saline. A nylon intravenous catheter (French gauge 6) is then fixed by its yellow end into the distal end of the catheter. The Foley catheter is then pulled gently down until the balloon sits snugly in the lower segment over the internal os. A 20-ml syringe containing 2 mg of dinoprostone is now connected and the instillation is given at the rate of 2 ml of the solution to the hour. Intervals exceeding an hour between instillation should not be allowed whatever the hour of day or night until the abortion process is complete or the catheter balloon is expelled, whichever is the sooner.

It is a good plan to insert, in series, a Millipore Swinnex 13 bacterial filter. Alternatively a Palmer pump can be used providing a continuous infusion starting at the rate of 240 minutes per inch of drive, increasing the rate according to response up to 160 minutes per inch. This is rather a clumsy type of pump for the purpose and others may prove more handy if available. The aim is to vary the rate from 0·9 ml up to 2·7 ml per hour. If the uterine response is not very satisfactory intravenous oxytocin can be given at the same time.

Unfortunately the patient is in for a thoroughly miserable day. Abortion may not occur for about 15 hours average, sometimes ranging over into the next day.

It will be noted that the catheter balloon is a fairly large one. Even so extrusion before abortion has occurred is very likely, whereupon a vaginal examination should be undertaken. At this point the membranes will be found bulging through the internal os, in which case abortion will proceed if necessary with the help of continued oxytocin. Too small a balloon may be passed too early and may have to be replaced with another. Clearly this technique has to be undertaken in hospital because almost two-thirds of the cases abort incompletely and retain the placenta sometimes with appreciable bleeding requiring evacuation of the retained products under general anaesthesia forthwith.

The method is clearly far from ideal but there is no perfect method of terminating pregnancy at this stage. The best that can be said for this particular technique is its safety. Perhaps even more important is that the operation is attended by less late sequelae than others. Cervical rupture either in the form of a lateral tear or a "bucket handle" has been reported from intra-amniotic prostaglandin but this complication does not appear to occur when the extra-amniotic route is chosen. This safety factor has got to be balanced against the obvious convenience of a single intra-amniotic injection through the abdominal wall, leaving the patient to get on with the abortion herself.[9]

The possibility of infection, though seldom serious, has to be borne in mind, and more or less contra-indicates the use of this technique in cases of cardiac disease. Fortunately the indications for terminating pregnancy in the middle trimester on cardiac grounds are very rare.

Fetal Monitoring during Late Pregnancy

It has been reckoned that in about 10 per cent of children with mental retardation the defects are attributable at least in part to antenatal and early postnatal complications which theoretically at least are avoidable. In fact the long-term consequences to the family of fetal death are slight compared with those of fetal damage particularly of the developing brain. The subject is therefore every bit as important as the study of perinatal mortality as already discussed in Chapter I. Even minor impairments in cerebral function can be commonly identified in children subjected to pre- and perinatal hazards.[8] The vulnerability of infants to similar adverse factors may vary. It is important to recognise those on which the greatest effort must be concentrated. This involves the obstetrician in the ability to recognise the case at risk.

Clinical Evidences

Here history counts for more than physical signs in alerting the physician, since history has an ugly trick of repeating itself.

Suspicion is aroused by previous abortion, especially if recurrent; fetal abnormality, of course; a previous dysmature or "small-for-dates" baby; one which was premature and if so for what reason; and even postmaturity may be significant. In this particular pregnancy the story of threatened abortion should not be ignored. The family history should be scrutinised for any instances of recognisable genetic defect, as well as known adverse disease, such as diabetes. On clinical examination, apart from eliminating maternal diseases, any discrepancy in size of the uterus as compared with the known dates calls for further inquiry. Both polyhydramnios and oligohydramnios may signify underlying fetal abnormality. Failure of the mother to gain weight throughout pregnancy may also indicate a fetus that is faring none too well. Furthermore poor socio-economic status of the mother does nothing to improve the welfare of her child.

The older primigravida who has been many years in attempting to achieve conception may not only prove to be a poor reproductive performer but the premium attached to her unborn child is loaded.

The vulnerability of the fetus in later pregnancy comes under three headings. Firstly, disorders of placental function. More is written and less is known about this than almost any subject except perhaps pre-eclamptic toxaemia. In the words of Klopper "placental insufficiency means many things to many men."[12] Placental function is not just a matter of oxygen transfer, but transfer of all other nutrient factors as well. It is also concerned with the passage of antibodies and with excretory function.

The subject of dysmaturity is dealt with very much more fully in a later chapter. The second vulnerability class concerns labour which is likewise dealt with elsewhere. Finally are the cases of congenital abnormality which still appear too often for the first time only at birth and sometimes after it.

Monitoring Methods in Late Pregnancy

The most generally available fetal monitoring techniques concern a variety of excretory tests, usually in 24-hour collections of urine but sometimes in serum (see later). Although there are more than about two dozen structurally related oestrogens in maternal urine, oestriol accounts for approximately 90 per cent. The consistent finding of low levels may signify an undergrown, dysmature baby, or postmaturity, but unfortunately is less reliable in diabetes. Low oestriol levels may also indicate poor maternal renal circulation, sometimes from postural causes, but more commonly from hypertensive states in which plasma levels however may build up because of poor renal clearance. Fetal adrenal hypoplasia, anencephaly and hydrocephalus may also be associated with low oestriol outputs because of poor fetal adrenal activity. Less commonly maternal steroid therapy may be the cause. In studying oestriol excretion one is making a "blanket cover survey" of fetal pituitary and adrenal function, placental function, and the ability of the mother to handle the products and to excrete them. However useful and available it is, oestriol estimation alone can never be fully definitive. Nevertheless it retains pride of place in most obstetrical units. Heat-stable alkaline phosphatase is produced only in the placenta and can be measured. It is recognised by the fact that it is not destroyed by incubation at 50–60° C. for thirty minutes. The level increases progressively from the 32nd week of pregnancy until term, but the individual variations are too wide to make it really useful.

Assays of human placental lactogen (HPL) in the plasma are available by radioimmunoassay and a kit is commercially available on the "do-it-yourself" principle. Serum levels rise from the 8th to the 32nd week of pregnancy and then flatten out until labour, disappearing within a few hours of delivery. The attraction of this approach lies in the fact that HPL is produced by the placenta itself although this may not mean as much as one would hope with regard to the placenta's ability to nourish the fetus.

The comparative usefulness of studying at-risk pregnancies by human placental lactogen, urinary oestriol and ultrasonic biparietal cephalometry has been undertaken in our own department and our present opinion is that cephalometry and oestriol assays combined together give the most reliable indication of intra-uterine growth retardation.[18] (Fig. 3.) It will be seen that our own practice is to chart biparietal growth curves simultaneously with oestriol excretion curves. The two together are indeed useful in recognising the fetus at risk from an unhealthy uterine environment.

Dysmaturity is of more than one type, as described in a later chapter,

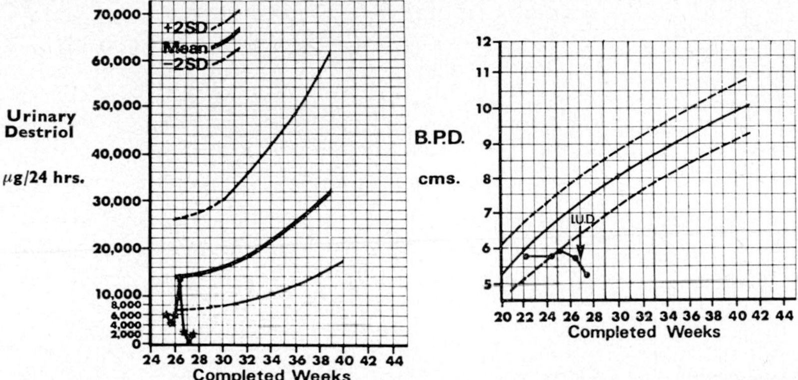

3/FIG. 3.—Fetal growth failure and intra-uterine death. Right-hand curve shows ultrasonic biparietal diameter measurements. Left-hand curve, urinary oestriol output.

but is a cause of associated mental retardation and other neurological handicap which may seriously reflect the standard of antenatal care.

Prediction of Fetal Distress in Labour

Some interest is now centered on a baby's ability to withstand the stresses of labour and to what extent this can be foreseen, in other words to forestall fetal distress before the need to treat it arises. A variety of provocative tests on the fetus with concomitant study of fetal heart changes has not so far yielded much encouragement to the clinician but it has been suggested in a prospective study[14] that consistently low levels of HPL around 4 µg per ml in the circulating blood between the 35th and 40th week of pregnancy may indicate a risk of approximately 70 per cent of fetal distress in subsequent labour, or of neonatal asphyxia. At the moment it does not appear likely that obstetric management in labour would be seriously modified by this finding in the absence of other evidences. This is hardly surprising since the causes of fetal distress in labour itself are numerous.

In conclusion, we are left with a largely uncharted sea of uncertainty. Without wishing however to appear unduly partisan it is suggested that the most direct approach is the study of the object of the exercise itself, namely the fetus, and this provides unlimited scope for future developments in sonar. In its approach towards the valley of the shadow of birth every child, as my friend Hellman has remarked, has the right not to be stillborn but wellborn. This concept is fundamental to human dignity.

GENETICS OF FETAL ABNORMALITY

by MALCOLM A. FERGUSON-SMITH, M.B., Ch.B., F.R.C.P. (Glas.), F.R.C.Path.

Professor of Medical Genetics, University of Glasgow, Honorary Consultant in Human Genetics, Royal Hospital for Sick Children, Glasgow

ACKNOWLEDGEMENT

The substance of this section is based in part on an article on Prenatal Diagnosis prepared for *The Practitioner* (Vol. **213,** pp. 655–666, 1974), and is reproduced here in modified form by kind permission of the Editor.

Spontaneous Abortion

It has long been suspected that faulty development of the ovum is an important cause of spontaneous abortion, but the relative parts played by genetic and environmental factors were unknown. The early studies have concentrated mainly on the careful histological examination of aborted embryos.[27] During recent years chromosome analysis of aborted material has demonstrated dramatically how frequently one class of genetic disorder, the chromosome aberrations, accounts for spontaneous abortions. It is now clear that at least 25 per cent of all spontaneous abortions have gross chromosomal aberrations detectable under the laboratory microscope,[23] and one suspects that genetic aberrations beyond the resolution of the microscope account for a significant proportion of the remainder. The types of chromosome abnormality present in these abortuses are in most instances similar to those found in liveborn infants with multiple developmental malformations. Thus the most frequent aberration is a missing sex chromosome, the 45,XO chromosome complement characteristic of most cases of Turner's syndrome, and is caused by a disorder of meiosis whereby the sex chromosome fails to be included in either the sperm or egg. XO conceptions account for 21 per cent of chromosomally abnormal abortions or 4 per cent of all spontaneous abortions. As the XO state occurs in rather more than 1 in 5000 liveborns, and assuming that 15 per cent of all pregnancies end in abortion, only 2·5 per cent of XO conceptions survive to term.

The second most frequent aberration found in spontaneous abortions seems to be triploidy, a situation where every chromosome is represented three times instead of twice in each cell in the embryo (Fig. 4), i.e., each cell has 69 instead of 46 chromosomes. This defect arises by the accident of double fertilisation of the ovum or by failure of extrusion of the second polar body. It occurs in about 17 per cent of chromosomally abnormal abortions (i.e. 3 per cent of all spontaneous abortions). Various types of chromosomal trisomy

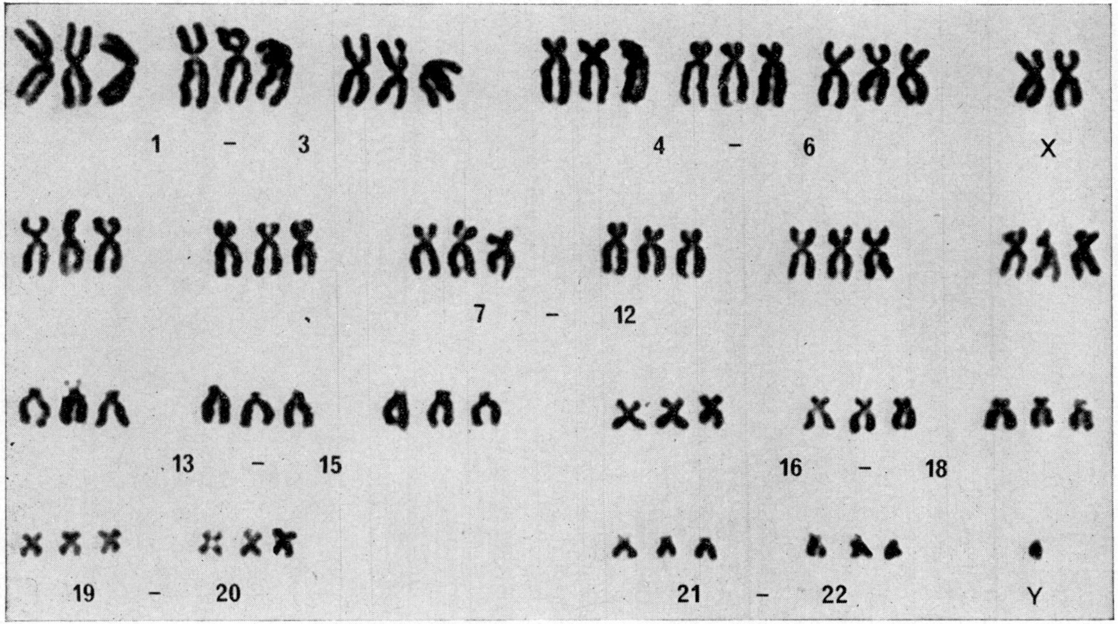

3/FIG. 4.—Chromosome analysis in a triploid cell cultured from an abortus of approximately 9 weeks gestation.

(where one chromosome only is present in triplicate) account for the majority of the remaining chromosomally abnormal abortions. These include the trisomy 21 of mongolism as well as the 13 and 18 trisomies which are well known in the newborn. Trisomy 16, which has probably only once been described in the liveborn, proves to be the commonest single type of trisomy in abortions.

It has been found that almost all the chromosomally abnormal abortions occur between the 8th and 16th week of gestation. Calculated in another way, the frequency of chromosome aberrations in abortuses in the first and second trimesters is 30 per cent and 11 per cent respectively; in other words, the earlier the abortion, the greater the incidence of chromosomal abnormality. Pathological examination of these conceptions shows that the embryo is absent in about a third and grossly malformed in most of the remainder. The interesting exceptions are the triploid embryos which seem to have comparatively few external malformations. Their abortion, typically around the sixth week, appears to be the result of defects of the placenta which is much larger than normal and typically shows a mild form of hydatidiform change.

There is currently much interest in factors which might predispose to chromosome aberrations in abortuses and data on such agents as infections with viruses and mycoplasma and exposure to irradiation and radiomimetic drugs are being accumulated. So far, only increased maternal age has been found to be a significant factor, and this operates only in the case of the trisomic abortions.

Habitual Abortion

A history of recurrent abortion is frequently found in families in which a structural chromosome abnormality or translocation is being transmitted. A translocation arises by the exchange of chromosome segments between the chromosomes of different pairs and is caused by agents such as irradiation which lead to chromosome breakage (Fig. 5). When both products of the translocation are present the total complement of genes is unchanged (although abnormally distributed), the translocation is said to be "balanced", and development is normal. However, the offspring of the carrier of a balanced translocation may inherit only one of the products of the translocation, in which case the total complement of genes is "unbalanced", and embryonic development is defective. Thus, the usual finding in these families is that one parent has the balanced translocation and a varying proportion of the pregnancies result in (a) normal offspring without the translocation, (b) normal offspring carrying the balanced translocation like the parent, (c) abnormal offspring with an unbalanced translocation, and (d) miscarriages.

These observations have prompted chromosome analysis in

several series of patients and their husbands who have a history of recurrent abortion. Rather surprisingly, these studies seldom demonstrate a significant chromosome aberration, and it is now thought that the part played by gross transmissible chromosome aberrations in the aetiology of habitual abortion is small, possibly in the order of less than 3 per cent.

Investigation for chromosomal abnormalities in obstetrics (as distinct from gynaecology) is, however, indicated in dysmature babies, especially those with developmental abnormalities affecting more than one system because, in a proportion, a chromosomal aberration in the baby may point to a transmissible defect in one or other parent which may influence the prognosis of future pregnancies. Parental translocation is, of course, a strong indication for prenatal chromosome analysis (*see below*).

Genetic Counselling

Following the birth of a malformed or severely handicapped child, the possibility should always be considered that the cause of the abnormality is genetic for there may be a high recurrence risk in future pregnancies. Even in the absence of a history of similarly affected relatives, it is important to look for a genetic cause and to establish a correct diagnosis so that an accurate genetic prognosis can be given to the parents. A great number of different rare dysmorphology syndromes, chromosomal syndromes and single-gene defects are now described in which it is possible to give firm advice about recurrence risks. Genetic Counselling Clinics are increasingly taking on responsibility for providing this information. However, in many cases the provision of a genetic prognosis is frustrated because all affected relatives are deceased and inadequate information is recorded about them. Where the cause of the fetal abnormality is in doubt it is therefore important to insist, whenever possible, on a full investigation including photography, X-ray examination, chromosome analysis and autopsy. It is not always appreciated that chromosome analysis can be performed post-mortem and that some 5 per cent of stillbirths have chromosome aberrations.

In many cases of fetal abnormality, for example spina bifida cystica, the cause is unknown and yet the genetic counsellor can give helpful information on recurrence in future pregnancies from empiric risk estimates. These estimates are based on the accumulated experience of similarly affected families.

One important aspect of a Genetic Counselling Clinic is that it has responsibility not only to the individual patient but to the whole family. The discovery of an inherited disorder in one member of a family imposes an obligation to ensure that there are no other family members who might be at risk and could benefit from genetic advice.

In some conditions, such as X-linked muscular dystrophy, the detection of family members at risk of producing affected children is made easier by the availability of tests for the carrier state.

Prenatal Diagnosis

Many mothers at risk of bearing handicapped children ask about the possibility of testing their pregnancy to make certain that the child that they are to deliver is free from handicap. For lethal and severe fetal abnormality detectable in early pregnancy, most parents are prepared to accept selective termination rather than run the risk of yet another severely handicapped child. Most of the medical profession are in sympathy with this view. It is argued, for example, that the majority of conceptions affected by severe chromosomal and neural tube defects are spontaneously aborted in the first trimester, and that selective abortion in the second trimester of similarly affected fetuses that have escaped spontaneous expulsion is a sensible form of medical management. However, it should be recognised that a decision on whether or not to have prenatal diagnosis and selective termination is one which has to be taken by parents themselves. Unfortunately, many patients who could benefit from this diagnostic facility are unaware that it is available to them.

There are 4 main groups of disorder which are detectable early enough in pregnancy to allow termination: these are:

Chromosome aberrations;
X-linked recessive disorders;
Certain inborn errors of metabolism;
Open neural-tube defects.

The two most common and important are mongolism (Down's syndrome, trisomy 21), and spina bifida cystica.

Mongolism

Between 1300 and 1500 mongol children are born in the United Kingdom each year. The majority have 47 chromosomes including an additional chromosome 21. In less than 3 per cent the chromosome abnormality is in the form of an unbalanced translocation. In this case the additional chromosome 21 is attached to another chromosome, usually chromosome 14 (Fig. 5). The majority of these translocations arise by new mutation, but a few are familial in that one of the parents has a balanced translocation, for example, only one normal chromosome 21, the other being translocated to chromosome 14.

The cause of trisomy 21 is unknown, but the risk of having a mongol child is much greater in older women. The incidence of mongolism among all births is about 1 in 600, but where the mother is 40 years

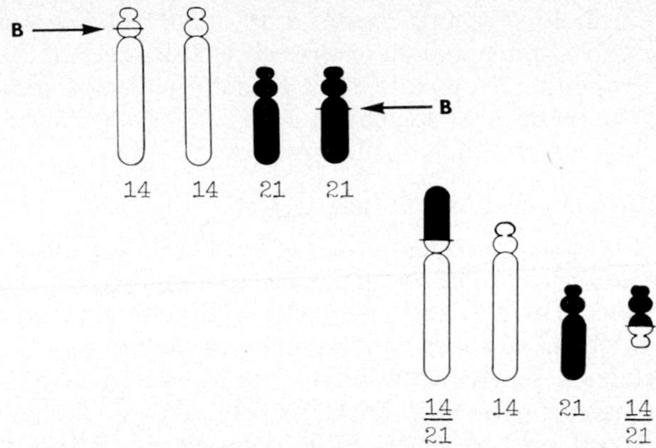

3/FIG. 5.—Diagram showing the origin of a translocation between two non-homologous chromosomes, numbers 14 and 21. Chromosome breakage had occurred at B and, by chance, the normal process of repair had occurred between the wrong fragments. This particular aberration is a cause of familial mongolism.

of age or over it is estimated at about 2·6 per cent, and 1·6 per cent at maternal ages between 35 and 39 years.[29] In other words, the incidence of mongolism could be halved if all babies were born before the mother was 35 years old. For the older woman in her late thirties therefore, and certainly in our service over the age of 37, there is much to be said for offering fetal chromosome analysis from amniotic cell cultures so that affected pregnancies can be detected and a decision made as to termination.

To a mother who has previously had a child with trisomy mongolism the risk of recurrence can cause acute anxiety, sufficient in fact to discourage further pregnancies even though the risk in this group is only about 1 per cent. Truly this is a most important indication for prenatal diagnosis if only for the humane consideration of being able to reassure the patient, although it is not likely to reduce the number of mongol births to any marked extent.

Mongolism is the most important chromosomal abnormality but it is not the only one. Trisomy 13, trisomy 18 and sex chromosome aberrations such as 47,XXY (Klinefelter syndrome) may be diagnosed prenatally by fetal chromosome analysis. Familial chromosome aberrations such as reciprocal translocations are rare but nevertheless important indications for such an analysis as the risk of unbalanced chromosome aberration and severe fetal abnormality is about 10 per cent. In Glasgow, our experience has been more fortunate than others, for of the 29 translocation cases that have already been studied in the last eight years, chromosome analysis of the fetus has shown a balanced carrier state in 12 and a normal chromosome complement in 15. The two fetuses with unbalanced chromosomes were aborted and the remainder were successfully delivered.

There is one major advantage of prenatal chromosome analysis over other prenatal tests inasmuch as a different technique is not required for each chromosomal disorder.

Spina Bifida and Open Neural-tube Defects

About 2000 cases of spina bifida are born each year in the United Kingdom, an incidence of about 2·4 per thousand births. Thanks to modern neonatal surgery and early closure of the spinal lesion and the use of the Holter valve to combat hydrocephalus, nearly half the affected children survive to adult life, but about half of those are severely handicapped with paralysis of varying degree, mental retardation and incontinence. In recognition of the poor quality of life of many of those that survive there is nowadays in most centres an attempt to select the patients most likely to benefit from active surgical intervention and other treatment. Severe hydrocephalus at birth, severe flaccid paraplegia, brain injury, kyphosis and other gross defects at birth all have a grave prognosis and discourage active treatment. Those infants who are not selected for treatment pose almost intolerable problems of management not only on parents but on doctors and nurses too. A reliable prenatal test for the more severe varieties of spina bifida and even more so the screening tests for detecting the condition in mothers who are not even suspected of being at risk can only be accepted as a major development, which if it were properly employed could help to reduce considerably the frequency of the most severely affected cases that survive their birth.

Anencephaly, iniencephaly and encephalocele are closely related to spina bifida and are grouped together collectively as neural-tube defects. Congenital hydrocephalus when it occurs without spina bifida is thought to be a separate condition. In spite of speculation the cause of these defects is still unknown. The incidence is higher in Ireland, the West of Scotland and South Wales than in the rest of this country. In Glasgow, for example, the incidences of spina bifida and anencephaly are each about 3 per 1000, whereas in the South of England they are 1·8 and 1·3 per 1000 respectively. There are geographical and seasonal differences and some association with occupational class which suggests possible environmental factors. Although a genetic component is suggested by family and twin studies, spina bifida is only likely to be prevented ultimately by recognising and removing the environmental factors.

After the birth of one child with a neural-tube defect, the risk of having another is about 1 in 20 and this rises to 1 in 8 after two such disasters. These daunting figures may discourage many families from having further children and for these there is clearly a great need for a reliable test in early pregnancy. This need has been met to a large extent by the work of Brock and Sutcliffe (1972)[4] who observed that in cases of anencephaly, amniotic fluid samples at 25 to 35 weeks gestation (in one case at 13 weeks gestation) showed that the level of alphafetoprotein (AFP) was significantly raised. AFP is a serum protein with a molecular weight of 64,000 which is formed in the fetal liver and yolk sac. It can diffuse through open spinal or cranial lesions and thus contaminate amniotic fluid. Following these observations Allan *et al.* (1973)[1] studied amniotic AFP prospectively in 20 mothers who had a history of one or more previous children with spina bifida or anencephaly and were therefore clearly at risk. In two of these pregnancies the AFP at 16 weeks gestation was ten times the mean normal level. Both fetuses were found, following termination, to have large open dorsolumbar myeloceles. So far, at the time of writing, over 700 pregnancies at risk have been tested in our genetics laboratory before the twentieth week of gestation. Of these, all 25 open lesions have been successfully identified in time to permit the option of termination of pregnancy; but there were 7 *closed* lesions which were not detected because there was no leakage of AFP into the amniotic fluid. The overall recurrence risk in this series was thus 4·5 per cent, and 21·9 per cent of the lesions were closed. Fortunately, most of the infants with closed defects seem to do well.

This prenatal diagnosis test is now in routine use in many centres and is applied in the case of mothers recognised to be at risk. The technique seems to be reliable although raised AFP levels have been found to be associated with intra-uterine death. False positive results have only occasionally been reported in normal pregnancies. Even the contamination of amniotic fluid with a little fetal blood in the course of amniocentesis does not, as a rule, produce levels of AFP such as are found in open neural-tube defects. In interpreting prenatal tests the gestational age of the pregnancy must be taken into account since the amniotic AFP level alters significantly, reaching a maximum concentration in the fetal serum at about 13 weeks.[26] This concentration falls off rapidly and is less than 2 per cent of the maximum by the thirty-fourth week. The total amount of fetal AFP increases until the twenty-seventh week of gestation. For example, the mean level of AFP in amniotic fluid at fourteen weeks is about $26{\cdot}0 \pm 95$ μg/ml and this falls to $17{\cdot}1 \pm 8{\cdot}5$ μg/ml at 16 weeks, further to $13{\cdot}6 \pm 7{\cdot}9$ μg/ml at 18 weeks and to $6{\cdot}7 \pm 3{\cdot}3$ μg/ml at 20 weeks. After 22 weeks the levels are so small that the "rocket" technique of assay is not senstive enough to detect them. The importance of knowing the maturity of a given pregnancy is therefore obvious.

Only in about 5 per cent of cases of spina bifida is there a history of another sibling affected by neural-tube defect. If therefore only mothers who have a previous history are tested the majority of cases will not be detected by this means. However, it has now been shown that neural-tube defects are often associated with raised levels of AFP in the maternal serum.[22] This opened up the exciting possibilities of screening cases in the hope of preventing not simply the second neural-tube disaster but the first as well. These concentrations in maternal serum are small and require sensitive radioimmunoassay technique to detect them. However, by this method we have confirmed that the mother's serum AFP is significantly elevated in each case of open spina bifida so far diagnosed by amniotic AFP levels. Prospective studies are now under way in many centres including Glasgow and this has led already to the identification of anencephaly and intra-uterine death in early pregnancy. When a raised maternal serum AFP is found an indication is provided for amniocentesis and more definitive amniotic AFP determination. False positives occur in 1·4 per cent of pregnancies in our series, and are frequently due to underestimating the gestation, to twins, or to missed abortions. Approximately 81 per cent of open spina bifida pregnancies and almost all anencephalies can be detected if the 98th percentile is used as the cut-off point and if screening is performed between 16 and 20 completed weeks gestation. Seventy-five per cent of false positives can be correctly identified by obstetric ultrasound, or excluded by repeating the serum AFP test, without recourse to amniocentesis, which is needed in only 0·63 per cent of pregnancies. Nearly half the amniocenteses yield liquor with elevated amniotic AFP due to fetal abnormality.

X-linked Recessive Disorders

The fetal sex can be determined in early pregnancy by analysis of X and Y chromatin in amniotic cell nuclei and incidentally in the course of chromosome analysis of amniotic cell cultures. This is valuable for the management of severe X-linked diseases. These disorders are not so common as mongolism and spina bifida, but are none the less important. Haemophilia and Duchenne muscular dystrophy are the best known of these X-linked conditions, both affecting only males and inherited through carrier females. In neither of these conditions can the affected male fetus be diagnosed prenatally and therefore the basis for selective termination has to rest simply on the diagnosis of male sex in the fetus. In only the most severe cases could haemophilia be regarded as a justifiable indication for this kind of selective liquidation. In the case of X-linked Duchenne muscular dystrophy a mother known to be a carrier may request termination of pregnancy in the knowledge that her fetus is male and has a fifty per cent chance of being affected with a crippling disease that will keep him in a wheel-chair by the age of ten years and kill him before he reaches the age of twenty. A female fetus of such a patient though not affected herself will have a fifty per cent chance of being a carrier and thus possibly passing on the genetic disorder to the next generation. This disturbing possibility is not legally accepted as grounds for termination. Until the specific prenatal test for this disorder is found mothers at risk of bearing a child with X-linked muscular dystrophy can only hope to have a normal, healthy baby provided it is a female. Until that day normal male fetuses may be sacrificed unnecessarily. At present, however, specific tests are available for only two sex-linked disorders, the Lesch-Nyhan syndrome of hyperuricaemia, mental retardation and self-mutilation and the Hunter form of mucopolysaccharidosis.

Autosomal Recessive Metabolic Diseases

Individually autosomal metabolic diseases are extremely rare but the number of such disorders collectively may affect a substantial number of individuals. In all such cases both parents carry one dose of the abnormal gene and consequently their affected children may inherit this gene from both of them so that the risk of occurrence in such families is 25 per cent.

Of the known metabolic disorders most are enzyme abnormalities and their diagnosis depends upon a biochemical assay of the enzyme in a sample of the patient's cells. Prenatal diagnosis is possible if the assay can be made on amniotic cell cultures. Already there are over sixty different disorders for which a prenatal test is now possible (Table 1). The number grows every month but unfortunately the more common autosomal recessive conditions such as cystic fibrosis (1 in 2000 livebirths) and phenylketonuria (1 in 10,000 livebirths) are not included in this list since no reliable prenatal tests are yet available.

At present the only way of recognising a pregnancy at risk of an autosomal recessive disease is, as in the case of chromosomal translocations, by the history of the previous birth of an affected child. Since the first disaster cannot be forestalled, the total reduction in individual cases in a community achieved by selective termination is small, even if such a service were available to everyone. More could be hoped in the way of reducing the number of affected children by identifying "matings at risk" before any children are conceived. This would require a reliable screening test for carriers and would have to be applied to all mothers attending the antenatal clinic and also to the husbands of those mothers found to be carriers. In theory at least, such a scheme could more or less eliminate a disease such as cystic fibrosis. The identification of "matings at risk" by population screening has only been successfully attempted so far in the case of

3/ TABLE 1

A LIST OF METABOLIC DISEASES FOR WHICH PRENATAL DIAGNOSIS IS POSSIBLE

Fabry's disease	Argininosuccinic aciduria
Farber's disease	Citrullinaemia
Gaucher's disease	Cystinosis
Generalised gangliosidosis	Disorder of isoleucine catabolism
Juvenile G_{M1} gangliosidosis	Histidinaemia
Juvenile G_{M2} gangliosidosis	Homocystinuria
Krabbe's disease	Hyperlysinaemia
Lactosyl ceramidosis	Hypervalinaemia
Metachromatic leucodystrophy	Isovaleric acidaemia
Niemann-Pick disease	Maple syrup urine disease
Refsum's disease	Methylmalonic aciduria
Sandhoff's disease	Ornithine-ketoacid transaminase deficiency
Tay-Sachs disease	Propionyl CoA carboxylase deficiency
Wolman's disease	Saccharopinuria
Hurler's syndrome	Adenosine deaminase deficiency
Hunter's syndrome	Gout (X-linked)
Maroteaux-Lamy syndrome	Lesch-Nyhan syndrome
Sanfilippo syndrome	Orotic aciduria
Scheie's syndrome	Acatalasaemia
CoA transferase deficiency	Congenital erythropoietic porphyria
Fucosidosis	Beta-glucuronidase deficiency
Galactosaemia	I-cell disease
Galactokinase deficiency	Lysosomal acid phosphatase deficiency
Glucose-6-phosphate dehydrogenase deficiency	Lysyl-protocollagen hydroxylase deficiency
Glycogen storage disease (Type II)	Methylene THF reductase deficiency
Glycogen storage disease (Type III)	Testicular feminisation
Glycogen storage disease (Type IV)	Vitamin B_{12} metabolic defect
Mannosidosis	Xeroderma pigmentosum
Phosphohexose isomerase deficiency	
Pyruvate decarboxylase deficiency	
Pyruvate dehydrogenase deficiency	

(After Littlefield *et al.*, 1974[29])

Tay-Sachs disease in the Jewish community in parts of Eastern United States (Kaback *et al.*, 1973). Tay-Sachs disease is very rare in the U.K. and suitable population screening tests are not available for the more common autosomal recessive conditions in this country.

Since the number of metabolic disorders which can be detected by enzyme assay of amniotic cell cultures is so large, but individually rare, it can be seen that it would be impossible for any single laboratory to gain enough expertise with each test to provide a comprehensive service. This would only be possible by collaboration between all laboratories who limited their tests and provided material to other given laboratories for specific assays as required. This already exists to some extent on an informal and even international basis.

Need for Amniocentesis

All the prenatal tests so far described depend on biochemical and/or cytological examination of amniotic fluid samples. Although the procedure is possible at 14 weeks, the best time is about 16 weeks gestation, when sufficient amniotic fluid is usually available to provide a 15/20 ml sample. Smaller amounts than 10 ml require longer to establish amniotic cell cultures and the results are therefore available that much later.

Since amniocentesis is not wholly without hazard it is only offered when there are grounds for suspecting a severe fetal disorder and not for such trivial reasons as choosing the sex of the offspring. It would hardly be logical to offer the test to parents if it was not coupled with the assurance that termination would be undertaken if serious abnormality were found and the request was made by them.

The risk of complications following amniocentesis is fortunately low enough not to dissuade mothers from seeking the assurance of such a test that the fetus is unaffected.

Biochemical and Cytological Tests

All samples of amniotic fluid are processed for chromosome analysis and amniotic AFP in our laboratory, whatever the primary indication. Already four chromosome aberrations and eight open neural-tube defects have been found in cases where neither of these conditions was suspected in the first place.

The amniotic fluid arrives at the laboratory in a sterile container and is processed as follows. Two to 3 ml are removed for X-chromatin analysis. Amniotic cells are separated from the fluid in a millipore filter, and fixed and stained by cresyl violet *in situ* on the filter. The proportion of amniotic cell nuclei containing X-chromatin can then be determined under a microscope. Only cells recognised as being fetal in origin are scored. From another small sample of the amniotic fluid, cells are removed by centrifugation, fixed in acetic alcohol fixative and air dried onto clean microscope slides, using a cytocentrifuge. Staining is now by quinacrine fluorescence and the cells are examined under the ultraviolet microscope for fluorescent Y-chromatin. The fetal sex must be determined by both these methods in all cases because maternal cells may rarely overgrow the amniotic cell culture.

The rest of the amniotic fluid is centrifuged and amniotic cell cultures are set up from the cell deposit.[27] Chromosome analysis is undertaken on the primary cultures, and subcultures are used for enzyme analysis.

Amniotic alphafetoprotein estimation is undertaken on the cell-free fluid, using the "rocket" method of counter immuno-electrophoresis.[1] The height of the rocket is directly proportional to the level of AFP in the sample which is calculated by reference to known standards set up along with the test fluids.

Other tests are still under development and include the use of genetic markers for the prenatal detection of autosomal dominant disorders due to genes which are known to be linked to the marker loci. Fetal blood sampling with the aid of the fetoscope has already been used in the prenatal diagnosis of the haemoglobinopathies.

In the future it may be possible to develop methods of treating amniotic cells so that genes normally expressed only in more differentiated tissues may be activated in amniotic cell cultures. This would open the door to the prenatal diagnosis of many more inborn errors, including phenylketonuria.

Ideally the prenatal diagnosis of abnormality should be made as early as possible in pregnancy, before the stage of viability and preferably before fetal movement is felt; in other words, the results should be available by 20–22 weeks gestation. This is possible with certainty in the case of fetal sexing and amniotic AFP since the results are available within 24 hours of amniocentesis. Chromosome analysis which requires amniotic cell culture can usually be reported within 13–18 days of securing a sample and a successful culture rate of 90 per cent is aimed at. It is usually evident by 7–10 days after initial amniocentesis whether a second amniotic sample is likely to be required.

Enzyme assays in autosomal recessive diseases require large numbers of cultured amniotic cells and this may require growth periods of from 4–6 weeks, with a still further week required for biochemical testing. It seems unlikely that any method will emerge for accelerating the growth of amniotic cell cultures and the solution may lie in the development of microassay techniques which require only a comparatively small number of cells.

In conclusion, it is suggested that antenatal diagnosis should be offered to mothers in the following categories (the risk of severe fetal abnormality being indicated within parenthesis).

1. Mothers of 40 years of age and over (3·6 per cent risk of mongolism or other gross chromosome aberration).
2. Mothers with a previous mongol child (1·2 per cent).
3. Mothers liable to have a chromosomally unbalanced child because of parental chromosome translocation (average 8·9 per cent).
4. Mothers with a previous child affected with a diagnosable autosomal recessive metabolic disorder (25 per cent).
5. Mothers with one or more children affected by a neural-tube defect (5 per cent).
6. Mothers who are known carriers of a severe X-linked recessive disorder (25 per cent).
7. Mothers found to have abnormally high serum alphafeto-protein levels during routine antenatal screening.
8. Mothers aged 35–39 years (1·4 per cent).

For those concerned about the cost of such a service it will be appreciated from even the most superficial cost-benefit analysis that this is only a fraction of the expense involved in looking after those tragic cases born with incurable disability due to chromosome abnormalities, lethal inborn errors of metabolism, or extensive spina bifida. The humane considerations are more compelling and these include a consideration of the interest of the family in terms of suffering, anxiety, illness and deprivation. Although prenatal diagnosis is in its infancy and still has its limitations, it is clear that it has an important part to play in the reduction of congenital disease now, and to an increasing extent in the future.

BIOCHEMISTRY IN OBSTETRICS

by ROBERT W. LOGAN, T.D., M.B., Ch.B., B.Sc., F.R.C.Path., F.R.C.P. (Glas.)

Senior Lecturer. University of Glasgow; Honorary Consultant Medical Biochemist, Queen Mother's Hospital, Glasgow

Biochemical Techniques in Obstetrics

The widespread availability of biochemical determinations has greatly altered the confidence with which assessment of the feto-placental unit can be made. As with all laboratory measurements, it is important to distinguish between the accuracy and precision of such biochemical techniques. Accuracy can be defined as the nearness of an analytical result to the true value. Precision is a measure of the reproducibility of the determination. It is possible, therefore, to have a very precise technique which will, however, consistently yield an inaccurate answer for the parameter in question. As a consequence of this, it is important that each laboratory constructs appropriate "normal ranges" for use when attempting to diagnose possible abnormality.

Methods of Measurement and Separation

No attempt will be made to provide an exhaustive list of the procedures available but the principles commonly employed will be discussed.

Colorimetry.—Methods based on treatment of samples with various reagents and measurement of colour developed at specific wavelengths form the basis of many of the techniques employed in biochemistry. Unfortunately, although colorimetry has proved to be satisfactory for many of the electrolyte and liver function tests commonly requested, it is not sufficiently sensitive for some of the hormonal determinations required. The Kober reaction (1931)[38] is, however, still widely employed in the estimation of urinary oestrogens in pregnancy.

Fluorimetry.—The great advantage of measurements involving fluorescence is the sensitivity offered. They are, however, subject to the disadvantage that unless adequate precautions are taken, specificity may be less than necessary. The principle involves activation of the material in solution by submitting it to a strong light of known wavelength. Absorption of some of this light is associated with emission of secondary light at a longer wavelength. By the use of suitable filters, it is possible to measure only the secondary light emitted, the intensity of which is directly related to the concentration of material being measured. A combination of fluorimetry with the Kober reaction has yielded methods for determining both urinary oestrogens[31] and plasma oestriol.[42]

Chromatography forms part of the art of the modern biochemist and involves the separation of the multiple constituents being studied. Among the compounds so investigated are included proteins, lipids, steroids, amino acids and carbohydrates.

Paper chromatography.—Following initial treatment and extraction from biological materials, the extract requiring fractionation is applied to a sheet of suitable paper using an appropriate solvent. Thereafter, migration of the components occurs at rates governed by their respective solubilities in the solvent system utilised. The materials are then located by various methods including colorimetry, fluorescence and radioactivity. One of the disadvantages of paper chromatography is that certain agents used in the chemical reactions would destroy the paper itself. In spite of this, however, partition chromatography using paper has been widely employed in clinical biochemistry.

Column chromatography.—By choice of material (cellulose, silica gel, alumina, etc.) and solvents (alcohol, benzene, hexane, etc.) separation of individual compounds can be effected by partition, adsorption or ion exchange. Fractionation of individual steroids such as oestriol, oestrone, oestradiol, pregnanediol and pregnanetriol may be accomplished. Formerly this formed an integral part of most of the methods developed to estimate these compounds but the requirement for increased sensitivity has led to their being superseded.

Thin-layer chromatography has been widely employed in biochemistry for the separation of steroids and lipids. Thin-layer separations resemble those on paper in some ways but the much wider choice of media means that separations by partition, adsorption, gel filtration and ion exchange can be performed by this technique. The special properties of thin layers also allow much shorter development times to be achieved. Either rigid glass plates or flexible polyester, aluminium foil or fibreglass may be coated with silica gel or other suitable adsorbent. The substances to be separated are then applied and the appropriate solvent system is allowed to run either up or down the plate. The various compounds migrate at different rates according to their solubilities in the solvent employed. Localisation of the materials is then accomplished by spraying the plate with suitable reagents and more exact quantitation may be achieved by elution of the spots and measurement colorimetrically or fluorimetrically. This technique has found widespread use in obstetrics in the determination of amniotic fluid lecithin and sphingomyelin contents.[37]

Gas-liquid chromatography has recently been introduced for the determination of many of the steroid hormones. Separations depend upon the partition of solute molecules between a liquid, supported on a suitable solid, and the gas flowing through the system. The technique involves extraction of the hydrolysed compounds from the sample using a suitable organic solvent. Thereafter, the solvent is evaporated to dryness and the material or some suitable derivative, is dissolved in a small volume of further solvent before application to the chromatographic column. An inert carrier gas, e.g. nitrogen, is then allowed to pass through the column which may either be retained at a constant temperature (isothermal) or may be subjected to a controlled increase in temperature. The vaporised samples are borne by the carrier gas (mobile phase) through the column which is packed with a non-volatile, high molecular weight liquid (stationary phase) such as a silicone polymer coating on inert material. Due to differences in solubility and electrical charge, the stationary liquid phase has a different retarding effect on the various components of the moving gas phase, thereby separating these components as they proceed through the column. Individual compounds emerge from the column at predictable time intervals and measurement follows detection by suitable means (flame ionisation, electron capture). Part of the procedure can be automated and both sensitivity and specificity are fairly good. One such method for the simultaneous determination of urinary pregnanediol and pregnanetriol has been described by Rahman (1974).[44] Another for the estimation of palmitic acid in amniotic fluid as a measure of fetal lung maturity has been developed by Warren *et al.* (1973).[50]

Competitive protein binding (CPB).—Such methods are based on the principle that the material, X, being measured, can be bound by some suitable protein, P. Provided that a radiolabelled form of X is available, *X, an assay system can be prepared where the equilibrium

$$\text{Protein-bound } {*X} \rightleftharpoons \text{free protein} + \text{free } {*X}$$

can be displaced to the right by addition of unlabelled X which has been extracted from the sample under investigation. This means that the quantity of radiolabelled *X which is protein bound will diminish according to the amount of X added from the sample being measured. Separation of the protein-bound isotope from the free isotope *X can be achieved by a variety of techniques (differential migration of bound and free fractions, adsorption methods, fractional precipitation, double-antibody method, solid-phase methods). By using known amounts of unlabelled material, a calibration curve can be constructed and patient samples can then be analysed.

This method has been employed for a variety of estimations including plasma oestriol[32,33] and plasma oestradiol.[42,43] The advantages of the method when suitably employed include sensitivity and specificity and at the same time the procedures are convenient for clinical usage.

In the assessment of thyroid function, serum thyroxine may also be estimated by a similar competitive protein-binding technique.

Radioimmunoassay (RIA).—Where ultrasensitivity is required, this method, or adaptations thereof, is the one of choice. As originally described, this technique was applied to the determination of protein or polypeptide hormones. It has, however, been extended to include many other classes of compound including oestrogens[35] and thyroid hormones. The prerequisites for the analytical system are:

1. Purified human antigen X or antigen-protein complex in the case of oestriol—16,17 dihemisuccinate linked to bovine serum albumin;
2. Potent antibody P developed against 1;
3. Pure radiolabelled human antigen *X (usually ^{125}I-labelled in the case of polypeptide hormones);
4. Means of separating protein-bound radiolabelled antigen PB*X from free radiolabelled antigen *X.

By a procedure similar to that employed in the competitive protein-binding assay, analysis of patient samples can be achieved by counting either the protein-bound or free radioactivity remaining after addition of the unlabelled antigen derived from the sample undergoing assay.

Radioimmunoassay is available for measurement of the pituitary and placental hormones FSH, LH, TSH, ACTH, HCG and HPL (HCS). A procedure has also been developed for determining the serum concentration of alphafetoprotein.

So, too, it is likely that with the difficulty of assessing protein-bound iodine results in pregnancy due to the increase occasioned by the increment in thyroid-binding globulin, radioimmunoassay will be increasingly used for thyroid assessment. Unequivocal evaluation of thyroid function in suspect cases should involve at least measurement of serum thyroxine (T_4), tri-iodothyronine (T_3) and TSH.

The great advantages of RIA are that, when carefully employed, it is associated with excellent sensitivity, specificity and accuracy, whilst being suitable for development for routine use.

Radial immunodiffusion is a technique involving the preparation of agarose in which antibodies to specific proteins are dissolved. To wells punched in the agarose are added known standards of the protein being measured together with samples of biological fluid obtained from patients. Around each well, concentric precipitation rings develop whose diameters are related to the protein concentration originally added. This method can be used to estimate a variety of proteins including albumin, α_2 macroglobulin, transferrin and the immunoglobulins, IgA, IgG and IgM. It has also been employed to estimate the alphafetoprotein content of amniotic fluid although in this case the sensitivity of the basic technique is barely suitable and such modifications as counter immunoelectrophoresis are necessary.[4] In this procedure, the advantage of the electrophoretic separation of proteins is combined with the sensitivity of detection accorded by using a monospecific antiserum prepared against alphafetoprotein.

Assessment of the Fetoplacental Unit

Various methods have been developed to monitor the function of the developing fetoplacental unit and it is important to realise that each technique is measuring a particular facet of the function. It is, therefore, not surprising that results obtained using different procedures may initially appear to yield conflicting information. The biochemical parameters which have been most widely employed to assess fetal development include:

Steroid hormones—oestrogens, pregnanediol;
Enzymes—oxytocinase, alkaline phosphatase (total and heat-stable);
Human placental lactogen—(HPL, HCS);

Human chorionic gonadotrophin—(HCG);
Alphafetoprotein (*AFP*);
Selenomethionine uptake.

In addition to these investigations, biochemical measurement of various substances in amniotic fluid, e.g. creatinine, lecithin and sphingomyelin has been used to predict fetal maturity.

3/TABLE 2

ORIGIN OF OESTRIOL IN MATERNAL URINE

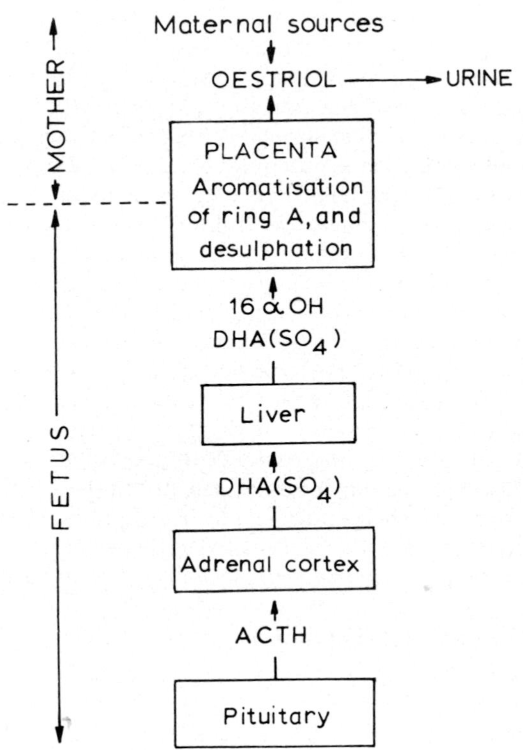

NB—Oestriol production demands the integrity of all the systems shown boxed.

Steroid hormones. Biosynthesis of the oestrogens, and in particular of oestriol, by the fetoplacental unit may be considered for simplicity as in Table 2.

It can be seen that oestriol output in the maternal urine depends upon integrity of each part of the biosynthetic chain and that a reduction in excretion does not necessarily indicate placental dysfunction. Such conditions as anencephaly with failure of pituitary development, congenital adrenal hypoplasia, congenital cirrhosis and placental sulphatase deficiency will result in a fall in maternal oestriol output. So, too, the administration of glucocorticoids in dosage greater than the equivalent of 75 mg cortisol per day can cause suppression of the fetal and maternal adrenal cortices with subsequent fall in urinary oestriol. Maternal ingestion of such drugs as ampicillin and mandelamine is also likely to occasion such falls in oestriol output without signifying fetal upset. Conversely, elevated output of oestriol in maternal urine may rarely be associated with congenital adrenal hyperplasia (where $DHA(SO_4)$ secretion is increased) although more often this is due to a large fetus or a multiple pregnancy.

The rationale for measuring oestriol rather than total oestrogens is based on the observation that, in the non-pregnant subject, oestriol forms only about 50 per cent of the total urinary oestrogen excretion whereas in late pregnancy, for the reasons already described, this percentage increases to 80 or greater. In spite of this theoretical advantage of oestriol measurement, it is the case that less specific methods estimating total urinary oestrogens provide useful information in evaluating fetal development. The choice of sample for analyses is also a matter for debate. It has been shown that, allowing for the precision of the technique of measurement and the wide physiological variation from day to day in healthy subjects, the coefficient of variation is 20 per cent for urinary oestriol measurement using urine collected over 24-hour periods. For a 48-hour urine the variation is 16 per cent, and for an 8-hour urine it is 30 per cent. Measurement of creatinine as well as oestrogen content in the urine affords a definite advantage in that the ratio oestrogen output:creatinine output obviates difficulties encountered with incomplete collection. Whether the convenience offered by determination of this ratio in casual rather than 24-hour urine collections will offset the disadvantage of the wider fluctuation in results which occurs, remains to be scientifically elucidated. What is clear is that single urinary oestriol values are of limited value in assessing fetal status and that repeated tests to determine the trend of results are of major importance.[30]

So, too, measurement of maternal plasma oestriol concentration yields an attractive means of obtaining current information regarding fetoplacental function and many of the protagonists of such analyses now decry urinary oestriol measurements as obsolete. Definitive evidence is still awaited, however, illustrating the clinical superiority of plasma oestriol measurements over those performed using urine. The great advantage of employing urine specimens is that methods exist where one technician can analyse 150 specimens in a working day, and in general, it is easier to obtain at least a casual specimen of urine than a venous blood sample.

Urinary pregnanediol is derived from the progesterone secreted by various tissues in the mother, placenta, and to a lesser extent, fetus. Whilst it can be a useful index of placental function, especially where spurious reasons exist for a low oestriol output, its use has been largely superseded by measurement of such materials as human placental lactogen (HPL).

Enzymes.—The placenta is known to secrete various enzymes and as such, measurement of the activity in maternal serum of alkaline phosphatase and oxytocinase reflects the function of the syncytio-trophoblast. In particular, serum alkaline phosphatase withstanding heating at 56° C or 60° C for 30 minutes (heat-stable) has been used as an index of the placental isoenzyme. Unfortunately, such techniques offer little information as to possible intra-uterine growth retardation and compare unfavourably with other parameters.[45]

HPL.—Originally called human placental lactogen (HPL) in 1961, this material is produced by the syncytiotrophoblast and has, as yet, an undefined physiological role. In 1967 at Sienna it was decided to alter its name to human chorionic somatotrophin (HCS), but in London in 1970 the original name (HPL) was reinstated.

HPL can be measured by radioimmunoassay using a sensitive, precise technique. One technician can analyse 400 serum specimens in a day and various studies have been performed to determine the value of HPL measurement either alone[47] or with other parameters.[18] Currently, it would appear that sequential determination of HPL is most useful during early pregnancy in predicting whether a threatened abortion is inevitable. In later pregnancy, measurement seems to offer a means of predicting unexpected fetal distress occurring during labour or asphyxia of the newborn child in pregnancies otherwise judged to be normal.

HCG.—The production of human chorionic gonadotrophin during pregnancy was first demonstrated biologically many years ago although it was not until much later that it was proved to be of placental and not of pituitary origin. Immunological and sensitive radioimmunoassay methods for its determination now exist and either the plasma or urinary content can be measured. The production of HCG by the placenta is maximal in the first trimester and a failure to show the normal increment may indicate that the pregnancy will not proceed to term. Unfortunately, determination of HCG in either urine or plasma has been of little value in assessing fetal status in later pregnancy. Whilst detection of increased HCG concentrations may be of value in the diagnosis of hydatidiform mole and choriocarcinoma, the main purpose for HCG determination remains as a diagnostic test of pregnancy.

Alphafetoprotein (AFP) is an oncofetoprotein which attains its highest concentration (2000 mg/l) in fetal serum at about the 12th week of intra-uterine life. Thereafter, its concentration declines slowly until at term it is about 20 mg/l. Conversely, the concentration in maternal serum during normal pregnancy rises from 15 μg/l at conception to 150 μg/l at 12–16 weeks and 500 μg/l at term. In later pregnancy, any condition causing fetal distress may result in an increase in the concentration of AFP in maternal serum and as such, its measurement has been used to predict fetal distress.[49] In amniotic fluid, the mean AFP concentration at 16 weeks is approximately 20 mg/l whereas at term, it has fallen to 70 μg/l, a fact which has been used in estimating gestational age.[48] At present, however, the most valuable feature of this protein is that during early pregnancy open neural-tube defects are associated with high levels of AFP in amniotic fluid. So, too, many of those cases also exhibit elevated AFP concentrations in samples of maternal serum and it has been estimated that routine screening of maternal blood samples obtained around 16–20 weeks could detect about 80 per cent of affected cases.[13] Elevated serum AFP also occurs in teratocarcinoma of the ovary or testis and recently an interesting paper has appeared describing its use in differentiating neonatal hepatitis from biliary atresia.[51]

Selenomethionine uptake.—Although not strictly a biochemical test, this technique employs radiolabelled methionine in which the sulphur of methionine has been replaced by ^{75}Se. The material is administered intravenously into the maternal circulation and, using suitably placed counters, the uptake by placenta and fetus is monitored.[36, 39] Whilst theoretically attractive, the results yielded by this test do not in general agree with other well established procedures and it has, therefore, been seldom employed in the management of "at risk" pregnancies.

Amniotic fluid.—Amniocentesis involves a slight risk to the fetus and mother but prior localisation of the placenta by ultrasound minimises the hazard. Samples of amniotic fluid taken early in pregnancy (15–16 weeks) tend to be used for genetic counselling whereas those taken after 30 weeks may be submitted for various biochemical estimations designed to assess fetal development. In both situations, the value of the information likely to be obtained must be carefully considered before undertaking the procedure. It has been shown that amniotic fluid creatinine and urea correlate with gestational age and in particular, with development of the fetal kidney. Attempts have been made to estimate gestational age by such analyses but even when using a computer-derived estimate based on various biochemical results, a prediction correct to within 2 weeks occurs in only 67 per cent of cases.[40] It is known that the tissues in the fetus develop at different rates and that an overall assessment of fetal maturity demands measurement of head size, skin development, bone development and development of lungs and kidneys. Perhaps the most important factor following birth is the maturity of the fetal lung and it has been shown by Gluck *et al.* (1971)[37] that measurement of amniotic fluid lecithin and sphingomyelin concentrations provides an excellent means of determining antenatally what fetal lung function will be following delivery. Assessment of lung maturity by this procedure is certainly more important than determining the actual gestational age since satisfactory lung function can be found after only 30 weeks of gestation whilst immature lung function with development of RDS may occasionally result in a term fetus.

It is certain that no one test will satisfactorily separate all normal pregnancies from those associated with intra-uterine growth retardation or some other abnormality. Currently the best results are obtained by using a combination of parameters among which figure prominently measurement of urinary oestriol and amniotic fluid lecithin/sphingomyelin or palmitic acid. When these results are associated with ultrasonic measurement of fetal biparietal diameter, the clinical value of the findings is greatly enhanced.

Fetal pH.—In 1962, Saling introduced the technique of assessing the acid-base status of the fetus using samples of capillary blood obtained from the fetal scalp during labour. Subsequent evaluation of this procedure during the first stage of labour[34] has shown that where labour is prolonged, or where there is meconium-staining, pH measurement on such blood samples taken at regular intervals can significantly reduce fetal mortality due to prolonged intra-uterine anoxia and acidosis. What is certain is that one normal pH reading obtained well before delivery in a difficult case will offer no guarantee that acidosis will not subsequently develop.

New biochemical procedures are constantly being investigated in an attempt to improve the management of the mother and fetus during pregnancy. Some of these techniques will be found to offer information of value to the clinician and it is expected that before long, some of the tests described will have been supplanted by those offering finer diagnostic discrimination.

REFERENCES

1. Allan, L. D., Ferguson-Smith, M. A., Donald, I., Sweet, E. M. and Gibson, A. A. M. (1973). *Lancet*, **2,** 522.
2. Ardran, G. M. and Kemp, F. H. (1972). *Brit. med. J.*, **4,** 422.
3. Bang, J. and Northeved, A. (1972). *Amer. J. Obstet. Gynec.* **114,** 599.
4. Brock, D. J. H. and Sutcliffe, R. G. (1972). *Lancet*, **2,** 197.
5. Brock, D. J. H., Bolton, H. E. and Monaghan, J. M. (1973). *Lancet*, **2,** 923.

6. Campbell, S. (1973). In: *Proceedings of the Fourth International Conference on Birth Defects, Vienna.* Ed. by A. G. Motulsky and W. Lenz. p. 240. Amsterdam: Excerpta Medica.
7. Claireaux, A. C. (1973). *Proc. roy. Soc. Med.*, **66,** 119.
8. Drillien, C. M. (1973). Scientific meeting of R.C.O.G., Dundee University, 30th March.
9. Fraser, I. S. (1974). *Brit. med. J.*, **4,** 404.
10. Hellman, L. M., Duffus, G. M., Donald, I. and Sunden, B. (1970). *Lancet*, **1,** 1133.
11. Hellman, L. M., Kobayashi, M. and Cromb, E. (1973). *Amer. J. Obstet. Gynec.*, **115,** 615.
12. Klopper, A. (1970). *Amer. J. Obstet. Gynec.*, **107,** 807.
13. *Lancet.* (1974). Editorial "Towards the prevention of spina bifida." **1,** 907.
14. Letchworth, A. T. and Chard, T. (1972). *Lancet.* **1,** 704.
15. Miller, A. W. F., Calder, A. A. and Macnaughton, M. C. (1972). *Lancet*, **2,** 5.
16. Mitchell, R. (1973). Scientific meeting of R.C.O.G. Dundee University, 30th March.
17. Roberts, G., Cassie, R. and Turnbull, A. C. (1971). *J. Obstet. Gynaec. Brit. Cwlth*, **78,** 634.
18. Robinson, H. P., Chatfield, W. R., Logan, R. W. and Hall, F. (1974). *Ann. clin. Biochem.*, **11,** 15.
19. Stein, Z., Susser, M. and Guterman, A. V. (1973). *Lancet*, **1,** 305.
20. Stewart, A. (1968). *Lancet*, **1,** 104.
21. Stewart, A. (1970). *Lancet*, **1,** 923.
22. Brock, D. J. H., Bolton, A. E. and Scrimgeour, J. B. (1974). *Lancet*, **1,** 767.
23. Carr, D. H. (1967). *Amer. J. Obstet. Gynec.*, **97,** 283.
24. Ferguson-Smith, M. A. (1974). *The Practitioner*, **213,** 655.
25. Ferguson-Smith, M. E., Ferguson-Smith, M. A., Nevin, N. C. and Stone, M. (1971). *Brit. med. J.*, **4,** 69.
26. Gitlin, D. and Boesman, M. (1966). *J. Clin. Invest.*, **45,** 1826.
27. Hertig, A. T. and Rock, J. (1949). *Amer. J. Obstet. Gynec.*, **38,** 968.
28. Kaback, M. M., Zaiger, R. S., Reynolds, L. W. and Sonneborn, M. (1973). In: *Proceedings of the Fourth International Conference on Birth Defects, Vienna.* Ed. by A. G. Motulsky and W. Lenz. p. 248. Amsterdam: Excerpta Medica.
29. Littlefield, J. W., Milunsky, A. and Atkins, L. (1973). In: *Proceedings of the Fourth International Conference on Birth Defects, Vienna.* Ed. by A. G. Motulsky and W. Lenz. p. 221. Amsterdam: Excerpta Medica.
30. Barnard, W. P. and Logan, R. W. (1972). *J. Obstet. Gynaec. Brit. Cwlth*, **79,** 1091.
31. Brown, J. B., MacLeod, S. G., Macnaughton, C., Smith, M. A. and Smyth, B. (1968). *J. Endocr.* **42,** 5.
32. Corker, C. S. and Naftolin, F. (1971). *J. Obstet. Gynaec. Brit. Cwlth*, **78,** 330.

33. CORNS, C. M., STEVENS, J. F. and MILLER, A. L. (1973). *Clin. chim. Acta*, **47**, 203.
34. GALLOWAY, R. K. (1970). *J. Obstet. Gynaec. Brit. Cwlth*, **77**, 587.
35. GURPIDE, E., GIEBENHAIN, M. E., TSENG, L. and KELLY, W. G. (1971). *Amer. J. Obstet. Gynec.*, **109**, 897.
36. GARROW, J. S. and DOUGLAS, C. P. (1968). *J. Obstet. Gynaec. Brit. Cwlth*, **75**, 1034.
37. GLUCK, L., KULOVICH, M. V., BORER, R. C., BRENNER, P. H., ANDERSON, G. G. and SPELLACY, W. N. (1971). *Amer. J. Obstet. Gynec.*, **109**, 440.
38. KOBER, S. (1931). *Biochem. Z.*, **239**, 209.
39. LEE, P. and GARROW, J. S. (1970). *J. Obstet. Gynaec. Brit. Cwlth*, **77**, 982.
40. MACVICAR, J., LOGAN, R. W. and BARNARD, W. P. (1973). *Scot. med. J.* **18**, 84.
41. MURPHY, B. E. P. (1968). *Canad. J. Biochem.*, **46**, 288.
42. NACHTIGALL, L., BISSET, M., HOGSANDER, U., SLAGLE, S. and LEVITZ, M. (1966). *J. Clin. Endocr.*, **26**, 941.
43. PRATT, J. J. VAN DER LINDEN, G., DOORENBAS, H. and WOLDRING, M. G. (1974). *Clin. chim. Acta*, **50**, 137.
44. RAHMAN, M. (1974). *Clin. chim. Acta*, **51**, 233.
45. ROBINSON, H. P., CHATFIELD, W. R., LOGAN, R. W., TWEEDIE, A. K. and BARNARD, W. P. (1973). *J. Obstet. Gynaec. Brit. Cwlth*, **80**, 230.
46. SALING, E. (1962). *Arch. Gynäk.*, **197**, 108.
47. SAXENA, B. N., EMERSON, K. and SELENKOW, H. A. (1969). *New Engl. J. Med.*, **281**, 225.
48. SEPPALA, M. and RUOSLAHTI, E. (1972). *Amer. J. Obstet. Gynec.*, **114**, 595.
49. SEPPALA, M. and RUOSLAHTI, E. (1973). *Amer. J. Obstet. Gynec.*, **115**, 48.
50. WARREN, C., ALLEN, J. T. and HOLTON, J. B. (1973). *Clin. chim. Acta*, **44**, 457.
51. ZELTZER, P. M., NEERHOUT, R. C., FONKALSRUD, E. W. and STIEHM, E. R. (1974). *Lancet*, **1**, 373.

CHAPTER IV

SPECIAL CASES

Four special types of case are discussed in this chapter: the elderly primigravida, the grand multipara, the patient with the bad obstetric history and the grossly obese.

THE ELDERLY PRIMIGRAVIDA

There is a general tendency to include in this category all women going through their first pregnancy over the age of 35, but this includes large numbers of women who in no sense deserve to be classed as elderly and who run a perfectly normal obstetrical course. Earlier papers discuss only women over the age of 40.[10, 11] Larger series more recently reported widen the definition to include age of 35 and over.[2]

Considering how common the problem is, it is surprising that the literature is not more replete with information on the subject, and it certainly deserves a review. There is no doubt that the elderly primigravida is somewhat more likely to encounter complications which are the result of the natural process of growing older, but even more important is the fact that her dwindling chances of further pregnancies put more of a premium on the present one. Furthermore, her endurance and her resistance to disease are not those of a woman in her early twenties, and she is therefore likely to require help earlier. A long history of antecedent infertility serves only to magnify this point. Notwithstanding all this, the majority of these patients, properly supervised, are capable of safe and successful pregnancy.

Complications of Pregnancy

A normal woman's fertility is at its maximum at about the age of 23, after which there is a gradual decline, so that by the age of 40 the chances of conception are greatly reduced. Having once conceived the elderly primigravida has a greater predisposition to abort, and the usual precautions as outlined in the chapter on abortion should be advised.

Within the limitations of our knowledge of the aetiology of pre-eclamptic toxaemia, one is hardly surprised at an increased incidence in the more elderly, because increasing age, of itself, favours hypertensive disease and reduces the resilience of the cardiovascular system as a whole.

Hyperemesis gravidarum is somewhat more common, but much

of this can be accounted for by the patient's very natural anxiety. Placental abruption may be favoured by folic acid deficiency, hypertensive disease or both, but increasing age rather than primiparity is likely to be the more dominant cause.

Because a patient is getting older she naturally has more time to develop gynaecological abnormalities, of which fibroids are likely to be the most common. In other respects pregnancy is not specifically complicated, although any general disease has added significance.

Complications of Labour

Premature labour is rather more likely.

The duration of labour tends to be increased by about 25 per cent on average. Much of this is due to the greater anxiety of the older woman facing labour for the first time, and some degree of inertia is common. Posterior positions of the occiput are very much more usual, while the effects are more troublesome, and in about a third of the cases labour is likely to be prolonged because of this malposition. Inertia is also particularly likely to complicate the case which has had labour induced, and the response to induction tends to be so unsatisfactory that one should have very good indications for embarking upon it. It is said that labour may be adversely influenced by the impaired joint mobility which comes with increasing years, but the significance of this is small compared with the functional activity of the uterus and the elasticity of the soft tissues of the birth canal.

Signs of maternal distress in labour, as might be expected, appear more readily in the older woman, so that delivery has to be more often assisted surgically; in fact, only 40 per cent of Miller's cases more than 40 years ago had spontaneous deliveries and 38 per cent required forceps. The Caesarean section rate was increased fourfold. This situation has not changed much in modern times and certainly the forceps will be required about twice or three times as often as in younger women.

The perineum and lower vagina do not stretch so well, so that episiotomy is often indicated and should be unhesitatingly employed.

The inertia of the first and second stages of labour is likely to obtrude into the third stage. Manual removal of the placenta is required more frequently, and the co-existence of fibroids makes this operation more likely.

Barring the direct results of surgical intervention, the puerperium is not abnormal, but breast feeding is only satisfactorily established in a minority.

Maternal and Fetal Mortality

The maternal mortality is only slightly higher, and this is in direct ratio to the appearance and nature of complications already described and the need for operative intervention. Under modern conditions this aspect of the problem has been reduced to very small proportions. The fetal mortality, however, gives no grounds for complacency, although the appalling figure of 26 per cent given by Miller over 40 years ago, the majority dying of intracranial haemorrhage after forceps delivery or breech extraction, has now been radically modified by the more ready use of Caesarean section. Nowadays stillbirths are still more common with increasing maternal age, the rate being about three times as high in primigravidae over 40 years of age as in young women in their teens or early twenties. Prematurity accounts for some of the increased mortality, but it is particularly tragic that in these cases the chances of fetal abnormality are unquestionably increased; moreover, the association of mongolism with elderly primiparity is well known although here, too, age is the more important factor.

Treatment

The elderly primigravida does not require any special surgical treatment on the grounds of age alone, but the need for detailed supervision both in pregnancy and labour is obvious. It is our practice to offer these patients amniocentesis to exclude (or to detect) a chromosome aberration. These patients should, therefore, be seen at more than usually frequent intervals throughout pregnancy and very early note taken of any signs of developing pre-eclamptic toxaemia.

The bony pelvis should be assessed and found to be above reproach before contemplating vaginal delivery, while the combination of malpresentation with elderly primiparity demands Caesarean section as an elective procedure. There is no place for trial of labour in the elderly primigravida. The relative indications for Caesarean section have to be extended, and for this reason an X-ray to exclude fetal abnormality in all these cases is necessary, as such a discovery is likely to modify treatment.

As has been said elsewhere, Caesarean section is no guarantee of live birth, and is not to be employed on grounds of elderly primiparity alone. The frequent unsatisfactory response to induction of labour has been commented upon already and the indications for it should be stringently met. If a patient's condition is bad enough to warrant induction at this age, there is a strong possibility that it warrants Caesarean section instead. The elderly primigravida should not be allowed more than a week's postmaturity at the most and induction, if undertaken, should be followed by Caesarean section within twenty-four hours if it misfires.

One fact needs stressing particularly. These patients are anxious and very unsure of their ability to deliver themselves safely. Sympathetic but firm, confident handling is therefore an essential part of treatment, and the patient should be encouraged to hope for normal delivery, and the attendant should conduct his vigilance without a trace of ceremony.

THE GRAND MULTIPARA

Nowadays grand multiparity is usually defined as applying to cases which have had five or more previous viable babies, although Barns (1953) and Feeney (1953) produced impressive papers restricted to women carrying their eighth pregnancy or over. Barns's cases numbered 306 and Feeney, at the Coombe Lying-in Hospital, in a two-year period, collected the astonishing number of 518 grand multiparae, including two cases, one in her 20th and the other in her 21st pregnancy, out of a total of 4115 deliveries, an incidence of grand multiparity of 12·6 per cent. In reviewing 136,000 deliveries in the Coombe Lying-In Hospital in Dublin over a 41-year period up to 1969, grand multiparae were found to amount to one tenth of the patients but to account for one third of the maternal deaths.[7]

Ever since Solomons in 1934 drew attention to what he called "the dangerous multipara", increasing cognisance has been taken of grand multiparity as a clinical entity in its own right. These patients are liable to a series of dramatic complications, all the more dangerous because they are often unsuspected, and, as will be seen, it is foolhardy to expect a woman who has had a long series of previous uneventful deliveries to maintain her unblemished record indefinitely.

Solomons pointed out that in child bearing, practice does not make perfect and indeed was impressed with the increased maternal mortality associated with grand multiparity. Today the penalty of death has receded, but formidable risks remain of a similar nature as before. The pooled results of several institutions over a short period of time are now available for assessing hazards which no single unit can nowadays supply, because very high degrees of parity are becoming less common. A study of over 5000 grand multiparae has been made through the American Obstetrical Statistical Co-operative,[8] covering women at least para seven and upwards, amounting to 4·3 per cent of all patients delivered in these institutions over a 3-year period. Over 60 per cent of the series was white, a fact which reduced the average age to under 35 in two-thirds. This increases the value of this report as it helps to reduce the adverse factor of age alone. In this series the incidence of anaemia was more than doubled, hypertensive disease, including pre-eclamptic toxaemia superimposed on chronic hypertension had an increased occurrence which could not be gainsaid, haemorrhage of all varieties before, during and after delivery was mainly doubled, uterine rupture trebled and the primary Caesarean section rate because of a wide variety of complications was as great as in less parous women.

Many factors operate to increase the hazards of high parity. For one thing the patient is getting older and her cardiovascular system is consequently less resilient, so that hypertensive disease is more manifest. Other general conditions which are part of the normal process of ageing are liable likewise to intrude themselves upon the clinical picture. Obesity, which is often gross in these cases, increases the dangers of childbearing, as is well known, and not the least reason for this is the difficulty of making an accurate examination.

Sociological factors play a very important part, for the majority of these patients are poor, overworked and tired. Many of them have never fully regained a good blood picture, and anaemia may dog them from one pregnancy to the next without respite. They tend to feed their numerous children at the expense of their own nutrition, so that they are consequently often very short of vitamins and first-class protein. They are too busy to attend to their health, and in a rapid succession of pregnancies and periods of lactation they are likely to become seriously depleted of calcium. It is small wonder, then, that dental fitness is unusual and their mouths are often full of useless and infected stumps.

With increasing weight and lumbar lordosis, the abdominal wall gives up the unequal struggle, and we have, therefore, the picture of a harassed woman who stands badly, walks badly, eats indifferently and cannot get enough sleep.

Complications of Pregnancy

The abortion rate is increased, but it is difficult to say how much of this is spontaneous as, undoubtedly, these women are driven in many cases to seek interference. Anaemia is so common in multiparous pregnancy that it should always be looked for and treated energetically. It is usually of the iron deficiency type but megaloblastic anaemia may supervene very rapidly because folic acid reserves are often low before the next pregnancy even starts. Every effort should be made to see that the patient's haemoglobin is at least 80 per cent before she approaches term. The method of achieving this will depend upon the time at one's disposal, and the choice lies between administering iron by mouth or by injection or, for those in more urgent need, by transfusion of packed cells. The women who faces labour with a haemoglobin of 65 per cent or less does so in real peril, and this matter is dealt with more fully elsewhere.

Hyperemesis is relatively uncommon in multiparous patients, but is far more significant and should always be taken seriously. It is so seldom neurotic that an organic origin must be diligently sought.

Hiatus hernia is more common than generally recognised in multiparae, and may give rise to dramatic symptoms in late pregnancy including haematemesis.

Hypertensive vascular disease comes increasingly into the picture with the patient's higher age group and, if present, necessitates prolonged periods of bed-rest during pregnancy. Termination of pregnancy in the worst cases is fairly widely practised in some centres; although we are of the opinion that with proper hospital supervision this should seldom be necessary. Nevertheless, the fetal prognosis is adversely affected; premature induction of labour is often necessary and these cases should not be allowed to become postmature. Unfortunately it is in just such cases of grand multiparity that the dates are most often in doubt. In spite of the increased incidence of hypertensive disease, pre-eclamptic toxaemia and eclampsia are no more common in grand multiparae, but the effects of eclampsia are more serious, and the mortality is raised because the patient is less well equipped than younger women to contend with them.

To the patient with a cardiac disability, high degrees of multiparity constitute a very definite additional risk. The patient, of course, is older, and therefore cardiac failure more likely. Although pregnancy may be regarded as only an incident in the progressive disease process, its advent may nevertheless be unwelcome.

As might be expected, any of the minor ailments of pregnancy are exaggerated, particularly such conditions as haemorrhoids and varicose veins, which may be very troublesome indeed.

Twin pregnancy is about three times as common in grand multiparity, and this fact can be partly explained by the patient's high degree of fertility. Placenta praevia likewise is more common in direct proportion to the patient's parity, and antepartum haemorrhage may be very sudden and profuse, so that its effects in the likely presence of iron deficiency anaemia are magnified.

Accidental antepartum haemorrhage is largely a complication of multiparity, and in 148 of Solomon's cases at the Rotunda Hospital no less than 130 were multiparous. In grand multiparity placental abruption is far more likely to complicate pre-eclamptic toxaemia or folic acid deficiency. This increases perinatal mortality too.

Malpresentations are very much more common, and are favoured by a pendulous abdomen and lordosis of the lumbar spine, and in any case it is usual for the head not to engage in the pelvis until the onset of labour.

Fortunately, fetal abnormality is no more common in grand multiparity, but *erythroblastosis fetalis* in the Rh iso-immunised case has an enhanced opportunity.

The onset of labour is commonly premature and, for this, associated sociological factors are largely to blame.

Complications in Labour

It is when we come to labour that the grand multipara is capable of exhibiting the greatest treachery. Feeney gave a very revealing list of complications in his 518 cases:

Breech presentation	33
Oblique lie	14
Presentation and prolapse of cord	14
Disproportion	14
Postpartum haemorrhage	71
Rupture of uterus	6
"Obstetric shock"	7
Precipitate labour	2

These observations deserve comment. Malpresentation, as already stated, is favoured by a pendulous abdomen together with the high angle of pelvic inclination resulting from associated lordosis of the spine. Even in cases in which the presentation is normal the head may remain free after the onset of labour, thereby favouring prolapse of the cord if the membranes rupture with a sudden gush of liquor. In many of these cases the lie is unstable, and treatment by external version and abdominal binder is ineffective.

Feeney's finding of no less than 14 cases of disproportion may at first seem surprising, as one is tempted to regard the pelvis of a highly parous patient as beyond question. Nothing could be more dangerous than such a complacent attitude. In the first place babies tend to get larger with successive pregnancies, and may consequently give rise to cephalopelvic disproportion for the first time. Occasionally contracted pelvis can secondarily occur in the adult quite apart from osteomalacia. In grand multiparity two things may reduce pelvic capacity: firstly, the increasing inclination of the pelvic brim already referred to, and, secondly, the occasional subluxation forwards of the sacrum upon the sacro-iliac joints so that the sacral promontory advances and the true conjugate is effectively reduced. Failure to recognise this condition may end in uterine rupture, especially in the presence of tumultuous pains. Pendulous abdomen together with occipitoposterior position of the fetus and undiagnosed brow presentation should always be kept in mind.

Uterine rupture constitutes one of the gravest risks of high parity, and it is important to realise that it may occur after only a short period of labour. Uterine contractions tend to be better coordinated and more forceful in multiparous labour, whereas the strength of the myometrium to resist rupture is by no means increased by successive pregnancies. The presence, moreover, of a larger size of baby than heretofore increases the strain, and the use of oxytocic drugs is more than usually dangerous in this respect. Even the closest supervision may not be able to prevent sudden and catastrophic uterine rupture.

The onset of uterine rupture does not always follow the classical textbook descriptions, and many cases are undoubtedly unrecognised and may be recorded as cases of postpartum haemorrhage or so-called "obstetric shock". A fuller description of uterine rupture is given in another chapter.

Postpartum haemorrhage is another real risk. This is an interesting matter, because the uterus seldom demonstrates an unwillingness to contract, and, in fact, haemorrhage may follow precipitate labour. It is suggested that the essential difference between contraction and retraction operates here, and that only the latter will protect a woman against postpartum haemorrhage. Now, where labour has been rapid, vigorous uterine contractions may cause early partial separation of the placenta, but the whole process has occurred too fast for retraction to catch up, so that bleeding may occur very early in the third stage. Furthermore, full retraction may be hampered by the increased quantities of elastic tissue in the myometrium, which is associated with high parity. Adherent placenta is also more common than in the primigravida. It follows, therefore, that the third stage is not to be lightly regarded, and unexplained bleeding or shock should always rouse a suspicion of spontaneous uterine rupture.

It is hardly surprising that Caesarean section is not infrequently employed in grand multiparity. The complications enumerated above demand it from time to time.

The puerperal morbidity rate is not increased except in so far as major complications may have arisen during labour.

Mortality

Maternal mortality rises appreciably in the higher degrees of parity. Solomons, 40 years ago, considered that the mortality rose progressively with each child after the fifth until by the tenth child the figure was five times the overall rate. In Eastman's series, rupture of the uterus accounted for a quarter of the deaths, chronic hypertensive disease for a fifth and placenta praevia for one-sixth. Parity of such degree is becoming less and less common even in Glasgow, so that it is hard to find comparable figures today.

The fetal mortality shows a somewhat similar curve. The neonatal death rate, however, is less markedly increased, and here the management of prematurity and better sociological conditions should improve the picture.

It goes without saying that in the light of the increased hazards to both mother and child, women who are expecting their fifth child or over must be delivered in hospital. It is agreed that this advice is not likely to be well received in all quarters, particularly by the patients, who are so tied up with their large families that they are unwilling to leave them even in the interests of personal safety. To many of them the advent of another confinement is no more serious apparently than an attack of toothache, but the doctor undertaking these cases should critically review the facilities at his disposal for coping with the occasional and dramatic catastrophe. A compromise is often sought by promising the patient dismissal from hospital within the first 48 hours after delivery. While this is obviously better than flat refusal to come into hospital at all, it should only be reluctantly conceded since these are the women most in need of decent postnatal care such as a modern attractive hospital can give.

THE BAD OBSTETRIC HISTORY

Recurrent *versus* Non-recurrent Factors

It is not uncommon for a particular case to be described as having a "bad obstetric history". The term requires clarifying, because it is often loosely used to signify that a woman has had previous disappointments in childbearing. In many cases there are no more than compassionate aspects as distinct from factors which are obstetrically relevant to the present pregnancy. In other words, the term ought really to be restricted to those patients in whom the obstetrical future is likely to be modified by the nature of the previous disaster. Certain factors may operate recurrently in successive pregnancies or their threat may influence one's management, and these will be considered in this section.

History-taking in obstetrics is every bit as important as in any other branch of medicine, and the fullest information should always be sought about previous deliveries and abortions. The parous woman bears in her history more information than clinical examination is likely to provide.

Any history of stillbirth demands enquiry, if necessary from the patient's previous attendant, as to whether it was a fresh case or macerated, whether labour had followed intra-uterine death or the baby had died in the process of delivery, whether the onset of labour was spontaneous or induced, and if the latter for what reason, the period of gestation, and the nature of any operative intervention. Necropsy details, especially of intracranial haemorrhage and tentorial tearing, are of the greatest importance, likewise the degree of moulding at birth. The weight of the child should be ascertained and the views of the patient's previous attendant obtained as to the cause of death. Likewise, in the case of neonatal death the maturity and weight should be known, the duration of life and the cause of death. A history of fetal deformity is significant and its exact nature should always be determined.

The duration of previous labour should be ascertained. Very prolonged labours and precipitate deliveries are relevant.

The indications for Caesarean section if done in the past are important; for example, if placenta praevia had been the reason, one would be less concerned about vaginal delivery next time, whereas disproportion or a failure of trial of labour makes the need for repeated sectioning more than probable. Above all, the integrity of the uterine scar must be in doubt if there is any history of puerperal sepsis. The standard of obstetrical notekeeping in this country has so greatly improved in recent years that the fullest information can nearly always be obtained on enquiry from sister hospitals, and registrars in answering these letters would do well to summarise all the above facts.

The subject of intra-uterine death always raises the question whether the same factors may not operate again. Where pre-eclamptic toxaemia was associated previously it does not necessarily follow that the patient will suffer a repetition, but the trickiest decisions are in those cases of recurrent intra-uterine death for no apparent cause shortly before term. For these the syndrome of "placental insufficiency" has been postulated. Every now and then one meets such a sequence, and it furnishes a very clear indication not only for a very general investigation but also for securing premature delivery before it is too late. Unfortunately reliable estimates of placental function still elude us. The clinical observation of "small-for-dates baby," namely, poor or absent maternal weight gain,[6] low oestriol excretion rates, vaginal cytological changes and poor growth curves as determined by sonar are all helpful indications but none, except perhaps the last (which is not yet generally available) is absolute.[3, 13, 14, 15]

In any case in which a previous disaster was associated with even so much as a suspicion of disproportion, it is worth while perusing the full notes of that labour and obtaining, if possible, the previous X-rays. It must be remembered that trials of labour fail more often because of uterine inertia than because of the dimensions of the bony pelvis, and the present pregnancy should be very critically considered in the light of this information before deciding as a matter of course that elective Caesarean section will be necessary.

A history of third-stage accidents is always relevant, and adherent placenta particularly tends to be recurrent. It is now general practice to recommend specialised hospital confinement in the case of any woman who has had a manual removal of the placenta or a postpartum haemorrhage in any previous labour.

Postmaturity is significant in obstetric history. In many patients it recurs apparently as a natural phenomenon. The size of the babies and the nature of any dystocia will indicate whether the patient can be safely allowed to overrun her dates this time.

The incidence of fetal abnormality climbs steeply with each instance. After one monster the chances next time are about six or eight times as great, and after two such consecutive disasters the chances of a third are in the region of 60 or 70 per cent. Any previous history, therefore, of fetal abnormality indicates the need for the taking of a straight X-ray. It is certain that the patient herself, who very naturally fears a repetition, deserves this reassurance.

The previous appearance of pre-eclamptic toxaemia or any hypertensive disorder indicates a closer supervision in this pregnancy. In respect of recurrence it will often appear that the case who has had full-blown eclampsia is in less danger than one who has had a long low-grade pre-eclampsia which has niggled on for many weeks.

Nephritis is an uncommon complication of pregnancy, but a past history is highly significant, and where there is doubt that this disease is still operative it is worth admitting the patient to hospital early in pregnancy for thorough assessment. Urological disorders are always noteworthy in the history. The more common types of urinary infection due to *E. coli* have a marked tendency to recur in the course of subsequent pregnancies, especially if the infection was not previously fully eradicated. More significant still is a history of genito-urinary tuberculosis. This is a matter which is dealt with more fully in the section on abnormalities of the urinary tract.

Previous injuries to the bladder, particularly vesicovaginal fistula of obstetrical origin, which have been successfully treated, demand Caesarean section rather than the risk of repeating this calamity, and a history of stress incontinence which has been successfully operated upon in most cases contra-indicates the local stresses of a subsequent vaginal delivery. Where, however, colporrhaphy has been performed for prolapse rather than for stress incontinence, the rules are less rigid, and the decision will depend largely upon one's assessment at term of the available capacity of the vaginal vault. This is often more important than the fact of previous amputation of the cervix.

Histories of third-degree tears and damage to the rectum are a sure indication for generous episiotomy as soon as the head gets anywhere near the pelvic floor. To allow the scar of a previous repair of this nature to give way would be wanton indeed, and on the second occasion one might be less lucky in curing the patient of the very terrible disability of rectal incontinence.

The fullest details should always be obtained of previous pregnancies and labours in cardiac cases. This will provide additional warning of the patient's liability to decompensate, and will to some extent determine the need for hospitalisation during the pregnancy.

The question of rhesus iso-immunisation is dealt with elsewhere. The likelihood of the present fetus being affected will be made almost cetain if, on genotyping, the patient's husband is found to be homozygous. Nevertheless, the severity of the disease in previous babies does not necessarily indicate a hopeless outlook for the future, and the possibilities of salvage have so greatly increased within recent years that sterilisation has ceased to feature as treatment in the worst affected cases.

Maternal syphilis as a cause of recurrent stillbirth hardly needs stressing these days when any doctor who omits a Wassermann reaction in pregnancy, whatever the social status of his patient, is almost guilty of culpable negligence. There can now be little excuse for this sort of disaster.

Lastly, a history of puerperal insanity raises a very difficult issue. The fear that this hideous complication of childbirth may recur is one that may well justify the termination of pregnancy, but the decision is essentially one for the expert psychiatrist. As a general rule psychiatric grounds for terminating pregnancy would be better met by admitting the patient to a mental institution and treating her illness or preventing her suicide rather than taking the illogical step of destroying her pregnancy.

The above short list shows that there is much to reckon with in good history-taking in obstetrics, and in a busy antenatal clinic it is so often below standard that some vital and relevant detail is often missed. The practice of entrusting this task to nurses who are not fully aware of the significance of all these points, and who therefore omit to make specific enquiry, is to be deplored, and it is not difficult as a rule to catch out one's house surgeon on such points as these. It might also be added as a point of minor importance that candidates in examinations often make a very bad showing on this aspect of their presentation of a clinical case, and may reveal a lack of experience by their emphasis on a host of irrelevant details at the expense of a proper assessment of the facts which really matter. This may count far more than the correct elicitation of physical signs.

GROSS OBESITY

If there is one thing that a woman dislikes more than fatness it is the means by which it can be controlled. Pregnancy provides a moratorium and a vigorous policy of weight reduction is likely to be suspended for the time being. It is the purpose of this section to review the possible effects of obesity on pregnancy and vice versa. Starting with the latter it is unlikely that pregnancy will make a fat woman thin unless something is very radically wrong such as uncontrolled hyperemesis or extreme malnutrition. A weight gain of up to 10 kg can be regarded as physiological in any pregnancy. Much of this can be accounted for by the weight of the fetus and placenta, liquor amnii, uterine mass, breast hypertrophy and physiological hydraemia. The remainder is made up mostly of water and to a lesser extent of fat. Theoretically most of this is got rid of by delivery and the diuresis which follows it.

Pregnancy *per se* is therefore not fattening, except temporarily, yet there are many women who fail to regain their figures after it is all over. It is claimed, however, that they have largely failed to regain their original eating habits. This is altogether understandable since the harassments of a new baby in the house, the "weariness, the fever and the fret" (Keats)[9] may undermine resolve or interest in herself for the time being. What is likely to follow in the ensuing years of multiparous child-rearing is a degradation in feeding standards for the mother with regard to protein because carbohydrates are so much cheaper and so much less trouble to prepare for the table. The role which child bearing and rearing has upon developing obesity therefore operates only indirectly by altering the circumstances and outlook of a considerable proportion of women.

The effects of obesity on the course and outcome of pregnancy may now be reviewed. The problem is such a common one that it is surprising that more has not been written about it since obstetricians do not regard it favourably. From the patient's own point of view pregnancy is likely to be a far more uncomfortable business than for a thinner woman and skin disorders, especially of the intertriginous variety, may be more troublesome. Oedema of the lower extremities is exaggerated which still further reduces comfortable mobility.

Dyspnoea on exertion or secondary to bronchitis has often more than nuisance value and the subjective effects of anaemia are magnified. But the most striking complicating factor in obese pregnancy is hypertension, both essential, so-called, and that due to superimposed pre-eclamptic toxaemia.

It is doubtful if obesity *per se* causes a high blood pressure but hypertension, overt or latent, is commonly associated with the obese type. To understand this association one would have to review the causes of obesity itself but apart from certain endocrine disorders such as pre-diabetes and pituitary dyscrasias which, in themselves, to some extent limit fertility, there is no doubt that to many otherwise healthy women obesity is a psychosomatic response to stress in life, as is hypertension too. The woman who finds little enough comfort in her husband may console herself with compulsive eating. This is what we call "eating for comfort". True, she will deny that she ever eats a proper meal, and the more the pity, but she does not admit to the constant nibbling throughout the day from her larder and kitchen shelves with an overwhelming taste for carbohydrates. The association between hypertension and obesity may therefore be based upon a common psychological background. To these people dietary restrictions are more in the nature of a spiritual exercise demanding default than a practical proposition.

In the series recorded by Emerson (1962) no less than one in five patients was overweight, yet the incidence of hypertension of 140/90 mm Hg and above at the beginning of pregnancy was seven times as high as in women of normal build. Likewise, pre-eclamptic toxaemia supervened more than four times as commonly. A further corollary is the markedly increased incidence of antepartum haemorrhage, especially the toxaemic accidental variety.

Malpresentation is, as might be expected, not only harder to detect but also harder to correct by external version and there is a greater need for antepartum radiology or sonar to exclude this and twins as well.

Labour is no better favoured by obesity. The need for surgical induction is commoner because of hypertension, pre-eclamptic toxaemia or postmaturity and labour is often tryingly inert and incoordinate. The babies are often much larger than clinical examination would lead one to expect and minor degrees of disproportion may only declare themselves by unsatisfactory labour. The need for operative delivery both by forceps and Caesarean section is about doubled (Emerson) and in the case of the latter, the fatness of the abdominal wall may discourage healing by first intention and postoperative chest complications may not only be troublesome of themselves, but, because of poor ventilation, may encourage venous stasis and thrombosis.

Postpartum haemorrhage is also more common (more than four times in Emerson's series) and veins are less accessible for transfusion. Lastly, obese women do not lactate as well as their thinner sisters. The babies of these patients have a higher perinatal mortality partly because of maternal hypertension and partly because of more difficult delivery.

For these reasons major degrees of obesity contribute an indication for hospital confinement. Increased vigilance for pre-eclamptic toxaemia is necessary and anaemia should be watched for at an early stage.

Appetite-killing drugs and tranquillisers are not recommended but a high-protein and fat and low-carbohydrate diet should be resolutely encouraged, preferably with the expert help of a dietitian. Diuretics and salt restriction are relatively useless and only make the patient more miserable than she need be.

At the first and most minor signs of supervening pre-eclamptic toxaemia the patient should be admitted to hospital, not forgetting that thin eclamptics are much easier to nurse and pull through than fat ones.

The traditional idea that fatness and jollity are associated is certainly not true in pregnancy and these women need sympathy and help not only to forestall the complications which they face but to rehabilitate their morale and self-respect.

REFERENCES

1. Barns, T. (1953). *Edinb. med. J.*, **60,** 28.
2. Booth, R. T. and Williams, G. L. (1964). *J. Obstet. Gynaec. Brit. Cwlth*, **71,** 249.
3. Donald, I. and Brown, T. G. (1961). *Brit. J. Radiol.*, **34,** 539.
4. Eastman, N. J. (1949). *N.Y. St. J. Med.*, **40,** 1708.
5. Emerson, E. G. (1962). *Brit. med. J.*, **2,** 516.
6. Feeney, J. K. (1953). *J. Irish med. Ass.*, **32,** 36.
7. Feeney, J. K. and Greene, A. T. (1970). *Brit. J. hosp, Med.*, **4,** 371.
8. Israel, L. S. and Blazar, A. J. (1965). *Amer. J. Obstet. Gynec.*, **91,** 326.
9. Keats, J. *Ode to a Nightingale.*
10. Miller, D. (1931/2). *Trans. Edinb. obstet. Soc.*, **52,** 161.
11. Nixon, W. C. W. (1931). *J. Obstet. Gynaec. Brit. Emp.*, **38,** 821.
12. Solomons, B. (1934). *Lancet*, **2,** 8.
13. Thompson, H. E., Holmes, J. H., Gottesfeld, K. A. and Taylor, E. S. (1965). *Amer. J. Obstet. Gynec.*, **92,** 44.
14. Willocks, J., Donald, I., Campbell, S. and Dunsmore, I. R. (1967). *J. Obstet. Gynaec. Brit. Cwlth*, **74,** 639.
15. Willocks, J., Donald, I., Duggan, T. C. and Day, N. (1964). *J. Obstet. Gynaec. Brit. Cwlth*, **71,** 11.

CHAPTER V

THE CARDIAC CASE

In the eyes of the physician, pregnancy comes as a temporary complication in the disease process of the patient's cardiac lesion, a process which, in any case, is likely to shorten life. The question at issue is how to prevent, as far as possible, the additional burden of the pregnant state from accelerating the rate of the patient's decline.

Fortunately, under good supervision, provided that the extra demands of pregnancy are satisfactorily met at the time, it should generally be possible for the patient to emerge from the experience of childbirth without any degradation in her cardiac condition, and this should be the obstetrician's aim. Any complication, however, is likely to increase cardiac strain, quite apart from that of delivery, and in this subject particularly prevention is better than cure.

As a cause of maternal mortality a relatively greater part is now taken by cardiac disease, but this is only one side of the picture. Postpartum invalidism is almost as important.[5]

Incidence of Cardiac Diseases in Pregnancy

This varies from centre to centre and depends largely upon the degree to which minor cardiac lesions are sought out and registered and also upon the subjective interpretation on the part of the doctor of the minor types of symptoms and signs which may appear at antenatal examination. MacRae, reviewing a total attendance of 29,713 patients at Queen Charlotte's Hospital, recorded the incidence as 0·8 per cent (225 cases). Of these, 13 had congenital lesions, nowadays commoner because of increased survival, and in the remainder a definite history of rheumatic disease was obtained in 91·1 per cent. In a more recent series of 500 cases in Glasgow in the years 1949–59 quoted by Sutherland and Bruce (1962) the incidence works out at 3·2 per cent of all pregnancies attending their unit. In more than a quarter of these cases no relevant rheumatic history was obtained.

With the progressive rise in social standards in Western communities the traditional preponderance of rheumatic heart disease is becoming progressively less, whereas congenital heart disease is as common as ever or more so. Barnes, reviewing a large series in the years 1968–71 at Queen Charlotte's and Hillingdon Hospitals, noted a fall in rheumatic heart disease in pregnancy to a quarter of the level which had been observed 20 years before. The position now is that rheumatic heart disease represents about 70 per cent of all cardiac problems instead of the traditional 90 per cent. Although the full-blown clinical picture of acute rheumatic fever in childhood is far less commonly seen nowadays, the milder clinical forms of rheumatic fever, which often go unrecognised in children, are just as capable as ever of damaging both the heart valves and the myocardium. It would appear that the response in the form of rheumatic carditis to streptococcal infections in childhood is a family defect and all patients, pregnant or not, who have a significant family history should be very carefully scrutinised from this point of view. The diagnosis of mitral stenosis was missed repeatedly in my own case, for example, until incipient failure and atrial fibrillation brought the matter to a head and it now appears that three generations of my own family have not escaped. The point to be made is that family history of rheumatic heart disease is even more commonly significant than a history of rheumatic fever or chorea in the patient herself.

Types of Cardiac Lesions

Of all forms of rheumatic heart disease mitral stenosis is easily the commonest and accounts for more than three-quarters of all cases. When combined with other types of valvular lesion the figure for mitral stenosis is even higher, and Barry[2] found it to be present in 247 out of his 266 cases. Aortic incompetence by itself is much less common and accounts for less than 10 per cent of the cases. Isolated aortic lesions are not in themselves worse than mitral lesions, and the nature of the valvular damage matters very much less than the state of the myocardium.

It is not surprising that rheumatic heart disease should form the main bulk of cases, considering the age of the patient and the point along the disease process at which the patient is likely to be fertile.

The four phases of rheumatic heart disease are as follows:

1. An initial infection manifested by carditis, polyarthritis, chorea or muscle and joint pains of varying degree, often overlooked.
2. Recrudescences, single or multiple, which, following on a haemolytic streptococcal infection, resemble the primary episode.
3. A latent or inactive phase lasting from puberty until the fourth of fifth decade.
4. The stage of diminishing cardiac reserve leading progressively to congestive failure and death.

It will be seen, therefore, that a patient is most likely to be pregnant during the third phase.

Other types of heart disease are found less often in pregnancy because of the factor of age incidence. Until recent years many cases of congenital heart disease, for example, did not live long enough or were not in sufficient health to marry and become pregnant, while hypertensive heart disease and syphilitic heart disease tend to belong to a later period of life.

Cardiomyopathy is increasingly recognised by physicians, and Conradsson and Werkö have noted it particularly amongst black women where it may present as cardiac failure in the last month of pregnancy or postpartum. The heart muscle is described at necropsy as soft with dilatation of all chambers. There is degeneration and hypertrophy of heart muscle to which mural thrombi may be adherent. This is a difficult diagnosis during life and from what I myself have observed it is aided by cardio-ultrasonography. In it the cardiogram is usually not characteristic. Left ventricular outflow obstruction is a common feature, likewise embolism. The ultimate prognosis is said to be worsened by pregnancy, especially in cases where there is permanent cardiac enlargement.

Atrial flutter and paroxysmal tachycardia are functional disorders which fortunately do not increase the risks of childbearing, but Barnes has pointed out that ectopic beats though common and not significant in pregnancy may, if mitral stenosis is present, presage the onset of atrial fibrillation.

Many cases only come to light as a result of antenatal examination, and Morgan Jones reported that approximately 40 per cent of patients with cardiac lesions were symptom-free before their pregnancies.

Physiology

While it should be one's endeavour to ensure that a patient's heart is no worse after pregnancy than it was before, there is no doubt that childbearing in no way confers any beneficial effect whatsoever upon a damaged heart. It would be as well, therefore, to review the nature of the additional temporary burden.

The circulatory strain is unpredictable, and during the long period over which it operates adjustment has to be made to certain basic physiological changes. Firstly, the heart has to deal with an increase in the volume of circulating blood. This increase is progressive, although it rises more steeply during the second half of pregnancy, and it is only reduced during the early part of the puerperium. The circulation of the enlarging and highly vascular uterus and placental site accounts only for some of this increase, and much of it is due to the fluid retention of pregnancy resulting in a hydraemic plethora. Plasma volume may increase by over 40 per cent but red cell volume only to half that extent, resulting therefore in haemodilution. Cardiac output is nowadays reckoned to increase by about 30 to 40 per cent but much of this increase occurs in early pregnancy and continues thereafter certainly up to the 28th week of pregnancy, although there may be some fall in the last eight weeks. Some of this may be due to supine inferior vena caval occlusion by the large uterus. The change in cardiac output in pregnancy is mainly achieved by an increase in stroke volume. The pregnant uterus acts rather like, an arteriovenous fistula which helps to reduce peripheral resistance. In labour, however, uterine contractions squeeze more blood into the circulation and raise the central venous pressure and increase the venous return with a rise in stroke volume as a result. Cardiac output however rapidly falls to non-pregnant levels during the puerperium.[22]

There is a considerable increase in body weight which inevitably means more work for the heart. This increase is due chiefly to water retention, but is caused also by the weight of the fetus, liquor and the enlarged uterus, and some increase in fat deposition is usual. Furthermore, the metabolic rate is increased out of proportion to the weight increase.

In the next place the heart, in the latter half of pregnancy, has to operate against certain mechanical disadvantages due to the enlarging uterus. This causes displacement and rotation of the heart and, to some extent, splints the diaphragm. Respiration is embarrassed and, as a result, the venous return is slowed down to the detriment of the heart's activity. In spite of the splinting of the diaphragm, however, the vital capacity is not decreased, because some compensation is provided by the increase in the diameter of the thoracic cage.

The above mechanical factors are probably the least important of all, because the changes so far recorded in cardiac activity appear at an earlier stage of pregnancy than could be accounted for by the factor of mechanical displacement by the uterus.

From a study of post-mortem material and from X-ray measurements of the heart in pregnancy it does not appear that the heart normally hypertrophies or dilates in any approximate ratio to the amount of work now demanded of it, and the question of existing cardiac reserve, therefore, is all-important (*cf.* Fig. 1).

The extra work which the heart has to do is partly compensated for by a lowering of blood viscosity, which reaches its lowest level between the 33rd and the 36th week.[13] There is also some reduction in the rate of blood flow as measured by such tests as the fluorescin method (arm to eye), while, in the lower part of the body, it is well known that the circulation is more stagnant. Pulse-rate changes are

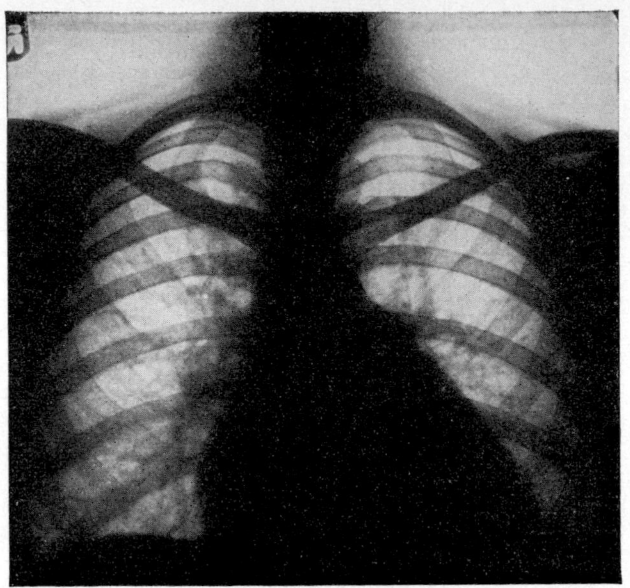

5/FIG. 1 (*a*).—Mitral stenosis and aortic incompetence at 36 weeks' gestation. Shows cardiac enlargement in the transverse diameter.

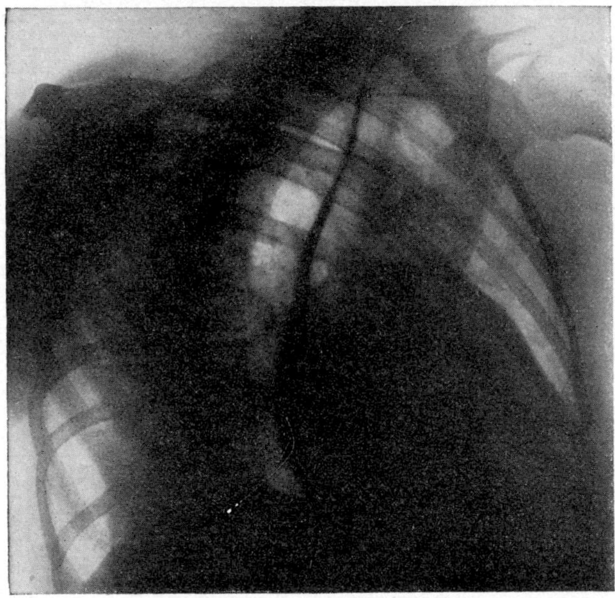

5/FIG. 1 (*b*).—Oblique view shows left atrium mainly involved. The pulmonary arteries are slightly prominent and so are the main pulmonary vessels.

not remarkable during pregnancy, although there is a slight tendency to quickening at the time of maximum cardiac output. The blood pressure alters only slightly, a small drop being characteristic during the middle of pregnancy.

In other words, in spite of some compensating factors, pregnancy inevitably involves the heart in increased effort. Most observers now agree that the main rise in cardiac output occurs during the first trimester and Kerr[16] has revised previously accepted figures by studying cardiac output by catheterisation techniques using the lateral recumbent position, as a result of which he reports cardiac output figures as averaging 6·1 litres per minute in the first trimester, 6·1 l/min in the second and 6·26 l/min in the 3rd trimester, and consequently disputes the previously accepted fall alleged to occur towards term. Using a femoral/inferior vena cava catheter at and during Caesarean section he demonstrated the adverse effect of the supine position upon venous return to the heart and the consequent lowering of cardiac output. This observation has led most of us to the practice of tilting the operating table in the left lateral direction to 15° during induction of the anaesthetic and at least until after the uterine contents have been emptied.[16, 17]

Using a dye-dilution technique, cardiac output has been estimated at Hammersmith in 30 women at monthly intervals during pregnancy and the puerperium,[33] a massive work involving the recording and calculation of over 1300 dye-dilution curves. This team has concluded that although cardiac output is increased in the first trimester, the maximum level is only reached between the 24th and 32nd week of pregnancy, thereafter declining to approach non-pregnant levels at term, with a further fall after delivery. As there is little increase in pulse rate, the increase in cardiac output is due to an increase in stroke volume. These findings are in agreement with what has been standard teaching for years.

The arguments as to methodology may continue but meantime most present-day clinicians treat their patients in the belief that there is an early increase in cardiac output, that the strain is worst by about the 32nd week, if not earlier, and that barring complications such as infections of all types, particularly respiratory, embolic phenomena and obstetrical complications in late pregnancy, the patient can look forward to some shedding of her cardiac load towards the end of pregnancy. Therefore, if the cardiac state is carefully assessed between the 28th and the 32nd week, one is in a position, barring complications, to make a reasonable estimate of how the heart will behave during labour.

The onset of pre-eclamptic toxaemia puts an additional load upon the heart, although this is not so in a patient suffering from essential hypertension. If, by some mischance, intra-uterine death of the fetus should occur, the heart is automatically relieved of some of its burden, even though the fetus is retained *in utero*.

To sum up, as far as cardiac function is concerned, a pregnant woman at rest is in a position similar to a non-pregnant woman doing moderate work.

THE RISKS OF PREGNANCY WITH HEART DISEASE

In recent years there has been a great reduction in mortality. This is not due to any revolutionary change in treatment but to the increased care with which these cases are supervised. Antibiotics, too, have played their part. Nevertheless under present conditions the patient with heart disease is at five times the risk of the normal patient.

What is particularly striking is the enormous difference in the mortality rate between the unbooked and the antenatally supervised cases, the mortality of the former being at least three times as high. Atrial fibrillation complicating pregnancy still has a very high mortality, and Morgan Jones[24] reported that 35 out of 85 such cases died. More recent figures given by Szekely and Snaith[32] in Newcastle upon Tyne still demonstrate the gravity of atrial fibrillation. In their cases the incidence of frank heart failure developing during pregnancy or shortly thereafter rose from 25 per cent in cases fibrillating before their pregnancy began to over 70 per cent in those who developed their fibrillation during pregnancy or the puerperium.

Because of the considerable risk of embolism occurring shortly after its onset, atrial fibrillation should be treated as a medical emergency. As a means of restoring sinus rhythm quinidine is now regarded as a very dangerous drug, and 2000-volt cardioversion is the favoured treatment by physicians. This involves a high-voltage shock applied externally to the chest wall using direct current, the shock being triggered by the QRS complex of the electrocardiogram. The effects are by no means permanent. Undoubtedly the most immediate hazard associated with attempts to restore sinus rhythm is that of cerebral embolism, and long-term anticoagulant therapy is the only means of protection. The patient should, of course, be adequately digitalised to prevent an uncontrollable tachycardia due to fibrillation which may precipitate her into cardiac failure.

Mitral stenosis and Eisenmenger's syndrome both produce pulmonary hypertension and have a higher mortality.[6] Deaths are often due to acute pulmonary oedema, although right-sided heart failure is the chief cause of death in non-pregnant cases. Mitral stenosis, by far the commonest lesion, greatly raises the pulmonary venous pressure which tends to localise the oedema to the lungs; in fact, plumonary oedema occurs as the commonest and most dramatic form of disaster, and may present as an acute emergency. Any cause of tachycardia, ranging from paroxysmal tachycardia to emotional or infective types of accelerated cardiac output, can precipitate acute pulmonary oedema by piling up blood behind the mitral valve.

During pregnancy itself the onset of an attack of acute rheumatism is a very serious risk and, superimposed upon a damaged heart, is far more likely to cause death than myocardial stress due to the presence of the valve lesion. Death may rapidly follow delivery in cases of active rheumatic carditis, and clinically the patient behaves as though in a state of acute obstetric shock.

A freshly superimposed endocarditis is a very real risk, and is to be suspected when a patient shows tachycardia at rest, dyspnoea, fever, oedema, anaemia and occasionally proteinuria. Subacute bacterial endocarditis occurs in about 1 per cent of cases, and apart from a persistent pyrexia and anaemia, splenic enlargement may be demonstrated and embolic phenomena may occur. Blood culture may be positive but may require repeated testing to detect it. In fatal cases fresh, very mushy vegetations may be found on the heart valves.

The danger of pulmonary embolism is somewhat increased, particularly if there has been interference such as Caesarean section.

It is interesting to note that death during the last eight weeks of pregnancy is uncommon. This is the period during which the load upon the heart is lightening. Death, too, during labour itself is uncommon, but it may occur suddenly during the next 24 hours or first few days of the puerperium. I often preach "the rule of fives" by which I mean that death may occur within 5 minutes, 5 hours, 5 days, 5 weeks or 5 months of delivery.

Causes of Death

Two-thirds of the deaths occur after delivery, and congestive cardiac failure and acute pulmonary oedema accounted for three-quarters of all cases in Haig and Gilchrist's series. Slightly more than half were found to have died within the first 24 hours after delivery and about one-third died within the next 4 days. Fortunately nowadays no single unit gets enough cases to produce more up-to-date statistics.

Bacterial endocarditis accounted for 15 per cent and peritonitis following Caesarean section for 4 per cent. Of the remaining 7 per cent, one case was attributable to acute rheumatic fever, another to an anaesthetic accident during the repair of a perineal laceration, and one to a mismatched blood transfusion. In cases dying a few days after delivery, more often than not fresh vegetations can be found upon the heart valves.

The mortality of acute pulmonary oedema in pregnancy is ten times as high according to Gilchrist (1962) as in cases of congestive cardiac failure. This complications cannot be foreseen by studies of exercise tolerance nor from the history, but a small heart with pulmonary hypertension and a tight mitral stenosis is the most dangerous in this respect.

Pulmonary Congestion and Acute Pulmonary Oedema

Right-sided heart failure usually comes on gradually and responds well to treatment in pregnancy, but acute pulmonary oedema is of rapid onset and is far more dramatically dangerous. It is particularly liable to occur suddenly a few hours or minutes after delivery, and is thought to be due to an overloading of the circulation with blood which would normally have been diverted through the placental site.

During pregnancy the signs of failure are often not to be found in engorgement of the neck veins, nor in ankle oedema of cardiac origin, but are demonstrated by increasing pulmonary congestion with attacks of paroxysmal dyspnoea. This last symptom usually accompanies acute exacerbations of pulmonary congestion. It is important therefore to watch the lung bases closely for evidences of pulmonary congestion, for this gives an index of the liability of the patient to develop acute pulmonary oedema which can be rapidly fatal. If moist sounds at the lung bases persist after coughing or deep breathing, they signify pulmonary congestion, confirmed by a typical "hilar moustache" on screening. This radiological appearance is due to increased pulmonary vascular markings. The following are the signs of increasing pulmonary congestion:

1. Dyspnoea. In severe cases paroxysmal attacks develop.
2. Persistent moist sounds at the lung bases.
3. Radiological signs of vascular congestion, especially in the hilar regions. Repeated screening of the chest for signs of early hilar congestion provides a good warning of failure (Fig. 2).
4. Haemoptysis. This is usually a very serious sign.
5. A diminution in the vital capacity.

The onset of acute pulmonary oedema can be precipitated not only by an upper respiratory infection, which is perhaps the commonest mechanism in the antenatal period, but also by anything which increases the output of the heart, particularly the right ventricle, above the level at which the mitral valve can accept and pass the volume of blood returning from the lungs. If this level is exceeded, pulmonary congestion and then pulmonary oedema rapidly build up due to back-pressure. Because the mitral valve cannot cope with greater volumes, it is imperative to reduce the right ventricular output to the pulmonary vascular bed in such cases, before the overloading becomes

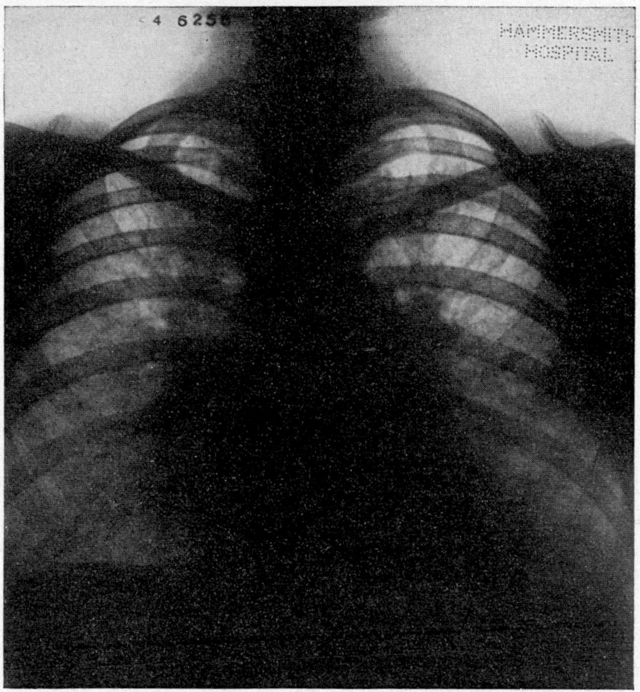

5/FIG. 2.—X-ray showing cardiac enlargement. Well-marked congestive changes showing incipient pulmonary oedema. Calcareous left hilar gland and calcareous focus in left mid-zone. Mitral stenosis.

irreversible and the capillaries have been rendered permeable by anoxia.

This kind of heart attack can, therefore, be precipitated by excitement or exertion or any other major cause of tachycardia in cases of "button-hole" mitral stenosis. Furthermore, tachycardia does not allow sufficient time for left ventricular filling. This mechanism is, in effect, not so very different from that which may obtain in the third stage of labour with the sudden shut-down of the uterine arteriovenous anastomosis although, in this case, a resultant increase in peripheral resistance has to be faced as well.

When acute pulmonary oedema occurs in the first half of pregnancy for no apparent reason apart from the known existence of mitral stenosis it is as well to consider coitus, in the usual dorsal position for the woman, as a possible cause. In a recent case of mine who twice had to be admitted for acute pulmonary oedema, and who for that reason was being considered for valvotomy, the true reason, as above, came to light and is obvious enough if one thinks of it. The use of the lateral position for coitus removes this hazard and in this case, after suitable advice, no further attacks occurred and she completed her pregnancy without mishap and without the need for valvotomy.

Acute pulmonary oedema may also be triggered off by an initial small pulmonary embolus, and I have seen such a case who greeted me normally one morning but who, a few minutes later and before I had completed my round, was in desperate straits with lungs rapidly becoming more oedematous every minute. She was dangerously ill for many days thereafter but recovered in time to deliver herself several weeks later. It is believed that a pulmonary embolus started the emergency.

Treatment of Acute Pulmonary Oedema

Minutes often count. The patient should be propped up at once and morphine 15 mg injected intravenously. Oxygen should be given, and in severe cases no time should be lost in carrying out venesection which can be dramatically life-saving if performed early enough and in time to relieve the overburdened pulmonary circulation. About 500–600 ml of blood should be let off as quickly as possible. This treatment requires courage and also the certainty that the patient's collapse, especially in labour, is not due to other causes; nor can it be employed in the presence of severe anaemia. Hanging the legs down over the edge of the bed and before the application of venous tourniquets may suffice for the less desperate cases. Until recently it was recommended that digoxin in large dosage of up to 1·5 mg should be injected intravenously and repeated, 0·5 mg six-hourly, until the patient was well digitalised, but a note of warning is necessary here. In so far as the condition may be entirely due to a button-hole mitral valve, such treatment could aggravate matters by increasing right ventricular output beyond the mitral valve's capacity, actually intensifying dyspnoea and pulmonary oedema.[19] In other cases, such as in "hypodynamic" ventricular states, digoxin may produce benefit since an improved left ventricular performance may reduce the right ventricular load provided the mitral valve is adequate to handle the volume.

The extent, therefore, to which digoxin may be prescribed is not easy to determine in any given case without the maximum foreknowledge of the cardiac pathology which is often lacking and we are now more cautious in the use of this powerful drug, being guided mainly by the degree of tachycardia and the need to control it.

These cases are often complicated by bronchospasm which aggravates their dyspnoea, and intravenous aminophylline (250 mg) may be of great help. We have also used amyl nitrite inhalations with short-lived but definite benefit.

As a temporary emergency measure, tourniquets can be applied to the limbs sufficiently tight to occlude venous return and therefore reduce the output of the right heart. This constitutes, in effect, a type of venesection without costing the patient blood which, perhaps through trauma for example, she may none too readily afford. Antibiotic cover with penicillin is also advisable.

These are among the most worrying cases to be encountered in modern obstetrics and in no instance is the patient likely to be out of acute danger for many hours, usually three or four days at least, so that one is often left wondering what next to do. By now an oxygen tent will have been set up and it is important to secure adequate rest with sedatives, to maintain digitalisation as long as persisting tachycardia indicates it and to promote diuresis with frusemide (Lasix) 40–80 mg which, by mouth, begins to be effective within two hours. Above all, respiratory tract infection is to be feared and we have, in this instance, a very valid indication for prophylactic penicillin therapy.

Differential Diagnosis and Assessment

It is easy to be mistaken, since even a healthy woman in pregnancy often produces symptoms and signs which are simply due to the physiological adjustments which the heart has to undertake to meet the new circulatory demands. The earlier in pregnancy that the diagnosis can be made the more likely is it to be accurate. Early diagnosis also makes for safe delivery. If one cannot be certain of the presence of a cardiac lesion in early pregnancy it is unlikely that the diagnosis will become any easier later on, because murmurs may become masked, and a rising diaphragm later confuses the clinical picture and assessment. Foreknowledge of the cardiac condition will enable one to decide whether later signs are due to cardiac disability or to exaggeration of the normal physiological changes of late pregnancy, and without it the assessment of right-sided heart failure becomes increasingly difficult as pregnancy advances.

A family history of rheumatic fever is very important. It is now recognised that this is a disease with a certain hereditary predisposition. I feel strongly about this because it has gone through three generations of my own family (predominantly redheads too) and in my own generation has affected three out of four siblings. Nowadays permanent cardiac damage can be prevented by daily prophylaxis with oral penicillin (125 mg twice a day). It stops the ravages of yet another streptococcal infection in a patient already sensitised. The initial sensitising infection is caused by the Group A beta haemolytic streptococcus and it is believed that it is subsequent infections which do the cardiac damage. Therefore infection is only one side of the aetiology, the patient's own sensitivity response being even more important. In deciding whether or not a patient has had rheumatic fever, and is therefore at risk, account has to be taken of certain diagnostic criteria, such as carditis producing murmurs at the time of the infection, cardiac enlargement, pericarditis and occasionally congestive cardiac failure. An arthritis flitting from joint to joint is almost diagnostic, likewise a true history of chorea. Subcutaneous nodules felt particularly over the extensor surfaces of elbows, knees or wrists and in the occipital region, or spinous processes of the vertebrae may have been noted. Less conclusive criteria of rheumatic fever are painful joints without objective findings of tenderness or limitation of movement, a prolonged P-R interval in electrocardiogram, an increased erythrocyte sedimentation rate or unexplained leucocytosis. The child so affected may have loss of weight and fatigue easily, is liable to an elevated sleeping pulse rate, sweating, pallor, anaemia and general malaise. Unfortunately only in the few instances where a doctor has known his patient for many years is the diagnosis of past rheumatic fever easy to establish. Furthermore the severity of the original infection bears no relationship to the extent of subsequent cardiac damage. The important thing is to recognise the cases at risk as indicated by such a history, including the family history, and never to forget that a rheumatic cardiac lesion may become apparent for the first time after an obstetrical catastrophe and not before it.

The signs of mitral stenosis in early pregnancy often alter as pregnancy advances and, moreover, mitral stenosis may be wrongly diagnosed because a physiological third sound in diastole may mimic a presystolic murmur. The first sound may also be split and produce the same impression. Towards the end of pregnancy the pulmonary second sound is often increased without any cardiac pathology, and apical systolic murmurs of no significance are common.

Breathlessness on exertion and oedema of the ankles are so common in normal pregnancy, occurring in about 30 per cent of healthy women, that they should not be regarded as evidence of heart disease unless other cardiac signs are present. This source of confusion would have been avoided if the heart condition had been properly assessed at the beginning of pregnancy.

A significant history should put one on guard, and Barry recommends that the heart should be examined at every antenatal visit if this is the case. The importance of auscultating the heart with the patient half turned on to her left side cannot be overstressed if significant mitral presystolic murmurs are not to be missed. A large number of patients are referred from the antenatal clinic to the cardiologist with a provisional diagnosis of heart disease but are in fact found to be normal.

Effort syndrome has to be distinguished. In this condition there is often submammary pain, dyspnoea, palpitations and premature systoles. The dyspnoea is not related specifically to exertion, but may come on even at rest or when the patient is psychologically upset. Morgan Jones found premature systoles in 15 out of 100 pregnant patients with heart disease, but by themselves they are not significant. They only "appear to disappear" on exertion because of tachycardia. Sinus arrhythmia is another common source of pulse irregularity and is physiological. A pulse rate of over 100 with a patient completely at rest, however, suggests cardiac pathology, and fibrillation denotes a severe lesion. Heart block is rather uncommon, and doubtful cases should always be subjected to electrocardiography.

Angina of effort is very rare in pregnancy, mainly because of the factor of age incidence.

The assessment of cardiac enlargement in pregnancy is notoriously difficult, because in normal cases the apex beat is displaced upwards into the fourth space and as far out as the mid-clavicular line or farther. Mensuration of the heart, to be accurate, should be undertaken as early in pregnancy as possible for this reason. Radiology also provides additional useful evidences of atrial enlargement by means of a barium swallow. Pulmonary venous congestion is very significant.

Anaemia, especially if there is a history of rheumatic fever, frequently confuses the issue because of itself it can produce many of the symptoms and signs of cardiac disability. If present in association with a heart lesion, the signs are greatly exaggerated. The routine estimation of the haemoglobin at the same time is essential. This is now standard practice with us in all patients and at every antenatal visit.

It is far more important to assess the heart's condition according to functional capacity than to the nature of the structural damage, and this grading is done according to the patient's tolerance to effort, the presence or history of atrial fibrillation and the existence of pulmonary venous congestion.

The procedure has now been almost universally adopted of grading cardiac disease in accordance with the New York Heart Association classification. This classification consists of four Grades, I, II, III and IV. Grade I cases have no limitation of activity. Signs but not symptoms are present. In Grade II, the patient has slight limitation under conditions of moderate activity. In Grade III, there are signs of incipient failure. Under circumstances of ordinary activity the patient suffers definite limitation. In Grade IV, there is complete limitation and signs of heart failure are present even at rest. Also included in Grade IV are patients who have any past history of cardiac failure and all cases of atrial fibrillation past or present. Atrial fibrillation is not an absolute bar to pregnancy, provided it can be controlled by digitalis, but it constitutes one of the most serious signs. Severe mitral stenosis however may be under-rated in the young and apparently healthy, who may at the moment be without subjective symptoms. Physical signs therefore, including particularly cardiac enlargement and diastolic murmurs or atrial fibrillation, cannot be shrugged off however well the patient may say she feels.

Prognosis

In the long run the nulliparous patient with heart disease fares no better in life than the parous woman, and the death rate, age for age, shows no difference between the two groups. To judge from statistics also, the death rate does not appear to be influenced by the number of pregnancies. There is, however, a fallacy in inferring too much from such figures, because the patient who manages to achieve a large number of pregnancies is likely to have a well-compensated heart lesion, and this will weight the figures unduly in favour of parity.

The prognosis depends utterly upon the thoroughness of medical supervision throughout pregnancy, during labour and after. For example, O'Driscoll and colleagues in Dublin[26] in a prospective study of rheumatic heart disease complicating pregnancy between the years 1948–56 reported the final outcome 5 to 13 years later of 385 mothers who achieved 539 pregnancies in this period. The only deaths in pregnancy or within a year afterwards occurred in patients who were admitted in cardiac failure having had no previous antenatal care whatsoever (7 cases), and of those who were traced subsequently in 1961 at the end of the longer follow-up period (94 per cent) 86 per cent were still living with an average age of 40·7 years and an average parity as regards viable infants of four. In no instance was therapeutic abortion carried out since this is regarded as a dangerous substitute for adequate care. Early diagnosis and thorough supervision can practically eliminate the immediate disasters, nor is the patient's life expectancy subsequently shortened, a point of view with which most of us would now agree.

In Sutherland and Bruce's series[31] the immediate death rate was 1·4 per cent and of the survivors more than half had no alteration in cardiac grading. Only 6·8 per cent suffered a sustained deterioration and in 17 per cent the patient's cardiac state was actually better when she was dismissed than when she first attended. The remainder suffered a temporary deterioration only.

It is quite certain that pregnancy never conferred any benefit upon a damaged heart although, at best, it may be no more than a temporary threat. Provided pregnancy is safely survived, the patient is often none the worse for it and life is not necessarily shortened.

One's most immediate concern therefore is the immediate progress in the course of the pregnancy under review, and this must take many factors into account. Above all, the functional capacity of the heart must head the list of prognostic criteria; in other words, the patient's cardiac grading. It will be remembered that these groups are related to the patient's response to normal activity. Exercise tolerance tests are not applicable, because the patient's apparent reactions are too much influenced by age, habits and training. There is a tendency for the patient to drop one grade during the course of her pregnancy, in other words, a Grade I case may easily become a Grade II or a Grade II may turn into a Grade III, although any complication, particularly infection, may precipitate failure in any group. On the whole, Grades I and II are good risks and Grades III and IV are bad.

A history of failure before pregnancy started, even though apparent recovery may have taken place, is a bad prognostic sign, and atrial fibrillation, as already stated, is the most serious sign of all. The nature or even the extent of valvular damage is of far less prognostic significance than the patient's functional grading, and the prognosis does not differ much between cases of mitral stenosis, for example, and aortic incompetence.

Age must be taken into account, because increasing years will place the patient, whether pregnant or not, nearer to ultimate failure, and for this reason the risk would appear to be doubled in patients after the age of 35, but only because the patient, in getting older, tends to occupy a lower functional grade.

Some guidance may be obtained from the history of how a patient fared in previous pregnancies, and other factors are the willingness of a patient to co-operate in submitting to in-patient care if necessary. Any complication of pregnancy doubles its significance in the case of the cardiac patient.

If a patient starts her pregnancy with no signs whatever of failure, she is unlikely to fail later in the absence of other complications, provided her lesion is not so gross as to make failure rapidly possible whether pregnant or not.

The prognosis is most fully revealed between the 28th and the 32nd week when the heart is shouldering its greatest load, and if the patient's condition is satisfactory then, the outlook for labour is very good. The need for assessing cardiac enlargement earlier in pregnancy has already been mentioned, and in most cases in which it can be unquestionably proven it is a bad prognostic sign.

Repeated Pregnancies

In subsequent pregnancies there is often a tendency for the patient to fall into a lower grade than that in which she passed her first pregnancy, but this to a large extent depends upon the care she gets, and much of the deterioration is due to the work involved in looking after such children as have already arrived. When cardiac breakdown occurs in later pregnancies, it most commonly does so with the third.

Fetal Prognosis

This is also influenced somewhat adversely, the neonatal death rate being slightly higher in patients with cardiac disease, mainly because of prematurity. Postmaturity tends not to be very common in cardiac disease, so that, fortunately, induction of labour seldom has to be undertaken on that account, but prematurity is definitely more common. Some of this may be due to the lower social grading as a general rule of patients with rheumatic heart disease, but certainly any failure during pregnancy enormously increases the hazard of premature labour supervening at what is now a most dangerous time and great effort must be directed towards getting the patient out of failure as much as getting her out of labour if possible. The two are a deadly combination. The fetal prognosis in cases of congenital heart disease, especially where there is cyanosis, is worse than in cases of rheumatic heart disease (see later).

Management during Pregnancy

The patient's cardiac grade should be decided during the first four months of pregnancy if possible, and management will depend upon the grade in which she is placed, but certain general principles are applicable to all of them. In the first place, ample rest should be secured and exertion permitted only to a degree which falls just short of producing dyspnoea. The lesser grades need only be seen monthly during the early part of pregnancy, but the more severe should preferably be seen every week, although the exertion of visits to the antenatal clinic must be taken into account. As far as possible steps should be taken to avoid infection, and any febrile illness should be taken seriously should it occur. There is much to be said for the prophylactic use of sulphonamides in small dosage, e.g. 0·5 g daily. During pregnancy failure is not as a rule unheralded, and a vigilant watch should be kept for its earliest signs, paying particular attention to the lung bases.

Cases in Grade I and II should have 12 hours in bed at night and, if possible, 2 hours' rest during the middle of the day; a home-help service is of enormous value in enabling a patient to carry out these instructions conscientiously. The patient should go to bed even for a very mild cold, because respiratory tract infections are more likely to precipitate failure than labour itself.

The patient should, of course, be weighed at every antenatal examination, and excessive weight gain should be restricted as far as possible by diet and reduced salt intake. More severe degrees of fluid-retention call for admission to hospital. Weight gain should not be allowed to exceed 0·6 kg in any one week since such a gain can and often does precede clinically detectable oedema.

Anaemia is one of the most common complications, which should be diagnosed early and vigorously treated.

Re-assessment of the patient's grade is carried out between the 28th and 32nd week, and any deterioration should thereupon be reversed by complete bed rest before labour becomes imminent. Cases in Grade III already have some signs of failure, and should be in hospital if necessary throughout pregnancy, while cases in Grade IV are in such peril that there should be no question of allowing them up and about.

It may seem curious that one advises admission to hospital during the last fortnight of pregnancy in cases in Grades I and II when this is the period when the heart is being gently but progressively relieved of some of its load, and it is popularly taught that one is aiming to rest the heart before labour starts. The chief reason, of course, is that the patient is far less likely to catch a respiratory tract infection if she is kept in hospital during that time, and if one should occur it can be spotted immediately and treated energetically. The standard practice of admission to hospital at or before the 38th week obviates the dangers of transporting such a case after labour has actually started. Certain types of influenza, e.g. Asian 'flu, of which there was an epidemic in West Scotland some years ago, proved very dangerous in pregnant patients with rheumatic heart disease and we had four maternal deaths from this ugly combination within the region over a short period of time.

The condition of the teeth should be attended to thoroughly, because there is some evidence that the risk of subacute bacterial endocarditis may thereby be reduced. If this dreaded complication occurs, it should be treated with massive doses of penicillin, and labour should be conducted under this protective "umbrella", which must be continued for at least two weeks into the puerperium.

There should be no root-filling or capping of teeth in cardiac cases for this very reason, whether pregnant or not. Dental extraction, under penicillin cover, is safer when filling alone will not suffice, and even fillings require prophylactic penicillin given intramuscularly, 1 g within half an hour of treatment starting. Oral penicillin V 250 mg twice a day should be continued thereafter for 3 days.

Subacute bacterial endocarditis is due to the *Streptococcus viridans* and vegetations are liable to form on any valve which is deformed either congenitally or by disease. The infection may lie dormant in the genital tract, but a particularly dangerous source is provided by dental roots and areas of dental caries. A patient who has a proven or suspected bacterial endocarditis should be put on to large doses of penicillin at once, starting with a loading dose of two million units, and while blood cultures are obtained the dental roots should be X-rayed. Extraction should only be undertaken with full antibiotic cover, preferably as soon as possible after the antibiotic has been started because although resistance to penicillin is uncommon, provided adequate dosage is maintained, occasionally the *Str. viridans* may require another potent antibiotic. If the patient is already receiving penicillin at the time a dental extraction is contemplated, it is as well to switch to another antibiotic, for example, erythromycin 300 mg by intramuscular injection about a quarter of an hour before the extraction is undertaken; an oral dose thereafter of 250 mg being maintained six-hourly for two or three days.

Cephaloridine (2 g intramuscularly) is also a good alternative and must be given unhesitatingly and repeated in 1 g injections 8- or 12-hourly (a) if penicillin resistance is suspected, (b) where major dental treatment is to be undertaken in a patient already on prophylactic penicillin, and (c) when the membranes rupture in the case of a patient already receiving penicillin, the objective being, as stated, to prevent the emergence of penicillin-resistant strains.

Apart from attention to teeth and such potential sources of infection, the patient's general health as regards diet, rest and fresh air should receive careful attention. Vitamins are often prescribed particularly the vitamin B complex and an adequate intake of calcium through milk is desirable. Urinary infections should be spotted early and eliminated as far as possible. Next to anaemia, preventive medicine here will yield one of the really big dividends in antenatal care.

The onset of pre-eclamptic toxaemia should be taken even more seriously than usual, not only because of the increased burden on the heart from the hypertension but also because of the increased fluid retention which is a part of that disease. Proteinuria may be due to pre-eclamptic toxaemia, cardiac failure, or both, or may be the first indication of urinary infection.

Occasionally and coincidentally hydramnios may complicate the picture and embarrass the patient's cardiac condition still further. This should be treated by abdominal paracentesis if bed rest and diuretics do not afford rapid relief.

Above all, failure must be controlled before labour starts, and in nearly every case this is possible. The instances of inability to do so are due to the onset of an unpredictable upper respiratory tract infection.

Recently, the question of surgical treatment of mitral stenosis by valvotomy has come under consideration, and in suitable cases the operation can be carried out at almost any stage of pregnancy.

O'Connell and Mulcahy[25] report a successful case at term. Certain criteria of suitability, however, have to be observed, and these, to some extent, restrict its application, namely, mitral stenosis should be of a severe degree with only a minor degree of associated mitral incompetence, the other valves should be almost normal, nor should there be any marked left ventricular enlargement. The operation has a very definite place as an emergency procedure in cases who continue in failure in spite of a fair trial of medical treatment, and Marshall and Pantridge[21] found the operation preferable to termination of pregnancy. The modern view is that operation is not made more dangerous by pregnancy and that the fetal chances are not worsened as compared with medically treated cases.

In my own practice I have never yet seen fit to recommend a case for mitral valvotomy during pregnancy and my attitude has somewhat hardened by having personally to undergo this operation myself. I found it a very disagreeable experience and would think more than twice before I subjected a pregnant women to it. It would be far better to carry out valvotomy as an elective procedure between pregnancies, as Gilchrist recommended,[10] so that the only cases in pregnancy which can fairly be considered are cases of emergency. Unfortunately the operation is likely to be disqualified or certainly made more dangerous by the very conditions most likely to give rise to the emergency, namely an acute respiratory infection or a pulmonary embolus.

The factor of age is very important and the advice is given that patients should complete their reproductive careers while still young, rather than waiting a long time between pregnancies because such delay does not improve their fitness for the next pregnancy, but merely gives them more time in which to get older and to deteriorate in accordance with the natural history of the disease.

Thanks to advances in open heart surgery, a new problem is being increasingly encountered in modern obstetrics, namely that of the woman who has either had a valve replaced by prosthesis or by a homograft, or who has had a congenital lesion surgically corrected. Pregnancy with a prosthetic valve is not regarded as an unacceptable hazard[18] but all patients with such valves live under the threat of embolism, as like as not cerebral, whether pregnant or not, male or female. Anticoagulant therapy must therefore be maintained. This raises its own problems in pregnancy, but the challenge is better met by continuing the pregnancy than by terminating it. Anticoagulation by oral drugs such as warfarin is maintained until within a fortnight of term or whenever labour is evidently imminent, whereupon it is necessary to change to heparin, which does not cross the placenta and does not expose the fetus to the danger of haemorrhage in the course of its birth. This heparin is either administered by thrice-daily intravenous injections or by continuous subcutaneous injection. (*See* section on thrombosis.) During the heparin treatment the clotting time should be maintained at at least twice normal levels. The general rules of withholding ergometrine in the third stage of labour in the absence of haemorrhage do not apply in these cases and it is better to prevent haemorrhage at this time by the standard dosage of 0·5 mg of ergometrine. When the immediate risk of haemorrhage has passed the warfarin cover is resumed forthwith. The effects of heparin can be immediately corrected by protamine sulphate, whereas those of warfarin and similar anticoagulants take many hours to reverse even with vitamin K_1.

While on oral anticoagulants during pregnancy it is necessary to monitor the dose much more frequently, for example weekly if there are any gastro-intestinal disturbances, which may upset anticoagulant intake or utilisation. Phenindione is nowadays regarded as less acceptable than warfarin because a few people show undue sensitivity to it. Advice has been given to listen regularly to the prosthesis for warning sounds of a thrombus breaking free but I have no experience of this physical sign I am glad to say.

The risk of subacute bacterial endocarditis is every bit as great with a prosthesis now as with any other type of intracardiac lesion. The need for antibiotic cover in labour therefore is as great too.

Onset of Failure

The patient should be admitted at once and kept in hospital for the rest of pregnancy. Bed rest must be absolute and fluid intake should be restricted. Sedatives should be liberally given and the patient should be digitalised, whether or not the heart is failing with irregular rhythm. To some extent digitalis is a cumulative drug, and overdosage can easily occur, the signs of which are nausea, vomiting, a tightness in the chest and a pulse rate lower than 60. In severe overdosage the beats may be coupled. Atrial fibrillation, of course, demands digitalis and anticoagulant therapy, preferably with warfarin, the dose being controlled by Thrombotest, must be established, because of the risk of embolism.

Smoking enormously increases the symptoms of pulmonary congestion, namely, sputum and cough, which exhausts the patient and aggravates the failure. We had one such case in a young woman who smoked secretly and managed to aim the cigarette ends through the window; for a time it appeared as though all our treatment was of no avail, until a one-eyed Matron visiting the hospital noticed the enormous collection on the path outside and drew the attention of the nursing staff to it. The patient, who besides her cardiac lesion had chronic bronchitis and emphysema, died some months after delivery smoking almost up to the end.

Diuresis with frusemide, 40 to 80 mg immediately, and maintained 6-hourly at first to secure a rapid diuresis is also an important part of the treatment. Loss of potassium, however, is likely to be severe and it is advisable, as soon as possible, to restrict the frusemide diuresis to alternate days at most, replenishing the potassium loss by Slow-K tablets or better still by effervescent potassium tablets such as Sando-K which upset the stomach less.

Frusemide is an effective but vicious diuretic, as I well know, and hydrochlorothiazide (50 mg) once or twice a day is almost as effective and certainly kinder.

On no account may obstetrical intervention be undertaken until the patient's cardiac failure is under control, although the situation may seem so grim that one may be tempted to interfere. To do so would simply seal the patient's fate. Once failure has been controlled, however, the need to intervene in the pregnancy has passed.

Termination of Pregnancy

There is some conflict of opinion here. Termination within the first trimester of pregnancy is less dangerous than formerly in these days of vacuum aspiration and wholesale abortion in early pregnancy but in fact there is seldom a straight indication for it. Barnes stated that since 1954 he had only recommended termination in one out of 535 cases of rheumatic heart disease (and she refused). For the patient who is not in cardiac failure there is no need to terminate and if she is in failure termination is next door to manslaughter. The latter point of view can only be supported if the patient can be persuaded to spend the whole of her pregnancy under supervision in hospital. To achieve this objective in Grade III cases I have adopted the practice of allowing the patient week-end "48-hour passes" to be spent quietly at home and thus we manage to secure at least 80 per cent supervision and at the same time maintain her morale. This policy has practically eliminated irregular dismissals and even the most homesick patients report back cheerfully early on Monday morning and none has so far let us down.

All are agreed that after the 12th week the risks of termination are greater than those of continued pregnancy and normal delivery at term, for abdominal hysterotomy will now be the method of choice and is certainly more dangerous than a natural vaginal delivery. Intra-uterine hypertonic saline or prostaglandins administered by either intra-amniotic or extra-amniotic routes carry too great a risk of infection to be countenanced and too often require evacuation of retained products. The problem arises in its most acute form when cardiac failure persists in spite of treatment, but in this dreadful dilemma it is as well to remember that termination of the pregnancy will be tantamount to driving the last nail into the patient's coffin, and should she die without termination one can only reflect that she could not have been saved in any case by operating. Certainly, as already indicated, valvotomy now offers a chance which, not long ago, few dared to take.

Open Heart Surgery during Pregnancy

This is a much more serious matter than valvotomy, a fact to which I can testify from personal experience. Involving as it does cardiopulmonary bypass with or without hypothermia, experience to date has not been large, but the outcome of 20 cases has been reviewed from a number of centres collectively.[35] One patient and her fetus died and a further six babies were lost as a result of premature labour. A similar number were lost as previable abortuses and the one baby who survived birth only to die in the neonatal period had multiple congenital abnormalities. These fetal results are of course appalling but one has to reflect that they are still less than the 100 per cent mortality which results from therapeutic abortion! This type of desperate surgery however is not more dangerous for the mother than if she were not pregnant, so that pregnancy *per se* is not in itself a contra-indication, where the operation is really needed.

Induction of Labour

This has little place in the management of the patient with heart disease alone. In the first place, it is seldom necessary because of the improvement which occurs in the patient's condition during the terminal weeks. The babies are usually rather small, and, as a rule, the more serious the case the more premature is labour likely to be. Quite apart from the fact that induction is unnecessary, it may be, positively dangerous. For one thing, it may misfire and a prolonged induction-delivery interval may result in infection or the need for Caesarean section, or both, which might otherwise never have been necessary. For another, the anxiety which it is likely to entail for the patient will do her cardiac condition nothing but harm. Induction may be indicated for other reasons, such as pre-eclamptic toxaemia in multiparae, but in primigravidae, particularly, an assessment of all the relevant risks may indicate Caesarean section as the safer course. Modern methods of induction combining escalating oxytocin dosage with amniotomy can now mitigate but not eliminate these hazards.

If surgical induction, in fact, has to be undertaken the risks of subacute bacterial endocarditis must be kept in mind and prophylactic penicillin should be started, as in the case of dental extractions, within half an hour before the operation, using a combination of soluble and long-acting penicillin, one to two million units by intramuscular injection, to prevent the emergence of penicillin-resistant strains of *Str. viridans* and thereafter maintaining penicillin coverage with longer-acting penicillins for at least four days after labour is safely over. If the patient is already on penicillin prophylaxis, cephaloridine should be given. In certain instances where a patient has been successfully treated for cardiac failure, one may be tempted to consider induction while the going is good, but this is worse than playing with fire, and one's energies should be devoted to preventing the onset of further failure.

Management of Labour

Because spontaneous normal labour is devoutly to be wished, every precaution should be taken in advance to ensure that such is possible. This will include an accurate assessment of the bony pelvis, for a strenuous labour due to disproportion cannot be countenanced, and a trial of labour is absolutely contra-indicated. Fortunately, in the majority of cases labour is fairly easy. Inertia is rare and the cervix appears to dilate with considerable ease, probably because it is more soft and vascular than usual because of venous congestion.

With proper nursing and supervision, the first stage of labour should not seriously strain the damaged heart. Penicillin, ½ mega unit, twice daily should be injected throughout labour and after the membranes rupture cephaloridine should be given (1 gram intramuscularly every 12 hours). Breathlessness and tachycardia are more often the result of worry and apprehension and the discomfort of labour rather than the efforts which labour entails. For this reason, sedation should be liberal and morphia is superior to other drugs. Cases in Grades I and II provide no problem in the first stage, which is conducted as usual, except that the patient should be kept in bed; nevertheless, supervision must not be relaxed. Cases in Grades III and IV should be propped up and be given digoxin. Where failure is pronounced, oxygen should be continuously administered and venesection may be required. In any case the patient should be immediately digitalised should the pulse rate rise above 110 or respirations above 24, for heart failure is far less likely to supervene in patients whose pulse and respiration rates remain below these levels during the first stage regardless of the nature of the cardiac condition.

The onset of failure in the first stage is a contra-indication rather than an indication for intervention in the form of Caesarean section, which would then tip the scales against the patient.

Epidural anaesthesia and assistance with the ventouse later, in the second stage, may obviate the need for desperate abdominal delivery. Fortunately, the average duration of labour is usually shortened in the cardiac case, and 8 hours in the first stage would be an average figure.

The Second Stage of Labour

This is the stage of effort, and effort on the part of the patient is at all costs to be avoided or curtailed. It is often taught that the forceps should be applied as soon as the cervix is fully dilated, but the risks of this and the possible need to induce anaesthesia are greater than a spontaneous rapid second stage. The forceps should not be used unless the patient is clearly unlikely to deliver herself within the next 20 minutes. A good rule is to start preparing the instruments and setting the trolley as soon as the patient is fully dilated in the hope that happily she may be already delivered by the time the preparations are completed. She should not be encouraged to bear down forcibly, and in many cases labour will be surprisingly easily terminated. As soon as the head is on the perineum, episiotomy is thoroughly worth while and greatly facilitates effortless delivery. Pudendal block is a very valuable type of anaesthesia, and caudal anaesthesia has also much to recommend it, alternatively "saddle-block" spinal anaesthesia. The forceps rate is naturally high in these cases and is usually over 25 per cent, while cases in Grade IV will, in the majority of instances, be delivered by the forceps unless labour is extremely rapid.

More recently the ventouse (vacuum extractor—see Chapter XIX) has come to prove its worth as an alternative to the use of forceps to curtail the duration and effort of the second stage. It involves considerably less disturbance to the patient and can be used without putting the patient's legs up in the lithotomy position. This is an enormous advantage because raising the legs increases the load on the heart. We now prefer to deliver with the ventouse than with forceps in these cases.

The Third Stage

This should never be hurried. In cases who are not on anticoagulant therapy the routine use of ergometrine is barred, as it will increase the heart's load by causing additional blood to be squeezed back into circulation, and it shuts down the uterine arteriovenous shunt. Ergometrine should not be used until 15 oz (420 ml) have been lost in the course of abnormal postpartum bleeding and when, or if, transfusion is necessary it is far more dangerous to give too much blood than too little. Many welcome a mild postpartum haemorrhage, but this is a wanton outlook, for who can be sure when haemorrhage starts whether it will end up by being a mild one? It is preferable to control the amount of blood removed from the patient's circulation by venesection where, following a bloodless delivery, the need to relieve the heart of its volumetric load is apparent. In the most severe grades, venesection will certainly go far towards preventing the onset of pulmonary oedema, and amounts of blood up to half a litre may be removed. Lastly, the suture of the episiotomy or laceration, if any, should be done always under local anaesthesia only, and it is seldom advisable to resort to general anaesthesia.

As soon as delivery is completed the patient should be propped up, given morphia and a supply of oxygen should be at hand throughout. Penicillin given throughout labour may materially reduce the hazard of subacute bacterial endocarditis.

The Place of Caesarean Section

Caesarean section takes a very poor second place as an alternative to normal delivery in these patients, and it is never indicated on cadiac grounds alone. The situation, however, is quite otherwise when labour is in any way complicated, and it is on the whole preferable to a difficult forceps delivery due to minor disproportion.

The mortality of Caesarean section is two or three times as high as that of vaginal delivery. One has to consider not only the strain of the operation itself but the effect upon the heart of the first few post-operative days. Cardiac output falls by about 40 per cent immediately after the operation while the patient is still under the anaesthetic, and it may not return to normal for three or four days. During this time the lung bases are often not well ventilated, a state of affairs greatly aggravated by any ileus, so that pulmonary oedema and failure may be precipitated. It is seldom that labour is prolonged in these cases, but when this uncommon complication occurs, Caesarean section offers the safer alternative. In the primigravid patient, Caesarean section is usually safer, for example in the pre-eclamptic case, than surgical induction, for reasons already stated, though this argument does not apply in the case of the experienced multipara.

Because it may be desirable to sterilise the patient, it might appear that there was something to be said for performing elective Caesarean section at the same time, but the need for sterilisation is never an indication for Caesarean section, and in any case the tubes can be dealt with far more simply through a very small incision under a local anaesthetic towards the end of the first week of the puerperium. The last time I carried out this apparently simple procedure, I, or rather the patient, was rewarded with subacute bacterial endocarditis which nearly killed her. It is, on the whole, safer to sterilise the patient after a few months if she can be trusted not to become pregnant again meanwhile—an unlikely hope in some patients. We now undertake the operation of sterilisation by means of a laparoscope.[30] Postnatal contraception for a period of three months can be achieved by simply injecting depot progesterone (e.g. Depo-Provera 150 mg). This operation electively carried out at a time convenient to the patient is a trivial one and obviates the need for laparotomy.

Caesarean section has a definite place in cardiac disease, but it is limited. It is, however, the only reasonably safe alternative to spontaneous or low forceps or ventouse delivery.

Puerperium

The first 12 hours after delivery are easily the most critical, because the right side of the heart suffers some overload with the diversion of blood which normally would have gone to the placental site and uterus. Signs of pulmonary congestion and oedema must be carefully watched for. Sedatives are liberally given in the first few days to reduce tachycardia, and the patient is not allowed out of bed until all signs of cardiac failure, if present, have disappeared.

Any infection in the puerperium, however mild, is taken seriously, and visitors should be restricted to the minimum possible, not only because they interfere with rest but because they may introduce respiratory tract infections. Breast feeding is contra-indicated in Grade IV cases and in most of those in Grade III, but it has to be remembered that the palaver of artificial feeding may put the mother to more strain, trouble and worry than breast feeding. Individual circumstances have to be taken into account. Oral anticoagulants contra-indicate breast feeding because of excretion in the milk. Oestrogens should preferably not be used for the suppression of lactation because they encourage fluid retention.

It is little use discharging a patient, fairly well at the end of three or four weeks in hospital, to home conditions which will undo all the good work done, and the patient's domestic circumstances should be understood before she is allowed home. It is now that home-help schemes play such an important part, for it is more necessary to relieve the postnatal cardiac case of domestic strain than a patient who has undergone an average major abdominal operation. A good follow-up system, therefore, outside as well as within the hospital is essential. These patients are often perversely fertile, and contraceptive instruction should not be delayed therefore, because they are often pregnant again within the twinkling of an eye.

Congenital Heart Disease

In so far as it is possible to compare them, cases of congenital heart disease tend, on the whole, to have a worse prognosis than cases with other cardiac lesions. Cases with ventricular septal defects and patent ductus arteriosus, however, usually do fairly well, and the prognosis is related far more to the degree of cyanosis than to the actual type of abnormality present.

As it happens, the grosser lesions tend to cause death before the patient has an opportunity of becoming pregnant, and gross cyanosis also prevents pregnancy. Coarctation of the aorta comes into a class of its own and will be discussed presently.

The danger of bacterial endocarditis is just as great in these cases during labour as in cases of rheumatic heart disease, and prophylactic penicillin is equally indicated in either case.

Kerr and Sodeman recorded 80 deliveries in 33 patients with congenital heart disease with the following incidence:

Atrial septal defect, 16
Inter-ventricular defect, 14
Patent ductus arteriosus, 18
Coarctation of the aorta, 11
Pulmonary stenosis, 12
Fallot's tetralogy, 3
Undiagnosed heart disease, 6

Of these, four patients developed congestive cardiac failure as a result of pregnancy and one died. Fifty pregnancies in 19 patients with severe cyanotic congenital heart disease were described from Sheffield[3] over a ten-year period without maternal death, nor was therapeutic abortion considered necessary.

Congenital heart block must be added to the above list and I have a case who has completed two successful pregnancies without incident and with a pulse rate which never under any circumstances exceeds 50 beats per minute.

In all, four cases of complete congenital heart block attended the Queen Mother's Hospital in one year.[14] Of these two went postmature and failed to respond to induction, one reached the forty-second week of gestation and was delivered by mid-cavity forceps delivery and the other, my own case, delivered spontaneously at the forty-first week. Postmaturity would seem therefore to be a feature of the condition unlike in rheumatic heart disease, but none of these cases suffered any disability apart from anxiety and a certain amount of dyspnoea, which was rapidly got under control by brief periods of rest in hospital.

The diagnosis of the congenital lesion is outside the scope of this book, but certain basic signs suggest such a lesion, namely the presence of cyanosis, a harsh basal murmur often with a thrill and evidences of cardiac enlargement. Where cyanosis is persistent or easily provoked, the prognosis is so much the worse. Serious degrees of right-left shunt in fact may demand surgical intervention in their own right, but the fetal mortality as indicated earlier is high because of abortion, prematurity, hypoxia and often congenital defects too.

The danger of subacute bacterial endocarditis is not dissimilar from that in rheumatic heart disease.

The indications for surgical correction of the defect are progressive failure to respond to treatment, particularly progressive deterioration in the first half of pregnancy, a history of deterioration in the previous pregnancy, or a Grade IV status in early pregnancy.[6] The best time for operation is said to be between 20 and 24 weeks if there is any choice in the matter.

Eisenmenger's syndrome consists of pulmonary hypertension with a raised pulmonary resistance together with a septal defect either atrial or ventricular or a patent ductus producing cyanosis with blood being shunted from right to left. This is a dangerous condition and according to the maternal mortality statistics for England and Wales there were 15 deaths between 1961 and 1969. For this condition Barnes[1] recommends early termination, but not in late pregnancy where the risk thereof would be greater.

Most of these cases are in considerable danger of sudden collapse following any rapid emptying of the pregnant uterus, and the blood pressure may swing widely during labour and be followed by hypotension. Precipitate delivery is, therefore, particularly dangerous. As might be expected, eclampsia enormously magnifies the risks.

Coarctation of the Aorta

This is not a common complication of pregnancy because of the short expectation of life. Modern cardiovascular surgery, however, is altering the picture. The dangers to the case that has not been previously surgically corrected consist of rupture of the aorta or cerebral haemorrhage, which may occur before or after delivery. For these reasons there has been a natural recommendation for routine Caesarean section at term. Four out of five cases reported by Rosenthal[29] died, two before and two after delivery. Our own limited experience has been happier.

The condition is more common than the literature would suggest, and the vast majority of the cases have not been reported; practically every obstetrician throughout the land has had some experience of it. The dangers have been overstressed in the past. If the femoral pulses were felt for in all cases who had severe hypertension in earlier pregnancy many more cases would come to light.

In addition to the dangers of aortic rupture, cerebral haemorrhage and subacute bacterial endocarditis, there is some risk of hypertensive encephalopathy, and acute circulatory failure may follow delivery. The incidence of pre-eclampsia does not appear to be increased, but of course when it occurs the added rise in blood pressure becomes especially dangerous.

In addition to the absence of femoral pulses, coarctation of the aorta is suggested by visible pulsation in the infra-scapular regions and along the medial borders of the scapulae. Although the systolic pressure is very high, the diastolic pressure is normal and pulsation cannot be felt in the lower extremities. If the blood pressure is now taken in the legs, the characteristic difference between arm and leg readings will clarify the diagnosis. Skiagrams show notching of the lower borders of the ribs. The left ventricle is enlarged and the ascending aorta may be seen dilated. An electrocardiogram shows left ventricular preponderance.

Pregnancy should be constantly supervised, preferably in hospital. This precaution will at least tend to keep the systolic pressure at the lowest level and the possible onset of pre-eclamptic toxaemia will be immediately noted.

The subject was fully reviewed by Pritchard (1953) who, in a study of 79 cases, including two of his own, found that mortality was not lower in Caesarean section (7·1 per cent) than in cases delivered vaginally (6·5 per cent). The conduct of such a case should follow the lines already given for other forms of heart disease, including the use of antibiotics in labour to reduce the hazard of subacute bacterial endocarditis or aortitis.

Surgical cure by aortic resection is nowadays not only feasible but likely to be successful. Although it can be undertaken during pregnancy it is best carried out between pregnancies and provides a sufficiently good prognosis to render sterilisation an unnecessary alternative.

Thyrotoxicosis

This is not a common complication of pregnancy, to some extent because of the impaired fertility of such patients. Pregnancy easily may confuse the diagnostic problem both on clinical and on laboratory grounds, since even a euthyroid pregnant patient may complain of tiredness, palpitation, dyspnoea and heat intolerance; she may even have moist hands and tachycardia, also thyroid enlargement, yet not be thyrotoxic. The serum PBI measures iodinated protein compounds of which T-4 forms the greater part and is normally raised in any case in pregnancy although values of over 9 μg per cent are suggestive. Radioiodine uptake tests are not only misleading but dangerous and the doubt is hard to resolve. Triiodothyronine (T-3) resin uptake levels, normally 25–35 per cent, are decreased in pregnancy because of the increase in TBG (thyrosine-binding-globulin) levels which provides more capacity for T-3 binding in competition with T-4 which binds more strongly. Consequently in pregnancy there is less T-3 left over for resin uptake.

A test for thyrotoxicosis however has emerged[28] based upon tyrosine tolerance. According to this test thyrotoxic patients have a higher-than-normal fasting concentration of tyrosine in the plasma and following the administration of L-tyrosine powder in a dose of 50 mg per kg body weight, the rise in subsequent plasma concentration is consistently higher than in the euthyroid. Pregnancy does not appear to alter tyrosine tolerance. Since most of our cases have already been diagnosed as thyrotoxic before presenting in pregnancy we lack experience of this test.

The general management of the patient during pregnancy and labour is on similar lines prescribed for cardiac cases, particular emphasis being laid upon adequate rest and the avoidance and prompt treatment of infection.

Unfortunately radio-iodine, so singularly successful in the non-pregnant, older patient, is absolutely contra-indicated in pregnancy because the isotope crosses the placenta and is concentrated in the fetal thyroid gland as well as in that of the mother.

The therapeutic choices therefore lie between antithyroid drugs and subtotal thyroidectomy and even if the latter were being contemplated it would still have to be preceded by a course of antithyroid drugs. There is even less reason to terminate pregnancy than in the case of cardiac disease.

The case for surgery has been well put by Hawe and Francis (1962) in Liverpool. They point out that antithyroid drugs cross the placenta and that thyroid function is depressed in the fetus as well as the mother who originally required the treatment. The depression of the fetal thyroid increases the production of fetal TSH so that hyperplasia of the gland may result in the formation of fetal goitre. Furthermore, the danger of induced cretinism is very real. The antithyroid drugs, moreover, are excreted in breast milk so that breast feeding is contra-indicated if the mother continues on treatment after delivery. Finally, nearly one-third of the Liverpool series who completed their pregnancies on drug treatment came ultimately to thyroidectomy which could have been just as safely and conveniently carried out during pregnancy. On the other hand all their cases treated surgically had live and healthy babies with one unrelated exception. Prophylactic replacement with thyroxine therapy was usually employed during the rest of pregnancy and the operation was preferably delayed until after the twelfth week to reduce the risk of abortion.

Crooks and his colleagues (1962) drew attention, however, to the difficulties and uncertainties of assessing the severity of thyrotoxicosis in pregnancy and the consequent dangers of such a radical and irreversible step as removing the major portion of a patient's thyroid gland. Certainly, clinical evidences alone are unreliable since physiological enlargement of the thyroid gland occurs in more than half of all pregnant women and increased pulse rate, diminished tolerance to heat, sweating and anxiety are common both to pregnancy and thyrotoxicosis. However, persistent tachycardia, especially while asleep, failure to gain weight in spite of a good appetite, and tremor and exophthalmos are significant.

Our own practice for many years has been to use antithyroid drugs in preference to surgery. The three main drugs used for the purpose are methyl thiouracil, carbimazole and potassium perchlorate.[7] We were doing very well with the last-mentioned of these, under the direction of Crooks before he departed to Aberdeen, but he has since drawn our attention to cases of aplastic anaemia reported in the literature which might reasonably be attributed to this drug.[4]

Most thyrotoxic pregnant patients do well on antithyroid drug therapy but control must be very thorough since the fetus is at even greater risk than the mother, namely abortion or premature stillbirth in the case of undertreatment and fetal goitre or cretinism from overtreatment.

It used to be the practice to suppress maternal thyroid function almost wholly with methyl thiouracil and then to cover this depression by giving thyroxine in controlled amounts to regulate maternal, metabolism and to prevent fetal goitre, but we now prefer to use the more potent synthetic drug carbimazole (called methimazole in U.S.A.) in the smallest amounts consistent with euthyroidism and not to prescribe thyroxine as well unless an acute phase of hypothyroidism occurs.

An initial dose of 30–40 mg daily is divided into 10 mg fractions. The dose is then progressively reduced after a fortnight until minimal amounts are being given in the second half of pregnancy. It is most important to space the doses evenly throughout each 24-hour period because the drug's action is short. The dosage is controlled by serum PBI estimations (protein bound iodine 127—non-radioactive) carried out on 10 ml samples of clotted blood from the patient. The euthyroid level in pregnancy to be aimed for is 6–9 μg per cent as against 4–8 μg in the non-pregnant.[34]

This scheme of treatment has the merit of simplicity and certainly eliminates the hazards of unnecessary surgery. Fears of congenital abnormalities have not been realized except goitre in the overtreated case which regresses spontaneously in the months following birth; the prognosis for drug-induced cretinism, however, is less certain and serves as a reminder that these cases should be simultaneously supervised by obstetrician and physician too.

REFERENCES

1. Barnes, C. G. (1974). *Medical Disorders in Obstetric Practice*, 4th edit. pp. 7, 11, 27. Oxford: Blackwell Scientific Publications.

2. BARRY, A. (1952). *Irish J. med. Sci.*, 6th series, October, p. 398.
3. BATSON, G. A. (1974). *J. Obstet. Gynaec. Brit. Cwlth*, **81,** 549.
4. BRITISH MEDICAL JOURNAL. (1961). Leading article. **1,** 1520.
5. CLAYTON, S. and ORAM, S. (1951). *Medical Disorders in Pregnancy.* London: Churchill.
6. CONRADSSON, T. A. and WERKÖ, L. (1974). *Progr. cardiovasc. Dis.*, **16,** 407.
7. CROOKS, J. (1957). *Postgrad. med. J.*, **33,** 322.
8. CROOKS, J. (1962). Personal communication.
9. CROOKS, J., KHAIR, S. A., MACGREGOR, A. G. and TURNBULL, A. C. (1962). *Brit. med. J.*, **2,** 1259.
10. GILCHRIST, A. R. (1962). *Cardiological Problems in Younger Women.* Lock Lecture, Royal Faculty of Physicians and Surgeons, Glasgow.
11. HAIG, D. C. and GILCHRIST, A. R. (1949). *Edinb. med. J.*, **56,** 55.
12. HAWE, P. and FRANCIS, H. H. (1962). *Brit. med. J.*, **2,** 817.
13. KELLAR, R. J. (1950). *Edinb. med. J.*, **57,** 27.
14. KENMURE, A. C. F. and CAMERON, A. J. V. (1967). *Brit. Heart J.*, **29,** 910.
15. KERR, A. and SODEMAN, W. A. (1951). *Amer. Heart J.*, **42,** 436.
16. KERR, M. G. (1968). *Brit. med. Bull.*, **24,** 19.
17. LEES, M. M., TAYLOR, S. H., SCOTT, D. B. and KERR, M. G. (1967). *J. Obstet. Gynaec. Brit. Cwlth*, **74,** 319.
18. MACDONALD, H. N. (1970). *J. Obstet. Gynaec. Brit. Cwlth*, **77,** 603.
19. MCMICHAEL, J. (1952). *Brit. med. J.*, **2,** 525.
20. MACRAE, D. J. (1948). *J. Obstet. Gynaec. Brit. Emp.*, **55,** 184.
21. MARSHALL, R. J. and PANTRIDGE, J. F. (1957). *Brit. med. J.*, **1,** 1097.
22. METCALFE, J. and URLAND, K. (1974). *Progr. cardiovasc. Dis.*, **16,** 363.
23. MORGAN JONES, A. (1944). *Postgrad. med. J.*, **20,** 176.
24. MORGAN JONES, A. (1952). *Practitioner*, **168,** 49.
25. O'CONNELL, T. C. J. and MULCAHY, R. (1955). *Brit. med. J.*, **1,** 1191.
26. O'DRISCOLL, K. M., COYLE, C. F. V. and DRURY, M. I. (1962). *Brit. med. J.*, **2,** 767.
27. PRITCHARD, J. A. (1953). *Obstet. gynec. Surv.*, **8,** 775.
28. RIVLIN, R. S., MELMAN, K. L. and SJOERDSMA, A. (1965). *New Engl. J. Med.*, **272,** 1143.
29. ROSENTHAL, L. (1955). *Brit. med. J.*, **1,** 16.
30. STEPTOE, P. C. (1967). *Laparoscopy in Gynaecology.* Edinburgh: Livingstone.
31. SUTHERLAND, A. M. and BRUCE, D. F. (1962). *J. Obstet. Gynaec. Brit. Cwlth*, **69,** 99.
32. SZEKELY, P. and SNAITH, L. (1961). *Brit. med. J.*, **1,** 1407.
33. WALTERS, W. A. W., MACGREGOR, W. G. and HILLS, M. (1966). *Clin. Sci.*, **30,** 1.
34. WILSON, G. M. (1967). *Prescribers' J.*, **7,** 1.
35. ZITNIK, R. S., BRANDENBURG, R. O., SHELDON, R. and WALTON, R. B. (1969). *Circulation*, **39–40,** Suppl. 1, 257.

CHAPTER VI

DIABETES MELLITUS

It is generally reckoned that there are over half a million diabetic people in the United Kingdom, although not all of that number are yet patients, that is to say diagnosed and under treatment. In this disease almost more than any other "events cast their shadow before".

In spite of this large number the incidence of diabetes mellitus in pregnancy is not likely to be more than one in seven hundred to a thousand births, so that an average-sized maternity hospital undertaking two-and-a-half to three thousand deliveries a year does not deal with even a dozen cases annually.

Statistics are therefore all the more worthwhile from units like that at King's College Hospital, London, which has traditionally attracted a large diabetic clientèle, amounting to more than 700 cases over a twenty-year period up to 1970. These cases did not include "latent diabetes", subclinical, or chemical diabetes.

Nevertheless perinatal mortality can be just as high in latent diabetes as in the declared and properly treated cases.

Varieties of the Diabetic Trait

In addition to the full-blown case of diabetes mellitus about which there can be no argument there are a number of subvarieties which should be recognised.

Firstly, one should regard as a potential diabetic any patient with parent or sibling so affected or having herself previously given birth to a baby weighing more than 4¼ kg. Family history should also include uncles, aunts and grandparents.

Latent diabetes is so-called because it is only manifest under stress, such as surgical operations or acute infections.

I can well recall the occasion during the war when I crawled from my sick bed with a massive carbuncle to the urine-testing room of my own sick quarters to test my own urine!

When the particular stress happens to be pregnancy itself, the term "gestational diabetes" is nowadays employed to indicate the patient who develops abnormal glucose tolerance during pregnancy, the test reverting to normal thereafter. This manifestation may be the first indication of diabetes yet to come in later years. Significantly, however, the perinatal mortality is characteristically increased. In chemical or subclinical diabetes the features of glycosuria and the symptoms of diabetes have not yet appeared, but glucose tolerance tests record the fate in store for her. Meanwhile the fetus is at risk *in utero*.

Maturity-onset diabetes is not of immediate concern to the obstetrician except for its prediabetic aspects which are not easily foreseen and which affect perinatal mortality adversely as well. It is the commonest type of diabetes when taking all ages into account, comprising about two-thirds of the diabetic physician's work load.[1] It arises in middle age, usually after child-bearing, and is associated with obesity and at the same time high levels of plasma insulin, unlike the adolescent type which is insulin-deficient.

The Effect of Diabetes upon Fertility

Before the discovery of insulin, and in the case of the uncontrolled diabetic, infertility was the rule. Many of these cases tend to have amenorrhoea and, in the pre-insulin era, only about 2 per cent of diabetic patients conceived. Increasing numbers of diabetics are now becoming pregnant, and the fertility rate is now 25–30 per cent. Therefore, testing the urine for sugar in the case of a woman complaining of sterility still remains an important part of the investigation.

Once a diabetic woman has become pregnant, her chances of a successful pregnancy depend almost wholly on the quality of her antenatal care. Unfortunately every physician today is still inclined to regard himself as an expert diabetic physician. The situation is worse still if the obstetrician fancies himself in this role.

GLYCOSURIA

We are concerned here with the case of the woman who, at the antenatal clinic, presents with a reducing substance in her urine. This, if present, is nearly always glucose and glucose-oxidase paper strip tests (Clinistix) are not only highly sensitive but are specific for glucose.[19] The chief point to settle is whether or not the presence of glucose in the urine denotes the existence of diabetes. If acetone is also present, it makes the diagnosis of diabetes more than probable, but in the majority of cases this is not found.

Glycosuria is commoner at some time or other in pregnancy the more often one looks for it; for instance in a series reported from Newport, Monmouthshire, over 9 per cent of 1500 cases showed glycosuria and when a series of 30 cases of pregnancy were tested round the clock, glycosuria was found in over 70 per cent, whereas the incidence in a control group was 13 per cent.[6] Certainly it would appear that unselected cases in pregnancy given a 50 g oral dose of glucose show a 90 per cent incidence of glycosuria by Clinistix testing. Since glycosuria, albeit in small amounts, is so commonly found at one time or another in pregnancy it is worth confirming or refuting by the simple expedient of testing a *second* fasting morning specimen of urine.[17] Fasting glycosuria, so found in pregnancy has a sinister significance even though glucose tolerance may be apparently normal.[18]

Glucose Tolerance Testing

During pregnancy the normal fasting blood sugar is lower than in the non-pregnant and is usually between 70–90 mg/100 ml, due to fetal consumption. In diabetic pregnancy the fasting blood sugar may exceed 120 mg/100 ml following the ingestion of 50 g of glucose disguised in a draught of about 300 ml of flavoured water. Thereafter capillary or venous blood sugar levels are estimated every half hour along with urine testing for 2½ hours.

In the normal pregnant woman there may be an initial sharp rise in glucose levels but it should not exceed 180 mg/100 ml. A higher rise, associated with a time lag of return to 120 mg of more than 2 hours denotes diabetes mellitus. The normal rate of fall is a little slower in pregnancy because the action of insulin is partly impeded by human placental lactogen.

As can be imagined there is quite a bit of a morning's work here and the test leaves room for improvement.

We ourselves are interested in a modified glucose tolerance test introduced by one of our members[10] which is very suitable for outpatient practice and involves simply the taking of a fasting venous blood specimen and a two-hour specimen following 50 g of glucose orally, and dispensing with urine testing. Using this test the criteria of the fasting blood sugar in the normal case should be less than 110 mg per cent and the two-hour specimen should not be more than 30 mg above the fasting level. If either figure is abnormal, then a full glucose tolerance test curve is done. The convenience of such an arrangement is very obvious, without loss of diagnostic accuracy.

Because standard glucose tolerance testing may be affected by the rate of absorbing the glucose administered and for the rapid screening of women at risk, the use of the intravenous method is advocated by Sutherland and Stowers in Aberdeen. Here 25 g of glucose is given intravenously, using heparinised syringes to avoid local venous complications. Also nausea and vomiting do not occur. False positive tests may be due to thiazide diuretics which cause hyperglycaemia and should be borne in mind.

Some such test of glucose tolerance as above should be undertaken in the case of all antenatal patients who have been delivered of a previous child weighing more than 4·25 kg, or in whom there is a significant family history, or in whom there has been a rapid increase in obesity at any period previously and lastly when glycosuria occurs more than once.

The commonest cause of glycosuria in pregnancy is a lowered renal threshold. In these cases the sugar tolerance curve is perfectly normal. This lowering of the renal threshold is a common physiological occurrence in normal pregnancy, but it occurs also in diabetes, and may make the latter much more difficult to control. The renal threshold usually falls between the third and the fifth month of pregnancy, and may remain at this low level until after delivery. The condition is of no pathological significance and no treatment is indicated.

A less common type of physiological glycosuria is that referred to by some as alimentary. It is due to a rapid absorption of carbohydrate from the gut, which produces, temporarily, a level of blood sugar above the renal threshold before the mechanism of storage has had time to take effect.

In any case of doubt, glucose tolerance testing must be carried out without more ado. At this moment, as I write, I am smarting for my failure to take notice of mild and temporary glycosuria many weeks ago in early pregnancy of one of my patients whose father is a known diabetic. Her own past obstetric history is unblemished and her antenatal course uneventful, but she has just been delivered of a large, macerated stillborn baby at term. Only a fortnight ago (after the fetal heart had stopped without warning) did I ascertain her glucose tolerance which showed a diabetic type of curve without frank diabetes. Had such a curve been demonstrated a few months ago premature induction might have saved the baby. Although not yet a diabetic she is likely to become so in a few years. This matter is discussed later.

In not a few cases the existence of diabetes only comes to light as a result of the patient's routine examination in pregnancy.

While it is important to diagnose diabetes if present as early as possible in pregnancy, for the positive reasons of being able to institute treatment early and to stave off some of the worst disasters, it is catastrophic to fail to make the diagnosis through omission to test the urine for sugar. A case so neglected may, a few weeks later, present in coma provoked by an acute infection or some other such complication.

Maternal Mortality

Before insulin was introduced there was an immediate maternal mortality of over 25 per cent of the cases who approached anywhere near term. A few of these died during pregnancy, but the majority in the puerperium. As many again died within the ensuing two years, so that the mortality, as the result of pregnancy in diabetes, was about 50 per cent. Today the maternal mortality should be less than 0·5 per cent, even this figure taking into account the attendant dangers of major surgery such as Caesarean section.

Fetal Mortality

Effect of Maternal Diabetes on the Baby

The longer a patient has suffered from diabetes the more hazardous does pregnancy become for both mother and child, particularly if the duration of the disease exceeds 25 years, and it depends to a large extent upon the pre-existence of vascular disease. Peel and Oakley, however, did not consider that fetal mortality is appreciably influenced by the duration of diabetes. White has drawn attention to the condition of the blood vessels of the mother in fetal prognosis, and reports that, where radiological evidence of calcification of blood vessels within the pelvis exists, the chances of fetal survival are no more than 10 per cent.

Unfortunately, the introduction of insulin has not conferred the same benefits upon the baby as it has upon the mother, and the fetal loss, due to intra-uterine and neonatal death, remains a challenge which fully justifies a specialised interest in the subject as at King's College Hospital.[3]

Peel states that intra-uterine fetal death is particularly liable to occur in cases where the diabetes is inadequately controlled, where hydramnios is marked, when the baby's size is clearly excessive, in hypertension and in the pre-diabetic state. One-third of his cases died *in utero* and well over half of them died shortly after birth. This was in marked contrast to the number of babies dying in a less well controlled series, in which almost half died *in utero*, a quarter died during labour, and a further quarter died in the neonatal period. It would appear, therefore, that treatment not only influences the gross fetal survival rate, but the period at which death occurs, and, in this matter, earlier termination of pregnancy has had a considerable effect. It is now generally agreed that the intra-uterine death rate rises progressively during the last six weeks of pregnancy.

In my own unit in Glasgow in four years we delivered thirty diabetic mothers with only two neonatal deaths and no stillbirths, a perinatal mortality of 6·7 per cent, and in both of these serious complicating factors operated, namely severe pre-eclamptic toxaemia in one and Rh haemolytic disease in the other. In the 700 cases at King's College Hospital already referred to, ninety per cent were established diabetics and in these the perinatal loss was 33 per cent when there were additional complications.

Otherwise the loss had been reduced to 16 per cent and is now reported to be lower still.[3]

The following factors influence the baby's chance of survival:

1. *Proper control of the maternal diabetes.* Although brief ketosis or hypoglycaemia seldom cause the death of the baby, diabetic coma is unquestionably dangerous.
2. *Pre-eclamptic toxaemia.* The occurrence of this complication more than doubles the fetal mortality in the case of diabetic pregnancy as compared with non-diabetic, and although it is only one of the causes of intra-uterine death, it is associated with a fetal loss of about 45 per cent.
3. *Essential hypertension.*
4. *Fetal abnormality.* The incidence here is very much higher and ranges from 4 to 6 per cent in different centres.
5. *Prematurity.* In a large number of cases labour is deliberately induced or Caesarean section performed some weeks before term, but in a significant number the spontaneous onset of premature labour also occurs.
6. *The existence of hydramnios.* Although frequently associated with fetal abnormality, it is present, to some degree, in all diabetic pregnancies. If severe, it may precipitate spontaneous premature labour, or it may call for treatment which incidentally brings pregnancy to an end. It is often to be regarded as a sinister sign and betokens a higher risk of fetal death.[4]
7. *The age of onset of the diabetes and the duration of the disease before pregnancy.* On the whole the younger the onset the worse the outlook.
8. *Dystocia.* This may occur during labour because the baby is unusually large. With proper obstetric supervision this factor should not operate.
9. *Asphyxia at birth.* These babies, especially after Caesarean section, may be very difficult to resuscitate. (See chapter on resuscitation of the newborn.)
10. *Fetal hypoglycaemia immediately after birth.* The blood sugar in normal babies is about 40 to 50 mg per cent during the first 24 hours of life, but in diabetic babies the level is often lower and may reach 25 mg per cent, which accentuates the tremendous difference from the conditions obtaining while still *in utero.* Before birth, the fetus tends to have a very high blood sugar comparable with that of its mother. Although it very quickly adjusts itself to its new environment, some degree of hyperinsulinism immediately after birth is likely to make itself felt because there is pancreatic islet cell hyperplasia.
11. *Atelectasis.* This is very common, and, as discussed in the chapter on resuscitation of the newborn, it may have something to do with the large quantities of fluid present in the stomach

at birth, especially after Caesarean section. The fluid is regurgitated and aspirated, and whereas the child begins by breathing fairly well, it develops cyanotic attacks a few hours afterwards and dies with atelectasis and the clinical picture of respiratory distress syndrome.

12. *Jaundice.* Jaundice may retard the child's progress from the second day onwards until it fades.

Most of the neonatal deaths occur within the first 48 hours, by far the larger number occurring within the first 12.

Lastly, there is an increased risk of neonatal infection, especially after vaginal delivery. Considering this formidable list of hazards, it is remarkable that the results are not worse.

The babies are so large for the period of gestation that they have in the past frequently been wrongly classed as postmature. In appearance, these babies at birth often look as fat as butter, for they are bloated and oedematous. Their behaviour is lethargic, and cyanotic attacks appear to occur with a sort of indolent ease. Both spleen and liver are usually enlarged, and in both these organs there is excessive haemopoiesis. The heart is also somewhat enlarged, and in the pancreas there is islet hyperplasia. Placental insufficiency is often postulated to account for these overgrown babies who die so readily *in utero* but this is almost impossible to establish from examination and histology of the placenta. Endometritis may be seen in biopsies of the placental bed but only in those diabetic cases complicated by pre-eclampsia or hypertension (Peel).

The very wide variation in fetal prospects shown by different workers only serves to emphasise the need for very close co-operation between physician, obstetrician, and paediatrician, and this factor, more than any other, must influence the results.

The Pre-diabetic State

Pre-diabetes can only be a retrospective diagnosis at present and wisdom is more likely to be demonstrated after the event than before.

Much interest has been focused upon the association of large babies and mothers who subsequently develop diabetes mellitus. While it has long been known that diabetic women tended to have large babies, it is only more recently that the association has been noticed in cases exhibiting a latent interval, often amounting to many years, before developing the disease. Kriss and Futcher noted that 77 per cent of 144 babies whose birth weights exceeded 4·7 kg were born to women who subsequently developed diabetes, and, where a family history of diabetes existed, they noted too that the babies tended to be larger. They regard birth weights of over 4·7 kg as significant, and it would appear that the average birth weight was greater in prediabetic cases than in those who had actually developed the disease.

The latent interval between the birth of such a child and the development of clinical diabetes may range up to 40 years, and Kriss and Futcher give the average as 24 years. What is even more important is that there is a higher fetal mortality during the maternal pre-diabetic state than normal, although the onset of true diabetes worsens the fetal outlook still further. Peel and Oakley quote a fetal loss of 23 per cent in pre-diabetic pregnancies, and Gilbert and Dunlop found that the over-all pre-diabetic fetal loss rate was twice as high as in non-diabetic pregnancy and three times as high in cases developing diabetes before the age of 45.

It also appears that the fetal mortality rate increases the nearer the mother is to developing the full-blown disease, and the loss is at its highest in the two years before its appearance, reaching a figure which is not worsened during the period of established diabetes. The pre-diabetic loss rate, however, gives no indication of the severity of the diabetes to follow.

At a superficial glance it would appear that the babies of prediabetic mothers have a higher birth weight than those born to frank diabetics, but it is not nowadays possible to make a comparison, since pregnancy is so commonly interrupted prematurely when the diagnosis is established.

Considering the high perinatal death rate in the phase of maternal pre-diabetes it would be useful if the diagnosis could be reliably established before catastrophe overtook the baby. To this end glucose tolerance curves are none too helpful although a tendency to the "lag" type of curve is often seen. Cortisone has a known diabetogenic activity and Fajans and Conn (1954) used this in developing the cortisone-stressed glucose tolerance test in the hope of unmasking the potential diabetic whose carbohydrate tolerance was still normal by ordinary standards. The technique which they devised was to carry out first a normal glucose tolerance test after a standard 300 g daily diet of carbohydrate for 3 days and then to repeat the test next day following a priming with 50 to 62·5 mg of cortisone orally administered 8½ and 2 hours before the same glucose load as before. They found not only a number of hitherto undiagnosed diabetics among the relatives of known diabetics, but also found a positive result to the cortisone-stressed tolerance test in no less than 24 per cent of these relatives of diabetics whose own diabetes had not yet declared itself.

Obstetricians as a whole, however, have not taken up the cortisone-stressed glucose tolerance test and Peel, for example, frankly regards it as unreliable and misleading. Certainly a family history and a history of large, stillborn babies is far more significant.

Although diabetes, as already mentioned, is a cause of infertility, this would not appear to be the case while the woman is still in the pre-diabetic state. It is now recognised as almost certain that excessive secretion of the growth factor by the anterior lobe of the pituitary is responsible for the combination of progressive maternal obesity, large babies, and the subsequent onset of diabetes. Certainly if women who have had babies weighing more than 4·7 kg are followed up for a number of years diabetes is likely to declare itself in a significant number.

Fitzgerald *et al.* (1961) in Birmingham studied 61 such cases and 20 were already diabetic within thirteen years and more than half those whose ages at the follow-up examination were over 45 years had abnormal glucose tolerance curves.

Growth Hormone and Diabetic Pregnancy

The role of the pituitary growth hormone has been studied by Young in relation to experimental diabetes. This worker, in the experimental extracts used, has not been able to demonstrate the separate existence of growth hormone, diabetogenic hormone, and pancreatotrophic hormone, and it seems that these three separate effects are merely related facets of the same substance.

The large size of the baby is not due to postmaturity, because, contrary to traditional belief, diabetic pregnancy is not often abnormally prolonged. Young has pointed out that for the growth hormone to operate, additional insulin together with an adequate blood sugar range must be produced by the pancreatic islets. This is produced either by the direct effect of the growth hormone upon the pancreas, thus increasing the production of insulin, or, he suggests, the growth hormone may antagonise the peripheral action of insulin, and may cause it to be utilised in the tissues at such a high rate that the level of insulin in the blood falls, and as a result the islets may be stimulated to produce even more.

The known hypertrophy of the fetal pancreatic islets in cases of maternal diabetes is due to hyperplasia of the beta cells and insulin is therefore more copiously produced in response to the high blood sugar levels obtaining both in mother and fetus *in utero*, so that carbohydrate utilisation and storage as fat leads to the characteristic fat overgrown baby of such a pregnancy. This hypothesis has been soundly confirmed by Baird and Farquhar (1962) who demonstrated the rise in neonatal plasma insulin-like activity (PIA) in response to a glucose load administered via the umbilical vein.

Now the rat's epiphyses do not fuse throughout life, and if given growth hormone it does not develop diabetes but grows larger. The same effect has been found in puppies and kittens, but if adult dogs and cats are given enough growth hormone for a long enough period of time, the rate of growth declines and diabetes makes its appearance. If, however, sufficient insulin is now given at the same time, the diabetes is controlled and the rate of growth is resumed. It is only when the pancreas is called upon to produce more insulin than it can achieve that diabetes occurs. So long as an animal is capable of continuing its growth under the stimulus of the growth hormone, diabetes does not develop, but if further growth, for example in the adult whose epiphyses are already fused, cannot continue beyond a certain point, then diabetes follows.

In other words, the growth hormone in the young animal produces growth and not diabetes, and Young was not able to induce diabetes by this method in pregnant animals, because the alternative result of extra growth was reflected in the development of the fetus. A small but continuous over-production of growth hormone, therefore, over a number of years demonstrates itself preferentially in the production of large babies and only later in the overt development of the diabetic state.

During pregnancy itself the hormones connected with placental function, namely oestrogen, progesterone, and chorionic gonadotrophin, were studied by Priscilla White, and Smith and Smith, but Peel suggested that any hormone imbalance is the result of failing placental function and not the cause of it.

An enquiry conducted by the Medical Research Council (1955) found that the perinatal mortality was practically the same whether stilboestrol and ethisterone were given or not and that there was very little difference in the other complications.

Maternal Complications

Pregnancy is liable to aggravate the diabetic condition, and it may bring it out of latency, since many cases do not declare themselves until pregnancy occurs. In diabetes, the patient is prematurely aged both physically and gynaecologically by vascular disease and threatened ovarian failure respectively. It is small wonder, therefore, that certain complications, notably pre-eclamptic toxaemia, are prone to occur.

As pregnancy advances, carbohydrate tolerance is reduced and insulin requirements usually tend to rise, especially after the sixth month until shortly before term, although in a few cases the reverse may obtain. The renal threshold is very often reduced, and the patient loses sugar through her urine in even greater quantities than before, with the result that acidosis more easily occurs. Under these circumstances, in combating acidosis with insulin, hypoglycaemia is very easily provoked, especially during the night, so that the patient becomes more and more difficult to stabilise. Any diabetic patient, therefore, who is likely to get hypoglycaemic reactions when not pregnant will now become much more vulnerable in this respect. Another feature of diabetic pregnancy is the increased liability to undue water retention, which is often associated with pre-eclamptic toxaemia and with the appearance of hydramnios.

Hydramnios, as previously stated, is almost invariably present in some degree, and is marked in about a quarter of the cases.

Pre-eclamptic toxaemia supervenes in about one case in every five and very greatly worsens the fetal prognosis. In a large proportion of cases it is a terminal event, and its incidence in diabetic pregnancy is inevitably reduced somewhat in those centres where pregnancy is deliberately interrupted at the 37th week. Frequently hydramnios and pre-eclamptic toxaemia are co-existent. The amniotic sugar level is always raised, although the level is not related directly to the amount of excess fluid. The reason for hydramnios is not certain, but it is possible that the baby, as a result of its own hyperglycaemia, passes more urine than usual, and the presence of the sugar within the amniotic fluid may irritate the amnion to produce increased amounts of liquor, quite apart from the factor of increased osmosis. Because of hydramnios, malpresentations are naturally more common, and likewise premature labour more readily occurs. As already stated, intra-uterine death becomes increasingly likely during the last four or five weeks of pregnancy.

Any acute intercurrent infection, notably pyelitis, in the course of pregnancy may have far-reaching consequences. Not only is the patient's resistance lower than that of the non-diabetic, but the control of her diabetes is immediately undermined, and she may get out of control and go into coma.

Diabetic retinopathy or nephropathy carry a very serious hazard to both mother and child.

The onset of labour is rarely postmature, and inertia frequently complicates its course. Difficulties may arise during labour due to the large size of the baby, and disproportion may prejudice the issue. Even after successful delivery of the head, large shoulders may obstruct safe delivery.

In the puerperium infection, too, may take a serious course, and full lactation is hard to achieve.

Management in Pregnancy

Provided that the patient is well controlled throughout pregnancy, the diabetic state is not permanently worsened. Unfortunately, many of these cases are hard to stabilise and constant supervision is necessary. It is often not possible to get the urine sugar-free, and in many cases it is undesirable, because hypoglycaemia readily occurs as a result of the associated lowering during pregnancy of the renal threshold to glucose, and the help of an experienced physician is invaluable in deciding not only the optimum dosage of insulin but the spacing of the injections.

Even in apparently well-controlled diabetes there are quite sharp alterations in blood sugar levels during each twenty-four hours. Hypoglycaemia is particularly likely to occur in the small hours of the morning.

The badly controlled case of glycosuria may lose up to 100 g glucose in a day and develop ketosis so that the carbohydrate intake has to be increased to not less than 200 g per day as well as increasing the insulin dosage and dividing its timing.

For the above reasons soluble insulin is to be preferred to the long-acting forms and changes in dosage are best made in small steps of 5 units at a time. Mixtures of soluble and isophane insulin are often suitable to provide night cover.

In the case requiring frequent blood sugar estimations, especially during the stabilisation process the Dextrostic glucose-oxidase test provides a rapid and useful method especially at night.

Insulin hardly crosses the placenta but oral hypoglycaemic agents do and may stimulate fetal pancreatic islet tissue. These oral diabetic drugs can be divided into two main groups, namely, the sulphonylureas and the diguanides. Two commonly used examples of the former are tolbutamide and chlorpropamide and their main action is to stimulate the release of endogenous insulin with possibly an increase in the viable beta cells of the pancreatic islets, hence the hypoglycaemic action. It also appears that the liver may be inhibited in its output of glucose. Clearly the sulphonylureas will only be useful in cases capable of producing insulin under the stimulus of such drugs and therefore the sulphonylureas are to some extent restricted to the middle-aged with diabetes of relatively recent onset. Diabetic patients with a history of ketosis do not respond well. The drugs of the sulphonylurea class vary in their biological half-life, from a few hours in the case of tolbutamide to about a couple of days in the case of chlorpropamide and the latter may accumulate dangerously if there is any element of renal failure. In addition to this there are toxic effects, mainly of a dyspeptic nature; very rarely marrow aplasia and intra-canalicular biliary stasis have been attributed to them. The diguanides work in a totally different manner by stimulating the uptake of glucose in muscle, rather than in fat, and there is increased production and accumulation of lactate and pyruvate. The blood sugar may be brought down but without preventing diabetic ketosis and again toxic dyspeptic side-effects may be caused. The main use of the diguanides (phenformin and metformin) is to supplement the action of the sulphonylureas and to assist in weight loss in the obese diabetic. Quite apart from their failure, even in combination, to prevent ketosis in diabetic patients who are already insulin-deficient, which is what we are commonly facing in obstetrics, control is very difficult to maintain and toxicity is readily incurred. Consequently our own view is that the oral hypoglycaemic drugs are far better replaced by proper insulin control during pregnancy.

There is no evidence that these drugs are teratogenic in humans. They are, in fact, said to have a place in the management of Asian pregnant diabetics who may have a different pattern of the disease with higher-than-normal plasma insulin levels.[1]

Ketoacidosis must at all costs be prevented since it is particularly lethal to the fetus.

The importance of diabetic control increases as pregnancy advances and beyond the 30th week it must be rigorous indeed to reduce the hyperglycaemia which stimulates fetal hyperinsulinism and so increases the fetal growth beyond the limits of placental reserve.

We now prefer to admit our diabetic mothers at the 30th week and certainly no later than the 32nd week so that this control can be maintained from day to day from then onwards; this is also made easier by securing more rest for the patient. Yet another advantage is the earlier detection of any rise of blood pressure. The aim of insulin control should be to maintain a blood sugar at least below 180 mg per cent, and down to less than 100 mg/100 ml before meals.

Infections should, so far as possible, be avoided, and when they occur should be treated seriously and energetically.

The diet should be generous and should provide 30 calories per kilogram of body weight a day, and the daily protein intake should not be less than 2 g per kilogram of body weight. The total daily intake of carbohydrate should not be less than 200 g, allowance being made for the needs of the baby's growth. It is often advisable to restrict sodium intake, especially in those cases in which the weight is rising unduly rapidly. Where there is evidence of undue water retention, frusemide 40 mg on alternate days should suffice.

The patient should be seen at fortnightly intervals throughout pregnancy until admission at the 30th week, and the blood pressure and urine should be examined at each visit. In every case an X-ray of the fetus should be taken, because the discovery of a fetal abnormality will influence the method of delivery. In cases allowed to proceed to spontaneous labour it is often found that insulin requirement falls a day or two before delivery.

Interruption of Pregnancy

There is practically no indication for therapeutic abortion except for retinopathy and diabetic nephropathy which carry a high perinatal mortality rate in any case as well as maternal hazard. In other respects, however bad the past obstetric history, skilful management should nowadays be fully effective. Sterilisation after delivery is seldom indicated except in cases demonstrating a permanently raised blood pressure.

After the 36th week of pregnancy the risk of intra-uterine death of the fetus overtakes that of neonatal death, and one has to strike a balance between leaving a baby in its unhealthy environment or challenging it to cope with prematurity, which it is ill-equipped to fight. Any set rule for determining when to deliver the child is to be deplored, although the majority of obstetricians favour interrupting the pregnancy at the end of the 37th week. A mistake about dates may involve risk of a disastrous degree of prematurity. In deciding the optimum time one should take into account the presence or absence of pre-eclamptic toxaemia, the degree of hydramnios, the severity of the diabetes, the facilities for coping with prematurity and the patient's age and her obstetric history; therefore, it will be seen that there is no rule-of-thumb method. Our present technique is to study the continuing rate of fetal growth by repeated biparietal cephalometry by sonar, which is carried out every few days. As long as there is continuing fetal growth we feel it can safely be assumed that intra-uterine fetal death is not likely to occur in the immediate future, but that as soon as the growth curve flattens off delivery should be effected within the next seven to ten days in order to forestall such a disaster. In this way we are able to avoid unnecessary premature delivery, so often the result of rule-of-thumb practice, and obtain the maximum degree of maturity consistent with intra-uterine survival.

The commonest cause of neonatal death is the respiratory distress syndrome with the formation of hyaline membrane within the lungs producing secondary atelectasis. The likelihood of this can be to some extent foreseen by estimating the lecithin/sphingomyelin ratio in amniotic fluid obtained by amniocentesis not more than 48 hours before delivery. Normally this ratio rises above 2:1 as pulmonary maturity is achieved and is progressive, but in diabetic pregnancy the ratio may fail to continue its rise and may even fall, indicating the need for immediate delivery.[23]

Even this test however can be invalidated in the presence of ketosis which serves still further to emphasise the need for absolute diabetic control and the availability of expert paediatric care.

The practice of early termination tends to transfer one's fetal deaths from the column of stillbirth to that of neonatal death, but nearly two-thirds of the intra-uterine deaths occur during the last four weeks of pregnancy, and this must weight one's decision. There is a tendency to reserve surgical induction for multiparous patients who have previously delivered themselves satisfactorily by the vaginal route. In the primigravida the induction-delivery interval is often prolonged at this stage of pregnancy with its increased hazards both maternal and particularly fetal, and, even when labour starts, it is frequently inert. In all severe diabetics, therefore, and in primigravidae and elderly patients, Caesarean section is being increasingly favoured as an elective procedure. Our own policy is to rupture the membranes and induce labour surgically, even in primigravidae, with the reservation that if labour is not well established within 12 hours Caesarean section will be undertaken without more ado.

As a result of this policy more than half our diabetics are now delivered vaginally and the section rate has been reduced to 46 per cent. Two recent cases thus achieved vaginal deliveries who had been delivered before by Caesarean section by more timid obstetricians elsewhere and we feel that, given very thorough supervision, the risks of a "trial of induction" are insignificant and the advantages of an expeditious labour to mother and child are well worth the attempt.

Labour

When the fetus is normal, vaginal delivery is only permissible if there is no obstetrical abnormality apart from the diabetes, and any case of suspected cephalopelvic disproportion should be delivered by Caesarean section. Trial of labour has no place in the management of the diabetic patient. Where there is fetal abnormality, vaginal delivery should, of course, be sought if possible. The above categorical statement about disproportion is occasioned by the fear of a prolonged labour. This complication, from whatever cause, is very dangerous to both mother and child. In any labour lasting more than 24 hours, diabetes becomes increasingly difficult to control because of poor carbohydrate intake, vomiting and dehydration, with the result that the patient may easily develop ketosis. There is a strong case for expediting labour with escalating oxytocin dosage, properly monitored. Epidural anaesthesia is also valuable.

Hypoglycaemia becomes a constant and recurring nuisance, and during labour the carbohydrate intake should be maintained by intravenous drip therapy, up to 10 g of glucose per hour. Any isophane insulin is omitted the night before. The insulin dosage is split up into small injections given every four hours. One should aim to keep blood glucose levels between 80–100 mg/100 ml by hourly estimations. Where the patient threatens to become unstable, 20 units of insulin may be injected and covered by 40 g of glucose. If the patient does develop diabetic ketosis it may be observed that her low pH may be associated with a low P_{CO_2} due to hyperpnoea. If this is the case 200 to 500 milliequivalents of sodium bicarbonate may be required by intravenous infusion (1 ml of 8·4 per cent sodium bicarbonate equals 1 mEq). An intravenous 8 per cent glucose drip should be maintained until the patient is later feeding by mouth.

Since the patient's stabilisation can be so easily undermined by infection, there is something to be said for the use of prophylactic chemotherapy unless labour shows signs of being fairly rapid. These cases are very worrying in labour and require unremitting supervision.

The baby at birth must be very competently handled, for it is oedematous, lethargic, premature, prone to atelectasis and usually has a full stomach. Mucus must be very thoroughly aspirated by a tube passed into the stomach, in order to remove its contents before they are regurgitated and aspirated. An incubator should be immediately available, and the baby should be carefully supervised, even though apparently normal, for the first 48 hours, because it is very liable to develop a cyanotic attack and die without warning, even though its initial condition appears good. A rapid weight loss in the first 2 days is a very welcome sign.

The cord is often very thick, and broad tape may be more suitable than plastic clamps.

Puerperium

There is a sharp fall in the patient's insulin requirements immediately after delivery, and she is very liable to hypoglycaemia at first. The insulin dosage will therefore have to be re-adjusted, and it will be found that very much less is required during the first 24 hours. Thereafter, the patient must be restabilised.

The morbidity rate is not directly increased, but the effects of infection are more serious when they occur.

It is usually hard to establish satisfactory lactation, and the majority of diabetic mothers fail within a few days. The baby also, because of its lethargy and prematurity, is less efficient at sucking, and this contributes to the disappointing result. The baby also suffers from an initial, although usually short-lived, hypoglycaemia although after the first few hours of life it comes to better terms with its new blood sugar level. Feeding within the first 2 days is far more dangerous than not feeding it, and we have now abandoned the routine use of glucose in the early days since it would appear to make little difference to survival chances. Above all, the baby has fluid to get rid of and it would be wanton to replace it at this stage, but acute hypoglycaemia must be watched for and promptly corrected by intravenous injection.

REFERENCES

1. ALLAN, J. W. (1975). Personal communication.
2. BAIRD, J. D. and FARQUHAR, J. W. (1962). *Lancet*, **1,** 71.
3. BRUDENELL, M. (1974). Address to Glasgow & West of Scotland Obstetrical Society.
4. CLAYTON, S. G. (1956). *J. Obstet. Gynaec. Brit. Emp.*, **63,** 532.
5. FAJANS, S. S. and CONN, J. W. (1954). *Diabetes*, **3,** 296.
6. FINE, J. (1967). *Brit. med. J.*, **1,** 205.
7. FITZGERALD, M. G., MALINS, J. M. and O'SULLIVAN, D. J. (1961). *Lancet*, **1,** 1250.
8. GILBERT, J. A. L. and DUNLOP, D. M. (1949). *Brit. med. J.*, **1,** 48.
9. KRISS, J. P. and FUTCHER, P. H. (1948). *J. clin. Endocr.*, **8,** 380.
10. LUNAN, B. (1967). Personal communication.
11. Medical Research Council on Diabetes and Pregnancy (1955). *Lancet*, **2,** 833.
12. PEEL, J. (1955). *Brit. med. J.*, **2,** 870.
13. PEEL, J. (1961). *Proc. roy. Soc. Med.*, **54,** 745.
14. PEEL, J. and OAKLEY, W. (1949). *Trans. 12th Brit. Congr. Obs. Gyn.*
15. SMITH, O. W. (1948). *Amer. J. Obstet. Gynec.*, **56,** 821.
16. SMITH, O. W. and SMITH, G. V. S. (1949). *Amer. J. Obstet. Gynec.*, **58,** 994.
17. SUTHERLAND, H. W., STOWERS, J. M. and MCKENZIE, C. (1970). *Lancet*, **1,** 1069.
18. SUTHERLAND, H. W. and STOWERS, J. M. (1975). *Carbohydrate Metabolism in Pregnancy and Newborn.* Edinburgh: Churchill Livingstone.
19. TUNBRIDGE, R. E., PALEY, R. G. and COULSON, D. (1956). *Brit. med. J.*, **2,** 588.
20. WHITE, P. (1945). *J. Amer. med. Ass.*, **128,** 181.
21. WHITE, P. (1947). *Med. Clin. N. Amer.*, **31,** 395.
22. WHITE, P. (1949). *Amer. J. Med.*, **7,** 609.
23. WHITFIELD, C. R., SPROULE, W. B. and BRUDENELL, M. (1973). *J. Obstet. Gynaec. Brit. Cwlth*, **80,** 918.
24. YOUNG, F. G. (1951). *J. clin. Endocr.*, **11,** 531.

CHAPTER VII

ANAEMIA AND PULMONARY TUBERCULOSIS

ANAEMIA

ANAEMIA may antedate conception; it is often aggravated by pregnancy, and the accidents of labour may perpetuate it. It is one of the prime concerns of antenatal care to forestall it, for the safety of labour and the puerperal state, to say nothing of future health, in very large measure depend upon the state of the patient's blood. So much importance, in fact, do we now attach to this matter that it is the practice in our hospital to estimate the haemoglobin at every antenatal visit which the patient makes throughout pregnancy. In this way the early signs of incipient anaemia and failure to respond to medication are picked up at a very early stage, leaving plenty of time to evaluate and correct any deficiency. This is a counsel of perfection and where it is not possible to have a technician from the haematology department in attendance at every clinic, as we have, at least four haemoglobin estimations should be carried out in pregnancy, namely, at first booking, then at about 24 to 26 weeks' gestation, then between the 32nd and 34th week and finally just before term. It is not many patients who get even that much surveillance and the more is the pity, since megaloblastic anaemia particularly can become very rapidly manifest and leave inadequate time to correct it, as will presently be discussed. It often takes almost as long to identify the nature of a given anaemia as it takes to correct it, yet there can be no more important aspect of antenatal care. The patient who has been in a chronic state of sub-health from anaemia has a poor myocardium to match and it is a dangerous form of optimism to reckon that the immediate correction of anaemia is going to be followed by an immediate increase in the resilience of the patient to withstand a traumatic or infected labour, for which adequate preparation should have been instituted long before.

Physiology

Pregnancy causes a state of hydraemic plethora; in other words, the total volume of blood is increased partly by dilution, and the haemoglobin is consequently reduced to a varying extent, occasionally as low as 80 per cent (approximately 12 g per 100 ml). Levels below this are pathological, and one should aim at raising the haemoglobin to 80 per cent or more if possible before delivery. The dilution picture is, however, normochromic and normocytic.

This phenomenon is commonly regarded as physiological, which is not the same thing as saying that it is either beneficial or even necessary. It can, in fact, be a positive danger by increasing the circulatory burden, for example, in cases of cardiac disease, and, because of the reduced oxygen-carrying power of diluted blood the fetus may be less efficiently oxygenated. Nor is hydraemia an invariable accompaniment of pregnancy and most of us would agree that the term "physiological anaemia of pregnancy" were better dropped in recognising that in nearly all women the condition can be corrected before term.[4, 12] In round figures the pregnancy demands for iron come to a total of about 900 mg of which about 500 to 600 mg go to the uterus and its contents. Somewhere between 150 and 200 mg are accounted for in an average blood loss at delivery and a similar amount is expended in lactation. On top of this there is an increased maternal haemoglobin mass of about 500 mg, the iron of which is returned to store after delivery. On the credit side, however, there is an average saving of about 225 mg as a result of the amenorrhoea throughout pregnancy, but this still leaves a total likely ultimate iron deficit of about 600 or 700 mg. It will be seen, therefore, that time is required for a reasonable diet to make good the iron overdraft of pregnancy and consequently if pregnancies succeed each other rapidly the patient is unlikely to "get out of the red".

Just how common iron deficiency is amongst the women of the United Kingdom has been reviewed in an average housing estate practice on the West side of Glasgow, which also included some suburban communities and some of the poorer industrial districts. In this practice frank iron deficiency anaemia was present in over 8 per cent of cases, but latent iron deficiency without anaemia was found in at least three times as many of the female population of all ages.[19, 26, 27] These figures were obtained in women who were not pregnant, but serve to show that a large proportion of the population start their pregnancies short of iron. The term "latent iron deficiency" (i.e. tissue depletion of iron without anaemia) is defined as a state in which the saturation of the total iron binding capacity is below 16 per cent, but in which the haemoglobin level is above 12 g per 100 ml, as stainable marrow-iron will not be found in cases in which the TIBC is below 16 per cent.

The commonest source of trouble in anaemic pregnancy is inadequate absorption of iron. The normal daily requirement for the gravid woman is about 20 mg of iron, even in cases in which the iron stores have not suffered depletion prior to pregnancy. The baby, especially in the later months of pregnancy, makes heavy demands upon maternal iron, and the average fetal requirements amount to about 375 mg. Unfortunately, the margin between the patient's requirements and the quantity of iron normally available in a reasonably good diet is a very narrow one, in fact, the average diet seldom contains more than about 15 mg a day. Of the total amount of iron in food, only a fraction (about 10 per cent) is available for absorption. Natural foods, such as liver, meat, peas, eggs and certain dried fruits, for example apricots, are good sources of iron. Phytic acid, present in brown bread, which also contains iron, tends to interfere with iron absorption by combining with iron to form insoluble salts. The presence of calcium in the diet, however, tends to divert some of this phytic acid effect. Iron absorption is favourably influenced by the presence of hydrochloric acid in the stomach; conversely, the absence of hydrochloric acid or the copious intake of alkaline powders tends to reduce it. Intestinal disorders, for example chronic diarrhoea, naturally interfere with iron absorption. The ferrous salts, as is well known, are far more readily absorbed than the ferric, and vitamin C, amongst other properties, has the power of reducing ferric to ferrous iron, hence the dietary value of fresh-grown vegetables. The therapeutic implications are therefore obvious.

In the formation of red cells an active bone marrow requires not

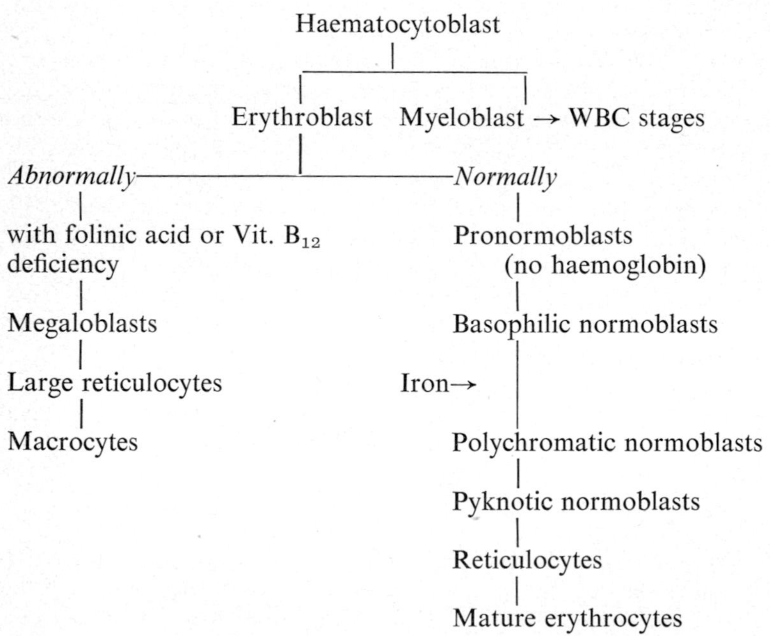

only iron and incidental traces of copper for haemoglobin formation, but also folic acid and vitamin B_{12}, vitamin C and nucleoprotein. The further role of vitamin C is to assist in the conversion of folic acid, derived from the vitamin B complex, into folinic acid, which is necessary for the synthesis of purines and pyrimidines which ultimately take part, with vitamin B_{12} (the haemopoietic principle), in the synthesis of nucleic acid and hence of nucleoprotein. The following diagram illustrates the level in haemopoiesis at which these dietetic factors operate.

Therefore it will be seen that a lack of folic acid gives rise to macrocytic or, as is now more usually described, "megaloblastic" anaemia. True pernicious anaemia is due to a lack of vitamin B_{12} and is rare in pregnancy.

After about four months the normal red cell disintegrates and the haemoglobin is broken down into haemosiderin and bile pigments.

Definitions

The following are some definitions:

The packed red cell volume (PCV) is the number of cubic centimetres of packed red cells per 100 ml of blood.

The mean corpuscular volume (MCV) is the average volume of one red cell in μm^3.

The mean corpuscular haemoglobin (MCH) is the average haemoglobin content of one red cell in picograms.

The mean corpuscular haemoglobin concentration (MCHC) is the mean or average haemoglobin concentration in percentage per unit volume of cells.

The difference between mean corpuscular haemoglobin (MCH) and mean corpuscular haemoglobin concentration (MCHC) should be clearly understood. The former measures the weight of haemoglobin in the average red corpuscle and expresses the result in parts of a gram (picogram); the latter (MCHC) indicates the concentration of haemoglobin in the average red cell, the ratio of weight of haemoglobin to the volume in which it is contained, and the result expressed in percentage. The distinction is an important one. In most types of anaemia, increases or decreases in the average size of the red corpuscles (MCV) are associated with corresponding increases or decreases in the weight of haemoglobin (MCH) carried in the corpuscles. The ratio of these to one another is indicated by the mean corpuscular haemoglobin concentration (MCHC).

The total iron binding capacity (TIBC) is represented by the level of unsaturated siderophyllin (transferrin) by serum iron and the saturation percentage is calculated from the ratio of serum iron to TIBC. In iron deficiency anaemia the serum iron may be only 60 μg per

100 ml and the TIBC might be as high as 400 μg of unsaturated siderophyllin per 100 ml. The ratio thus of Fe/TIBC × 100 would give a saturation percentage of

$$\frac{60}{400} \times 100 = 15 \text{ per cent.}$$

Normal Values

RBC 5 million/mm^3
Hb 14·8 g/100 ml
Reticulocytes 0·2 per cent
PCV (haematocrit) 39–42 per cent
MCV 78–94 μm^3
MCH 27–32 pg
MCHC 30 per cent (28–34 per cent)
Serum iron 60–120 μg/100 ml (level varies sharply during the day, falling in the later part and also in infection)
TIBC 325–400 μg/100 ml
Ratio Fe/TIBC (saturation) 30 per cent.

Examples.—In iron deficiency anaemia (hypochromic microcytic) the reduction in red cell volume and haemoglobin content is characteristically more marked than reduction in the number of red cells. MCHC is reduced.

Table of Equivalents

Hb per cent	*Hb g/100 ml*	*Hb per cent*	*Hb g/100 ml*
10	1·5	70	10·3
15	2·2	75	11·1
20	3·0	80	11·8
25	3·7	85	12·6
30	4·4	90	13·3
35	5·2	95	14·1
40	5·9	100	14·8
45	6·6	105	15·5
50	7·4	110	16·3
55	8·1	115	17·0
60	8·9	120	17·8
65	9·6		

In megaloblastic anaemia (macrocytic) the red cells are increased in volume, the mean corpuscular haemoglobin is proportionally increased, and there is an increase in the size and haemoglobin content of the red cells roughly inversely proportional to the number of cells. The mean corpuscular haemoglobin concentration remains fairly normal throughout or may be slightly reduced.

In normocytic anaemia the number of red cells is reduced without any or at most a slight increase in MCV, and the MCH and MCHC are normal throughout.

Clinically one may classify the anaemias associated with pregnancy as:

1. **Iron deficiency**
2. **Megaloblastic**
3. **Haemolytic**
4. **Secondary**, for example to repeated bleeding, chronic infection, Hodgkin's disease, etc.
5. **Aplastic varieties**
6. **Haemoglobinopathies**

Iron Deficiency Anaemia

This is the commonest type and, depending upon the social grades of patients, may be found in up to nearly a quarter of all pregnancies. Multiparity, previous menorrhagia and subnutrition favour its origin. It may be due to dietary insufficiency or to interferences with iron absorption. In the latter respect the digestive upsets which are common in pregnancy frequently operate adversely. Achlorhydria, too, if present, discourages absorption.

The importance of chronic infection in the aetiology of iron deficiency anaemia must not be overlooked and this is particularly true of chronic and apparently latent pyelonephritis. In fact a urinary infection may present as a case of apparently refractory anaemia and is more than twice as common in anaemic patients as in controls in spite of administering prophylactic iron and folic acid routinely in pregnancy.[18] In such cases appropriate antibacterial therapy is first necessary before a response to haematinics can be expected. The mechanism for this is not clear, but it must be a clinical observation common to all of us. One should not be put off by the absence of urinary symptoms as this type of infection is asymptomatic in about 90 per cent of cases.

More than one of the above types of anaemia may co-exist and, of course, their effects are additive.

In iron deficiency anaemia the blood picture shows both a low haemoglobin and a reduced packed cell volume, the colour index is less than unity, and the MCV and MCHC are both reduced. In other words, the picture is characteristically microcytic and hypochromic. New cells are being generated at the normal rate, and the reticulocyte count shows little deviation from normal. The cells, besides being smaller than usual, are of unequal sizes and staining (anisocytosis and polychromasia). There is no undue haemolysis, and the serum bilirubin is not increased. The bone marrow is normoblastic in character.

In our clinic in Glasgow less than 50 per cent of patients come to the antenatal clinic with a haemoglobin over 10 g/100 ml.[36] It is our practice to divide our antenatal cases from the point of view of anaemia into three groups—(1) those with haemoglobin levels above 12 g who, in our experience, have usually maintained their haematological wellbeing on a rechecking at the 34th to 36th week of pregnancy; (2) those with haemoglobin levels between 10 and 12 g (about 30 per cent of patients). These require routine iron by mouth and rechecking throughout pregnancy to make sure that they are not losing ground or failing to take their pills; (3) those who present with levels below 10 g per cent. These are referred to a special haematological clinic for intensive therapy and supervision. It would appear that the second group with levels between 10 and 12 g are cases who, though not yet ill, are of the low-iron-reserve group and who will almost certainly deteriorate under the demands of pregnancy unless prophylactic measures are taken forthwith to stop the drift.

The symptoms are often not very pronounced, but when present consist of fatigue, dyspnoea, palpitations, loss of appetite and digestive upset, and the patient usually demonstrates pallor of the mucous membranes and, in severe cases, a considerable degree of oedema, mainly of the lower extremities.

The treatment consists in making good the iron which the patient lacks, and the method will depend upon the time available before delivery. Provided one has at least ten weeks' grace and the anaemia is not severe, a satisfactory result can be obtained by oral medication, and there are many satisfactory preparations of ferrous salts now available. Ferrous sulphate (0·2 g tablets) is the cheapest of these and is suitable for most patients, but the more expensive ferrous gluconate, fumarate and succinate may produce less epigastric discomfort, nausea, vomiting and constipation in the minority who cannot tolerate ferrous sulphate. Preparations of ferrous succinate to which succinic acid has been added are absorbed better than others it is believed, because the transport of iron across the mucosal cells is facilitated by the addition of succinic acid. Most symptoms of intolerance to iron are more related to the dose of elemental iron itself than the actual preparation and therefore the daily dose of ferrous sulphate, for example, should not exceed three 200 mg tablets, taken during or after a meal. Increasing the dosage does not improve the haematological response and adverse side-effects may well demand a reduction. Ferrous fumarate being a rather drably coloured brown tablet is less dangerous if it gets into the hands of small children, as it is not so likely to be mistaken for a sweet. If acute iron poisoning occurs in a child who has got hold of iron tablets the danger is very real and calls for immediate treatment with desferrioxamine mesylate (Desferal) which, as a powerful iron chelator, may be life-saving. An intravenous infusion of this substance should be given at once in a dose of 20 ml in saline per kg every six hours for the next 24 to 48 hours; if for any reason such an infusion cannot be given immediately, an intramuscular injection of 1 g of desferrioxamine mesylate should be given meanwhile, the stomach should be washed out and 5 to 12 g of the same substance in half a litre of saline should be left in the stomach.

For cases in which the need for iron in pregnancy is more pressing, saccharated iron oxide preparations were introduced a few years ago for intravenous injection. This was a very important step forward in the treatment of iron deficiency states but these substances are not without their risks. For example, a test dose is always necessary first since alarming collapse and other sensitivity reactions such as dizziness, dyspnoea, vomiting and backache occur in about 5 per cent of cases even with careful selection.[35] Furthermore, the darkness of these solutions makes it difficult to check that the point of the syringe needle is in the lumen of the vein and a perivenous injection is very irritant to the tissues. For these reasons a solution suitable for intramuscular injection was gladly welcomed when it first appeared in the form of iron dextran complex (Imferon). It had hitherto been impossible to administer iron parenterally without the penality of toxicity from the ionised metal and this difficulty was first overcome by binding ferric hydroxide to carbohydrates to form substances of a high molecular weight. Intramuscular iron dextran came in for extensive and enthusiastic use at the hands of all of us, since very favourable results were reported with an incidence of reactions in less than 0·5 per cent in some hundreds of cases.[37] A serious disadvantage, however, was the discoloration of the overlying skin so that the patient looked as though she had been beaten black and blue. This staining lasted a very long time, usually some years, although it was possible to reduce it by skilful technique such as the Z-technique which involves pulling the tissues laterally while the needle is being inserted so that the needle track, and therefore the track of back leakage, is zig-zagged. A further refinement is to inject a small quantity of saline down the needle before withdrawing it.

The enthusiasm for parenteral iron however is steadily diminishing as it is fairly widely recognised that the increase in haemoglobin concentration is only marginally accelerated as compared with oral medication. One of the commonest troubles is that the patient is not taking her iron and the easiest way to find out is to inquire of her about the colour of her stools. If she reports that they are normal instead of black, one can be certain that she is not, in fact, taking her iron tablets.

Intramuscular iron therapy received a setback in popularity with reports that sarcoma could be induced at the site of intramuscular injection in rats subjected to massive doses of iron dextran complex (Imferon),[34] a finding confirmed in both rats and mice a year later.

Fortunately at about this time an iron-sorbitol citric-acid-complex (iron sorbitol) came on the market with the trade name Jectofer. The molecule of this substance is smaller than the iron dextran molecule and is therefore more rapidly absorbed, so greatly reducing the possible hazards of local irritation at the injection site and the possibility of sarcomatous reaction. Various workers were quick to investigate the absorption and clearance rates from the site of injection by labelling the iron sorbitol with radioiron.[33, 41] It was found that the mean half-time for clearance at the injection site was 46 minutes in iron-deficient patients and 174 minutes in controls and that clearance from the site was almost complete in ten days. Also in treating iron-deficient subjects and comparing them with cases similarly investigated after iron dextran injection, it was found that all the iron had been removed from the injection site within ten hours in the case of iron sorbitol whereas between 17 and 45 per cent of the radioactive iron was still at the injection site at the end of 20 days in the cases treated with iron dextran. This persistence at the injection site would appear to be a function of the respective molecular weights. There is, of course, wastage in the case of iron sorbitol due to loss of about 30 per cent in the urine,[38] but this does not matter provided it is taken into account in deciding on dosage.

Iron sorbitol (Jectofer) contains 50 mg of elemental iron per ml and is supplied in ampoules of 2 ml. The recommended dose is 1·5 mg of iron per kilogram of body weight, given daily, or on alternate days, so an adult weighing approximately 70 kg would receive one ampoule (100 mg of iron) in a single dose. It takes about 200 mg of iron in women to raise the haemoglobin value by 1 g per 100 ml of blood, or 350 mg of iron to raise the haemoglobin level by 100 per cent in rough figures. The total dose should be calculated to compensate for the haemoglobin deficit and the makers recommend an additional amount to replenish iron stores, certainly not less than 250 mg. A course of 10 to 20 injections is usual. The drug is very well tolerated and does not discolour the skin. In our experience we have had no untoward reactions. Since instituting the policy of estimating the haemoglobin at every antenatal visit, however, and full and early prophylaxis with oral prophylaxis, the need for parenteral iron including Jectofer has dropped astonishingly in our antenatal practice.

In a comparison of oral, intramuscular and intravenous routes of iron administration, ferrous succinate by mouth was found to be just as effective as the other two methods, though not so rapid in pregnancy.

Even parenteral iron, however, is not effective at once in raising the haemoglobin level for at least two weeks, but an earlier indication of a favourable response can often be seen in a reticulocyte count which may exceed 12 per cent.

The absence of a response is an indication for full investigation, even marrow biopsy, rather than the blind repetition of intramuscular injections.

The iron dextran preparation Imferon, originally designed for intramuscular use, came back into popularity in the form of total dose intravenous iron infusion, introduced in 1963.[2] In this treatment the total iron requirements are supplied over a matter of several hours in one dose calculated on the formula, *total dose in iron in mg equals the weight in pounds* × *the haemoglobin deficit in percentage* × 0·3. The dose is given in solution diluted to 5 per cent in normal saline, or 5 per cent dextrose, immediately before setting up the infusion with additional precautions of cleaning the skin of the arm with ether soap and without alcohol, and the administration of an antihistamine orally, thirty minutes before starting. The infusion itself is very cautiously started for the first quarter to half hour at a rate of only ten drops a minute initially.[3] There is a particular value in this crash type of treatment in cases of severe iron deficiency associated with abortion, who, after evacuation of the uterus, have a trick of disappearing and not coming back for follow-up. Certainly we ourselves have found more use for total dose iron infusion in gynaecological practice, including cases of anaemia from abortion and women with recurrent menorrhagia heading for hysterectomy, than in obstetrical practice. Unfortunately there are frequently troublesome complications from total dose iron infusion, such as a very painful arm from local phlebitis and, in pregnancy particularly, there seems to be a tendency to severe and alarming reactions demanding resuscitation. No less than seven out of 150 cases so treated come into this alarming category.[8] The series quoted here from Hull is possibly exceptional. A possible explanation[25] is that the cases had an unsuspected folic acid deficiency which was unmasked and that treatment with oral iron before the infusion was given had triggered off a sensitivity reaction. The value and the hazards of total iron transfusion may continue to be debated and our own practice is to reserve the treatment as already stated for gynaecological cases and not as a form of crash treatment in pregnancy. Furthermore parenteral iron should not be given without first proving the existence of iron deficiency by estimating the serum Fe/TIBC ratio to be less than 20 per cent and aggressive iron therapy is positively contra-indicated where there is iron overload, for example in thalassaemia.

The maximum haemoglobin response to this treatment does not appear for between four to nine weeks, so that if the treatment is not started until the last month of pregnancy there may be insufficient time to raise the haemoglobin to a safe level (10 g) before delivery. Under such circumstances blood transfusion, usually with packed cells, should be given; if labour has already started, however, and the anaemia is severe, transfusion may cause a rigor in which the fetus may die. In such desperate and late cases it is probably safer to keep a saline or glucose drip running during labour, with ergometrine and cross-matched blood to hand in case of postpartum haemorrhage.

Severe Anaemia late in Pregnancy

This problem, with labour imminent, is an ugly one. Such cases are already on the verge of circulatory failure and a transfusion of any appreciable quantity of blood may throw an immediate and fatal burden upon a myocardium that cannot cope with it. In West Africa, for example, the effects of malnutrition, particularly in respect of iron and folic acid, are aggravated by haemolysis due to malaria and sickle-cell anaemia with a further contribution from ankylostomiasis. In the Lagos district of Nigeria the incidence of anaemia, that is to say with a haemoglobin below 10 g per 100 ml is over 65 per cent, which is more than three times the incidence in Glasgow; nor is it necessarily related to multiparity because primigravidae appear to be even more afflicted. Furthermore the incidence of megaloblastic anaemia is high and adds very greatly to the severity of the effects of sickle-cell anaemia.[30] Anaemia accounts for over 20 per cent of all maternal deaths. In Ibadan, Nigeria, congestive cardiac failure is present in about a third of the cases.[14] It would appear that the lower the haematocrit reading (and PCV levels of less than 8 per cent are not uncommon) the more likely is the patient to die of congestive cardiac failure.

As a means of countering this desperate situation, without adding to the total blood volume load, Fullerton and Turner described a technique of partial exchange transfusion. The procedure is not actually an exchange transfusion in the literal sense since that would require truly enormous quantities of blood, but their aim is to transfuse up to $1\frac{1}{2}$ litres of concentrated red cells simultaneously removing the same volume of blood plus 100 to 200 millilitres from the opposite femoral vein, so that the patient ends up with a deficit in blood volume but with an enormous improvement in oxygen-carrying capacity. This procedure is now adopted in all patients with a PCV of under 13 per cent, even as late as the second stage of labour. A pump is necessary to maintain negative pressure to ensure reliable withdrawal. The needles, tubing and syringes are siliconed and the patient is heparinised. Infusion and venesection proceed simultaneously with the outflow rate exceeding the infusion rate, at least for the first half litre, so that the benefit of the reduced blood volume will be felt by the heart at once. With good organisation they were able to carry out the operation in less than twenty minutes and the immediate effect is dramatic—the patient recovering consciousness from coma and now able to withstand operative procedures. The mortality was thus reduced from 20 per cent to under 3 per cent in well over 400 cases.

This is clearly a life-saving procedure for cases presenting in a truly desperate state and in the United Kingdom it is rarely necessary, but our limited experience confirms all that is claimed for it. The simultaneous use of a powerful diuretic such as frusemide helps to maintain a negative fluid balance. These patients who have usually been anaemic for a long time have pronounced myocardial ischaemia, which may be accompanied by a great increase in heart size, and at necropsy the weight of the heart is increased and the myocardium is described as having "a thrush breast" appearance. Transfusion even of packed cells without using the exchange technique can kill by precipitating further cardiac failure with pulmonary oedema. A further report from Durban, South Africa, confirms the safety of exchange transfusion. In dealing with patients with a haemoglobin below 4·4 g per 100 ml (30 per cent) the indications for this operation are given as:

1. All cases of cardiac failure due to severe anaemia;
2. All cases of severe anaemia facing urgent operation;
3. Pregnant patients with severe anaemia whatever the type who are approaching term.[31]

What is perhaps the most important advantage is that the patient can be more or less made safe within a matter of just over 20 minutes by exchange transfusion as compared with at least three days following conventional packed cell infusion. Unfortunately the amount of blood that has to be used is considerable and an ingenious suggestion has been made that the blood already withdrawn from the patient should be centrifuged in a special apparatus and spun at 1200 r.p.m. for twenty minutes and then, after withdrawing the serum, the remaining packed cells are reinfused into the patient. This type of plasmaphaeresis may indeed save a great volume of cells which are obviously acceptable to the patient.[32]

Megaloblastic Anaemia

We once thought, not so very long ago, that megaloblastic anaemia was uncommon in this country and there are some who still do. Incidence figures of one in two thousand pregnancies have often been quoted, but in recent years the incidence works out in Glasgow, for example, at between 2 and 4 per cent of all pregnancies. The figure is considerably higher in parts of the world where nutrition is worse and especially where haemolytic factors either congenital or parasitic operate. It is particularly common in West Africa and Fullerton and Watson-Williams (1962) found megaloblastic erythropoiesis in the majority of patients whose initial haemoglobin in pregnancy was less than 7 g per 100 ml. The association of haemolysis due to malaria with megaloblastic anaemia is well known, but these workers have drawn attention to other types of haemolysis as being likewise responsible particularly, for example, haemoglobin SC disease. Although this variety of sickle-cell anaemia accounted for less than 10 per cent of their cases in Ibadan they hoped by this study to explain the development of megaloblastic anaemia in all patients who suffer from haemolytic conditions as a primary cause of their anaemia. They found that folic acid clearance was very rapid even before megaloblastic anaemia appeared and they reckoned that when the rate of red cell destruction is about twice normal, the compensatory marrow hyperplasia, together with the demands of the fetus, rapidly exhaust the available supplies of folic acid whereupon erythropoiesis becomes megaloblastic. Once this develops, anaemia rapidly progresses thereafter. The more usual causes, however, are a deficient supply of folic acid in the diet or defective absorption as in cases of tropical sprue.

The increased demands of pregnancy and particularly of twin pregnancy are well demonstrated by the more rapid clearance of injected folic acid from the plasma in pregnancy.[5] This has nothing to do with the absorption of vitamin B_{12}, which is usually normal in pregnancy. This substance also has a very long storage life.

Addisonian anaemia is therefore very uncommon in pregnancy. There are two additional reasons for this; firstly, it is rare at the age of childbearing and, secondly, such cases are usually infertile.

What is astonishing is the infrequency of cases of megaloblastic anaemia reported from the United States. In Brooklyn, for example, it has been reckoned that folic acid deficiency is frequent during the last trimester of pregnancy amongst the lower social groups, yet megaloblastic anaemia of pregnancy remains exceedingly rare and it is suggested that there must be additional factors operating.[39] One wonders whether American views on the incidence will change in time as our own have recently.

A megaloblastic form of erythropoiesis is one thing (and marrow samples taken from an unselected group of pregnant patients show an incidence of this of about 25 per cent[40]), but a true megaloblastic anaemia of clinical significance is about one-tenth of that figure: in other words most laboratory tests will reveal the tendency long before it becomes clinically significant. There is accumulating evidence to indicate that the average British diet is not equal to the demands of pregnancy, which are considerably in excess of the generally recognised 50 μg per day required in the non-pregnant state. A good deal of work has therefore been done to arrive at some sensible estimate of how much extra folic acid should be supplied in pregnancy. The picture is further complicated by the fact that diagnostic criteria are uncertain, hence there is very marked variation in the accepted incidence of the condition and we cannot do more than supply our own standards which, over the last few years, have served us so well. There can be no doubt that iron deficiency itself may conceal the morphological evidence of megaloblastic anaemia and may of itself be a factor in the aetiology of the folic acid deficiency state.[6] It is thus that the correction of the iron deficiency only at this point brings to light the underlying associated folic acid deficiency as well. An extensive trial was therefore undertaken at the Queen Mother's Hospital to find the optimum folic acid supplement which would effectively eliminate folic acid deficiency later on in pregnancy. The technique employed in this review was to investigate the fasting serum folate levels in the second and fourth day postpartum in a consecutive series of 350 patients from groups who had been allocated at random to different supplementary doses of folic acid. A dietary assessment was also undertaken at the same time. The results were compared with an accepted normal range in the non-pregnant, namely 2·8 to 8 ng/ml. Marrow biopsy has now been given up except in the most inexplicable cases. For one thing the results are little better than an observation of the criteria presently to be described and, secondly, the process itself is inconvenient and often very painful to the patient. Marrow biopsy from the iliac crest is considerably better in this respect than from the sternum where pain can be very severe and one of my residents once had the shattering experience of going straight through into the heart. She withdrew the needle in a hurry and fortunately all was well.

In the survey referred to, the postpartum period was chosen for measuring the serum folate because the lowest levels associated with pregnancy are demonstrated at this time due to the combined demands of the fetus and blood loss at delivery; also, as is well known, many cases of latent megaloblastic anaemia are first manifested after delivery in the immediate puerperium and not before it. Now, while, as already mentioned, the lowest non-pregnant adult serum folate value is 2·8 ng/ml, 75 per cent of the patients who fitted our criteria for the diagnosis of megaloblastic anaemia had levels below 2·5 ng/ml. It appeared from this survey of an average Glasgow population, with a diet which is clearly inadequate in all but the most favoured social classes, that a supplement of approximately 300 μg a day is necessary to prevent a major fall in postpartum serum folate level and it is now our practice to prescribe this supplement in all cases, on the argument that it is insufficient to be wasteful and not a big enough dose to mask a vitamin B_{12} deficiency.[42]

If, for example, in a woman over 35 there is any element of doubt that one may be missing a case of Addisonian pernicious anaemia, one can be reasonably certain of excluding the condition by finding free gastric hydrochloric acid, but quite a number of pregnant women, especially those who are folic-acid-deficient and anaemic in any case, have an incidental gastric achlorhydria although this is not histamine-fast and furthermore tends not to persist after delivery.

Criteria for the Diagnosis of Macrocytic or Megaloblastic Anaemia[42]

The haemoglobin level must be below 10 g per cent, and at least two of the following features, sought for in films of the buffy coat layer, must be present:

(*a*) More than 4 per cent of the neutrophil polymorphs must have 5 or more lobes;
(*b*) Orthochromatic macrocytes must be present with diameters exceeding 12 μm;
(*c*) Howell-Jolly bodies (which are residual nuclear inclusion bodies within the erythrocytes) are demonstrable (Fig. 1);
(*d*) Nucleated red cells, that is to say normoblasts showing premature haemoglobinisation for their stage of nuclear development are found;
(*e*) Macropolycytes may be present. These are giant polymorphs within the buffy coat layer.

These findings have been supported by the study of a thousand serum folate estimations. Results from Montreal are similar, where a good correlation between the appearance of segmentation of the neutrophils in peripheral blood has been confirmed by marrow examination where, of course, the very earliest changes might be expected. Marrow biopsy is therefore now a rare operation in our hospital and reserved for the determination of other types of anaemia.

The clinical picture is that of a woman, usually in the later part of pregnancy, who demonstrates a fairly severe anaemia which has failed to respond to a genuine intake of iron, including parenteral therapy. Twins may be present and clearly here the increased demands of folic acid for such a pregnancy are responsible. What is less easy to explain is the common association of hydramnios with megaloblastic anaemia as well. Signs of pre-eclamptic toxaemia may often be present; in fact in one reported series[17] all three signs of hypertension, albuminuria and oedema were found in 14 per cent of

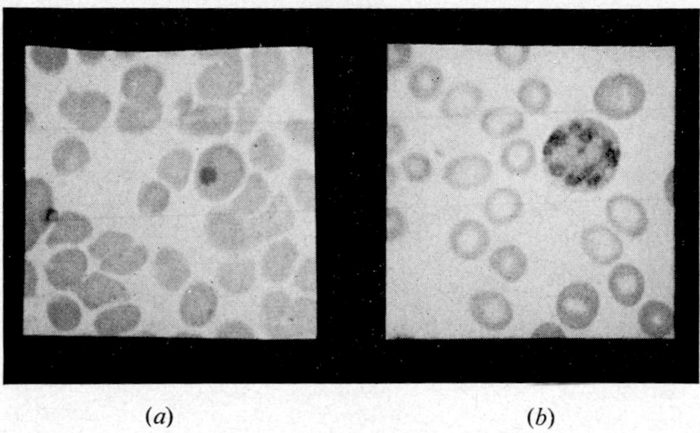

(*a*) (*b*)

7/FIG. 1.—Megaloblastic anaemia—blood film.
(*a*) Howell-Jolly residual nuclear inclusion bodies within erythrocytes.
(*b*) Hypersegmented neutrophil.

(By courtesy of Dr M. L. N. Willoughby.)

cases with megaloblastic anaemia, as against an overall incidence of 6 per cent of cases of pre-eclamptic toxaemia in Dublin.

Because of the key role of folic acid in DNA synthesis, so readily demonstrable within the marrow, it is interesting to consider other parts of the body where rapidly proliferating cells might show the effects of such deficiency, and for this reason cervical epithelial cells have been studied with this mechanism in view.[29] In fact a number of characteristic cytological changes have been thus described which reverted to normal when the patient was successfully treated with folic acid. Since other cells within the body are also in the process of active proliferation and equally dependent upon DNA synthesis, an observation of this sort sets one thinking about possible wider effects elsewhere, but, so far, experimental evidences are lacking.

In severe cases the spleen and occasionally the liver may be enlarged and there may be purpuric spots. Signs of congestive cardiac failure may be present and I myself have seen more than one case of jaundice, which was probably a contributory factor. The severity of the disease may vary from the apparently iron-resistant case to a woman acutely ill in whom the differential diagnosis may be quite difficult. There may be a misleading history of pernicious anaemia in other members of the family. There is often atrophic glossitis but neurological lesions never.

Of one practical point one can be reasonably certain, namely, if the haemoglobin drops sharply after a normal delivery, in which the blood loss has been minimal, the case is almost certain to prove on proper examination to be one of folic acid deficiency. This must be put right over the next three months by iron and folic acid.

Epileptic patients on anticonvulsant drugs which interfere with folic acid metabolism such as phenytoin, phenobarbitone or primidone, are liable to develop megaloblastic anaemia, and the prolonged use of sulphonamides may have a like effect.

It has also been suggested that the prolonged taking of oral contraceptives before pregnancy may have reduced folate stores by interfering with absorption.

Diagnosis of Achlorhydria

A particularly useful ward procedure is the Azuresin diagnostic test (Squibb) better known as Diagnex Blue. This test determines the presence or absence of free hydrochloric acid in the stomach without any special equipment. It depends upon the liberation of an indicator material (azure A) from a cation exchange resin, by the action of free gastric hydrochloric acid. This indicator is then absorbed from the stomach and excreted in the urine two hours later where its blueness can be seen and compared with a colour comparator supplied in each box of the test material. The test is valid except in cases of pyloric obstruction, severe hepatic or renal disease, in severe vomiting or marked dehydration or after partial or total gastrectomy, for obvious reasons.

The exclusion of achlorhydria, besides ruling out a diagnosis of pernicious anaemia, puts carcinoma of the stomach out of the differential diagnosis as well. These conditions are admittedly very rare in pregnancy but that fact would not diminish the catastrophe of missing them.

FIGLU test.—This test was all the rage and an enormous amount of unnecessary work was undertaken in carrying it out in the early 1960s. The enthusiasm for the test has now almost totally evaporated, and we seldom employ it. Nevertheless it is based upon a very important recognition of the biochemical pathways in the conversion of folic acid to folinic acid which is the really active principle, a deficiency of which is revealed in the faulty metabolism of histidine to the end product glutamic acid. The term FIGLU is short for formimino glutamic acid.

Histidine normally breaks down to FIGLU which is converted to glutamic acid only if sufficient folic acid is present.

Now in pregnancy there is an increased histidine breakdown load which may reveal a latent folic acid deficiency. This same deficiency, by failure to make possible the full conversion of FIGLU to glutamic acid, is thus revealed by a persistence of FIGLU excreted in the urine.[24]

The FIGLU excretion test provides an indirect means of demonstrating folic acid deficiency but does not indicate whether the deficiency is due to a dietary lack, malabsorption, increased utilisation, for example in twins, disorders of fat absorption with associated steatorrhoea in which absorption of vitamin B_{12} may also be unsatisfactory, or the increased demands of a marrow having to cope with pathological degrees of haemolysis.

Another of the disadvantages of the FIGLU test is that it is too often positive without clinically significant degrees of megaloblastic anaemia in pregnancy. In other words it would appear too sensitive. The probable reasons are that there is a different type of absorption of folic acid in pregnancy and there is increased utilisation of histidine in pregnancy which makes the test so much less useful than in the non-pregnant state, and a growing number of reports regard an estimate of serum folic acid levels as a better guide to the type of erythropoiesis.[7] (Serum levels in normal pregnancy may fall to 3·0–7·5 ng/ml.) There now seems fairly general agreement that the urinary excretion of formimino glutamic acid is not only unsatisfactory as a test for folic acid deficiency in pregnancy but is within normal limits in half the patients who, in fact, have the actual disease.

Prophylactic Folic Acid Therapy

This is much debated. There are many units which give folic acid treatment in addition to iron as a blind routine, on the argument that it cannot do harm and that pernicious anaemia and carcinoma of the stomach are unlikely to be missed and are too rare anyway in pregnancy to bother about. In parts of the world where megaloblastic anaemia is very prevalent and the consequences acute and where laboratory facilities are limited there may be something to be said for this view, but there is no excuse for it in this country and least of all in teaching units. On general principles all routine treatment, as a substitute for intelligent investigation and thought, is to be condemned. Such a process can only lead to slovenly thinking in the first instance and presently to no thinking at all and we would end up knowing even less than we did before about folic acid metabolism and no one would suggest that there is not a great deal still to learn. Unnecessary treatment also involves unnecessary expense and some patients may not wholly escape the implication that there is something abnormal to treat. Finally there is a danger that we may be treating laboratory data rather than patients.[44]

Notwithstanding all this there is much to be said for treating any acute anaemia presenting in the last month of pregnancy with empirical folic acid as well as with iron sorbitol while awaiting results of investigations, since time is short. The same argument applies in all cases of twins since time may be shorter than one thinks due to the possible onset of premature labour.[17] No case of megaloblastic anaemia, however, should be put on to folic acid therapy without at least the Diagnex Blue test to exclude achlorhydria. Any case in whom the reticulocyte response and rise in haemoglobin level is not apparent within ten days should have a full haematological investigation.

There would appear to be more than a possible relationship between folic acid deficiency and abruptio placentae[21] and that such a deficiency may be an aetiological factor in fetal malformation and recurrent abortion,[22, 28] although there is still room for debate on these subjects.

The decision to use a dietary supplement of folic acid in pregnancy depends upon the type of population with which one is dealing and at least in Glasgow, as in other centres, an attempt has been made to assess the deficit. In our own practice we have found that in a survey of over three and a half thousand patients, randomly allocated to different supplementation groups, treated with differing doses of folic acid supplements and checked by the postpartum serum folate level, a minimum daily requirement of 300 μg/day was sufficient to protect the vast majority of the patients.[43] For this reason we now prescribe in all our antenatal clinics one tablet each day of Ferrograd Folic which contains 105 mg of elemental iron plus 350 micrograms of folic acid. Gastric irritation is minimal with this preparation, thanks to its slow release of iron. These supplementary requirements might vary with different types of population and in different parts of the world and would be well worth estimating before prescribing on a large scale.

Megaloblastic anaemia of pregnancy may continue for up to five months into the postnatal period and occasionally may only first come to light in the puerperium, often provoked out of latency by haemorrhage at delivery. The usual time of onset, however, is between the fifth and seventh months of pregnancy. Anorexia and vomiting may confuse the differential diagnosis which includes leukaemic states.

Most types of clinically full-blown megaloblastic anaemia can cause the patient's death far more readily than is the case with iron deficiency anaemia, and treatment should be energetic. This consists of a liberal diet, folic acid in daily doses ranging from 15 to 30 mg by mouth and, of course, parenteral iron, for example iron sorbitol, in cases seriously deficient in iron as well. Folic acid treatment should be maintained for four weeks after delivery.

This treatment can restore a normal blood picture within five weeks but the danger of even a small antepartum haemorrhage in the uncorrected state should be keenly recognised and treated by transfusion. In fact haemorrhage is the main if not the only indication for transfusion in this type of anaemia.[13] Transfusion given before investigation may wreck the chances of accurate diagnosis.

Thrombocytopenic purpura is an uncommon complication of

pregnancy, but an impressive series of 44 pregnancies in cases of the idiopathic form of the disease have been reported from Manchester[20] without maternal fatality. Thirty-eight of the pregnancies were in women who had undergone previous splenectomy. In one, the operation was undertaken in pregnancy, and in another during the puerperium; the remaining four had not undergone splenectomy either before or after delivery and it would appear that the maternal risk is not great if splenectomy has already been carried out before pregnancy. The danger is greater in women still with their spleens *in situ*, and the operation itself in the course of pregnancy is hazardous and should not be considered in any case unless adrenal cortical steroid therapy has already failed. The expulsive efforts of the second stage may encourage purpuric haemorrhages which may also involve the brain and should, therefore, be eliminated by the timely application of forceps. As might be expected, haemorrhage at Caesarean section or from genital tract lacerations occurred in a quarter of the cases in this series. About 18 per cent of the live-born babies showed purpuric manifestations with thrombocytopenia lasting up to twelve weeks, even in mothers who had apparently been cured by previous splenectomy. If, in fact, the thrombocytopenia is due to the destruction of platelets by circulating autoimmune antibodies, which may be capable of crossing the placenta, this curious neonatal liability to the disease, thus passively acquired, seems understandable in a baby, which, unlike its mother, has a normally functioning spleen. A platelet count should therefore be done on all infants of mothers with a history of thrombocytopenic purpura, even though previously cured by splenectomy.

The other varieties of anaemia, such as the aplastic varieties and the haemolytic anaemias, will not be discussed further in this chapter, as they are in no way peculiar to pregnancy, but the role of sepsis in favouring anaemia should not be overlooked, and its proper control is essential for healthy haemopoiesis. The transfusion of packed cells, besides helping the patient to cope with her sepsis, will often permanently benefit her anaemic state.

Effects of Anaemia on Pregnancy and Labour

The abortion and prematurity rates are somewhat increased, but it is nevertheless surprising how well the majority of fetuses manage to survive in cases of quite considerable anaemia. Practically all the complications of pregnancy are aggravated quantitatively by anaemia, and, in particular, the patient with a cardiac lesion suffers from greatly increased dyspnoea.

Labour is not materially influenced by anaemia, and inertia is no more common, but the accidents of labour, especially those involving haemorrhage or shock, are rendered correspondingly more serious, and the patient who comes into labour with a haemoglobin level of less than 9·6 g (65%) is at serious risk in this respect. Her ability to cope with infection in the puerperium is much undermined by anaemia, and her recovery in the postnatal period will be greatly retarded to the extent that she may now face years of chronic subhealth.

HAEMOGLOBINOPATHIES

There are a large number of variants of the haemoglobin molecule, some of which are particularly common in certain populations such as West Africans and Mediterranean seaboard races. Haemoglobin itself is a conjugated protein with a molecular weight of about 68 thousand, which contains a globin fraction bound to 4 haem molecules. Abnormalities affecting the synthesis of the haem part of the molecule are responsible for the porphyrias, which need not concern us further here. The haemoglobinopathies are concerned with disorders within the polypeptide chains which comprise the globin fraction. There are four possible chains, namely alpha, beta, gamma and delta, but most haemoglobin in normal adult blood has, within the globin molecule, a pair of alpha and a pair of beta chains and is called Hb A ($\alpha_2\beta_2$).

This applies to over 90 per cent of the haemoglobin and up to 3 per cent has two delta chains instead of the two beta chains and is known as Hb A_2 ($\alpha_2\delta_2$).

Fetal haemoglobin (Hb F) has a globin portion consisting of 2 alpha and 2 gamma chains ($\alpha_2\gamma_2$). This accounts for about 80 per cent of the haemoglobin in cord blood at term. This fetal haemoglobin is gradually replaced by the normal adult haemoglobin (Hb A) over the first year of life.

Two classes of abnormality can result in a decreased proportion of the normal adult haemoglobin A in later life; the thalassaemia syndromes and the haemoglobinopathies. In beta thalassaemia there is an impaired synthesis of beta chains, resulting in a low concentration of normal Hb A ($\alpha_2\beta_2$) with a compensatory increase in Hb F ($\alpha_2\gamma_2$) and/or Hb A_2 ($\alpha_2\delta_2$). A rare form of alpha thalassaemia also exists, where there is impairment of alpha chains. This form affects the newborn, unlike beta-thalassaemia, since alpha but not beta chains are present in Hb F. On the other hand when the Hb A molecule is replaced in whole or in part by a pathological haemoglobin because of abnormal polypeptide chains not to be found in normal globin, one is faced with a haemoglobinopathy, viz. a qualitative rather than quantitative abnormality of Hb A synthesis. These pathological polypeptide changes are, in fact, due to substitution alterations in the amino acid residue; for example substitution of the amino acid valine for glutamic acid results in the structural difference between sickle-cell (Hb S) and normal haemoglobin and because glutamic acid has a different electrical charge from valine, starch-gel electrophoresis is capable of separating and distinguishing the two. Sickle-cell haemoglobin also crystallises out readily in blood which is reduced after giving up its oxygen and the red cell envelope is consequently distorted, hence the term "sickling". Blood viscosity increases at the same time and vessels may become blocked with thrombosis and likewise haemolysis may occur. In haemoglobin C (Hb C) lysine takes the place of the glutamic acid radicle.

These abnormal haemoglobins are also genetically determined and the blood of an individual may be either heterozygous or homozygous. For instance if the sickle-cell gene is inherited from both parents, the child has the full-blown sickle-cell disease, (SS) whereas, in the heterozygous, sickling does not normally occur because there is enough normal haemoglobin in each red cell to prevent it. The heterozygous state produces what is called the sickle-cell trait.

The heterozygotes with the sickle-cell trait are said to have considerable resistance to malaria and therefore the trait is common in parts of the world where malaria has been traditionally rife.

There are quantitative variations in the amounts of abnormal haemoglobin in any given case and in the case of sickle-cell anaemia about three-quarters of the haemoglobin is made up of the S-type, namely homozygous (SS), whereas in the sickle-cell trait more than half the haemoglobin may be of the Hb A variety. The laws of Mendelian inheritance apply.

The most commonly encountered abnormal haemoglobins are S, C, D and E. These abnormalities reside in the beta chain and, therefore, do not become manifest in the neonatal period. They may also exist in a variety of combinations including mixed syndromes with the thalassaemias. The anaemia in non-sickling haemoglobinopathies (i.e. C, D, E) is usually very mild unless in combinations with thalassaemia.

The thalassaemias are a somewhat different class as already explained because here there is an abnormal quantitative relationship between the different types of haemoglobin which can be found in normal blood, namely Hb A, Hb A_2 and Hb F. In thalassaemia minor (heterozygous form) the disease is not normally severe. In thalassaemia major (homozygous form) the disease is much more severe.

Until recently the haemoglobinopathies were no more than a haematological curiosity in British obstetric practice, but with the enormous influx of immigrants, especially from West Africa and the West Indies, they demand more recognition, and any case of refractory anaemia in a patient coming from these parts of the world and also from races on the Mediterranean seaboard should be investigated. Furthermore thalassaemia is being more frequently found amongst patients of apparently British stock. Thalassaemia and most haemoglobinopathies are likely to present as refractory hypochromic anaemias during pregnancy, with target cells in the blood film, a constant reticulocytosis and a fasting serum iron level higher than the degree of hypochromia would suggest. In the more severe forms they may present as a haemolytic or aplastic crisis or, in the case of Hb S, manifest thrombotic incidents.

The haematological features of the anaemia should raise the possibility of thalassaemia or haemoglobinopathy the precise variety of which may require family studies and the application of techniques only available in specialised centres. Demonstration of the presence of Hb S, however, is a simpler matter, depending upon its unusual physical characteristics already mentioned. By mixing a drop of blood with a reducing agent such as sodium dithionite and sealing the coverslip, sickling may be seen under the microscope in 20 minutes if the test is positive.[1] It is now our routine practice to screen all African patients for Hb S at antenatal booking by mixing a drop of blood (0·02 ml) with a sickle-cell reagent solution consisting of buffer to which is added sodium dithionite which reduces the oxygen content, produces the sickling phenomenon by crystallisation and turns the mixture cloudy. The major method, however, of identifying abnormal haemoglobins is by starch-gel electrophoresis. Fresh heparinised blood (10–20 ml) is required for this type of investigation.

The clinical effects of the haemoglobinopathies are first of all to reduce fertility. In fact the death rate amongst children in severe cases is high and abortion is said to be more common. In sickle-cell disease (haemoglobin SS) the patient is recurrently affected in two very damaging ways, namely haemolytic crises and crises of infarction, and in between these crises she continues with chronic haemolytic anaemia with some degree of jaundice and miserable health. The bone marrow endeavours to compensate by increased erythropoiesis and there is usually reticulocytosis. Stores of folic acid may, therefore, be exhausted and the patient never really becomes well between one crisis and the next. Infarction may strike in any part of the body and produce pain anywhere and even intracranial catastrophes, whereas the haemolytic crises produce jaundice and fever. Infection may precipitate haemolysis and infarction may be encouraged by circulatory stasis and local acidosis. Sickle-cell haemoglobin C disease (SC) is less severe than full-blown sickle-cell (SS). In fact the SC case may suffer no more than moderate ill health until pregnancy precipitates haemolytic or infarctive crises, particularly in the last trimester or in the postpartum period. Any exposure to hypoxia, e.g. inexpert anaesthesia or high-altitude flying in inadequately pressurised aircraft may precipitate Hb S crystallisation and therefore sickling in the red cells. Crises due to haemolysis or infarction are more common in the later weeks of pregnancy.

The picture is a dismal one inasmuch as there is clearly no specific treatment; but transfusion may tide a patient over a crisis and a higher-than-usual dose of prophylactic folic acid should be given to meet increased requirements. Delivery should be covered by antibiotics to prevent triggering off a further haemolytic crisis. These patients therefore call for what Bannerman and White have described as "maximal obstetric care".

PULMONARY TUBERCULOSIS

In recent years our attitude has changed from that which regarded pregnancy as a disaster in the course of the disease. This, however, does not mean that the complication is less important. On the contrary, the more hopeful attitude depends absolutely upon adequate supervision being available.

Routine chest radiography in pregnancy is less popular now because of radiation hazards, but immigrant patients, especially Pakistanis, who have a high incidence, should be screened. Nor should full chest radiography be withheld from the case whose history, or where contact with the disease, demand it.

Effects of Pregnancy on the Disease

Edge (1952) from the Brompton Hospital concluded that pregnancy in general had no dramatic effect upon the course of the disease. Cohen (1946) also reported on 177 cases of pulmonary tuberculosis in pregnancy with a long follow-up of 120, and he likewise concluded that pregnancy and labour rarely harm the pulmonary disease and pregnancy is no more than an incident in the disease process. The proviso is always made, however, that adequate treatment and supervision are instituted, not only through pregnancy and labour but in the even more important postnatal period. It is in the latter that mischief is most often evident, and the added work and fatigue of looking after a fretful baby can be more serious than the effects of pregnancy and labour added together.

It might be expected that the rise in the level of the diaphragm in pregnancy would be bound to affect the pulmonary lesion in one direction or another by reducing lung capacity, but this is compensated for by the increased width which occurs in the thoracic dimensions. The increased metabolic effort on the part of the patient should be offset by greater periods of rest. The outlook, of course, is immeasurably worse when there is associated tuberculous laryngitis, but this would apply whether the patient was pregnant or not.

A death rate of up to 30 per cent in five years was not unusual in former years in women of childbearing age who were sputum positive, whether pregnancy supervened or not. Modern antituberculous chemotherapy has transformed what was once a gloomy long-term outlook.

What has been said above is all very well provided pregnancy itself is normal in other respects and there are no obstetrical complications, but when these are present the tuberculous patient is clearly at greater risk. Hyperemesis is indeed a serious complication and requires very urgent and energetic treatment. Trial of labour has only a limited place, anaesthesia must be judiciously selected and administered.

Conversely, the presence of pulmonary tuberculosis has, on the whole, little effect on pregnancy itself, although if the disease is active there is a slight tendency for the patient to go into premature labour.

The modern outlook for the patient has been summarised on a question-and-answer basis in a report of the Joint Paediatrics and Obstetrics Committee of the Joint Tuberculosis Council (1958) and confirms the above reassuring change of outlook, even breast feeding being encouraged in non-infective cases.

Management

The problem is primarily sociological. Overwork, overcrowding, fatigue and malnutrition are far greater enemies of the patient's chances than her pregnancy. Her medical treatment should follow the same lines as would have been adopted were she not pregnant, with rather more emphasis on necessary periods of hospitalisation. The cornerstone of treatment, of course, is antituberculous chemotherapy. Although streptomycin crosses the placenta, ototoxic effects have not yet been reported in the babies. Major surgery is preferably confined at present to the first half of pregnancy or, better still, deferred if possible until the postnatal period, relying meanwhile on chemotherapy. Antenatal supervision should be as thorough as it is for the patient with a cardiac lesion, and periods of hospitalisation during pregnancy should be unhesitatingly recommended on even minor obstetrical indications. In any case, it is wise, as in the cardiac case, to admit the patient to hospital for 10 to 14 days before delivery. This not only improves supervision but guarantees adequate rest.

Treatment in labour largely follows the same lines as in cases of cardiac disease, with the same attention to the patient's general condition. Caesarean section should only be employed where there are obstetrical indications, and its use is not to be recommended simply as a means of furnishing an opportunity to sterilise the patient at the same time. The second stage should not be allowed to be strenuous, and the forceps should be used whenever it appears that spontaneous delivery cannot take place without effort.

It used to be thought that the changes in abdominal anatomy following delivery would have a deleterious effect upon the pulmonary lesion as a result of the sudden lowering of the diaphragm. As it so happens, however, there is no immediate diaphragmatic descent, and the old idea of inducing a pneumoperitoneum immediately after delivery, in order to keep the diaphragm up, has now been abandoned. Without paralysis of the phrenic nerve it is quite difficult anyway to alter the level of the diaphragm, and filling the peritoneal cavity with air simply bulges the flabby abdominal wall and, at the very least, merely increases the patient's discomfort.

Care of the Baby

Congenital tuberculosis in the baby is extremely rare, but the chances that it will contract the infection during the first few months of life are very great. To separate the mother from her child may be theoretically desirable but is often not feasible. Nevertheless, until recently there was no other method of protecting a child from this deadly hazard, since a baby has no natural immunity to tuberculosis. In underdeveloped countries where artificial feeding is dangerous because of gastro-enteritis and where neglect of the young in any hands other than the mother's is by no means uncommon, segregation of the babies from their mothers has its own peculiar dangers. Dormer and colleagues (1959) working in a Bantu tuberculosis unit of 1000 beds in Durban found the mortality of babies born there to be appallingly high as a consequence of separation from their mothers—for example, in one year 15 out of 17 died. They therefore decided to keep the mothers and babies together and to protect the babies with isoniazid meanwhile, even though some of the mothers were sputum positive and all were nursed together in thirty-bedded wards. The dosage they gave was 25 mg of isoniazid in syrup twice a day by mouth, increasing after 6 months to 50 mg twice a day. There were no adverse effects and the babies remained Mantoux negative. Unfortunately the babies had still to face their primary infection as soon as the isoniazid prophylaxis was stopped after discharge home and these workers suggested the possibility of immunising the babies with isoniazid-resistant BCG vaccine, but gave no record of having done so. This has since been carried out by Gaisford and Griffiths in Manchester. Here, separation of mother and baby has been dispensed with, provided the mother does not suffer from isoniazid-resistant tuberculosis, and the baby is protected with isoniazid and at the same time immunised with an isoniazid-resistant BCG vaccine. It would not be rational to give the normal freeze-dried BCG vaccine as the concurrent isoniazid would ruin the effect, but it was found that the isoniazid-resistant vaccine was just as potent, and produced satisfactory tuberculin conversion without complications. Isoniazid prophylaxis is, of course, maintained until the tuberculin test becomes positive.

Breast feeding is definitely contra-indicated in all cases of activity of the tuberculosis process. Recently achieved quiescence of the lesion is also a contra-indication.

In the soundly healed case there is no objection on pulmonary grounds to breast feeding. Indeed, the labour involved in preparing artificial feeds can often be more tiresome than breast feeding. Artificial feeding for the single-handed mother can be a real strain, but if adequate help in the home is available the advantages are considerable.

These patients are far more likely to break down as a result of overwork and fatigue while the baby is still very young than because of the alleged strain of pregnancy, labour and lactation, and it is an essential part of postnatal treatment to ensure that the patient receives all the domestic help that her condition demands. As in the cardiac case, the home-help service can be of great value.

Therapeutic Abortion

The more carefully pregnant patients with pulmonary tuberculosis are reviewed, and the more thoroughly they are treated, the less often will termination of pregnancy be called for. The indications for this type of intervention are mainly sociological and, medically speaking, they cannot for that reason be regarded as wholly genuine. The ideal answer to the problem is to attend to the patient's social circumstances rather than to destroy a potentially healthy baby. Unfortunately this is a counsel of perfection, like ridding the world of slums and poverty. The highly multiparous patient suffering from the disease may often be found to be living in conditions of such irredeemable squalor that one may occasionally be forced, in the interests of expedition, to terminate and sterilise simply to preserve the patient as a functioning social unit for the sake of her numerous existing children.

The risks of therapeutic abortion, whether by the vaginal or by the abdominal route, are every bit as great as the risks of a continuing pregnancy, and the prognosis in either instance has to be viewed against the general five-year mortality in all patients, whether pregnant or not. Termination does not appear to influence the outlook significantly, nor is the course of the disease appreciably altered.

The patient with quiescent and arrested disease is only at slight risk in any case, and where the disease is active the only indication for termination is gross inadequacy of available supervision, a state of affairs which should not be admitted in any civilised community.

If the patient is well enough to benefit hypothetically from termination, she does not need it, and if her condition is so bad that she apparently requires abortion, she is too ill to recover after it.

Future Pregnancies

It is generally held that it is better for the patient to avoid pregnancy until quiescence is assured for about two years, in order to obviate the possible risks of subsequent breakdown inherent in the rigours of infant rearing. In the past, victims of this disease have been traditionally advised to postpone marriage and pregnancy, but pregnancy should be discouraged only after very careful consideration, and only in cases where there would appear to be a reasonable prospect of arresting the disease in the very near future. Much will depend upon the social and domestic circumstances of the girl and her husband and the availability of additional help in the home.

REFERENCES

1. Bannerman, R. H. O. and White, J. C. (1957). *J. Obstet. Gynaec. Brit. Emp.*, **64,** 682.
2. Basu, S. K. (1963). *Lancet.* **1,** 1430.
3. Bonnar, J. (1965). *Brit. med. J.*, **2,** 1030.
4. Camilleri, A. (1958). *J. Obstet. Gynaec. Brit. Emp.*, **65,** 266.
5. Chanarin, I., MacGibbon, B. M., O'Sullivan, W. J. and Mollin, D. L. (1959). *Lancet*, **2,** 634.
6. Chanarin, I., Rothman, Doreen and Berry, Valerie (1965). *Brit. med. J.*, **1,** 480.
7. Chisholm, Morag and Sharp, A. A. (1964). *Brit. med. J.*, **2,** 1366.
8. Clay, Barbara, Rosenburg, B., Sampson, Nanita and Samuels, S. I. (1965). *Brit. med. J.*, **1,** 29.
9. Cohen, R. C. (1946). *Brit. J. Tuberc.*, **40,** 10.
10. Dormer, B. A., Harrison, I., Swart, J. A. and Vidor, S. R. (1959). *Lancet*, **2,** 902.
11. Edge, J. R. (1952). *Brit. med. J.*, **1,** 845.
12. Fisher, M. and Biggs, R. (1955). *Brit. med. J.*, **1,** 385.
13. Forshaw, J. W. B., Jones, A. T., Chisholm, W. N. and McGinly, W. K. (1957). *J. Obstet. Gynaec. Brit. Emp.*, **64,** 255.
14. Fullerton, W. T. and Turner, A. G. (1962). *Lancet.* **1,** 75.
15. Fullerton, W. T. and Watson-Williams, E. J. (1962). *Brit. J. Obstet. Gynaec. Brit. Cwlth*, **69,** 729.
16. Gaisford, W. and Griffiths, M. I. (1961). *Brit. med. J.*, **1,** 1500.
17. Gatenby, P. B. B. and Lillie, E. W. (1960). *Brit. med. J.*, **2,** 1111.
18. Giles, C. and Brown, J. A. H. (1962). *Brit. med. J.*, **2,** 10.
19. Goldberg, A. (1967). Personal communication.
20. Heys, R. F. (1966). *J. Obstet. Gynaec. Brit. Cwlth*, **73,** 205.

21. HIBBARD, B. M. and HIBBARD, E. D. (1963). *Brit. med. J.*, **2,** 1430.
22. HIBBARD, E. D. and SMITHELLS, R. W. (1965). *Lancet.* **1,** 1254.
23. Joint Tuberculosis Council (1958). *Antenatal and Obstetric Care of Tuberculous Patients and Measures to Safeguard their Infants.* Bovey Tracy: Joint Tuberc. Counc.
24. KNOWLES, J. P., PRANKERD, T. A. J. and WESTALL, R. G. (1960). *Lancet*, **2,** 347.
25. LANE, R. S. and SCOTT, JEAN M. (1965). *Brit. med. J.*, **1,** 449.
26. LOWENSTEIN, L., HSIEH, Y. S., BRUNTON, L., DE LEEUW, M. K. M. and COOPER, B. A. (1962). *Postgrad. Med.*, **31,** 72.
27. MCFARLANE, D. B., PINKERTON, P. H., DAGG, J. H. and GOLDBERG, A. (1967). *Brit. J. Haemat.*, **13,** 790.
28. MARTIN, J. D. and DAVIS, R. E. (1964). *J. Obstet. Gynaec. Brit. Cwlth*, **71,** 400.
29. VAN NIEKERK, W. A. (1966). *Acta. Cytol.* (*Philad.*), **10,** 67.
30. OJO, O. A. (1965). *J. trop. Med. Hyg.*, **68,** 32.
31. PHILPOTT, R. H., FOSTER, N. E. G. and CRICHTON, D. (1966). *Brit. med. J.*, **2,** 1630.
32. POWLEY, P. H. (1965). *Brit. med. J.*, **1,** 1068.
33. PRINGLE, A., GOLDBERG, A., MACDONALD, E. and JOHNSTON, S. (1962). *Lancet.* **2,** 749.
34. RICHMOND, H. G. (1959). *Brit. med. J.*, **1,** 947.
35. ROSS, I. P. (1957). *Lancet*, **2,** 77.
36. SCOTT, J. M. (1962). *Postgrad. med. J.*, **38,** 202.
37. SCOTT, J. M. and GOVAN, A. D. T. (1954). *Brit. med. J.*, **2,** 1257.
38. SCOTT, JEAN M. (1963). *Brit. med. J.*, **2,** 354.
39. SOLOMONS, E., LEE, S. L., WASSERMANN, M. and MALKIN, J. (1962). *J. Obstet. Gynaec. Brit. Cwlth*, **69,** 724.
40. BRITISH MEDICAL JOURNAL (1964). Today's drugs, **2,** 1348.
41. WETHERLEY-MEIN, G., BUCHANAN, J. G., GLASS, U. H. and PEARCE, L. C. (1962). *Brit. med. J.*, **1,** 1796.
42. WILLOUGHBY, M. L. N. and JEWELL, F. J. (1966). *Brit. med. J.*, **2,** 1568.
43. WILLOUGHBY, M. L. N. (1967). *Brit. J. Haemat.*, **13,** 503.
44. WITTS, L. J. (1962). *J. Obstet. Gynaec. Brit. Cwlth*, **69,** 714.

CHAPTER VIII

GENERAL DISTURBANCES

ACUTE ABDOMINAL PAIN

THERE are many pitfalls in differential diagnosis in cases of acute abdominal pain. In some, pregnancy is merely incidental, for example appendicitis, torsion of an ovarian cyst, volvulus and intestinal obstruction, acute cholecystitis and the perforation of a hollow viscus. Others may be due directly to some abnormality of the gravid state, such as abruptio placentae, uterine rupture, pre-eclamptic toxaemia, degeneration of a myoma, pyelitis (more common in pregnancy than out of it), septic abortion, angular pregnancy, pregnancy in a rudimentary horn, and acute retention of urine due, for example, to a retroverted gravid uterus.

Many of these diagnoses are dealt with under their appropriate chapters, but it is as well to remember the above list. The first relevant matter is to know that the patient is pregnant, and as a corollary the stage of gestation. The following diagnoses are more applicable to early pregnancy: ectopic gestation, pregnancy in a rudimentary horn and angular pregnancy, torsion of an ovarian cyst (which is more liable to occur in the earlier months and after delivery rather than in late pregnancy), and septic abortion.

Angular pregnancy is a very rare condition. Munro Kerr, in his *Operative Obstetrics*, described his personal experiences of six cases. Severe pain is a predominant feature; there is tender asymmetry of the uterus in the cornual region, and a marked tendency to abort. The case usually presents between the 12th and 20th weeks, and in the few which go to term the placenta may be retained in the cornual pocket, in which region morbid adhesion is a definite possibility. This pocket may be very thin and uterine rupture easily provoked.

Pregnancy in a rudimentary horn is simply a variety of ectopic gestation, and is usually diagnosed as such in these cases. Much will depend on the state of development of the horn, but rupture is most likely to occur between the 4th and 5th months.

The accidents to ovarian cysts have been fully dealt with elsewhere.

Cases of septic abortion are a great snare. Often the products of conception have not been passed, and in these circumstances it is most unusual for the case not to be of criminal interference. The history, therefore, may be very unreliable. As an example, some years ago I had a patient with pyrexia, abdominal pain, blood-stained purulent vaginal discharge, and a very tender uterus whose fundus was at the level of the umbilicus. She passed later a necrotic fetus of about 20 weeks' development which was extensively lacerated. Interference was stoutly denied. She made a good recovery with intensive anti-gas infection treatment. It is, incidentally, as well to keep a very careful watch for urinary suppression in these cases.

In acute degeneration in a myoma the pain and tenderness are localised at the site of the tumour and the diagnosis will depend upon recognising its existence.

Pre-eclamptic toxaemia, as a source of acute abdominal pain, can easily be missed out in writing examination answers, but in clinical, practice with a proper examination, which in any case includes testing the urine and blood pressure, the diagnosis would hardly be overlooked. One of the most important differential diagnoses is, of course, that of acute appendicitis. It can also be one of the most difficult. To some extent the rather serious prognosis in this complication of pregnancy is due to the fact that the diagnosis is often too long delayed; furthermore, the omentum cannot so readily reach and wall off the inflamed appendix and, therefore, intraperitoneal rupture and spill may occur earlier. This is particularly so in later pregnancy when the diagnosis is also harder to make. So many of the other causes of acute abdominal pain in pregnancy call for a conservative attitude without laparotomy that, as a result, operation is undertaken too late and, to make matters worse, recovery is often complicated by abortion or premature labour. In the series of 25 cases quoted by Black (1960), in which there was one maternal death, there were five abortions and four premature labours with three neonatal deaths.

The appendix is displaced upwards from its normal position, and examination of the abdomen is hampered by the presence of the gravid uterus, which masks abdominal guarding and the elicitation of many of the well-known clinical signs. The important thing is to remember the possibility of appendicitis and not to temporise in attempting a concrete diagnosis in cases of acute abdominal pain. A maternal death in my own experience was due to just this mistake. The issue was confused by the known existence of pre-eclamptic toxaemia, an apparently tender uterus and an absent fetal heart; there was also slight vaginal bleeding. The blood pressure dropped sharply and the patient's condition became rapidly grave. The diagnosis of abruptio placentae was made, and only after a delay of several hours, during which time the patient's condition progressively deteriorated, was the decision to operate reached. The patient died of a perforated appendix while the arrangements were being made.

In general it has to be admitted that the graver the patient's condition and the more acute the illness, the harder does differential diagnosis become.

JAUNDICE

Jaundice in pregnancy may be due to any of the following:

1. Virus hepatitis
   (*a*) Infectious hepatitis, and
   (*b*) Homologous serum jaundice
2. Drugs
3. Pre-eclamptic toxaemia and eclampsia
4. Acholuric jaundice
5. Gall-stones
6. Infective mononucleosis
7. "Recurrent jaundice of pregnancy"
8. Acute fatty atrophy
9. Neglected hyperemesis
10. Weil's disease
11. Cirrhosis
12. Carcinoma of the head of the pancreas

The last three are very rare in pregnancy.

Jaundice in pregnancy is a very disturbing symptom or sign because of the ugly possibilities which it may indicate and the differential diagnosis is by no means easy. The following tests are now regarded as the most useful in helping one to arrive at the correct differential diagnosis which, nevertheless, can often only be made in retrospect.

	Normal ranges
Serum bilirubin	0·2–1·2 mg/100 ml
Serum glutamic oxaloacetic transaminase (SGOT) *also named* Aspartate transaminase (AsT)	up to 40 iu/litre
Serum glutamic pyruvic transaminase (SGPT) *also named* Alanine transaminase (AlT)	up to 35 iu/litre
Alkaline phosphatase	3–13 King-Armstrong units/100 ml
Prothrombin (Quick one-stage)	10–14 seconds
Owren thrombotest	70–100% of standard normal
Serum albumin/globulin ratio	1·5–2

Other tests, though less useful:

Thymol turbidity	0–4 units
Flocculation	0
Urobilinogen in urine	0–4 mg/24 hr

Isocitrate dehydrogenase	1–3·5 iu/litre
Serum iron	80–160 μg/100 ml

The transaminases (SGOT and SGPT or AsT and AlT) are likely to be as high as 250–1000 iu/litre in viral hepatitis. They are also raised in drug necrosis, congestive cardiac failure and shock, sometimes with infective mononucleosis complicated by jaundice and rarely with gall-stones. Isocitrate dehydrogenase, however, is normal in the latter. Alkaline phosphatase is raised in extrahepatic obstructive jaundice but is very much lower in most viral types of hepatitis and in cirrhosis.

Virus Hepatitis

The transaminase is very high because this is an acute disease, although the degree of jaundice is not proportional to the transaminase levels. Of the two, SGPT is usually higher than SGOT and is the more indicative of viral hepatitis. The serum levels of these enzymes may reach 250–1000 iu/litre. Cirrhosis has much lower levels being a chronic disease.

Obstructive jaundice can be ruled out if the alkaline phosphatase level is not greatly raised because this enzyme is excreted in the bile.

The erythrocyte sedimentation rate is lower than 10 mm in the first hour in about a quarter of the patients whereas most other causes of jaundice produce a high sedimentation rate. Thymol turbidity level is not particularly raised.

The clinical picture is more or less the same as in the non-pregnant case, but the differential diagnosis is, of course, harder, especially in the presence of albuminuria which is common also to the pre-eclamptic state. The urine darkens first and the bilirubin rises before clinical jaundice is evident. The stools become pale and the duration of the disease is longer in the older patients. The sources of infection are believed to be by droplet and food. In cases of marked malnutrition the disease is likely to run a more vicious course and the worst cases may be associated with acute yellow atrophy. The mortality, however, is the same as in the non-pregnant woman and is very low indeed and there is no indication for terminating the pregnancy, in fact the operation may be dangerous at such a time. A temporary passive immunity may be obtained by giving gamma globulin but considering the favourable prognosis there is very little need for it, except in the seriously undernourished and therefore vulnerable patient.

As in any severe infectious illness during pregnancy, abortion or premature labour may ensue. In a series of 34 cases in which 30 were followed up[1] there was one maternal death, one case of residual cirrhosis of the liver and in 28 recovery was complete, but labour was premature in no less than 8, with two neonatal deaths, and spontaneous abortion occurred in another two. Being a virus infection, the question naturally arises of the possible effect upon fetal development and it is generally considered that the baby is not affected,[33] although in one of my own cases, in which the infection occurred in early pregnancy, the baby showed a mild degree of hemi-hypertrophy, a rare condition. The question is by no means settled.

Homologous serum jaundice.—This may be contracted from blood or from plasma transfusion or by direct inoculation of the virus with syringes and needles used for venepuncture, even for finger or ear pricking in order to obtain small samples of blood, and it is now the practice in antenatal clinics to use disposable materials entirely. The disease is not the same as virus hepatitis because it differs immunologically. Also the incubation period is very much longer and the virus is not found in the stools of the patient. The virus is often associated with a serum antigen known as Australia antigen which can be identified serologically and by electron microscopy. Although it usually disappears from the blood of hepatitis sufferers within a few months, some patients silently carry the Australia antigen for years. This carrier state now calls for screening of all blood donated for transfusion.

It is a complication of pregnancy much to be feared and we have had one maternal death in our practice which was probably due to this disease contracted in the above manner. This was before the institution of disposable materials in collecting blood samples. Hitherto syringes and needles had been boiled or autoclaved, but neither of these procedures may be sufficient to render the instruments safe.

It is surprising that more diseases are not transmitted by blood transfusion; in fact the four principal instances are hepatitis, syphilis, malaria and brucellosis.

Hepatitis is the most important and common, and it is reckoned that a patient receiving two units of blood is exposed to a risk of about 0·8 per cent[9] although nowadays more thorough screening is likely to reduce the hazard well below this figure which dates from 1966.

Large-pool plasma puts the risk up to nearly 12 per cent but with small-pool plasma, prepared from less than 10 bottles, the figure is 1·3 per cent. Massive blood transfusion therefore carries a distinct hazard. By no means are all cases due to a previous transfusion traced, because of the long incubation period which varies up to 160 days before the appearance of jaundice. When homologous serum jaundice does occur, however, the disease runs a fiercer course than the oridinary viral hepatitis referred to earlier, and apart from nausea, vomiting and anorexia, there may be joint pains and skin rashes. In favourable cases the illness may burn itself out in about 30 days but there is an appreciable mortality, seven deaths being reported in a series of 134 cases in 1949. In blood donation centres a history of jaundice is a reason for rejecting the donor, but even this precaution does not eliminate the risk because about one in 200 healthy donors harbours the virus in his blood stream. The risks of malaria and syphilis transmission can be forestalled by examination of the blood and serology of the potential donor, although in the case of syphilis it is very unlikely that active spirochaetes would survive for more than two or three days in stored blood.

Drugs

Until chloroform became taboo as an anaesthetic in pregnancy and labour many cases of jaundice were often attributed, probably correctly, to this agent. The danger was greatest when the anaesthetic had to be repeatedly induced in the course of a complicated labour. Personally I have not seen such a case now for over thirty years. There are two main groups of drugs which are now regarded as causes of jaundice:

(*a*) those which mimic hepatitis, e.g. PAS and isoniazid (SGOT levels start to rise above 20 iu/litre and before jaundice appears) and

(*b*) those that produce an intrahepatic obstruction, e.g. the phenothiazines, the promazines, diabenase. Methyl testosterone and anabolic agents. Lastly, arsenic—an unlikely medicament these days.

The alkaline phosphatase level is raised, and transaminase too, and isocitrate dehydrogenase (ICD) is a very sensitive index of drug damage to liver cells.

Pre-eclamptic Toxaemia and Eclampsia

Jaundice may appear as a manifestation of the pre-eclamptic state and some cases of severe eclampsia may indeed become jaundiced. Jaundice may also appear terminally in severe and neglected cases of hyperemesis.

Acholuric Jaundice

Acholuric jaundice may complicate pregnancy; the diseases is familial and there is abnormal fragility of the red cells.

Gall-stones

These are not common as causes of pregnant jaundice in this country, but in the better-fed parts of the world on the other side of the Atlantic the condition is very much more common. Parity is a

8/TABLE 1 JAUNDICE IN PREGNANCY

	Transaminase	*Isocitrate dehydrogenase*	*Alkaline phosphatase*	*Thymol turbidity*	*Prothrombin time*	*ESR*	*WBC*
Virus and Serum Jaundice	+ + + +	+ + +	± (< 30)	+	Prolonged	Low	Normal
Drugs, e.g. Chlorpromazine	+ +	+ + +	+ + (> 30)	Normal	Normal	Normal	Often low
Pre-eclampsia	Normal	Normal	Normal or slightly raised	±	Normal	Normal	Normal
Acholuric (congenital spherocytosis)	Normal or slightly raised	Normal or slightly raised	Normal	±	Normal	Normal	Normal
Gall-stones and Obstructive Jaundice	Normal, rarely raised	Normal	+++ (>30)	Normal	Normal	Slightly raised	Slightly raised
Infective Mononucleosis	++	++	+	+	±	+	Normal
Recurrent jaundice of pregnancy	Normal	Normal	++	Normal	Prolonged	+	
Acute fatty degeneration	Low	Low	±	+	Prolonged	Low	++
Cirrhosis	+	+	+ (<30)	++	++	++	Normal or low

factor in the aetiology of gall-stones, and less than 10 per cent of sufferers have not borne children. A raised blood cholesterol is often associated with gall-stones, and it has to be remembered that figures of 300 to 400 mg per cent are not uncommon in pregnancy. The pressure in the gall bladder area of the fetal head in breech presentation may stimulate the pain of gall-stones, but when jaundice is also present it is worth remembering the possibility of cholelithiasis. The alkaline phosphatase levels are usually very high.

Infective Mononucleosis

In these cases jaundice is not usually severe. The alkaline phosphatase level is moderately raised, and the transaminase levels are unlikely to rise above 150 iu/litre. The diagnosis is made on other grounds, such as Paul-Bunnell testing.

"Recurrent Jaundice of Pregnancy"

I have not encountered such a case myself but in 33 patients with jaundice during pregnancy seen at the Rotunda Hospital over a 9-year period 3 were in this category[29] and the pathological condition appeared to be one of intra-hepatic cholestasis. The urine is dark and the stools are pale. The disease is usually at its worst during the last 4 months of pregnancy and the jaundice and pruritus may for a time be actually worse in the immediate puerperium before recovery. Premature labour and postpartum haemorrhage due to vitamin K deficiency are possible complications. There is usually no maternal or fetal mortality. The condition recurs in each succeeding pregnancy and is obstructive in type. It is a familial condition and generalised pruritus is a prominent clinical feature and may appear two or three weeks before jaundice. The transaminase levels are normal and the disease clears up after each pregnancy with normal cholangiographic appearances. It is thought to be due to a latent enzymatic defect.

Acute Fatty Atrophy

This has a very high mortality, usually well over 80 per cent. Ninety per cent of the cases occur during the last trimester and a few in the postpartum period. The patients present with vomiting and haematemesis and in two-thirds there is severe epigastric pain. Headache is severe in about half the cases and jaundice and coma supervene within a fortnight. The condition would appear to be a separate clinical entity in its own right and Sheehan (1940) described six cases in four hundred maternal deaths. The cause is not known but very severe shrinkage of the liver occurs without histological evidence of inflammatory reaction or necrosis, yet only the cells around the portal tracts remain normal in appearance. The white cell count is raised to about 18,000 to 20,000 per mm^3, bilirubin, of course, is raised, but, unlike virus hepatitis, there is only a slight rise in transaminase levels. If these levels are reduced one can assume that the liver is incapable of producing them, which is a further bad prognostic sign. The prothrombin time is prolonged, the serum albumin levels are low and there is reduced erythrocyte sedimentation rate. The liver shows a massive fatty necrosis and may weigh only about 800 to 850 g (normal 1200 to 1500 g). It is red and mushy. Fat is laid down both in the centrilobular areas and between the cells. The cytoplasm of the liver cells is foamy in appearance and replaced with fat in multiple small droplets involving all the parenchymatous cells. There is an increase in Kupffer cells. With the condition there is often an associated low nephron necrosis, the renal tubular cells being replaced with fat and renal failure supervenes, with rising creatinine and blood urea levels. Pancreatitis is often associated. Sometimes fat emboli appear in the lungs and the ovaries contain haemorrhagic cysts. The postpartum milder cases may survive and, in those that do, recovery of hepatic function is complete.

The treatment of jaundice in pregnancy, apart from dealing with any specific cause, is on general lines. The patient's appetite is at first impaired, but as soon as possible a diet rich in carbohydrate and later in protein and vitamin B complex is necessary, with the exclusion, as far as possible, of fat. It is also worth administering vitamin K_1 because of the likely association of hypoprothrombinaemia. This may be particularly important from the baby's point of view should premature labour ensue.

CHOREA GRAVIDARUM

Fortunately, this is not a common complication of pregnancy. Beresford and Graham (1950) reviewed the subject fully, having collected details of 127 hitherto unpublished cases from British hospitals and added 3 more of their own. They estimated the incidence at approximately 1 in 3000, but today it is rarer still.

The clinical picture may vary from the very mild to the manic, and is characterised by restlessness and inco-ordinate, non-purposive and non-repetitive movements. Grimacing is noteworthy, and the jack-in-the-box tongue sign characteristic. General hypotonia and emotional lability are also features.

The majority of cases give a history of previous attacks of chorea or rheumatism, and the former may have appeared in earlier pregnancies, since the gravid state seems to favour recrudescences. The main precipitating causes of the present attack are worry and, occasionally, intercurrent infection.

Approximately one in three of the patients have clinical evidence of a cardiac lesion, and of those who die and come to necropsy carditis is found in the great majority.

About a third of the cases, however, give no history of either previous chorea or rheumatism. As a rule the disease subsides fairly soon after delivery and can often be controlled meanwhile by adequate rest, isolation and supervision.

The maternal mortality naturally varies with the severity of the case, but is influenced by the co-existence of a cardiac lesion and the tendency to develop bronchopneumonia. Neglected cases of the manic type may die of exhaustion. The fetal mortality is mainly influenced by the possibility of premature labour or the need to intervene and terminate the pregnancy.

The differential diagnosis rests between Huntingdon's chorea and hysteria. In the former there is a later age incidence and usually a family history, while in the latter other stigmata of hysteria are usually present.

The main complications are the development of an acute psychosis, which takes the form either of profound confusion or of mania, and may even necessitate supervision in a padded cell. Secondly, acute carditis and pericarditis may supervene and prove fatal.

The treatment consists in hospitalisation and the enforcement of absolute rest in isolation. Sedatives should be given liberally, and in the manic varieties it may be necessary to administer paraldehyde 5 ml intramuscularly. Hyoscine 0·5 mg has also been used with varying success. Promazine by mouth, 50 mg 8-hourly, in the severe and uncontrollable case can be of dramatic benefit.[10] The diet should be liberal and a watch maintained for the development of an active cardiac lesion. With good nursing and supervision it is often possible to bring the case under control, but in severe cases the question of terminating pregnancy arises. This is a serious step, because the patient is already ill enough as it is; nevertheless, occasionally it may be the only course to adopt. There is much to be said for sterilising the patient at the same time because of her proneness to suffer a recurrence of the disease in subsequent pregnancies.

VIRUS DISEASES IN PREGNANCY

The extent to which virus diseases contracted in pregnancy may damage the unborn fetus varies from the trivial to the ultra severe. It was Gregg (1941) who first noted an association between congenital cataract and a history of rubella in early pregnancy. Many of these cases had also congenital cardiac lesions. The epidemic of rubella in question, which had taken place in Australia, was of a very severe variety. Nevertheless, since attention was first directed towards this complication of pregnancy, more cases of associated fetal defect have come to light.

Retrospective analysis is difficult, because the diagnosis of rubella, made many months later after delivery, is often open to question. In Gregg's series of cases in Australia the position was more clear-cut. He described 78 cases of congenital cataract which was obvious from birth and as a rule bilateral; two-thirds of the cases had microphthalmia. All but 10 of the mothers of these affected infants had a definite history of rubella, usually within the first or second month of pregnancy.

Prospective studies are now available on which to assess the risks and it is quite clear that the likelihood of major congenital abnormality in the fetus depends upon the time of attack by the rubella virus. For instance, in one large analysis[36] involving 222 live births in patients contracting rubella in the first trimester of pregnancy, major abnormalities were found in 61 per cent, in the case of the first four weeks, in 26 per cent in the second four weeks and in only 8 per cent in the third. In other words, the earlier in pregnancy, the worse the damage. Mental deficiency and deafness are not usually immediately obvious at birth, so that a longer follow up is necessary to assess the true hazard and as spontaneous abortion and stillbirth are also common complications, especially in mothers developing rubella within the first eight weeks, the chances of a healthy infant, completely undamaged, are about 35 per cent. If the children of such affected pregnancies are followed up to the tenth year of life and over, the findings in surviving children at this age indicate major abnormalities in about 15 per cent, in more than half of whom there is more than one abnormality, and minor abnormalities in a further 16 per cent, with again more than half with more than one defect.[40] Ninety-two per cent of this later series, however, were attending ordinary schools, even though some required hearing aids or speech therapy.

It is clear that much so-called mental backwardness may be more apparent than real and related to some handicapping lesion such as deaf-mutism which, even in educated households, may not be recognised for the first few years of the child's life.

The rubella virus can be isolated from placental and fetal tissues many weeks after the initial attack and would appear to act by a direct destructive effect upon dividing tissue cells rather than by producing chromosome abnormalities. It is even possible for the nursing staff to be infected by the congenital presence and excretion of rubella virus in babies surviving birth after a pregnancy infected much earlier, in fact it has been found up to eight months later in urine and stools and from throat washings, and may be isolated from many tissues at autopsy.[6] The case has even been described of virus being still present in the lens of a child, almost three years old, operated on for congenital cataract.[26]

Taking fetal abnormality as a whole, virus diseases make only a small, though serious, contribution to the problem.

The Survey instituted by the Ministry of Health covered a very large, nation-wide survey, conducted prospectively into the possible effects of not only rubella but other virus infections during pregnancy.[25] In the case of rubella, records were available for an analysis of 578 pregnancies so complicated, in 202 of which the disease had occurred during the first twelve weeks. There were also 103 pregnancies complicated by measles, 298 by chickenpox, 501 by mumps, 33 by poliomyelitis and 166 by influenza. These were matched against a control series of 5700 selected on the basis of all babies born on a certain date. This enquiry extended throughout England, Scotland and Wales during 1950 to 1957 and the results are nothing like as depressing as previous accounts would have suggested. In the first place it would appear that infection after the 16th week certainly (and after the 12th week probably) does not affect the fetus, but the death rate *in utero* and up to two years of age is more than doubled when rubella is contracted within the first trimester. Furthermore, the abnormality rate is very much worse, the incidence of congenital heart disease being 4·7 per cent, as against 0·2 per cent in the control series, cataract 4·7 against, 0·04 per cent, deafness 3 per cent (0·08) with probable deafness in a slightly greater number. The incidence of mental deficiency was about quadrupled to the figure of 1·8 per cent, as against 0·4 per cent. There was also an increased incidence of pyloric stenosis. Of the children who lived beyond the age of three years nearly 20 per cent had impaired hearing.

In a similar but smaller series quoted from Australia[30] the total incidence of all malformations added up to 26 per cent and one child in fifty was severely retarded mentally.

Although there was a suggestion that measles might raise the incidence of infant deaths and malformations the figures were not very conclusive. The other virus infections appeared to be very much less important as causes of abnormality although there was a higher death rate in cases of maternal influenza and poliomyelitis.

The importance of influenza is less easy to assess because of inaccuracies in diagnosis, but in the year 1957 to 1958 there was an epidemic of Asian influenza in Dublin of some severity in which 663 pregnant women contracting the disease were analysed.[11] The congenital deformity rate was about two-and-a-half times that of the control group and the abnormalities were noted to be mainly of the central nervous system, particularly anencephaly.

As vaccination against smallpox involves inflicting the patient with a virus disease deliberately, there has naturally been some debate about the advisability of undertaking this in the early months. The general consensus of opinion is that the procedure is safe, although primary vaccination may result in temporary but severe pyrexial illness in the mother which might increase the risk of abortion. On the other hand the risks both to the mother and the baby of the patient contracting smallpox, however, are so horrifying that there should be no hesitation in advising vaccination even in the earliest months of pregnancy in the case of a patient who has been actually exposed. Acting on general principles, therefore, one would be inclined to recommend that vaccination be postponed, especially if it is primary, to the second and third trimesters, unless there are special reasons. The dangers from secondary vaccination are minimal.

In the present state of our knowledge, therefore, it would appear that the rubella virus stands out as the principal if not quite the main offender; the teratogenic effects of other viruses are still not widely

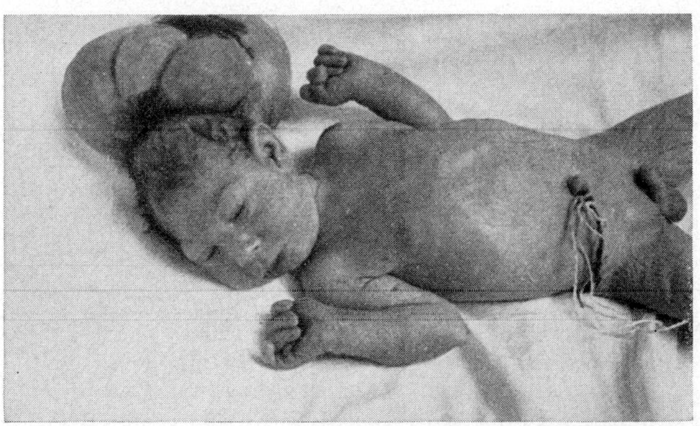

8/FIG. 1.—Large meningocele.

recognised and a confidently reassuring attitude should be taken with the patient exposed to the other exanthemata.

There is a correlation between the time of onset of the infection in pregnancy and the period of gestation at which embryonic development is most rapid and, therefore, presumably most vulnerable, and this too selects the particular structure most likely to suffer damage. Once differentiation has taken place a particular organ ceases to be susceptible to rubella. Furthermore, rubella might so damage the embryo as to reduce its chances of being born alive. The following abnormalities are likely to be encountered either singly or in combination:

Deaf mutism
Mental deficiency
Microcephaly
Congenital cardiac lesions
Cataract
Cleft palate
Spina bifida, etc. (Fig. 1)
Pyloric stenosis.

The cardiac lesions encountered include patent ductus, patent foramen ovale and interventricular septal defect. In the ears of deaf mutes the organ of Corti is absent.

A very severe epidemic of rubella swept the United States in 1964 with a noticeable increase in the type and extent of damage done to unborn babies, and as a result of this epidemic there has been described the "expanded rubella syndrome".

Expanded rubella syndrome.—The following further clinical features may be encountered[34]

Thrombocytopenia (100 per cent of cases)
Purpuric lesions
Growth retardation (78 per cent)
Hepatosplenomegaly
Central nervous system changes, including increased CSF protein, a full fontanelle and osseous manifestations (84 per cent).

The osseous manifestations as demonstrated on X-ray consist of a large anterior fontanelle and in the metaphyses of the femora and tibiae near the knee joint there is an altered trabecular pattern with linear areas of longitudinal radiotranslucency, contrasted with areas of increased bone density. There may also be radiotranslucency parallel to the growth plate. These lesions are said to be reversible.

Another report quotes a 33 per cent incidence of long-bone X-ray changes as described above and, furthermore, over half the babies were of retarded development, weighing less than 2500 g at birth.[31]

This is a formidable list of possible misfortunes, and the patient who contracts a virus infection, particularly rubella, within the first three months of pregnancy is undoubtedly exposed to the risk of tragedy.

It goes without saying that women in early pregnancy should avoid, as far as possible, contact with virus infections, and the compulsory notification of cases of rubella would make a difference. Strangely enough the severity of fetal malformation is not directly related to the severity of the clinical disease in the mother and quite minor infections might pass unnoticed. To the woman who believes she has been exposed to the risk of rubella and who has no idea of whether or not she is susceptible, the mental anguish can be very great and various methods have been tried serologically to assess whether the patient has an immunity to the disease or whether, in fact, the disease has been recently contracted. This problem may be solved, by demonstrating a rise in haemagglutination-inhibiting antibodies (HIA) whose level alters sharply early in the disease. It is this rise in antibody which helps to distinguish the patient already immune from rubella from one who has been recently infected and from such a calculation it should be possible to assess the risk to this particular pregnancy. The finding of complement-fixing antibodies, which do not persist so long, also indicates a recent infection. The earliest immunoglobulins (IgM) to be found after the primary stimulus have a very high molecular weight, but these immunoglobulins are replaced within a few weeks by those of a lower molecular weight (IgG and IgA). New methods are described from St. Thomas's Hospital[2, 3] which have been devised for distinguishing the two by haemagglutination-inhibition tests, titrating early and late convalescent sera before and after treating the sera with 2-mercaptoethanol, which is a sulphydryl-reducing compound that breaks down the IgM immunoglobulins. The amount of IgM immunoglobulin is therefore revealed by the difference between the level found in a control specimen from the patient compared with another treated with 2-mercaptoethanol. The discrepancy would appear to be most marked during the first few days of the illness, thereby proving beyond doubt the existence of a very recent infection. Clearly the test should be carried out at an early stage of infection, but may help to confirm or allay fears that pregnancy may be adversely affected. The test is claimed to be both simple and rapid and may determine treatment.

Occasionally, one gets requests for termination of a given pregnancy simply because there is a story that a child of a woman further down the street has developed German measles, hardly a reason for liquidation of a pregnancy which may be perfectly normal however real the maternal anxiety. Fortunately the majority of women in the population have immunity to the disease already without being aware of having had it before. Serological testing as above should put the matter beyond doubt. Attempts may be made to confer a temporary passive immunity by the use of gamma globulin, in an injected dose of 1500 mg, repeated within a week if the absence of antibody is confirmed. The value of this prophylactic passive immunotherapy, however, is doubted in many quarters.[32]

Rubella Vaccination

About 80 per cent of young women during reproductive life are already immune to rubella, whether there is a positive history of infection or not. The remaining 20 per cent are at real risk which it is now being attempted to eliminate. Rubella vaccination employs attenuated but nevertheless living virus and is undesirable during early pregnancy and there is the danger that it may be given inadvertently to a woman who was not aware that she was already pregnant,[22, 24] or that she may become pregnant during the ensuing sixty days through failure to take proper contraceptive measures.

Ideally no woman should enter the reproductive phase of her life still susceptible to rubella. A policy of vaccination of all schoolgirls between the ages of 11 and 13 is now fully under way. Above this age it is not considered advisable to vaccinate against rubella without first screening to indicate the need for it since the vaccine, given unnecessarily, may have teratogenic effects upon an unexpected pregnancy, which in any case should be avoided for at least two months thereafter.

We are now much interested in vaccinating recently delivered women who are found to be still susceptible to rubella and covering them against the risk of the disease for the first few months by combining the procedure with injected depot progesterone such as medroxyprogesterone acetate.[37]

Seronegative members of the medical and nursing staff, especially in obstetrical and gynaecological units may be at special risk of contracting and transmitting the infection and might, with advantage, be offered vaccination.[12]

Apart from pregnancy or the immediate risk of it, the most important contra-indication is current corticosteroid therapy.

The Abortion Law in the United Kingdom which legalises the termination of pregnancy when there is a "substantial" risk of "serious" handicap to the child does not, in fact, define the level at which action should be taken and is therefore really of very little help to the patient or the clinician whose individual conscience alone can guide them, bearing in mind always that the policy of termination, on the offchance of fetal abnormality, means that many a potentially normal baby will be sacrificed.

Other live virus vaccines in pregnancy.—As a general rule, living though attenuated virus vaccines should not be given in the first trimester of pregnancy unless epidemic conditions threaten, mainly in overseas areas.

Herpes Gestationis

This curious condition has a tendency to recur in subsequent pregnancies at an earlier stage each time. Fortunately with modern corticosteroid therapy the patient can usually be kept under control and neither she nor the fetus may come to permanent harm.[35, 43]

High doses of prednisone, for example, may be required, and the patient is liable to collapse under the stress of labour unless adequate corticosteroid therapy is maintained. She must, of course, be delivered in hospital under full specialist care, both obstetrical and dermatological. With these provisos there is no need to terminate pregnancy nor to advise the patient against further child-bearing.

Lupus Erythematosus

This curious disease is thought at present to result from an interaction of genetic factors and viral infection.[20] Moreover it is nine times as common in women as in men and its incidence chiefly straddles the reproductive period of life. It is usually regarded as a rare complication of pregnancy. However in the past we have had no less than four such cases in the Queen Mother's Hospital simultaneously. I do not imagine that our experience is unique. One of the four cases died undelivered.

There are two main types of lupus erythematosus, namely the discoid and the systemic.[27] The discoid disease is chronic and the lesion affects mainly the skin, including a scaly erythema of butterfly distribution over the cheeks and the bridge of the nose. The palms of the hands show a violaceous erythema and there are sometimes mottled haemorrhages on the pulps of the toes. Patches of permanent alopecia of uneven distribution are common. The condition, whether the patient is pregnant or not, is essentially benign, although photosensitivity and unfavourable reactions occur to certain drugs like sulphonamide and hydrallazine. About 5 per cent of these cases go on to develop the full-blown variety of the systemic disease.

Systemic lupus erythematosus is an ugly complication of pregnancy. It is a multisystem disease and according to the American Rheumatism Association there are no less than fourteen criteria of which the concurrent appearance of at least four qualifies for the diagnosis of SLE. Of these the most important, from the point of view of pregnancy, are proteinuria of over 3·5 g/day associated with renal involvement, neuropsychiatric disorders, progressive anaemia and leukopenia. These worsen the prognosis.

Usually the pregnant sufferer presents with the disease already diagnosed earlier and there remain only the problems of treatment, for what it is worth, and of prognosis, which is very unpredictable.[42]

A year or two ago one of our undiagnosed cases presented with massive proteinuria and unaccountable pyrexia and it was some time before the correct diagnosis was made.

The basic pathology is a liquefaction of the basal layer of the skin with degeneration of the dermis but, apart from the liver, the viscera are also likely to show immunohistochemical changes, particularly the kidney.

The diagnosis is made on the basis of serological findings such as antinuclear antibody (ANF) in titre higher than 1:64, DNA-binding capacity, estimated by radioimmunoassay (a result of over 30 per cent being significant), and the presence of LE cells. These are polymorphonuclear leucocytes which have "swallowed whole" or phagocytosed a lymphocyte so that the original nucleus is squashed out towards the periphery of the cell. This phenomenon is due to LE factor, a gamma globulin which is an antibody to deoxyribonucleoprotein present in the patient's serum and can produce this effect *in vitro*.

Provided the disease is in a quiescent state, patients do no worse in pregnancy than they otherwise would but exacerbations, particularly with renal involvement, are dangerous, and termination of pregnancy in the very earliest stage may have to be considered. Although corticosteroids may be life-saving in controlling exacerbations they are less effective at coping with renal involvement.

Another serious complication of this disease in pregnancy is progressive anaemia and I have watched a patient's haemoglobin sink in a few months from 10 g to little more than 4 g per 100 ml. Transfusion even of washed red cells is hazardous and infection vies with the need for prednisolone and likely sensitivity to antibiotic cover.

A series of 41 patients with a total of 104 pregnancies have been described by Madsen and Anderson but more than half of these were of the discoid variety. Even so the abortion and premature delivery rates were high, 17 per cent and 23 per cent respectively. Pre-eclampsia and eclampsia were also trebled in incidence. One of our own cases developed apparently fulminating eclampsia but she also had malaria as well which further complicated the diagnosis. She died.

In the series of 33 pregnancies in 21 patients reported by Garsenstein *et al.* it was noted that exacerbations of systemic lupus erythematosus were liable to occur in the first half of pregnancy and in the first eight weeks after delivery. There were four maternal deaths, three of whom had extensive renal involvement as did the fourth who died in spite of termination of pregnancy within the first trimester. Only 58 per cent of the 33 pregnancies resulted in a live baby and corticosteroids did not appear to have influenced the fetal prognosis. However the maternal prognosis was just as grim in a comparable series of women who were not pregnant.

It would thus appear that pregnancy is no more than an incident, albeit an ugly one, in the course of a progressive and dangerous disease.

Antenatal Thrombosis

The commonest variety of this complication of pregnancy is in veins already varicose. The condition can produce a great deal of discomfort and misery in pregnancy and seldom gets the treatment it deserves. Varicose veins themselves nearly always get worse, usually because of neglect to a large extent. Any varicosities in the legs noted at first booking should receive attention before and not after worsening. The best way to prevent aggravation of the condition is to make sure that the patient gets adequate rest during the day, with her feet up; but this is impossible for most women, therefore she must be advised against prolonged periods of standing, especially in the second half of pregnancy. Support from outside, in mild cases, can be obtained by rolling several pairs of stockings, one on top of the other, onto the legs and for this stockings which have already got holes and are not worth repairing are admirable. In more severe cases elastic stockings coming well up the thigh should be obtained at an early stage. Needless to say these supports should be applied while the patient is still in bed and before her feet are put to the ground; in other words before swelling has had time to occur and not after.

In spite of all these precautions, however, the condition may deteriorate surprisingly. The reluctance of surgeons to operate or to inject these veins with sclerosing fluids is due to the high rate of failure in pregnancy and the comforting reflection (at least comforting to the surgeon) that the condition will improve after pregnancy is all over; but it may well be necessary to treat by the injection of sclerosing agents, using the empty vein technique.

At the Rotunda Hospital in Dublin this miserable condition gets more of the attention it deserves and an enormous experience has been acquired. The aim of the treatment here is "to prevent abnormal pressure and retrograde flow from the deep to the superficial venous system." For this purpose a great deal of trouble is taken identifying the sites of incompetence by a careful clinical examination. The empty vein technique is used, with the defective leg raised in the air and, by digital compression, a segment of affected vein being isolated and emptied of blood before injection of sclerosing fluid is undertaken. The substance used is half to one ml of sodium tetradecyl as a sclerosant; it is held there by the fingers while the syringe is removed. Thereupon an Elastocrepe bandage is applied with a Sorbo rubber pad placed over the injection site. Multiple injections are carried out in this way and then the whole limb bandaged. Further treatments may have to be given. Compression has to be maintained for some weeks until fibrosis definitely occludes the offending vein.[15] One has only to visit Dublin to be impressed with the success of this care.

It is suggested that attention to venous inadequacy of this sort will reduce the incidence of antepartum thrombo-embolism.

Pulmonary Embolism

When antepartum pulmonary embolism occurs the situation is one of great urgency. The immediate necessity is to relieve pain and anxiety with an opiate and put the patient immediately onto intravenous heparin. The quoted incidence of thrombo-embolic disease is not more than somewhere between 0·018 and 0·29 per 100 deliveries. A recent appreciable rise has been reported from Dundee[4] but some of this may have been due to an increased awareness of the possibility of the diagnosis. Needless to say previous taking of the contraceptive pill has come in for the usual speculation.

Once the diagnosis of pulmonary thrombo-embolism is made, or even suspected, an injection of 15,000 units of heparin intravenously should be given as soon as possible in order to initiate anticoagulation, and this should be followed up with 10,000 units six-hourly for at least the next 48 hours. The choice of anticoagulant therapy varies between 4 alternatives.[45]

1. Heparin only, by intermittent injection or continuous intravenous infusion, at a rate of 10,000 units every 6 hours;
2. Heparin to start with, converting as soon as possible to phenindione or warfarin;
3. Phenindione alone;
4. Phenindione alone at the beginning, with conversion to heparin when delivery is thought to be imminent.

Because of the urgency of the situation there is little point in the last two alternatives. Of the above drugs only heparin does not cross the placenta because of its high molecular weight and if the case is deemed severe enough to justify anticoagulation then the danger is here and now and not in 36 or 48 hours time by which time the oral anticoagulants will have had time to take effect. Of the oral anticoagulants my own personal preference is for warfarin since I have been living on it myself for many years. The only nuisance is that it takes the best part of a fortnight to obtain a stable dose, which may vary between 8 mg and 10 mg in a day. This should be controlled with frequent thrombotesting, aiming at a figure between 8 and 15 per cent of normal. Heparin control is by estimation of clotting time.

The more common problem is the case who develops an obviously superficial thrombophlebitis, usually in a vein previously varicose, and in whom the danger of pulmonary thrombo-embolism is very slight. To go to the length of full anticoagulant therapy often appears in these cases to be unnecessary. So long as one can be sure that the thrombosis is entirely superficial, that it is not extending and that there is no question of signs of deep thrombosis such as oedema of the lower leg or a positive Homan's sign, it may be sufficient simply to elevate the foot of the bed and await developments; but if there is the slightest doubt there should be no hesitation in giving heparin forthwith and reviewing the situation within 48 hours. The danger of the oral anticoagulants is that they cross the placenta and should labour ensue—and this can never be fully foreseen—not only is the patient at risk from haemorrhage herself but the baby too, and the latter may be liable to neonatal haemorrhagic disease, more especially if it is premature. It takes many hours to reverse the effects of oral anticoagulants with vitamin K_1 injections whereas heparin can be instantly reversed by protamine sulphate, a dose of 1 ml being reckoned to neutralise 1000 units of heparin, bearing in mind that the effective dose within the circulation will depend upon the time since the last intravenous injection.

Operations undertaken for the relief of varicose veins are likely to produce their biggest benefit by the necessary rest entailed post-operatively and are therefore seldom performed.

Pain and disability can unquestionably be shortened by intravenous heparin maintained in standard dosage over a period of at least three days, by which time the danger of embolism or of further spread of the condition should have passed. Bandaging with ichthyol solutions is a time-honoured ritual which is more impressive in the picturesque mess it produces than actually beneficial. Heparin is recommended as the drug of choice for several reasons; firstly its action is immediate; secondly, with its molecular weight of 16 thousand it does not cross the placenta and therefore is perfectly safe for the fetus; and thirdly, its effects are short-lived and can be quickly countered should the patient go into labour. Admittedly the more superficial the affected vein, the less likely is thrombo-embolism to occur, but this does not justify a casual attitude. With adequate treatment starting with 20,000 units, for example, followed by about 10,000 every six hours intravenously, or, maintained, better still, by intravenous drip, so as to prolong the clotting time to 20 minutes, it will be found that the thrombotic process does not extend and the pain disappears very quickly.[17]

The slower-acting anticoagulants given orally, namely warfarin and phenindione, are less suitable because their effect is slow and because they cross the placenta and may produce or aggravate fetal hypoprothrombinaemia with a dangerous tendency to haemorrhagic disease should labour ensue while the fetus is still affected by the drug.[21] The danger can be minimised by the timely injection of vitamin K_1 (Konakion) 10–20 mg slowly to the mother by the intravenous route and before delivery actually takes place.

Fatal pulmonary embolism, which may occur antenatally and is becoming a more prominent cause of maternal death nowadays, can thus be prevented by anticoagulants. Therefore, thrombosis superficial or deep should not go untreated.

VOMITING, HIATUS HERNIA AND HEARTBURN

by WALLACE BARR, M.B., B.Sc., F.R.C.S. (Glas.), F.R.C.O.G.,
Gynaecologist, Western Infirmary, Glasgow, and Obstetrician, Queen Mother's Hospital, Glasgow

Vomiting

This is one of the most common of all the tribulations of the first trimester. It generally occurs during the early part of pregnancy and in many instances precedes the first missed menstrual period. For many, it is a minor complaint to which they are resigned but to others the anticipation of an uneventful pregnancy may be rudely shattered by weeks of intense discomfort with associated domestic upheaval and inconvenience.

Uncontrollable vomiting has shown a remarkable decline over recent decades and in the following table are shown the figures obtained from the records of the Glasgow Royal Maternity Hospital for three comparable five-year periods since 1936.

	1936–40	1946–50	1956–60
Total births in hospital	16,532	16,326	17,759
Admissions for hyperemesis gravidarum	396 (2·4%)	168 (1·0%)	97 (0·6%)
Termination of pregnancy	33	4	nil
Maternal deaths	15 (12 after termination)	nil	nil

The number of cases of hyperemesis admitted to the Queen Mother's Hospital has nowadays fallen to an insignificant trickle.

It is difficult to explain this diminishing incidence of severe hyperemesis gravidarum but some at least of the credit must be given to the newer drugs which have recently become available, and many patients now seek advice earlier in the pregnancy, and thanks to earlier booking are able to shed any psychological load more readily.

Family planning has also helped to reduce the number of unwelcome pregnancies.

Aetiology

Our ignorance of the cause is almost as striking as the success which nearly always attends treatment. The condition is commoner in first than in subsequent pregnancies and it has also been found that women who have nausea and vomiting in their first pregnancy are more likely to have symptoms again in later pregnancies: there is no relationship between maternal age and the incidence of hyperemesis gravidarum. It is safer to classify cases according to the severity of the vomiting than to use the old division into toxic and neurotic varieties. This is not only obsolete but dangerous too, as the diagnosis of neurosis may engender a regrettable complacency regarding the outcome of the condition.

In all cases and especially those of acute onset it is essential to exclude organic disease of extra-uterine origin such as appendicitis, gastro-enteritis, intestinal obstruction, peptic ulcer, twisted ovarian cyst, cerebral tumour, fulminating pre-eclamptic toxaemia, pyelitis and uraemia. Hydatidiform mole should also be excluded.

Only when these have been excluded, and not before, may one contemplate the many nebulous and ill-substantiated theories which have been conjured up to explain this curious condition. There are still those who think that the vomiting may be reflexly engendered by some pelvic abnormality, such as retroversion of the gravid uterus. The anatomy of the reflex arc is of doubtful authenticity, however, and the cures obtained by correcting the malposition are just as likely to be due to suggestion. Vitamin-deficiency states and carbohydrate deficiences have also been put forward as possible aetiological factors, but they are more likely to be effects than causes.

Fitzgerald (1956) in a discussion on the epidemiology of hyperemesis gravidarum points out that its incidence and severity in Aberdeen and North-east Scotland was significantly diminished during the last war and the immediate post-war years, the assumption being that the major problems engendered by war conditions allowed the patient less time to worry about personal affairs. Few will deny that the psychogenic factor is of prime importance and it is probable that the many adjustments demanded by the newly-pregnant woman impose a mild condition of stress coupled with an irrationally exaggerated fear of the obstetric hazards confronting her, especially that of producing an abnormal child. These factors, superimposed upon the subtle physiological accompaniments of reduced gastric secretion and motility, provide a much more likely cause for the condition than the hitherto fashionable explanation that vomiting constitutes a symbolic rejection by the mother of her pregnancy.

Pathology and Biochemical Changes

There are no specific morbid anatomical findings and the changes described by Sheehan (1939) in the liver, heart, kidneys and central nervous system are common to all cases of severe malnutrition whatever the cause. The lesions in the brain stem resembling Wernicke's encephalopathy are probably due to vitamin B_1 deficiency.

The biochemical changes which occur can also be attributed to chronic starvation and are not specific to hyperemesis. There is a loss of water and salt with consequent haemoconcentration and reduction of urinary chlorides. Extracellular fluid is diminished and plasma, sodium and chloride are reduced. Ketosis occurs and the blood urea is elevated as a result of the disturbance in nitrogen metabolism. Potassium deficiency soon follows, as potassium is not stored by the normal adult and rapid loss occurs in the vomit and in the increased renal excretion. This hypokalaemia may cause further vomiting, which, together with liver damage, sets up a vicious circle difficult or impossible to break.

Clinical Features

The insidious change from the mild to the severe state has constantly to be watched for. So long as she is not losing weight appreciably, has a clean, moist tongue and no acetone in her urine, there is little cause for concern even if she protests that she vomits every morsel of food swallowed. As her condition deteriorates, the pulse rate starts to rise and blood pressure falls, the tongue becomes dry and furred while the breath smells strongly of acetone. Emaciation supervenes with dramatic speed, the urine becomes concentrated and in addition to acetone may contain albumin and bile with chlorides greatly diminished or absent. Epigastric tenderness is frequently noted. In the later stages the temperature starts to rise, jaundice supervenes and haematemesis may occur. She becomes apathetic and drowsy or confused and euphoric. Squint, diplopia and nystagmus may be noted and retinal haemorrhages appear. Various palsies develop and there may be great tenderness in the legs together with other signs of peripheral neutritis. Ultimately Wernicke's encephalopathy becomes fully established and the patient usually dies in coma.

Treatment

In early cases, simple dietetic measures will often be effective and should be given a trial before resorting to the countless proprietary and often expensive remedies advertised by the drug manufacturers. Constipation should be corrected and small carbohydrate meals taken frequently, while all greasy foods should be avoided. When the sickness has a well-defined morning incidence the time-honoured piece of toast or cream cracker taken before rising is often helpful.

Of the drugs to be employed, the antihistamines and vitamin B_6 preparations are often of value. Since Dougray (1949) first recommended the use of mepyramine maleate (Anthisan) and promethazine hydrochloride (Phenergan), many other antihistamines have appeared of which dimenhydrinate (Dramamine) and promethazine theoclate (Avomine) are among the most effective. Meclozine dihydrochloride (also an antihistamine) is now combined with pyridoxine (Ancoloxin) since, rightly or wrongly, pyridoxine deficiency is believed to occur in hyperemesis gravidarum. Debendox, too, enjoys a reputation for efficiency.

Because the thalidomide disaster focused attention on the possible dangers of prescribing, during early pregnancy, drugs whose exact action on the developing fetus is not known, some evidence has been produced to suggest that certain anti-emetic drugs may possibly have teratogenic effects. The matter remains *sub judice* and until the issue has been finally resolved, it is suggested that the greatest discrimination is employed in the exhibition of any drug prescribed during the early stages of pregnancy (Barr, 1963). For the severe case the only place for the patient is a hospital bed where, out of the range of all visitors, including her husband, she very often recovers abruptly without further treatment. The attitude of the nurse in attendance is important and the ideal approach is one of firm competence allied with tactful understanding. A fluid balance chart is kept and the blood pressure recorded at least twice daily.

If the vomiting does not immediately cease, all feeding by mouth is stopped, the lost fluids and chlorides are made good by intravenous infusion and ketosis is combated with glucose. Glucose 4·3 per cent in 0·18 per cent saline should be used and one should aim to administer at least 3 litres in 24 hours. Ten units of insulin may with advantage be added to each half-litre of glucose solution to encourage the intracellular shift of potassium ions and to increase glycogen storage. In addition, adequate sedation is obtained with the help of Sparine 50 mg by injection. Oral hygiene is attended to with mouth washes, and only when ketosis and dehydration have been overcome, and the patient has stopped vomiting, are fluids given by mouth in small and often repeated quantities. The patient then gradually proceeds to solids, and it is indeed unusual for this treatment not to succeed within a very few days. To prevent neuropathy, injections of vitamin B_1 (aneurine) and B_6 (pyridoxine hydrochloride) 100 mg are given daily.

Therapeutic Abortion

If the patient fails to respond to the above energetic treatment therapeutic abortion has to be considered, especially in multiparae, in whom vomiting often has a more sinister significance. The decision to operate is easily too long delayed, in which case death may be precipitated rather than prevented. The following are the indications for therapeutic abortion:

1. Jaundice;
2. Persistent albuminuria;
3. Polyneuritis and neurological signs;
4. Temperature consistently above 38° C (100·4° F) and a pulse remaining above 100;
5. The onset of psychosis, although Sheehan rather hinted that abortion precipitates death in these cases.

It is nowadays so rarely that pregnancy has to be interrupted that one is very naturally reluctant to take such drastic action, but to operate too late is just as bad as not operating at all. The method of termination will vary according to circumstances but there is much to be said for abdominal hysterotomy, possibly under regional anaesthesia.

Vomiting in Late Pregnancy

No case of vomiting occurring during the later weeks of pregnancy should be disregarded and a full investigation should always be undertaken as it may be a symptom of sinister import. We have seen a case of acute liver failure present only with retching and occasional vomiting followed rapidly by jaundice, severe hypotension, coma and death within 48 hours. Urinary infection is the most common cause of vomiting in late pregnancy and a clean specimen of urine should be examined in all cases for the presence of pus cells and organisms. Other causes are pre-eclamptic toxaemia, and occasionally acute hydramnios. Extraneous causes such as intestinal obstruction, gastro-enteritis, cholecystitis, appendicitis and red degeneration in a fibroid should also be excluded.

Hiatus Hernia

Hiatus hernia is a well recognised cause of gastro-intestinal upset during pregnancy and it is quite remarkable how published figures have shown that this condition, which was thought to be a rare one, is nowadays almost commonplace. Mixson and Woloshin (1956) found 31 cases in 360 pregnancies selected at random.

We ourselves found a low incidence and in 85 patients with heartburn and nausea during pregnancy only 4 showed hiatus hernia on X-ray examination with barium.

It appears to be much commoner in multiparae, presumably due to the increasing size of the diaphragmatic gap. The symptoms are usually due to reflux oesophagitis and the competence or otherwise of the lower oesophageal sphincter is more important in producing symptoms than the degree to which the stomach lies above or below the diaphragm.

Many cases go through pregnancy and labour uneventfully and many more are never diagnosed, but occasionally symptoms are severe. In most cases the chief complaint is intractable heartburn, unrelieved by alkalis or other medication and aggravated by the recumbent posture. In others vomiting is the main feature and a few of these go on to haematemesis. In the third and by far the smallest group, the clinical picture is one of severe and sudden onset, epigastric pain being associated with shock, dyspnoea and often cyanosis. This may be due to "spillover" disease of the lung—the result of aspiration of material from the hernia itself or from an oesophagus obstructed by stricture.

Treatment in the vast majority of cases is conservative and consists of frequent small meals, sleeping in a propped-up position, sedation as required and the use of alkalis if they provide any relief. Mucaine (*vide infra*) may also be of value in this condition. Powerful bearing down during the second stage tends to aggravate the condition and should be avoided by the timely application of forceps.

After delivery, although the symptoms usually clear up within a few days, Sutherland *et al.* (1956) reported that the hernia persists in 36 per cent of cases.

HEARTBURN

This is one of the minor disorders of pregnancy and its unfortunate victims seldom get much sympathy, but frequently, by disturbing sleep and appetite, it lowers morale and promotes a chronic depression out of all proportion to its severity. Moreover, it is extremely common and in our experience nearly 45 per cent of patients suffer from heartburn during pregnancy severely enough to compel them to seek relief.

It is almost certainly due to regurgitation of gastric content on lying down or stooping, and by screening patients with barium in the stomach we have been able to demonstrate such regurgitation in 64 of 85 patients with heartburn. In an overall analysis of 624 cases (Barr, 1958) it was found to bear little relationship to gastric acidity and hiatus hernia accounted for only 6 per cent of the cases X-rayed. Age and parity were not significant aetiological factors, nor was there any apparent association with nausea and vomiting of pregnancy, constipation or previous digestive disorders, and since it usually comes on during the first trimester encroachment upon the abdominal cavity by the enlarging uterus is not likely to be a factor. There was however a striking relationship to posture and no fewer than 92·3 per cent of cases found that lying down, bending or stooping, initiated an attack.

Using an inflated balloon in the stomach attached to tambour and recording drum, gastric motility during pregnancy was investigated and it was found in patients with heartburn that there is a significant reduction in gastric tonus rhythm, although peristaltic activity and emptying time remain unaltered. This reduced tone which is shared by the muscle of the lower oesophagus is probably responsible for regurgitation.

Treatment in the first instance is by alkalis which give relief in about half of all cases, especially if combined with a sensible dietary regime. Mucaine (oxethazaine, a topical anaesthetic agent, in combination with aluminium hydroxide gel and magnesium hydroxide) enjoys considerable success in severe cases. The recommended dose is 1 or 2 teaspoonfuls 15 minutes before meals. It should not be washed down straightaway with a drink as this may diminish the effect. Granules of Gaviscon (5 g single-dose cachets) chewed thoroughly after meals produce a colloidal gel of alginic acid which is viscous and floats on top of gastric fluids and coats and thereby protects the oesophageal mucosa. Gastrocote tablets have a similar action. In those which do not respond to such simple measures, the value of Prostigmin, first suggested by Williams (1941), is beyond doubt and Bower (1961) found that 76 per cent of patients unrelieved by alkalis obtained relief for an average period of about five days from an injection of Prostigmin. In about half these cases the effect was thought to be due to a genuine pharmacological action and in the remainder, to suggestion. In our opinion it is not necessary to administer it by injection and we have been obtaining a cure rate of more than 80 per cent with pyridostigmine (Mestinon) in a dosage of 16 mg given by mouth four times daily. It is somewhat slower in onset than Prostigmin but longer acting.

Ptyalism

This is not a common complaint but can be very distressing. It is regarded as a variant of hyperemesis gravidarum but without its biochemical sequelae. It may well have a psychosomatic origin and treatment, usually unsuccessful, may be tried in the form of sedation and anticholinergic drugs such as Pro-Banthine. Removal to a hospital environment may also help. Hypnosis may be tried but I have no experience of it. Any coexisting oral pathology should be eliminated.

REFERENCES

1. Adams, R. A. and Coombes, B. (1965). *J. Amer. med. Ass.*, **192,** 195.
2. Banatvala, J. E., Best, J. M., Kennedy, E. A., Smith, E. A. and Spence, M. E. (1967). *Brit. med. J.*, **2,** 285.
3. Banatvala, J. E., Best, J. M., Bertrand, J., Bowner, N. A. and Hudson, S. M. (1970). *Brit. med. J.*, **3,** 247.
4. Barr, W. (1958). *J. Obstet. Gynaec. Brit. Emp.*, **65,** 1019.
5. Barr, W. (1963). *Prescriber's J.*, **3,** 3.
6. Bellanti, J. A., Artenstein, M. S., Olson, L. S., Benscher, E. L., Luers, C. E. and Milstead, K. S. (1965). *Amer. J. Dis. Child.*, **110,** 464.
7. Beresford, O. D. and Graham, A. M. (1950). *J. Obstet. Gynaec. Brit. Emp.*, **57,** 616.
7A. Black, W. P. (1960). *Brit. med. J.*, **1,** 1938.
8. Bower, D. (1961). *J. Obstet. Gynaec. Brit. Cwlth*, **68,** 846.
9. British Medical Journal. (1966). Editorial. **2,** 426.
10. Campbell, A. J. M. and Henderson, J. (1959). *Scot. med. J.*, **4,** 128.
11. Coffey, V. P. and Jessop, W. J. E. (1959). *Lancet*, **2,** 935.
12. Department of Health and Social Security (1972). *Immunization against Infectious Diseases*. H.M.S.O.
13. Dougray, T. (1949). *Brit. med. J.*, **2,** 1081.

14. DUNCAN, I. D. and COYLE, M. G. (1971). *J. Obstet. Gynaec. Brit. Cwlth*, **78,** 904.
15. FEGAN, W. G. and FITZGERALD, D. E. (1966). *J. Obstet. Gynaec. Brit. Cwlth*, **73,** 222.
16. FITZGERALD, J. P. B. (1956). *Lancet*. **1,** 660.
17. FLESSA, H. C., KAPSTROM, A. B., GLUECK, H. I. and WILL, J. J. (1965). *Amer. J. Obstet. Gynec.*, **93,** 570.
18. GARSENSTEIN, M., POLLAK, V. E. and KARK, R. M. (1962). *New Engl. J. Med.*, **267,** 165.
19. GREGG, H. M. (1941). *Trans. ophthal. Soc. Aust.*, **3,** 35.
20. HUGHES, G. V. (1974). *Brit. J. hosp. Med.*, **12,** 309.
21. KRAUS, A. P., PERLOW, S. and SINGER, K. (1949). *J. Amer. med. Ass.*, **139,** 758.
22. LEVINE, M. M., EDSALL, G. and BRUCE-IHWATT, L. J. (1974). *Lancet*, **2,** 34.
23. MADSEN, J. R. and ANDERSON, G. V. (1961). *Obstet. and Gynec.*, **18,** 492.
24. MAIR, H. and BUCHAN, A. R. (1972). *Brit. med. J.*, **4,** 271.
25. MANSON, M. M., LOGAN, W. P. D. and LUZ, R. M. (1960). *Rubella and other Virus Infections in Pregnancy*. Min. of Health Reports on Public Health and Medical Subjects, No. 101.
26. MENSER, M. A., HARLEY, J. D., HERTZBERG, R., DORMAN, D. C. and MURPHY, A. M. (1967). *Lancet.*, **2,** 387.
27. MILNE, J. A. (1975). Personal communication.
28. MIXSON, W. T. and WOLOSHIN, H. S. (1956). *Obstet. and Gynec.*, **8,** 249.
29. MOORE, H. C. (1963). *Lancet*, **2,** 57.
30. PITT, D. B. (1961). *Med. J. Aust.*, **1,** 881.
31. PLOTKIN, S. A., OSKI, F. A., HARTNETT, E. M., HERVADA, A. R., FRIEDMAN, S. and GOWING, JEAN (1965). *Pediatrics*, **67,** 182.
32. Public Health Laboratory Service Working Party on Rubella (1970). *Brit. med. J.* **1,** 497.
33. ROTH, L. G. (1953). *Amer. J. med. Sci.*, **225,** 139.
34. RUDOLPH, A. J., SINGLETON, E. B., ROSENBERG, H. S., SINGER, D. B. and PHILLIPS, C. A. (1965). *Amer. J. Dis. Child.*, **110,** 428.
35. RUSSELL, B. and THORNE, N. A. (1957). *Brit. J. Derm.*, **69,** 339.
36. SALLOMI, S. J. (1966). *Obstet. and Gynec.*, **27,** 252.
37. SHARP, D. S. and MACDONALD, H. (1973). *Brit. med. J.*, **4,** 443.
38. SHEEHAN, H. L. (1939). *J. Obstet. Gynaec. Brit. Emp.*, **46,** 681.
39. SHEEHAN, H. L. (1940). *J. Obstet. Gynaec. Brit. Emp.*, **47,** 49.
40. SHERIDAN, M. D. (1964). *Brit. med. J.*, **2,** 536.
41. SUTHERLAND, C. G., ATKINSON, J. C., BROGDON, B. G., CROW, N. E. and BROWN, W. E. (1956). *Obstet. and Gynec.*, **8,** 261.
42. TAYLOR, R. T. (1970). *Brit. J. hosp. Med.*, **4,** 653.
43. VICKERS, H. R. (1964). *Practitioner*, **192,** 639.
44. WILLIAMS, N. H. (1941). *Amer. J. Obstet. Gynec.*, **42,** 814.
45. WINGFIELD, J. G. (1969). *J. Obstet. Gynaec. Brit. Cwlth*, **76,** 518.

CHAPTER IX

LOCAL ABNORMALITIES

In this chapter a variety of conditions occurring in the pelvic viscera is dealt with, as it affects the practising obstetrician.

CONGENITAL UTERINE ABNORMALITIES

The many different degrees of imperfect Mullerian development, fusion or canalisation, seldom trouble the practitioner because the grosser forms of uterine maldevelopment prevent pregnancy in the first place, and of the cases who conceive the majority run an uneventful course and deliver themselves without undue difficulty. It is reckoned that two out of every thousand women have a sufficiently severe degree of congenital uterine deformity to interfere with pregnancy.[17] From the practical point of view there is little point in describing all the varieties of uterine abnormality, which are of more anatomical than obstetrical interest, but if one appreciates how the Mullerian ducts from each side fuse together and become canalised it will at once be seen that a particular structural abnormality is simply a matter of degree in the embryological process. All degrees may be encountered, from the subseptate uterus at one end of the scale to the completely double uterus and cervix at the other (Fig. 1). Neither of these two extremes gives any trouble as a rule, but intermediate stages may do so. Where there is a full septum in the uterus the fetus must perforce lie in the uterine axis longitudinally, but lesser degrees favour a transverse lie, so that one pole of the fetus lies in each half of the uterus. The incomplete septum also prevents version. About 12 per cent of cases of transverse lie are reckoned to be associated with a subseptate uterus[9] and they are even more liable to inertia in labour. It would appear that the lower uterine segment may resist expansion. Retention of the placenta and atonic postpartum haemorrhage are also more likely to occur. The bicornuate uterus with the single cervix is by no means uncommon, and occasionally the placenta may occupy one chamber and the fetus the other, an arrangement which prejudices the safety of the third stage of labour, inasmuch as a placenta so situated is liable to be retained and may be difficult to remove.

One tends to think of a bicornuate uterus with its two horns sticking symmetrically upwards and outwards like a donkey's ears, but usually there is a good deal of inequality and asymmetry and a tendency for one of the horns to flop backwards, in which case it may become trapped below the pelvic brim and prevent the engagement of the presenting part or even obstruct labour. In this position it is of course very vulnerable, and lochial drainage is likely to be inadequate. It is easy to see how torsion of the whole uterus may be favoured by the presence of a sizable non-gravid horn.

In the occasional case which gives trouble the clinical diagnosis is by no means easy unless hysterography has provided foreknowledge of the condition. Other pelvic tumours have to be distinguished and, earlier in pregnancy of course, the question of ectopic pregnancy enters into the differential diagnosis.

It is often a more serious matter when one of the horns of a bicornuate uterus happens to be rudimentary. This may become the site of a pregnancy, and its walls are in no condition to withstand its growth, so that acute rupture with intraperitoneal bleeding is very likely. In other cases the rudimentary horn has only a very narrow connection with the cervical canal or perhaps none at all, so that blood collecting within its lumen cannot be discharged and an acute haematometra develops. There is a fairly common association of congenital uterine abnormalities with other urogenital defects. In other words, the discovery of one freak indicates a search for others.

As already hinted, many of these cases go through their obstetrical

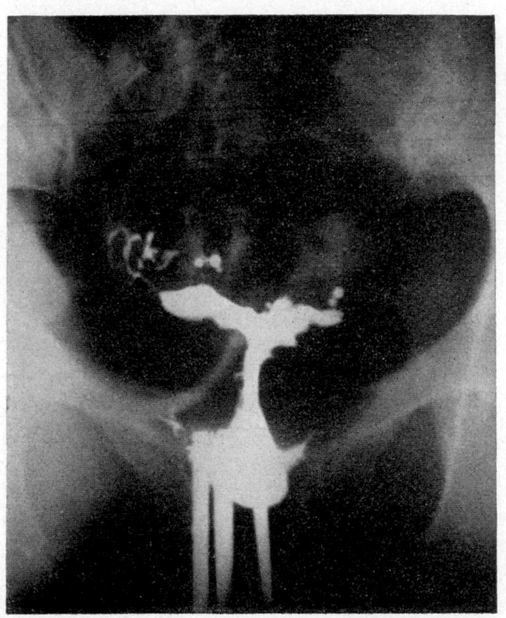

9/FIG. 1.—Double uterus. Hysterosalpingogram.
(By courtesy of Dr Pecker, Lambeth Hospital.)

careers sometimes undiagnosed and often without trouble, and provided a woman proves herself capable of conceiving, an optimistic prognosis can usually be given. When seen for the first time in pregnancy, in the absence of a double cervix, which can be ascertained with certainty, one should be very cautious of diagnosing congenital uterine abnormality because of apparent uterine asymmetry, which is common in the early months of pregnancy. The diagnosis is usually made between pregnancies, and hysterography is invaluable; but it should be pointed out that the case who delivers herself without any trouble should not be subjected to such an investigation purely to satisfy a point of academic interest.

Certain adverse effects upon pregnancy are well recognised. In reviewing a series of 42 pregnancies occurring in association with congenital uterine abnormalities MacGregor (1957) observed that 19 ended in abortion, and of the remaining 23 pregnancies premature labour occurred in 5 and the presentation was unstable in 8. In 5 instances manual removal of the placenta was necessary. Out of the 23 pregnancies reaching the stage of viability 4 babies were lost. Although the maternal and fetal accident rate is high, especially from cord prolapse and placenta praevia, it will depend upon the completeness or otherwise of congenital abnormality, thus illustrating the paradox that the more trivial anatomical abnormalities are, for that very reason, the more treacherous.

Congenital Vaginal Abnormalities

A completely double vagina with a longitudinal septum may occur and seldom gives any trouble; in fact, Munro Kerr and Chassar Moir stated that the more complete the malformation the less likely is dystocia. A septate vagina, however, may hold up delivery, but the amount of birth canal room can only be properly assessed towards term after the distensibility of the soft parts has had full time to develop.

Congenital strictures of the vagina are far more serious and may occur at any level in the Mullerian system, in other words in the upper three-quarters of the vagina. This abnormality again is due to imperfect canalisation. Occasionally the vaginal vault may be perfectly patent and the stricture may occur at the junction of the upper third and lower two-thirds. I once had a case with such a stricture which was barely adequate to allow the discharge of menstrual blood and caused an obstructive type of dysmenorrhoea, yet the passage of a spermatozoon must have been possible, for she became pregnant. The condition was not recognised until she went into labour at another hospital. She was delivered by Caesarean section and the true state of affairs assessed at the time. I then did a modified Mc-

Indoe type of operation with Thiersch graft which relieved her dysmenorrhoea and was structurally fairly satisfactory, although some vaginal narrowing was still palpable on follow-up examination. She again became pregnant and I delivered her by Caesarean section as I was doubtful of the capacity of the vagina to allow the passage of the fetus. However, in her third pregnancy she was delivered *per vias naturales*. It is impossible to assess the obstetrical importance of these strictures early in pregnancy, as the ensuing months may produce a remarkable change, so that with the softening up of the vagina the stricture may be no longer palpable. In the case of traumatic strictures, for example after plastic repair operations for prolapse, a vaginal or cervical stricture tends to be more dangerous; in fact, it is the narrowing of the vaginal vault that often occurs which is of even more importance than the actual state of the cervix, so that obstruction to delivery occurs at a particularly dangerous point with regard to the safety of the bladder.

Less common vaginal abnormalities in obstetrical practice are rectovaginal and vesicovaginal fistulae. Their mere presence, after all, discourages the opportunity for conception; nevertheless, should the patient conceive, normal delivery commonly occurs, although in the case of rectrovaginal fistulae the danger of complete perineal rupture is very great.

RETROVERSION

The importance of retroversion has, in the past, been greatly overestimated, for about one in every ten women has a retroverted uterus which is not necessarily of any pathological significance. Its discovery on routine examination in an otherwise normal patient, therefore, calls for no active measures. Retroversion has been found in 5·5 per cent of all primigravidae before the 12th week of pregnancy and in 6·5 per cent of multiparae.[2] Provided the retroverted uterus is both mobile and not tender on palpation, the likelihood is that no obstetrical trouble will ensue, and that, as the uterus enlarges, the malposition will naturally correct itself. It has been said that retroversion aggravates the severity of hyperemesis if present, but it is probable that the psychological effect of its manipulative correction does more to cure the patient of this symptom than the correction itself. There is no doubt, however, that women with retroversion conceive a little less easily than when the uterus is in the normal position, mainly because after coitus the cervix points away from the seminal pool in the posterior fornix, and all of us can recall instances in which conception has followed correction or advice to adopt a different position during coitus or immediately after. Symptoms from retroversion in pregnancy do not normally arise until incarceration within the pelvis threatens.

Retroversion is also regarded as being a possible aetiological factor in early abortion, although there is little convincing statistical evidence of this; but coitus, in the early months of pregnancy, may, by direct trauma, precipitate miscarriage in a retroverted uterus predisposed to abort. Where the patient has already had one or two previous abortions and is now found to be pregnant again with retroversion, it is naturally prudent to advise her to abstain, at least until pregnancy has safely reached the 16th week.

Incarceration of the gravid uterus does not occur until after the third month, when the uterus has become large enough to fill the pelvic cavity. Normally by the 12th week the uterus should have already risen so that the fundus is palpable per abdomen, but where this has not occurred it is as well to see the patient at more frequent intervals and to be on the lookout for incarceration, which may produce symptoms as early as the 13th week. The symptoms of incarceration are mainly due to effects upon the bladder. A short period of frequency gives way to dysuria and finally to acute retention of urine. Oedema in the region of the bladder neck adds its effects to those of mechanical compression and neuromuscular inco-ordination from the great elongation of the anterior vaginal wall and the structures that lead to it, so that the onset of retention is usually sudden and is followed by overflow incontinence.

Fortunately this dangerous mishap is rather uncommon. Decompression of the bladder by catheterisation is an urgent necessity if it is to be saved from the risks of rupture, sloughing and almost ineradicable infection. For the time being the pregnancy is ignored and all attention is given to the bladder, which must be kept empty. In the majority of cases the uterus undergoes spontaneous correction within the course of 48 hours. To encourage this correction the patient should be told to lie as much as possible semi-prone or in an exaggerated Sims' position.

The problem arises when spontaneous correction does not occur. With the uterus continually enlarging, one of two things must happen: either the anterior wall will sacculate, thus permitting the pregnancy to enlarge into the abdomen, or the patient will abort, the bladder meanwhile continuing at risk until either of these solutions has occurred. Since neither is desirable, intervention is indicated after two days of catheter drainage of the bladder. An attempt is made, therefore, by manipulation, to correct the retroversion, and for this the genupectoral position of the patient is ideal but complicates the giving of an aesthetic should it be necessary. It will often be found easier to push up the fundus by steering it to one side or other of the sacral promontory. The cervix should not be pulled upon with a vulsellum because it tears very easily in the gravid state and is often quite difficult to expose owing to its very displaced position. A finger in the rectum will often succeed where vaginal manipulation fails. This operation should be done under the influence of morphia at least, and it carries with it a fairly high risk of provoking abortion. It is for this reason that 48 hours is allowed to elapse initially in the hope of spontaneous correction.

Very rarely, the uterus remains incarcerated because of the presence of adhesions in the depths of the pelvis. The combination of circumstances is rare, because such cases are usually infertile. Nevertheless, when all attempts at correction have failed and the bladder has remained for many days on continuous or regular catheter regime, the question of laparotomy and division of adhesions will arise. This will ultimately succeed in dealing with the condition except in the rarest instances, where abdominal hysterotomy is necessary.

The diagnosis of retroversion in pregnancy is not usually difficult. The soft, boggy, pulsatile body of the uterus is easily felt through the posterior fornix on bimanual examination; however, it may be mistaken for an ovarian cyst and vice versa. This is an important matter, because, as mentioned later, ovarian cysts demand surgical removal. Careful palpation, if necessary under an anaesthetic, will distinguish uterine body from ovarian tumour. An even more serious mistake is to diagnose the tense, hard, over-distended bladder in incarcerated retroversion as a uterine swelling and to ignore the true state of affairs. These patients in their acute illness are often at the same time threatening to abort and are bleeding per vaginam.

A posterior wall fibroid may be confused with a retroverted gravid uterus, and in fact it may be difficult to decide in pregnancy which swelling is fundus and which fibroid. Provided no urinary symptoms are developing, however, the case calls only for observation.

The most important differential diagnosis is that of pelvic haematocele due to ectopic pregnancy, and tenderness may prevent adequate clinical examination. The confusion will only arise in the case of the retroverted gravid uterus which is threatening to abort or is already the seat of infection as a result of abortion.

The treatment of gravid retroversion, in the absence of symptoms due to incarceration, is much debated, but the modern tendency is, if possible, not to interfere. Postural treatment by the use of the exaggerated Sims' position is worth encouraging; the patient should be advised against allowing her bladder to become over-filled, and abstinence from intercourse will reduce the risks of miscarriage. Cases in which manipulation is successful would probably have corrected themselves later spontaneously, and those in which it is difficult carry a high abortion risk. Some favour the use of a rubber-ring pessary, which is supposed, by its constant pressure upon the retroverted uterine body, to encourage correction, but it is probable that these cases, too, owe their cure to Nature rather than to the treatment.

Pendulous Belly

Acute anteversion of the gravid uterus occurs with pendulous belly. The condition is usually due to a weak abdominal wall, with wide divarication of the recti between which the uterus herniates. A marked lordosis of the spine is usually associated and, in fact, is necessary if the patient is going to maintain her balance. In a few cases the distance between xiphisternum and symphysis pubis may be so greatly reduced by kyphosis of the thoracic spine that the pregnant uterus can find room for itself only in extreme forward displacement. If the uterus is grossly over-distended, for example by twins or hydramnios, gravity too plays a part in accentuating pendulous belly. Malpresentations are naturally more common in these cases, but since most of the patients owe their poor abdominal walls to high degrees of parity, the reason for malpresentation will be seen to lie as much in parity as in abnormal uterine position.

The condition has considerable nuisance value and makes the patient extremely uncomfortable, puts additional stresses upon her back and sacro-iliac joints and greatly increases her fatigue during pregnancy. The remedy is to supply a properly designed corset.

Prolapse in Pregnancy

Minor degrees of this are fairly common and may be associated with stress incontinence, but severe degrees seldom complicate pregnancy. The worst forms are those of acute onset following some sudden rise in intra-abdominal pressure. The trouble and inconvenience which a patient may experience are fortunately short-lived and limited to the earlier weeks of pregnancy since, as soon as the volume of the uterus exceeds that of the pelvic cavity, prolapse becomes impossible. Palliative treatment only is necessary, therefore, and a ring pessary usually suffices to supply the necessary support below; but where the perineum is markedly deficient the patient may have trouble in retaining it, in which case rest in bed is the only alternative.

Torsion of Uterus

Minor degrees of rotation of the uterus about its longitudinal axis are physiological, but acute torsion is an uncommon accident and does not occur in the case of an anatomically normal uterus. It is favoured by associated mechanical factors such as the presence of fibroids or a bicornuate condition of the uterus. The case presents as an acute abdomen, and in many respects the symptoms resemble those of ectopic gestation if the accident occurs in early pregnancy, while in the later months the condition resembles abruptio placentae with severe pain, shock and a hard and very tender uterus. The decision to open the abdomen is more likely to be made on the grounds of a misdiagnosis than because one recognises the condition clinically, and in any case the diagnosis will not be confirmed until laparotomy. Without operation the case may well deliver herself of a dead fetus and continue to be classified as a case of placental abruption.

FIBROIDS AND PREGNANCY

Although fibroids are found in about 20 per cent of all women who come to necropsy, their association with pregnancy is very much less common, and in hospital practice occurs in somewhere between 0·5 per cent and 1 per cent of cases. The reason for this is that the majority of pregnancies occur within age groups below that of the development of fibroids. Fibroids, particularly if submucous, may cause infertility. Alternatively, the very conditions which give rise to fibroids, which are as yet not fully understood, may in themselves be the primary cause of the patient's failure to conceive. It is, nevertheless, reasonable to perform myomectomy in a patient complaining of infertility.

In the majority of cases the presence of fibroids does not complicate pregnancy, but in others there is an increased tendency to abort. Much depends upon the mechanical influence of the position of the fibroid. If it is placed posteriorly and of a size sufficient to catch below the sacral promontory, incarceration may occur within the pelvis.

The commonest complication is the onset of acute degeneration, usually of the red variety, which may occur either in the second half of pregnancy or during the puerperium. It is only the larger fibroids, with their precarious blood supply, that are liable to degenerate acutely. Cystic degeneration of a fibroid is less common. The condition is characterised by the onset of abdominal pain of all grades of severity. Vomiting is frequently associated, and both temperature and pulse are likely to be raised. The tongue is often dirty and the patient looks ill. On examination, the most characteristic feature is the localisation of maximal tenderness to the actual site of the fibroid. The diagnosis of acute degeneration in a fibroid in pregnancy is enormously assisted by foreknowledge of the tumour's existence. In mild cases the symptoms subside after a few days, but in severe cases the patient may present the features of an acute abdominal emergency, and may require morphia to control her pain. Provided one can be certain of the diagnosis, a conservative attitude is nearly always worth while, and treatment consists of the use of pain-relieving drugs, a light or fluid diet and good nursing. Usually within ten days the patient's condition has improved out of all recognition and only in exceptional instances is it necessary to operate.

Uterine torsion may be provoked by a fibroid, as has already been mentioned.

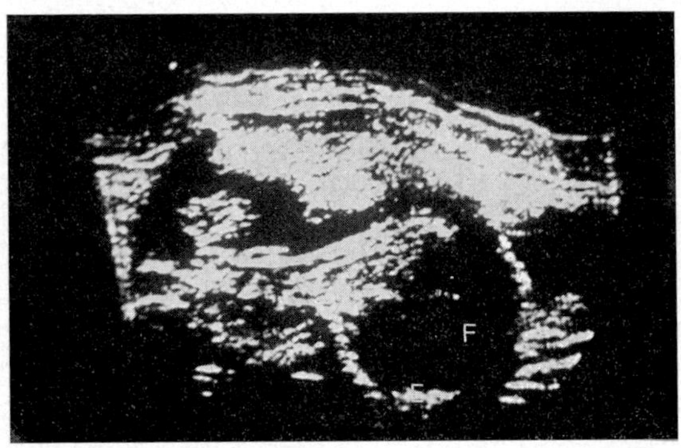

9/FIG. 2.—Large fibroid (F) in lower pole of uterus, filling pelvic cavity, in association with pregnancy of 15 weeks. Longitudinal section, cephalad to left.

Accidental haemorrhage is more common in association with fibroids, and occasionally it may be difficult to be certain how much of a patient's symptoms are due to abruptio placentae and how much to degeneration in a fibroid.

Malpresentations and all their associated complications may be caused by fibroids situated below the presenting part. When seeing a patient early in pregnancy it may appear that a fibroid is bound to give trouble, and yet, as the weeks go by, most of the tumours rise safely into the abdomen and one may often have difficulty in identifying them by palpation later on. This is because fibroids are often much softened in the course of pregnancy and tend to become more discoid and flattened in shape.

Cervical fibroids, or fibroids very low in the uterine wall, may, however, remain below the presenting part as pregnancy advances and may threaten to obstruct labour. Now there is a great difference between such a fibroid anteriorly placed and one situated behind the uterine canal. The former has a far better opportunity of being drawn up out of the pelvis after the onset of labour than a posterior tumour which tends to get trapped within the pelvis. It is, therefore, usually possible to make a shrewd guess about the likelihood of a fibroid obstructing labour before its onset by observing whether the fibroid is posterior or not, and in the case of the anterior tumour still within the pelvis at the end of pregnancy it is often worthwhile, other circumstances being favourable, to give labour a chance under close observation.

The onset of premature labour is a not uncommon risk especially in cases of large multiple fibroids in which the sheer size of the uterus makes it mechanically difficult for the patient to hold her pregnancy until term.

In labour itself, provided no fibroid continues to occupy the pelvis and provided there is no malpresentation, progress is usually unhindered. Nevertheless, the incidence of inertia is higher, especially if any appreciable proportion of the uterine wall is occupied by fibroid and therefore unable to contribute to the expulsive efforts of the rest of the uterus.

More commonly, troubles are encountered in the third stage with a definitely increased incidence of postpartum haemorrhage, partly due to interference with the retractile power of the uterus. When the placenta happens to be sited over a fibroid, there is often a defective decidual reaction so that it is liable to be, partially at least, morbidily adherent, thus necessitating manual removal. Very rarely a fibroid situated at the fundus of the uterus may, for mechanical reasons, precipitate uterine inversion.

During the puerperium involution is retarded by fibroids, the lochial loss tends to be greater, and secondary postpartum haemorrhage may occur in a few cases. For a variety of reasons, including degeneration of the fibroid, a possibly associated anaemia, a prolonged and inert labour, or because of the need for intra-uterine interference, the puerperium is more likely to be morbid.

Quite often during the puerperium a persistent low-grade pyrexia is attributable to degeneration in a fibroid, and I recall one case in which fever continued for some weeks until I removed a large necrotic fibroid by myomectomy, after which the patient's fever subsided.

So far we have mainly considered the manner in which fibroids may affect pregnancy, delivery and thereafter; but pregnancy is not without its effect upon fibroids. On the whole these effects tend to be beneficial inasmuch as they discourage growth, and simple atrophy commonly occurs postpartum, so that a fibroid which, earlier on, was felt with ease may be quite hard to find a few weeks after delivery. Red degeneration has already been mentioned, but this is a much more acute process than simple atrophy. A subserous pedunculated fibroid may become twisted and give rise to acute symptoms. Less commonly a fibroid becomes infected.

Diagnosis

The diagnosis of fibroids in pregnancy is by no means always easy unless the tumour is discrete. Apparent asymmetry in early pregnancy has already been mentioned, and for this reason fibroids are quite often diagnosed when they do not exist. Fibroids never cause amenorrhoea, and any woman who has come to hospital for myomectomy or hysterectomy and whose period is only a few days overdue should be suspected of having become pregnant if disaster is to be avoided. The consistency of a fibroid is, of course, much harder than that of the gravid uterus, but even so one can be misled. I well recall a young patient in my wards who was admitted for myomectomy for a mass of fibroids the size of a 32-weeks pregnancy, one of which was degenerating. Her expected period was overdue on admission so we awaited confirmation of the diagnosis of pregnancy. She thereupon started to bleed intermittently and the urinary pregnancy tests remained equivocal. Ultrasonography, however, presently showed fetal echoes at the top of the tumour mass and was therefore discredited—unjustly. After a few demoralising weeks the body, but not the head or the placenta of a 14-weeks fetus was passed through an invisible cervix so high up in the left anterolateral fornix that two attempts at exploration of the cavity (whose whereabouts could not be foretold) had to be abandoned. There followed a period of sepsis and fortunately only minor bleedings while the situation was got under control with antibiotics, after which I gave up the unequal struggle to preserve her reproductive function and performed hysterectomy. The head was never found but numerous submucous fibroids were clustered around above the internal os, any one of which might have tempted a convincing pull with ovum forceps had I been able to introduce such an instrument. Having preached for years that any non-malignant uterus capable of implanting a pregnancy deserves conservation I had to eat my words—not for the first time.

A retroverted gravid uterus has to be distinguished from a fibroid situated posteriorly. The size of the uterus may make one suspect a fibroid when in actual fact the case is one of twin pregnancy, and vice versa. An ectopic pregnancy with pelvic haematocele is less likely to be confused with a fibroid if one bears in mind that the margins of a haematocele are usually not very discrete. An ovarian tumour must be distinguished from a fibroid in the differential diagnosis because the treatment of the former is laparotomy and removal, while with the latter conservative measures are indicated. Lastly, the non-gravid half of a variety of double uterus may be clinically indistinguishable from a fibroid.

Treatment

In the non-pregnant state any fibroid exceeding in size that of a tennis ball is usually worth removing in order to forestall further growth or possible acute degeneration, unless the patient is already proceeding without trouble through the menopause. Cases of infertility and recurrent abortion indicate removal of the fibroid by myomectomy. One need have little fear of myomectomy scar rupture in subsequent pregnancy and labour, even though it has been necessary to open the cavity of the uterus, and Gemmell (1936) reported no case of such rupture in his own series, and observed that a study of the literature furnished rather few instances.

When fibroids are diagnosed for the first time in pregnancy, the indications for their removal are infrequent. Firstly, the operation is seldom necessary because the uterus has demonstrated its functional ability by conception; secondly, the operation is extremely bloody because of the great vascularity of the uterus and thirdly, it is quite liable to be followed by abortion. One may have fears for the integrity of the scar in labour within the next few months, although these are usually groundless, but one of the chief difficulties is to procure satisfactory haemostasis in the course of the operation, so that one may be faced with the choice of two unpleasant alternatives, namely to close the abdomen in the presence of a persistent ooze, or to proceed to hysterectomy. In either case one would wish never to have started the operation. Only acute torsion and the rarest and most refractory varieties of acute degeneration, or impaction of a fibroid in the pelvis, causing acute retention of urine, are likely to provide sufficient grounds for undertaking myomectomy in pregnancy.

There are other less cast-iron indications, such as the presence of fibroids so large that it is reckoned that the patient's only hope of prolonging pregnancy to the point of viability lies in myomectomy. The safest time for operating is between the 16th and 20th weeks, as abortion is less likely to complicate convalescence at this time. It might be added here that abortion shortly after myomectomy is fraught with danger, especially if the products of conception are retained, because sepsis is thereby enhanced and magnified. Blood loss in the course of the operation can be very brisk and cannot be in any way minimised by the use of a myomectomy clamp, for obvious reasons, so that a supply of blood for transfusion should be at hand. Another technical difficulty is provided by the softness of the tissues, which may cause the sutures to cut out. One is further handicapped by trying throughout to handle the uterus as little as possible for fear of provoking abortion. It will, therefore, be clear that the indications for myomectomy in pregnancy must be overwhelming before one embarks on what may prove a very dangerous operation.

In the course of performing Caesarean section it is naturally tempting to avail oneself of the opportunity of removing a fibroid at the same time. Caesarean myomectomy, however, is an indefensible operation, and I have seen near disasters follow it both from haemorrhage and from severe puerperal peritonitis. The only possible exception is the case of a subserous pedunculated fibroid with a stalk so narrow as to be capable of direct ligation with one stitch. Even though the fibroid presents directly in the line of the uterine incision, the temptation should be resisted and the uterus should be entered at a safer point. Caesarean hysterectomy is vastly preferable to Caesarean myomectomy, but fibroids do not often provide a satisfactory excuse for such radical surgery because the uterus, which has proved itself capable of carrying a pregnancy so far, is a uterus worth conserving. If, however, Caesarean hysterectomy is necessary, and such cases are indeed few, the total operation is preferable to the subtotal on general gynaecological principles. Nevertheless, it is often surprising how much of the cervix manages to get left behind, as revealed at postnatal examination.

During the puerperium, myomectomy may be indicated because of persistent illness from degeneration or, for example, from torsion, but in any case it is better to put off the operation as long as possible in order to minimise the risks of sepsis. It goes without saying, therefore, that the best time to remove fibroids is some months after delivery, when involution is complete. The exercise of this forbearance will, in many instances, abolish the need for operating at all.

CARCINOMA OF THE CERVIX

Carcinoma of the cervix is by no means rare in pregnancy, although its incidence is reduced by the discouragement which its presence offers to conception. Munro Kerr many years ago reported an incidence of 1 in 2000 pregnancies at the Glasgow Royal Maternity Hospital, but this figure is on the pessimistic side for the country as a whole. Most people are agreed that the presence of pregnancy worsens the prognosis, and that the growth develops more rapidly as a result of the increased blood supply. Furthermore, blood-borne metastasis is encouraged, thereby making the case less amenable to irradiation and surgery. These impressions, based usually upon a too limited personal experience, are not borne out by Kinch (1961) who reviewed 705 cases followed up over a five-year period and compared with a series of non-pregnant women matched for age. Kinch found in fact that the overall 5-year prognosis was the same in both groups but he noted a greater liability to rapid dissemination in stage I cases in pregnancy for which he largely blamed the disturbance of vaginal delivery which he does not favour. The outlook is further worsened by the likelihood of severe haemorrhage accompanying abortion or delivery, and the opportunities for postabortum and puerperal sepsis are multiplied by the presence of a growth which is inevitably somewhat necrotic and infected.

The patient presents with bleeding which may be profuse and, to a lesser extent, with discharge, and for this reason a diagnosis of threatened abortion is likely to be made in the first instance. The importance, therefore, of making a pelvic examination and inspecting the cervix if bleeding persists for more than five to seven days is obvious. In the later trimester of pregnancy the examination should, of course, be restricted as far as possible to inspecting the cervix by speculum for fear that the case may be one of placenta praevia.

There may be some difficulty in deciding that a lesion on the cervix is a carcinoma. Hardness of the suspected portion is very characteristic, because in pregnancy no area of the cervix should demonstrate hardness. Cervical biopsy is essential if there is the slightest doubt. Bleeding may be rather free as a result of this, and it should, therefore, only be carried out after admission to hospital. Even after biopsy the diagnosis may be uncertain, since the pregnant cervix can play some very dangerous histological tricks, encouraging a false positive diagnosis, particularly in the case of columnar cell tissue. One of our cases at Hammersmith Hospital proved to be of extraordinary interest and doubt.[13] The patient in question demonstrated apparent adenocarcinoma of the cervix in two successive pregnancies, in a cervix which was normal in the intervening months. I myself saw this case some years later, when frank invasive malignancy had developed in the vaginal vault long after hysterectomy. The services of a very experienced pathologist should always be sought before committing oneself to this diagnosis and the very radical treatment necessarily involved, and I bitterly remember performing Wertheim's hysterectomy on a case so diagnosed on cervical biopsy in a pregnant patient in whom the diagnosis was not substantiated by full histological examination of the excised uterus.

Lastly, carcinoma of the cervix occurring late in pregnancy may present as a case of apparent placenta praevia, and for this reason, amongst others, whenever possible an examination under anaesthesia should be performed before carrying out Caesarean section, as otherwise the true diagnosis may be overlooked until routine examination of the pelvic organs is made much later (Fig. 3).

Carcinoma *in situ* of Cervix

The development of pre-invasive malignant change in cervical epithelium (carcinoma *in situ*) in pregnancy is a matter of great

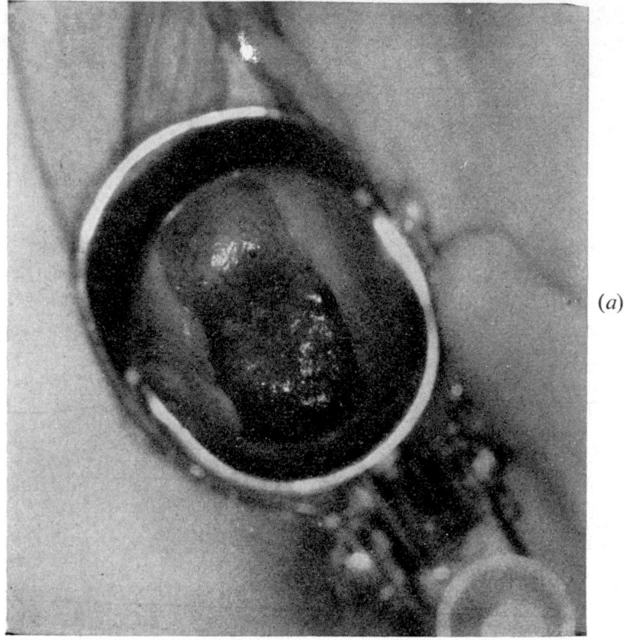

(*a*)

9/Fig. 3

(*a*) Carcinoma *in situ* in pregnancy. Aborted spontaneously. Papanicolaou smears positive. Extended hysterectomy with removal of appendages. Has since done well.

(*b*) (*opposite*). Showing dedifferentiation and mitoses (H and E × 346).

(*c*) (*opposite*). Shows carcinoma *in situ*, same case. The underlying cervical stroma shows a marked inflammatory infiltrate with lymphoid hyperplasia (H and E × 136).

interest and controversy and it is not yet certain to what extent such lesions regress between pregnancies, but Kinch refers to the rapidly dying impression that the stage O lesion as diagnosed during pregnancy is an "evanescent situation".

The practice of taking routine Papanicolaou smears in early pregnancy is growing faster than its demonstrable value. Its main use is to exclude invasive cancer of the cervix which can usually be spotted on proper clinical examination. The diagnosis of pre-invasive carcinoma of the cervix at this stage in pregnancy is both worrying and to some extent futile as the management of the pregnancy should not be altered thereby. There is a tendency here for the tail to wag the dog and a positive or suspicious smear should not be acted upon surgically at once, but a repeat smear should be taken. Better still is the method devised by Faulds in Carlisle[4] of taking a sponge

(b)

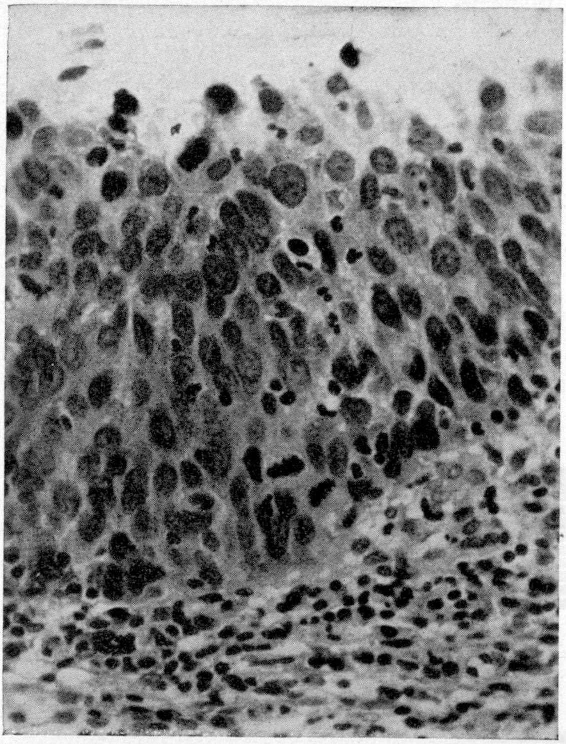

(c)

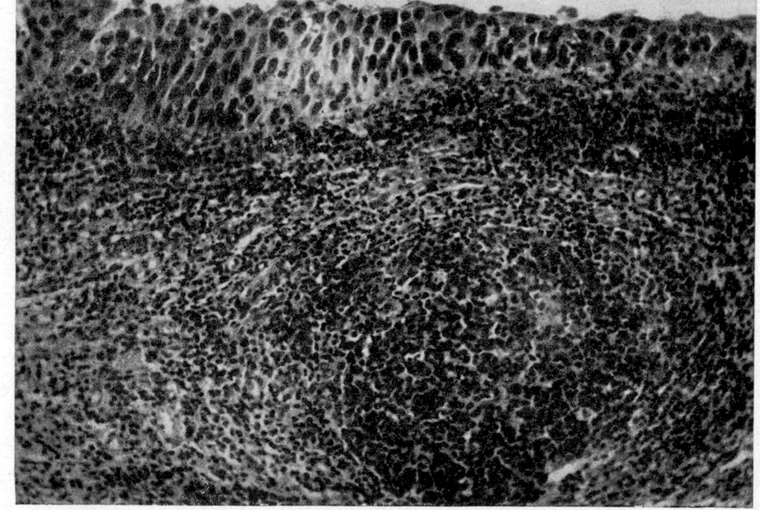

(FIG. 3 *b* and *c* by courtesy of Dr J. E. Duncan Taylor)

biopsy as is now our practice in our gynaecology department. This technique has replaced the use of the Ayre spatula, is very simple, and merely involves the use of small chopped up pieces of polythene sponge bought from Woolworths and allowed to dry hard. The little chunk of sponge is held in a vulsellum and after exposure of the cervix with a speculum, a corner of the sponge is pushed into the external os and rotated through 360°. With this sponge a cytological smear can be made and the sponge itself dropped into a bottle of fixative. The whole piece can now be paraffin blocked and sectioned, providing a very useful microhistological specimen, which enormously reduces the incidence of equivocal smear results which may easily cause unnecessary alarm and despondency. If the result of such a test is still positive or equivocal, one has no option but to undertake a proper cone biopsy of the cervix. This must be done in hospital because of the danger of bleeding due to the associated pregnancy for which the standard methods of electrocoagulation or packing tightly, particularly the latter, are likely to be rewarded by the onset of abortion. I have attempted to minimise blood loss by trying to tighten a soft rubber catheter round the cervix, gripped between the jaws of an artery forceps, rather like a venous tourniquet, but it is difficult to get the catheter applied high enough unless the cervix can be pulled well down, and furthermore the cervix itself "crinkles" (as after a Shirodkar suture) making it difficult to perform a neat biopsy. It is far better, in fact, to make the cone biopsy with a fistula-type knife blade starting from behind and working forwards, and ignoring the bleeding until the specimen has been fully obtained. I am not very fond of underrunning sutures in the pregnant cervix and sometimes the number of bleeding points is too numerous to control by this means. Faced with this situation the best method of arresting the bleeding is to apply sponge forceps, commonly two pairs, from outside the cervix over both anterior and posterior lips, so that the raw bleeding surfaces are compressed together. A few minutes of this will usually stop the bleeding but, if not, the forceps can be reapplied and the patient sent back to the ward with them still on the cervix, to be removed an hour or so later. This is a simple method which does not expose the patient to the same risk of abortion. There is a growing opinion that far too much radical treatment is employed in cases of cervical carcinoma *in situ* and as many of the women are nowhere near the end of their reproductive lives a conservative attitude towards the type of surgical attack, if any, is well worth considering in the interests of future pregnancies.

Green, in fact, who has long pleaded for moderation in this respect has reported a series of 60 pregnancies in New Zealand occurring in patients previously treated, some by ring biopsy, that is to say less than 2 cm, and a larger number by cone biopsy, namely of more than

2 cm. It would appear that the more radical cone biopsy influences the course of subsequent pregnancy because out of 30 patients so treated no less than eight aborted, five had premature labours and all three term labours with cervical dystocia were in patients who had had cone biopsy. Thus with 16 out of 30 patients previously coned the incidence of complication was more than 50 per cent as compared with 2 out of 17 ring biopsy cases. This is a big penalty to pay for what should be really a diagnostic procedure. This is bad enough, but when one considers how often hysterectomy is undertaken for what is, after all, a precancerous lesion in a young woman, the picture is even worse, and demonstrates how often in modern medicine the investigation and treatment are worse than the original disease. This is not to deny the importance of watching these cases closely, but is a plea for staving off the more radical forms of surgical attack, at least until the young woman has completed her childbearing. In McLaren's series of 141 patients treated by conisation and follow-up for carcinoma *in situ* or marked basal cell dysplasia, the procedure was reckoned adequate for both diagnosis and treatment in all but 14, but even so it is recommended that the patient must be followed up indefinitely, both clinically and cytologically. Sooner or later the patient begins to realise what she is being watched for, of course, and will not be happy until the uterus has been removed, and one cannot help feeling that she might have been lucky had the diagnosis been made just a little later in her life. In this last-mentioned series there were 39 pregnancies in 25 of the patients, with 3 abortions, one case of premature rupture of the membranes and one case of cervical stenosis.

In my own view a case so diagnosed and treated should be encouraged to complete her desired score in child bearing before the age of 35, after which her hysterectomy may be the only means of peace of mind for both her and her doctor and perhaps, most definitely of all, her husband. Needless to say, all such deliveries, after these operations on the cervix must, be undertaken in hospital because of the risk of cervical stenosis or damage in labour, and postnatal follow up must be thorough.

Treatment of carcinoma of the cervix.—This involves one of the most difficult decisions in all obstetrics. The case for Wertheim's hysterectomy is a strong one in gravid carcinoma of the cervix. The operation is likely to cause considerable blood loss, but is facilitated technically by the great ease with which the tissues can be stripped. Because the growth is likely to declare itself fairly early the chances of encountering an operable stage are correspondingly greater. The case first diagnosed late in pregnancy may with some justification be denied treatment for a short while in the hope of securing a viable child, but except in these borderline instances the pregnancy will have to be disregarded and treatment started with the minimum of delay. Late in pregnancy the alternatives are to perform Caesarean section followed within ten days by irradiation or, preferably, Wertheim's Caesarean hysterectomy. The latter is preferred, because the puerperium may be infected after Caesarean section, and the presence of sepsis may delay the start of radium treatment. The employment of subtotal hysterectomy at the time of Caesarean section has been advocated by some in order to reduce the hazard of infection and to ensure the prompt institution of radium treatment, but this is not recommended, because stump irradiation is very much less satisfactory than when proper cavitary application can be included, as in the usual techniques.

In the earlier part of pregnancy the choice lies between Wertheim's hysterectomy, abdominal hysterotomy followed by irradiation, or irradiation given first. The first method is preferred, the second involves delay in treatment and has the same objections as Caesarean section followed by irradiation mentioned above. The application of radium in the first instance with the pregnancy still *in situ* has much to recommend, it, but it carries with it a very great danger of precipitating abortion at a most disadvantageous time. The technique of applying the radium should be very cautious, only the vaginal vault being packed, and the gauze plugging to hold the radium in place must be most gently inserted to prevent this complication. I once had to perform an emergency Wertheim's hysterectomy in the middle of the night on a patient four and a half months pregnant, who had started to abort and exsanguinate herself rapidly as a result of radium applied the previous day. She made a good recovery, but died about fifteen months later from multiple blood-borne metastases. Many would nowadays prefer to treat with supervoltage X-rays first. This will be followed by intra-uterine fetal death and abortion after which radium can be applied. This is a sound alternative to radical surgery.

Attempts are sometimes made to leave the pregnancy undisturbed and to confine treatment to radium. The effects of this on the fetus are difficult to forecast, but are likely to be very damaging, especially in the early months of pregnancy, and may result in such conditions as microcephaly. In the later months the effects are less obvious, but at the very least an area of baldness is probable.

Other Lesions of the Cervix

The most important of these, from the obstetrical point of view, is the scarring of the cervix which may follow previous amputation, for example in the course of a Manchester repair for prolapse and after deep cauterisation of the cervix for cervicitis. The latter is a notorious offender in this respect, and is far more likely to interfere with dilatation in labour than the operation of diathermy conisation. I recall having to perform Caesarean section on a para 4 with an unblemished obstetrical record but who had had cervical cautery. There was cross-union between anterior and posterior lips of the cervix together with scarring and no dilatation took place in spite of three weeks postmaturity with several abortive attempts at labour, a hind-water induction carried out "blind" and with great difficulty two and a half days earlier and a fairly determined oxytocin drip. In fairness to myself I should point out that I only saw her a short time before her section! The cervix felt even worse from above at operation than from below and scissors were used from above to divide the band, followed by dilatation to secure lochial drainage. It is useless to assess the ability of the cervix to dilate until it has been put to the test of labour, but the possibility of cervical dystocia should be borne in mind in any patient with a history of these operations. Labour, following a previous Manchester repair, is far more likely to be obstructed by scarring of the vagina in the vault than by cicatricial rigidity of the cervix. Needless to say, all patients who have had previous operations on the cervix or repairs of prolapse should be delivered in hospital. The Caesarean section rate thereafter is likely to be high (18 out of 100 cases reviewed by Hunter and 23 per cent in the series of 156 cases reviewed by Averill). If the previous operation had been undertaken for stress incontinence, the case for Caesarean section is even stronger since none would gladly risk a recurrence. Nevertheless, the physiological effects of pregnancy without those of labour can undermine the result of a previous repair and elective section is no guarantee against recurrent loss of urinary control or prolapse.

Labour should be conducted with great vigilance. Any reluctance on the part of the cervix to dilate or any palpable rigidity of the cervix found on vaginal examination is warning enough of an impending split to justify Caesarean section. If vaginal delivery takes place, prophylactic episiotomy is obligatory.

Previous high amputation of the cervix or deep cervical laceration, as mentioned in the chapter on abortion, are causes of recurrent miscarriage.

Cervicitis, so common in gynaecological practice, gives surprisingly little trouble in obstetrics. Discharge is seldom troublesome, but there is the possibility of slight bleeding, especially after intercourse, so that the patient may be admitted for observation for either threatened abortion or for undiagnosed antepartum haemorrhage. The routine inspection of the cervix by speculum should clarify the diagnosis, but there may be doubt about the possibility of carcinoma, in which case biopsy of the cervix is essential. Cervicitis is preferably not treated during pregnancy; for one thing it is seldom necessary. There is no serious objection to superficial cautery of a cervical erosion, but the case likely to benefit from such trivial treatment is unlikely to need it anyway. It is always worth doing bacterial cultures of the cervical secretions in cases of obvious cervicitis, if only to indicate the appropriate chemotherapy following labour.

Cervical polyps can cause intermittent bleeding during pregnancy, and for this reason their removal may be advisable. Avulsion of a polyp may be followed by persistent bleeding, and it is, therefore, better to admit the patient before twisting it off. The bleeding will stop readily with the use of styptics and gentle local pressure with gauze, coupled with an injection of morphia.

Discharge in Pregnancy

This is a farily common symptom, and an increase in vaginal transudate is physiological in pregnancy. In these cases microscopic examination of the wet specimen will reveal large numbers of well-cornified squames and very few pus cells. For this no treatment is indicated. A purulent discharge, however, may be due to gonorrhoea, which calls for proper bacteriological confirmation before smothering the diagnosis with antibiotics.

Trichomonas vaginitis is not uncommon in pregnancy, but fortunately it responds, in most cases, to the usual proprietary pessary treatments rather more readily than in the non-pregnant state. Occasionally it causes a bloodstained discharge in later pregnancy and may, in fact, present as a case of mild antepartum haemorrhage. The diagnosis should be apparent, however, on routine speculum examination and microscopy of a wet smear.

Metronidazole (Flagyl) is amazingly effective in stamping out this very recurrent and occasionally persistent infection. Given by mouth in 200 mg tablets three times a day for seven to ten days it succeeds at the first attempt in over 80 per cent of cases (and, in fact, has enabled us to close down our leucorrhoea clinic in my gynaecological unit and to absorb the work in other more general clinics). The persistent and recurrent cases are usually due to reinfection by coitus from the male partner unless he is treated at the same time and the use of a condom insisted upon for at least a month.

Local treatment with proprietary pessaries such as clotrimazole (Canesten) 100 mg pessaries and the cream of the same substance is preferred by us in pregnancy before resorting to metronidazole, especially in early pregnancy. Although reports so far indicate no harmful effect on pregnant women or their babies one is reminded by the thalidomide disaster to think twice before prescribing systemic drugs which are even remotely capable of causing a drop in polymorph count, and 3 out of 41 of the cases (non-pregnant) investigated by Rodin *et al.* (1960) for possible toxic effects showed a fall to 1500 per mm^3 which is at the very bottom of normality even though the counts rose smartly after withdrawal. The efficacy of metronidazole is by no means diminished in pregnancy and in a series from Washington, D.C., of 206 pregnancies[15] the cure rate was even higher than what we normally expect, but over 15 per cent recurred until the husbands were concomitantly treated. Since there is no placental barrier to the passage of metronidazole into the fetus uneasiness about possible teratogenic effect continues, but still without proof.

In this series the abortion and prematurity rate overall were the same, as was also the incidence of fetal abnormality, but if analysis is restricted to treatment given in the first trimester of pregnancy then this series showed that there were no less than 4 fetal abnormalities, although there was little similarity between any of them. This would be much higher than expected. Our own preference is still, therefore, to withhold all metronidazole during the period of organogenesis within the first 11 weeks of pregnancy. Later the drug can be prescribed with confidence.

A severe discharge may be associated with a very distressing crop of vulval warts (condylomata acuminata) which are due to a specific virus operating in an area first sensitised by a discharge of almost any type. The primary treatment is of the underlying discharge and the warts may be treated by the local application to their surfaces of podophylin (25 per cent) on one or more occasions. The surrounding skin should be protected by Vaseline. They tend to clear up after delivery but if persisting are best removed by the diathermy cutting loop postnatally.

Vaginitis due to *Candida albicans* (*monilia albicans*) is relatively more common in pregnancy than *trichomonas vaginitis* and is favoured by the very acid state of the vagina (Fig. 4). In moniliasis the patient complains predominantly of pruritus vulvae and secondarily of vaginal discharge, and the vulva may become extensively excoriated and eczematised. The diagnosis can be easily clinched by a simple culture at room temperature on Nickerson's medium (Ortho) for five days. No special apparatus is required and a positive culture shows black colonies on naked-eye inspection. This condition can be extremely distressing and resistant to treatment, although it usually clears fairly rapidly after pregnancy is over. These patients show a remarkable tendency to become sensitised to a wide variety of local applications, and 0·5 per cent aqueous gentian violet still remains a safe stand-by in treatment. It is applied daily, if necessary, in the form of a paint. The condition will improve almost immediately with gentain violet, but recurrences up to the time of delivery are by no means uncommon. The most severe cases, accompanied by serious degrees of eczematisation of vulva and thighs, should be admitted to hospital, where the condition will often be found to clear up in half the time taken with ambulant treatment.

Nystatin (Nystan-Squibb), a substance isolated from *Streptomyces noursei*, has been found to inhibit mycelial growth and its clinical

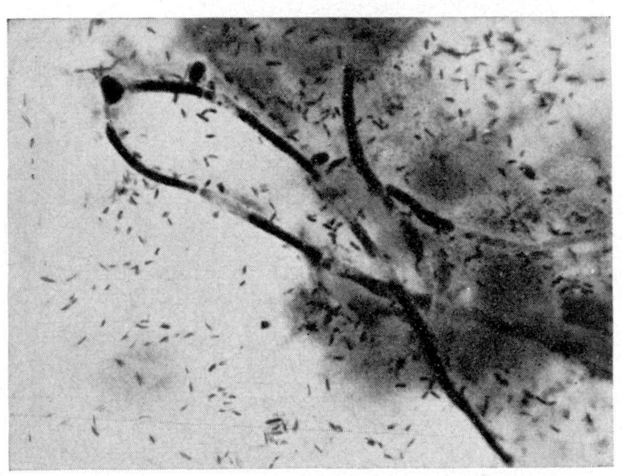

9/FIG. 4.—*Candida albicans* (× 750).
(By courtesy of the late Prof. I. Lominski)

efficacy in vulvovaginal moniliasis has been fully demonstrated by Barr (1957). Fungilin (amphotericin B) is similarly effective.

The relief afforded by properly used nystatin pessaries in these cases is truly dramatic within a few hours and relapses are relatively infrequent. The preparation is colourless and spares the patient the inconvenience of clothing and bed linen indelibly soiled with the depressing colour which gentian violet always spreads.

Cases which persist after delivery are usually due to reinfection by the husband who may have a monilial balanitis or a scrotocrural dermatitis or the source may be in the patient's intestinal canal and peri-anal region. In the former case the husband should use an ointment containing amphotericin B (Fungilin-Squibb) and pay close attention to genital and digital hygiene and use a condom at coitus. My latest personal preference in a growing list of highly effective proprietary preparations is Canesten applied locally in pessary and ointment form and I have not yet encountered sensitivity reactions. In the case of intestinal reinfection, which can be very intractable, especially if antibiotics have destroyed the normal bacteriology of the gut, Mycostatin 500,000 units orally t.i.d. can be prescribed.

In the postnatal period the cervix may harbour the infection for a long time. This is best dealt with by diathermy conisation of the endocervix.

OVARIAN TUMOURS

Ovarian tumours are common at all stages of reproductive life, and their discovery in pregnancy is not surprising. The commonest varieties are dermoids, pseudomucinous cysts and simple serous cysts. Pregnancy renders the patient particularly susceptible to the risk of complications occurring in the tumour itself. Torsion of the cyst is an ever-present risk, especially in the puerperium, when the rapid change in the anatomical relations of the pelvic viscera, combined with the lax abdominal musculature, particularly favours twisting. Ovarian cysts may also rupture, especially in the course of labour, or they may, from mechanical pressure, undergo necrosis and infection. Likewise, haemorrhage may occur into the substance of the tumour. Apart from these complications the tumour may suffer incarceration within the pelvis, possibly causing acute retention of urine as in the case of the incarcerated retroverted gravid uterus. Their presence within the pelvis also favours malpresentation and may obstruct labour. Very large cysts can add enormously to abdominal distension as pregnancy advances, so that the patient is hardly able to get about. (Fig. 5.)

One can never be certain that an ovarian tumour is not malignant

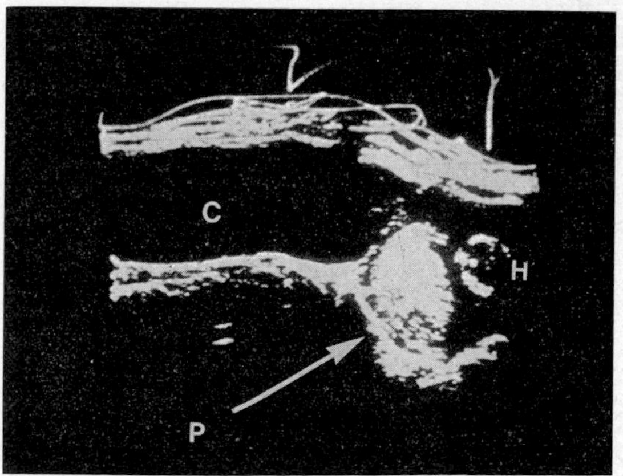

9/FIG. 5.—Huge ovarian cyst and 14 weeks cyesis. The vertical marks in the abdominal wall indicate the level of the umbilicus in the centre and symphisis pubis to right. The upper margin of the cyst (to the left) cannot be seen, because it is out of range. Patient presented clinically as a case "large for dates". (From *Diagnostic Ultrasound*, 1974. Ed. D. L. King, by courtesy of C. V. Mosby Co.)

until it has been inspected, so that, whether pregnant or not, at any time in life a patient with an ovarian tumour requires laparotomy.

The diagnosis is not difficult if the tumour can be palpated separately from the uterus. Ultrasonography may reveal a cyst lying alongside the gravid uterus with its fetal echoes and so clinch the

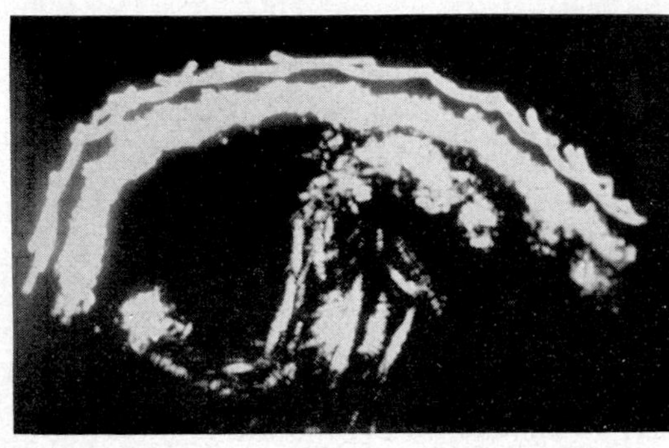

9/FIG. 6.—Ultrasonogram. Transverse section of pregnancy showing large ovarian cyst on left and fetal echoes on right. (By courtesy of the Editor, *Brit. J. Radiol.*)

diagnosis beyond all doubt (Fig. 6). The following conditions enter into the differential diagnosis:

1. The retroverted gravid uterus may be hard to distinguish from an ovarian cyst in the pelvis, especially when the bladder is distended and painful, but examination after the passage of a catheter should help to resolve the diagnosis. My own record for a "cyst" which vanished on catheterisation is 105 fluid ounces, almost 2 litres.
2. A haematocele, either in the pouch of Douglas or peritubal, may simulate ovarian cyst, but its margins are less discrete and definite than in the case of an ovarian tumour.
3. Fibroids in pregnancy, when pedunculated, may be soft enough to give the impression of being cystic (the distinction is important, because the treatment of fibroids in pregnancy is, if possible conservative).

Other less common sources of confusion are:

4. A double uterus.
5. A uterus distended by hydramnios.

In the early months a perfectly normal pregnancy may yet have such uterine asymmetry that at first one may be inclined to think that the patient has an ovarian cyst, but again careful examination should distinguish the two. Ultrasonography is invaulable, of course, but in the absence of this modern diagnostic aid, the demands made upon careful palpation are all the greater. Sometimes it is possible to discern a groove between the fundus of the gravid uterus and an ovarian cyst if the patient is placed in the head down Trendelenburg position.[7]

An X-ray of the abdomen is usually worth taking when an ovarian cyst is found in pregnancy, because a tooth may show up and indicate the diagnosis of a dermoid straight away (Fig. 7). Many cases have

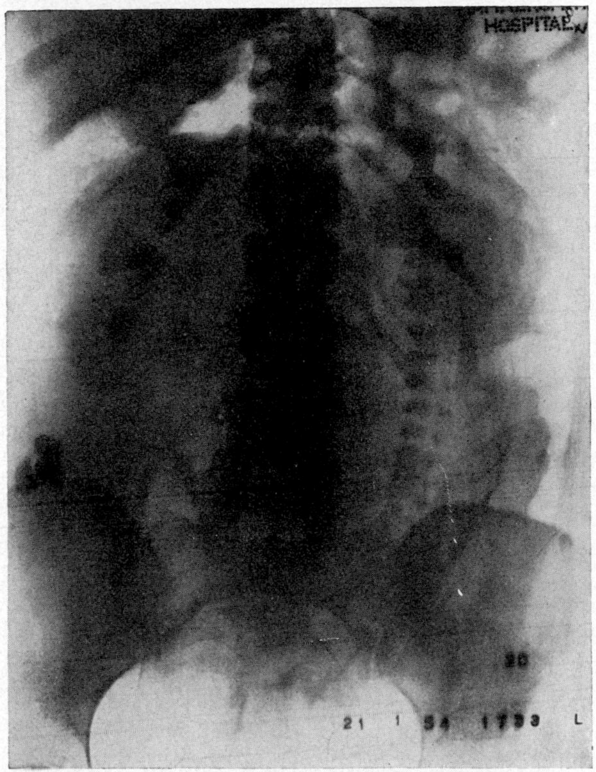

9/Fig. 7.—Dermoid in pregnancy revealed by tooth. Found incidentally in course of IVP. Proved at operation to be a parasitic cyst.
(By courtesy of Prof. R. E. Steiner).

no symptoms when first seen, and the tumour is only diagnosed on routine pelvic examination. This constitutes one of the principal indications for examining the patient per vaginam in early pregnancy. Later on the cyst may not be so easily identified once it has escaped from the pelvic cavity.

Treatment of Ovarian Cysts in Pregnancy

Elective operation is better than being forced to perform laparotomy in the face of emergency caused by a complication in the cyst, because there is a strong likelihood that the patient will abort after such emergency surgery. The absolute reasons for operating have already been made clear, and this matter brooks no argument. The only debatable point is the optimum time for doing so. The ideal time is about the 18th week, because the risk of post-operative abortion is thereby much reduced. In the case of a cyst within the pelvis, to delay much after this time would make access to it very difficult because of the size of the uterus. As a matter of practical fact, however, the correct time for operating is "now".

If the cyst is discovered within the last five weeks of pregnancy, one has the choice of removing it there and then (which is preferable, since who can say before laparotomy, except in the case of a radiologically proved dermoid, that an ovarian cyst is benign) and leaving the patient to go spontaneously into labour, or of waiting until term and performing Casarean section and removal of the cyst at the same time. If the tumour is discovered right at the end of pregnancy the last of these alternatives is the only sensible choice. It may be argued that at term it is better to remove the cyst and then allow the patient to continue with her labour in order to save a scar in the uterus, but this is sheer inhumanity. Munro Kerr and Chassar Moir stated "one procedure is quite unthinkable, to perform ovariotomy and allow the labour to continue after that operation".

A previously undiagnosed cyst may come in for some very rough handling during the third stage of labour in the belief that it represents the uterine fundus. It is true that the cyst may not be observed until after the patient is delivered, and because of the great liability to torsion, infection and formation of adhesions in the puerperium, it is better to operate fairly soon and before these complications have a chance to develop. (Fig. 8.)

In operating, wherever possible, and especially in the case of dermoids, an attempt should be made to resect the cyst conservatively,

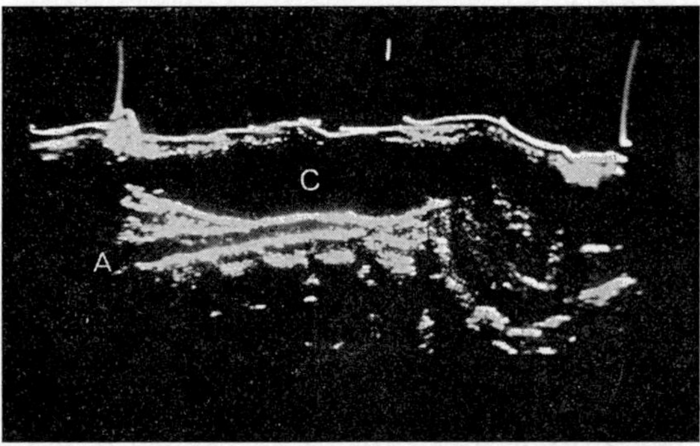

9/Fig. 8.—Large puerperal cyst (C). Longitudinal section. Note aorta (A).

and preserve the remainder of the ovary. The patient, after all, has demonstrated by her pregnancy the integrity of the rest of her pelvic organs, and they deserve to be conserved as far as possible.

REFERENCES

1. AVERILL, L. C. L. (1955). *J. Obstet. Gynaec. Brit. Emp.*, **62,** 421.
2. BARNES, H. F. (1947). *Brit. med. J.*, **1,** 169.
3. BARR, W. (1957). *Practitioner*, **178,** 616.
4. FAULDS, J. S. (1964). *Lancet*, **1,** 655.
5. GEMMELL, A. A. (1936). *J. Obstet. Gynaec. Brit. Emp.*, **43,** 715.
6. GREEN, G. H. (1966). *J. Obstet. Gynaec. Brit. Cwlth*, **73,** 897.
7. HINGORANI, VERA (1966). *J. Obstet. Gynaec. Brit. Cwlth*, **73,** 155.
8. HUNTER, J. W. A. (1955). *J. Obstet. Gynaec. Brit. Emp.*, **62,** 809.
9. HUNTER, W. (1960). *Brit. med. J.*, **2,** 1124.
10. KINCH, R. A. H. (1961). *Amer. J. Obstet. Gynec.*, **82,** 45.
11. MACGREGOR, W. G. (1957). *J. Obstet. Gynaec. Brit. Emp.*, **64,** 888.
12. MCLAREN, H. C. (1967). *J. Obstet. Gynaec. Brit. Cwlth*, **74,** 487.
13. MARTIN, R. T. and KENNY, MEAVE (1950). *J. Obstet. Gynaec. Brit. Emp.*, **74,** 487.
14. MOIR, J. C. (1964). *Munro Kerr's Operative Obstetrics*, 7th edit. London: Baillière, Tindall and Cox.
15. PETERSON, W. F., STAUCH, F. E. and RYDER, CONSTANCE D. (1966). *Amer. J. Obstet. Gynec.*, **94,** 343.
16. RODIN, P., KING, A. J., NICOL, C. S. and BARROW, J. (1960). *Brit. J. vener. Dis.*, **36,** 147.
17. WILSON, D. C. and HARRIS, G. H. (1961). *J. Obstet. Gynaec. Brit. Cwlth*, **68,** 841.

CHAPTER X

HYPERTENSION AND ECLAMPSIA IN PREGNANCY

by R. J. WEIR, M.D., F.R.C.P. (Glasg.)

Consultant Physician, Western Infirmary and Gartnavel General Hospital, Glasgow; Honorary Clinical Lecturer, University of Glasgow. (Previously Consultant Physician with MRC Blood Pressure Unit, Western Infirmary, Glasgow.)

HYPERTENSION

HYPERTENSION in pregnancy is still associated with increased maternal and fetal mortality and morbidity, and regular reliable measurement of blood pressure from early gestation is therefore of great importance. High blood pressure is a sign, not a disease—it is an indication that an increase has occurred in cardiac output or, more commonly in disease states, in total peripheral resistance. These vascular changes can arise in a number of conditions which may have different effects on the outcome of pregnancy both for the mother and for the child. Correct management of the individual woman with raised blood pressure will therefore depend on the identification of the underlying cause of the high pressure where this is possible.

Blood Pressure Measurement

The conventional sphygomomanometer is quite suitable for routine clinical use. The woman should be as relaxed as possible with her forearm horizontal and well supported and her upper arm level with her heart. She should be in the sitting position, either in a chair or in bed. The cuff should be long enough to encircle the arm, should be applied firmly without creasing, and inflated and deflated smoothly.

Although there is a wide variation, the disappearance of the *Korotkoff* sounds (Phase V) appears to correlate better with direct intra-arterial measurement of diastolic pressure than the muffling or fading of the sounds (Phase IV) (Raftery and Ward, 1968) and readings based on the clear-cut disappearance of the sounds are generally more reproducible when measurements are made by different clinical staff. However the recording either of Phase IV or Phase V readings as diastolic pressure varies from hospital to hospital and even within the same hospital. It is therefore important to standardise this procedure throughout the Obstetric Unit for nurses, doctors and students, preferably recording both phases. This variability of practice should also be kept in mind when comparing blood pressure data between different Obstetric Units.

Automatic recorders capable of making repeated regular measurement of blood pressure have been developed in the past few years (Labarthe *et al.*, 1973). These are of particular advantage in the labour room or intensive care unit.

Normal and Abnormal Blood Pressure

Arterial pressure varies over a wide range in normal non-pregnant individuals and during a 24-hour period of continuous recording the highest levels are often twice the lowest (Bevan *et al.*, 1969). Large changes occur during exercise, conversation, mental arithmetic, defaecation, copulation and sleep (Bevan *et al.*, 1969) and progressively lower values are found as the subject becomes familiar with her surroundings (Armitage and Rose, 1966). Blood pressure varies widely in different communities or even in different parts of the same community (Hawthorne *et al.*, 1969) and it may be associated with increased dietary sodium and obesity (Evans and Rose, 1971). It is well known that blood pressure tends to increase with age (Pickering, 1968).

In a large population blood pressure values are distributed continuously with no borderline between "normal" and "abnormal" groups and Pickering (1968) has suggested that high blood pressure is a "disease of degree" and not a "disease of kind", i.e. the higher the pressure the greater the risk and the lower the pressure the lower the risk. In clinical practice, however, it is helpful to designate an arbitrary level above which the subject is considered to be at greater risk than the average person of the same age and sex, and in whom treatment to lower the blood pressure must be considered. Because it is arbitrary, numerous such levels have been suggested but the one most commonly used in clinical (including obstetric) practice is 140/90. Evidence is as yet scanty that treatment of a non-pregnant patient with a diastolic pressure between 90 and 110 mm Hg will significantly affect the long-term survival, but there is no doubt that lowering the blood pressure is of benefit when the diastolic pressure is persistently greater than 110 mm Hg (Evans and Rose, 1971). Generally, non-pregnant females appear to be at less risk than males for any given age and blood pressure (Pickering, 1968).

In most women both systolic and diastolic blood pressures fall a little in the first 6 months of pregnancy then rise to pre-pregnancy levels before term (MacGillivray *et al.*, 1969). This fall in early and mid-pregnancy may also occur in women with pre-existing hypertension and the rise to previous hypertensive levels in late gestation may be interpreted as "pre-eclampsia" if there is no record of blood pressure early in pregnancy or before conception. Measurement of the blood pressure at the woman's earliest antenatal visit is therefore important.

Although in general women appear to tolerate high blood pressure better than men, this is not the case if the woman is pregnant. Pickering (1968) has shown that the development of accelerated (malignant) phase hypertension, with its complications of acute left ventricular failure, hypertensive encephalopathy and cerebral haemorrhage, is associated with very high levels of blood pressure (diastolic usually greater than 130 mm Hg) in the non-pregnant subject. In pregnancy these complications may occur at a much lower diastolic pressure (e.g. 110 to 120 mm Hg) and eclampsia can accompany diastolic pressures of 90 to 110 mm Hg. The response of the blood pressure to pregnancy and the critical level for the development of complications appears to vary in different parts of the world (Davies, 1971).

Causes of Hypertension in Pregnancy

A. Hypertension before 24 Weeks' Gestation

The finding of hypertension (i.e. sustained blood pressure over 140/90 or more) before the 24th week of gestation usually signifies that the blood pressure has been raised before the pregnancy has developed, i.e. the woman has *pre-existing hypertension*. In obstetric departments this is often called "essential hypertension", but this term is too vague. In such a case it is important to classify the cause of the hypertension as listed in Table I, as the prognosis for the mother and the child may be variably affected according to the aetiology of the raised pressure. It must be remembered that some of these diseases may become clinically apparent for the first time at any stage during pregnancy, with an associated rise in blood pressure levels which had been previously normal.

B. Hypertension after 24 Weeks' Gestation

When faced with the problem of a woman with persistently elevated blood pressure (i.e. 140/90 or greater) after the 24th week of gestation, the following questions must be asked:

1. What was the blood pressure earlier in the pregnancy?
2. What was the blood pressure before this pregnancy?
3. What was the blood pressure during and after any previous pregnancies?

If the blood pressure has been recorded as "normal" (i.e. less than 140/90) before and in the first 12 weeks of the present pregnancy then it is very likely that the woman has *pregnancy-induced hypertension*. This will be confirmed by a return of the blood pressure to previous normal levels in the postpartum period. It should be remembered, however, that some of the diseases listed in Table I may develop in the last months of pregnancy and the associated rise in blood pressure may mimic pregnancy-induced hypertension.

10/TABLE 1

CLASSIFICATION OF HYPERTENSION IN PREGNANCY

A Pregnancy-induced hypertension, i.e. pregnancy with superimposed hypertension arising after the 24th week of gestation and returning to normal in the postpartum period.

B Pre-existing hypertension, with superimposed pregnancy i.e. blood pressure raised before and in the early weeks of pregnancy and persisting after the postpartum period:

1. Essential (idiopathic primary) hypertension—cause unknown;
2. Renal hypertension due to renal artery stenosis, glomerulonephritis, pyelonephritis, interstitial nephritis (analgesics, diabetes, gout), polycystic disease, tuberculosis, neoplasm and rarer congenital lesions;
3. Adrenal causes: Phaeochromocytoma;
Cushing's syndrome;
Primary hyperaldosteronism (Conn's syndrome);
4. Connective tissue diseases e.g. polyarteritis nodosa, systemic lupus erythematosus, scleroderma;
5. Coarctation of aorta.

If high blood pressure found in the early months of pregnancy has shown a further marked rise after the 24th week, then the woman is likely to have *pre-existing hypertension with superimposed pregnancy-induced hypertension*. The outlook for the mother and especially for the child may be profoundly affected by this development.

PREGNANCY-INDUCED HYPERTENSION

DEFINITION

Pregnancy-induced hypertension is diagnosed when a woman with previously normal blood pressure shows a sustained rise of pressure to 140/90 or more on at least two occasions, 24 hours apart, after the 24th week of gestation, in the absence of evidence of an underlying cause for the hypertension (as listed in Table 1).

It has already been pointed out that raised blood pressure in the general population is a state of graded risk, i.e. that a definition of abnormal blood pressure is arbitrary. The same holds true for high blood pressure in pregnancy and it must be recognised that the level of 140/90 is an arbitrary one, albeit based on the experience of clinical practice that complications are more likely to occur above this level.

Pregnancy-induced hypertension may be subdivided into mild and severe forms:

(*a*) mild—sustained blood pressure between 140/90 and 160/100, with the woman resting in bed;
(*b*) severe—sustained blood pressure of 160/100 or more, with the woman resting in bed.

In many women with blood pressure levels of 160/100 or more there is an accompanying proteinuria which is considered to be clinically significant in a concentration of 0·3 g/litre or greater. The appearances of such proteinuria, in the absence of a urinary tract infection, indicates more serious renal involvement in the hypertensive process (or perhaps the development of a significant renal lesion for the first time) and implies that the pregnancy is now at definite risk, i.e. it is the stage of pre-eclampsia.

Incidence

Because of variation in definition it is not possible to compare accurately the incidence of pregnancy-induced hypertension—or pre-eclampsia—from one centre with another. It is useful, however, to look at the figures for one centre alone where definitions have not changed over a number of years. In the Queen Mother's Hospital, Glasgow the following definitions have been used until recently:

Mild pre-eclampsia—blood pressure between 140/90 and 160/100 after 20th week of gestation, with no proteinuria.
Severe pre-eclampsia—blood pressure greater than 160/100 after 20th week of gestation, with oedema and proteinuria.

The incidence of these conditions over 8 years was as follows:

	1964–65	1966–67	1968–69	1970–71
Mild	708 (14·8%)	428 (7·4%)	895 (14·9%)	395 (7·2%)
Severe	132 (2·8%)	112 (2·0%)	92 (1·5%)	94 (1·7%)
Total number of cases with pregnancy-induced hypertension	840 (17·6%)	540 (9·4%)	987 (16·4%)	489 (8·9%)

The figures in parenthesis indicate the percentage of cases of the total births in the hospital.

In this one centre, then, the incidence of pregnancy-induced hypertension has fluctuated over an 8-year period but there appears to have been a mild sustained fall in the number of cases with blood pressure greater than 160/100 and accompanying proteinuria, i.e. pre-eclampsia. Other centres and countries, using different definitions, have also reported a decreasing incidence of pre-eclampsia and severe hypertension in late pregnancy.

Predisposing Factors

A number of social, genetic, medical and obstetric conditions carry an increased risk of a woman's developing pregnancy-induced hypertension and pre-eclampsia.

Social and economic.—Pregnancy-induced hypertension is more likely to occur in women in the poorer and underprivileged communities. This appears to be due to a combination of poor dietary habits with ignorance and apathy leading to poor antenatal care. Failure to consult a doctor early in pregnancy is an important factor in the high incidence of this condition among unmarried mothers. The incidence appears to be lower in smokers than non-smokers, but when hypertension does develop in a pregnant woman who smokes the fetal outlook is worse than for hypertension alone (Duffus and MacGillivray, 1968).

Genetic.—Women with pregnancy-induced hypertension are more likely to have female relatives with a similar condition than are women with normal blood pressure during pregnancy (Adams and Finlayson, 1961). A greater incidence of hypertension occurring outwith pregnancy in female relatives of these women has been found (Adams and Finlayson, 1961) although other studies have not confirmed this (Solan *et al.*, 1970).

Medical.—Pre-existing hypertension from any cause listed in Table I appears to predispose to the development of superimposed pregnancy-induced hypertension in the last 3 months of gestation. Women with chronic renal disease with or without associated hypertension and women with clinical or latent diabetes mellitus, are also more likely to develop raised blood pressure in the last trimester.

Obstetric.—A multiple pregnancy (e.g. twins, triplets) carries a greater risk of pregnancy-induced hypertension than a pregnancy with a single fetus. Hydramnios also is a predisposing factor. The gaining of excessive weight in mid-pregnancy is often followed by high blood pressure in the later weeks. Whether the weight gain is related to sodium and fluid retention and whether it plays a causative role in the change of pressure or is an accompanying earlier feature of the underlying disease process remains controversial (Vedra and Pavlikova, 1969). It has been suggested that a normotensive woman at 28 to 32 weeks' gestation is likely to develop hypertension later in pregnancy if her diastolic blood pressure rises by 20 mm Hg or more within 5 minutes after changing from the left lateral to the supine position (Gant *et al.*, 1974) but this has not been confirmed (Weir *et al.*, unpublished data). Women with rhesus isoimmunisation are susceptible to raised blood pressure in later pregnancy but, as discussed elsewhere, this condition is much less common now. Cases with hydatidiform mole may develop hypertension which subsides when the trophoblastic tissue is removed, but this of course is not strictly within the definition of pregnancy-induced hypertension as outlined earlier.

Many obstetricians consider that pre-eclampsia is a disease only of the primigravid woman. There is no doubt that this condition arises much more frequently in a first than in subsequent pregnancies, but multiparous women are also seen with high blood pressure which has developed after the 24th week of gestation and which returns to normal levels after the postpartum period, i.e. they fulfil the criteria for the definition of pregnancy-induced hypertension. A multiparous woman with a previous history of raised blood pressure in late pregnancy which has settled postpartum appears to be at greater risk of further episodes of raised blood pressure during subsequent pregnancies than her normotensive counterpart, especially if she has also had accompanying proteinuria.

Clinical Examination

Most women with hypertension in late pregnancy have no symptoms or signs attributable to the raised blood pressure unless the condition has deteriorated to the stage of impending eclampsia (see later).

Specific questions to be asked are:

Is there a previous history of high blood pressure?

Was the blood pressure normal or high during any previous pregnancies? If high, did it return to normal after the postpartum period?

Has she ever taken the oral contraceptive pill and if so was her blood pressure normal or high while taking this?

Is there a previous history of kidney disease (e.g. "pyelitis", "cystitis", "chill in the bladder", "infection in the urine") which might suggest renal hypertension?

Before the pregnancy did she have polyuria and/or nocturia? This would indicate possible chronic renal failure.

Had she noticed marked weakness of her limbs? This, often accompanied by nocturia and polyuria, is a symptom of hypokalaemia due to hyperaldosteronism, either primary (Conn's syndrome), or secondary to severe hypertension or excessive diuretic therapy.

Is there any disturbance of her visual fields, as may occur in Cushing's syndrome?

Has she had any episodes of severe sweating perhaps accompanied by headache, palpitation, chest tightness, pallor and panic? These are the symptoms of excess catecholamine production as found in phaeochromocytoma.

Symptoms of blurred vision and severe generalised or occipital headache are very suggestive of accelerated (malignant) phase hypertension and impending eclampsia. This demands immediate treatment, as will be discussed later.

Some women will have had excessive weight gain for several weeks before the high blood pressure has been found and this group will often have evidence of more than the trace of oedema which may normally be expected in pregnancy, i.e. they may have generalised oedema affecting the face, hands and ankles. They may also complain or more exertional dyspnoea than expected for the length of gestation but examination of the respiratory system is usually normal.

On *physical examination* particular attention should be paid to the apex beat; if this is displaced to the left and heaving in character, it is likely that the woman has long-standing hypertension. The second sound at the aortic area may then be accentuated. A physiological aortic systolic flow murmur occurs frequently in normal pregnancy. A systolic murmur heard between the scapulae and accompanied by collateral arteries suggests coarctation of the aorta and this will be confirmed by finding delayed and diminished pulsation of the femoral arteries. Palpation of the femoral pulses is therefore mandatory in every case of hypertension.

Bimanual palpation of the loins will detect kidney enlargement (e.g. polycystic disease of the kidneys) although this may be more difficult to carry out satisfactorily in the last weeks of gestation. The systolic bruit heard in some cases of renal artery stenosis is best listened for in pregnant women over the renal areas posteriorly.

Ophthalmoscopic examination of the optic fundi is an essential part of the examination of every hypertensive patient as this is the only site in the body where the effects of high blood pressure on the smaller blood vessels can be visualised and assessed. In most women with pregnancy-induced hypertension the optic fundi show no abnormality. Some, especially those with evidence of excessive fluid retention, may have retinal oedema. If there has been long-standing pre-existing hypertension the arterioles may show silver-wiring and tortuosity and in more severe cases arteriovenous nipping. The presence of exudates and haemorrhages is a very serious sign indicating the development of accelerated (malignant) phase hypertension which is accompanied in its florid form by bilateral papilloedema.

In addition to the measurement of blood pressure at each antenatal visit, the urine should be routinely tested for protein and glucose. Both tests are now rapidly and easily performed using the Albustix and Clinistix methods respectively. Clinically significant albuminuria is present when the Albustix shows a + reaction, i.e. 30 mg/100 ml or 0·3 g/litre. Generally the approximate amount of albumin in the urine can be estimated by the Albustix method. If more detailed quantitation is required from day to day, the Esbach's method on a sample from a 24-hour collection of urine is still of practical value although this is now being superseded by more accurate turbidometric techniques. Estimation of the different urinary protein fractions by immunoelectrophoresis (Kelly and McEwan, 1973) is of interest but does not appear to have a place in day-to-day practical management.

If protein is found in the urine, it is important to exclude a urinary tract infection which may be present in spite of the lack of symptoms of dysuria, increased frequency of micturition or loin pain. In the absence of a urinary tract infection, the finding of proteinuria is of serious prognostic importance to the outcome of the pregnancy. The triad of very high blood pressure, severe generalised oedema and marked proteinuria carries an especially grave significance and implies that the woman is in the severe stage of pre-eclampsia and that eclampsia is imminent.

Laboratory Investigations

Tests of fetal growth and maturity.—These are essential in the management of hypertension in the last trimester particularly with regard to the timing of induction of labour or Caesarean section. They are fully discussed elsewhere.

Urine microscopy and culture.—Mention has already been made of the importance of excluding a urinary tract infection when proteinuria has been discovered. This is usually performed by obtaining a mid-stream specimen of urine, examining this microscopically for cells, casts and organisms, and plating it out on a culture medium. On a satisfactory mid-stream specimen (i.e. with as little contamination as possible) a bacterial count of 100,000/mm^3 or greater is considered to indicate significant infection, especially when there is an accompanying significant white-cell count in the urine. Bacterial counts between 10,000/mm^3 and 100,000/mm^3 are of borderline significance and a further urine sample should then be obtained. Counts of less than 100,000/mm^3 are unlikely to indicate active infection. The recently introduced dipculture technique should improve the reliability of urine culture and lead to speedier reporting of results and initiation of the correct antibiotic therapy (McAllister, 1973). The presence of a urinary tract infection in a woman with hypertension in pregnancy does not, of course, signify that these two conditions are related. However, if urine culture is positive in a woman who has clinical evidence of long-standing hypertension then the possibility of chronic pyelonephritis must be considered even in the absence of renal tract symptoms.

Serum urea and creatinine.—The lower levels of serum urea and creatinine in normal pregnant women compared with non-pregnant subjects reflect the increased glomerular filtration rate which occurs during normal gestation (Hytten and Leitch, 1971). In pregnancy-induced hypertension, especially if associated with proteinuria, the serum levels are higher than in normal pregnancy although usually within the normal non-pregnant range. Levels above this range suggest underlying chronic renal impairment either as a cause or as a result of pre-existing hypertension. An acute rise in blood urea may occur in acute renal failure which sometimes accompanies eclampsia (see later).

Serum electrolytes.—Serum sodium and potassium concentrations are generally lower in normal pregnancy than in normal non-pregnant women. The administration of potassium-losing diuretics will aggravate this (see later). Persistent plasma levels of potassium below 3·0 mmol/litre in a hypertensive pregnant woman who is not taking diuretics are suggestive of hyperaldosteronism. This may be secondary to renal or accelerated phase hypertension, or may be due to a primary adrenal lesion, either an adenoma or hyperplasia. Measurement of plasma aldosterone concentration is not diagnostically helpful in pregnancy as it is usually raised in this situation (see later). Plasma renin concentration is also usually high in normal pregnancy but a level in the lower part of the normal non-pregnant range in association with hypokalaemia and very high concentration of aldosterone would be very suggestive of primary hyperaldosteronism (Conn's syndrome).

Serum uric acid.—Like the blood urea this is lower in normal pregnant women than in non-pregnant women due to increased renal clearance (Hytten and Leitch, 1971). It is usually raised in the stage of pre-eclampsia, and a rising level in a woman with high blood pressure in the last trimester may be an indication of impaired fetal prognosis (Beilin *et al.*, 1974).

Creatinine clearance.—This is an indirect measurement of glomerular filtration rate and is generally high in normal pregnancy (Hytten and Leitch, 1971). Pregnancy-induced hypertension, especially with proteinuria, is associated with a creatinine clearance lower than in normal pregnancy but usually within the normal non-pregnant range. When the serum creatinine is raised measurement of the creatinine clearance should be performed on a 24-hour urine collection. This will establish to some extent the degree of renal failure and when performed serially it is also useful as an index of change in renal function.

Urinary catecholamines.—The presence of a catecholamine-producing tumour such as a phaeochromocytoma is suggested by the characteristic symptoms described earlier, but such tumours may rarely occur without these symptoms. Biochemical confirmation is obtained by finding increased 24-hour urinary levels of the metabolites of adrenaline and noradrenaline, i.e. metadrenaline, normetadrenaline and vanillylmandelic acid (VMA). Drugs such as methyldopa should be stopped for at least 48 hours before making these measurements, and dietary items such as bananas and cocoa should be avoided before urinary VMA is assayed. Urinary catecholamines should be measured only if the symptoms are suspicious of phaeochromocytoma or if the blood pressure is fluctuating widely or is persistently very high and difficult to control.

Electrocardiogram.—This is not necessary in every case of hypertension in pregnancy but should be performed when the blood pressure is persistently very high or if there is clinical evidence of left ventricular hypertrophy, cardiac failure or an arrhythmia.

Blood film and platelet count.—The haemoglobin should be checked frequently in every pregnant woman. If she is severely hypertensive and has symptoms of severe pre-eclampsia (see later) there may be evidence of reduced platelets, increased reticulocytes and abnormally shaped red cells, i.e. microangiopathic haemolytic anaemia. This carries a grave risk to the mother until the pregnancy is terminated.

Serum and urinary fibrin degradation products and other coagulation studies.—Increased levels of fibrin degradation products (FDPs) imply disseminated intravascular coagulation which occurs to a variable degree in all cases which have deteriorated to the stage of severe pre-eclampsia. Microangiopathic haemolytic anaemia is associated with this process and where this is suspected, on examination of a blood film, then plasma or urinary FDP levels may be estimated. Depending upon the local laboratory facilities other coagulation studies may also be carried out, i.e. estimation of circulating Factor V, VII etc.

Management

All pregnant women should have their blood pressure checked regularly from as early as possible in gestation. When the blood pressure is found to be raised at the surgery or antenatal clinic, where possible the women should be allowed to rest quietly for about 30 minutes and the blood pressure then measured again. It was pointed out earlier that blood pressure normally fluctuates over a wide range throughout the day. Raised levels associated with rushing, anxiety and tension in unfamiliar surroundings occur no less frequently in pregnancy than in normal non-pregnant women and it is not unexpected, therefore, that some women will have rather high levels of blood pressure initially. Many of these women will have normal readings after resting quietly for 30 minutes, especially if the doctor and nurse take time to talk to them about any problems and are able to allay any anxieties.

If a woman in the last trimester has a blood pressure of 140/90 or more after a period of rest then she should be admitted to the antenatal ward for further assessment and rest. In many cases the pressure will settle within a few days after admission. This may be due to a relaxation of nervous tension associated with home or work, but may also be due to the physiological effect of bed rest on blood pressure in pregnancy (Hytten and Leitch, 1971). In some cases excess tension and anxiety may appear to be causing a marked lability of blood pressure and the administration of diazepam, chlordiazepoxide or barbiturates in such cases may be of value. These women can usually be discharged after several days, to be followed up at the antenatal clinic at weekly or two-weekly intervals.

Of more concern is the woman whose blood pressure fails to settle after several days of rest with or without mild sedation, i.e. she appears to have established pregnancy-induced hypertension. The concern is greater if there is associated proteinuria. Management in such a case is determined by the stage of gestation and by the apparent maturity of the fetus as judged by clinical, ultrasound and biochemical methods which are described elsewhere.

If the length of gestation is 38 weeks or more and the fetus appears to be normal size and maturity, then elective induction of labour should be carried out. This is of more urgency if there is accompanying proteinuria. Apart from ensuring very adequate analgesia and possibly administering mild sedation, induction of labour should be performed as described for the normotensive pregnancy (see Chapter XVI). Hypotensive drugs are not usually required in this situation but may be needed if the diastolic pressure rises to over 110 mm Hg or symptoms of impending eclampsia develop.

In cases with pregnancy-induced hypertension before the 38th week, the pregnancy should be maintained as long as possible to ensure adequate growth and maturity of the child. Hypotensive drugs should be given in cases with proteinuria or with diastolic levels greater than 110 mm Hg. If proteinuria is progressive, if the blood pressure is uncontrolled and if early symptoms and signs of impending eclampsia develop, then intervention is required in the mother's interests and labour should be induced.

Newer techniques, such as the measurement of the sphyngomyelin: lecithin ratio on samples of liquor, are now adding a more precise dimension to the assessment of fetal maturity (see Chapter XVI) and the obstetrician is now more prepared to carry out an earlier induction of labour if these tests are satisfactory. Also modern paediatric techniques have revolutionised the concept of very early delivery and, where continuation of the pregnancy constitutes a serious maternal risk, it is now possible to induce labour even as early as the 32nd week and still have a reasonable chance of delivering and maintaining a viable child.

Women with severe pregnancy-induced hypertension before the 32nd week present a very difficult problem. The fetus is barely viable at this stage and yet continuation of the pregnancy is risky for both mother and child. Rest in hospital, sedation if required and control of blood pressure by hypotensive drugs offer the only means of maintaining the pregnancy for the several vital weeks necessary to allow further critical improvement in fetal growth and maturity. Not infrequently, however, these measures are insufficient and intrauterine death occurs or the pregnancy has to be terminated on account of maternal deterioration with impending eclampsia.

From the foregoing, it will be appreciated that termination of pregnancy, either by spontaneous delivery or by artifical induction, is the only adequate cure for pregnancy-induced hypertension. Other measures, such as rest, sedation and hypotensive drug therapy, are merely aids to control the blood pressure while the pregnancy is allowed to proceed to a stage where the child is of sufficient maturity to survive.

Hypotensive Therapy

In general, the drugs used to lower blood pressure in non-pregnant situations are also suitable in pregnancy-induced hypertension. It must be remembered, however, that these drugs act to reduce blood pressure by interference with one or other of the normal mechanisms of blood pressure control and that this will involve some disturbance of physiological functions with resulting side-effects of varying severity. An additional important factor to take into account in pregnancy is the possible effect of such drugs on the placental circulation and the fetus.

Details of the hypotensive drugs which may be used in pregnancy are given at the end of this chapter.

Where the blood pressure is at levels which, in pregnancy, may be associated with complications such as eclampsia, left ventricular failure or stroke, it is mandatory to reduce such a pressure as soon as possible. In the very acute situation, intravenous diazoxide or hydrallazine seem to be the drugs of choice. Where there is rather less urgency, adequate doses of oral methyldopa or clonidine are preferable in the recumbent hypertensive patient, keeping oral diazoxide and hydrallazine as reserve drugs for use if the blood pressure does not come under satisfactory control within a few days. Adequate controlled trials in such a situation are extremely difficult, but it does seem likely that maternal mortality and morbidity have been influenced in part by controlling the blood pressure. Whether the risks to the fetus have been reduced is debatable.

The case for treating the pregnant woman with a blood pressure less than 110 mm Hg in late pregnancy is controversial. If there is associated proteinuria the woman is more likely to develop hypertensive complications and oral hypotensive drugs should be given until induction of labour is possible. If there is no proteinuria and the woman has no symptoms, there is no satisfactory evidence that the administration of a hypotensive drug will influence the outcome of the pregnancy; rest with regular monitoring of blood pressure, weight, urinary protein and fetal growth are, of course, essential.

ECLAMPSIA

Eclampsia is the term used to describe the clinical condition of convulsions associated with pregnancy and may occur before, during or after labour (Table II). Convulsions more than one week after delivery are unlikely to be due to eclampsia.

Eclampsia is almost always associated with hypertension and proteinuria. The blood pressure is usually very high but convulsions can occasionally occur with diastolic pressures between 90 and 100 mm Hg. Proteinuria may be as much as 15–20 g/day, when it is usually accompanied by severe generalised oedema; in occasional cases, however, there may be very little urinary protein or oedema.

The incidence and mortality of eclampsia has fallen dramatically over the past 5 decades. This is likely to be due to better antenatal care associated with improved social and economic conditions. The woman now most at risk is the teenage primigravida with a concealed pregnancy. However, any woman with hypertension after the 24th week of gestation is a potential candidate for eclampsia and this is especially so if the hypertension is accompanied by proteinuria, excessive weight gain and severe oedema.

Premonitory Symptoms and Signs of Eclampsia

Eclampsia is impending when the following are present:

1. Headache—usually generalised but may be localised to the

occipital and occasionally to the frontal area. It is persistent and often severe.

2. Visual disturbance—blurring of vision and photophobia are important symptoms. Examination of the optic fundi will show marked retinal oedema and in the severe stages haemorrhages, exudates and papilloedema may also be present.
3. Restlessness and agitation.
4. Epigastric discomfort, nausea and vomiting.
5. Oliguria.
6. Increasing laboratory evidence of disseminated intravascular coagulation.

Management of Impending Eclampsia

The main aim of management in the pre-eclamptic stage is to prevent eclamptic seizures. When a woman develops the symptoms and signs of impending eclampsia at home she should be kept in bed, sedated (e.g. sodium amytal 200 mg or diazepam 10 mg) and subsequently transferred as soon and as gently as possible to the intensive care area of the local obstetric hospital. She should be accompanied by a doctor or a member of the flying squad for this journey. She should be nursed in a *quiet, darkened room*, the *sedation* repeated as necessary and hypotensive *drug therapy* initiated. Oral therapy may be sufficient, e.g. methyldopa 500 mg followed by 250 mg t.i.d.; clonidine 0·3 mg followed by 0·2 mg t.i.d.; hydrallazine 50 mg followed by 25 mg t.i.d. The dose may then require to be increased according to the blood pressure response. Severely hypertensive cases may require intravenous diazoxide 150–300 mg or hydrallazine 20 mg, subsequently repeating the injection after 30 or 60 minutes or introducing oral therapy depending upon the response.

If there is gross oedema, frusemide should be given orally in a dose of 40 mg daily, increasing this to 80 or 120 mg daily depending upon the response. An intravenous line should be set up with a slow infusion of 5 per cent dextrose to maintain patency—this is initially mainly a precautionary measure to be used if intravenous therapy is urgently required. In severe cases a central venous line may be helpful to detect early evidence of cardiac failure.

Blood pressure, fluid balance, proteinuria and degree of restlessness should be monitored regularly. In most cases the situation should be improved after 24 to 48 hours. Once the condition is stabilised the pregnancy should be terminated by induction or Caesarean section.

If the condition fails to improve, i.e. if the headaches, visual disturbance and restlessness worsen and especially if early twitching of the face or limbs occur, then *anticonvulsant therapy* should be started. This should be initiated without waiting until a full-blown eclamptic seizure has occurred.

Anticonvulsants suitable for this situation are:

Chlormethiazole (*Heminevrin*).—Intravenous infusion of 30–50 ml Heminevrin 0·8 per cent (8 mg per ml) at an initial rate of 4 ml (60 drops) per minute until the patient feels drowsy. The exact dose depends on the patient's response. Maintain the drip rate at around 1 ml (15 drops) per minute, increasing the rate if restlessness occurs or decreasing it if the woman appears to be too drowsy. (References: Duffus *et al.*, 1969; Varma 1972.)

Diazepam (*Valium*).—Intravenous infusion of 0·15–0·20 mg/kg body weight. Adjust the rate of infusion according to the patient's response. (References: Lean *et al.*, 1968; Joyce and Kenyon, 1972; Ruoss, 1974.)

Tribromethol (*Avertin*).—This drug is unfortunately no longer available.

Magnesium sulphate.—4 g in a 20 per cent solution given intravenously over 5 minutes; or intravenous infusion of 1 g hourly; or 10 g in a 50 per cent solution given intramuscularly every 4 hours. (References: Pritchard and Stone, 1967; Speroff, 1973.)

All of these drugs have a mild but variable hypotensive effect which is of advantage in this situation. However, in excess they will cause deepening of unconsciousness and coma, with the hazards of maternal and fetal respiratory depression, anoxia, cardiac depression and circulatory failure. It is mandatory therefore, that a nurse be in constant attendance. If necessary an oral airway should be inserted and an aspirator should be immediately available.

Morphine, pethidine, promazine and amytal have all been used to treat impending and established eclampsia, either singly or in varying combinations. They are more likely to cause maternal and fetal respiratory depression and seem to have little advantage over the drugs already discussed.

The Eclamptic Seizure

In the majority of cases the convulsions are preceded by some or all of the symptoms and signs discussed above but they may also occur suddenly with no warning. The seizure is similar to that occurring in grand mal epilepsy with premonitory slight twitching of the face and limbs leading into the generalised tonic and clonic stages and followed by coma. There may be only one convulsion—this is usually associated with labour. More commonly the fits recur at irregular intervals, and in severe cases they may take place in rapid succession—status eclampticus.

The general condition of the woman may not be greatly affected by infrequent seizures. Repeated convulsions, however, lead to a rapid deterioration with cyanosis, tachycardia, pyrexia, deepening coma and death. The onset of eclampsia presages a poor outcome for the fetus unless the seizures are controlled quickly. Intra-uterine death may occur and the immediate neonatal mortality rate is high due to intra-uterine anoxia, cerebral haemorrhage or prematurity.

The immediate management of an eclamptic fit is a matter of nursing technique, as a member of the nursing staff rather than a doctor is more likely to be present at the time a fit commences. The nurse should insert, if possible, a gag between the patient's teeth (an airway may be already present), turn the woman on her side and give oxygen while awaiting the arrival of the doctor. The principle involved is to maintain a clear airway and reduce anoxia.

A most effective way of aborting a fit is to give a small dose of pentothal intravenously, just sufficient to stop the convulsion. One of the anticonvulsants discussed above can then be administered to prevent a recurrence of seizures. Failure of the above regime to control the convulsions may necessitate the use of complete anaesthesia, muscle relaxants and assisted ventilation. Intravenous heparin has been used in cases with severe disseminated intravascular coagulation (Brain *et al.*, 1967) but the response to this is difficult to evaluate; results seem to be very variable and the procedure itself is not without danger in an already critical situation.

Raised Blood Pressure during Labour

It has been pointed our earlier that any stressful situation may cause a rise of blood pressure. The stress of labour is no exception especially in the more apprehensive woman, and it is therefore not unexpected to find some rise of blood pressure at this time in an otherwise normal pregnancy. Sympathetic reassurance and guidance combined with adequate analgesia are all that is required in this situation and the blood pressure will settle rapidly after delivery.

However, if the blood pressure maintains a high level and is associated with the appearance of proteinuria, headache, visual disturbance or marked restlessness (i.e. the symptoms of impending eclampsia) then hypotensive therapy must be given as well as adequate sedation and prophylactic anticonvulsant therapy.

Lumbar epidural analgesia is of value in women with raised blood pressure before or during labour (Moir *et al.*, 1972). It gives potent localised analgesia with no complications of respiratory depression and has a significant hypotensive effect. Combined with an anticonvulsant in the severe case, it provides balanced therapy and avoids the use of narcotics in high doses. There is no evidence of any deleterious effect on the fetus.

Blood Pressure after Delivery

In most cases of pregnancy-induced hypertension, the blood pressure, and proteinuria and oedema if present, settle rapidly within several days after delivery. If hypotensive drugs have been needed the dose can usually be quickly reduced, the women often being discharged requiring no hypotensive therapy. If the blood pressure remains satisfactory at the postnatal clinic then no further follow-up is necessary unless there has been some evidence of a pre-existing lesion which has been unmasked by the pregnancy.

In a few cases the blood pressure fails to settle satisfactorily after delivery. If the diastolic pressure is less than 110 mm Hg, such women can be discharged without treatment; if it is greater than this, a hypotensive drug should be given and the patient discharged when the pressure falls consistently below this level. These women must then be seen frequently at the out-patient clinic and the blood pressure would be expected to settle gradually over the next few weeks or months. If it has not returned to normal after six months, the diagnosis of "pregnancy-induced" hypertension must be reviewed and a further search made for an underlying renal or endocrine lesion.

Uncommonly the blood pressure rises for the first time in the first few days after delivery—"postpartum hypertension". The reasons for this are not clear, but most cases settle spontaneously within several days or weeks and only rarely is a hypotensive drug required. These women should be followed up at the out-patient clinic as outlined above.

Maternal Complications

Short-term Complications

These are uncommon but potentially lethal, especially if several complications arise in the same individual.

1. Eclampsia. This has already been discussed in detail.
2. Cerebrovascular accident—usually intracerebral haemorrhage, occasionally ruptured intracranial aneurysm or cerebral thrombosis. This may be fatal or the woman may be left with a residual neurological deficit such as hemiplegia, dysphasia or visual disturbance.
3. Accidental haemorrhage. Abruptio placentae is an important complication of hypertension in pregnancy and a massive unheralded bleed can have disastrous consequences.
4. Acute left ventricular failure with pulmonary oedema.
5. Acute renal failure.

6. Micro-angiopathic haemolytic anaemia (haemolytic uraemic syndrome). The patient usually has evidence of severe widespread intravascular coagulation which may be associated with eclampsia, renal failure, hepatic failure, cerebral thrombosis and circulatory collapse.
7. Side-effects of drug therapy (see later).

The incidence of maternal complications of pregnancy-induced hypertension in the Queen Mother's Hospital between 1964 and 1971 was:

	1964–65	1966–67	1968–69	1970–71
No. of cases	840	540	987	489
Eclampsia	12 (1·4%)	4 (0·7%)	6 (0·6%)	3 (0·6%)
Antepartum haemorrhage (not placenta praevia)	13 (1·5%)	6 (1·1%)	39 (4·0%)	14 (2·9%)
Maternal mortality	1	0	0	0

(percentages are of number of cases of pregnancy-induced hypertension)

Since 1964, therefore, this hospital has recorded a decrease in cases of eclampsia but an increase in women with antepartum haemorrhage associated with hypertension.

The Enquiry into Maternal Deaths in Scotland for the years 1965–1971 (Scottish Home and Health Department, 1974) has reported the following statistics:

Deaths from pre-eclamptic toxaemia	8
Deaths from eclamptic toxaemia	9
TOTAL	17

Of these:

71% were less than 25 years of age and in Classes 4 and 5 of the Registrar General's Social Classification;
59% occurred in a first pregnancy;
29% were unmarried;
35% were not booked for admission to a Maternity Unit.

The young unmarried primigravida with a concealed pregnancy is therefore most at risk.

Causes of death were reported as:

Cerebrovascular accident	8
Pulmonary oedema	4
Renal failure	3
Hepatorenal failure	1
Adrenal failure	1

Long-term Complications

Eclampsia which has occurred in a woman with no previous history of hypertension does not appear to be associated with residual hypertension or increased late mortality or morbidity. If it has been superimposed on pre-existing hypertension, then the blood pressure will remain high after delivery and the woman will be liable to the complications which accompany such a level of blood pressure, i.e. the occurrence of eclampsia does not influence the long-term outcome of pre-existing hypertension (Chesley *et al.*, 1968).

10/TABLE 2

ECLAMPSIA IN QUEEN MOTHER'S HOSPITAL

		1964–65	1966–67	1968–69	1970–71
No. of cases		12	7	6	6
% of total births		0·25	0·12	0·10	0·11
Age	less than 21	6	1	4	3
	21–34	5	5	2	1
	more than 34	1	1	0	2
Parity	0	9	6	4	4
	1+	3	1	2	2
Relation to labour	Antenatal	3	2	1	2
	First stage	1	4	0	0
	Second stage	5	0	1	1
	Postpartum	3	1	4	3
Maternal Mortality		0	0	0	0
Stillbirths		2	1	1	2
Neonatal deaths		1	0	0	1
Total fetal loss		3	1	1	3

About 25 per cent of women who have pregnancy-induced hypertension will have a rise of blood pressure in a subsequent normotensive pregnancy. The likelihood of further episodes of pregnancy-induced hypertension is much higher if the woman has had severe hypertension with proteinuria in two or more preceding pregnancies, especially if these have been associated with intra-uterine deaths or abruptions. Such women must be watched extremely carefully after the 24th week, preferably with constant hospital in-patient observation, frequent monitoring of fetal development and as early an induction of labour as possible.

The evidence to date suggests that hypertension and proteinuria induced solely by pregnancy and with no other apparent cause, do not appear to predispose to sustained hypertension or renal impairment in later life. (Adams and MacGillivray 1961; Chesley *et al.*,

1968), although this has been disputed (Gibson and Platt, 1959; Epstein, 1964). However, pregnancy in some women may unmask a latent genetic tendency to hypertension which settles after delivery but recurs permanently later. Such women usually have a strong family history of raised blood pressure (Adams and MacGillivray, 1961).

Fetal Complications

The improvement in maternal morbidity and mortality has not been paralleled by improved statistics for the child.

Complications which may arise are:

1. Intra-uterine death.
2. Poor intra-uterine growth—associated with "placental insufficiency".

Neither of these complications appears to be related to the actual level of blood pressure. Of more importance is the duration of the hypertension and the presence of proteinuria (Leather *et al.*, 1968; Walters, 1966).

3. Immaturity and prematurity—with associated hazards of neonatal death and pulmonary, renal and hepatic dysfunction. Early labour may occur spontaneously, for example in placental abruption; it is more likely to be due to artifical induction in the maternal interest. Recently introduced tests of fetal respiratory function such as the lecithin: sphyngomyelin ratio are likely to be of value in predicting more accurately the maturity of the fetus and therefore of influencing the timing of induction.
4. Brain damage, e.g. cerebral palsy. This is likely to be due to anoxia associated with (*a*) poor placental blood flow, (*b*) maternal hypoxia induced by eclampsia or excessive therapy with sedatives and anticonvulsants, (*c*) prolonged and difficult labour.
5. Side-effects of hypotensive drugs, e.g. intestinal ileus, thrombocytopenia, pancreatitis.

The incidence of fetal mortality associated with pregnancy-induced hypertension at the Queen Mother's Hospital for the years 1964–1971 was:

	1964–65	1966–67	1968–69	1970–71
No. of cases of pregnancy-induced hypertension	840	540	987	489
Stillbirths	24 (2·9%)	16 (3·0%)	21 (2·1%)	29 (5·9%)
Neonatal deaths	9 (1·1%)	7 (1·3%)	8 (0·8%)	7 (1·4%)
	33 (4·0%)	23 (4·3%)	29 (2·9%)	36 (7·3%)

In these 7 years, there has been no improvement, and perhaps a deterioration, in fetal mortality in hypertensive pregnant women. This is in agreement with data from Edinburgh for the period 1949 to 1963 (Thomson, 1969). The reasons for these disappointing figures are not clear.

PATHOLOGY

Because of the low maternal mortality of pregnancy-induced hypertension, post-mortem examinations are few and are limited mainly to the severely hypertensive and eclamptic patient. The placenta, of course can be examined in every case. Renal biopsies have been performed during pregnancy and immediately after delivery in some centres, but there is no clinical justification for these procedures unless an underlying renal lesion is strongly suspected which might influence management.

Placenta and Uterus

Comparisons of placentas from normal and hypertensive pregnancies have shown an increased incidence of infarcts, haematomas, congestion of chorionic villi, proliferative endarteritis and degeneration in the hypertensive group (Salvatore, 1968). The degree of these changes is roughly proportional to the clinical severity of the disease.

In normal pregnancy the spiral arteries are progressively converted to large tortuous channels by replacement of the musculo-elastic wall with a mixture of fibrinoid material and fibrous tissue. Organisation of mural thrombi results in intimal thickening. The basal arteries are relatively unaffected, perhaps showing some muscular hyperplasia or a loss of elastic tissue (Robertson *et al.*, 1975).

In pre-eclampsia and eclampsia changes occur in both the basal and spiral arteries. There appears to be a distinct vascular lesion characterised by fibrinoid necrosis and infiltration of the damaged vessel with foam cells and round cells. These vascular lesions could result in the reduction of intervillous blood flow, the placental lesions and some of the fetal complications which are found in this condition, and their extent and severity are proportional to the clinical severity of this disease (Robertson *et al.*, 1975).

Kidney

Pregnancy-induced hypertension appears to have a characteristic renal lesion not usually found in other clinical states. Electron-microscopy studies of biopsy material have shown glomerular endothelial swelling, obliteration of capillary lumina, subendothelial deposits, and enlargement of mesangial cells; basement membrane is normal and foot processes are discrete (Thomson *et al.*, 1972).

Fluorescence microscopy of the glomeruli shows deposition of fibrin, IgM and IgG in proportion to the severity of the clinical disease; both afferent and efferent arterioles contain complement, which may also be found within glomeruli in severe cases (Petrucco *et al.*, 1974).

These lesions are distributed patchily throughout the kidneys and vary even within a single glomerulus. Their incidence and severity generally match the clinical condition, but they persist in spite of adequate control of blood pressure. They are no longer present when biopsies are taken three months after delivery (Petrucco *et al.*, 1974). These pathological changes are in keeping with the reduced renal blood flow and glomerular filtration rate which are found in this condition (Klopper, 1964).

Other Organs

Changes in organs other than placenta, uterus and kidney have been demonstrated only in the severe cases, which have come to autopsy. There is usually evidence of disseminated intravascular coagulation, with thrombi of the arterioles and associated ischaemia, necrosis and haemorrhage.

The brain may show multiple petechial haemorrhages or larger haemorrhages in the cortex, pons or mid-brain. Multiple haemorrhages of varying size occur in the liver and in the portal regions and if they become large and confluent necrosis occurs. Subendocardial petechial haemorrhages may be present in the myocardium and the left ventricle may be dilated if acute left ventricular failure has occurred. The lungs may demonstrate pulmonary oedema. Haemorrhages and necrosis of the adrenal glands are particularly likely if there has been a profound circulatory collapse.

AETIOLOGY

Many theories have been advanced for the rise of blood pressure and frequently associated proteinuria which occurs in some women in late pregnancy. Some of these theories have failed to stand up to further investigation, others have shown conflicting results by different workers, and none has yet explained all the changes in this condition. As Boyd has stated, pre-eclampsia remains "die Krankheit der Theorien"—the disease of theories.

Uterine and Placental Ischaemia

Perhaps the commonest and most long-standing theory has been that of uterine and placental ischaemia (Young, 1914; Page, 1953). The functional changes of reduced uterine artery flow (Assali *et al.*,

1964) and choriodecidual blood flow (Dixon *et al.*, 1963) are consistent with the pathological changes already described. Interference with the placental circulation in animals may result in an elevation of blood pressure which is not dependent upon intact kidneys (Cavanagh *et al.*, 1972) and a circulating pressor substance has been found in animals following a reduction of placental circulation (Berger and Boucek, 1964). In the human, arteriography has revealed a decreased blood supply to the pregnant uterus in hypertensive compared with normotensive women (Bieniarz *et al.*, 1969). Whether this is a cause or a result of the raised blood pressure remains undecided—the latter seems more likely on present evidence.

Secretion of a Pressor Agent

The presence of a pressor agent in the circulation of a woman with pregnancy-induced hypertension is an attractive hypothesis, whether due to placental or renal ischaemia or other factors. It is of interest therefore that a slight rise of blood pressure has been demonstrated on reinfusing after delivery blood drawn from women with pre-eclampsia (Pirani and MacGillivray, 1975). The nature of such a pressor material (if it exists) is as yet unknown.

Women with pre-eclampsia have urinary concentrations of catecholamines similar to their normal counterparts (Pekkarinen and Castren, 1968) but to date there has been no satisfactory comparison of plasma levels between hypertensive and normotensive pregnant women.

In normal pregnancy the circulating levels of renin, renin-substrate and angiotensin II are raised, for reasons which remain unclear (Weir *et al.*, 1975). Women with pregnancy-induced hypertension, however, have significantly lower levels of these substances, plasma angiotensin II concentration being in the lower part of the normal non-pregnant range in such cases (Weir *et al.*, 1973).

Peripheral resistance is higher in hypertensive compared with normotensive pregnancies (Ginsburg and Duncan, 1967) and there is an increased vascular sensitivity to infused noradrenaline and angiotensin (Talledo *et al.*, 1966). As early as 18–22 weeks' gestation a greater pressor response to infused angiotensin II has been demonstrated in normotensive women who subsequently develop hypertension in later pregnancy (Gant *et al.*, 1973). The pressor response of angiotensin II is known to be enhanced in states of sodium excess (Brown *et al.*, 1971); it is possible, therefore, that the lower circulating levels of angiotensin II in pregnancy-induced hypertension may be having a greater vasoconstrictor effect on blood vessels which are more sensitive than normal due to increased concentration of sodium in the extracellular mucopolysaccharides of the arterial wall (Harris, 1970).

Hormones affecting Sodium and Fluid Balance

A number of workers consider that pre-eclampsia is associated with greater sodium retention than normal pregnancy (Finnerty, 1964; Chesley, 1966) but others have found a relatively greater retention of water than of sodium, with a lower plasma volume (MacGillivray, 1961; Hytten and Thomson, 1968) and cardiac output (Smith, 1970).

The adrenal corticosteroids aldosterone, corticosterone, deoxycorticosterone (DOC) and cortisol are all raised during normal gestation, with similar or lower levels in pregnancy-induced hypertension (Weir *et al.*, 1973 and 1975; Brown *et al.*, 1972; Galvao-Teles and Burke, 1973). Part of this increase, especially in the case of cortisol, is due to the increased protein-binding capacity of the plasma which occurs in pregnancy (Hytten and Leitch, 1971). More has to be learnt about unbound circulating levels of these steroids in hypertensive pregnancy and about the lesser known corticosteroids and their metabolites using the more sensitive assays which are gradually being introduced.

The production of progesterone and oestrogens increase steadily throughout normal gestation (Hytten and Leitch, 1971) and in general women with pregnancy-induced hypertension show similar or lower levels of these hormones (Said *et al.*, 1973; Kreikenbaum *et al.*, 1974). Prolactin secretion is increased in normal pregnancy (Fournier *et al.*, 1974) and appears to be further increased in hypertensive pregnant women with proteinuria (Redman *et al.*, 1975). Human placental lactogen (HPL) or human chorionic somatomammotrophin (HCS) shows a gradual rise in normal pregnancy with relatively lower levels in hypertensive pregnancy (Lindberg and Nilsson, 1973; Kreikenbaum *et al.*, 1974). The plasma concentrations of arginine vasopressin (antidiuretic hormone, ADH) are raised equally in both groups (Weir, 1975).

Abnormal Placentation

Compared with normal women, women destined to develop pre-eclampsia may have a poorer physiological response to the development of the placenta. There appears to be a halt in the development of trophoblastic invasion of the spiral arteries, resulting in a diminished blood supply to the placenta and fetus, and the retention of the capacity to react to vasomotor stimuli (Robertson *et al.*, 1975).

Nutritional Deficiency

Impaired intake and synthesis of proteins has been suggested as a cause of pre-eclampsia (Brewer, 1966; Kramer, 1973). Although this could influence the degree of oedema, there is no satisfactory evidence that deficiency of proteins or vitamins plays any part in the pathogenesis of pregnancy-induced hypertension (Davies, 1971).

Renal Dysfunction

It has been claimed that stretching of the uterine muscle can stimulate a uterorenal reflex with resulting renal cortical ischaemia and increased renin activity (Sophian, 1972), but there is no satisfactory evidence for this. It does seem likely, however, that the kidney plays some role in this disease, in view of the apparently specific pathological changes which occur. The glomerular lesion would explain the selective proteinuria (Kelly and McEwan, 1973) but renin and angiotensin II are not increased and the question of excessive sodium retention remains debatable—the reason for the raised blood pressure is therefore not yet adequately explained.

The cause of this renal lesion has also not yet been elucidated. It may be the result of intravascular coagulation caused perhaps by some substance released from the placenta and therefore part of a disseminated vascular disturbance. Alternatively, it may be the result of an immunological reaction.

Intravascular Coagulation

Compared with normotensive pregnancies, severe cases of pre-eclampsia have raised Factor VIII, increased cryofibrinogen, reduced platelet counts, lower plasminogen and increased serum and urinary levels of fibrinogen degradation products (Bonnar *et al.*, 1971; Howie *et al.*, personal communication). The extent of these changes is roughly proportional to the clinical severity of the disease. Soluble fibrin complexes are also circulating in pre-eclamptic women (McKillop and Prentice, personal communication).

Some of the features of this condition could be explained by a glomerular reaction to the circulating fibrin, but other mechanisms such as the release of vaso-active materials from the action of thrombin on platelets and fibrinogen may play a role. The basic cause of the disseminated coagulation is unexplained.

Immunological Mechanisms

There may be an antigenic relationship between the placenta and the kidney (Boss 1965; Curzen 1968) and the pathological lesions found in the placenta in cases of pregnancy-induced hypertension bear some similarity to those found in kidneys rejected after transplantation (Robertson *et al.*, 1975). The fluorescent microscopy studies of renal biopsies mentioned earlier (Petrucco *et al.*, 1974) are in keeping with an immune mechanism affecting the kidneys. There is, therefore, some evidence to support a disturbed immunology in women with this condition, and it has been suggested that there may be a deficient immune response of the mother to the fetus (Beer, 1975).

PREGNANCY WITH PRE-EXISTING HYPERTENSION

Definition

A pregnant woman is diagnosed as having pre-existing hypertension if the blood pressure is known to have been 140/90 or over before pregnancy or is found to be consistently at or above this level before the 24th week of gestation. It will remain high after the postpartum period.

Classification

The possible causes of pre-existing hypertension are listed in Table 1. "Essential" hypertension, although the commonest type, is not the sole cause of pre-existing hypertension, and this term should be used only in cases where there is no evidence of any other causative lesion.

Incidence

The figures for the Queen Mother's Hospital over an 8-year period were as follows:

	1964/65	1966/67	1968/69	1970/71
Total number	78	150	94	80
% total births	1·6%	2·7%	1·6%	1·5%

Clinical Examination and Laboratory Investigations

These have already been discussed in detail in the section on pregnancy-induced hypertension.

Where the hypertension has been known to exist before the pregnancy it is likely that a full investigation, including chest X-ray and intravenous pyelogram, has already been performed. In such cases the relevant data can be obtained from the previous records and it may not be necessary to repeat these investigations in the Obstetric Unit.

MANAGEMENT

"Essential" Hypertension

A hypertensive woman who becomes pregnant should be seen at frequent intervals from early pregnancy. If she has not required hypotensive drugs before conception it is unlikely that she will require these during her pregnancy unless the blood pressure rises further in the last trimester. Such a patient should be seen at monthly intervals until the 20th week of gestation and then at two-weekly intervals thereafter.

If hypotensive drugs have been necessary before pregnancy the requirements for these may change considerably during the first six months of gestation when the blood pressure may show the physiological drop seen in normotensive women. The continuing administration of adrenergic- or ganglion-blocking drugs at this time may result in marked postural hypotension and the dose will have to be reduced accordingly. Such women should be seen at one- or two-weekly intervals during this time.

In many women with pre-existing hypertension the blood pressure becomes more easily controlled during early and mid-pregnancy, then rises to previous levels in late pregnancy, with no apparent deleterious effect on the mother or child. However a hypertensive woman who becomes pregnant is more prone than her normotensive counterpart to develop high levels of blood pressure and proteinuria in the last trimester, i.e. she runs a greater hazard of developing the complication of pre-eclampsia and eclampsia. After the 24th week of gestation, therefore, the blood pressure, urine and weight should be checked at one- or two-weekly intervals and the woman admitted to the ward for rest, sedation and added hypotensive therapy if necessary. The management at this stage is similar to that already described for pregnancy-induced hypertension.

After delivery, these women should be seen regularly to monitor the changes in blood pressure and adjust the hypotensive therapy if required.

Other Causes of Hypertension

Specific treatment of a lesion causing hypertension is occasionally required during gestation.

Renal.—The advisability of renal artery reconstruction or unilateral nephrectomy should be considered after the postpartum period and a decision will depend upon the ease of control of the blood pressure and the functional severity of the underlying renal lesion. A patient with chronic nephritis may show little or no deterioration during pregnancy, but a very low glomerular filtration rate as shown by a low creatinine clearance is associated with a poor fetal prognosis. An exacerbation of chronic pyelonephritis should be treated with an appropriate antibiotic.

Women with *connective tissue disorders* may already be under treatment with steroids or immunosuppressive agents and such patients are less likely to conceive. If pregnancy does occur, early termination must be considered in the context of the severity of the lesion, its complications and the long-term prognosis. If the pregnancy is allowed to continue, immunosuppressive therapy should be stopped and the dose of steroids monitored carefully according to the clinical condition of the patient.

Women with *Cushing's syndrome* are unlikely to conceive because of the associated infertility and amenorrhoea. If pregnancy does occur there is a high risk of abortion or stillbirth and partial or total adrenalectomy is usually necessary, followed by replacement therapy with cortisone. Such a procedure is compatible with a continuing pregnancy to term. Occasional cases have been reported in which the pregnancy has proceeded to full term without surgical intervention (Grimes *et al.*, 1973).

Primary hyperaldosteronism (*Conn's syndrome*) is a rare complication of pregnancy. It can be associated with a normal obstetric course with the delivery of a normal full-term infant (Gordon *et al.*, 1967). Symptoms of severe hypokalaemia such as profound muscle weakness may necessitate surgical intervention, although the aldosterone antagonist spironolactone might be expected to counteract the effects of excessive circulating aldosterone and possibly delay surgery until after delivery.

Untreated *phaeochromocytoma* in pregnancy carries a high maternal and fetal mortality and surgical removal is urgently indicated as soon as the diagnosis is made (Smith, 1973). If the fetus is mature enough this can be combined with Caesarean section. Before and during surgery, the effects of the excessive production of catecholamines should be reduced by giving an alpha-blocking drug (e.g. phenoxybenzamine) and a beta-blocking drug (e.g. propranolol).

In addition to its effect on the mother's blood pressure *coarctation of the aorta* may be associated with diminished renal and placental blood flow thus compromising the fetus. If this uncommon condition is diagnosed early in pregnancy, surgical correction should be advised. When found later in pregnancy a decision regarding surgery will depend upon the maternal blood pressure and the growth of the fetus. If these are satisfactory then it may be possible to maintain the pregnancy until the fetus is mature and viable.

HYPOTENSIVE DRUGS USED IN PREGNANCY

Guanidine Sympathetic Blockers

The three main drugs of this group—guanethidine, bethanidine and debrisoquine—lower blood pressure by interfering with transmission in sympathetic adrenergic nerves. Guanethidine also depletes peripheral nerve stores of noradrenaline. These agents interfere with the normal circulatory adjustments which occur on standing and on exertion; consequently they produce a distinct fall in arterial pressure on standing and often an even more marked fall during exercise.

Guanethidine (dose 20 mg to 100 mg daily) has a prolonged action, the effect lasting more than 24 hours. This is advantageous in that only one daily dose is necessary, but has the disadvantage in that rapid adjustments of dose cannot be made, and hypotension may be troublesome in the early morning. Looseness of the bowels, urgency of defaecation or diarrhoea are not uncommon with guanethidine, possibly because of unopposed parasympathetic activity.

Bethanidine and *debrisoquine* have briefer actions than guanethidine, being given 8- or 12-hourly in a total daily dose of 20 mg to 120 mg. They rarely cause disturbance of bowel function and in this respect are preferable to guanethidine.

In an acute hypertensive crisis, as may be found in eclampsia, guanethidine may be given intramuscularly or by *slow* intravenous infusion (N.B. rapid intravenous injection may provoke a *hypertensive* response). One injection of 10–20 mg will generally cause a fall of blood pressure within 30 minutes which reaches a maximum in 1–2 hours and is maintained for 4–6 hours. If a further injection of 10–20 mg is thought necessary then 3 hours should be allowed to elapse between doses.

Maternal side-effects, which are usually mild and transient, include headache, faintness, muscle weakness and nasal stuffiness. Marked postural hypotension with faintness indicates excessive dosage. The hypotensive action of these drugs may be enhanced by anaesthetic agents—therefore it is wise to stop guanethidine for 24 hours and bethanidine and debrisoquine for 8–12 hours before induction or Caesarean section. Fetal intestinal ileus is a potential side-effect of these drugs, but there is no evidence of other specific toxic effects to the fetus.

(References to use in pregnancy: Michael, 1972; Athanassiadis *et al.*, 1966.)

Methyldopa is metabolised to alpha-methyl-noradrenaline which accumulates and partly replaces noradrenaline in peripheral nerve endings, thus interfering with the vasoconstrictor effect of noradrenaline. Methyldopa is much less dependent upon posture for its effect than guanethidine, bethanidine or debrisoquine and is therefore of particular value in treating patients who are recumbent. It is given in an initial dose of 250 mg b.d. rising gradually to 1 g t.i.d. (3 g daily) according to the response. Where necessary methyldopa can be given by intravenous infusion over 30–60 minutes in a dose of 250 to 1000 mg (5 to 20 ml) added to 100 ml of 5 per cent dextrose. An effective dose will produce a fall in blood pressure within 4–6 hours, lasting 10–16 hours.

Diarrhoea is a rare complication but bradycardia, skin rashes, unpleasant dreams, drowsiness and depression are common and intense lethargy may be troublesome. A positive direct Coombs' test is a frequent finding but autoimmune haemolytic anaemia occurs rarely. Fetal side-effects do not appear to be common, apart from possible intestinal ileus.

(References to use in pregnancy: Hans and Kopelman, 1964; Kincaid-Smith *et al.*, 1966.)

Clonidine is thought to have both central and peripheral sites of action with an initial central reduction of sympathetic outflow and a more long-term reduction of responsiveness of peripheral vessels to sympathetic stimulation. Like methyldopa, it is not dependent upon posture for its effect and is therefore of particular value in recumbent patients. It is given orally at an initial dose of 0·1 mg t.i.d. increasing gradually to 0·6 mg t.i.d. (1·8 mg daily) depending upon the blood pressure response. In a hypertensive crisis clonidine can be given by slow intravenous injection (rapid injection may cause a transient pressor effect) in a dose of 0·15–0·30 mg (1 ml to 2 ml) diluted in normal saline or 5 per cent dextrose. An effect is usually seen within 10 minutes, reaches a maximum at about 30–60 minutes and lasts about 3–6 hours.

Side-effects are rather similar to those of methyldopa and include particularly drowsiness, depression and bradycardia and less frequently headaches, nocturnal unrest, dryness of the mouth and Raynaud's phenomena. Fetal side-effects have not been reported.

(References to use in pregnancy: Johnston and Aickin, 1971.)

Beta-adrenergic Blockers

This group of drugs appears to lower blood pressure by reducing sympathetic nervous stimulation to the heart with resulting reduction in force of myocardial contraction and cardiac output. Suppression of circulating renin and angiotensin II may also play a part. The effect is largely unrelated to posture and they are therefore effective in recumbent patients.

The drugs in this group which are at present used most commonly are propranolol (dose 40 mg b.d. to 320 mg t.i.d.) and oxprenolol (dose 80 mg b.d. to 320 mg b.d.). More recent and less well established preparations are pindolol, sotalol, timolol, tolamol and metoprolol. It is claimed that some of these drugs are more cardioselective than others (i.e. that they block the beta-1-receptors in the heart but not the beta-2-receptors in the bronchi) but the value of such selectivity remains to be established in the clinical situation. No intravenous or intramuscular preparations are available for the treatment of acute hypertension.

Because of their blocking effect on the bronchodilator beta-2-receptors, bronchospasm is an important complication and these drugs should not be used in a woman with a history of asthma or chronic bronchitis. Nor should they be used in cases with heart block (bradycardia is a constant feature of treatment), or untreated heart failure. Carbohydrate metabolism is also affected to some extent and the control of a diabetic patient may have to be altered. Beta blockers alter the response to stress and should be withdrawn 24 hours before induction or Caesarean section. If emergency anaesthesia is required, anaesthetic agents causing myocardial depression should be avoided (i.e. ether, chloroform, cyclopropane and trichloroethylene) and atropine given to counteract excessive bradycardia. Provided these drugs are not used in the situations described, they are remarkable free of other side-effects and are very well tolerated in most cases. They may however, cause premature uterine contractions. and in high dosage may be associated with depressed fetal respiration.

(References to use in pregnancy: Levitan *et al.*, 1973.)

Diuretics

Natriuretic drugs have a mild hypotensive action with little postural effect. Their use is limited to the milder forms of hypertension but they are valuable adjuncts to more powerful drugs where control of the pressure is difficult or side-effects are troublesome. Diuretics are also required in those patients in whom blood pressure reduction leads to concomitant fluid retention and have a definite place in the treatment of a woman with pregnancy-induced hypertension associated with severe oedema.

The most widely used are the benzothiadiazines, e.g. bendrofluazide (5–10 mg daily), hydrochlorothiazide (25–100 mg daily), cyclopenthiazide (0·5–1·0 mg daily). The more potent diuretic frusemide (dose 40 mg to 120 mg daily) should be reserved for cases with very severe oedema or acute cardiac failure. Increased excretion of potassium may aggravate the mild hypokalaemia associated with pregnancy and a potassium supplement should be given routinely, e.g. Slow-K 600 mg t.i.d. Carbohydrate tolerance may be impaired and control of diabetes therefore affected. Hyperuricaemia may occur and pancreatitis is a rare complication. In pregnancy a serious potential side-effect may be a further reduction in plasma volume which is already lower in the hypertensive compared to the normotensive pregnant woman. This could result in a reduced placental blood flow to the deteriment of the fetus. Reported side-effects in the fetus include thrombocytopenia and hyponatraemia.

Spironolactone (dose 25–50 mg q.i.d.) is a diuretic with a mild non-specific hypotensive effect which, because of its anti-aldosterone effect, does not cause excessive urinary potassium loss and therefore does not require added potassium supplements. It may cause maternal epigastric discomfort and constipation but fetal side-effects have not been reported. It is, of course, the specific drug treatment for hyperaldosteronism. The use of other diuretics which do not cause hypokalaemia (e.g. amiloride, triamterine) has not yet been reported in pregnancy.

(References to the use of diuretics as hypotensive agents in pregnancy: Anderson, 1970; Lindheimer and Katz, 1973; Clark *et al.*, 1972; Kraus *et al.*, 1966.)

Autonomic Ganglion Blockers

Drugs which act by blocking transmission at autonomic ganglia have a powerful hypotensive action, but their use is limited because of the associated parasympathetic block which may lead to constipation, ileus, urinary retention and paralysis of visual accommodation. These complications may also affect the fetus. The ganglion blockers are now usually reserved for the parenteral treatment of an acute hypertensive crisis as may be found in impending or established eclampsia. For example, pentolinium may be given slowly intravenously in an initial dose of 2 mg with further injections at 10 minute intervals, the dose being gradually increased until the desired hypotensive effect is achieved. As its hypotensive action is mainly postural, it may be necessary to tilt the bed to obtain the full effect.

Vasodilators

In emergencies requiring rapid lowering of the arterial pressure, intravenous vasodilators may be helpful and have some advantages over the ganglion-blocker pentolinium, especially as they are less dependent on a postural effect. Diazoxide, the non-diuretic analogue of chlorothiazide, may be given as a single intravenous dose of 150–300 mg following which there may be a substantial lowering of blood pressure for two or more hours. Hydrallazine also may be given slowly intravenously in a dose of 20 mg with onset of action in about 15 minutes. Both drugs may cause tachycardia, but it is claimed that they do not reduce renal or placental blood flow, unlike most of the other hypotensive agents.

Diazoxide (dose 50–100 mg t.i.d.) and *hydrallazine* (dose 25–100 mg b.d.) may be used orally in the treatment of hypertension in pregnancy, but have potentially serious side-effects when used for longer than a week or two. Both may cause marked sodium and fluid retention requiring the additional administration of a diuretic. Diazoxide may seriously and rapidly disturb carbohydrate tolerance with resulting diabetes mellitus which requires a hypoglycaemic drug for control. Other side-effects of hydrallazine are palpitation, flushing, headache, nausea and skin eruptions; rarely with prolonged use of a large dose a syndrome similar to systemic lupus erythematosus may develop. Although little has been reported in this regard it would seem possible the fetus could be detrimentally involved in some of these reactions; alopecia and delayed fetal bone growth have been reported when diazoxide has been given.

Generally, these drugs should be reserved for the uncommon cases of severe hypertension which either fail to respond to less potent hypotensive agents or which require rapid control of the pressure. (References to the use of these drugs in pregnancy are: diazoxide—Pohl *et al.*, 1972; Milner and Chouksey, 1972; Michael, 1972; hydrallazine—Joyce and Kenyon, 1972; Ruoss, 1974; Ratnam *et al.*, 1971.)

Miscellaneous Hypotensive Drugs

Reserpine depletes stores of noradrenaline in nerve endings and probably also has a central depressant effect. Alone it has only a mild hypotensive action but it may sometimes be a useful adjunct to other drugs. Doses greater than 0·5 mg daily are inadvisable because of the risk of severe mental depression. Nasal obstruction, respiratory depression and disturbance of temperature regulation may occur in the fetus.

Veratrum alkaloids act on the baroreceptors and provoke a reflex fall in blood pressure with accompanying bradycardia. They are rarely used in non-pregnant situations but some obstetricians still use puroverine intravenously to control blood pressure in eclampsia. Vomiting may be troublesome and there is no satisfactory evidence that it has any advantages over other rapidly acting hypotensive drugs. (Reference: Ratnam *et al.*, 1971).

REFERENCES

1. Adams, E. M. and Finlayson, A. (1961). *Lancet*, **2,** 1375.
2. Adams, E. M. and MacGillivray, I. (1961). *Lancet*, **2,** 1373.
3. Anderson, J. B. (1970). *Acta paediat. scand.*, **59,** 659.
4. Armitage, P. and Rose, G. A. (1966). *Clin. Sci.*, **30,** 325.
5. Assali, N. S., Holm, L. W. and Parker, H. R. (1964). *Circulation*, **30,** Suppl. 2, 53.
6. Athanassiadis, D., Cranston, W. I., Juel-Jensen, B. E. and Oliver, D. O. (1966). *Brit. med. J.*, **2,** 732.
7. Beer, A. E. (1975). *Europ. J. Obstet. Gynec. Reprod. Biol.*, **5,** 135.
8. Beilin, L. J., Redman, C. W. G. and Bonnar, J. (1974). In: *Tenth Symposium on Advanced Medicine*. Ed. J. G. G. Ledingham. p. 1. London: Pitman Medical.
9. Berger, M. and Boucek, R. J. (1964). *Amer. J. Obstet. Gynec.*, **89,** 230.
10. Bevan, A. T., Honour, A. J. and Stott, F. H. (1969). *Clin. Sci.*, **36,** 329.
11. Bieniarz, J., Yoshida, T., Romero-salinas, G., Curuchet, E., Caldeyro-Barcia, R. and Crottogini, J. J. (1969). *Amer. J. Obstet. Gynec.*, **103,** 19.
12. Bonnar, J., McNicol, G. P. and Douglas, A. S. (1971). *Brit. med. J.*, **2,** 12.
13. Boss, J. H. (1965). *Amer. J. Obstet. Gynec.*, **93,** 574.

14. BRAIN, M. C., KUAH, K. B. and DIXON, H. G. (1967). *J. Obstet. Gynaec. Brit. Cwlth*, **74**, 702.
15. BREWER, T. H. (1966). In: *Metabolic Toxaemia of Late Pregnancy. A disease of malnutrition*. Springfield, Illinois: Thomas.
16. BROWN, J. J., FRASER, R., LEVER, A. F. and ROBERTSON, J. I. S. (1971). *Abstr. Wld Med.*, **45**, 549.
17. BROWN, R. D., STROTT, C. A. and LIDDLE, G. W. (1972). *J. clin. Endocr.*, **35**, 736.
18. CAVANAGH, D., PAPANENI, S. R., TUNG, K., LAMONT, W. G. (1972). *Obstet. and Gynec.*, **39**, 637.
19. CHESLEY, L. C. (1966). *Amer. J. Obstet. Gynec.*, **95**, 127.
20. CHESLEY, L. C., ANNITTO, J. E. and COSGROVE, R. A. (1968). *Amer. J. Obstet. Gynec.*, **101**, 886.
21. CLARK, A. D., SEVITT, L. H. and HAWKINS, D. F. (1972). *Lancet*, **1**, 35.
22. CURZEN, P. (1968). *J. Obstet. Gynaec. Brit. Cwlth*, **75**, 1128.
23. DAVIES, A. M. (1971). *Israel J. med. Sci.*, **7**, 751.
24. DIXON, H. G., BROWNE, J. C. MCC. and DAVEY, D. A. (1963). *Lancet*, **2**, 369.
25. DUFFUS, G. M. and MACGILLIVRAY, I. (1968). *Lancet*, **1**, 994.
26. DUFFUS, G. M., TUNSTALL, M. E., CONDIE, R. G. and MACGILLIVRAY, I. (1969). *J. Obstet. Gynaec. Brit. Cwlth*, **76**, 645.
27. EPSTEIN, F. H. (1964). *New Engl. J. Med.*, **271**, 391.
28. EVANS, J. G. and ROSE, G. (1971). *Brit. med. Bull.*, **27**, 37.
29. FINNERTY, F. A. (1964). *Circulation*, **30**, Suppl. 2, 63.
30. FOURNIER, P. J. R., DESJARDINS, P. D. and FRIESEN, H. G. (1974). *Amer. J. Obstet. Gynec.*, **118**, 337.
31. GALVO-TELES, A. and BURKE, C. W. (1973). *Lancet*, **1**, 737.
32. GANT, N., CHAND, S., WORLEY, R. J., WHALLEY, P. J., CROSBY, U. D. and MACDONALD, P. C. (1974). *Amer. J. Obstet. Gynec.*, **120**, 1.
33. GANT, N., DALEY, G. L., CHAND, S., WHALLEY, P. J. and MACDONALD, P. C. (1973). *J. clin. Invest.*, **52**, 2682.
34. GIBSON, G. B. and PLATT, R. (1959). *Brit. med. J.*, **2**, 159.
35. GINSBERG, J. and DUNCAN, S. L. B. (1967). *Cardiovasc. Res.*, **1**, 356.
36. GORDON, R. D., FISHMAN, L. M. and LIDDLE, G. W. (1967). *J. clin. Endocr.*, **27**, 385.
37. GRIMES, E. M., ELWIN, N., FAYES, J. and MILLER, G. L. (1973). *Obstet. and Gynec.*, **42**, 550.
38. HANS, S. F. and KOPELMAN, H. (1964). *Brit. med. J.*, **1**, 736.
39. HARRIS, G. S. (1970). *Circulat. Res.*, **27**, Suppl. II, 91.
40. HAWTHORNE, V. M., GILLIS, C. R., LORIMER, A. R., CALVERT, F. R. and WALKER, T. J. (1969). *Brit. med. J.*, **4**, 651.
41. HYTTEN, F. E. and LEITCH, I. (1971). In: *The Physiology of Human Pregnancy*. Second edit. Oxford: Blackwell Scientific Publications.
42. HYTTEN, F. E. and THOMSON, A. M. (1968). *Brit. med. Bull.*, **24**, 15.
43. JOHNSTON, C. I. and AICKIN, D. R. (1971). *Med. J. Aust.*, **2**, 132.
44. JOYCE, D. N. and KENYON, V. G. (1972). *J. Obstet. Gynaec. Brit. Cwlth*, **79**, 250.
45. KELLY, A. M. and MCEWAN, H. P. (1973). *J. Obstet. Gynaec. Brit. Cwlth*, **80**, 520.

46. KINCAID-SMITH, P., BULLEN, M. and MILLS, J. (1966). *Brit. med. J.*, **1**, 274.
47. KLOPPER, A. (1964). *Lancet*, **2**, 565.
48. KRAMER, M. E. (1973). *New. Engl. J. Med.*, **289**, 45.
49. KRAUS, G. W., MARCHESE, J. R. and YEN, S. S. C. (1966). *J. Amer. med. Ass.*, **198**, 1150.
50. KREIKENBAUM, K., ELSAESSER, F. and HÄHN, N. (1974). *Acta. endocr.* (Kbh) Suppl. **184**, 116.
51. LABARTHE, D. R., HAWKINS, C. M. and REMINGTON, R. D. (1973). *Amer. J. Cardiol.*, **32**, 546.
52. LEAN, T. H., RATNAM, S. S. and SIVASAMBOO, R. (1968). *J. Obstet. Gynaec. Brit. Cwlth*, **75**, 856.
53. LEATHER, H. M., HUMPHREYS, D. M., BAKER, P. and CHADD, M. A. (1968). *Lancet*, **2**, 488.
54. LEVITAN, A. A. and MARION, J. C. (1973). *Amer. J. Cardiol.*, **32**, 247.
55. LINDBERG, B. S. and NILSSON, B. A. (1973). *J. Obstet. Gynaec. Brit. Cwlth*, **80**, 1046.
56. LINDHEIMER, M. and KATZ, A. I. (1973). *New Engl. J. Med.*, **288**, 891.
57. MCALLISTER, T. (1973). *Nephron*, **11**, 123.
58. MACGILLIVRAY, I. (1961). *Path. Microbiol.*, **24**, 639.
59. MACGILLIVRAY, I., ROSE, G. A. and ROWE, B. (1969). *Clin. Sci.*, **37**, 395.
60. MICHAEL, C. A. (1972). *Aust. N.Z. J. Obstet. Gynaec.*, **12**, 48.
61. MILNER, R. D. G. and CHOUKSEY, S. K. (1972). *Arch. Dis. Childh.*, **47**, 537.
62. MOIR, D. D., VICTOR-RODRIGUES, L. and WILLOCKS, J. (1972). *J. Obstet. Gynaec. Brit. Cwlth*, **79**, 465.
63. PAGE, E. W. (1953). In: *The Hypertensive Disorders of Pregnancy*. Springfield, Illinois: Thomas.
64. PEKKARINEN, A. and CASTREN, O. (1968). *Ann. Chir. Gynaec. Fenn.*, **57**, 373.
65. PETRUCCO, D. M., THOMSON, N. M., LAWRENCE, J. R. and WELDON, M. W. (1974). *Brit. med. J.*, **1**, 473.
66. PICKERING, G. (1968). *High Blood Pressure*. Second Edit. London: Churchill.
67. PIRANI, B. B. K. and MACGILLIVRAY, I. (1975). *Amer. J. Obstet. Gynec.*, **121**, 221.
68. POHL, J. E. F., THURSTON, H., DAVIS, D. and MORGAN, M. Y. (1972). *Brit. med. J.*, **2**, 568.
69. PRITCHARD, J. A. and STONE, S. R. (1967). *Amer. J. Obstet. Gynec.*, **99**, 754.
70. RAFTERY, E. B. and WARD, A. P. (1968). *Cardiovasc. Res.*, **2**, 210.
71. RATNAM, S. S., LEAN, T. H. and SIVASAMBOO, R. (1971). *Aust. N.Z. J. Obstet. Gynaec.*, **11**, 78.
72. REDMAN, C. W. G., BONNAR, J., BEILIN, L. J. and MCNEILLY, A. S. (1975). *Brit. med. J.*, **1**, 304.
73. ROBERTSON, W. B., BROSENS, I. and DIXON, G. (1975). *Europ. J. Obstet. Gynaec. Reprod. Biol.*, **5**, 47.
74. RUOSS, C. (1974), *S. Afr. med. J.*, **48**, 1459.

75. SAID, S., JOHANSSON, E. D. B. and GEMZELL, C. (1973). *J. Obstet. Gynaec. Brit. Cwlth*, **80,** 542.
76. SALVATORE, C. A. (1968). *Amer. J. Obstet. Gynec.*, **102,** 347.
77. SLOAN, W. C., FLOREY, C. D. V., ACHESON, R. M. and KESSNER, D. M. (1970). *Amer. J. Epidem.*, **91,** 553.
78. SMITH, A. M. (1973). *J. Obstet. Gynaec. Brit. Cwlth*, **80,** 848.
79. SMITH, R. W. (1970). *Amer. J. Obstet. Gynec.*, **107,** 979.
80. SOPHIAN, J. (1972). In: *Pregnancy Nephropathy*, Vol. II, London: Butterworths.
81. SPEROFF, L. (1973). *Amer. J. Cardiol.*, **32,** 582.
82. TALLEDO, D. E., RHODES, K. and LIVINGSTON, E. (1966). *Amer. J. Obstet. Gynec.*, **96,** 141.
83. THOMSON, D., PATERSON, W. G., SMART, G. E., MACDONALD, M. K. and ROBSON, J. S. (1972). *J. Obstet. Gynaec. Brit. Cwlth*, **79,** 311.
84. THOMSON, J. (1969). *Scot. med. J.*, **14,** 89.
85. VARMA, T., (1972). *J. Obstet. Gynaec. Brit. Cwlth*, **79** 513.
86. VEDRA, B. and PAVLIKOVA, E. (1969). *J. Obstet. Gynaec. Brit. Cwlth*, **76,** 873.
87. WALTERS, W. A. W. (1966). *Lancet*, **2,** 1214.
88. WEIT, R. J. (1975). *Europ. J. Obstet. Gynec. Reprod. Biol.*, **5,** 75.
89. WEIR, R. J., BROWN, J. J., FRASER, R., KRASZEWSKI, A., LEVER, A. F., MCILWAINE, G. M., MORTON, J. J., ROBERTSON, J. I. S. and TREE, M. (1973). *Lancet*, **1,** 291.
90. WEIR, R. J., BROWN, J. J., FRASER, R., LEVER, A. F., LOGAN, R. W., MCILWAINE, G. M., MORTON, J. J., ROBERTSON, J. I. S. and TREE, M. (1975). *J. clin. Endocr.*, **40,** 108.
91. YOUNG, J. (1914). *Proc. roy. Soc. Med.*, **7,** 307.

CHAPTER XI

URINARY COMPLICATIONS

THE urinary system derives no benefit from pregnancy and occasionally the reverse. Certain physiological and anatomical changes occur as a result of pregnancy which may bring latent pathology to light or may encourage the development of a fresh urological handicap. In a previously healthy woman, control of micturition may be undermined, and subsequently recurring attacks of urinary infection originate in the urinary stasis which is an inevitable part of normal physiology in pregnancy.

Anatomical and Physiological Changes[2, 3]

Atony and dilatation of the renal pelves and ureters occurs, and the latter are not only displaced somewhat laterally in the abdominal portion of their course, but are liable to develop kinks. Fortunately, the ureteric dilatation is to some extent compensated for by smooth-muscle hypertrophy. This effect is partly due to hormonal influences and partly due to the mechanical pressure exerted by the enlarging uterus, and the changes are, therefore, more marked on the right side than the left because of the usual right obliquity of the uterine axis, the protection which the sigmoid colon and its mesentery afford to the left ureter, and the fact that the right ureter crosses the common iliac vessels at a more abrupt angle than its partner. These differences in pressure effects are, therefore, most noticeable at the level of the pelvic brim.

Some degree of ureteric kinking is very common in pregnancy, occurring most often just below the renal pelvis and at the lower part of the upper third of each ureter.

Urinary stasis is greatest between the 20th and 24th weeks, and although the mechanical effects of the enlarging uterus continue to operate right up to term, stasis lessens somewhat in the second half of pregnancy, thanks mainly to the muscular hypertrophy of the ureteric walls. Ureteric dilatation is only partly to blame for stasis which often persists for months after delivery, and although dilatation occurs in the multipara, stasis is much less common, possibly because of her more lax abdominal musculature.

Progesterone is mainly responsible for ureteric dilatation and urinary stasis by reducing ureteric tone and peristalsis, so that the capacity of the renal pelvis and ureters is greatly increased from the usual 6–15 ml to four times that amount. The rising level of oestrogen, however, as pregnancy advances, is believed to encourage smooth-muscle hypertrophy and, consequently, ureteric tone.

Since the ureter in pregnancy is less sensitive than normal to the usual stimuli, only a high fluid intake and consequently a high fluid output will encourage it to exert a healthy peristalsis. The implications, therefore, in the treatment of pyelitis are obvious, since stasis and bad drainage must inevitably aggravate and prolong the illness.

The bladder is an accommodating organ, and, after an initial protest in the form of frequency due to the local pressure of the enlarging uterus within the pelvis during the first twelve weeks, it settles down to the rest of pregnancy and merely develops an increased volume tolerance which reaches its maximum at the 8th month. It again becomes irritable towards the end of pregnancy with the descent of the presenting part, and occasionally stress incontinence may be a troublesome symptom. It is during labour, however, that the bladder and urethra may suffer their real ordeal. It is not true that in labour the bladder becomes a wholly abdominal organ with elongation of the urethra and displacement of the bladder neck above the symphysis pubis. Radiological studies[40] in labour indicate that, although the bladder neck is displaced closer behind the symphysis, it is not in fact drawn up. Such displacement as occurs is most marked in mid-cavity dystocia, and depends not upon the degree of cervical dilatation nor the stretching of the lower uterine segment, but purely on the descent and tight fit of the presenting part. In other words, there is no escape for the bladder neck in hard labour from its potentially dangerous position behind the symphysis pubis, and this accounts for the usual position of obstetrical vesicovaginal fistulae.

During pregnancy the ability of the bladder to empty itself is usually complete, in marked contrast to its state during the early days of the puerperium, when the recently acquired tolerance of the bladder to large quantities of urine is liable to be aggravated by traumatic bruising and mucosal congestion, so that retention commonly occurs and encourages puerperal urinary sepsis.

Renal Function

The patient who presents in pregnancy with clearly impaired renal function is not common. Chronic nephritis, as generally understood in medicine, is almost a rarity in obstetrics. It is far more often that renal function tests will be invoked to explain some incidental complication developing later in pregnancy. Unfortunately there is no overall test which will give all the answers.

The **blood urea levels** do not begin to indicate renal pathology until disease is very far advanced. The normal level of blood urea in pregnancy is very much lower than out of it and, in fact, figures over 20 mg per cent (3·3 mmol/l) are regarded as significant. At the other end of the scale in full-blown uraemia the levels do not reflect the full extent of renal damage.

The **water excretion test** has a certain limited value in areas lacking laboratory facilities, but again is crude and may be highly inconvenient for the patient. After a night's deprivation of water, the specific gravity of the urine should be normally as high as 1025, although abnormal constituents such as protein may confuse the result. If the patient then drinks a litre of water, 800 ml should be recovered in the urine within the next four hours if the kidneys are normal. With such a diuresis the specific gravity should go down to as low as 1002 but, where the kidneys are defective, these wide variations in specific gravity will not be achieved and there will be a tendency for the figure not to deviate from 1010.

Moles, Millimoles and Micromoles

Henceforward all laboratories in the civilised Western world will report their findings in SI Units (Système International d'Unités). Like a large slum family all sleeping in one bed, when father says "Turn" we all turn. This is almost the ultimate in metrication. For this purpose the reference volume for all concentrations is the litre (not 100 ml or even the old cc or ml).

The mole is the amount of a substance with a mass equal to its molecular weight expressed in grams, for example 40 in the case of calcium or 12 in the case of elementary carbon entities.

The biological activity of a substance is related very closely to the concentration of molecules or ions present so this method of reporting applies not only to ions but to non-ionised substance as well and therefore sensibly supersedes the old equivalent or milliequivalent standards.

For example, the molecular weight of glucose ($C_6H_{12}O_6$) is 180. A glucose concentration of 90 mg/100 ml as previously expressed would therefore be 0·9 g/litre which, when divided by the molecular weight of glucose (180), would be 0·005 moles/litre or better expressed as 5 millimoles/litre (5 mmol/l).

The system is not yet applicable to proteins of unknown molecular weight except in so far as their biologically active constituents may be concerned. Likewise haemoglobin concentrations will continue to be expressed as g/100 ml or g/dl.

Most of us clinicians who go about in a slight biochemical daze have a set of very rough-and-ready rules in the absence of conversion tables in our pockets, which we apply to certain substances with which we are familiar. For example oestriol, where a concentration previously recognised in mg/100 ml simply has the figure multiplied by 3·5 to provide an approximate answer to µmol/l.

Naturally, different conversion factors have to be applied to different substances. Younger generations will have the new units from studentship onwards.

The **urea clearance test** has enjoyed a long innings but has now been superseded by the creatinine clearance test.

The **creatinine clearance test** is now much more popular as a routine method because creatinine levels in the plasma do not alter as much as plasma urea levels do and because one is not faced with a comparable problem of reabsorption in the tubules. Furthermore the dietary intake of protein does not alter the level of plasma creatinine as happens in the case of urea. The blood urea level does not start to rise until long after the creatinine clearance rate shows a marked reduction and simultaneous plots of creatinine clearance against plasma urea show the former to be a far more sensitive index.[47] The creatinine clearance test normally lies between 130 and 170 ml/min in pregnancy. Great care must be taken in recording the exact amount of urine passed per minute, which depends upon strict technique of collection and on the patient emptying her bladder completely. Our practice is to collect an accurate 24-hour urine specimen and to send this together with a specimen of serum taken during that period of creatinine estimation. If specimens are collected over a long period of time, the addition of a few crystals of thymol to the collected urine will act as a suitable chemical preservative. Clearance is

$$\frac{U_c \times V}{P_c}$$

where U_c = urine concentration of creatinine, V = volume of urine per minute, and P_c = plasma concentration of creatinine.

Osmolarity and Osmolality

These are not quite the same thing.

Osmolarity refers, for example, to one mole of a substance, i.e. its molecular weight in grams, being made up with water to a total volume of 1 litre, whereas osmolality would imply adding one mole to one kg (litre) of water and the resulting volume would exceed a litre by an amount depending on the volume of the dissolved substances.

Renal function may be expressed in terms of osmolality by measuring the ratio of urine osmolality divided by the plasma osmolality. Normally in dehydration the ratio should certainly exceed 1·7 and may often attain 3 when urine osmolality attains 1200 milliosmoles/kg water. Conversely, in overhydration it may be considerably less than unity when urine osmolality may fall to less than 50 milliosmoles/kg water.

The measurements for this ratio are made in milliosmoles/kg (litre) of water and are indicated simply by determining the degree of depression of the freezing point which is related, as is the osmolality, to the number of particles in solution.

Infection of the Urinary Tract

Although the term "pyelitis" is commonly used, the infection is seldom confined to the renal pelvis, but often involves the renal parenchyma as well as ureters and bladder. In fact, the severity of the patient's constitutional disturbance depends mainly upon the level in the urinary tract at which the infection operates. Nevertheless, in deference to long-established usage, the term pyelitis will be retained.

Chief among the aetiological factors is urinary stasis, which, as already explained, is part of the normal physiology of pregnancy, but this operates more in primigravidae than in multiparae, and the incidence of the disease is, therefore, higher in the former. A previous history of urinary infection is significant, and this includes attacks of pyelitis in infancy as well as similar complications in earlier pregnancies. Urinary infection demonstrates the iceberg phenomenon in which the greater body of ice lies below the clinical surface and the ice appears above the surface only in peaks of provocation. Pregnancy is such a provocation. The chances of pyelitis developing during any given pregnancy are doubled in cases who have a history of previous infection.[19, 25] Bacilluria is common in pregnancy, quite apart from clinical disease. Kass (1957) defined bacteriuria as the presence of more than 100,000 bacteria per ml, which is grossly in excess of what could be found by contamination provided the urine is examined at once or frozen solid since urine is a surprisingly good culture medium. The suggestion is that the urinary tract is likely to be damaged to some extent by previous infection and is, therefore, more susceptible to a recurrence. Structural abnormalities, for example hydronephrosis, urinary calculus, etc., both encourage infection and certainly discourage its elimination (Figs. 1 and 2).

Intestinal stasis is probably not a very serious factor in itself, but since constipation is more often due to an inadequate fluid intake than anything else, the resultant urinary stasis is more likely to be the direct cause in these cases.

Infection may reach the urinary tract either directly by the regurgitation of infected urine up the ureter from the bladder, which, however, is more common in the puerperium than during pregnancy, or

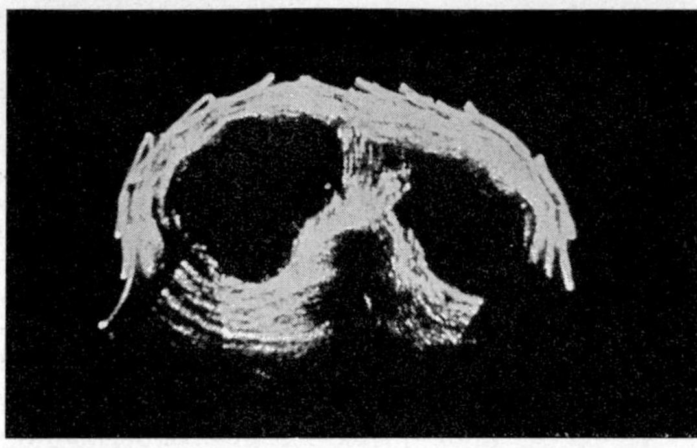

11/Fig. 1.—Ultrasonogram (transverse section) of massive bilateral hydronephrosis, five days after abdominal hysterotomy at 22 weeks gestation to enable reconstructive genito-urinary surgery to be carried out.

it may be blood borne, or, thirdly, it may reach the renal pelvis by the lymphatic route either from the neighbouring colon, particularly the ascending colon on the right side, or from the bladder via the periureteral lymphatics.

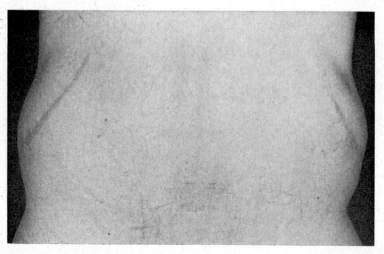

11/Fig. 2.—Same case two pregnancies later. Dorsal view of renal swellings. Previous bilateral operations had failed to ameliorate the condition and pregnancy was precariously maintained in both subsequent instances until Caesarean section near term. After the delivery of her second baby (both living) she accepted sterilisation. The kidneys by now were enormous and consisted of no more than a cortical rind, thinly surrounding enormously dilated renal pelves. She did well.

Asymptomatic Bacteriuria

The significance of bacteriuria as a source of trouble during this particular pregnancy and of later morbidity is worth reviewing at this stage. It is reckoned that in about 5 per cent of all necropsies, pyelonephritis is a major contributory cause of death and that there is at least some evidence of infection of the kidneys in about 20 per cent of all female post-mortem studies. Although women as a rule live longer than men, their kidneys are nevertheless more vulnerable. The main source of trouble in men lies in the complications of prostatic enlargement.

In the life history of women there is no doubt that symptoms of pyelonephritis become less and less severe with each successive attack. It is possible that a kidney once infected never fully regains its health and that the dangers of latent or persistent subclinical infection deserve wider recognition. Radiology may be of limited help by showing enlarged kidneys or calyceal abnormalities, but the fundamental test of latent infection depends upon a demonstration of an abnormal number of bacteria, usually coliforms, in a fresh specimen of urine. Gladys Dodds found bacteriuria present in 11 per cent of all pregnant women very many years ago, and in our hospital in Glasgow the incidence of asymptomatic bacteriuria in early pregnancy was found to be 4·6 per unit,[34] and of these 16 per unit developed clinical urinary tract infection as against a 4 per cent incidence for the whole hospital. If the case for routine screening of all women in early pregnancy is accepted, the load upon departments of bacteriology is daunting indeed. A large proportion of patients never come within range of a proper bacteriological department and for these the practice of posting off a possibly highly contaminated midstream specimen to the laboratory, either incubating warmly in the husband's pocket, or mislaid in the post, is a poor substitute for sending the patient herself to hospital, there to produce a fresh specimen. Yet even specimens collected in hospital, have a trick of lying around for a dangerously long time if they are not discarded without trace, a phenomenon by no means unknown even in the best of departments. What is often forgotten is that urine is a splendid culture medium for most of the bacteria likely to infect it.[1] Pregnant urine is an even more suitable culture medium than the non-pregnant, because the pH is commonly higher than 6 whereas it is only at lower and more acid levels that the growth of *E. coli* is inhibited—so much for the traditional futility of making the urine more alkaline with potassium citrate as a form of treatment! If one adds to this the fact that clinicians tend to work longer than the office hours of most laboratory staff, it can readily be seen that a specimen not received before about 3 o'clock in the afternoon may well get bacteriologically out of hand waiting for the next morning, or perhaps even a Monday morning or Tuesday following a Bank Holiday, unless it is refrigerated meanwhile at 4° C.

With proper instruction (and if necessary supervision), by a midwife a proper "clean catch" midstream specimen of urine is obtained by sponging and wiping clean the vulva with a tissue, or in our case with the help of a bidet, and then separating the labia, initiating micturition and catching the midstream in a sterile, wide-mouthed jar or honeypot. Obviously antiseptics are not used.

Into this midstream specimen a Uricult slide is dipped and shaken before replacing in its sterile container. The Uricult slide is coated on both sides with culture medium and the little outfit is incubated at body temperature overnight or for at least 16 hours. A density pattern chart is then referred to when viewing the bacterial colonies next day, which dispenses with the need to count actual colonies.

Counts of less than 10^4/ml can safely be accepted as due to contamination while counts over 10^5/ml indicate infection. Only now need the bacteriologist be troubled to identify the offending organism, usually coliform, and its antibiotic sensitivity.

Where there is need to confirm the diagnosis of a significant degree of bacteriuria, there is much to be said for aspirating the urine suprapubically through a fine-bore needle,[5, 38] rather than subjecting the patient to the now recognised hazards of wanton catheterisation.[20, 42] The value, however, of screening for asymptomatic bacteriuria has been enormously enhanced by the simple Uricult technique without straining laboratory resources.

Investigations designed to find the site of urinary tract infection by ureteric catheterisation have indicated that the kidney substance itself is the source in about half the patients and that the affected side or sides usually show some radiological evidence as well.[23]

What is somewhat depressing is that those who are found to have bacteriuria in early pregnancy will, if untreated, persist with the condition throughout pregnancy and into the puerperium. Apart from the risk of an acute flare-up already mentioned, an important series from Melbourne[32] shows that the incidence of prematurity is strikingly increased to 13·3 per cent in the bacteriuric as against only 5 per cent of those with clear urines, i.e. with less than the statutory number of 100,000 bacteria per ml, and furthermore that fetal loss and pre-eclamptic toxaemia were also commoner. This Australian work also showed that these figures were not affected by the treatment of the bacteriuria in pregnancy; from which the very reasonable deduction was drawn that bacteriuria of itself is not harmful but simply reveals underlying chronic renal disease which itself was responsible for the complications—in other words that the bacteriuria is an effect and not a cause.

Estimates of the incidence of pyelitis in pregnancy vary according to the criteria employed, but 2 per cent is a fairly conservative figure.

In over 90 per cent of cases *E. coli* is the responsible organism, though in chronic forms of the disease other organisms are commonly associated. A mixed bag of other organisms also comes into the picture during the puerperium, for example *B. proteus*, *B. aerogenes*, *Str. faecalis*, *Staph. pyogenes* and *Ps. pyocyaneus*, the last, together with typhoid and paratyphoid bacilli, being uncommon. Rarely the gonococcus may be responsible.

Clinically the disease has an acute onset, often with rigors, abdominal pain, vomiting, and pain in the back, particularly in the costovertebral angle. A temperature of 39·5° C is common, while it may occasionally be as high as 40·5° C and the patient looks ill, with flushed cheeks and dirty tongue. Deep breathing is often painful, and a dry cough may be troublesome. The pain, in its distribution, tends to be referred in accordance with the situation of the naturally occurring ureteric kinks. Bladder symptoms, in the form of frequency and dysuria, may co-exist or may precede the attack, but are commonly absent. On examining the abdomen, the most characteristic feature is tenderness in the loin and particularly in the costovertebral angle. Abdominal rigidity is usually not marked but is very variable. Urinary output is reduced, at first due to inflammatory congestion and oedema of the ureters in addition to dehydration, and the urine is strongly acid. The finding of large numbers of pus cells and organisms settles the diagnosis. It must be remembered, however, that pus may not be found in the urine for the first forty-eight hours due to temporary ureteric blockage.

Signs and symptoms occur more often on the right than on the left, even though the infection may be bilateral. Bowel sounds are usually audible, and the uterus, apart from referred and apparent tenderness, does not reveal clinical abnormality.

The differential diagnosis is chiefly concerned with acute appendicitis, which fortunately is not a common complication of pregnancy. In the case of appendicitis, vomiting is more usual, the initial temperature is lower, rigors are absent, and tenderness is more marked laterally at the level of the umbilicus rather than in the costovertebral angle. Rigidity, in so far as it can be assessed, is more marked, the pulse is relatively faster and urine examination is negative.

Retroplacental haemorrhage also comes into the differential diagnosis. In this instance, the patient is not febrile, the tenderness is restricted to the uterus or some part of it, the uterus is often tense, and although protein may be present in the urine, pus cells are unlikely. Some cases of pyelitis of pregnancy present with hyperemesis, and the urinary source of the trouble may be overlooked unless the patient is properly examined. A urinary calculus may produce acute symptoms, but is also often associated with a urinary infection.

Pneumonia and pleurisy can easily be mistaken for pyelitis and vice versa, hence the importance of examining the urine under the microscope.

Less acute cases of pyelitis may present with only mild pain and pyrexia and are more difficult to diagnose; in fact, one may first become aware of the condition by the presence of protein in the urine due to pyuria. Chronic pyelonephritis may present as refractory iron deficient anaemia.

The role of pyelography in assessing these cases is reserved for those in whom the infection persists in spite of treatment or in whom it recurs. By its use, an underlying aetiological factor may be unearthed. Its employment during the acute phase of the disease is contra-indicated, as it is undesirable to deprive the patient of fluid in order to secure clear-cut radiographs. If there is nitrogen retention, the dye is unlikely to be satisfactorily excreted, but otherwise pyelitis does not contra-indicate intravenous pyelography, when this is considered necessary. Sonar is increasingly useful and often eliminates the need for X-radiography.

Prophylaxis

To the patient with a history of previous recurrent attacks of urinary infection, prophylactic measures are often worth while. In these cases bacteriuria, as defined above, should be sought in a freshly collected midstream specimen of urine. In high-risk cases a powerful attempt should be made to eliminate the bacilluria by treatment with long-acting sulphonamides or nitrofurantoin, or, if necessary, by both. It would appear that by securing a sterile urine while the infection is still latent and not clinically manifest the renal parenchyma is likely to be spared yet another inflammatory insult and that this may make an appreciable difference to the patient's renal prognosis in middle-age and later life.

In the case which, though having an infected urine, remains symptom-free there is much to be said for short, one-week courses of treatment in the first instance and then re-examining. The emergence of drug-resistant faecal organisms is less likely but longer-term treatment should be given where there is no response. Much unnecessary treatment can be saved by this sort of surveillance.

Most strains of *E. coli* outside hospitals are sensitive to the sulphonamides, unlike infections contracted for example by catheterisation within hospital, but sulphonamide-resistant strains are more likely in gynaecological departments than in separate maternity units where, in my experience, this type of cross-infection is much, less likely to occur.

In our own practice the most frequently used sulphonamide is sulphadimidine. The initial oral dose is 2 g followed by 1 g 6-hourly.

There are three main long-acting sulphonamides, namely, sulphamethoxypyridazine (Lederkyn or Midicel), sulphaphenazole (Orisulf) and sulphadimethoxine (Madribon). Their action is bacteriostatic and interferes with the utilisation of para-aminobenzoic acid. They are very slowly excreted, hence their prolonged action, but they are less useful for acute infections since they are readily inactivated in plasma by becoming protein bound. However, sulphadimethoxine is excreted as a very soluble glycuronide and is therefore probably the most useful in the long-term prophylaxis of *E. coli* urinary infections. The dose is 0·5 to 1 g daily in a single dose. Not only will such ambulant treatment reduce the chances of an acute infection developing but may succeed in sterilising the urine at least for many months to come. Resistant cases may respond equally well to nitrofurantoin therapy.

Other very useful second-line drugs which are more expensive, but are highly effective in accordance with sensitivity testing, are ampicillin, cephalexin and nalidixic acid.

Trimethoprim sulphamethoxazole (Septrin) which is so successful in gynaecological practice is, alas, contra-indicated in pregnancy by the manufacturers because of hypothetical teratogenic risk, although the *British National Formulary* gives no such warning.

The dangers of catheterisation in women are now becoming increasingly recognised. Kass reckoned that the likelihood of subsequent bacteriuria was somewhere between 2 and 4 per cent after a single catheterisation. There is no such thing as a totally sterile catheterisation and a bladder that has already been once infected is readily infected again.[27, 28, 29, 36, 45] To us in Glasgow it also became apparent that the infection rate is likely to be related to the number of catheterisations and that indwelling catheters in particular are the worst offenders of the lot. We also incriminated the soft rubber catheter wielded by a nurse with naked, wet hands.[20, 42] The only excuse now for using a catheter is as a therapeutic measure, for example, before the application of foreceps or at some other obstetrical operation. This need cannot be eliminated because of the known interference with uterine activity which a full bladder causes, but the danger of cross-infection in a properly isolated maternity hospital is very much less than in the case of a gynaecological unit where the patients are subjected to a much greater risk of hospital strains of resistant organisms.

The Glasgow method described by Paterson *et al.* of catheterising with clean, dry, but not necessarily sterile hands, using a solid catheter held only by the hilt and instilling 60 ml of aqueous chlorhexidine (1:5000), but without the wetting agents in commercial

Hibitane (which may provoke haematuria) has been found to reduce the infection very materially in obstetric patients. Even more effective, and now preferred by us, is the instillation into the bladder before withdrawing the catheter of 10 ml of 2·5 per cent noxytiolin which almost halves the risks of infection.[39]

Of all the prophylactic measures which may be adopted during pregnancy, a satisfactory daily intake of fluid is the most important.

Latent Urinary Infection

Once a urinary infection, always a urinary infection. It is very doubtful if the kidney ever wholly recovers from a previous infection and a lifelong subclinical, chronic interstitial pyelonephritis is the likely result. Such a kidney in times of stress, for example, in pregnancy or the puerperium and after genito-urinary operations such as repairs for prolapse, is then very liable openly to declare its chronic infection. What is much more serious is that hypertension in later life may be due to this factor and the condition may ultimately shorten life. By the time renal excretion tests are positive, already about 80 per cent of the renal parenchyma has been damaged beyond repair.

Treatment

Once an acute attack of pyelitis has developed, the patient should be put to bed, and fluid intake should be sufficient to ensure the passage of not less than 1500 ml a day because dehydration, which is otherwise likely to occur, encourages urinary stasis. In the early stages of the disease the diet should consist only of milk, fruit juices and carbohydrates. Often the patient can be made more comfortable and drainage of the infected renal pelvis assisted by making her lie on the unaffected side. An aperient is given and, if the temperature is very high, tepid sponging may be necessary, especially since hyperpyrexia may cause intra-uterine fetal death. Potassium citrate and sodium bicarbonate are said to increase the efficiency of sulphonamides. Since Meave Kenny in 1937 introduced sulphonamides in the treatment of pyelitis in pregnancy and the puerperium, they have become our main therapeutic standby. In standard dosage they produce an improvement in the patient's condition within 48 hours. The more soluble preparations, such as sulphadimidine are efficiently excreted and concentrated in the urine.

If improvement is not obtained with this treatment by the time 30 g of such sulphonamides have been given, it is dangerous to persist blindly without a fuller urological investigation to identify, the underlying cause or insensitive organisms. The early hazards of such treatment are anuria from crystallisation, skin rashes and other sensitisation phenomena, to say nothing of nausea and vomiting which are common indeed.

After more than ten days' treatment on full dosage of sulphonamides there is the further danger of granuloleucopenia, aplastic anaemia and thrombocytopenia.

A sustained temperature for more than a week often indicates ureteric blockage, which is preventing drainage of the infected renal pelvis. It is in these rare cases that ureteric catheterisation is called for, and nowadays the need for this must be very rare indeed.

Organisms which prove to be insensitive to sulphonamides should be identified by culture, and their sensitivity to different antibiotics should be assessed in order to determine appropriate antibiotic treatment. Even the *E. coli* now shows, from time to time, an unexpected resistance.[27] This is particularly likely to occur if the urine is not rapidly made sterile by the first chemotherapeutic or antibiotic attack. Empirical treatment with the antibiotics is therefore not only likely to be ineffective but may breed resistant strains of organisms, prolong the illness, prejudice later cure and at the same time distract attention from the need to eliminate underlying genito-urinary pathology, for example hydronephrosis, calculus or tuberculosis. Furthermore, the prolonged and indiscriminate use of broad-spectrum antibiotics may make the patient more sick than the original illness with nausea, vomiting, diarrhoea and occasionally intestinal moniliasis or staphylococcal enterocolitis.

Before embarking therefore upon anything more drastic in the treatment of urinary infection than a five-day course of sulphonamide, full sensitivity reports should be obtained from the bacteriologist.

The tetracyclines are now taboo in pregnancy because of their adverse effects on the baby's teeth. Liver damage in the mother is another possible complication following high dosage. Nitrofurantoin (Furadantin) produces a very rapid and effective antibacterial concentration in the urine and because of its safety and absence of toxicity, enjoys wide popularity. It is given by mouth 100 mg q.d.s. in five-day courses. Ampicillin where bacteriologically appropriate has a notable advantage in parenchymatous lesions because of the high levels of concentration achieved in tissue as well as in urine.[7]

Certain organisms infecting the urinary tract are notoriously difficult to eradicate. The *B. proteus* for example is capable of developing resistance within a day or two. Nalidixic acid (Negram) may prove useful against *B. proteus* as well as other common urinary pathogens and would appear to be reasonably free of toxic side-effects. The usual dosage is 1 g, four times daily, for a five-day course. *Ps. pyocyanea* which is a very refractory organism, fortunately uncommon in obstetrics, responds well to colistin methane sulphonate (Colomycin) given by intramuscular injection 120 mg 8-hourly.[21] Another line of attack on these very difficult infections is Polymyxin B sulphate (Aerosporin 250,000 units by intramuscular injection four-hourly for four days).

The emergence of resistant strains in chronic urinary infections treated with antibiotics can be considerably postponed by the combined use of two antibiotics, to both of which the organisms have previously been shown to be sensitive. This is because of the much smaller statistical chance of a doubly resistant variant emerging.

Termination of pregnancy on account of urinary infection is now very rare and is restricted to cases in which only one kidney is present or functionally active and in which a severe degree of infection threatens to undermine what is left of renal function. The tuberculous kidney comes into a separate class.

One should not be satisfied with merely obtaining symptomatic relief for the patient, but a genuine attempt should be made to sterilise the urine by thorough treatment before term and certainly before the patient starts another pregnancy. In spite of modern treatment, however, the recurrence rate in the same pregnancy is high, and it is likely to complicate the puerperium in about 10 per cent of cases. In other respects the maternal prognosis is good, although even after apparently adequate chemotherapy the urine is likely to yield a positive culture several months later in a significant number.[26] Patients suffering from cardiac diseases are at greater risk because the acute infection may precipitate cardiac failure, and diabetics very easily get out of control, as with any acute infection, and are liable to go into diabetic coma. The fetal prognosis is, to some extent, adversely affected by the risk of abortion, premature labour or intrauterine death as the result of hyperpyrexia.

Puerperal Pyelitis

Urinary stasis in the upper tract is less of a factor after delivery, but the bladder is likely to be insensitive and guilty of retention, so that puerperal cystitis, together with residual urine, encourages an ascending urinary infection. Stagnant urine in the first days of the puerperium is liable to be regurgitated past a temporarily incompetent ureterovesical meatus. There is therefore great danger in using parasympathomimetic drugs.

Even normal uncomplicated labour in patients with previously sterile urine has been found to be followed by significant bacteriuria in 12 per cent by the fifth day of the puerperium. Catheterisation during labour significantly increases the incidence.

The organisms encountered after delivery, though more varied, are predominently coliforms, proteus and faecal streptococci. Puerperal screening and appropriate treatment are therefore worth while.[12]

Pyelitis in the puerperium is much more common than in pregnancy, and represents one of the chief causes of puerperal pyrexia. Characteristically, fever does not appear before the end of the first week unless the urine was already infected at the time of delivery. Localising symptoms are often absent, and although cystitis is present in the majority of cases, the patient complains of no urinary symptoms at all. Loin tenderness or pain are hardly ever to be found in such cases at this time. The treatment follows the same lines as in pregnancy pyelitis.

It is not usually too difficult to sterilise the urine, at least temporarily, in cases of acute urinary infection, provided the appropriate antibiotic is given in a course lasting from 5 to 10 days, but the chances of recrudescent infection are very high. Apart from the risk of recurrence in pregnancy the reality of a chronic infection may only come to light postnatally. This raises the question of how long chemotherapy should be maintained, as even 6 months' low-dose treatment with a suitable antibiotic may fail to produce a permanent effect. In such cases a very full search must be made for some persisting cause, such as vesicoureteric reflux or structural abnormality of the urinary tract. Even so the best efforts may be rewarded with no more than a 10 per cent permanent cure in the well-established chronic case.

Retention

This is occasionally hysterical, but in early pregnancy the commonest cause is incarceration of the retroverted gravid uterus or an impacted pelvic tumour. The subject has been dealt with fully in the chapter on local abnormalities, under "retroversion". Retention may be masked by apparent incontinence which is due to overflow. The characteristic time of onset is about the 13th or 14th week of pregnancy and the physical signs as described should make the diagnosis obvious enough.

Retention does not again complicate the obstetrical picture until labour is well advanced. It can now be very troublesome and interfere with progress and uterine activity, and repeated catheterisation may be necessary. Neglect in labour of the bladder which is incapable of emptying itself, quite apart from the other penalties, is simply asking for cystitis in the puerperium.

After delivery, bladder tone is always diminished, and there is great tolerance of large quantities of retained urine, so that the puerperal patient can hold up to a litre of urine without feeling any urgent desire to micturate. Labial lacerations and perineal sutures reflexly discourage micturition, and bruising and oedema of the bladder neck interfere with it in the first few days. The patient should therefore be firmly encouraged to perform, and if she fails to pass her water within the first 20 hours after delivery she should be catheterised. Catheterisation is both safer and more certain than the use of drugs, such as carbachol and doryl, which are often ineffective or may encourage the regurgitation of stagnant urine up the dilated ureters. One of the great arguments in favour of early rising in the puerperium is the more thorough spontaneous emptying of the bladder thereby encouraged. Puerperal catheterisation is now a rare ritual in our department. The relief afforded by hot-water bathing over a bidet, now a standard amenity, does much to help the patient with perineal discomfort and inability to relax the bladder sphincters.

Finally, the height of the fundus must only be recorded after one is satisfied that the bladder is empty, because a full bladder raises the level of the fundus and consequently gives the impression that involution is not proceeding normally.

Haematuria

The vesical causes of haematuria include trauma, especially after difficult delivery or Caesarean section, haemorrhagic cystitis, varicosities within the bladder, papilloma and stone. Cystoscopy will clear up doubtful cases.

The source of blood in the urine when it originates in the upper urinary tract is not always so clearly defined. There is a not uncommon type of haematuria which results from no recognisable pathology, appears to be peculiar to pregnancy, and clears up after delivery. This condition is sometimes due to the pregnancy engorgement of superficial veins in the region of the renal pyramids. Crabtree[14, 15] suggested that this may be due to oestrogens, and mentioned the case of haemorrhagic cystitis resulting from massive stilboestrol dosage.

Renal tuberculosis is one of the most important causes of haematuria and should be thought of first (see later). Other causes include renal infarction, papilloma, hydronephrosis, polycystic kidney and calculus. Haematuria also occurs in acute and chronic nephritis, and blood cells in the urine are often found in cases of severe hyperemesis and renal cortical necrosis.

Tuberculosis of the Urinary Tract

It is years now since I have seen a case of this very serious complication of pregnancy but less fortunate parts of the world may still encounter it and it therefore merits description. It has always been regarded as more serious even than pulmonary tuberculosis. Childbearing favours a miliary spread of the disease, either in pregnancy or in the puerperium; a chronic infection may become active and a unilateral case may be converted into one that is bilateral. Tuberculous cystitis develops readily, and tuberculous pyonephrosis may occur.

One is often confronted with the problem of a patient who has already had one kidney removed because of tuberculosis and who has

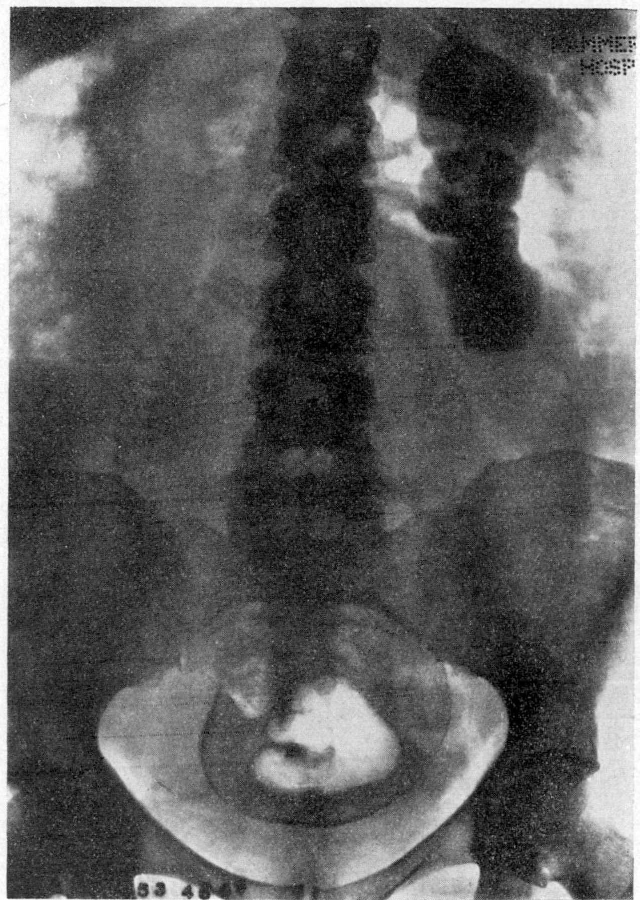

11/FIG. 3.—Calcified tuberculous pyonephrosis. Gestation 37 weeks. (By courtesy of Prof. R. E. Steiner.)

now become pregnant. Although she may be regarded as apparently cured, it is vital to assess the health of the remaining kidney, and pregnancy is absolutely contra-indicated unless one is reasonably certain that the other kidney is free from the infection (Fig. 3). Even then, the advent of the common or garden type of pyelitis in the remaining kidney affects the outlook sufficiently to warrant considering termination of the pregnancy. Fortunately, the advent of streptomycin and chemotherapy has brightened the outlook. Any woman who has had a kidney removed for tuberculosis should avoid pregnancy for a minimum of three years, in order to enable follow-up examination to be conclusively reassuring. With these provisos, the prognosis of pregnancy following successful nephrectomy would appear to be good.[24]

The symptoms are often indefinite, but haematuria or a pyelitis which is resistant to the usual sulphonamide and potassium citrate treatment should raise one's suspicions. Red blood cells are nearly always present on microscopic examination of the urine, and proteinuria may be of greater degree than one normally encounters in *E. coli* pyelitis. A sterile pyuria is very significant. The presence of the tubercle bacillus is often overshadowed by secondary invasion by other organisms, and guinea-pig inoculation may be necessary to identify it. Cystoscopy will clarify the diagnosis where there is bladder involvement or characteristic signs at the ureteric orifice. Intravenous pyelograms, though very necessary, are often difficult to interpret, but provided there is an adequate secretion of dye there may be noted abnormalities of the calyces, ureteric rigidity and less lateral displacement of the ureter than is usual in pregnancy.

Once the diagnosis of active renal tuberculosis is made, termination of pregnancy may be considered in order to save the lesion from becoming bilateral. Nephrectomy is then performed later. This is far safer than performing nephrectomy and allowing the pregnancy to continue, because then one cannot adequately prevent the infection from spreading to the other side. Whether pregnancy is terminated or not, treatment with anti-tuberculous chemotherapy should be conscientously maintained.

Structural Abnormalities of the Urinary Tract

There may be congenital absence or hypoplasia of one kidney, the kidney may be congenitally cystic, ectopic or horse-shoe. Other abnormalities include cases of double ureter and bifid renal pelvis and aberrant renal vessels. The majority of these cases pass through pregnancy and delivery without trouble, and many are only diagnosed because of a full urological investigation necessitated by the persistence of an infection. The case of single kidney following nephrectomy has to be considered in the light of the indications for which the original nephrectomy was done, for example, renal tuberculosis.

Hydronephrosis is bound to be aggravated by pregnancy, but one should be chary of diagnosing hydronephrosis for the first time in

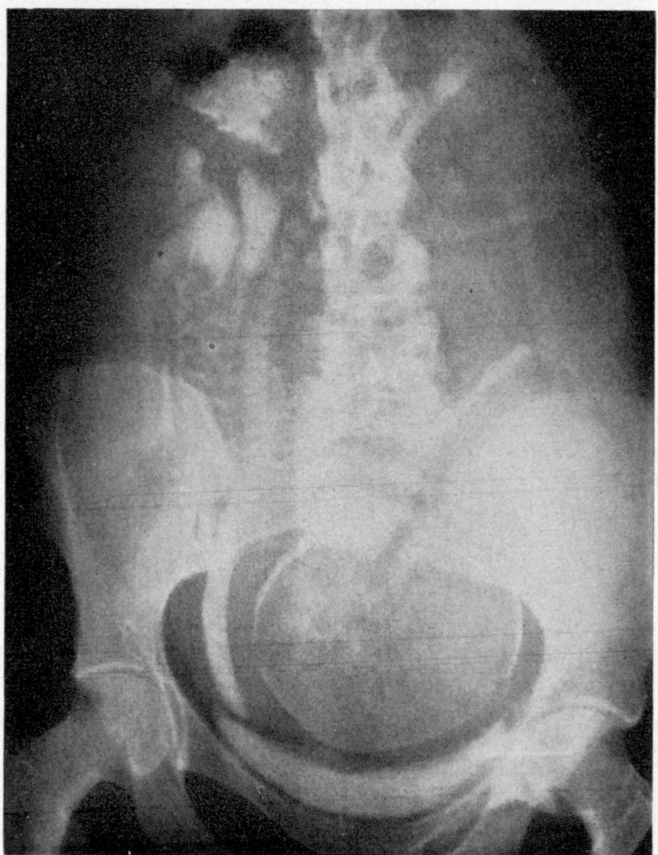

11/FIG. 4.—Right duplex kidney with tuberculous pyonephrosis of the upper component. Both components are still functioning.
(By courtesy of Dr Ellis Barnett.)

pregnancy because of the physiological dilatation of the renal pelvis which normally occurs. These remarks, of course, do not apply to gross cases. Whatever the reason for which previous nephrectomy was performed, the functional capacity of the remaining kidney should be carefully assessed, and serious notice should be taken of any complicating pyelitis during pregnancy, however mild.

Polycystic disease of the kidneys is an uncommon complication of pregnancy, partly because such cases are not very fertile, but in recent years we have had two such cases in our unit, one of which is illustrated in Figs. 6(*a*) and 7(*b*). Pregnancy only indirectly worsens what is in any case a bad ultimate prognosis and there is seldom any advantage to be gained by terminating it, since deterioration is inevitably a matter of time. The immediate risks, however, are a superimposed urinary infection to which these patients are liable and which must be watched for and treated early and energetically. Hypertension is also a likely complication and must be taken very seriously. Prolonged periods of hospitalisation during pregnancy are likely to be needed for either or both of these reasons and the chances of a successful pregnancy are largely determined by the degree of renal failure present.

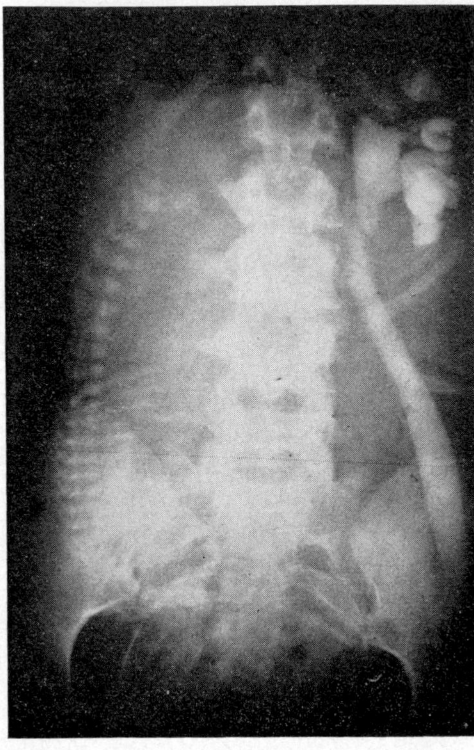

11/FIG. 5 (*a*).—INTRAVENOUS PYELOGRAM

Non-functioning right kidney due to chronic infection.

CALCULI

These are not common in pregnancy mainly because of age incidence. Stones in the bladder are very rare. In the upper urinary tract calculi not only encourage infection, but may be responsible for its persistence (Fig. 7).

Pain is complained of more frequently during the first half of pregnancy than the latter half, mainly because the physiological dilatation of the upper tract in pregnancy accommodates the stone more comfortably. Haematuria is variable and often absent. The

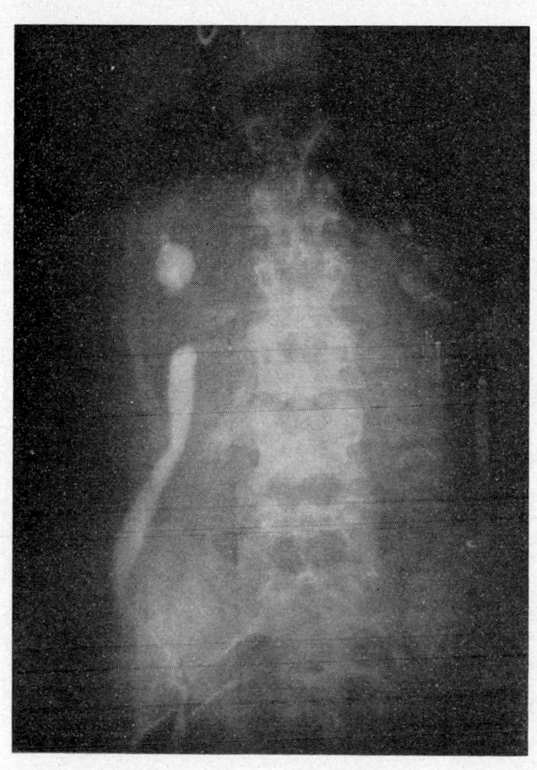

11/FIG. 5 (*b*).—RETROGRADE PYELOGRAM

Same case as Fig. 5 (*a*). Ureter is dilated up to the renal pelvis which does not, however, show the usual dilatation of pregnancy. In the kidney there is only a blob of dye representing the dilated calyces. Suggests a chronically infected right kidney shrivelling in size.
(Figs. 5 *a* and *b* by courtesy of Mr W. S. Mack.)

diagnosis usually comes to light in the course of full urinary investigation because of persistent infection. The best time to remove a calculus is between pregnancies, especially in the patient who manages to go through her pregnancy without trouble. Nevertheless, there is much to be said for removing at once a calculus which first comes to notice during the early months, before ureteric dilatation allows it to slip down the ureter, which it is likely to lodge at the level of the pelvic brim and be difficult to reach surgically because of the bulk of the gravid uterus. If the stone is first discovered in the latter half of pregnancy, it is best to temporise if possible and remove it in the postnatal period; but when active steps are called for in late pregnancy on account of severity of symptoms, there is much to be said for draining the renal pelvis by nephrostomy until after delivery.

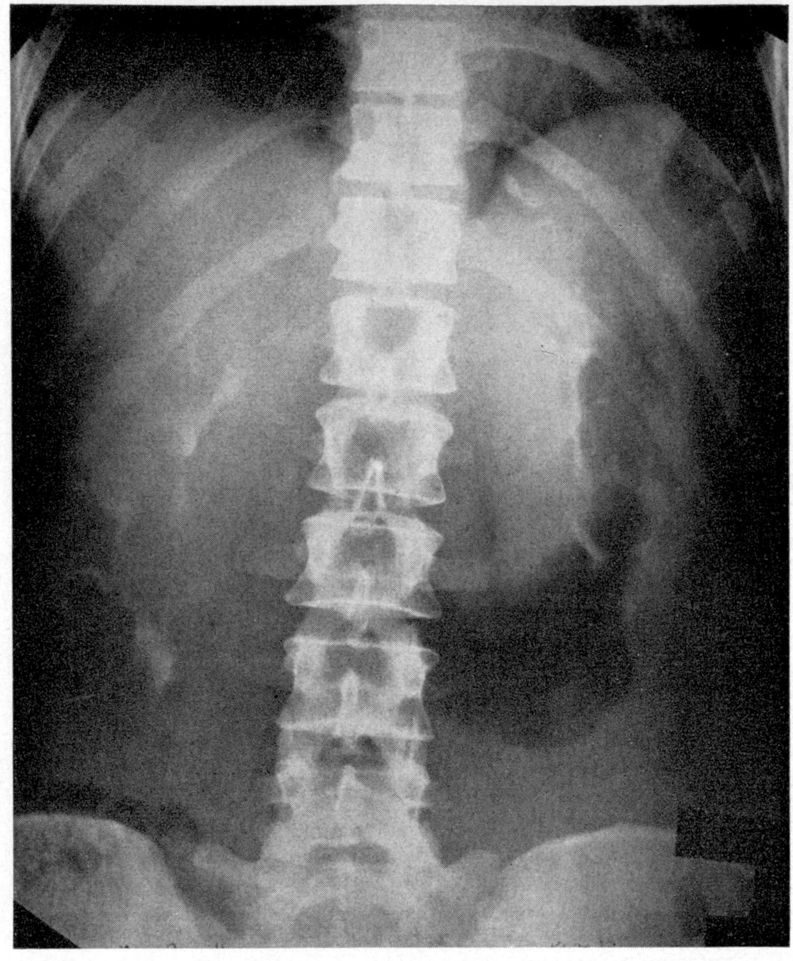

11/Fig. 6 (*a*).—Polycystic disease of kidneys—non-pregnant. IVP at 20′.
(By courtesy of Dr J. Innes.)

OLIGURIA AND ANURIA

Urinary suppression is an extremely grave sign, and it is necessary, if possible, to deduce into which of the two main pathological classes the case falls. These classes are, on the one hand, cases of acute cortical necrosis and, on the other, those of acute tubular nephrosis. Suffice it to remark here that clinically, cortical necrosis greatly resembles anuria due to other causes, but there is a world of difference in the prognosis, inasmuch as it is almost invariably fatal.

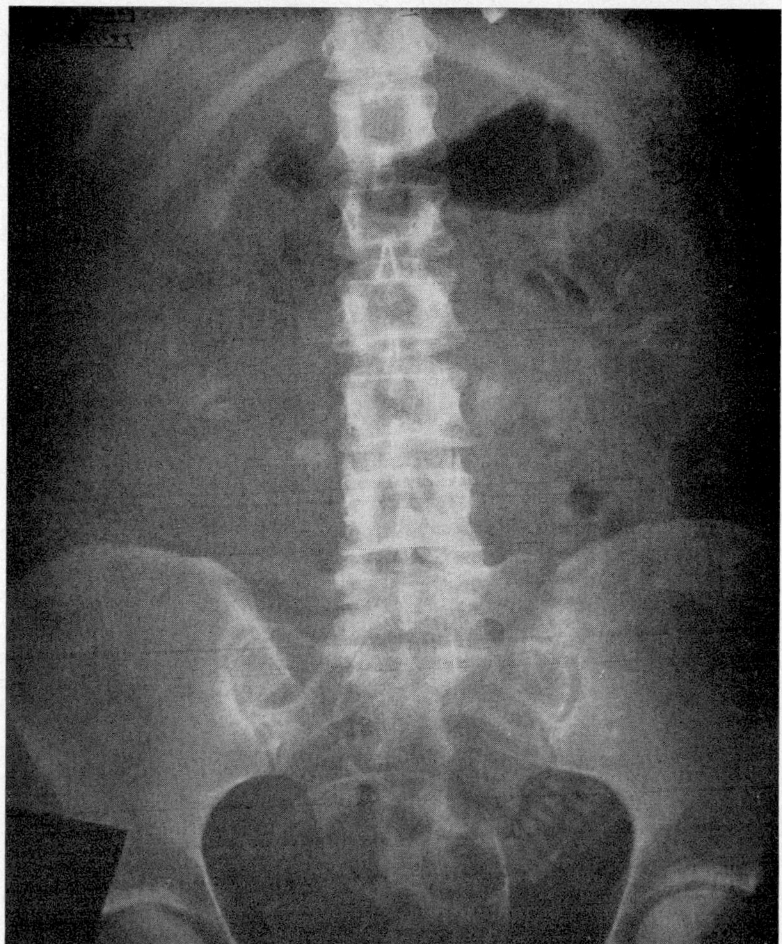

11/Fig. 6 (*b*).—Polycystic disease of kidneys in pregnancy. IVP at 40′. Same case. Both kidneys markedly enlarged. Calyces spidery and elongated with calcified glands on right. Some calyces show smooth concavities due to cyst distortion.

(By courtesy of Dr Ellis Barnett.)

The great difference between cortical necrosis and acute tubular nephrosis lies in the irreparable damage which occurs in the former, while in the latter recovery will occur in time provided that the patient can be prevented meanwhile from dying of uraemia or from the effects of injudicious treatment. Even in these days when haemodialysis is almost commonplace the gravity of acute renal failure of

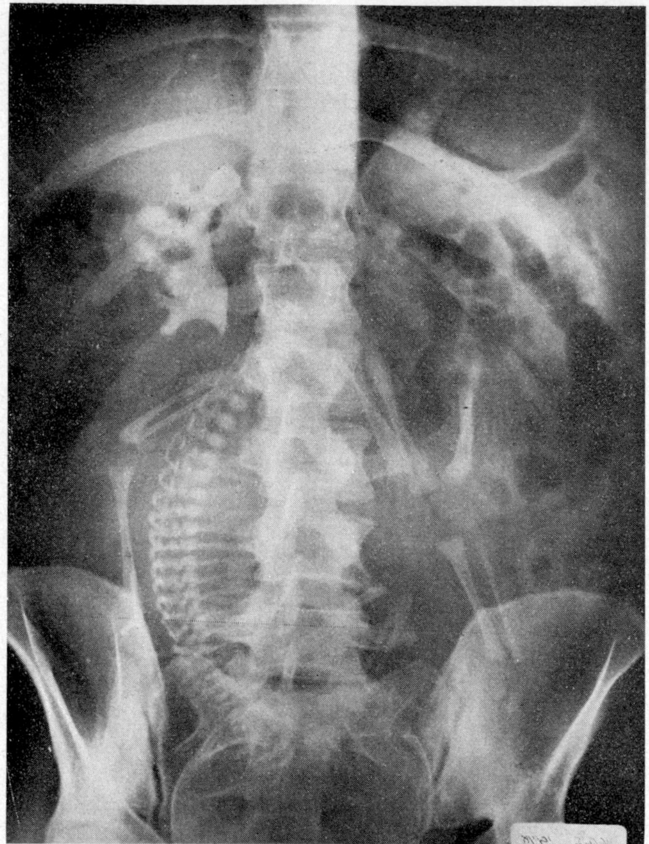

11/Fig. 7.—Staghorn calculus in right renal pelvis. Recurrent urinary tract infection in pregnancy.

obstetric origin should not be underestimated, and the mortality would appear to differ according to whether the renal failure occurs in the first half of pregnancy (mainly due to induced abortion) or those in the last trimester often complicated by pre-eclamptic toxaemia. These findings were brought to light by a study of a series of 70 patients with renal failure, all of whom had required some form of dialysis, and excluding all those that recovered or died without being dialysed.[46] Of the former group, i.e. in early pregnancy, 27 per cent died and 8 out of the 11 deaths were directly attributable to infection which had occurred either after recovery from renal failure or at a time when the fluid and electrolyte disturbances were under control. The infections were mainly clostridial or staphylococcal. What is particularly interesting is that no patient in this abortion group died with evidence of irreversible renal damage. Surgical intervention was eschewed because of the danger of converting a local infection to a general one and in conformity with more or less universal practice today, but because of the deadly significance of infection, particularly some gas-forming organisms, a policy of full doses of penicillin and ampicillin together was advocated as soon as swabs had been taken for culture and sensitivity testing. Of the cases of renal failure in late pregnancy the mortality was much worse at 45 per cent and at autopsy more than half were found to have renal cortical necrosis. The main causes were pre-eclamptic toxaemia, eclampsia, abruptio placentae and postpartum haemorrhage. Infection in these cases played a very much smaller part and there was also the factor of hepatic necrosis and one disaster from the complications of haemodialysis. In other words, one is dealing with a different pathology. Of those that were dialysed, not all by any means received the treatment on an artificial kidney machine, but peritoneal dialysis found increasing favour among the later cases in the group. This method was recommended for daily use and it was claimed that it permitted very efficient removal of excess sodium and water, allowing a smooth control of blood chemistry. It also allowed unrestricted fluid intake and Hammersmith workers have come to regard this as the method of choice, haemodialysis being reserved only for cases in which technical failure prevents the peritoneal route.

Acute Cortical Necrosis

Although this condition has been described in connection with specific fevers and dioxan poisoning, for all practical considerations it will be found that its association with pregnancy is almost invariable, and its relationship with eclampsia, the pre-eclamptic state and retroplacental haemorrhage is well known.

Pathology

A narrow band of cortex immediately beneath the capsule and portions in the region of the junction of cortex and medulla are the only parts of the cortex to survive, being able to derive their blood supply from sources other than the usual glomerular afferent vessels which undergo hyaline necrosis. These latter are the intralobular arterioles and their branches, and they are to be found widely dilated with small points of rupture and perivascular haemorrhages (Fig. 8). Small thrombi may occur within the lumina. The necrosis is primarily the result of ischaemia whether it be due, as Trueta *et al.* (1947) asserted, to a shunt mechanism whereby renal blood flow is diverted from the cortical nephrons to the juxtamedullary nephrons by a

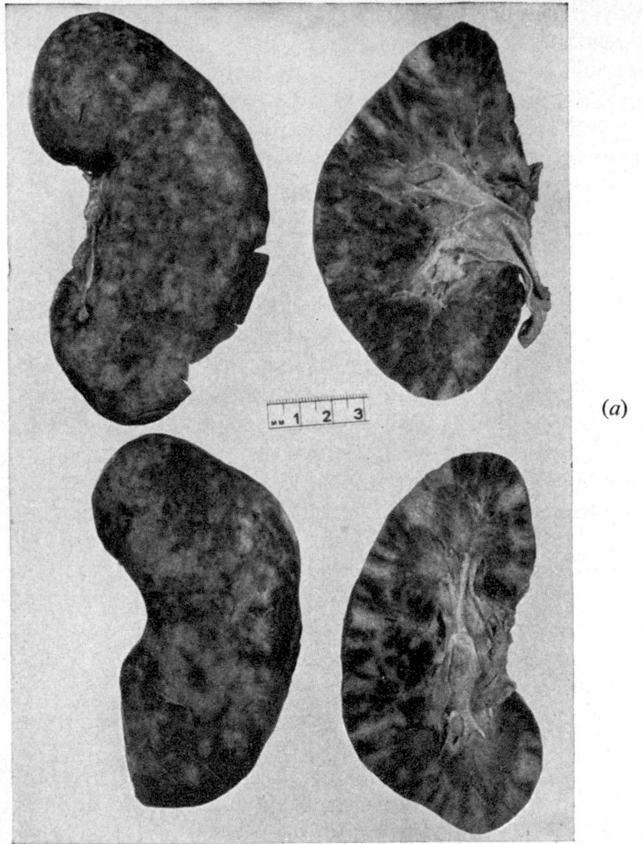

(*a*)

11/Fig. 8.

(*a*) Acute cortical necrosis of kidneys.

(*b*) Bilateral cortical necrosis of kidneys. Infarcted cortex showing an enormously distended thrombosed interlobular artery giving off two afferent glomerular arterioles. (× 40.)

(*c*) Bilateral cortical necrosis of kidneys. Oedematous congested renal capsule separated by a thin hyperaemic zone infiltrated with polymorphs from underlying infarcted cortex. (× 60.)

(By courtesy of Prof. I. Doniach and Dr H. Walker, and the Editor, *J. Obstet. Gynaec. Brit. Cwlth.*)

reflex spasm of the interlobular arteries supplying the former, followed by their later vasoparalysis and dilatation; or whether, as De Navasquez (1935) stated, vasoparalysis occurs in the first place due to some operative toxin which so retards circulation as to produce necrosis. Young (1942) considered that autolysis in the separated and ischaemic placenta may supply such an agent.

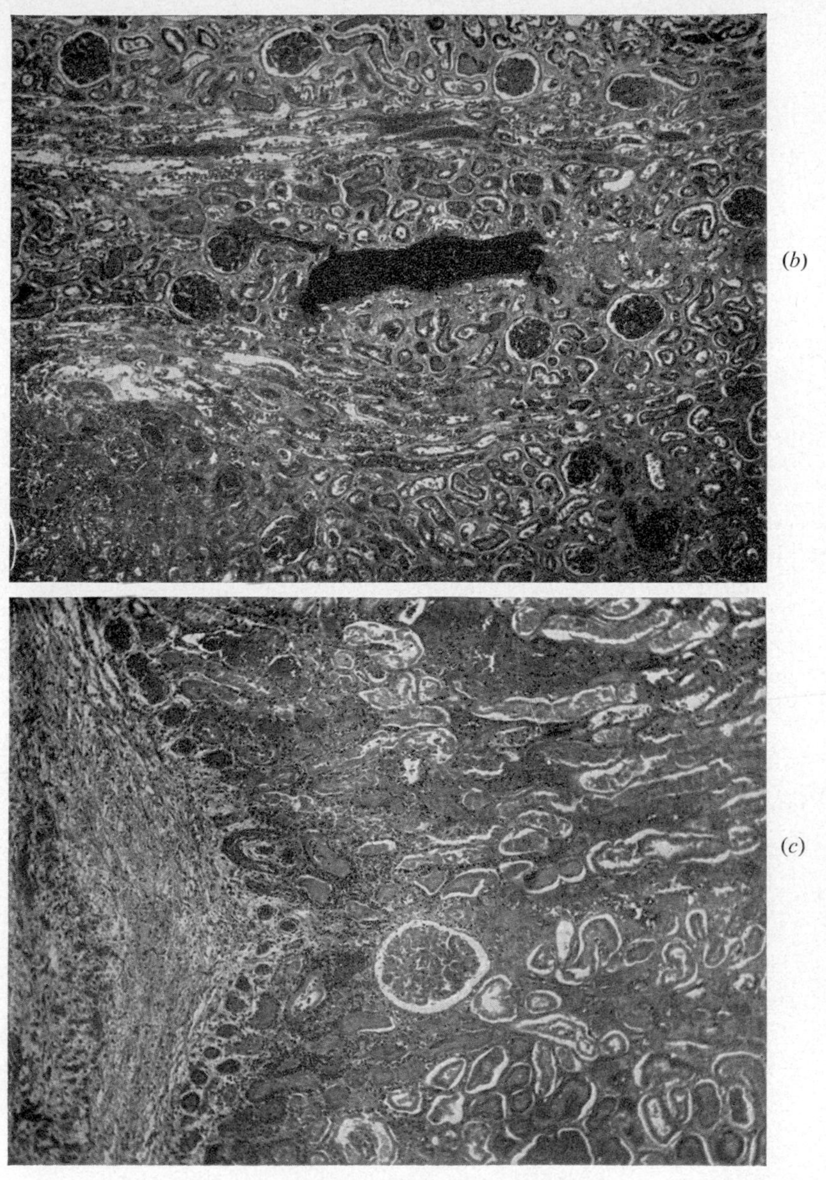

(b)

(c)

11/Fig. 8. (*see opposite*)

(see opposite)

The glomerular afferent vessels are end arteries, and damage is irrevocable, hence the ultimate issue.

ACUTE TUBULAR NEPHROSIS

Bull (1950) pointed out the striking clinical uniformity in this condition despite the wide variety of causes, ranging from shock to acute poisoning, and the pathological picture of acute necrosis is common to all.

The cases were divided (Dible, 1950) into those with pigment deposition and those without. Instances of the former include mismatched blood transfusion, transfusion of haemolysed, stale or overheated blood, intravascular haemolysis from any cause, blackwater fever, circulating myohaemoglobin as in the crush syndrome, cases of haemolysis resulting from criminal abortion using intra-uterine soap solution injections, which is a common practice today, quinine poisoning and *Cl. welchii* septicaemia, in which the exotoxin is haemolysing. Those cases without pigment include protracted shock from any cause, producing severe hypotension, as may occur, for example, in induced abortion or very traumatic delivery. Acute septicaemia may also be a cause. The average duration of the oliguric phase (to 1 litre of urine) is about nine days.

It is to be noted here that a systolic blood pressure which remains for long below 75 mm Hg is insufficient to produce secretion of urine in the absence of diuretic substances.

In all the above, recovery is to be sought and is possible, provided the case is correctly understood and treated.

Cases of oliguria resulting from acute nephritis, malignant hypertension and sulphonamide crystal obstruction have different mechanisms and do not belong to this class.

Pathology

In the first 30 hours the kidney is congested and the cortex appears full of blood. The lesion begins in Henle's tubules, especially in the intermediate zone, involving particularly the ascending limb and second convoluted tubule, and is fully developed after 48 hours. It is essentially degenerative in type.

Thereafter pigment, either myohaemoglobin or a haemolytic blood derivative, appears in the tubular casts, especially in the second convoluted tubule, though the whole nephron is to some extent affected with collections of necrotic cellular debris (Fig. 9).

After five or six days local inflammatory changes supervene, chiefly in the boundary zone, and finally some degree of fibrosis remains.

Pigment deposition is held to be a secondary phenomenon rather than the cause (Dible, 1950) as, in all cases, the tubular casts are not at first pigmented, though the later presence of pigment worsens the outlook because of its own toxic action. According to Darmady (1950) renal failure is not due to tubular blockage with pigment casts, as can be proved by microdissection of the nephron.

Death commonly occurs in about a week, but the full pathological picture would probably be seen more often if many candidates for the condition did not first die from additional causes such as sepsis, haemorrhage, shock and cardiac failure.

Toxic damage or primary ischaemia are the likely initial causes, and regarding the latter Bull (1950) does not consider, as some do, that the Trueta or Oxford "shunt" mechanism is responsible. His investigations have shown that the renal blood flow, at any rate in the human species, is markedly reduced and the blood removed by catheterisation of the renal vein is very low in oxygen content, thus differing from experimentally produced shunts in animals. Bull, in fact, considers that there occurs a passive fluid diffusion through damaged tubular walls, which leads to increased intrarenal tension, thereby compressing the capillary vessels and retarding circulation still further. This low renal blood flow persists in spite of a normal cardiac outflow which may be restored to the rest of the body, and remains peculiar to the kidneys, and cannot, therefore, be relieved by extrarenal agencies. If the Trueta shunt were still operative, splanchnic block or spinal analgesia would abolish it, but none of Bull's eight cases so treated did in fact respond. This does not disprove the existence of the shunt earlier. The tension within the kidney is "splinted" by the relatively rigid vascular stroma rather than by the renal capsule, and for this reason decapsulation of the kidney is unlikely to be effective.

Any apparently successful results to such treatment (which are, therefore, without rational foundation) must be viewed in the light of possibilities of spontaneous recovery.

Clinical Picture

Bull distinguished four definite phases. Firstly, there is the phase of abrupt onset sometimes preceded by a short-lived diuresis. Secondly, there follows the oliguric or anuric phase which may last from a few hours up to three weeks. Thirdly comes the early diuretic phase in which errors of treatment can ruin what is now a good prognosis. In this phase tubular reabsorptive function is delayed for a period proportional to the duration of the oliguric phase, and an important loss of sodium, potassium and chloride ions is likely to occur if this danger is not met. In the fourth or later diuretic phase tubular function returns and catches up with the already established glomerular activity. It is to be noted that in the second phase both glomerular and tubular function are absent as a result of reduced renal circulation, and the above-mentioned ions tend to accumulate, and in the case of potassium this may be highly dangerous. Treatment has to be modified, therefore, as the different phases of the process are recognised.

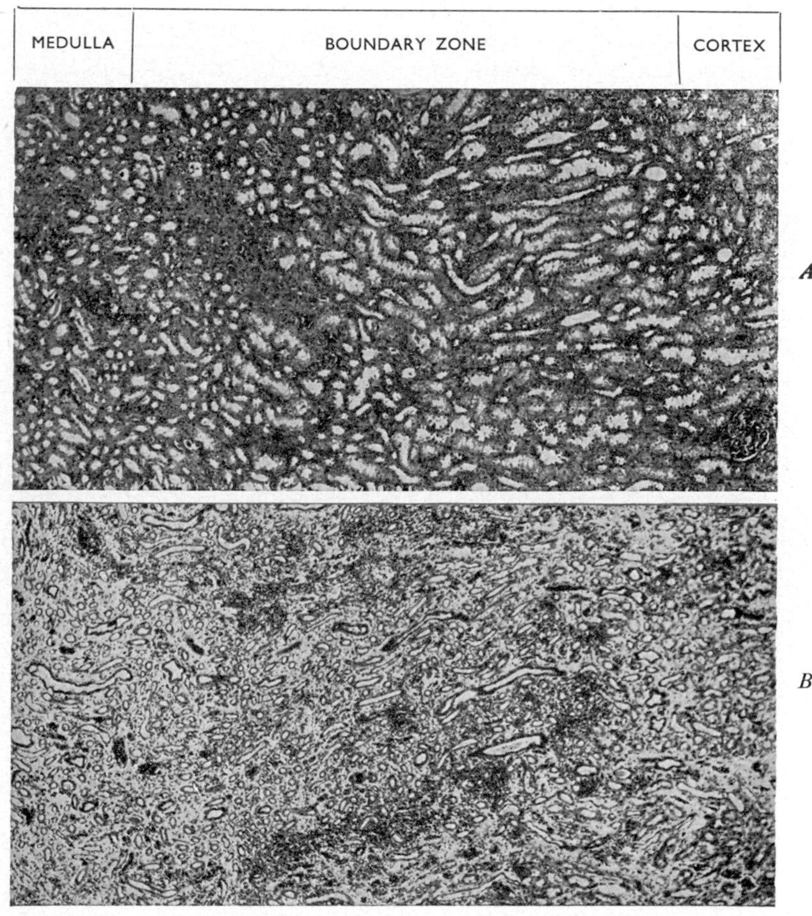

11/FIG. 9 (*a*).—Boundary zones of (*A*) normal and (*B*) anuric kidneys, showing degenerate and atrophic tubules, oedema and fibrosis of the intercellular tissue and widespread cellular infiltration. ($\times$ 36.)

A

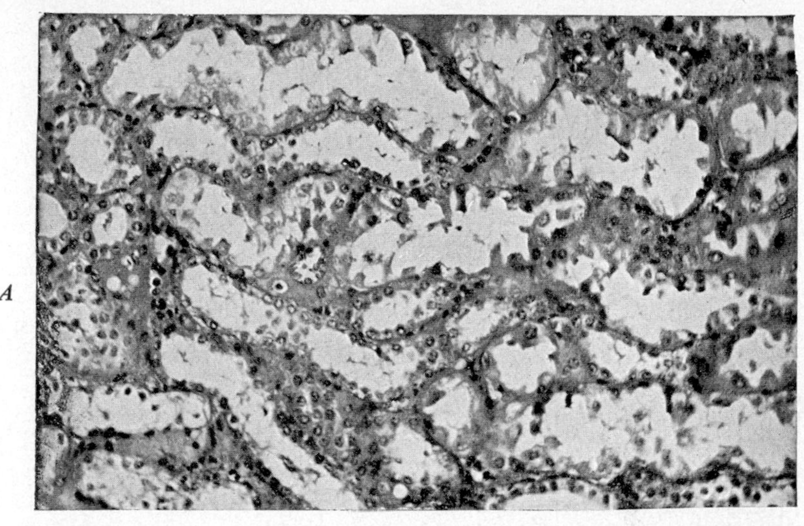

B

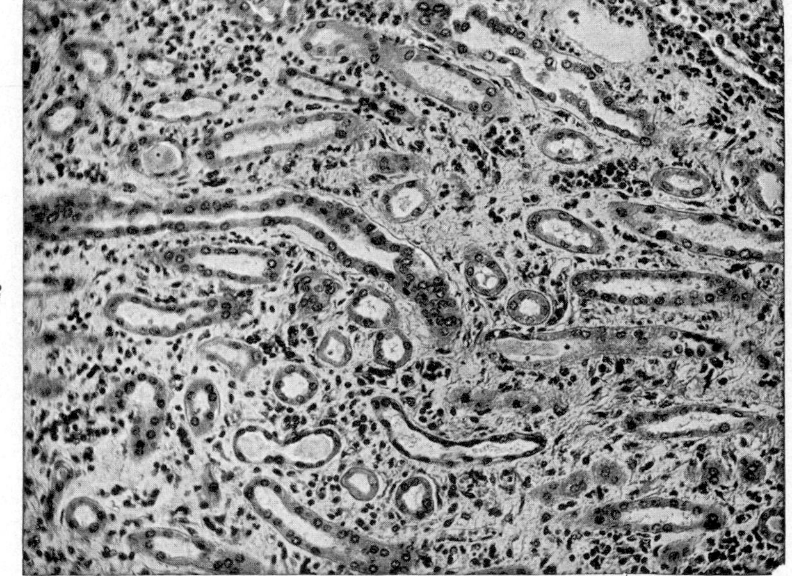

11/Fig. 9 (*b*).—High-power view of fields seen in preceding figure. (× 160.)

(Fig. 9 *a* and *b* from *Hadfield's Recent Advances in Pathology* by courtesy of Prof. J. H. Dible and J. & A. Churchill.)

Treatment

It goes without saying that any case in whom oliguria does not resolve spontaneously within 48 hours should be transferred to a renal unit; in fact the sooner the better.

It is now believed that there is initially a stage of functional renal failure before organic blockage of the renal tubules becomes established and it is during this very early stage when emergency treatment with mannitol may nip the process in the bud. Mannitol is a polyhydric alcohol, is inert, is rapidly excreted and is relatively non-toxic. Nevertheless if given over a long period it can produce necrosis. Its effect is thought not to be due to osmosis but to lowering of blood viscosity and renal vascular resistance. It is also believed to dilate the afferent arterioles to the glomeruli.

Oliguria after a surgical or obstetrical insult may be due either to post-operative dehydration or to renal shut-down and the stimulation of antidiuretic hormone from the posterior lobe of the pituitary may also play a part. It is important to be able to distinguish the two clinically, as dehydration simply requires intravenous fluid whereas renal shut-down requires the reverse. The distinction is simply made by estimating the ratio of the urinary urea over blood urea. If this is high it suggests occult dehydration but if it is low, i.e. below 14, it suggests renal functional failure for which the treatment is immediate infusion intravenously of 100 ml of 20 per cent mannitol, i.e. 20 g. This should be given very slowly,[35, 37] taking about 10 minutes over the injection. If the treatment is going to be successful there will be a diuresis within the hour, but if the hourly urine excretion does not increase by at least 50 per cent within two hours, the treatment may be repeated once. Further failure now indicates major organic renal damage. The strength of solution should not exceed 20 per cent because of the danger of crystallisation and repeated or overdosage may precipitate congestive cardiac failure because of the rapid increase in extracellular volume which results.

The main use of mannitol is simply as an emergency prophylaxis, which must be applied within the first 48 hours of oliguria if it is going to be effective. It will achieve nothing once organic pathological changes within the kidneys have set in.

On no account should mannitol be mixed with a blood transfusion drip because it will cause crenation of the red cells which may be irreversible and hence cause agglutination.[43] This is another reason for giving the injection very slowly in case it achieves the same unpleasant effect within the lumen of the vein.

On the biochemical side three facets have to be considered, namely those of water, mineral, and nitrogen imbalance, of which the last is the least important, although we still use the term "uraemia" in describing the patient's deterioration.

Many cases are actually killed with water. Lattimer (1945) pointed out that the body was not a tank into which water could be forced until it finally burst out through the kidneys, yet, until recently, overhydration was common in incorrectly treated patients who were driven into an oedematous condition, with bulging neck veins, cardiac dilatation, gallop rhythm, liver enlargement and crepitations at the lung bases, in fact, a state of cardiac failure. In addition, drowsiness, twitchings and coma can be provoked by water retention. Lattimer found that of his 33 anuric cases none died where the fluid intake was less than 2 litres a day, whereas 75 per cent of those to whom over $3\frac{1}{2}$ litres were given succumbed.

Mineral loss occurs only to a minor extent during the anuric stage and then only through faeces, vomit and sweat; that due to vomiting can be simply replaced. Any diet at this stage should be free, or nearly so, of electrolytes. The danger of building up a high potassium level is enormously increased by administering such apparently harmless drugs as potassium citrate, while it must be remembered that many bottled fruit drinks and coffee contain enough potassium to jeopardise recovery. When early diuresis starts in the third phase, however, electrolyte loss must be quantitatively replaced.

The level of blood urea naturally rises during oliguria, but urea itself is not toxic, although other end-products of protein breakdown may well be, and an accumulation of potassium ions occurs in the body from both exogenous and endogenous protein metabolism. Borst (1948) advised that endogenous protein catabolism can be reduced to a minimum in cases on a non-protein diet by ensuring an adequate number of calories by giving a high-carbohydrate diet. However, a limited protein intake can be overdone and in the end will produce the undesirable effects of hypoalbuminaemic oedema, anaemia and asthenia; but these late effects are confined to chronic cases of uraemia rather than the condition under discussion.

Infection has a disastrous effect in stimulating protein catabolism, and must be controlled by antibiotics, bearing in mind that those that are excreted in the urine may accumulate excessively during anuria and after the first few days the dose should be drastically cut.

Renal dialysis has today transformed the situation but a brief historical account is worth while as I well recall the first beginnings of rational treatment of this deadly complication. In fact I think it was the fourth successful case which we sent to Bull at a time when it was unheard of for an arrogant London teaching hospital to refer such difficult cases to Hammersmith Hospital. Their first dialysis machine was a home-made affair which looked like a clothes-drying frame wound round with polythene tubing and immersed in a huge domestic bath tub full of dialysing solution.

Our patient recovered whereas we would almost certainly have killed her with 5 per cent glucose infusions as was then the practice.

The scheme of treatment originally advocated by Bull and his colleagues was firstly, during the anuric phase, to limit water intake to 1000 ml in 24 hours, which approximately replaced the daily loss through the lungs, skin and faeces. All vomited material was collected, filtered and returned through a nasal stomach tube. This replaced lost electrolytes. Later a daily water intake of 1000 ml plus the previous day's measure of urinary output came to be regarded as excessive, and the basic figure was reduced from a litre to 500 ml. Barr and Chambers (1958), in a very full and detailed scheme of treatment, recommend the immediate stopping of all oral feeding and fluids and the administration by intragastric tube of 500–700 ml of 50 per cent glucose per 24 hours, plus 500 mg ascorbic acid and vitamin B complex preparation. The original peanut oil mixture devised by Bull was superseded by carbohydrate feeding only.

To meet the double difficulty of restricting the fluid intake and yet maintaining the high carbohydrate provision without producing thrombosis in a vein, Evans *et al.* (1953) recommended a drip of 1 litre a day of 40 per cent glucose directly into the superior vena cava using a cardiac catheter, a method based on that of de Kayser in Holland. This provided a daily intake of 1600 calories. Additional water could be given by mouth or in the drip in amounts equal to the previous day's urinary output, if any. The fact of placing the end of the catheter within a very large blood channel like the vena cava enables the irritant effect of the concentrated glucose solution to be sufficiently diluted by the large volume of blood flowing past. Heparin (10,000 units per 500 ml) had to be added, even so, to the caval drip. We then came to use more commonly the inferior vena cava for this type of administration as recommended by Scott Russell *et al.* (1954), the cannula being introduced through the upper end of the internal saphenous vein under rigid aseptic conditions. The drip had never to be allowed to stop, even momentarily, for fear of clotting and a reserve supply had to be available through a Y-piece connection to maintain the flow, however slowly, while the bottles were being changed. One such polythene catheter usually managed to serve for about a week or more. The treatment certainly had the advantage of leaving one in no doubt about what was going into the patient, whereas absorption through an intragastric drip was more problematical.

Today the method of controlling calorie and fluid intake has been simplified even further by replacing glucose with 20 per cent fructose, of which 600 ml are now given intravenously daily without the need for catheterising the inferior vena cava. The fluid volume is increased by the amount of urine passed or fluid vomited in the course of the previous day. When all danger of vomiting, however, has ceased the patient may take concentrated solutions of sugar in control quantities and in palatable form such as Lucozade.

Parsons and McCracken (1959) recommend the synthetic anabolic steroid norethandrolone (Nilevar) in dosage of 30 mg a day because of its ability to reduce protein catabolism and thereby to reduce or postpone the need for artificial kidney dialysis.

Under this scheme the blood urea would only rise about 17 mg per cent a day in the first week and 10 mg per cent in the second and thereafter, whereas in patients treated otherwise the daily rise in blood urea might exceed 50 mg per cent. In other words this treatment was one of playing for time—time for kidney function to recover before uraemia carries off the patient.

When diuresis starts, in addition to replacing electrolytes quantitatively the procedure is to add water to the basic ration in the same quantity as the previous day's urinary output, and when the diuresis exceeds 1 litre per diem, the drip feed may be discontinued and a low-protein diet commenced. The blood urea does not start to fall until a diuresis of at least 1 litre is achieved, as the urine filtrate during the third phase is, as yet, too dilute to rid the body of sufficient quantities.

If the haemoglobin level is at any time below 70 per cent, transfusion of packed red cells is given, as anaemia of itself reduces renal function.

In severe cases it may be anything up to four weeks before the kidneys begin to excrete urine, which shows what this treatment can achieve. Bull[9, 10, 11] frequently found himself initially handicapped by receiving cases that had been ill-advisedly waterlogged with glucose-saline intravenous therapy (personal communication).

As a rule the rise in serum potassium is not marked under the above regime and, if present, can to some extent be offset by giving 50 units insulin. This encourages the transfer of potassium, together with the glycogen thus formed, within the cell, where it is harmless. Nevertheless, cardiac arrest due to hyperkalaemia is still a potent cause of death and, where the potassium levels cannot adequately be controlled as above, an ion exchange resin may be used as a temporary expedient pending artificial kidney dialysis.

These resins do not affect the rise in blood urea but help to control the serum potassium levels. They act within the lumen of the intestine and are by no means rapid. Unfortunately in obstetrical anuria, hyperkalaemia may quickly assume emergency proportions requiring even more urgent treatment short of dialysis. In fact in the seriously ill case one may have little enough time even to wait for electrolyte balance studies. The quickest method of deciding treatment is to undertake electrocardiography, because the signs are, if anything, more important than high biochemical levels, to which the degree of cardiac danger is not directly related.

The signs of dangerous hyperkalaemia are as follows:

Gross peaking of the T-waves;
absent P-waves;
widening of QRS complex to 0·2 seconds.

Under these circumstances treatment is urgent with either 10 per cent calcium chloride intravenously, up to 60 ml given slowly over 5 minutes, or 10 per cent calcium gluconate (60 ml). The effect on the ECG is almost immediate. Calcium chloride is possibly more potent than calcium gluconate because the calcium is completely ionised, but the gluconate solution which is also adequate is less dangerous from the point of view of tissue necrosis due to perivenous extravasation. In either case the intravenous injection should be given very slowly with continuous electrocardiographic monitoring and should be stopped as soon as the ECG appearances indicate improvement.[13]

During the diuretic phase the rapid loss of potassium may be serious. To some extent this can be made good by giving fruit juices, but if the loss is urgent potassium chloride 5 g in a day can be given by mouth.

Electrolyte levels must be estimated twice daily and corrected quantitatively where possible. Barr and Chambers give warning of the additional danger of calcium depletion in prolonged treatment and recommend calcium gluconate if the serum calcium falls seriously.

It goes without saying that all cases of anuria should be transferred, as soon as possible, to centres where the necessary biochemical investigations can be undertaken daily and where facilities for dialysis exist. Dialysis is no longer the dangerous and formidable procedure of only a few years ago. In fact, it is no longer a last and desperate resort but the treatment of choice in cases of anuria lasting more than a week.

The following are nowadays accepted as the indications for artificial kidney dialysis:

1. Serum potassium higher than 6·5 mEq/l (mmol/l);
2. Electrocardiogram showing widening of the QRS complex;
3. Acidosis with bicarbonate reserve below 15 mEq/l (mmol/l);
4. Blood urea more than 50 mmol/l (300 mg/100 ml);
5. Mental changes and confusion;
6. Vomiting in spite of drip treatment (see above).

N.B. Potassium and bicarbonate are monovalent and therefore mmol/l and mEq/l are the same.

By the time twitching, fits and a falling blood pressure are observed it can be said that dialysis has been too long delayed. About six hours' treatment with the artificial kidney will restore an almost normal blood urea and electrolyte state which will tide the patient over for many more days and thus allow more time for the recovery of renal function.

REFERENCES

1. Asscher, A. W., Sussman, M., Waters, W. E., Denis, R. H. and Chick, Susan (1966). *Lancet*, **2**, 1037.
2. Baird, D. (1935). *J. Obstet. Gynaec. Brit. Emp.*, **42**, 577, 774.
3. Baird, D. (1936). *J. Obstet. Gynaec. Brit. Emp.*, **43**, 1, 435.
4. Barr, J. S. and Chambers, J. W. (1958). *Scot. med. J.*, **3**, 123.
5. Beard, R. W., McCoy, D. R., Newton, J. R. and Clayton, S. G. (1965). *Lancet*, **2**, 610.
6. Borst, J. G. C. (1948). *Lancet*, **1**, 824.
7. Brumfitt, W., Percival, A. and Carter, M. J. (1962). *Lancet*, **1**, 130.
8. Bull, G. M. (1950). *Brit. med. J.*, **1**, 1263.
9. Bull, G. M. (1954). *Proc. roy. Soc. Med.*, **45**, 848.
10. Bull, G. M., Bywaters, E. G. L. and Joekes, A. M. (1950). In: *Modern Trends in Obstetrics and Gynaecology*. London: Butterworth.
11. Bull, G. M., Joekes, A. M. and Lowe, K. G. (1949). *Lancet*, **2**, 229.
12. Carty, M. J., Chatfield, W. R. and McAllister, T. A. (1974). *Current Research & Medical Opinion*, **2**, 351.
13. Chamberlain, M. J. (1964). *Lancet*, **1**, 464.
14. Crabtree, E. G. (1942). *Urological Diseases of Pregnancy*. Boston: Little, Brown.
15. Crabtree, E. G. (1944). *J. Amer. med. Ass.*, **126**, 810.
16. Darmady, E. M. (1950). *Brit. med. J.*, **1**, 1263.
17. De Navasquez, S. (1935). *J. Path. Bact.*, **41**, 385.
18. Dible, J. (1950). *Brit. med. J.*, **1**, 1262.
19. Dodds, Gladys (1931). *J. Obstet. Gynaec. Brit. Emp.*, **38**, 773.
20. Donald, I., Barr, W. and McGarry, J. A. (1962). *J. Obstet. Gynaec. Brit. Cwlth*, **69**, 837.
21. Edgar, W. M. and Dickinson, K. M. (1962). *Lancet*, **2**, 739.
22. Evans, B. M., Hughes Jones, N. C., Milne, M. D. and Yellowlees, H. (1953). *Lancet*, **2**, 791.
23. Fairley, K. F., Bond, A. G. and Adey, F. D. (1966). *Lancet*, **1**, 939.
24. Felding, C. (1964). *Acta obstet. gynec. scand.*, **43**, 152.
25. Gabe, J. (1945). *Proc. roy. Soc. Med.*, **38**, 653.
26. Garrod, L. P., Shooter, R. A. and Curwen, M. P. (1954). *Brit. med. J.*, **2**, 1003.
27. Gillespie, W. A. (1956). *Proc. roy. Soc. Med.*, **49**, 1045.
28. Gillespie, W. A., Lennon, G. G., Linton, K. B. and Slade, N. (1962). *Brit. med. J.*, **2**, 13.
29. Gillespie, W. A., Linton, K. B., Miller, A. and Slade, N. (1961). *J. clin. Path.*, **13**, 187.
30. Kass, E. H. (1957). *Arch. intern. Med.*, **100**, 709.
31. Kenny, Meave, Johnston, F. D., Haebler, T. Van and Miles, A. A. (1937). *Lancet*, **2**, 119.
32. Kincaid-Smith, Priscilla and Bullen, Margaret (1956). *Lancet*, **1**, 1144.
33. Lattimer, J. K. (1945). *J. Urol. (Baltimore)*, **54**, 312.
34. Lawson, D. H. and Millar, A. W. F. (1971). *Lancet*, **1**, 9.

35. LINDSAY, R. M., LINTON, A. L. and LONGLAND, C. J. (1965). *Lancet*, **1**, 978.
36. LINTON, K. B. and GILLESPIE, W. A. (1962). *J. Obstet. Gynaec. Brit. Cwlth*, **69**, 845.
37. LUKE, R. G., LINTON, A. L., BRIGGS, J. D. and KENNEDY, A. C. (1963). *Lancet*, **1**, 980
38. McFADYEN, I. R. and EYKYN, S. J. (1968). *Lancet*, **1**, 1112.
39. McFADYEN, I. R. and SIMMONS, S. C. (1968). *J. Obstet. Gynaec. Brit. Cwlth*, **75**, 871.
40. MALPAS, P., JEFFCOATE, T. N. A. and LISTER, URSULA M. (1949). *J. Obstet. Gynaec. Brit. Emp.*, **56**, 949.
41. PARSONS, F. M. and McCRACKEN, B. H. (1959). *Brit. med. J.*, **1**, 740.
42. PATERSON, M. L., BARR, W. and MACDONALD, S. (1960). *J. Obstet. Gynaec. Brit. Emp.*, **67**, 394.
43. ROBERTS, B. E. and SMITH, P. H. (1966). *Lancet*, **2**, 421.
44. RUSSELL, C. S., DEWHURST, C. J. and BRACE, J. C. (1954). *Lancet*, **1**, 902.
45. SLADE, N. and LINTON, K. B. (1960). *Brit. J. Urol.*, **32**, 416.
46. SMITH, K., BROWNE, J. C. M., SHACKMAN, R. and WRONG, O. M. (1965). *Lancet*, **2**, 351.
47. STILL, B. M. (1966). *Proc. roy. Soc. Med.*, **59**, 157.
48. TRUETA, J., BARCLAY, A. E., DANIEL, P. M., FRANKLIN, K. J. and PRICHARD, M. M. L. (1947). *Studies of the Renal Circulation*. Oxford: Blackwell Scientific Publications.
49. YOUNG, J. (1942). *Brit. med. J.*, **2**, 715.

CHAPTER XII

TWINS AND HYDRAMNIOS

TWINS

TWIN pregnancy is due either to the fertilisation of two separate ova, in which case the twins are called binovular, or from the division of one fertilised ovum into two separate embryos, which are thus uniovular. The former are five or six times as common as the latter. As might be expected, uniovular twins are like two beans out of the same pod and are always of the same sex, whereas binovular twins bear only fraternal resemblance to each other.

Where two ova are thus fertilised it is usual for them to be produced simultaneously from one Graafian follicle, so that only one corpus luteum is present. Such twins have completely distinct sets of membranes of their own, so that the membranous septum between the two amniotic sacs consists of the amnion and chorion of one fetus, then the chorion and amnion of the other, and the two placentae, although contiguous in 9 out of 10 cases, are nevertheless

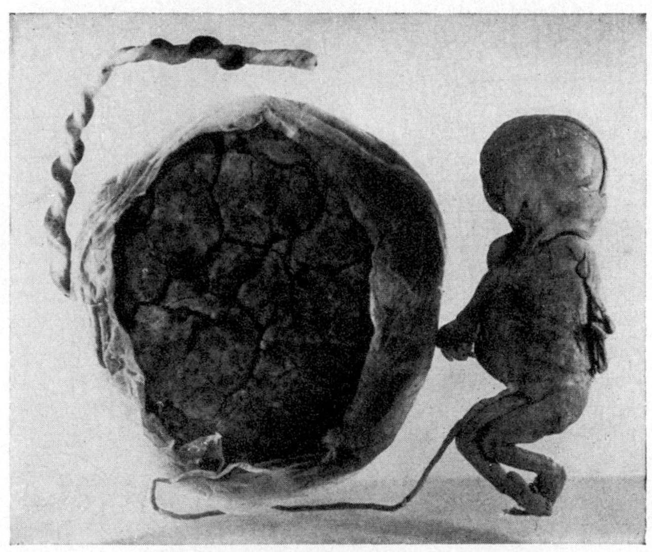

12/FIG. 1.—Fetus papyraceous.
(By courtesy of Dr E. W. L. Thompson and R.C.O.G. Museum.)

(*a*)

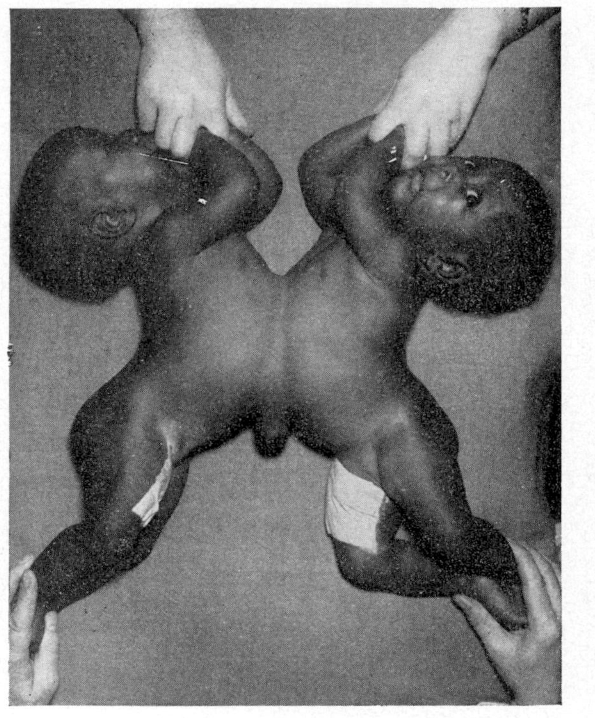

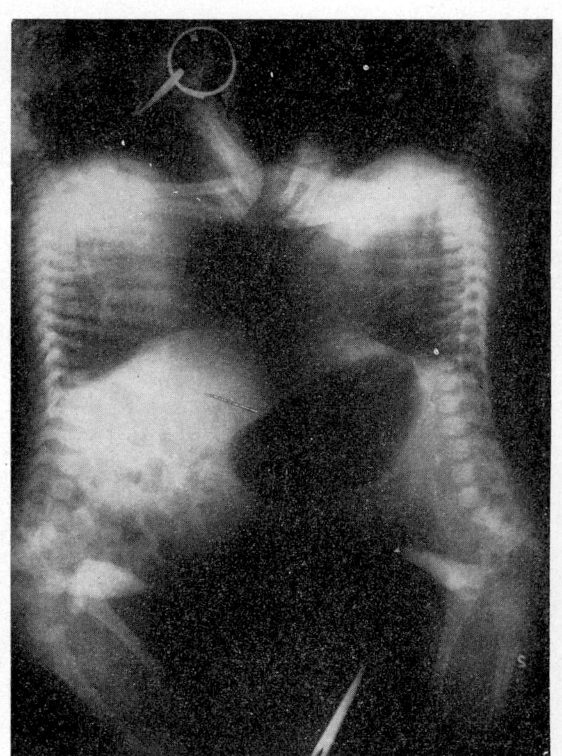

(*b*)

12/FIG. 2 (*a*) and (*b*).—Siamese twins of Kano.
(By courtesy of the late Prof. Ian Aird and the Editor, *Brit. med. J.*)

structurally separate and their circulations are practically always distinct from each other. In uniovular twins the double placenta, though not entirely common to both, has a varying degree of anastomotic circulation, and the membranous septum between the two

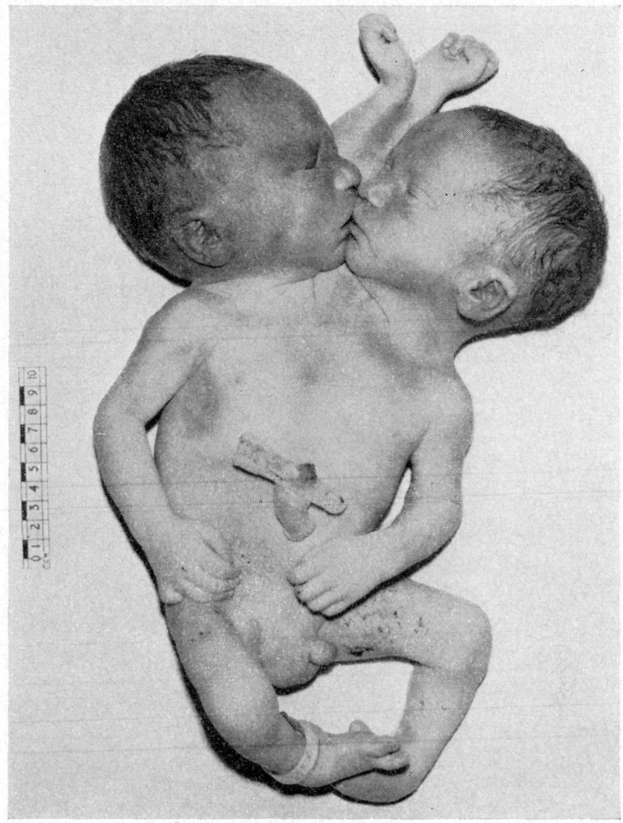

12/FIG. 3 (*a*).

fetal sacs, provided it has not been broken down, consists only of the two layers of amnion, one from each fetus.

Instead of the terms uniovular and binovular, therefore, it is also common to use the terms monochorionic and dichorionic. Careful inspection of the septum between two amniotic sacs often leads to mistakes however, which histological section would place beyond all doubt, because the chorion shows up well. This sort of information may be valuable one day as uniovular twins can in later life share a certain amount of transplantation surgery between them without fear of rejection.

All the above would be of little more than academic interest were it not for the fact that certain well-known disadvantages operate in the case of uniovular twins. For instance, intra-uterine death of one

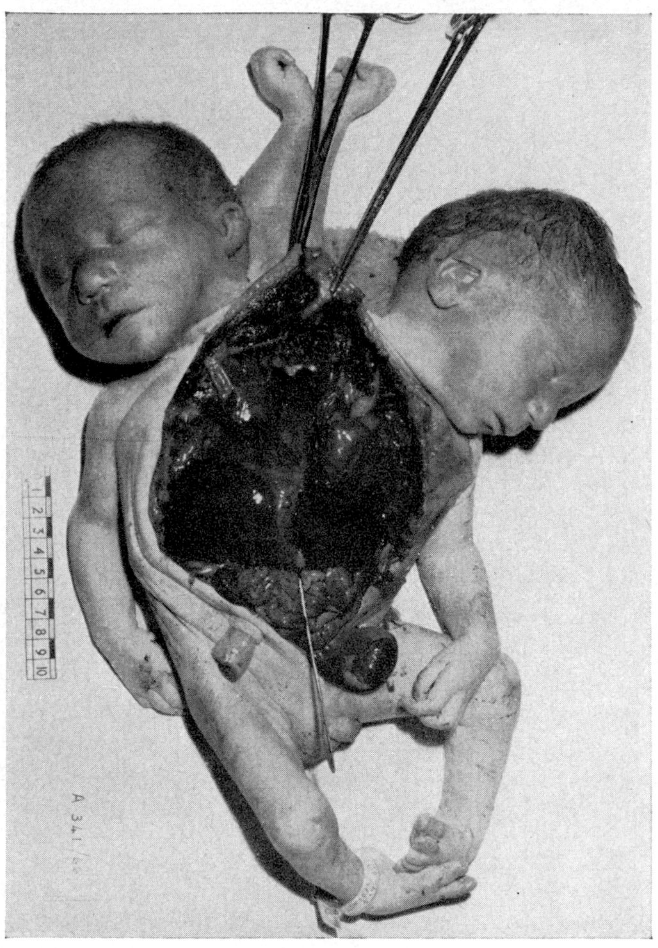

12/FIG. 3 (*b*).

fetus is not uncommon, and if it takes place relatively early in pregnancy, the dead fetus is usually retained *in utero* as a shrivelled and compressed object; hence its name, fetus papyraceous or compressus (Fig. 1). It is finally expelled with its surviving brother at delivery. It is thought that this phenomenon may be due to the overpowering of the circulation of the unsuccessful fetus by the more powerful cardiac output of the survivor through the placental anastomosis. On a lesser scale it is possible for one uniovular twin to

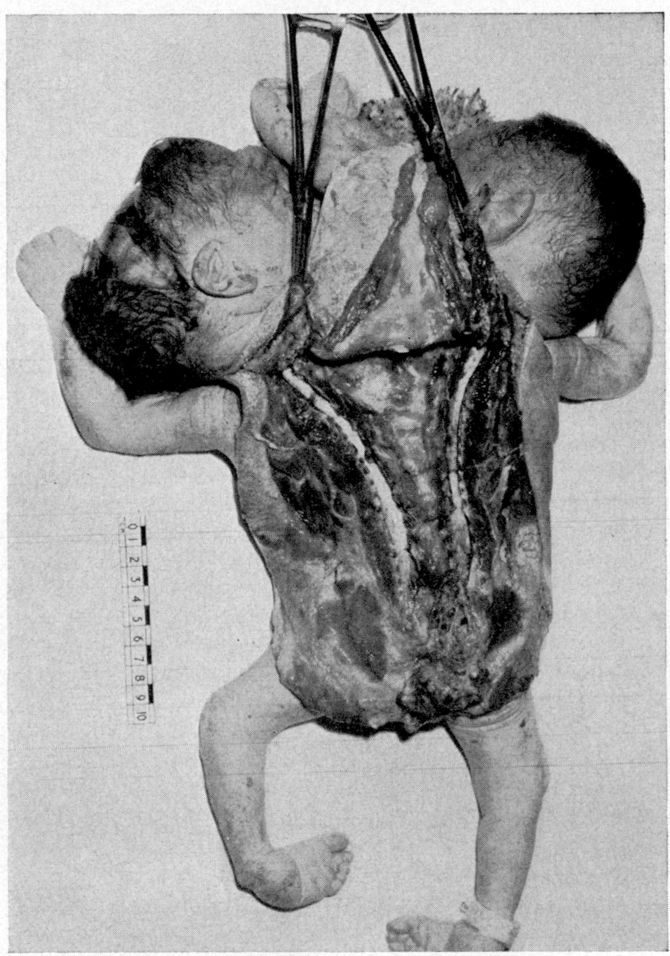

12/FIG. 3 (*c*).

exsanguinate itself into the circulation of the other, producing polycythaemia. Kerr (1959) reported four such cases occurring within three years at the Glasgow Royal Maternity Hospital. In two of them transfusion was required for the anaemic twin.

One can only speculate about the origin of uniovular twins, but this phenomenon may be due to some minor arrest in the very early development of the fertilised ovum, so that the embryonic streak divides by a sort of binary fission. In rare instances this division may not be complete, and all manner of double monsters, for example thoracopagus and Siamese twins, may result (Figs. 2 and 3). The

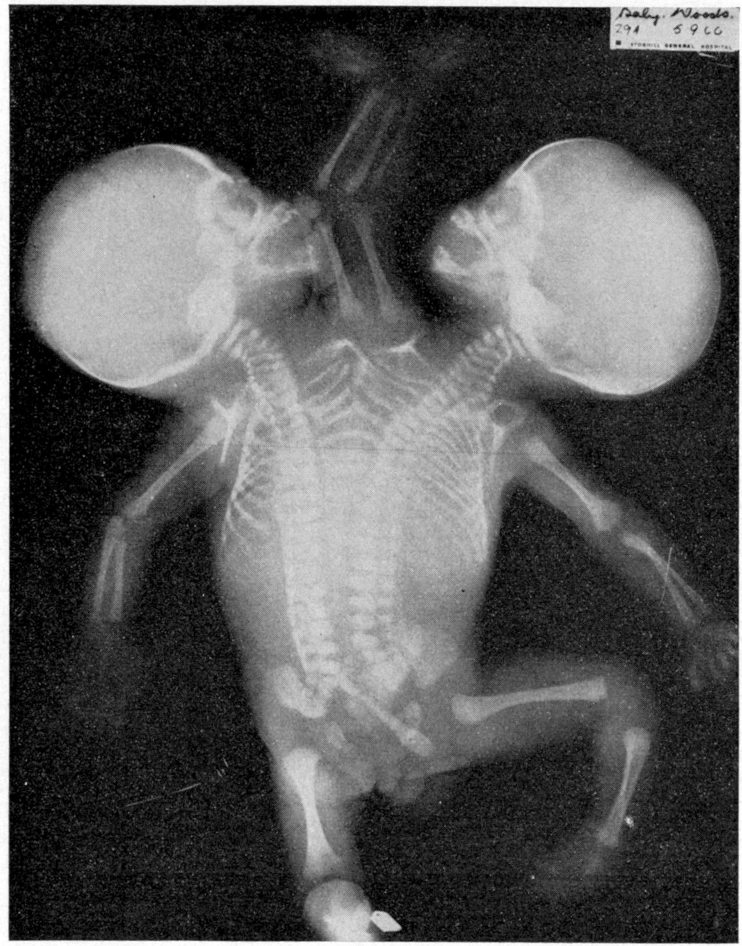

12/Fig. 3 (*d*).

12/Figs. 3 (*a*), (*b*), (*c*) and (*d*).—Siamese twins delivered at 36½ weeks gestation. Their existence was unsuspected until after the spontaneous delivery of the first head when difficulty with delivery of the shoulders was encountered. At this point the second head was found on examination. Delivery was completed with an intact perineum! The monster survived only a few minutes.

(By courtesy of Dr R. M. Still and Mr Waldie, Stobhill Hospital, Glasgow.)

incidence of fetal abnormality is higher in uniovular twins, and may be due to something in the nature of this mechanism or to a blood circulation overpowered by the stronger fetus.

Hydramnios, although associated with twins of both varieties, is relatively more often found in the uniovular variety, and tends to occur with the larger twin, whose greater cardiac output results in increased renal excretory activity.

Superfecundation and superfetation are freak occurrences, more often than not of doubtful authenticity. In the first, fertilisation of

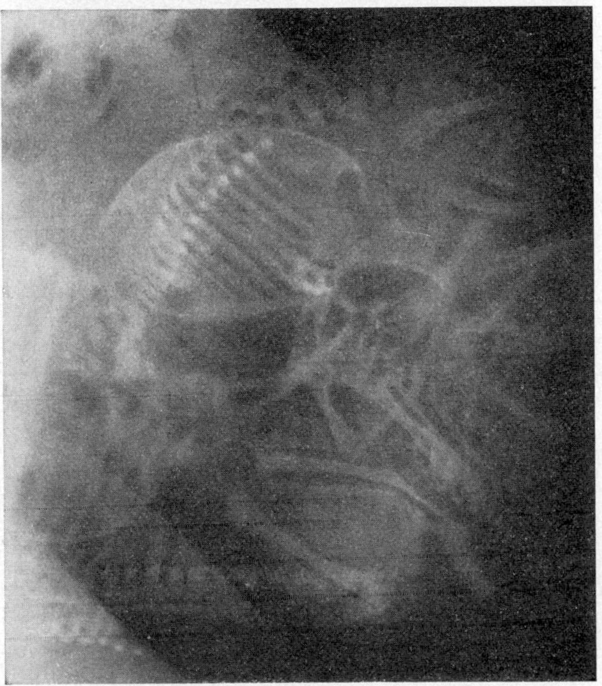

12/FIG. 4.—Triplets.
(By courtesy of Dr J. W. McLaren.)

two separate ova occurs during the same intermenstrual period by separate acts of coitus. In superfetation credulity is stretched a great deal farther, because the twins are derived from separate ovulations as well as separate acts of coitus during different intermenstrual periods, as a result of which a woman may simultaneously carry two fetuses of markedly different gestational ages. In theory such a phenomenon is mechanically feasible up to about the 12th week, after which the fusion of the decidua vera and decidua reflexa should make it impossible, except in the case of a double uterus.

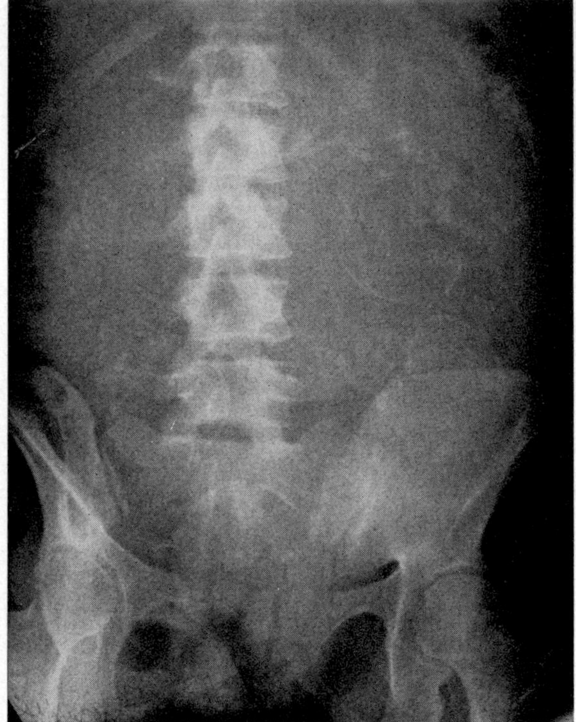

12/Fig. 5.—Quadruplets.
(By courtesy of Dr Ellis Barnett.)

Twins tend to run in families, and heredity plays a very important part. Oddly enough, paternal as well as maternal influences may be responsible.

The incidence of twinning varies with race, with population, with fertility and with age, and is more often encountered in fertile negro populations than among the white races. Moreover, as women get older they become less likely to have twins, in spite of the fact that multiple pregnancy is commoner in multiparae. The average incidence of twins, therefore, works out at about 1 in 80 pregnancies. The variations in different parts of the world are mainly composed of differences in the binovular incidence.

Triplets occur no more than about once in every 8000 pregnancies, and quadruplets about once in every three-quarters of a million (Figs. 4 and 5). Quintuplets are a very extreme rarity, of which the Dionne sisters were by no means the only cases, although they were remarkable for their survival. The highest score yet recorded for a human litter is six.

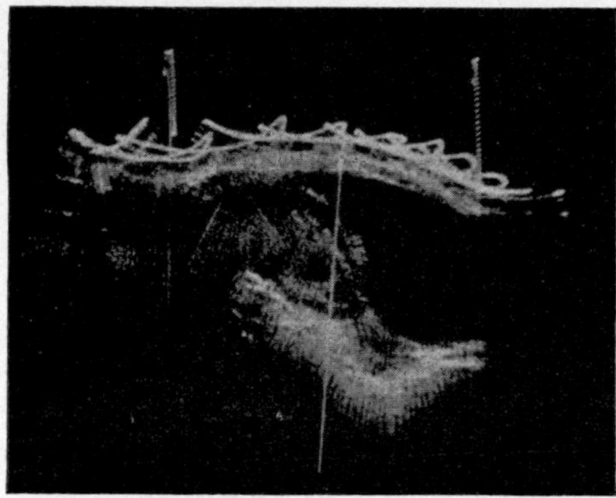

12/FIG. 6.—Ultrasonogram. Twin gestation sacs (indicated by white intermediate vertical line) found at eight weeks gestation although urine tests for pregnancy hitherto negative. L.S. behind moderately full bladder to the right.

(By courtesy of the Editor, *Brit. J. Radiol.*)

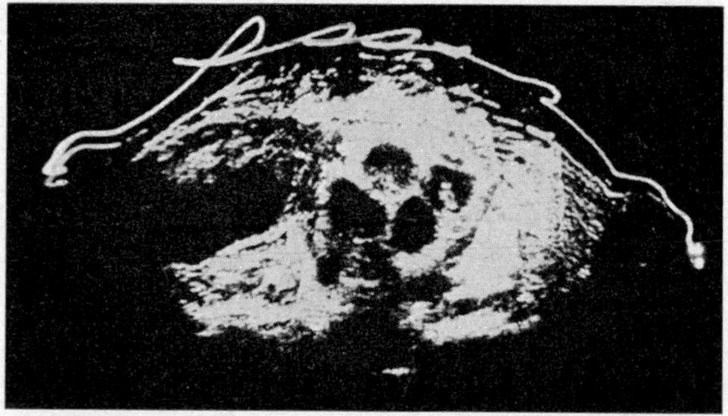

12/FIG. 7 (*a*).—Ultrasonogram taken at 9 weeks estimated menstrual age to show a transverse section of the uterus in its long axis and five gestation sacs. The probe has been moved across the abdomen transversely at a 20° tilt to the vertical. An embryonic echo is visible in sacs 1, 2, and 5. An ovarian cyst can be identified lateral to the uterus.

(By courtesy of Prof. Stuart Campbell and the Editor, *Lancet*.)

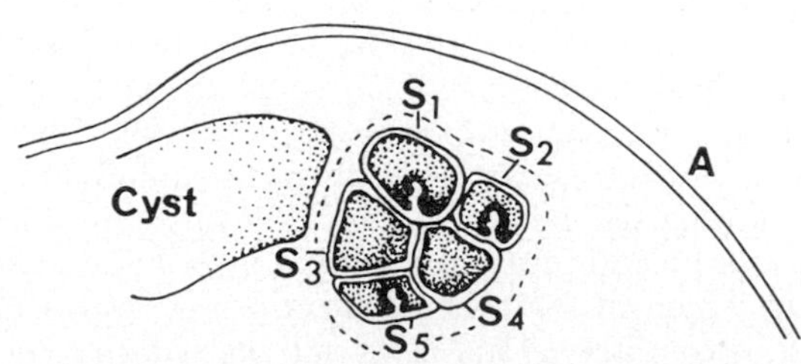

12/FIG. 7 (*b*).—Explanatory diagram. A = Abdominal wall. S = Gestation sac.

The technique of stimulating ovulation with human pituitary gonadotrophin is liable to result in high-litter pregnancies unless very careful control is undertaken. This is a dangerous situation, of course, because of the very high rate of abortion and prematurity, with only disappointment and possibly hazard to life at the end to reward it. Occasionally, however, a successful pregnancy, for example, quintuplets, following such treatment with human pituitary gonadotrophin, may be successful[13] but the human race was not designed to breed on this scale.

In spite of full endocrinological and biochemical control of gonadotrophic drugs, which may require adjustment over two or more years, this type of tragedy may still occur.

Early warning, however, of an excessive human litter has been strikingly achieved at Queen Charlotte's Hospital, London, by sonar diagnosis of quintuplets at nine weeks gestation (Fig. 7). Hospitalisation and careful prophylaxis against a lethal degree of prematurity resulted in the successful delivery by Caesarean section and survival of all five.[3] A truly remarkable feat!

Incidentally anovulatory infertility treated by clomiphene does not appear to carry the same risk of excessive multiple pregnancy, but cystic enlargement of the ovaries has to be watched for.

Diagnosis

In spite of all the emphasis which the textbooks lay upon the clinical signs of multiple pregnancy, the only sure diagnosis rests upon sonar (ultrasonography) or an adequate X-ray sufficiently late in pregnancy. Unfortunately X-rays are seldom reliable much before the 16th week, even if then, and depend upon the calcification of the fetal skeleton to reveal the existence of twins. Sonar wins here and this is now our standard technique for screening the uterus which is large for dates, to confirm or exclude a suspicion of twins.[7, 8, 9] In very early pregnancy the diagnosis depends upon the demonstration of twin gestation sacs, using the full bladder technique.[10] So far we have not been able to diagnose twins under $7\frac{1}{2}$ weeks from the last menstrual period. Later, from the 14th week onwards, the heads of the fetuses are discernible and throughout the rest of pregnancy the diagnosis of twins is made by finding two heads. The only pitfall is to mistake a transverse section of a fetal thorax for a head, but this should be eliminated by scanning in at least two different dimensions and so confirming the existence of both heads (Fig. 8).[18]

An even more certain way of avoiding a mistaken diagnosis of a second head when, in fact, the echogram is a sectional view of a fetal thorax, is to observe fetal heart activity within it, either by the ultrasonic Doppler method, or in earlier cases by ultrasonic time/

motion study (Chapter XXIX). This kind of cardiac activity, needless to say, cannot be demonstrated in a "suspected" fetal head.[11]

Nevertheless the final exclusion of triplets is not easy by sonar because of its present limitation to two-dimensional scanning only and later on in pregnancy a radiograph may be necessary.

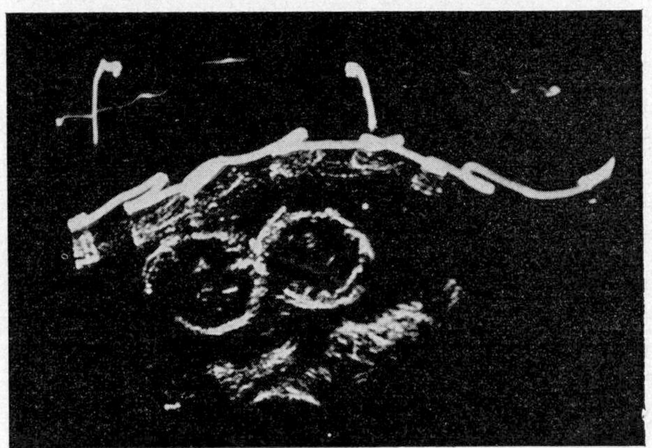

12/FIG. 8.—Ultrasonogram. Twin heads. Gestation period 22 weeks.

An additional advantage of sonar for the diagnosis of twins is that it eliminates the hazard of irradiation with X-rays and is serviceable at an earlier stage in pregnancy than standard radiography; but perhaps most important of all is the fact that both heads can be measured and it can be ascertained which of the two is the larger, the first-coming or the second-coming head. The advantages of the first head being the larger are considerable, and may influence one in the method of delivery of the second twin. For instance, to be caught with the second twin with a larger head, held up by an inadequately dilated cervix had one but foreseen it, might have encouraged delivery by the vertex, assisted if necessary by the ventouse. It is therefore our standard practice now to measure both heads well in advance of labour so as to know what to expect.

If it appears either by radiology or sonar that one baby is very much smaller than the other, a suspicion of intra-uterine death of the smaller is already aroused (Fig. 9).

The uterus is always larger than would correspond to the period of gestation, but this sign can be very misleading. If two heads can be palpated so much the better, but one should in these cases be satisfied about at least one other pole, namely a breech, before diagnosing the presence of two heads; in other words, at least three poles should be felt. An apparent multiplicity of limbs is often said to be suggestive of twins, but this can be deceptive. The hearing of a fetal heart in two separate places separated by a silent area is not conclusive unless two observers listening simultaneously note a discrepancy in fetal heart rates of at least 10 beats a minute. Personally I have yet to make this diagnosis by such a futile method.

Hydramnios suggests the possibility of the co-existence of twins because of the very frequent association of the two. In any case,

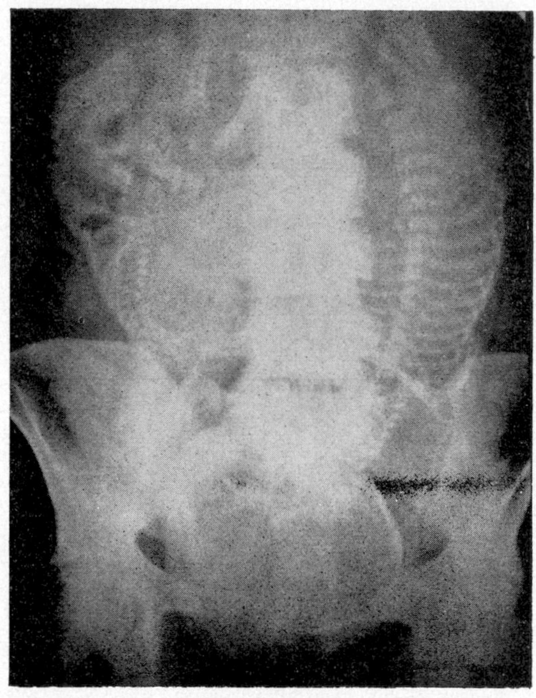

12/FIG. 9.—Twins. One baby on left of picture very much smaller than the other and already dead.

whether hydramnios or multiple pregnancy is suspected, an X-ray should be obtained, firstly to exclude fetal abnormality, which is commonly present in cases of hydramnios, and secondly to determine the number of fetuses and their presentations. Even though one is clinically certain with every good reason that a patient has twins, there is little credit in making the diagnosis if the patient subsequently delivers herself of three, and the diagnosis of triplets without the help of radiography is highly improbable. If a fairly acute degree of hydramnios occurs relatively early on, the chances of uniovular twins being present are indeed worth considering.

Effects of Twins upon Pregnancy

In some respects the complication rate is undoubtedly higher, and there is everything to be said for booking such a patient for hospital delivery as a matter of course.

During pregnancy the patient will require more than usually adequate periods of daily rest, and her diet will require supervision to ensure a sufficient intake of extra vitamins, calcium and iron, all of which tend, in these cases, to fall short of requirements. Iron supplements are almost always necessary and folic acid deficiency is common enough in twin pregnancy to make megaloblastic anaemia a fairly frequent complication and to justify prophylactic folic acid therapy (see Chapter VII).

Because of the increased uterine enlargement, all the usual pressure signs and symptoms are likely to be increased, and these include oedema of the legs, occasionally of the vulva and abdominal wall, and increasing shortness of breath as pregnancy proceeds. Hyperemesis when it occurs is often severe. A natural predisposition to varicose veins may become an established disability.

The incidence of pre-eclamptic toxaemia and eclampsia with twins is greatly increased, and for this reason antenatal supervision should be conducted at relatively more frequent intervals than in the case of single pregnancy. A woman can hardly have pre-eclamptic toxaemia without being pregnant, and whatever factors operate in producing this disorder, they are certainly magnified in the patient who is doubly pregnant.

Because of the large size of the placenta its site is liable to overlap on to the lower uterine segment, thus producing varying degrees of placenta praevia with antepartum haemorrhage as a result. Accidental haemorrhage, too, is more common, partly because of the increased incidence of pre-eclamptic toxaemia and, it is now believed, partly due to an association with folic acid deficiency, although the mechanism is not yet understood.

As has been mentioned already, hydramnios is more common, especially in the case of uniovular twins, and fetal abnormality in one of the two frequently occurs. The combination of plural pregnancy and hydramnios, even though mild, causes a degree of uterine overdistension sufficient to provoke the onset of premature labour in at least a third of the cases.

It is now increasingly our practice to admit cases of twins to hospital from about the 30th to the 34th week of pregnancy in order to reduce the prematurity risk, although the timing of prophylactic admission is determined more by the girth than the actual period of gestation, and there is no doubt that this counsel of perfection pays dividends. Prematurity, after all, is still responsible for the largest class of neonatal deaths, and hospitalisation over the critical period as above thus contributes to a lowering in neonatal mortality.

Presentation of the Fetuses

The following is a list in order of frequency:

1. Vertex, vertex
2. Vertex, breech
3. Breech, vertex
4. Breech, breech
5. Vertex, transverse.

The remaining possible combinations are too uncommon to be worth listing, the least common of all being the double transverse position.

LABOUR

An anaesthetist should always be present throughout the second and third stages of all viable twin deliveries, prepared to induce an anaesthetic at a minute's notice.

Labour is usually normal, but it is as well to be on the look-out for trouble. Because of the overdistension of the uterus there is some tendency towards uterine inertia, but this is to a certain extent offset by the smallness of the babies as a result of prematurity. Post-maturity with twins, incidentally, is very uncommon. If it appears that overdistension is handicapping uterine function, especially in association with hydramnios, it is worth relieving it by puncture of the forewaters, provided the lie of the first child is longitudinal. Hindwater rupture is inadvisable because the second sac may be thereby drained instead of the first. This may not only interfere with longitudinal alignment of the second twin in the second stage of labour but may also precipitate fetal distress in it as well. The membranes tend to rupture early, and it is a good rule to perform vaginal examination as soon as this occurs to ensure that the cord has not been washed down, and to satisfy oneself as to the identity and engagement of the presenting part. Provided this is either breech or vertex, no further action is required for the time being, but otherwise treatment appropriate to the particular malpresentation will be necessary. If the first child presents by anything other than the vertex, it is as well to conduct the first stage in bed and to withhold an enema in order to preserve the membranes as long as possible.

When labour is premature an episiotomy should be performed in good time during the second stage in order to save the head from damage, particularly if the first child presents by the breech. In this last instance the aftercoming head cannot be assisted in delivery by suprapubic pressure because the second twin, of course, is in the way, and the forceps should be ready for immediate use if necessary. The complication of locked twins preventing delivery of the first child captures the imagination of every student but is exceedingly rare. Here, the aftercoming head of the first child is prevented from entering the pelvis by the presentation of the head of the second child. Anaesthesia must be immediately induced and the treatment has to be both very prompt and lucky if the first child is to be saved, and consists in pushing the second head out of the way so that the first head can enter the brim—by no means an easy manoeuvre if the babies are of any reasonable size. More often the attempt fails or can only be made too late, and the first child dies of asphyxia, in which case the treatment is to decapitate the first child, deliver the body and retrieve the head after delivery of the second twin.

If the babies are small and the pelvis large, a more elegant alternative has been described by Begg who successfully delivered alive all four babies in two cases of locked twins occurring within three months of each other.[1] He managed to extract the head of the second twin past the first with Kielland's forceps thereafter extracting the aftercoming head of the first child by jaw and shoulder traction. If the first child is still alive, this should certainly be attempted in preference to decapitation if attempts at disimpaction have not been successful in the first place.

Rather more common, but still rare, is collision of heads at the brim, in which neither head will make way for the other. For this the treatment is simply to push one of the heads up and out of the way.

After the first child has been born the cord is divided between two ligatures. Every textbook makes much of this because of the risk of a second uniovular twin bleeding to death through the placental anastomotic circulation and cord of the first, but the practice of dividing the cord between clamps or ligatures is so universal in every delivery that it hardly needs stressing.

The Second Twin

After the delivery of the first child the first step is to palpate the abdomen and to ensure that the lie of the second child is longitudinal, if necessary performing external version. It is important that, on the return of contractions, the second bag of membranes should not rupture with the child in an uncorrected transverse position, for in that case the cord or an arm, or both, might prolapse.

There now follows a brief period of waiting for the contractions to return. Provided there is no maternal haemorrhage meanwhile, all that has to be done is to observe the fetal heart of the second twin in order to detect signs of fetal distress, which, of course, demands immediate intervention.

The placentae nearly always come together after the delivery of the second twin. Occasionally, however, the first placenta is extruded, often to the accompaniment of bleeding, with the second twin still unborn. Under these circumstances the second bag of waters should be ruptured and the remaining child delivered in order to empty the uterus and arrest haemorrhage by uterine retraction.

All of us have long recognised that the second twin is at far greater risk than the first; in fact a review of the literature shows that the increase to the hazard is of the order of about 50 per cent.[2] Failure to correct malpresentation by external cephalic version is one cause, but prolonged hypoxia jeopardises the second baby's chances the longer the interval between delivery of the first and second. Any general anaesthesia given for the delivery of the first twin has longer in which to affect the second, and wherever possible anaesthesia should be restricted to regional methods for the first and instantly available by a general technique for the second.

The use of epidural anaesthesia in twin deliveries has its own peculiar hazards. Firstly, it is commonly held that the uterus may clamp down too tightly on the second twin and endanger it, but more important is the sharp reduction in blood pressure which may be associated with epidural and spinal anaesthesia. Tipping the patient's head downwards may be all very well to maintain maternal cerebral circulation, but does not help placental circulation, which normally carries a double requirement load. Epidural and spinal anaesthesia therefore require a very close watch upon maternal blood pressure, bearing in mind the needs of two fetuses rather than one.

The second twin, for as long as it remains *in utero* after the first has been expelled, continues at risk due to reduction in uteroplacental circulation, and fetal distress must be watched for vigilantly and anticipated by early delivery rather than late.

A waiting period of half an hour used to be recommended, provided there was no bleeding and no fetal distress unless contractions returned earlier. Most of us are now agreed that this delay is not only unwise but excessive. After all, the cervix is fully dilated, and if one were conducting a normal single delivery one would rupture the membranes forthwith. The same argument applies to the second twin and it is now our practice to push the presenting part of the second twin into the pelvis about five minutes after the separation of the first and to rupture the membranes there and then. If delivery does not occur within a further ten minutes we proceed to operative delivery forthwith while the undelivered child is still well. Macdonald (1962) in a review of 500 consecutive cases in Glasgow showed that this practice not only lowers the complication rate but does not even encounter uterine inertia, as was once thought. If the presenting part is not well in the pelvis, or in any case if there is hydramnios, the cord may easily prolapse with membrane rupture and a look-out for this should be kept. Should this happen the child should be extracted forthwith, otherwise natural delivery is allowed to proceed.

If a general anaesthetic has been necessary in the course of delivery of the first child, one has a choice of action. The older teaching was to discontinue it while awaiting the arrival of the second. The modern practice, however, is to rupture the second amniotic sac at once, to insert the hand and perform internal podalic version and breech extraction.

This type of version is both safe and easy because of the newly-found room available. The latter type of treatment is also to be preferred to rupturing the second sac and failing to push the head well into the pelvis, usually because of a deflexion attitude of the fetus. The temptation to press on with the delivery by high forceps extraction must be resisted. Having manoeuvred oneself into this ugly dilemma with the second head high and the membranes newly ruptured, it is still better to perform internal version before it is too late, rather than awaiting spontaneous descent of the presenting part or embarking upon what may prove to be a hazardous and difficult high forceps delivery, in spite of the small size of the baby. The ventouse, or vacuum extractor, has, however, proved a useful alternative in our unit and is infinitely to be preferred to high forceps application, especially if the cervix is attempting to shut down. Its use leads to an easy and gentle delivery without general anaesthesia and with full co-operation from the patient and her stimulated uterus.

In such cases the traditional method of internal version and breech extraction may prove hazardous if the cervix is not fully dilated or if the second twin is unexpectedly larger than the first.[14]

The *third stage* of labour is undoubtedly the most dangerous in twin delivery. For several reasons the risks of postpartum haemorrhage are enhanced: firstly, because the very size of the double placenta may delay its spontaneous expulsion; secondly, the placental site is larger in area and therefore capable of more profuse bleeding; thirdly, the placental site may partially occupy the lower uterine segment where retraction is inefficient; and fourthly, the uterus may demonstrate a marked degree of inertia following its recent over-distension. A syringe already loaded with ergometrine should therefore be at hand, and the intravenous injection of 0·25 mg after the birth of the second twin is increasingly used as a prophylactic measure against postpartum haemorrhage.

It occasionally happens that ergometrine is given at the end of the second stage to a woman in whom the presence of twins has been hitherto unsuspected, and this risk constitutes one of the few serious objections to this excellent routine practice in normal labour. If such a mistake is made, the risks to the undiagnosed twin are very great as a result of uterine spasm, and the child should be extracted at once.

The treatment of any postpartum haemorrhage should be prompt and energetic, and whether or not ergometrine is used before the delivery of the placenta, half a milligramme of ergometrine should certainly be injected intramuscularly at the completion of the third stage in all cases of twins in order to maintain uterine retraction. The uterus is very liable to soften after a twin delivery and to fill with blood, and it is not really safe to relax vigilance for 4 hours after delivery. The patient should certainly not be left without first expressing any clots of blood which may have accumulated within the uterine cavity.

Triplets

The problems are similar to those of twins but considerably magnified, particularly the risks of premature labour. Admission from the 28th week of pregnancy is therefore desirable if reasonable maturity is to be achieved.

It is particularly inadvisable to waste much time between the births of each child and as soon as breech or vertex of the next appears in the pelvis the membranes should be ruptured artificially. If neither pole presents, then internal version and breech extraction should be carried out forthwith.

The use of a slow running oxytocin drip is an admirable precaution throughout the second and third stages of such cases in order to discourage any inertia or undue hold-ups. I watched the Glasgow quadruplets being delivered in splendid succession, placentae and all, in 28 minutes with a well-regulated drip, and postpartum bleeding was minimal.

Prognosis and Aftercare

The maternal prognosis is somewhat adversely influenced by the complications of pregnancy already enumerated, for example pre-eclamptic toxaemia and antepartum haemorrhage, but even more so by the dangers of postpartum haemorrhage and collapse. As a result, puerperal morbidity is to some extent increased.

The fetal prognosis is worse than in single delivery mainly because of prematurity. To a lesser extent the influence of malpresentation and the treatment thereof is also a factor to which cord prolapse, too, may contribute adversely. Intra-uterine death, especially in the case of one of uniovular twins, also occurs from time to time. Fetal distress in the second child during the second stage of labour often results in the aspiration of liquor and meconium because of asphyxia due to retraction at the placental site, and possible placental separation, so that the second child is frequently more in need of clearance of the upper air passages than the first.

Lastly, twins may be more difficult to rear than single infants, because the maternal milk supply is often inadequate for both, and rickets and anaemia are commoner, because during pregnancy the increased demands for iron and calcium may not have been fully met.

HYDRAMNIOS

The official name for this condition is "polyhydramnios" but the word hydramnios is universally used.

The degree to which an excessive amount of liquor should be regarded as pathological is not mathematically fixed, and in normal cases the amount varies, increasing a little in the third trimester as compared with the second.[5] The usual range is from 300 to 800 ml and is determined by a dilution technique, injecting sodium aminohippurate at amniocentesis and analysing liquor samples by spectrophotometry.[6] Liquor volumes exceeding 1500 ml are abnormal.

Sonar examination provides a characteristic picture with large "blob" echo patterns within copious clear areas representing liquor (Fig. 13*c*). In the second and third trimesters of pregnancy the head can always be found by sonar examination; in fact so confident are we that in a case of hydramnios in which the head cannot be found by this technique we are prepared to diagnose anencephaly.

Congenital malformations of the central nervous system, including anencephaly and spina bifida, are more likely to appear again in subsequent pregnancy than in the normal case. I have had one patient with three anencephalic fetuses and no living children. A second patient, by a variety of male partners, produced three babies with spina bifida all of whom had ultimately died and another surviving baby with ectopia vesicae and incontinence of urine, and who, at the age of 42, became pregnant by yet another man to whom she was not married. The substantial risk that this further pregnancy would end in an abnormal fetus drove me reluctantly to terminate the pregnancy and with somewhat less reluctance to sterilise her. Another high spinal deformity was found in the fetus.

For purposes of genetic counselling it has been suggested by Carter and Roberts[4] that the risk after two children with central nervous system malformations in England runs at about one in eight (see Chapter III).

Although the term is often loosely used to account for a uterus larger than would correspond to the period of gestation, because of the amount of liquor present, it should really be restricted to those cases in which undue pressure symptoms or malpresentations occur as a result.

The causes of hydramnios are still to some extent obscure, although many complicating conditions are associated with excess liquor. Even the source of normal amounts of liquor is open to some questions, but it would appear that hydramnios may owe its origin to maternal or fetal causes or both.

Whatever the source of excessive liquor, it does not, as a rule, noticeably differ in composition from normal cases. Hydramnios is commoner in multiparae than in primigravidae.

Some of the maternal conditions more likely to be associated with hydramnios are pre-eclamptic toxaemia, congestive cardiac failure and diabetes. In the case of the last mentioned, it is thought that the presence of sugar in the liquor may irritate the amnion to produce excessive quantities.

Of the fetal causes of hydramnios, the association of twins, especially uniovular, is noteworthy. Gross fetal abnormality is a prominent aetiological factor, with anencephaly predominating (Figs. 10 and 11). For a time it was thought that potato blight might be a factor[16] and would explain the higher incidence of anencephaly amongst the potato-eating populations of Ireland and the West of Scotland but this tentative view is now discounted.[17] The reputed inability of the anencephalic fetus to swallow and therefore to absorb liquor into its circulation is said to be the cause here, and for the same reason hydramnios may be associated with oesophageal atresia. To a lesser extent other types of gross fetal abnormality, for example spina bifida and hydrocephalus, are associated with hydramnios (Fig. 12).

Other associated fetal conditions are hydrops fetalis and the very rare condition of chorioangioma, a small tumour growing from a single villus and consisting of hyperplasia of blood vessels and connective tissue. Syphilis is not nowadays regarded as an aetiological factor.

The clinical picture will depend upon the degree of hydramnios and the rapidity of its onset. Acute hydramnios is so rare that F. J. Browne considered that every case encountered was worth reporting in the literature, but subacute varieties are by no means uncommon. Hydramnios occurring in mid-pregnancy should always arouse a suspicion of uniovular twins. The slower the development of the condition the less is the patient likely to complain. The acute variety may present many of the features of an acute abdominal catastrophe, the uterus being hard and tender and causing the patient great distress, so that the picture may resemble abruptio placentae.

In the usual cases of gradual onset the patient may complain of an unmanageable girth, shortness of breath, considerable digestive discomfort, oedema of the lower extremities, and increasingly troublesome varicose veins. Occasionally hydramnios can cause hyperemesis in late pregnancy, and I have seen a highly parous patient prostrated with vomiting due to this cause, with ketone bodies in her urine, and finally suffering repeated haematemesis. Hiatus hernia may well have been a complicating factor but was not proven. Following the surgical induction of labour and delivery, her condition dramatically improved. In mild cases the fetus can be freely ballotted and a fluid thrill is present. In more severe cases, however, palpation of the fetus may be very unsatisfactory, and it is most difficult to hear the fetal heart. Malpresentations are common, the lie may be unstable, and if the vertex presents the head is likely to be high.

The differential diagnosis is concerned firstly with multiple pregnancy. As has been repeatedly stated, all cases of hydramnios should have an X-ray as a matter of course, not only to determine the presence of twins but also to detect the possible presence of gross

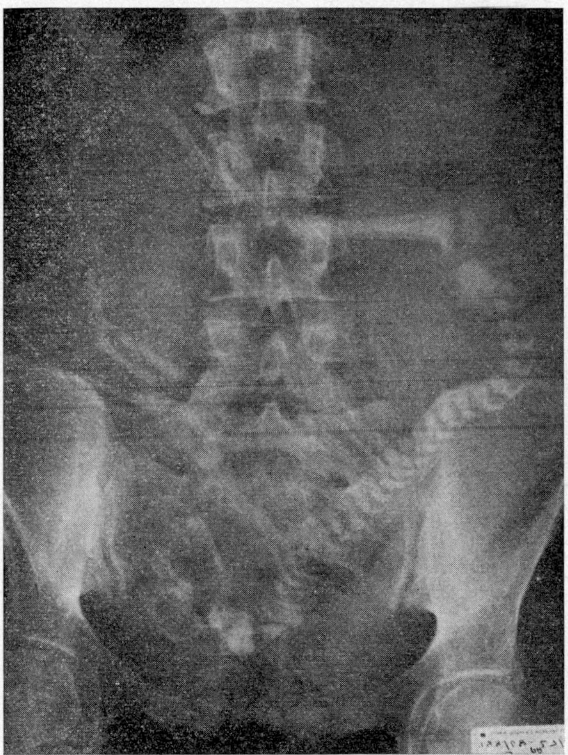

12/Fig. 10.—Anencephaly with gross lumbar kyphosis and spina bifida. (By courtesy of Dr E. M. Sweet.)

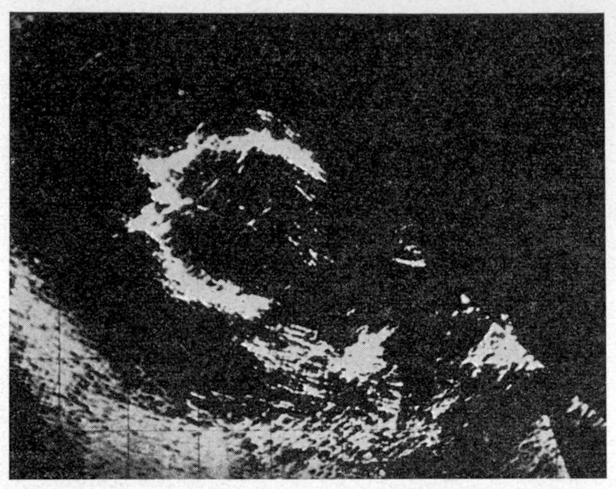

12/FIG. 11.—Gross open spinal defect and hydramnios. Ultrasonogram of fetal trunk in transverse section.

(By courtesy of Prof. Stuart Campbell.)

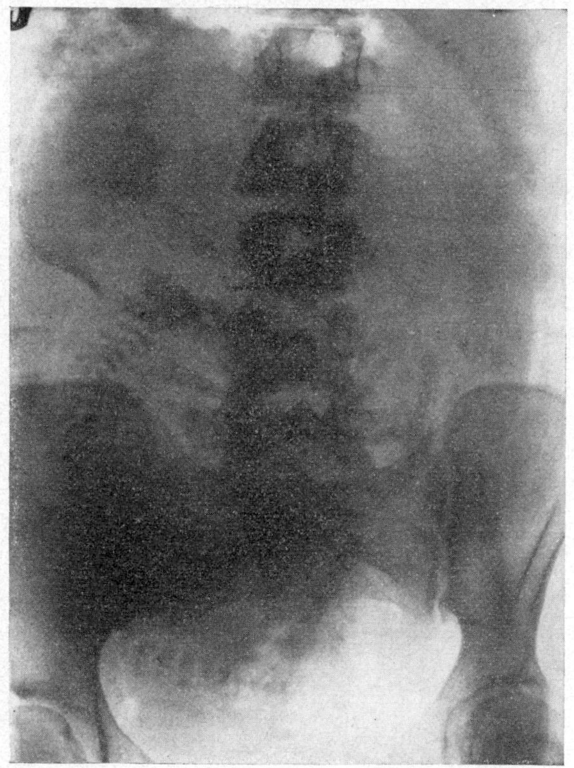

12/FIG. 12.—Hydrocephalus and spina bifida.

(By courtesy of Prof. R. E. Steiner.)

fetal abnormality. If no fetal abnormality is demonstrated radiologically a further X-ray should be taken after rupture of the membranes, because abnormality is now more readily demonstrated and its recognition might discourage Caesarean section if fetal interests should subsequently appear to indicate it. The usefulness of sonar in examining the patient who is "larger than dates" is now beyond all doubt and is routinely employed by us. Not only will such an examination determine that the patient's dates may be wrong, because the fetal head size gives a very good estimate of maturity, but the question of twins, hydramnios, associated ovarian cysts or fibroids, or even the very full bladder are readily distinguished from each other (Fig. 13).

Using sonar the diagnosis of hydatidiform mole in the abnormally enlarged uterus is easiest of all (see Chapter II).

An ovarian cyst may resemble pregnancy with hydramnios, but careful examination should distinguish the two conditions. There is a well-known story about a London gynaecologist who tried hard and unsuccessfully to induce labour with bougies in a case of ovarian cyst! In my own unit an erstwhile junior colleague diagnosed intrauterine fetal death because of absent fetal heart sounds and because "the head" (actually a loculus of a mucinous cystadenoma) failed to show signs of growth on repeated ultrasonography. After three unrewarding oxytocin induction attempts I took over the case and carried out an uneventful ovarian cystectomy.

An ovarian cyst displaces the uterus and pushes the cervix downwards, whereas in hydramnios the lower segment has to ride above the pelvic brim so that the cervix is consequently drawn up. Obesity may confuse the diagnosis of an ovarian cyst in association with pregnancy by making it difficult to palpate the sulcus between cyst and uterus. Examples of two-dimensional ultrasonograms differentiating causes of undue abdominal enlargement in pregnancy are shown in Fig. 13.

A full bladder may be mistaken for hydramnios, but this mistake is not likely to be made provided the possibility is thought of. Lastly, hydatidiform mole, by causing undue uterine enlargement, may suggest hydramnios, but in this case there is usually some bleeding, the patient is ill, no fetal parts can be ballotted, there is no fluid thrill, and pre-eclamptic toxaemia is more often present.

If the condition is bad enough to warrant treatment, putting the patient to bed is undoubtedly the most important measure. In many cases the excess quantity of liquor appears to diminish as pregnancy advances. Binders have been recommended, but as usual are almost worse than useless and merely increase the patient's misery. It is only when fetal abnormality is present, or in the unusual instances of great severity, that the question of removal of some of the excess liquor arises. As an alternative, labour may be deliberately induced.

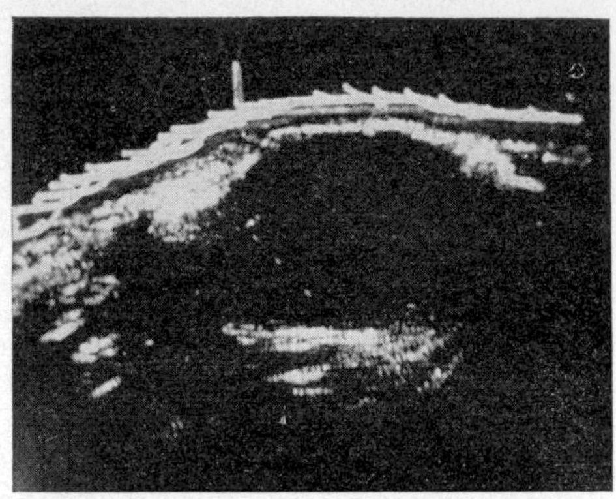

12/Fig. 13 (*a*).—Longitudinal section of abdomen. Umbilicus marked on the surface with a notch. Shows a large ovarian cyst cranialwards (to right) and fetal echoes to the left.

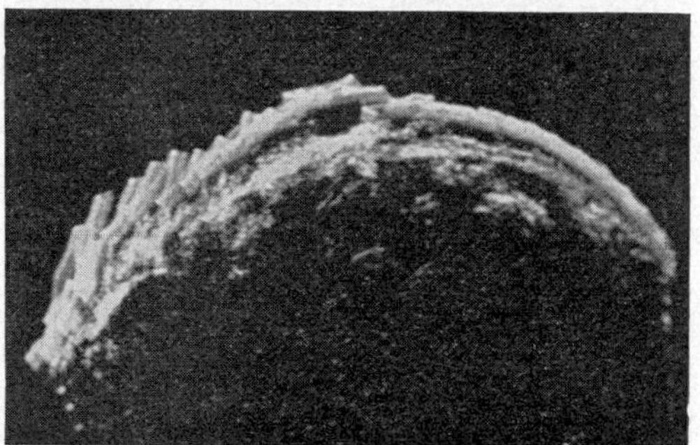

12/Fig. 13 (*b*).—Transverse section of normal though protuberant abdomen. Bowel echoes prevent deeper penetration. Not pregnant.

(By courtesy of the Editor, *Brit. J. Radiol.*)

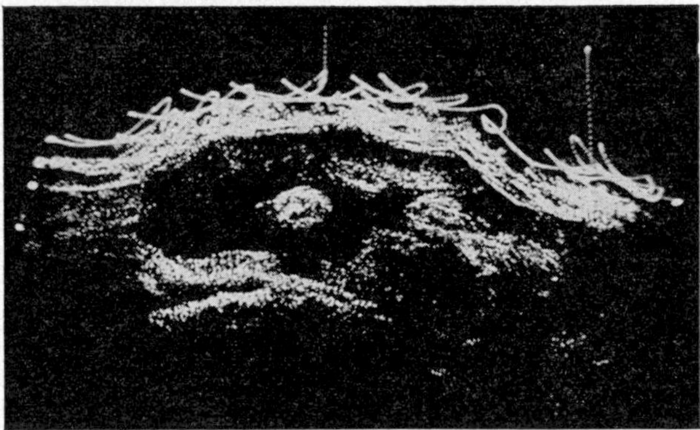

12/Fig. 13 (*c*).—Transverse section of hydramnios. In the centre is a sectional view of the body of an anencephalic fetus. The enormous distension of the amniotic sac is well shown.

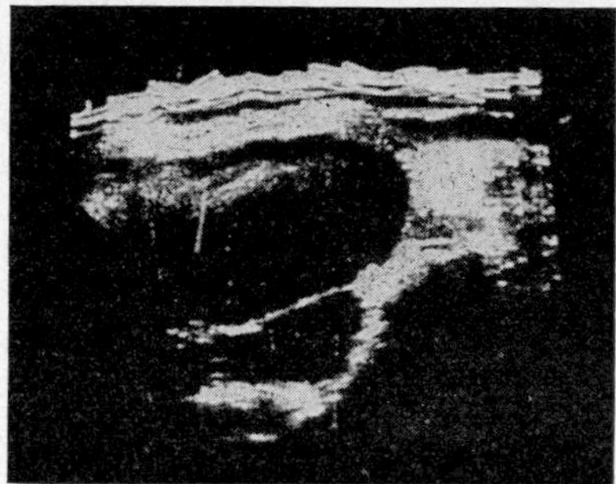

12/FIG. 13 (*d*).—Longitudinal section (cranialwards to the right). Shows very distended bladder with empty, non-gravid, anteverted uterus lying behind it.

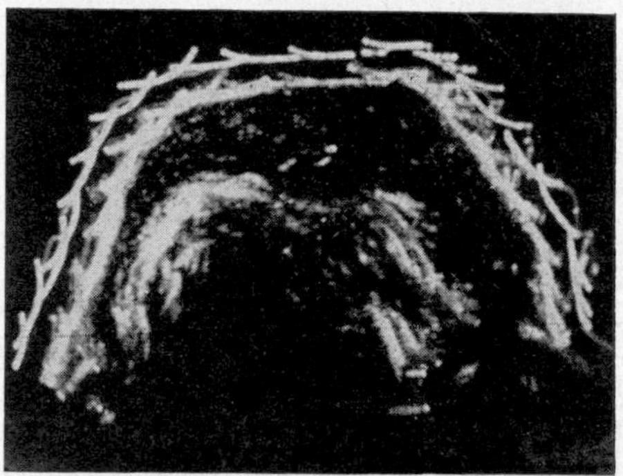

12/FIG. 13 (*e*).—Transverse section of pregnant diabetic uterus at 32 weeks gestation. Shows hydramnios and huge baby. (Caesarean section two weeks later: baby weighed 5·5 kg or 12 lb.)

The trouble about removing liquor is that the amount removed is liable to be quickly replaced, and the onset of labour is more often than not precipitated. One has the alternative choice of tapping through the abdominal wall (after catheterisation) or of performing high puncture of the membranes with a Drew-Smythe catheter, which usually results in accidental forewater amniotomy at the same time. Nowadays we seldom employ amniocentesis without first localising the placenta by ultrasonic placentography.[10] If bloodstained liquor appears, it should be tested for fetal haemoglobin at once (see Chapter III) to identify its source. I recall a case of haemo-amnion due to fetal haemorrhage in which the source was identified by this test and immediate Caesarean section secured a live birth. At operation a lacerated artery was found on the fetal surface of the placenta. It follows, therefore, that radiologically demonstrable fetal abnormality should be ascertained before interfering, Caesarean section in such a case being ruled out.

When draining liquor gradually in a case of hydramnios through a fine needle inserted through the abdominal wall and connected by a length of narrow tubing to a suitably enclosed receptacle to prevent infection, it is often a helpful plan to thread over the tubing and apply to the abdominal wall the tin core of a wide roll of adhesive strapping. This simple device helps to keep the needle in place and at right angles to the abdominal wall. A very safe and gradual decompression can thus be achieved.

If it is decided in any case to induce labour deliberately, high membrane puncture should be performed first, in order to give the presenting part an opportunity to settle into the pelvis before rupturing the forewaters. This simple precaution reduces the chances of the cord prolapsing. Often the forewaters are accidentally ruptured in the process, but an attempt should be made if possible to control the rate of loss since abruptio placentae with severe accidental haemorrhage may follow the sudden release of large quantities of liquor amnii. A late colleague of mine was once reckless enough to rupture the membranes in the patient's own house in a case of gross hydramnios and complained that he put the fire out. When anencephaly is associated with hydramnios there should be no hesitation in inducing labour by artificial rupture of the membranes. These cases do not fail to go into labour provided that the period of gestation is not less than thirty-four weeks. At earlier stages oxytocin infusion or prostaglandins may be required to expedite delivery.

Labour is usually normal, but may be complicated by uterine inertia, in which case hindwater rupture may enable the uterus to operate to better mechanical advantage. The patient should be nursed in bed during the first stage, until it is certain that the presenting part has settled well into the pelvic cavity, and a vaginal examination is indicated as soon as the membranes rupture to exclude the presence of a prolapsed cord. Labour may be complicated by malpresentation in this sort of case, and external version during labour may deal with the situation. Treatment appropriate to the nature of the malpresentation (if any) may be called for.

There is a hazard peculiar to anencephaly which I have personally encountered and which resulted in the death of the mother. As not infrequently happens, labour was postmature. The small "head" went readily through the cervix and provoked very strong expulsive contractions long before full dilatation of the cervix. The baby's body was very large (over 4 kg) with correspondingly wide shoulders which ruptured the lower segment extensively. She completed her own delivery and the first sign of trouble was a brisk postpartum haemorrhage followed immediately by cardiac arrest. Crash transfusion and internal cardiac massage failed after many hours to revive her. This tragedy serves to remind one of the ugly combination of anencephaly and postmaturity especially in the grand multipara.

Lastly, the risk of postpartum haemorrhage, though not as great as in the case of twins, is a very distinct possibility, and ergometrine should be immediately available, if needed, for intravenous injection.

After birth the baby should be tested for oesophageal atresia by the passage of a soft rubber catheter into the stomach. Failure indicates immediate further investigation since the surgical prognosis depends upon prompt recognition.

REFERENCES

1. Begg, H. (1970). *Proc. roy. Soc. Med.*, **63,** 1052.
2. Camilleri, A. P. (1963). *J. Obstet. Gynaec. Brit. Cwlth*, **70,** 258.
3. Campbell, S. and Dewhurst, C. J. (1970). *Lancet*, **1,** 101.
4. Carter, C. O. and Roberts, J. A. F. (1967). *Lancet*, **1,** 306.
5. Charles, D., Jacoby, Hannah, E. and Burgess, Florence (1965). *Amer. J. Obstet. Gynec.*, **93,** 1042.
6. Charles, D. and Jacoby, Hannah E. (1966). *Amer. J. Obstet. Gynec.*, **95,** 266.
7. Donald, I. and Brown, T. G. (1961). *Brit. J. Radiol.*, **34,** 539.
8. Donald, I. (1965). *Amer. J. Obstet. Gynec.*, **93,** 935.
9. Donald, I. (1965). *J. Obstet. Gynaec. Brit. Cwlth*, **72,** 907.
10. Donald, I. and Abdulla, U. (1967). *Brit. J. Radiol.*, **40,** 604.
11. Donald, I. (1974). *Amer. J. Obstet. Gynec.*, **118,** 299.
12. Kerr, M. M. (1959). *Brit. med. J.*, **1,** 902.
13. Liggins, G. C. and Ibbertson, H. K. (1966). *Lancet*, **1,** 114.
14. Lillie, E. W. (1962). *Brit. med. J.*, **1,** 940.
15. Macdonald, R. R. (1962). *Brit. med. J.*, **1,** 518.
16. Renwick, J. W. (1972). *Brit. J. prev. soc. Med.*, **26,** 67.
17. Smith, C., Watt, M., Boyd, A. E. W. and Holmes, J. C. (1973). *Lancet*, **1,** 269.
18. Sunden, B. (1964). *Acta obstet. gynec. scand.*, **43,** Suppl. 6.

CHAPTER XIII

BREECH PRESENTATION

". . . and don't forget, if you find a head which is deeply engaged it may not be there at all."

Irish midwifery tutor

WHEN any part of the fetus other than the vertex presents the case is one of malpresentation. From the baby's point of view, though not the most dangerous, breech is the most common form of malpresentation, of which there are three types, namely the complete breech with both legs flexed, the frank breech with both legs extended, and the footling or half breech in which one of the legs is extended. The frank breech is much more frequently seen in practice and is by far the more usual variety in primigravidae. The complete breech is most likely to be encountered only in the multiparous.

The breech presents in some 2 to 3 per cent of all women at the onset of labour but the incidence varies with the type of institution, its policies towards prophylactic version and the type of patient dealt with. Curiously nevertheless the figure is much the same even in units where prophylactic external version is falling into disuse.[5] The incidence at the Queen Mother's Hospital in 1975 was 2·8 per cent.

Aetiology

This is often a matter for speculation, nevertheless certain facts are significant. For example Vartan long ago pointed out that at 30 weeks gestation the breech presents in one out of every four women examined.[13] Certainly prematurity is associated with a higher incidence of breech presentation. At about 34 weeks the fetus in the majority of cases turns a somersault and the cause of the persistent breech presentation must be something which prevents this spontaneous version. So often in the past the cause has been given as something which prevents engagement of the head in the pelvis, but this is now thought to be unlikely because the head in any case does not normally engage until some time after spontaneous version should have taken place. The oft-quoted and time-honoured conditions such as contracted pelvis and placenta praevia and space-occupying lesions in the pelvis are found in only about 7 per cent of breech presentations, and even by this reckoning the factor of prematurity should be taken into account.

Vartan noted that spontaneous version failed to occur most frequently when the legs were extended. Multiple pregnancy accounts for many instances but no mechanical factor whatever can be found in about quarter of the cases. The presence of a second twin within the uterus naturally can prevent version but the main factor is extended legs which splint the fetal trunk and prevent flexion of the child which is necessary before it can pass the transverse axis of the uterus. The reason for the legs being extended at this time of possible spontaneous version is not yet known although there are plausible explanations. The baby that is presenting as a breech during the last ten weeks of pregnancy is always kicking with its legs and especially where the liquor is scanty it quite suddenly reaches a stage and a size at which it fails to draw back one or both its legs which thereupon remain extended. The resulting breech presentation because of splinting is thereby confirmed. One is reminded of the small child in the habit of putting its head through railings who does it just once too often and one day it finds its head too large to be got back. This theory fits in with the well-known increased frequency of extended legs preventing spontaneous version in the primigravida, especially because of the increased uterine tone in this class of patient. It is submitted that extension of the legs is a fortuitous phenomenon which happens in a small percentage of cases to coincide with failure to achieve spontaneous cephalic version. Certainly extended legs are not often seen in X-rays when the vertex is presenting.

In summary, a breech presentation is found either when the onset of labour is premature or at term when some factor in the past prevented spontaneous version. Of these extended legs and multiple pregnancy are the most important. Nevertheless a proportion cannot be explained. Stephenson however suggested that a cornual fundal insertion of the placenta is responsible in some of these remaining cases and showed by radiology that this type of placental insertion is common in breech presentations. It is an observation which I have not yet made myself by sonar.

The Dangers of Breech Delivery

The frank breech with extended legs forms a very satisfactory wedge-shaped presenting part so that the first stage should never be prolonged and if it is the outlook for successful delivery is greatly worsened. Theoretically the complete breech might cause a more prolonged first stage of labour but this is seldom the case because the patient is usually multiparous and the uterus therefore more efficient. The risks to the mother therefore are mainly those of injudicious treatment.

It is the baby who suffers most. Fetal mortalities have to be corrected for prematurity and fetal abnormalities. It is unlikely that mortality figures quoted by good units will be improved upon in the future and very often these corrected figures, which may vary between 1 and 3 per cent,[4] are influenced not only by the question of maturity but by proper selection of cases allowed to undergo breech delivery. Macerated stillbirths of course should not be included in mortality figures. Caesarean section has undoubtedly influenced present results but compared with a precisely similar series of vertex deliveries breech delivery is still more dangerous for the baby.

Quite apart from mortality the question of morbidity is more significant still. If the validity of Apgar scoring at birth is accepted, then undoubtedly breech deliveries come out of it badly and the hazards of permanent damage have to be reckoned with.[2, 3, 11] The most prominent cause of fresh fetal stillbirth is asphyxia because the head is delivered too slowly. By the time the head enters the pelvis the cord is obstructed. Furthermore placental circulation is likely to have come practically to a stop due to retraction and until the mouth and nose are delivered the baby is unable to breathe. Respiratory attempts can be seen commonly while the baby's mouth and nose are still plastered against the posterior vaginal wall, a sure sign that an airway must be established as soon as possible, at least to the child's mouth. This can sometimes be achieved by the use of the blade of a Sims speculum.

Another common cause of fetal death is intracranial haemorrhage due to the head being delivered too quickly. In normal vertex delivery the head has plenty of time in its passage through the pelvis to undergo a gradual process of moulding. In breech delivery the head must pass through the pelvis in not more than ten minutes and such a speedy passage of the head, even in a normal vertex delivery, can cause death.

Minor degrees of disproportion may not be recognised until too late because the fetal head cannot be used as a clinical pelvimeter.

Prolapse of the cord is not common with breech with extended legs but is quite likely to occur on membrane rupture with the complete breech and should always be sought for by pelvic examination. Apart from asphyxia and intracranial haemorrhage there are other appreciable fetal hazards. For instance the abdominal viscera, particularly the liver, which is badly protected by the thoracic cage at this stage of life, can be damaged by grasping the abdomen, and fractures of the femur and humerus may occur in the course of delivering legs and arms respectively; likewise there may be separation of epiphyses. Two kinds of nerve palsy may also be incurred; the commonest is Erb's palsy, due to traction on the upper elements of the brachial plexus and, less commonly, Klumpke's paralysis, due to extraction efforts to deliver an extended arm. In the case of the male child the fetal gonads may suffer haemorrhage and oedema and there is some current speculation about this as a possible cause of subsequent male infertility.

Antenatal Management

External cephalic version has had a traditional role during the latter weeks of pregnancy. The high fetal mortality of breech delivery in the past encouraged every effort to prevent it by version although this in itself carries a small risk. The risk however is negligible when performed without anaesthesia but when the patient herself is anaesthetised and unable to protect herself against the use of undue force, there is a definite fetal hazard, commonly due to separation of the placenta and consequent antepartum haemorrhage. The purpose of general anaesthesia is to achieve the relaxation necessary in the woman with a muscular and tense abdominal wall. Its purpose is definitely not to permit the use of greater force. We have now practically abandoned the use of version under anaesthesia and prefer to allow the patient to spend some hours in hospital lying quietly, if necessary with the foot of the bed blocked up so as to help disengage the breech. In the case of the anxious patient an intravenous injection of no more than 5 mg of diazepam may be sufficient to achieve the necessary relaxation. Another hazard of external cephalic version is that the patient may go into premature labour and babies may be lost from this cause. It is said that a true knot may be tied in the cord by the operation of external cephalic version, but I do not believe this since it takes more than a 180° turn to tie a knot in any material. Nevertheless it is commonly blamed.

As a general rule the fetus tends to undergo spontaneous version at or before the 34th week of pregnancy and it is my practice only to attempt version as early as 32 weeks if the baby can be turned with very light manipulations in the antenatal clinic, in which case it was probably not necessary anyway. However a more emphatic attempt may justifiably be made at 34 weeks since from now onwards external version is going to become increasingly difficult. Version undertaken at this time, if followed by a recurrence of the malpresentation, is commonly due to failure to complete the turning in the first place. If the patient persists with a breech presentation at the 36th week it is allowable to make a really determined attempt, if necessary with diazepam and an overnight stay in hospital before the operation.

Causes of Failure of External Version

Commonly the baby may have been allowed to grow too large and the liquor may be too scanty to permit version. A deeply engaged breech may also be difficult to disimpact and unless it can be convincingly lifted out towards one or other iliac fossa the chances of successful version are minimal. The difficulties are mainly confined to cases of extended legs due to splinting of the fetal trunk.

Another common source of difficulty is a tight abdominal wall, particularly with an apprehensive patient. In some cases the head is inaccessible under the right costal margin. This is usually in cases in which the baby has been allowed to grow too large. Other causes of failure are obesity, fibroids, and congenital abnormalities of the uterus, for example, septate and subseptate. An unduly short cord is usually included in the list, although I am sceptical about this, but I recognise that the dangers of placental separation are likely to be increased thereby.

Contra-indications to Version

These include all hypertensive states including pre-eclamptic toxaemia because of the risk of abruptio placentae. Likewise any case that has had an antepartum haemorrhage is in danger of further bleeding. If, furthermore, the placenta were known to be praevia in site, as discovered previously by sonar as would be the case in my department, we would consider attempts at version absolutely contra-indicated. Twins not only contra-indicate version but the operation is likely to fail. Where there is hydrocephalus it is most undesirable to perform version because these cases are more easily delivered by the breech than by any other method since perforating the after-coming head is such an easy operation.

A history of previous Caesarean section raises a debatable issue. If such a scar is unable to withstand version it would probably be unable to withstand subsequent labour in any case, but where puerperal convalescence had been perfectly normal following section version is safe, provided the operation can be carried out easily.

If there is the slightest doubt about the diagnosis of the presentation or the presence or otherwise of hydrocephalus, the case must be more fully examined, nowadays preferably by sonar which will confirm the malpresentation and also give an indication of the head size, but in units not so equipped an X-ray photograph may be necessary. Needless to say this examination should be undertaken as late as possible before the attempted version. Fibroids are commonly mistaken for fetal heads and vice versa, especially by the inexperienced and those seeing the patient for the first time. Many years ago one of our residents spent an unprofitable part of a morning trying to perform external version on a fundal myoma.

Apart from the onset of premature labour the fetus itself may show signs of stress with slowing of the fetal heart, especially if much force has been used. Having completed version and heard an irregular, slow fetal heart, it is commonly taught that the fetus should be immediately reverted to its original malpresentation, although personally I have never done this but have waited anxiously for a few minutes and observed the fetal heart recover spontaneously.

Much more sinister is antepartum haemorrhage, and an examination should always be made between the patient's legs before allowing her to leave the couch.

Technique of External Cephalic Version

It is often a good plan, if the slightest difficulty is encountered, to tip the head downwards to about 15° of Trendelenburg's position. This helps to disimpact the deeply engaged frank breech. Some people favour vaginal manipulations to help push it out of the pelvis although we seldom resort to this nowadays. Powder is now sprinkled over the abdominal wall because otherwise the mother's skin can get very red and sore in the course of the operation. With the woman in this position and as relaxed as possible and with full explanation and reassurance the breech is pushed with the right hand into the iliac fossa which has been occupied by the fetal back. In other words it is best to turn with the fetus head first, following its own nose. With the left hand the head is sought and gently pressed towards the other hand in order to flex the whole body. All movements should be gentle and unhurried and, furthermore, sustained. The transverse axis of the uterus is nearly always shorter than the crown-rump length of the fetus, therefore flexion is essential and this is where extended legs may defeat one.

In cases of difficulty it is a very good plan to get a second pair of hands on the job, so that steady pressure can be maintained on one or other pole of the baby waiting for a spontaneous kick on the baby's part which will often greatly assist rotation. The important thing is not to allow the breech to re-engage in the pelvis which will defeat the whole exercise. Once past the transverse diameter of the uterus the baby will take up a cephalic presentation with very little further manipulation but it is nearly always impossible to push the head into the pelvis at this stage because the lower uterine segment is not yet ready to accommodate it and furthermore the head is not yet sufficiently flexed. The patient should, of course, be seen in a week to make sure that the malpresentation has not recurred.

The fetal heartbeat should be counted after completion of the version as already mentioned. The possibility of a short cord as the cause of fetal bradycardia, although it cannot be confirmed at the time, might be a reasonable encouragement to restore the malpresentation, but it would take at least several minutes of fetal heartbeats below 100 per minute without any sign of recovery to convince me of the need for it.

If bleeding should be provoked, the patient must be kept on the couch until transferred to a stretcher, admitted forthwith and treated as a case of antepartum haemorrhage with all the usual precautions.

If the above technique fails an attempt to rotate the baby in the opposite direction may succeed. But it is usually fairly clear by the time two attempts have failed that it is useless to persist, nor is it particularly kind, and the patient should be seen in a week's time. Commonly the baby will have "taken the hint" and will now present by the vertex without further ado. If any abdominal pain is encountered, the patient should be detained in hospital under observation. Uterine rupture is most unlikely in a primigravida but the possibility of a small retroplacental haematoma has to be borne in mind. Twenty-five years ago it was common to undertake cephalic version at least once in the course of an antenatal clinic but nowadays a more conservative attitude is maintained. Breech delivery is no longer as hazardous to the fetus as formerly because even in the case of the multipara the task is less and less left to the inexperienced and there is good case selection.

There is a considerable failure rate to version under anaesthesia and the fetal mortality is by no means negligible (1 per cent) but while the patient is still under the influence of an anaesthetic a very comprehensive assessment of the capacity of the maternal pelvis should be made since any question of even minor disproportion will modify one's attitude in favour of Caesarean section.

X-ray pelvimetry is now out of fashion because of the known ionising hazard to the mother and also to the fetus since its gonads will be in the line of fire, hence the importance of a very sound clinical examination. However, we attach increasing importance to ultrasonic cephalometry. Naturally the multipara with a history of rapid and normal delivery of a good-sized baby may put the size of her pelvis beyond question, but otherwise my preference is to observe the growth of the fetal biparietal diameter and as soon as it reaches 9·5 cm to consider delivery by induction of labour. The hazards progressively mount as the head enlarges beyond this point and I would only be discouraged from inducing labour by the unlikely presence of a very adverse lecithin:sphingomyelin ratio. In this event it might be preferable to allow the baby to continue growing *in utero* and to deliver by Caesarean section as an elective procedure.

The fetal prognosis is inversely related to fetal birth weight and even more to fetal head size. The combination of postmaturity, scanty liquor and a large baby is nowadays unacceptable for breech delivery.

Management of Breech Delivery

The fresh stillbirth rate in breech delivery has fallen to its present low levels thanks not only to better and more experienced management but also to the greater use of Caesarean section wherever there are combined indications even of the most slender sort; for example, a maternal age in the late thirties, a bad obstetric history or any suspicion of even minor disproportion. Consequently the Caesarean section rate in breech presentations may be as high as 30 per cent; in our case 50 per cent in 1975.

The number of primiparae and multiparae were approximately the same, 37 and 39 respectively.

I was surprised to find so high an incidence of Caesarean section in breech presentation in our own hospital and I am therefore very grateful to Dr M. S. Mehta, one of the junior members of my staff, for his analysis of a year's results (1975). Out of a total of 76 breech presentations, no less than 38 (50 per cent) were delivered by Caesarean section and of these the indications were often multiple.

Associated conditions leading to delivery by Caesarean section

Small pelvis	4
Maternal age above 30, and primigravid	4
Hypertension	3
Previous Caesarean section	4
Bad obstetric history	3
Intra-uterine growth retardation	2
Cord prolapse	1
Prolonged 1st stage	2
Previous cervical tear	1
Bicornuate uterus	2
Purposes of sterilisation (a doubtful indication)	1
	27

It will be noticed that out of these cases three required Caesarean section because labour developed complications.

Elective Caesarean section had, as can be seen, already been decided on in 24 cases because of more than one indication, but spontaneous labour began in 45 cases and labour was surgically induced in seven.

The policy may sound radical but the results speak for themselves. There were only seven stillbirths and no neonatal deaths, yielding a total perinatal mortality of 9·2 per cent uncorrected. Of these seven stillbirths, two were grossly premature, two had congenital fetal abnormalities, one was grossly affected with Rh haemolytic disease, one was macerated, and one was associated with abruptio placentae, so it can be seen that there were no unavoidable perinatal disasters in this series. It is felt therefore that this analysis gives us no cause to regret our policy.

Birth weights in excess of 3 kg confer no advantage whatsoever on the baby delivered by the breech, even if the pelvis is normal, and as the birth weight rises, so the mortality goes up by leaps and bounds, hence our enthusiasm for meticulous monitoring by sonar antenatally, which may indicate induction at or before term in some cases.

The best method of induction is by rupture of the forewaters, combined with an oxytocin drip. There is no danger of prolapse of the cord with extended breech presentations any more than with a well-applied vertex but the complete breech may more easily allow the cord to prolapse. Prolapse of the cord indicates immediate delivery by Caesarean section, hence it is our policy always to carry out amniotomy in one of our operating theatres fully equipped with the necessary pre-sterilised packs of instruments.

With proper monitoring as to fetal head size, mistakes about maturity should not occur and the remaining risk from now on is that of a prolonged inert labour with the added hazard of mounting infection. This is a situation which is no longer tolerated and it is best to cut one's losses and deliver by Caesarean section in that event.

The first stage of labour is managed normally. Any first stage of desultory labour lasting more than 20 hours is likely to end up in a hazardous situation with a larger baby than anticipated, or a smaller pelvis, and the penalty of an asphyxiated and possibly damaged child. Trial of labour in breech presentation is not and cannot be a trial of the passage of the fetal head through the pelvis since the answer would come too late, but is really a trial of uterine action, and any sign of uterine dysfunction should alert one to the need for abdominal delivery before it is too late.

There is often difficulty in knowing when a woman enters the second stage since the pointed breech may protrude some distance through a cervix insufficiently dilated to allow the head to pass later. We regard it as prudent therefore never to consider that the second stage has started until the anterior buttock is well and truly visible. In the case of a male fetus the scrotum may be so oedematous that it presents at the vulva some time before full dilatation and I have known a colleague, senior to myself, diagnose ruptured uterus on the strength of this since the halves of the scrotum felt like prolapsed intestine. To the great merriment of the chief, who was summoned urgently, the buttocks were delivered spontaneously just as the patient was being moved to the operating theatre.

Premature diagnosis of full dilatation leading to attempts to deliver the baby through an incompletely dilated cervix will lead not only to extended arms but also to difficulty in delivery of the head. This is the commonest fault in breech delivery. While the fetal condition remains good, the longer one can put off intervention the better. If the onset of labour has been spontaneous there is little to be gained by rupturing the membranes before at least half dilatation, by which time the uterus is likely to continue to behave itself properly, but it is a particular moment to watch out for prolapse of the cord and careful preliminary vaginal examination should be undertaken through the forewaters to exclude cord presentation.

An anaesthetist should always be present during the second stage of labour and when this point has unquestionably been reached the woman is encouraged to make voluntary expulsive efforts in any position most comfortable to herself. She should not be put into the lithotomy position until the posterior buttock is seen to be distending the perineum. Now during a contraction, the breech will be seen to be making its characteristic "climb up the perineum". This is the time for performing episiotomy. It should be undertaken in all primigravid and most multigravid breech deliveries, firstly because it eliminates the obstruction caused by the perineum and thus straightens the curve of the birth canal through which the fetal trunk has to bend before it can be delivered and secondly because during delivery of the head much of the pressure acting upon it is eliminated. Episiotomy should not be deferred until later mainly because if further manipulations become necessary during delivery they are usually needed quickly and to carry out episiotomy at this time is highly inconvenient and sometimes difficult. Putting the hand through the vulva when the fetal trunk is already occupying the orifice will almost certainly result in any ugly tear. Episiotomy is always done after infiltration with local anaesthetic although our preference is for a formal pudendal block since the latter will allow manipulations if necessary at a higher level in the vagina.

With the performance of episiotomy the breech will now begin to pass through the outlet, usually "climbing up" to a lesser extent. Nothing at this stage should be done to help it, nor should any attempt be made to disentangle the legs until at least the umbilicus is seen. Now is the time for real self control.

When the umbilicus is born it is permissible for the first time to touch the child, disengage its extended legs and pull down a loop of cord which may be on quite a stretch. The body now tends to flop downwards and the back, up to now facing obliquely, should be encouraged to look directly upwards. It is most important never to allow the ventral surface of a child's body to turn upwards at this stage or urgent corrective manipulations will have to be undertaken. During this part of delivery the midwife should have her hand on the fundus of the uterus, not only to notice the presence of each contraction but to follow the descent of the head, and by keeping a slight but steady pressure on the uterine fundus she may help thereby to prevent extension of the arms.

The points of the scapulae of the baby will presently be visible and this is the time, and not before, to look for the presence of arms folded across the chest. Normally they will be found there and can be easily flipped out at this stage. With the bearing down effort from the mother the child is now born to its neck.

The head has not yet entered the pelvis but from now on it will do so and compress the umbilical cord. From this point not more than ten minutes should elapse before the child is in a position to breathe. Conversely it is important not to hurry the passage of the head through the pelvis. There is a very natural temptation to employ the jaw flexion and shoulder traction manoeuvre variously described by Mauriceau, Smellie and Veit to draw the head into flexion and thus through the brim of the pelvis but this should not be necessary in the presence of progressive descent. In any case if this manoeuvre has to be used it is better to press the fingers on the facial maxillae of the baby than on its possibly limp jaw in order to increase flexion of the head.

The more usual method described by Burns is to allow the baby to hang by its own weight from the vulva, the woman being in the lithotomy position. This in itself will encourage flexion of the head and the body is seen to drop slowly, aided if necessary by some suprapubic pressure to help its descent.

Failure of the head to descend usually means that one has misjudged the case and it is larger than anticipated or it has become seriously deflexed, in which case the Mauriceau-Smellie-Veit type of manoeuvre may be employed to encourage the head to enter the pelvis in the transverse diameter where there is more room for it and then to assist delivery after the head has properly entered the pelvis and with the occiput now facing forwards.

The delivery of the head should not be attempted until the nape of the child's neck becomes visible, as indicated by the hairs of the fetal scalp. The obstetrician, now standing with his back to the patient's left leg, takes the child's legs in his right hand. Then, exerting a firm outward force he draws the child over the maternal pubis, the fetal head being finally delivered by movement of flexion. The left hand of the obstetrician must be used to guard the perineum and at the same time prevent the head from emerging too quickly. As soon as the mouth and nose of the baby are free, the baby can now breathe and it is a good plan to pause while the suction apparatus clears the airways to remove debris from nose and mouth. The head from now on should be delivered slowly and carefully (Fig. 1).

The position of the obstetrician described prevents the use of undue force while swinging the baby up over the mother's abdomen. Nevertheless it is necessary to pull the child outwards a little in order to encourage flexion and for the head instead of the neck to pivot, as it should, on the underside of the pubis. Failure of this manoeuvre

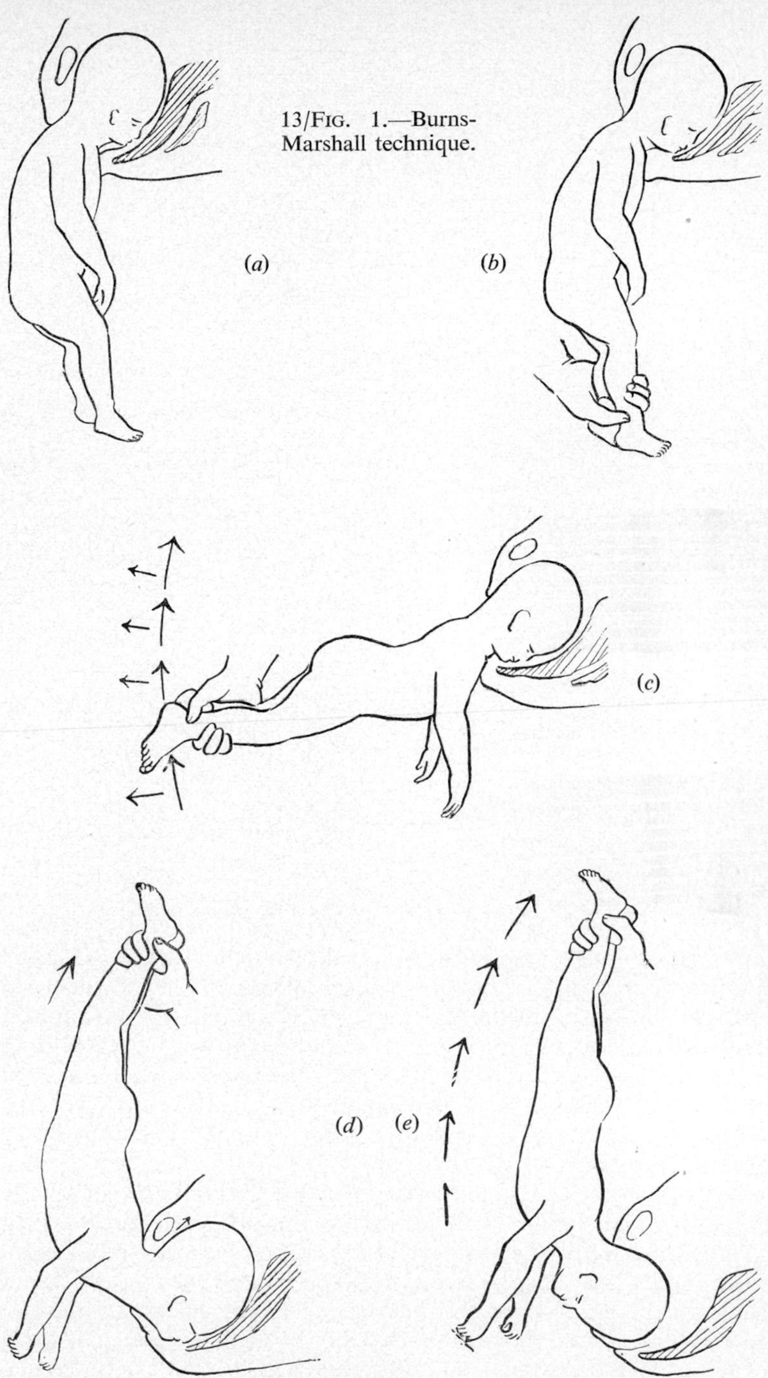

13/Fig. 1.—Burns-Marshall technique.

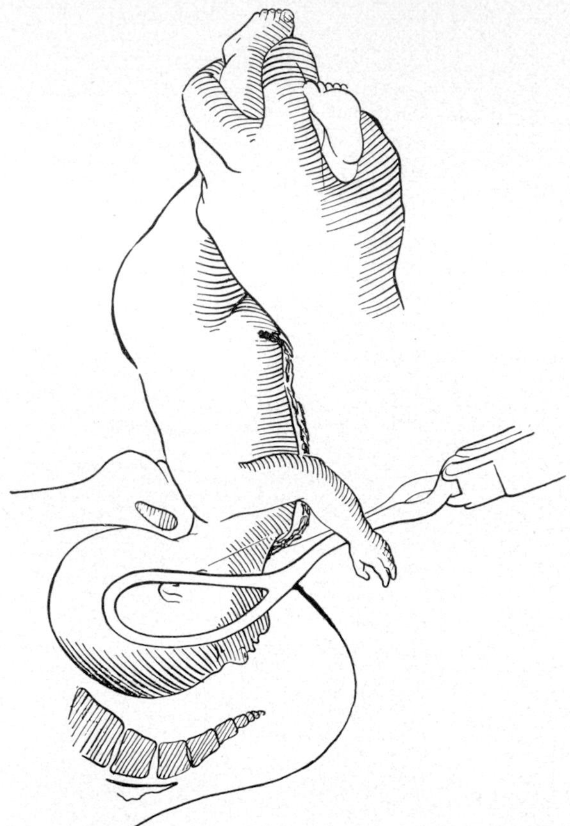

13/Fig. 2.—Forceps applied to the aftercoming head.

with inability to get at least the mouth and nose into the fresh air will find one now with less time in which to deliver the head safely and either a Mauriceau-Smellie-Veit manoeuvre or preferably the application of forceps will be required. If anaesthesia is needed it will have to be supplied quickly, hence the need for having an anaesthetist present in the second stage. The patient at this stage is unlikely to be very co-operative and the rapid induction of anaesthesia may make all the difference.

Delivery of the aftercoming head which does not come simply by the Burns manoeuvre as described is best achieved with forceps which can control the delivery. Instruments such as the Wrigley short forceps may relieve some of the pressure from the fetal head. However this necessitates another pair of hands unless the midwife guarding the fundus can also hold the baby's legs (Fig. 2). The body of the child however should not be lifted higher than necessary to apply the forceps as this encourages extension of the head in the birth canal. Of our 38 cases delivered *per vaginam* the forceps was applied to the aftercoming head in six (16 per cent).

Alternative Bracht Method of Delivery

This has been well described by Jotkowitz and Picton.[6] The difference here is that the mother is not put in the lithotomy position but remains in the dorsal position. As soon as the fetal sacrum rotates to the anterior position the downward pull of gravity on the baby's trunk is prevented by grasping each side of the baby's pelvic girdle with the thumbs over the backs of its thighs and assisting the full extension of the fetal spine at the delivery of the arms, aided by moderate suprapubic pressure. At this point the head will have entered the pelvis and, maintaining this attitude of extreme extension of the fetal trunk, the head, protected by forceps if possible, is delivered through the outlet as before. This technique can of course be used with the patient in the lithotomy position as long as the principle of resisting the downward pull of gravity is maintained, the baby being allowed to arch up over the maternal symphysis pubis by uterine and maternal forces. The difference here, be it noted, is that there is no leaving the baby to hang downwards by its neck until the hairline at the nape is visible.

The Third Stage

This is usually very quick in breech delivery and often the placenta comes out on top of the baby's head. In other respects the rules of conduct in the third stage are applied as usual.

Complications During Breech Delivery

Delay in Descent of the Breech

In the past this has been attributed to inability of the extended breech to undergo the lateral flexion of the trunk necessary to negotiate the curvature of the birth canal. This however is a rare phenomenon in the absence of disproportion. In the ugly event of the extended breech failing to descend properly into the pelvis until the anterior buttock becomes visible, full dilatation having unquestionably occurred, one is likely to be faced with the problem of an oversized baby. The curvature of the human birth canal can to some extent be eliminated by episiotomy but I am very distrustful of the breech that fails properly to descend. In the old days under general anaesthesia it was common practice to disimpact the breech and, as the old phrase went, "break it up" by inserting the hand, following the anterior thigh up to the knee, and then down to the appropriate ankle and pulling down a leg. This kind of veterinary procedure naturally carried a high fetal mortality. It may help to insinuate a finger into the anterior groin or preferably both groins and exert gentle traction but this can be very difficult with a large baby since it is hard to get the finger between the anterior aspect of the child's thigh and the abdominal wall. Traction anyway by this method is likely to encourage separation of an epiphysis. The use of the breech hook is all very well in the case of a child known to be dead but if used on a living child is almost certain to inflict serious injury, which however is still preferable to a fresh stillbirth. Such an instrument is seldom likely to be available on the rare occasion when one might want it.

Pulling down a leg, preferably the anterior, is not as easy as it sounds with a large baby and a smallish pelvis and considerable force may sometimes be necessary to reach the ankle before exerting traction. The situation of course is different in the case of delivering a second twin with membranes freshly ruptured and plenty of room. The difficulty about bringing down the anterior leg of the fetus in the kind of case here being described, and which in any event would have been better delivered by Caesarean section, is that the anterior buttock must be pushed up to the level of the top of the symphysis pubis before the popliteal fossa can be properly reached, the leg flexed and the foot slowly extracted in order to bring the thigh down through the pelvis. Only one leg needs to be brought down in this kind of case and the delivery proceeds as a breech extraction. This kind of delivery is only permissible in situations where facilities for Caesarean section do not exist.

Extended Arms

When the umbilicus is born and the fetal back has rotated upwards a finger can be passed up the posterior vaginal wall looking for the arms across the chest, in which case they can be flipped out very easily, but if they cannot so be found it can be assumed that they are extended and no time should be lost in bringing them down. Preferably an anaesthetic should be rapidly induced and the body of the fetus is pulled to the side opposite to what was its posterior arm and slightly upwards. The operator's hand (the episiotomy having long since been made) can now pass up the child's body to reach the shoulder and then the fingers work along the arm to the crook of the elbow. Flexion of the elbow can thus be produced and the arm brought down in front of the face of the baby. A similar procedure can now be carried out on the other side, but it is vital that no traction be employed until the elbow has been reached and properly flexed; otherwise the humerus is likely to be fractured. It is easier to go for the posterior arm first as there is more room in the hollow of the sacrum. This is the old and traditional method and one which I recall with considerable distaste because with a large baby and a small pelvis there is little enough room for the fetal thorax and the hand in the cavity of the pelvis at the same time. Nuchal displacement of the arm is very rare but this is dealt with by rotating the fetus towards that arm, which helps to sweep it across the baby's own face whence it can be brought down. I always used to preach that failure to bring down arms in the absence of disproportion was usually due to timidity but the need for brutish activity has largely been replaced now by the Løvset manoeuvre.

Løvset Manoeuvre

In 1937 Løvset described a method of dealing with extended arms which does not entail so much manipulation nor necessarily an anaesthetic. He pointed out that the posterior shoulder will be below the promontory of the sacrum when the anterior shoulder is above the symphysis pubis. Therefore, when the inferior angle of the anterior scapula is seen the baby is pulled gently downwards and at the same time rotated so that the back looks upwards, and the rotation is continued so that the posterior shoulder turns and, being in the pelvis already, is seen under the symphysis pubis. Turning the child in the opposite direction will now bring the erstwhile anterior shoulder under the symphysis pubis. The technique is seen in the accompanying sketches. It is easy to learn and works where the arm is extended or nuchally displaced. Similarly it can be used if disproportion is such that manual manipulations are difficult. Løvset claimed that he had no failures[7] (Fig. 3).

Difficulty in Descent of the Head

This can only be due to disproportion, if flexion is encouraged as already suggested. Having got into this uncomfortable situation the obstetrician can now only resort to brute force. Either the head can be drawn into the pelvis by strong jaw and shoulder traction (or preferably the jaw pressure being replaced by pressure on the fetal maxillary bones) or the forceps can be applied to the head above the pelvic brim. The latter is very bad practice. If the head cannot be made to enter the brim then almost certainly the baby will by now be dead and the best treatment is perforation. In fact the impossibility of adequate treatment at this stage, if the head is too big for the pelvis, makes us even more likely to ensure that disproportion is not present before embarking on a breech delivery.

Almost as a corollary it follows that breech presentation is easily the most favourable method of delivery in cases of hydrocephaly because the aftercoming head is so easily deflated. Unfortunately the diagnosis cannot be made with certainty as a general rule in vertex presentations in time to undertake external podalic version. Internal podalic version with a large hydrocephalus in order to secure,

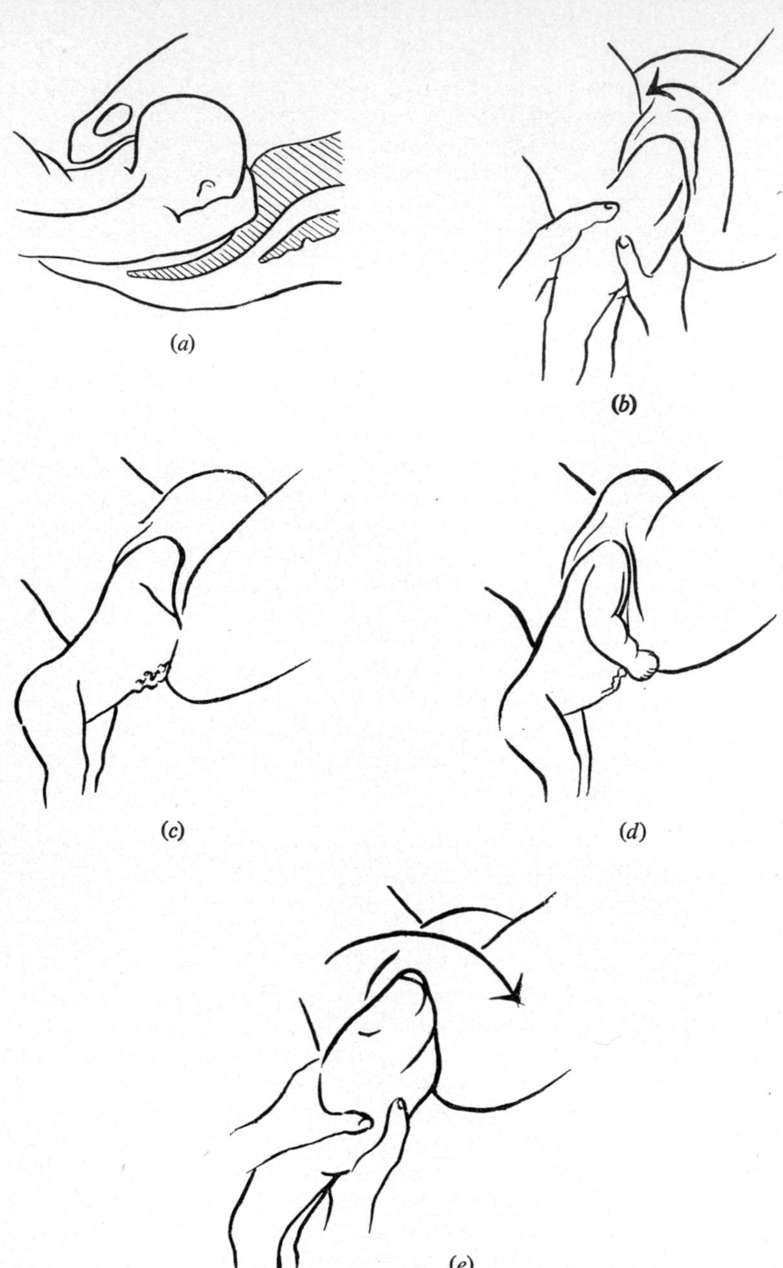

13/Fig. 3.—Løvset manoeuvre.
(Figs. 1–3 drawn by Miss Pat Burrows, and by courtesy of the Editor, *J. Obstet. Gynaec. Brit. Emp.*)

hopefully, an easy breech delivery can easily result in a ruptured uterus as I have found to my own cost. Where the baby is dead and the after-coming head is too large to remove safely without undue force, the delivery is proceeded with until the body and arms are delivered. The body is then pulled down and a transverse incision is made over the highest available cervical spine of the fetus. A straight metal catheter can then be introduced into the spinal canal and thrust through the foramen magnum to drain the excess cerebrospinal fluid. This operation is made much easier if a spina bifida is present which is often the case. After deflation of the hydrocephalic head delivery is quickly completed. Perforation through the occiput is also an easy operation.

It is true that some authorities now favour a little more traction in the delivery of a breech presentation as against the policy of non-intervention preached above. The results are so good that they cannot be ignored and obviously the important factor is the experience of the operator. This is, however, a different thing from breech extraction which Macafee (1956) insisted was dangerous and only to be done if absolutely necessary.

Finally it is noteworthy that in published series of breech mortality the figure in the case of the multiparous is sometimes as bad as that in primigravidae. It is felt that until recent years too casual a view was taken of the safety of breech delivery even for the experienced multipara. Here too experience counts.

REFERENCES

1. Burns, J. W. (1934). *J. Obstet. Gynaec. Brit. Emp.*, **41,** 923.
2. Dalrymple, I. J. (1965). *Clinical Report, Rotunda Hospital, Dublin*, **20.**
3. Donald, I. (1966). *Proc. roy. Soc. Med.*, **59,** 184.
4. Hall, J. E., *et al.* (1965). *Amer. J. Obstet. Gynec.*, **91,** 665.
5. Hay, D. (1959). *J. Obstet. Gynaec. Brit. Emp.*, **66,** 529.
6. Jotkowitz, M. W. and Picton, F. C. R. (1970). *Aust. N.Z. J. Obstet. Gynaec.*, **10,** 151.
7. Løvset, J. (1937). *J. Obstet. Gynaec. Brit. Emp.*, **44,** 696.
8. Macafee, C. H. G. (1956). *Med. Press*, **236,** 268.
9. Marshall, C. McI. (1934). *J. Obstet. Gynaec. Brit. Emp.*, **41,** 930.
10. Stevenson, C. S. (1951). *Amer. J. Obstet. Gynec.*, **62,** 488.
11. Todd, W. D. *et al.* (1963). *Obstet. and Gynec.*, **22,** 583.
12. Vartan, C. K. (1940). *Lancet*, **1,** 595.
13. Vartan, C. K. (1945). *J. Obstet. Gynaec. Brit. Emp.*, **52,** 417.

CHAPTER XIV

FACE AND BROW PRESENTATION SHOULDER PRESENTATION PROLAPSE OF THE CORD

THE other malpresentations consist of face, brow and shoulder. Stories of "neck presentation" following avulsion of the head are more apocryphal than real. In fact I only know of one instance and that was in the case of an extremely macerated fetus.

Most are agreed that disproportion under one guise or another is the most important aetiological factor.[3] Face and brow presentations occur often as the end result of a posterior position of the occiput in a borderline pelvis, and mento-anterior positions are at least as common as mento-posterior positions. The cause is a mechanical one in which deflexion already present is increased by uterine action pushing from above while the occiput is prevented from descending into the pelvis. This mechanism certainly occurs in a flat pelvis, especially if the fetal back is to the right and the uterus has its usual inclination to the right. In such cases the head pivots on its parietal eminences and extension results. When the malpresentation by this mechanism occurs in the course of labour it is said to be secondary, whereas when it is present before the onset of labour it is classed as primary.

Even when the occiput is anterior in position the presentation may become a brow or a face by a similar mechanism of extension when there is disproportion either from an unduly large baby or a contracted pelvis.

Shoulder presentations which are the end result of a persistent oblique or transverse lie of the fetus may represent an extreme result of inability of the head, or even the breech, to engage in the pelvis due to gross mechanical factors such as an extremely contracted or deformed pelvis or a very large child. At the other end of the scale gross degrees of prematurity may favour any sort of malpresentation.

Not only is disproportion a possible cause of malpresentation in general but the same is true of multiparity because of the lack of abdominal wall tone. I can personally recall the treacherous case of a multiparous woman with only a minor degree of contracted pelvis who developed an unsuspected brow presentation and in labour the first indication of trouble was a rising pulse rate whereupon it suddenly became apparent that she had ruptured her uterus, without any of the traditional warning signs. Shock was extreme and she did not survive. Multiparity in association with malpresentation cannot be taken lightly, especially in the case having tumultuous contractions.

Another cause of malpresentation is hydramnios, which, as in the case of prematurity, allows undue mobility of the fetus.

Both face and brow presentations raise the possibility of an associated fetal abnormality which should be sought for by radiography (Fig. 1). An anencephalic fetus can only present by the face if the head is the lower presenting pole. Tumours of the anterior aspect of the fetal neck may, on rare occasions, cause a primary face presentation (Fig. 2) and it is said that coils of cord round the neck may cause extension of the head to a brow or face presentation. A dead and macerated fetus may be so flaccid that any malpresentation can occur.

The site of insertion of the placenta may have a considerable effect on the presentation of the fetus.[8, 9] This may alter the shape of the amniotic cavity in such a way that an oblique or transverse lie results (Fig. 3). Even more serious is when the placenta which is praevia prevents engagement of a fetal pole as a presenting part and causes a transverse or oblique lie. This is particularly liable to occur in multiparae and is an indication nowadays for Caesarean section rather than the traditional haemorrhagic procedures of long ago such as bipolar podalic version. I have never used this except in cases of obvious previability. The same may apply when the fetus is already dead and therefore there are no fetal interests to consider. In such cases one's primary concern is the treatment of maternal haemorrhage.

The septate or subseptate uterus can be a cause of transverse lie especially to be thought of in the primigravida who so presents, the head lying in one half of the uterus and the breech in the other.

The multipara who demonstrates delay in labour with a high presenting part in spite of apparently good uterine contractions should always be suspected of having either an undiagnosed brow presentation or some fetal abnormality.

In more than half the cases of face and brow presentation none of the simple explanations given above apply and it is thought that many of these are primary cases, being present before the onset of labour with no exciting cause. Long ago Gibberd pointed out that the uterus cannot, by its constraining walls, have much effect on fetal attitude, as well-flexed babies are frequently seen in cases even of gross hydramnios. Therefore, the tone of the fetal muscles must be responsible for the position and attitude of the baby *in utero* and this depends particularly on the balance between flexor and extensor muscle tone. Gibberd considered that a primary face or brow presentation can result from excessive extensor tone and this tone could come on and pass off at odd times during pregnancy. Consequently

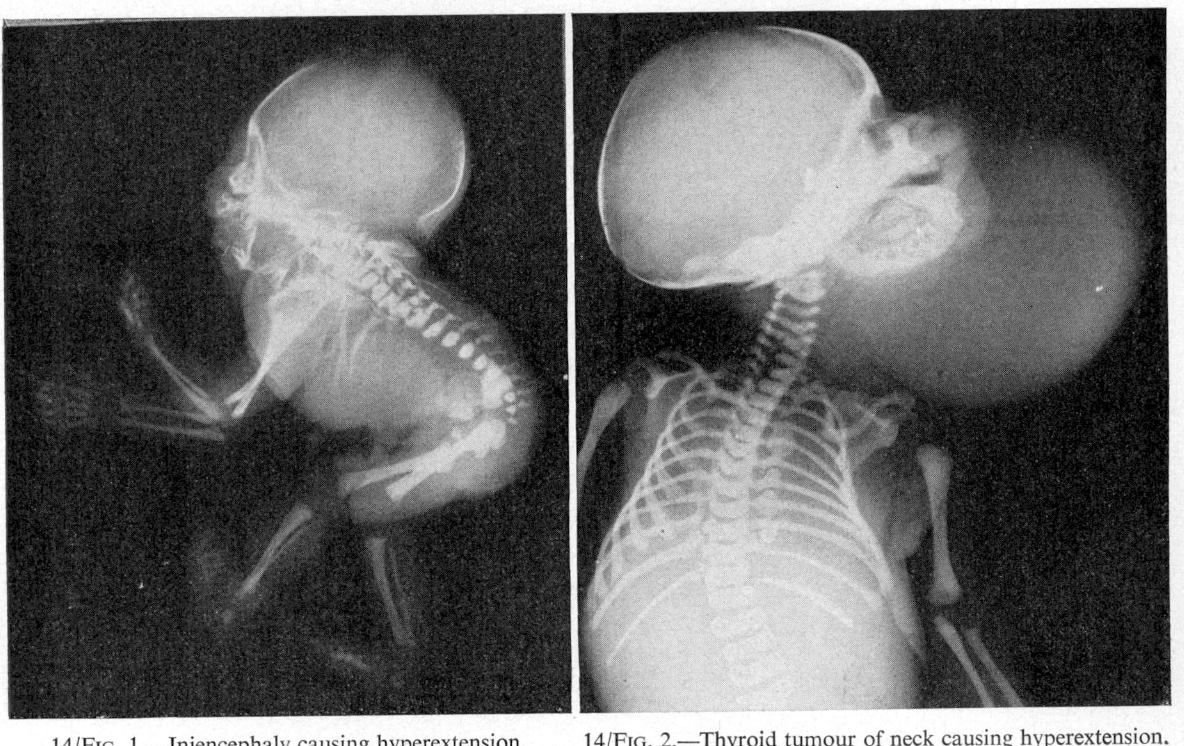

14/FIG. 1.—Iniencephaly causing hyperextension. 14/FIG. 2.—Thyroid tumour of neck causing hyperextension.
(Figs. 1 and 2 by courtesy of Dr Ellis Barnett.)

in many cases it is unrecognised. In others an X-ray photograph may show an obvious face presentation before labour and yet the child be delivered normally as a vertex presentation. In other words the excess extensor tone has passed off. In some cases the extensor tone persists even after delivery and may take several days to disappear.

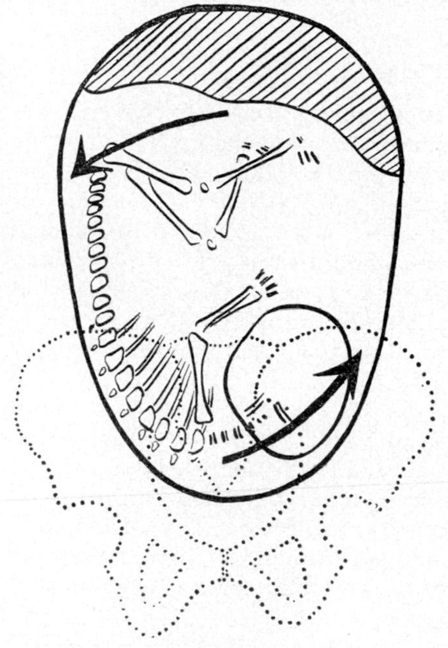

14/Fig. 3.—Aetiology of oblique lie. (By courtesy of Dr C. S. Stevenson and the Editor, *Amer. J. Obstet. Gynec.*)

Labour

As a general rule the untreated case with a malpresentation tends to face a long labour unless grossly premature. In the case of persistent mento-posterior position and brow presentations with a normal-sized baby such cases cannot in fact deliver themselves, and likewise, delivery is not possible with an unreduced shoulder presentation in a baby that has reached viable size.

Even however in cases of mento-anterior position, which is much more favourable, the second stage of labour is likely to be especially prolonged. The cause of the malpresentation of course may increase the length of labour in its own right. The membranes usually rupture early in labour and this is a moment when a vaginal examination must be immediately undertaken because of the very strong likelihood of prolapse of the cord.

As long as the membranes remain intact one has time to make up one's mind how to deal with the case or to observe what happens, and everything therefore is done to preserve the membranes intact. To this end the patient is kept in bed during the first stage of labour and in the favourable type of case malpresentation may correct itself spontaneously. Much will depend upon the relative size of the baby and the maternal pelvis as well as uterine activity.

Provided the case has been properly assessed, and in our view this would include sonar localisation of the placenta, one can afford to adopt a wait-and-see policy until the membranes rupture. Thereafter one may have to be prepared to act fairly quickly and should be in a position to do so. In other words operating facilities must be at hand.

Alas, all too frequently the malpresentation is only found during labour; in fact it may have occurred during labour itself and this is particularly true of the treacherous brow presentation.

FACE PRESENTATION

The incidence is said to be about one in every 600 deliveries but the real bulk is made up of anencephalic fetuses. According to the most recent analysis by my colleague Dr Mehta, for 1975 in the Queen Mother's Hospital the incidence was one in 445, one-third of which were delivered spontaneously, another third by manual rotation and forceps extraction, and the remaining third by Caesarean section. The condition is not dangerous provided it is recognised and appropriately treated. Perinatal mortality is of course most heavily influenced by the associated incidence of prematurity and anencephaly or other fetal abnormality.

There should be no hesitation in carrying out intrapartum radiography when in doubt, not only to assess the severity of deflection, etc., but also, and more important still, to exclude fetal abnormality, since the performance of Caesarean section only to produce a monster child is hardly good obstetric practice. Incidentally good quality X-rays may demonstrate visible calcification in thyroid tumours causing primary face presentation. The fetal spine should be very carefully scrutinised for signs of defect.

Diagnosis

It is not easy to recognise a face presentation by abdominal palpation alone. It is said that the marked protuberance of the occiput on the same side as the fetal back strongly suggests the diagnosis, but often, in fact more usually, the fetal chest in its attitude of hypertension is mistaken for the back. More often than not the diagnosis becomes obvious only on radiography because of an extremely deep and palpable sulcus between occiput and fetal back (Fig. 4). Vaginal examination in labour is the time when the diagnosis is most commonly confirmed.[2] There are snags even here because if the presenting part is high and the cervix only slightly dilated, a face presentation may easily be mistaken for a breech and vice versa. But when advance has taken place and the cervix has become more dilated the face presentation will provide the evidence of the alveolar margins and mouth, the nose and the supra-orbital ridges, the last being particularly indicative. The nose could on occasion be mistaken for a penis,

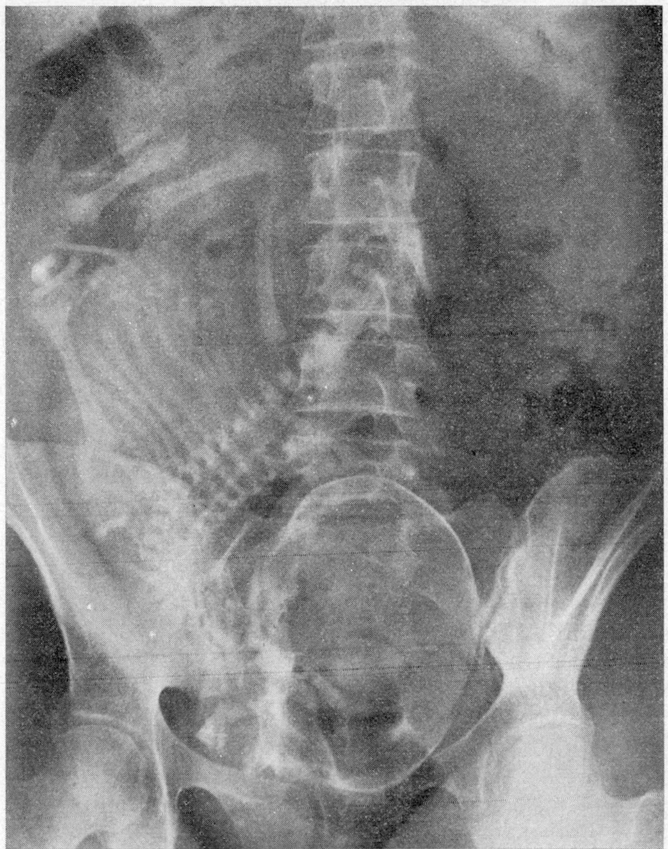

14/FIG. 4.—Primary face presentation.
(By courtesy of Dr David Purdie.)

but the anus and the mouth are unlikely to be confused. It is important at this stage to confirm that the head is fully extended to the face-prone position, and is not much more treacherously a case of brow presentation; hence the importance of examining the mouth and chin very carefully.

Management

Spontaneous delivery can occur with mento-anterior face presentation although the second stage may be prolonged. The diameter of engagement in such cases is the submento-bregmatic which is no greater than the suboccipito-bregmatic but delivery is not so easy as in the case of the vertex because the facial bones do not mould in the same way as the cranial vault. More than half the cases of mento-anterior position achieve spontaneous delivery and the others can be delivered by forceps. Obviously there is no place for the ventouse here.

Mento-posterior positions are very serious unless spontaneous rotation to the mento-anterior position occurs at latest by the earliest part of the second stage of labour. Otherwise the mento-posterior position becomes persistent and confirmed and labour inevitably becomes obstructed.

In managing cases of face presentation, having excluded all the aforementioned adverse causes and being satisfied that the pelvis is adequate, spontaneous labour can be allowed to proceed under supervision. Although the malpresentation may correct itself spontaneously before labour really gets under way, once it has started spontaneous rectification is unlikely, but normal progress is still worth anticipating. Should delay occur, however, even in the first stage of labour and with the membranes ruptured more than six hours, provided the child is normal, Caesarean section may be the wisest course. The treatment of long ago involving internal or bipolar podalic version is in my experience very dangerous and carries the risk of a uterine rupture. Methods have been described of flexing the head by abdominal manipulation but these never work and attempts to correct face presentation before full dilatation by combined internal and external manipulation are not likely to succeed, require deep anaesthesia, may be associated with fetal distress and end up with a more hazardous Caesarean section in the end. The problem really becomes acute when one knows that the fetus is abnormal in which case every attempt must be made to wait for full dilatation and delivery per vaginam.

Delivery of the fully rotated mento-anterior face presentation with forceps is not difficult but a generous episiotomy may be necessary. In the case of the mento-posterior position which does not correct itself spontaneously at the beginning of the second stage, operative intervention must be undertaken sooner rather than later. The best treatment then is manual rotation or the use of Kielland's forceps to a mento-anterior position although there are some who still recommend attempting to rectify the malpresentation to occipito-anterior by flexing the head and then applying the forceps. The danger is that one may be left with a brow presentation and therefore be worse off than before. When rotating a mento-posterior position with Kielland's forceps it may be found that rotation occurs more easily at a lower level in the pelvis than in the case of occipito-posterior positions when the vertex presents. If the rotation is unsuccessful, deeper anaesthesia is now required and the presenting part must be disimpacted and pushed up to the level of the pelvic brim using the whole hand. At this level it may be possibly flexed with the external hand assisting by pushing on the fetal chest, thereby securing rectification to the vertex presentation. If an assistant can pull the breech in the opposite direction to the force on the chest, fetal flexion will thereby be assisted. With the help of disimpaction it may be possible to convert the position to mento-anterior but in this kind of case one is often dealing with a large baby and a none-too-generous pelvis and these internal manipulations should not be persisted with in case of difficulty. It is better to deliver by Caesarean section.

In the case however where the baby is already dead, for example in a case of neglected persistent mento-posterior position, the safest procedure is to perforate through the orbital fossa; thereafter delivery with the help of a cephalotribe is not usually difficult, provided the procedure is unhurried.

The case of persistent mento-posterior position that cannot be corrected is likely to be so large that forcible delivery with forceps in the unreduced position is hazardous and likely to involve a third-degree tear of the maternal rectum at the very least.

BROW PRESENTATION

The average incidence is usually quoted as about once in three thousand deliveries. In the Queen Mother's Hospital, however, the incidence was one in 934 in 1971, and one in 449 in 1973, whereas there were no cases in 1975.

In brow presentation the largest of the fetal head diameters, namely the mento-vertical, attempts to engage, and descent is impossible with an average baby and pelvis. Nevertheless from time to time one sees some remarkable spontaneous deliveries in the experienced multipara who has a cavernous pelvic cavity and a baby of no more than normal size. The history of a patient's previous labours may give one cause to hope. Very premature babies may be delivered with the brow presenting.

In the majority of cases the head remains well above the brim in labour and interference becomes necessary.

Diagnosis

Abdominal palpation is even less certain than in the case of diagnosing face presentation. The head feels large and of course is not engaged. As with face presentations the diagnosis before labour is usually made by radiography. This may have been undertaken because the head may feel so big as to raise the question of possible hydrocephalus.

Vaginal examination must be undertaken, as in all cases where there is lack of advance of the presenting part in spite of reasonable uterine activity. The diagnosis may at first be very difficult if the presenting part is high, as it usually is, and there is as yet no cervical dilatation, but once the cervix has begun to dilate the points to note are the root of the nose, the supra-orbital ridges and the anterior fontanelle. These landmarks must be identified before the diagnosis can be made on clinical grounds. Caput formation very readily occurs and sometimes the diagnosis has to rest on radiographic evidence. Any multipara who demonstrates delay in labour with the head above the brim should be suspected of having a brow presentation until the contrary is proven. Even a history of previous large babies should not lull one into a false sense of security. The grand multipara is particularly at risk of ruptured uterus but the presence of a full bladder can produce just such a situation of high deflexed head even in spite of good uterine contractions, and often I have seen the so-called arrested labour in multiparous brow presentation delivered in a matter of minutes following the passage of a catheter into the bladder.

Treatment

If the diagnosis is made by X-ray taken before the beginning of labour it is best to await events since labour commonly proceeds normally with the vertex or occasionally the face presenting. But however the diagnosis is made, after the onset of labour and after the membranes have ruptured treatment should not be delayed, as a natural outcome is unlikely unless the head immediately flexes or extends and descends into the pelvis. As with all malpresentations, vaginal examination has to be undertaken at this time to exclude prolapse of the cord.

The onset of obstructed labour particularly in the multiparous can be very rapid in the neglected case. There is no hope now of successfully undertaking internal or bipolar podalic version. If the baby is alive Caesarean section is the obviously sensible treatment. However once while awaiting preparations for Caesarean section in a multipara with a very good history of passing babies weighing more than 4 kg in three-hour labours I applied the ventouse to the brow and secured a surprisingly easy delivery before the operating theatre and my colleague who was about to carry out the operation were even ready. In this instance I was influenced by the excellence of the woman's past obstetric history. Attempts to deliver by forceps in the unreduced brow position are totally unjustifiable.

If full, or nearly full, dilatation has been reached, there is a case for manual rectification to a face if the chin is anterior, or to a vertex, whichever is the easier, pushing down the head and following immediately with the application of forceps; but this manoeuvre should not be attempted if the woman has been in long and neglected labour.

If the baby is already dead, one is in a real quandary because of one's reluctance to inflict Caesarean section only to present the mother with a dead baby. Internal version is likely to be hazardous because of possible uterine rupture and one is left with the alternative of a destructive operation which in this instance can be full of pitfalls. Perforation of the head which is still high is made more difficult by not being able to obtain perpendicular access to the fetal skull and the point of the perforator must therefore be very carefully controlled. Cephalotripsy and cranioclasm require the sort of skill which the present day obstetrician lacks. I have always found the three-bladed combined cranioclast and cephalotribe quite exceptionally heavy, but nevertheless effective, especially if one allows time for its weight to exert traction to achieve slow and gentle delivery. The important thing about this type of destructive operation is to attempt to spare the maternal tissues from trauma and not to hurry the delivery.

This is the ugly sort of situation which has now become a very rare phenomenon in enlightened obstetric practice.

SHOULDER PRESENTATION

This is associated with a transverse or oblique lie, the latter description being usually the correct state of affairs, as the fetus seldom lies directly across the uterus; in fact I have only seen this in a case of extreme tuberculous dorsal kyphosis in which the distance between symphysis pubis and xiphisternum was so reduced that the child had no other possible position in which to lie. It is our usual practice to classify any case of oblique lie in which the head is above the level of the umbilicus as in fact a breech presentation, for such it is likely to turn out to be in labour. Otherwise the head is more likely to occupy one or other iliac fossa. It is a state of affairs often found at some time in the antenatal period and is very much more commonly seen in multiparae because of the laxity of the abdominal wall and uterine tone. Tumours in the pelvis preventing engagement of the presenting part are almost as likely to cause an oblique lie as a very high head, likewise placenta praevia may discourage engagement and cause the malpresentation.

One talks therefore more of an oblique lie than a shoulder presentation, the latter term being reserved for the situation after labour has already started.

Diagnosis

The very shape of the abdomen is abnormal and may raise the suspicion of an oblique lie, as the fundus is low and the uterus is spread across the abdomen. On palpation there is nothing in or over the brim of the pelvis and the head is found laterally and usually identifiable in one or other iliac fossa. In the rare cases seen nowadays for the first time late in labour all the signs of obstructed labour will be present and almost certainly the cord, or an arm, or the fetal ribs and a scapula will be noted lying across the internal os which is seldom fully dilated.

UNSTABLE LIE

It is appropriate here to consider the important and relatively common problem of unstable lie discovered late in pregnancy before considering the treatment of shoulder presentation in labour as such. In the absence of pelvic tumours, uterine structural abnormalities and fetal abnormality, the patient is almost certainly multiparous, very often a grand multipara. The presentation of the fetus is found to be different each time the patient is examined. Disproportion in such a case is an unlikely cause to consider since the history of previous labours is likely to have excluded it. At each antenatal visit the presentation is corrected by external version, which is nearly always easy, but malpresentation nevertheless repeatedly recurs, particularly if there is associated hydramnios. As term approaches, i.e. from 38 weeks gestation onwards, the problem arises that the patient may go into spontaneous and rapid labour at home with the malpresentation uncorrected. It may occur while she is out shopping. I always tell my students that the manager's office in Marks & Spencers is not a suitable place for obstetric emergencies. In actual truth I have never had this happen to one of my patients, the nearest being the case of a woman who sat on a chair at the entrance of Woolworths as blood poured down her legs while awaiting the arrival of an ambulance, the other customers having to avoid tripping over her with their shopping bags and small children. Her laconic comment was, "Doctor, I felt such a fool." To guard against this emergency in domiciliary practice it is wisest to admit the woman to hospital so that immediate action could be taken should she go into labour and the membranes rupture.

Once in hospital at least she is safe and my preferred policy is to await the spontaneous onset of labour in the hope that the malpresentation and instability of the fetus may be corrected thereby and during this wait the exact position of the placenta is identified by sonar. Failing these facilities soft-tissue radiography should be undertaken and the possibility of fetal abnormality may then come to light. There is no harm in repeatedly correcting the malpresentation by external version but until the uterus shows some interest in contracting and develops the necessary tone one cannot tell what is going to happen. The nearer to term one can get, the more likely is spontaneous correction and an uneventful labour to ensue. But occasionally the membranes rupture first while the fetus is lying obliquely and the cord may immediately prolapse. When this occurs at the onset of labour there is only one safe treatment for the baby and that is immediate Caesarean section.

To the multiparous patient with family responsibilities at home this period of inactivity in hospital may be very irksome. From the obstetrical point of view however one of the great nuisances is that these cases tend to become postmature. Now admittedly in the highly parous patient maturity may frequently be in doubt since the menstrual history is commonly unreliable, but in these days of sonar examination this should meanwhile be resolved. Many years ago before these facilities were available I once applied this conservative principle doggedly for six weeks; ultimately our nerve broke and we induced labour, and she rapidly produced a baby weighing more than 10 lb ($4\frac{1}{2}$ kg). Nowadays we much prefer the Birmingham method of stabilising induction which avoids in such cases the long-recognised hazards of an increased fetal mortality associated with postmaturity, which increase could otherwise be lowered only by resorting to Caesarean section.[6]

The success of stabilising induction depends entirely upon securing uterine activity at the same time as amniotomy is undertaken and this really the basis of treatment.[4] Once we are satisfied that the patient is unquestionably more than 38 weeks pregnant she is admitted to the labour ward, the presentation is checked and external cephalic version undertaken if necessary. An infusion of oxytocin is then set up with a dosage which escalates until uterine contractions are well established. During this time it is essential to see that the cephalic presentation is maintained. Once the uterus has been contracting regularly for at least an hour, as shown by tocography, a vaginal examination is made in the operating theatre with an anaesthetist in attendance. The pelvic capacity is again assessed and both placenta praevia and cord presentation must be excluded. There now follows one of the rather infrequent present-day indications for using a Drew Smythe catheter, having undertaken a digital "membrane sweep" of the lower segment. Sufficient amniotic fluid is removed from the hindwaters to stabilise the cephalic presentation. Once the head is properly applied to the lower segment, the forewaters are then ruptured encouraging at the same time the vertex to descend and making quite sure of course that the cord does not prolapse. The case is thereafter conducted as with elective induction for any other reason. The important feature of this treatment, be it noted, is that uterine activity is fully maintained in order to prevent the recurrence of the malpresentation which, with the membranes now ruptured and the cervix already beginning to dilate, would only otherwise be rewarded with cord prolapse.

This practice of stabilising induction towards the end of pregnancy gets over the hazards of postmaturity and reduces the need for Caesarean section.

Treatment of Shoulder Presentation

This depends upon the dilatation of the cervix, the tone of the uterus, how long the membranes have been ruptured, and the condition of the baby, especially including the degree of prematurity. When the shoulder presents the arm must inevitably prolapse sooner or later. Any hope of spontaneous labour from now on, except in the grossly previable, cannot be entertained, and the therapeutic alternatives lie between internal or bipolar podalic version, Caesarean section, or decapitation in the case of the baby already dead. External cephalic version is only worth considering if the membranes are not already ruptured. The commonest instance of this, of course, is in the case of the second twin which is lying obliquely, in which case amniotomy is likely to be followed by spontaneous delivery.

Internal or bipolar version should never be considered if the membranes have been ruptured even as long as an hour, or if the uterus does not relax well between contractions. Caesarean section will therefore nearly always be the method of choice if the baby is still alive and gives by far the best results to mother and child. A very small, premature baby may be delivered by spontaneous evolution, which I have only witnessed once with a baby that survived it. The uterus was contracting very strongly and I watched the ribs present at the vulva followed finally by the breech and legs, after which the second arm and the aftercoming head came easily, but the child was very small. Spontaneous expulsion simply applies to a totally previable fetus, usually dead, which comes out more or less doubled up in any position.

In the neglected case of shoulder presentation with prolapsed arm in which the baby is already dead, decapitation is the treatment of choice. The traditional method is to exert strong pull on the prolapsed arm in order to bring the neck as low down as possible to make it more accessible and then to use a Ramsbottom's hook which has a rounded end and a sharp instead of a serrated edge. The position of the back and head having been ascertained the hook is passed along the palm of the hand until its end is above the fetal neck, meanwhile pulling the neck as low as possible. The hook is then rotated backwards through a right angle so as to bring the cutting edge across the neck. The tissues are then severed, partly by a sawing motion, the end of the hook always being guarded by the finger in order to avoid damage to maternal soft tissues, but most of the cutting in fact can be most safely done with strong scissors from below. An even better method is to use a wire saw of the Gigli type, which can be passed over the neck by means of a thimble sort of device and then to decapitate not merely through the neck but to sever right through the axilla of the prolapsed arm. This leaves the decapitated head still attached to the prolapsed arm and prevents the escape of the head into the uterus and its subsequent extraction is that much easier.[1] If this precaution is not taken and routine decapitation through the neck is being employed, there may be difficulty in securing the head which has to be hooked down with a finger in the mouth. Although some authorities have recommended the use of a crotchet hook, I have no personal experience of this.

PROLAPSE OF THE CORD

This is associated with anything that prevents the presenting part from fitting closely into the lower uterine segment and thus shutting off the forewaters from the hindwaters. It is commoner therefore in multiparae, in cases of hydramnios, twins, prematurity, disproportion and, most important of all, in malpresentations. It is rare in the extended breech which fits the lower segment very snugly. Prolapse of the cord is also favoured by an unduly long cord, or more often a first-degree placenta praevia of battledore or velamentous type in which the cord commonly enters at the lower pole of the placenta. The placenta itself in this situation may be the original cause of the high head or malpresentation. Prolapse of the cord occurs about once in every four hundred deliveries.

Before the membranes rupture the diagnosis of presentation of the cord can be made if one is sufficiently fortunate to feel this pulsating structure through the intact membranes, in which case prolapse can be guaranteed the minute the membranes go and the emergency demands immediate Caesarean section. More commonly the diagnosis of prolapsed cord is only made on vaginal examination which has usually been done as a routine at the beginning of labour or after amniotomy, or after spontaneous rupture of the membranes in any case where the presenting part remains high.

In most cases, except in flexed breech presentations, the cord, having prolapsed, is likely to be pinched between the presenting part and the pelvic brim and the blood flow within it therefore becomes restricted or obstructed. But, as most obstetricians recognise, fetal death can occur even if there is no pressure on the cord; in fact the presenting part may be prevented by vaginal manipulation from descending and yet the cord may cease to pulsate. Rhodes (1956) suggested that spasm of the cord vessels may be as important a cause of fetal death as actual mechanical blockage. If this is so, and there is experimental evidence to support it, then the likelihood of its occurrence may be much greater and the fetal prognosis therefore much graver if the cord is actually allowed to prolapse outside the vagina and suffer a loss of temperature. Furthermore handling of the cord may also cause spasm in which case efforts to replace it can do little good. In any event the outlook for the fetus is bad unless delivery is prompt. In other words prolapse of the cord at full dilatation followed by immediate delivery with forceps may save the baby from an asphyxial death. The maternal risks are simply those of the intervention designed to save the baby.

Treatment

If the cord is found to have already ceased pulsating when first found, no treatment will be of any avail, but if however it is still pulsating, the patient should at once be placed in such a position that gravity will help to lessen the pressure of the presenting part on the cord. Traditionally the knee-elbow position is usually mentioned, but this is very tiring and irksome for the patient and hardly suitable for transport from home to hospital. It is more practical therefore to put her into an exaggerated Sims' position and at the same time to raise the foot of the stretcher. This is first-aid treatment and is only to allow time for more radical measures. If the prolapsed cord has not yet emerged from the vagina, it is important to prevent it doing so by applying a firm vulval pad since exposure to cold if it prolapses outside the vulva may quickly extinguish pulsations. An ingenious method of dealing with this emergency is described by Vago and involves the well-known physiological principle that a full bladder inhibits uterine contractions. The technique therefore is to insert a No. 16 Foley catheter with a 5 ml balloon into the urinary bladder and to introduce rapidly from 500 to 750 ml of normal saline, by means of an infusion set, after which the balloon is inflated and the catheter clamped, the patient being kept in a moderate Trendelenburg position. Enough saline is inserted into the bladder to show the signs of vesical distension suprapubically. The distended bladder keeps the presenting part high and relieves pressure on the cord without the necessity for the fingers of the assistant to remain in the vagina for a lengthy period, and uterine contractions are inhibited or temporarily disappear altogether. This allows time for preparations for Caesarean section. I have no personal experience of this method but obviously the cord must at all times be kept within the warmth of the vagina. One must bear in mind the possibility that there may be some associated abnormality which demands treatment in its own right, but if we are confronted with the problem of prolapsed cord not otherwise complicated, the cases are divided into those in which the cervix is fully dilated, or nearly so, and those where the cervix has only just started to dilate. In the former case immediate delivery by forceps is preferable to the ventouse which takes longer to apply, but care must be taken to avoid including the cord inside the forceps blades. Breech extraction is appropriate when the breech presents and, finally, if the head is very high immediately after the membranes have ruptured and when the cord prolapses, internal version and breech extraction may be the treatment of choice. When the cervix is not fully dilated, however, the choice lies between replacement of the cord and Caesarean section. Replacement of the cord is only feasible if the cervix is at least half-dilated and in the case of a long cord is likely to fail or be followed by recurrence. Many stupid methods have been advocated in the past, such as catheters with curious loops on top of them, but the only one that I have found of any use is to wrap the cord in a large piece of sterile rolled gauze and then under an anaesthetic gently to replace the whole bundle above the presenting part. After this the presenting part is pushed into the pelvis and further labour encouraged if necessary with the help of oxytocin. This sometimes works but is a very poor alternative to Caesarean section. It is worth considering if the child's viability is otherwise in doubt. The fear of performing section for a dead baby can and should be minimised by auscultating the fetal heart immediately before operating. Obviously, if at this time the heart sounds are already absent or very irregular, it is hardly justifiable to expose the mother to the operative risk with so little likelihood of a surviving child.

It occasionally happens that the cord prolapses immediately following forewater rupture in the induction of labour. This is one of the reasons why we always undertake this simple procedure in an operating theatre fully equipped for immediate Caesarean section and this precaution has on occasion saved life.

REFERENCES

1. CARTY, M. (1974). Personal communication.
2. CUCCO, U. P. (1966). *Amer. J. Obstet. Gynec.*, **94,** 1085.
3. DEDE, J. A. and FRIEDMAN, E. A. (1963). *Amer. J. Obstet. Gynec.*, **87,** 515.
4. EDWARDS, R. L. and NICHOLSON, H. O. (1969). *J. Obstet. Gynaec. Brit. Cwlth*, **76,** 713.
5. GIBBERD, G. F. (1939). *Proc. roy. Soc. Med.*, **32,** 1223.
6. MACGREGOR, W. G. (1964). *J. Obstet. Gynaec. Brit. Cwlth*, **71,** 237.
7. RHODES, P. (1956). *Proc. roy. Soc. Med.*, **49,** 937.
8. STEVENSON, C. S. (1949). *Amer. J. Obstet. Gynec.*, **58,** 432.
9. STEVENSON, C. S. (1951). *Amer. J. Obstet. Gynec.*, **62,** 488.
10. VAGO, T. (1970). *Amer. J. Obstet. Gynec.*, **107,** 967.

CHAPTER XV

ANTEPARTUM HAEMORRHAGE

MANAGEMENT AND DIAGNOSIS

THIS is one of the complications of pregnancy which very often has to be managed before it can be diagnosed, and an attempt will be made in this chapter to present the subject and its difficulties roughly in the chronological order in which they will greet the practitioner. Most books give an account of the signs and symptoms, diagnosis and treatment of placenta praevia on the one hand and accidental haemorrhage on the other, but this is of little help or guidance to the doctor who, for the moment, does not know which variety he is dealing with. This chapter, therefore, will start with the patient who presents with a story of bleeding only. After all, this is the commonest way in which these cases are encountered, and, for the moment, we will leave aside all those cases who present with the additional symptoms of pain, tenderness, or shock, which cannot be accounted for by the amount of blood lost; in order to keep the issues clear, we will defer consideration of abruptio placentae, other intra-abdominal lesions associated with the onset of premature labour, and "show".

It is often difficult to distinguish between a show and an antepartum haemorrhage, and, indeed, many so-called large shows at the beginning of labour are in fact due to placental separation and may furnish the only evidence of, for example, a low-lying placenta. The distinction between show and antepartum haemorrhage can only be made somewhat arbitrarily on the amount of blood lost.

For bleeding to qualify for the term antepartum haemorrhage, its origin should be restricted to a portion of the placental site, but since this fact cannot be known when the case first presents it is more practical to refer to all cases of bleeding from any part of the genital tract as cases of antepartum haemorrhage, provided pregnancy has reached the 28th week. Bleeding earlier than this is called abortion, of one variety or another, threatened or inevitable. The arbitrary dividing line at 28 weeks between antepartum haemorrhage and abortion represents the earliest accepted chances of fetal viability.

It was Rigby in the 18th century who first distinguished between cases of antepartum haemorrhage where the placenta was normally situated and those in which the placenta was situated, in whole or in part, in the lower uterine segment, and the importance of his observation lies in the fact that the latter type of haemorrhage is inevitable and is therefore liable to recur until the woman is safely delivered. From Rigby's day until our own this classification has continued, but it is no longer regarded as wholly satisfactory, because far too many cases of antepartum haemorrhage cannot be explained. In fact, in many cases it can never be proven whether or not the bleeding came from the placental site. It will, therefore, be realised that bleeding appearing at the vulva may be due to:

1. Placenta praevia;
2. Abruptio placentae;
3. Extraplacental incidental sources;
4. Vasa praevia;
5. Undetermined origin;
6. Small recurrent antepartum haemorrhages that may be associated with a circumvallate placenta. In such cases the uterus is "small for dates" with a small baby, a well-engaged presenting part and a normally placed placental site (Macafee, 1960).

In considering the different varieties of antepartum bleeding mentioned above, it still has to be recognised that fetal risks are increased in all cases of antepartum bleeding whatever the type. Numerically the undetermined are an important group and fetal mortality in fact has been shown to be higher in these than in cases of proven placenta praevia.[4] In our own hospital in the period 1964–69 we had 307 cases of antepartum haemorrhage of uncertain origin with 311 babies and the fetal mortality in this group was 14·2 per cent. The majority of perinatal deaths however occurred among the 52 cases in this group who weighed less than 2·5 kg, so that prematurity would appear to be the most serious source of fetal loss. Obviously, premature induction of labour would not have saved those who were already premature.[53]

A case can only really be diagnosed as having placenta praevia by feeling or seeing the placenta or by one of the newer methods demonstrating its presence wholly or partly over the lower uterine segment. Even the term "lower uterine segment", however, is not universally agreed. There are, for example, a few who say that the lower uterine segment is not properly developed until labour actually starts. There are three definitions, as follows:

1. The physiological definition: "It is that part of the uterus which passively stretches in labour and takes hardly any active, contractile part in the expulsion of the fetus." The importance of this definition lies in the word "stretches". In stretching, the placenta comes adrift from its attachment much as a postage stamp would come off a piece of elastic if the latter were stretched.

This type of haemorrhage is inevitable, because the lower uterine segment must sooner or later start to stretch.

2. The anatomical definition: "It is that part of the uterus which lies below the level at which the peritoneum on the anterior surface of the uterus ceases to be intimately applied to the uterus, and is reflected via the uterovesical fold on to the dome of the bladder." This definition only serves at laparotomy, as, for example, in performing Caesarean section.
3. Metric definition: "It is that portion of the uterus which towards term lies within three inches (7·5 cm) of the internal os." This is a rough-and-ready definition, but it is the one of most practical value in diagnosis, because it represents the distance over which the uterine cavity can be explored by the examining finger passed through the cervix. Therefore, if no placenta can be felt, one can be reasonably certain that the case is not one of placenta praevia.

The diagnosis of abruptio placentae is open to a good deal of error. In recording such a diagnosis, evidences of placental changes following separation and haemorrhage should be sought after delivery, though it will often be found that, following quite severe haemorrhages, no trace can be found by examining the placenta.

The abruptio group should be subdivided into cases of bleeding associated with pre-eclamptic toxaemia, hypertension or renal disease, as against those in which no such toxic association is present.

Premature separation of a normally situated placenta occurs no more than once in 133 non-toxaemic pregnancies, while with toxaemia the incidence rises to 1 in 18, and in eclampsia to 1 in 3. The aetiological significance of pre-eclamptic toxaemia becomes obvious. Often there is no more than a record of a systolic blood pressure of 150 mm Hg or more, occurring some time before the antepartum haemorrhage.

Macafee[25, 26] tabulated 341 cases of antepartum haemorrhage as follows:

1. Placenta praevia, 108;
2. Toxic cases, 83;
3. Extraplacental local causes, 18;
4. Unclassified, 132.

In a further series of 395 cases he was unable to trace the origin of the haemorrhage in 163. It will be appreciated, therefore, that the so-called unclassified group forms one of the largest classes. One of the important things about this indeterminate class is that it accounts for almost half of the fetal wastage. The risks to the fetus in placenta praevia are obvious, but it is only now becoming recognised that the baby is at even greater risk when the source of antepartum bleeding is not determinable.

There is, of course, no particular reason why pre-eclamptic toxaemia should not be associated with placenta praevia any more than with other pregnancies, and its incidental presence should not put one off the scent. Even though the case proves to be one of placenta praevia, there is no doubt that the addition of pre-eclamptic toxaemia greatly increases the fetal risks. Rigby's classification, although it was an important step, has rather helped to cloud the issue, and it is important to recognise that any true case of antepartum haemorrhage, of whichever variety, involves greater risk of stillbirth or neonatal death.

PLACENTA PRAEVIA

The incidence of this condition is approximately 1 in 200, but since the majority of these cases find their way into hospital, the published figures of maternity units exaggerate the incidence in pregnancies throughout the country. It is much more common in multiparae, although 20 per cent occur in primigravidae; but multiparous pregnancy is very much more common than first pregnancies and the factor of multiparity has probably been overstressed. More cases occur in the first pregnancy, however, than in any other subsequent pregnancy, for example the fourth or the fifth, and this fact encourages one to question the generally accepted factors said to predispose to placenta praevia. This incidence definitely increases over the age of 35 years.

It is probable that, as a result of some local aberration in uterine blood supply, the distinction between the areas of chorion frondosum and chorion laeve does not occur in the normal situation and the developing ovum comes to derive its nourishment from a lower region of the uterus than is customary. We are now in a position to demonstrate this phenomenon by sonar (Fig. 1) (see Chapter XXIX). The decidual reaction in the lower uterine segment is often inadequate, and this false secondary type of implantation may be defective, so that abortion occurs. Many of these cases, in fact, never reach the degree of maturity which would qualify them for the title of placenta praevia. Moreover, because of the local inadequacy of the decidua, patchy areas of morbid adhesion may occur and complicate the third stage of labour.

The incidence of placenta praevia is, of course, increased in multiple pregnancy, since the placental site, because of its size, has a greater chance of encroaching on to the lower uterine segment. Whatever the factor responsible for the development of placenta praevia, there is no doubt that the grand multipara runs a greater risk of this complication.

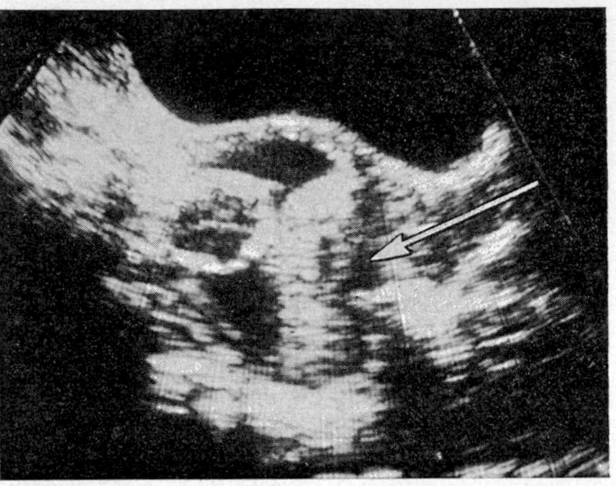

15/FIG. 1.—Ultrasonogram in longitudinal section. Placenta (arrow) situated over the cervix (to R). Fetal head, 16 weeks gestation, at fundus of uterus. History of bleeding.

Degrees of Placenta Praevia

There are four degrees (also called "types"):

1. The placenta encroaches on the lower uterine segment, but does not reach as far as the os.

In these minor degrees there is often a disproportionate amount of blood loss from what is known as marginal sinus bleeding following separation of the lower edge of the placenta, thus exposing a small localised area of the placental site. The amount of blood lost is not necessarily related to the area of placental separation.

2. The placenta reaches to the os, but does not cover it.
3. The placenta covers the os by reaching across to the farther margin, but ceases to do so as the cervix dilates.
4. The placenta covers the os to such a degree that even dilatation of the cervix does not bring its margin clear.

In the majority of cases the placenta mainly lies on either the anterior or the posterior wall. The latter is slightly more common and is also more dangerous because it discourages engagement of the head more readily, and the placenta is likely to be compressed in labour.

Steps to be Taken when First Seen

If word is received that a patient, still in her own home, has had an antepartum haemorrhage, she should be instructed on no account to come to the hospital, or to the doctor's surgery, until visited and until proper arrangements for her transport can be made. She should be told to remain in bed and instructed not to clear up sheets, etc., soiled by blood. This will, at least, give the doctor or midwife a chance of estimating how much blood has been lost. She should be visited as soon as possible and her general condition noted.

This is a curious but natural tendency on the part of those in attendance on the patient to clean her up before the doctor's arrival, so that traces of blood from thighs and legs have already been removed. When a patient finds herself bleeding in bed, her first reaction is to jump out of it and stand on the floor, so that blood runs down her legs and collects on the soles of her feet and between her toes.[36] Professor Parks of Washington, D.C., who, as far as I know, first made this observation, happened to be visiting the Queen Mother's Hospital one day and saw a woman recently admitted by the flying squad with antepartum haemorrhage. He immediately asked whether the nursing staff thought she had lost more or less than 150 ml of blood. He thereupon pulled back the bedclothes from her feet and legs which looked impeccably clean, and demonstrated the clotted blood still on the soles of her feet and between her toes, signifying a very sizeable haemorrhage. His triumph was almost as great as the consternation of my nurses.

If she arrives at the antenatal clinic either bleeding or with a history of having bled recently, she should be persuaded to remain in hospital and not to go home to pack her things. Patients are often reluctant to take this advice because, from their own point of view, they usually feel perfectly well; they are in no pain and the haemorrhage has often been no more than slight, and not a few will, in their own minds, rightly attribute it to the effects of coitus. The significance of antepartum bleeding, however, cannot be dismissed on the grounds of recent coitus, because placenta praevia bleeding is particularly easily provoked thereby.

If the patient is still bleeding when first seen she should, in the first instance, be given 15 mg morphia by injection and put to bed. Only the briefest examination is called for at this stage, but it will include the recording of blood pressure and pulse and any general signs of exsanguination. The abdominal wall is only lightly palpated, mainly to exclude the presence of any areas of uterine tenderness or to observe the presence of rhythmical contractions signifying the onset of labour or a hard consistency indicating abruptio placentae. The fetal heart is auscultated, and the urine, if necessary a catheter specimen, is examined for the presence of albumen. By now the injection of morphia already given will have begun to take effect. The same procedure is to be followed if the patient is first seen in her own home, and neither in clinic nor in private dwelling is any form of pelvic examination permissible.

If the patient is bleeding seriously at home it is far safer to send for flying squad assistance from a neighbouring hospital than to send the patient in before the necessary restorative treatment. One such case "posted in" to us by her doctor, continued bleeding on the journey and became so shocked that she could not be got over the doorstep alive but died as she was being lifted out of the ambulance. She should, of course, have been properly sedated and liberally transfused first until fit to make the journey.

Many general practitioners feel that, on being summoned by a midwife to a case of antepartum bleeding, they are not making much of a contribution to treatment by restricting their activities to arranging admission to hospital on a telephone. But the more experienced will realise the great value of such forbearance.

This is one of the emergencies in which the administration of morphia before admission is not only permissible but positively indicated, and a note to the effect that this drug has been given should accompany the patient. A clean vulval pad should be applied, abdominal binders should be eschewed and the patient's clothing should be disturbed as little as possible before transfer.

While awaiting admission, a history can now be taken, particular note being made of the presence or absence of any associated pain, when movements were last felt and what the patient was doing at the time when the bleeding first occurred. In many cases of placenta praevia bleeding the patient will state that the first thing she noticed was that the sheets were damp with blood or that the bleeding started during a visit to the toilet.

All cases of bleeding per vaginam should be admitted for observation and, in the vast majority, expectant treatment is employed in the first instance unless the bleeding is very severe or labour is actually in progress.

Reason for Admission of all Cases of Antepartum Haemorrhage

Since many patients are unwilling to go to hospital, it is as well to be conversant with the reasons for insisting. Firstly, every case of antepartum haemorrhage is to be regarded as due to placenta praevia until the contrary has been proven, because, in this event, further bleeding is bound to occur sooner or later and none can predict its severity. Even the smallest initial warning haemorrhage may be the herald of a loss so catastrophic as to cause not only the baby's death but that of the mother as well, and only a properly equipped institution is in a position to deal adequately with such an emergency.

Let us discuss the likely fate of the untreated case. Admittedly, she will most probably deliver herself ultimately in a variable state of exsanguination, although a small number would die from haemorrhage before delivery. Labour, moreover, would probably be premature, and in all but the lesser degrees of placenta praevia the child would be stillborn. In delivering herself, the placenta would be likely to come adrift completely before the delivery of the child and to present first at the vulva. Malpresentation too is common in placenta praevia, and the complications of this have to be added to the process of labour. If she failed to deliver herself of the placenta at the same time as the baby, it is more than likely that the placenta would remain partially detached within the uterus and cause still further bleeding. Even though she survives the second stage of labour, postpartum haemorrhage, not necessarily excessive, might prove more than her exsanguinated condition could stand. Lastly, having negotiated all these hazards, she would now find herself a ready prey to puerperal sepsis because of her anaemia. This sequence of events is not uncommon in outlying parts of the world where medical aid is not readily available.

Maternal and Fetal Mortality

Until recently, antepartum haemorrhage came fourth in the list of causes of maternal death. Much of this is preventable with proper antenatal supervision and institutional care. The majority of deaths from placenta praevia are due to mismanagement. Macafee, more than anyone else in this country, demonstrated what can be done in this respect by achieving a maternal mortality of 0·57 per cent in contrast to the previously accepted figures of 6 or 7 per cent. The fetal mortality was also impressively reduced from over 50 per cent to 23·5 per cent (1945). In his later series of 200 cases there was no maternal death and nowadays the fetal mortality should not exceed about 10 per cent and much of this may be due to prematurity.

One of the commonest causes of death in cases of antepartum haemorrhage, whether placenta praevia or accidental, is postpartum haemorrhage, for even a small loss of blood after delivery may tip the scales against an exhausted, shocked and exsanguinated patient. Areas of morbid adhesion of the placenta (placenta accreta) in the lower uterine segment are not uncommon in placenta praevia and can cause very dangerous postpartum bleeding[30] and even without difficulties of separation, bleeding can be very free. Another common cause of death is puerperal sepsis, to which the patient is particularly prone as a result of the interference which may have been occasioned in the course of delivering her and as a result of her diminished resistance to infection from anaemia. These patients often succumb to shock, operative or otherwise, the effects of which again are magnified by blood loss and, finally, both shock and haemorrhage invite the possibility of tubular nephrosis of the kidneys, so that the patient may die of anuria. The case of toxic accidental haemorrhage (abruptio) runs the additional risks of acute cortical necrosis of the kidneys and the possibility of eclampsia.

The reduced maternal mortality in recent years is mainly attributable, firstly to the increased use of blood transfusion, secondly to effective chemotherapy, thirdly to a better understanding of the management of shock, fourthly to the more rational management of anuria, and lastly to the abandonment of many of the older practices which, in the past, made midwifery such a blood-and-thunder subject.

All types of antepartum haemorrhage jeopardise the fetus, but, in the case of placenta praevia, the increased use of Caesarean section, preceded by expectant treatment as advocated by Macafee, has been universally adopted and Stallworthy as long ago as 1951 declared that it should be our aim to reduce maternal mortality to nil and the fetal mortality to less than 10 per cent.

Causes of Fetal Death

1. *Intra-uterine asphyxia*, due to placental separation, howsoever caused. This is the commonest mechanism, but hypotension in the mother, as a result either of haemorrhage or shock, may also starve the fetus of oxygen. In toxic antepartum haemorrhage the reduced maternal placental circulation, as a result of pre-eclampsia, also plays a part.
2. *The hazards of delivery*. Malpresentation, if present, confers its own penalties, particularly in the case of the premature infant who is very prone to intracranial haemorrhage, especially in breech delivery.
3. *Prematurity*. This, too, takes its toll, and the modern expectant treatment of placenta praevia has gone a long way towards minimising this hazard.
4. *Fetal abnormality*. This is more common in placenta praevia, and Macafee quoted a 3·4 per cent incidence. The most likely forms are spina bifida, hydrocephalus and anencephaly.
5. *Atelectasis neonatorum*. This is very commonly associated with prematurity, particularly with a history of antepartum haemorrhage.
6. *Hyaline membrane*. This condition is really a sub-variety of atelectasis neonatorum, and is dealt with more fully in the chapter on prematurity.
7. *Fetal exsanguination*. Usually ruptured vasa praevia are responsible for the fetal blood loss which does not have to be large to kill the baby or to make it seriously anaemic. The foolish use of hindwater rupture as a method of surgical induction of labour in cases of placenta praevia producing a "bloody tap",

is another potent source of this trouble. The possibility that the bleeding may be of fetal origin must be determined or eliminated at once. Fortunately this can be carried out within about 20 minutes by the alkali denaturation test for fetal haemoglobin, as described in the chapter on "Induction".[31]

Normally the fetal abnormality rate is not more than 0·94 per cent, so that it will be seen that the incidence is more than trebled in placenta praevia. Most of the neonatal deaths are due to prematurity with its associated risks, particularly atelectasis and intracranial haemorrhage, and lastly fetal abnormality.

There are certain special dangers, apart from injudicious treatment, which confront the fetus in placenta praevia in the course of vaginal delivery, and these are associated with battledore insertion of the cord, which is by no means uncommon and may even take the form of a velamentous insertion (Fig. 2). When, as is very often the case, the insertion is at the lower pole of the placenta, the fetal mortality is greatly increased, even with placenta praevia of only first degree. This combination of circumstances is even more dangerous if the placenta is situated posteriorly and encourages the acceptance of Stallworthy's term, the "dangerous low-lying placenta".

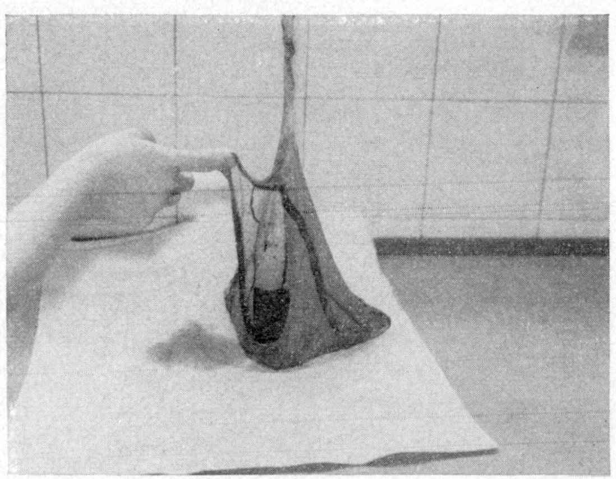

15/FIG. 2.—Velamentous insertion of the cord. This baby had the good fortune to escape through a rent between the large fetal vessels running in the membranes. Otherwise rapid fetal exsanguination would have occurred.

MANAGEMENT ON ADMISSION

Macafee's great contribution lay in his advocacy of expectant treatment, thereby reducing prematurity. As a rule, the first haemorrhage is not lethal either to the mother or the child, particularly in the case of the primigravida, and with morphia and rest in bed it presently ceases in practically every case. The separated area of placenta becomes infarcted and the maternal vessels supplying the exposed portion of the placental site thrombose. Provided too great an area of placenta is not detached, that is to say more than about a third, the fetus readjusts itself and probably some compensatory mechanism, if given time, meets its oxygen requirements. For this reason, small repeated haemorrhages are far less dangerous than single large ones. The words "if given time" are important, and hence unwarranted interference may defeat the process. The first warning haemorrhage is not an indication necessarily for active investigation, which is almost bound to provoke the need for immediate treatment. Diagnosis must, therefore, be deferred.

The first step to be taken in hospital is to ensure that the patient's blood group and Rh grouping is known and that a supply of compatible blood is available for transfusion at any moment. It is safer to keep the patient strictly in bed, not to allow her to have a bath and to forbid visits to the toilet, at least for three days after the cessation of bleeding.

The colour of the blood appearing at the vulva is noted, and its increasing darkness will reassure one that no fresh bleeding is occurring.

If on examination of the abdomen it is found that a malpresentation is present, no steps must be taken to correct it by external version.

The haemoglobin is estimated on admission and again read two or three days later to assess firstly the patient's general blood state, and secondly the anaemia which will be manifested at the second reading by haemodilution. No vaginal examination nor even a rectal examination may yet be made. The fetal heart is auscultated, the blood pressure is recorded twice daily, and the urine is examined every day for protein unless the specimen is contaminated with blood, in which case a clean swab specimen is tested.

It is important that the admitting officer or house surgeon on the ward should inform the consultant in charge of the patient's admission, rather than act upon his own initiative. Provided fresh bleeding does not occur, the patient is left alone for five days at least before proceeding further, during which period no purgative should be given. Locking of the toilet door is particularly dangerous and I know of one tragic case in which the first sign of trouble was the sight of blood winding its way across the floor and down the stairs from under a locked lavatory door, the patient herself being unconscious and in no position to call out for help. She lost her twins.

It is commonly taught that a speculum should be passed on admission and the cervix inspected, but with this practice we strongly disagree except in the very mildest cases of bleeding. For one thing if there is any appreciable amount of blood in the vagina, it will not be possible to see the cervix without resort to mopping, which in itself may be almost as bad as a full vaginal examination. Secondly, further bleeding may be provoked. Where the bleeding amounts to no more than a slight stain, however, a cautious speculum examination is often worthwhile, because it may not be possible later to ascertain whether the blood was issuing from the cervical canal or otherwise. In most cases, therefore, speculum examination is deferred until five days after the cessation of bleeding. This is done in order to exclude lesions of the cervix and vaginal vault which might have been the source. A large Fergusson speculum is admirable for the purpose.

After the first few days, the patient may be allowed to go outside to the lavatory. It is the fear of severe, inevitable and recurrent haemorrhage which necessitates this cautious attitude as long as the existence of placenta praevia remains a possibility.

Soft-tissue X-ray placentography may be undertaken at any time from the 34th week onwards (see later). This may not only determine the site of the placenta but may help to exclude fetal abnormality, or twins with which placenta praevia is more frequently associated. An assessment of fetal maturity may also be made at the same time. Ultrasonic localisation of the placenta can be undertaken several weeks earlier and with us has become standard practice. The discovery of a fetal abnormality will render further expectant treatment somewhat pointless, and will make one loath to deliver the patient by Caesarean section, although in fourth-degree placenta praevia this is the only safe method of delivery.

Any anaemia should be appropriately corrected during the patient's wait in hospital, so that intervention, if and when it has to be undertaken, is performed under optimum conditions.

There now follows a very irksome period of waiting. Not a few, for domestic reasons, will refuse to remain any longer in hospital and will take their discharge on their own responsibility. This is very understandable, and one cannot do more than advise them at least of some of the risks and the steps to be taken if they materialise, but on no account should a patient's desire to leave hospital precipitate one into trying to exclude the presence of placenta praevia at this stage by vaginal examination. For one thing, it is impossible to be certain without passing a finger through the cervix, which at this stage is unthinkable, and, for another, one's curiosity in those very cases where it was most warranted will provoke the very disaster against which one is trying to insure the patient.

As it is, the patient may have to spend many weeks of apparently fruitless imprisonment in hospital, only to find at the end that there was no placenta praevia after all. This is a serious matter, but in the present state of our knowledge the rule can only be broken in face of the risk of an occasional disaster. The end results of this expectant treatment speak for themselves, but they are achieved at a great price in inconvenience to the patient, and not infrequently we are prepared to take a chance on the patient who has a deeply engaged vertex and a history of very slight bleeding on one occasion only. Deep engagement of the head does not, of course, completely exclude placenta praevia, but makes it very much less likely. An increasing number of major obstetrical units are now equipped with sonar and with a good service the diagnosis of placenta praevia can be confidently excluded.

In the absence of modern diagnostic facilities this period of waiting and observation is maintained until the 38th week, that is to say until the question of prematurity no longer applies, and the patient is then examined under an anaesthetic as described below.

Should bleeding not cease within a few hours of admission, or should it at any time become profuse, expectant treatment is out of place. If the patient is already in labour she should be examined under an anaesthetic, in an operating theatre prepared to undertake immediate Caesarean section should the findings indicate it. It may be found, for example, that the patient is farther on in labour than expected and that the cervix is already appreciably dilated, in which case artificial rupture of the membranes or pulling down a leg may meet the case, especially in a multiparous patient. But this carries a prohibitive fetal mortality rate and may cause deep lacerations of the cervix and more haemorrhage and shock ultimately than the procedure is designed to prevent. It is only worth considering if the fetus is already dead or if the patient is parous with a cervix at least 3 fingerbreadths dilated and where the child is either grossly premature or deformed. Even after pulling down the leg through the vulval outlet it is better to await spontaneous delivery with just sufficient light traction to stop further bleeding rather than to hurry it by unnecessary and dangerous manipulation. If, however, the patient is not in labour and bleeding continues or is profuse at any time and shows no signs of abating, it is safer, provided that the fetal heart is still present, to omit the diagnostic examination and to proceed forthwith to Caesarean section in the interests chiefly of the child. The importance, therefore, of having previously excluded fetal abnormality by X-ray is now obvious. Lastly, if bleeding continues as described above and there is strong presumptive evidence that the baby is already dead, morphia and a blood transfusion should be given in a determined attempt to encourage its arrest. If, in fact, the baby is dead, the bleeding almost certainly will stop in due course, but if not, more active measures, however unwelcome, may have to be undertaken. Personally, I have not yet been confronted with this last situation, but I would be prepared to consider artificial rupture of the membranes under general anaesthesia in the first instance preferable to Caesarean section with a dead fetus.

So far we have only considered the patients who have actually bled, but it must be remembered that a certain number of cases of placenta praevia do not bleed until the cervix starts to dilate or vaginal interference is undertaken. The possible existence of the condition, therefore, should not be forgotten in the course of obstetrical examination, particularly in cases of otherwise unexplained variable lie.

Incidental and Extraplacental Causes of Bleeding

It is to be assumed that bleeding is coming from a portion of exposed placental site unless or until some lesion of the cervix or vagina can be found on speculum examination to account for it. It has already been noted that this examination is usually deferred until five days after bleeding has stopped, but this rule is broken if bleeding persists, or in cases in which it is very slight, and it is hoped to avail oneself of the opportunity of identifying its site of origin before all traces have disappeared.

Most important of the incidental causes is carcinoma of the cervix, which is by no means rare and has a very serious prognosis, since it grows with great rapidity. By observing the above rules, diagnosis will not be delayed more than a few days at the most. The appearance of the cervix is fairly characteristic, and certainly not by any stretch of imagination will it ever look normal. Friable and vascular growth will be seen which bleeds very readily on touching, and a small portion should be removed for biopsy. Microscopy of sections of the cervix in pregnancy can play notorious tricks on an inexperienced pathologist, who can be misled into wrongly diagnosing maligant disease.

Cervical erosions are a fairly common cause of blood-staining in pregnancy, but the haemorrhage is never more than slight. Although the erosion bleeds on gentle swabbing, it is not friable and, in any doubtful case a small portion should be removed for microscopy. Radical treatment of an erosion is not possible during pregnancy for obvious reasons, and there is no danger in the condition. Nevertheless, some employ superficial cautery as a temporary measure. It does no good.

Cervical polyps, both mucous and fibroadenomatous, are occasional causes of slight bleeding, while fibroid polyps, rarely, may be found. The last-mentioned are very uncommon because their very existence tends to discourage conception. One is tempted to avulse such polyps by twisting, but this should never be done in the out-patient department, firstly because, as already stated, the examination should only take place in hospital, and secondly because bleeding may continue from the base after removal. This will always stop in time, but the possibility is enough to discourage one from dealing with polyps in an out-patient clinic.

Varicosities may bleed quite profusely on occasion, especially if traumatised. They are usually situated at the introitus or at the lower end of the vagina, although occasionally they may be found in the vaginal vault. Local gentle pressure will quickly arrest the bleeding.

Occasionally a well-marked vaginitis, particularly trichomonas infection, is found to account for slight bleeding, but usually there is an associated discharge as well. In 16 out of Murdoch's 339 cases a lesion on the cervix or marked vaginitis was responsible for the blood loss.

Many so-called shows of blood are due to rupture of the small vessels in the lower segment decidua, which bleed when the overlying chorion is disturbed in the course of stretching of the segment. This mechanism also accounts for the slight amount of bleeding which often occurs when one passes a finger through the cervix and sweeps the membranes from the uterine wall, as, for example, in surgical induction of labour. Lastly, in a few cases there is a marked decidual reaction in the upper portion of the endo-cervix from which a small blood loss can be provoked by minor trauma.

The history of recent coitus is of very little help in clarifying the diagnosis, since all varieties of antepartum bleeding can be provoked thereby.

Attempts at Provisional Diagnosis

Without the aid of special methods and of examination under anaesthesia, it is only possible to guess in deciding whether the case is one of abruptio placentae or placenta praevia. The history is of only partial assistance. Characteristically, bleeding from placenta praevia is unrelated to activity on the part of the patient and often takes place at night. It is absolutely painless. The only symptoms which can be attributed to placenta praevia are those resulting directly from haemorrhage and no others. The fact that a patient associates the bleeding with activity or coitus, or that haemorrhage may have followed external version, does nothing to exclude placenta praevia. Further presumptive evidences of this condition are afforded by the fact that bleeding is often recurrent, although recurrence is not by any means restricted to placenta praevia.

With placenta praevia, the patient's general condition is directly related to the amount of blood actually lost. The uterus is normally relaxed and soft, so that fetal parts are readily palpable and no areas of tenderness can be found. In about a third of the cases, malpresentation will be observed, and in the remainder the head is usually not engaged. Often, however, a placenta praevia is very thin: under these circumstances the head may be able to settle in the pelvis, but it is very rare for it to do so deeply. A useful measure is to listen to the fetal heart at the same time as endeavouring to force the head into the pelvis. If, in doing so, it is found that the fetal heart becomes slow or irregular, it strongly suggests that the baby's oxygen supply is being pressed upon. This sign is very often found, according to Stallworthy, in cases of posterior placenta praevia, especially with a low insertion of the cord. It bodes ill for the baby in the course of a vaginal delivery, even though the placenta praevia may be only of the first or second degree, and, of itself, is a sound indication for deciding upon elective Caesarean section. I have often observed this sign, however, in women in whom there was no such abnormality and in whom perfectly safe and normal delivery, without fetal distress, took place later and I agree with Percival (1959) who reckons that any fetal heart rate will slow if the head is pushed hard enough regardless of placental situation. The sign, nevertheless, encourages one to carry out placental localisation by one specialised technique or another. Lastly, signs of pre-eclamptic toxaemia should be looked for. The association of this complication is no commoner than usual in placenta praevia, but in cases of abruptio placentae it will be found in approximately one-third of the cases. Not only is the presence of toxaemia a pointer in the diagnosis, but because of its own inherent risks, both to mother and child, its discovery may determine treatment.

Bleeding from torn vasa praevia is impossible to diagnose before delivery without special alkali denaturation tests to determine the presence of fetal haemoglobin, and is necessarily of small amount. In this instance it is the fetus and not the mother that is losing blood. The condition occurs as a result of velamentous insertion of the cord in association with placenta praevia. The baby may bleed to death before delivery, and there is no doubt that if, in the course of examination under an anaesthetic, pulsating vessels synchronous with the fetal heart are palpated through the cervix, the child should be delivered by Caesarean section, so great is its peril. It is, unfortunately, rare for one to have the luck to make this diagnosis in time to prevent the death of the child.

Localisation of the Placenta

Considering how often a patient has to be kept in hospital for no other reason than that she *might* have placenta praevia, it is natural that great efforts are being made on methods to identify the position of the placental site, short of adopting the obvious measure of passing the finger through the cervix and feeling it, a procedure which, as already stated, must be deferred until the last two or three weeks of pregnancy.

Radio-isotope Localisation of the Placenta

This method was first used by Browne and Veall (1953) at Hammersmith. Radiosodium in a dosage, which would not now be acceptable, of 50 microcuries was injected intravenously and, with the help of a Geiger-Müller counter, revealed the large collections of blood which would normally be found in the placental site as well as the liver and heart. Since that time a number of others have used this as a localising method, e.g. Hibbard (1962) using ^{132}I, but in nearly all units soft-tissue placentography has proved itself more popular. The isotope technique is not without its pitfalls especially when the placenta is situated wholly posteriorly and therefore less accessible to gamma-ray counting and because the lower dosages which are to-day acceptable are often insufficient to compete with natural background interference.

Certainly ^{132}I is a more suitable isotope of iodine than the more traditional ^{131}I with its much longer half-life of a matter of days instead of a few hours; consequently there is no need to block the thyroid of mother or baby with Lugol's iodine and the radiation dose is acceptably low. One nuisance, however, is that the ^{132}I has to be prepared fresh from tellurium, thus calling for facilities which are by no means universally available.

Technetium 99 is a more acceptable isotope for the same purpose and is said to involve the fetal gonads in no more than one to two weeks natural background radiation dose and about one hundredth that of a single X-ray exposure. It has the advantage of being rapidly excreted in the bladder urine, but this in itself may, by producing a high count at the lower pole of the uterus, tend towards a false diagnosis of placenta praevia. Radiochromium (^{51}Cr) labelled red cells, from donor or patient, can also be used and the isotope does not cross the placenta.

All isotope methods have one thing in common, namely, reliance upon the identification of a pool of maternal blood from which to infer the placental site. They also require the available services of hospital physicists at weekends too. The isotopes have to be ordered and dispensed, and permission to use them has to be obtained through the Medical Research Council; nor can the method be used on an occasional or casual basis and therefore its use is restricted to units with a reasonably large and stable turnover; in other words the occasional case cannot be undertaken without planning and it is for reasons such as these that the radioisotope methods of locating the placenta have only a limited acceptance, mainly confined to large services with other interests in nuclear medicine as well. I must admit to some prejudice myself, but, to our practised eyes, a well taken ultrasonic placentogram with its clean edges and positive identifiability in the majority of cases, seems greatly preferable to the fluffy mess which sometimes passes for an isotope localisation.[7]

Soft-tissue Radiography

This is a more generally available method which has been employed with increasing success during the last 20 years, although it is not yet universally reliable. As Chassar Moir has pointed out, the radio-opacity of the placenta differs very little, if at all, from that of uterine wall and liquor amnii, so that it requires skilful exposure to reveal it (Fig. 3).[5, 6, 15, 41, 42, 43] Occasionally there is a sufficient

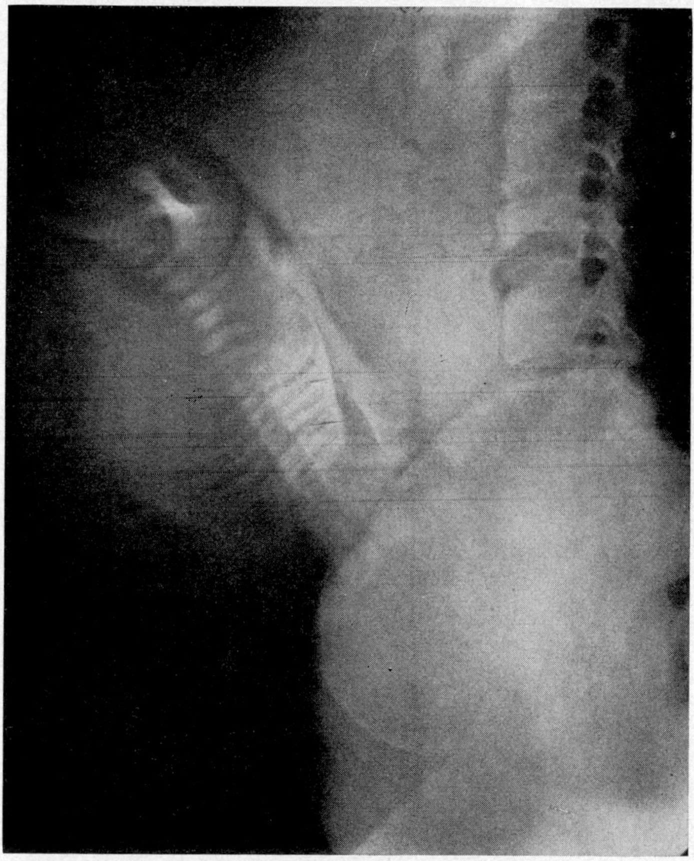

15/Fig. 3.—Soft-tissue radiography. Placenta localised in upper segment posteriorly.

degree of calcification in the placenta to make its localisation an obvious matter, but this is unusual. The accuracy of soft-tissue radiography is adversely affected by gross obesity, hydramnios and twins, for obvious technical reasons.

This method is best employed after the beginning of the 34th week before which it may be unreliable.

Arteriography

Of all radiological methods this is probably by far the most accurate and, carried out in highly specialised units, gives excellent results with minimum hazard. The necessary expertise, however, is not by any means widely distributed and the procedure has the status of a minor surgical operation at least, since it involves retrograde cannulation of the aorta usually by the Seldinger technique via the femoral artery.[12]

Infra-red Thermography

This is a wholly nonsensical method of locating the placenta. It is based on the old idea of localising maternal blood pools to signify the placental site, but differs from the common-sense of gamma-ray-emitting isotopes in relying upon the theory that the overlying skin of the abdominal wall would emanate more heat from an area overlying the placenta and incidentally fat abdominal wall, peritoneum and uterine musculature. The method seems to have crept into the textbook literature without verification. We at least undertook a large trial[29] in a series of 150 patients, and found it useless.

Ultrasonic Placentography

Ultrasonic localisation of the placenta can be undertaken several weeks earlier and, with us, this method has become standard practice.[9, 10]

If one is possessed of a two-dimensional B-scan apparatus (and I predict that the day will come when all diagnostic units are so equipped) localisation of the placenta by sonar has enormous advantages. For one thing the patient is in no way disturbed and can be examined even in her bed. All that is necessary is to switch on the machine and smear the abdominal wall with olive oil, and the results can be obtained within a few minutes. A small quantity of urine in the bladder is a help in delineating the lower pole of the uterus and its relationship to the presenting part (Fig. 4). The apparatus must be very expertly adjusted but the placenta shows up first of all as a space-occupying structure which gradually fills with speckles from in front backwards as the time-varied gain-setting of the machine is increased. Furthermore with correct positioning of the scanning direction the fetal surface can be revealed as a characteristic white line. We only resort to other methods of placentography if clinical evidences throw doubt upon the ultrasonic diagnosis. Some care is necessary in adjusting the apparatus in accordance with the obesity or otherwise of the patient's abdominal wall and it is a wise precaution to take 2-dimensional ultrasonograms in longitudinal,

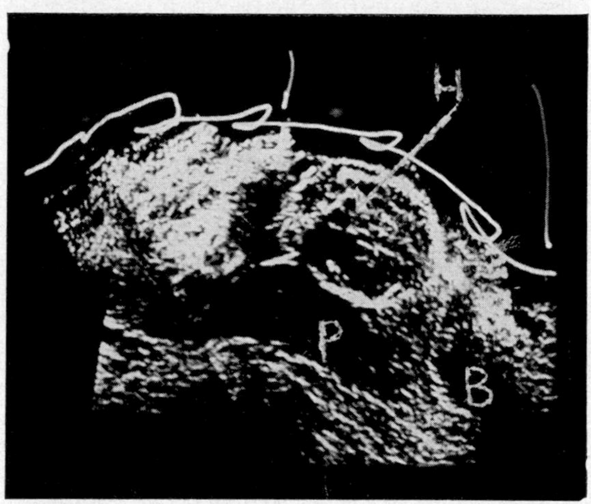

15/FIG. 4.—Posterior placenta praevia, type II, at 37 weeks gestation. Ultrasonogram in longitudinal section, cranialwards to left, confirmed at Caesarean section.

B = Bladder;
H = Fetal head;
P = Placenta.

transverse and, if necessary, oblique section before jumping to conclusions.[9, 10, 14]

To the practical physician no diagnostic method is as reliable as the use of the God-given digit which, unfortunately, must await the maturity of the 38th week. Nevertheless there is great value in knowing rather than suspecting that a placenta is in fact praevia, or conversely that it is safely situated in the upper segment.[7]

Where placenta praevia can be confidently excluded and where bleeding has been slight and has not recurred, it is permissible to allow the patient home from hospital, at least until the 38th week. So far we have not had cause to regret this procedure and from the patient's point of view it saves much unnecessary and tedious hospitalisation. In the large series quoted by Crawford and Sutherland (1961) there was a very material difference in antenatal hospitalisation before delivery or vaginal examination without increasing perinatal mortality, which is the acid test. It is, therefore, our practice to confirm or eliminate the diagnosis of placenta praevia as soon as possible and to review the advisability of allowing the patient home at least until the 38th week. If there is any doubt about the position of the placenta or the bleeding has recurred or is more than slight, then we consider it reckless to allow the patient out of our sight. In quite a significant number of patients, nothing further happens and the cause of bleeding is never finally explained. It might be argued that it was unnecessary to readmit them at the 38th week for examination, but we feel that this is a wise plan because any bleeding from, or damage to, the placental site must to some extent have damaged the baby's chances and we are more than ever inclined to take the opportunity not only of checking the accuracy of the placentography, which is usually well over 90 per cent, but we usually rupture the membranes and induce labour at the same time for fear that the baby may outstrip the reserve of an already damaged placenta, whether it be praevia or normally situated.

Notwithstanding the increasing reliance which so many units, including our own, are placing upon this method Macafee (1960) stated that in his hospital placentography had not been carried out for years. He evidently regarded it as both unnecessary and dangerously misleading. If one is going to take this attitude one must do as he did and keep the patients in hospital until safely delivered. It rather depends upon how much store one places on the woman's liberty to be out and about during pregnancy and whether one is prepared to accept with equanimity and in retrospect an unnecessary period of incarceration within an antenatal ward. Safety may be purchased at too high a price.

Accuracy in placental localisation by sonar increases with the experience of the operator, the quality of his apparatus, and the amount of liquor present in the amniotic cavity. In my view the earlier in pregnancy the placenta is localised the more certain is the diagnosis of the true position of the placenta at the time of the examination. We have nevertheless frequently observed that a placenta which appears to be praevia even at mid-pregnancy, at which time the diagnosis is not correctly allowable but is nevertheless the mechanism in a history of maternal bleeding, such a praevia position may gradually be converted to the upper uterine segment by what King in New York calls "placental migration".[21] I am more inclined to regard this as due to the development of the lower uterine segment in later pregnancy. Such a case showing ultrasonic evidences of a possibly culpable implantation site of the placenta is worth re-examining from time to time, so that this favourable turn of events can be observed. Conversely I cannot recall having seen a case in which the placenta was clearly identified in the upper segment in early pregnancy subsequently turning out to occupy a praevia position. This reassuring information may be very valuable if for some other reason the patient presents with bleeding in later pregnancy.[8]

The identification of the white line of the fetal surface first noted by Kobayashi and his colleagues in New York undoubtedly helps to locate the limits of the placenta with great precision. Accuracy figures have improved upon our own of 94 per cent in 1966 and the literature is replete with better and better results.[22, 40]

The preference for sonar as the means of localising the placenta is rapidly becoming general but I feel strongly that this should be achieved by the means of standard 2-dimensional pulsed echo technique as described in the chapter on sonar and not by the use of Doppler machines, whatever their manufacturers may claim. It is not sufficient to diagnose or exclude placenta praevia by listening to the Doppler effect caused by the movement of circulating blood. The diagnosis is far too serious, and the method is far too imprecise to be trusted.

By comparison soft-tissue radiography (see Figs. 5 to 10) requires a very high standard of radiography and is only obtainable in the sort of unit which ought to be equipped with sonar in any case.

Exclusion of placenta praevia is easiest in the presence of a vertex presentation. A breech presentation introduces difficulties unless the subcutaneous fat around the buttocks is well developed. A transverse lie creates even more difficulty. But no matter what the presentation the basic principles outlined still apply.

In spite of high-grade radiography, soft-tissue techniques provide many pitfalls with which to reckon. Firstly, the placenta may be too thinned out to contribute much of a significant shadow between the fetal outline and the uterine wall. Secondly, the coexistence of hydramnios spoils definition and confuses the diagnosis. Thirdly, the lax abdominal wall, as in the case of a multipara, may allow the unengaged head too much mobility to permit of a reliable assessment. Fourthly, the presence of any pelvic tumour will, of course, vitiate the results. In the next place it may not be possible to obtain a true profile view of the placenta, especially if there is uterine obliquity or rotation, and finally, in any but vertex presentations the X-rays are very much less reliable.

It has been suggested[38, 51] that the hazards attendant upon encountering a major degree of placenta praevia when exploring the lower uterine segment with the finger can be eliminated altogether if the radiological or ultrasonic diagnosis is accepted. Pelvic arteriography, once so definitive,[47] has now been abandoned because of the radiation and technical hazards.

Examination under Anaesthesia at the 38th Week

Let us assume that a patient has now reached the 38th week of pregnancy without further serious blood loss. One has the choice of continuing the supervision in hospital until she goes spontaneously into labour at term, with the question of placenta praevia still in doubt, or of making the diagnosis by vaginal examination. The latter course is usually to be preferred, because if, in fact, placenta praevia is present in severe degree, there is little to be gained by sitting any longer on a volcano. On the other hand, fetal interests may be best served in cases of earlier abruptio placentae by artificial rupture of the membranes at the 38th week, because of the higher incidence of stillbirth already discussed.

The examination is conducted in an operating theatre, where the instruments are all laid out in readiness for Caesarean section should it be necessary. A slow saline drip should be set up in advance. Compatible blood should be available for immediate use if required, and the anaesthetic should be such as will permit proceeding to

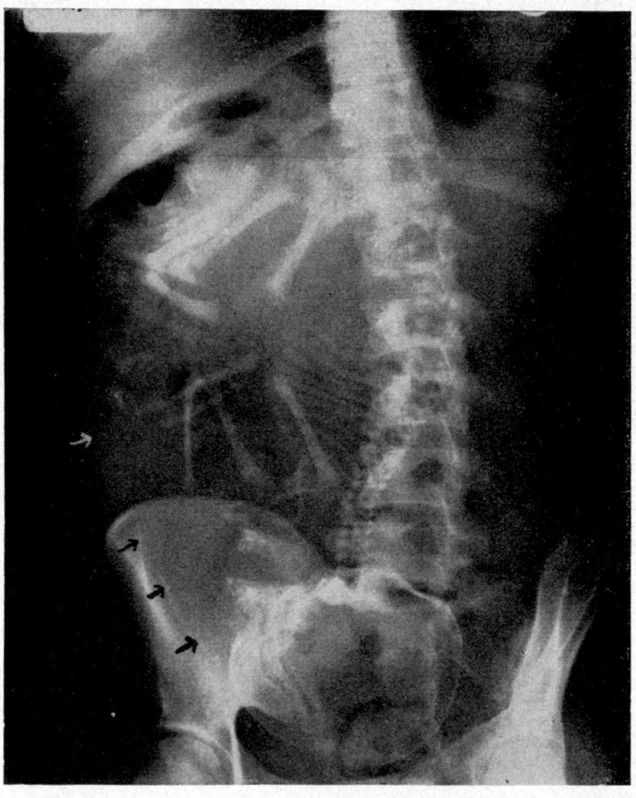

15/Fig. 5.—Placental calcification. Fine filigree calcification in the placenta which is implanted on the right lateral uterine wall.

operation without further delay. It is better not to put the patient in the lithotomy position. I have been badly caught out with a massive haemorrhage which was provoked in this position and valuable seconds were lost in replacing the patient's legs on the operating

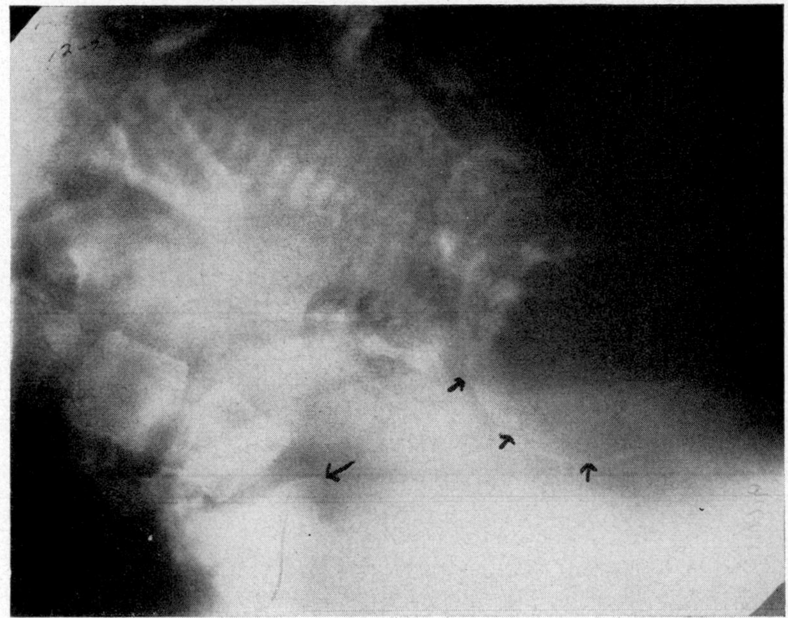

15/FIG. 6.—Semi-inclined view. Posterior placenta praevia. Note the failure of the presenting part to descend into close relationship to the sacral promontory.

table. For the same reason an assistant should be standing by, ready gloved, to open the abdomen while the surgeon changes his own gown and gloves, in order to save precious time and blood. If haemorrhage is really profuse it is tempting to dispense with the examination under anaesthesia altogether and proceed forthwith to Caesarean section. Occasionally I have been in that much of a hurry, but I can recall a case in which the haemorrhage was, in fact, coming from some large, torn varicose veins just inside the introitus that were fortunately observed before proceeding to a section which would have been wholly inappropriate.

Our own rules about working only in operating theatres for all surgical procedures, however minor, including, of course, all cases of antepartum bleeding whatsoever the diagnosis, was on one occasion disastrously ignored by a junior colleague who had excellent clinical reasons for diagnosing abruptio placentae and set out to rupture the

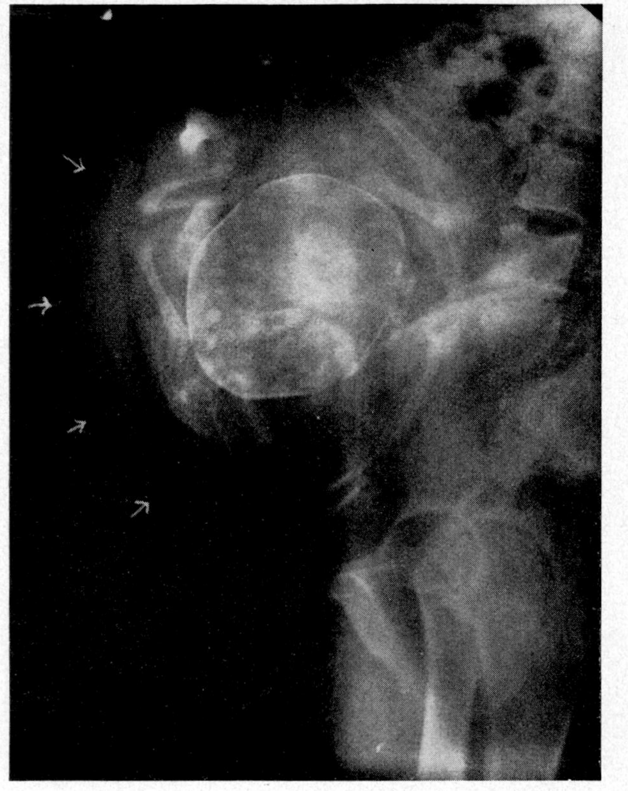

15/Fig. 7.—Normal anterior placenta. No placenta praevia. Fetus lies transversely.

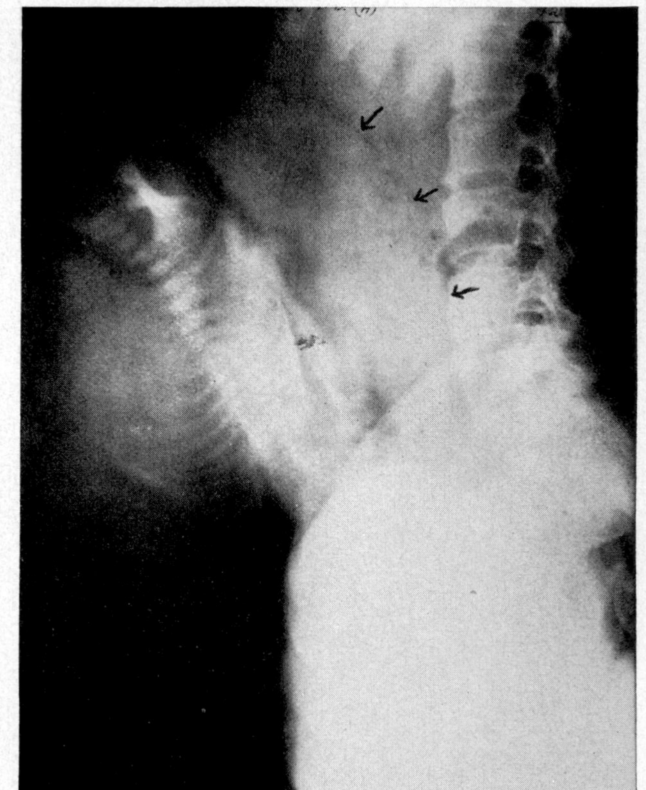

15/Fig. 8.—Normal posterior placenta. No placenta praevia.

membranes in one of our small normal delivery rooms, in which surgical procedures are forbidden. He was greeted with such torrential haemorrhage from placenta praevia that the patient had a cardiac arrest within a minute or two and before any kind of effective action

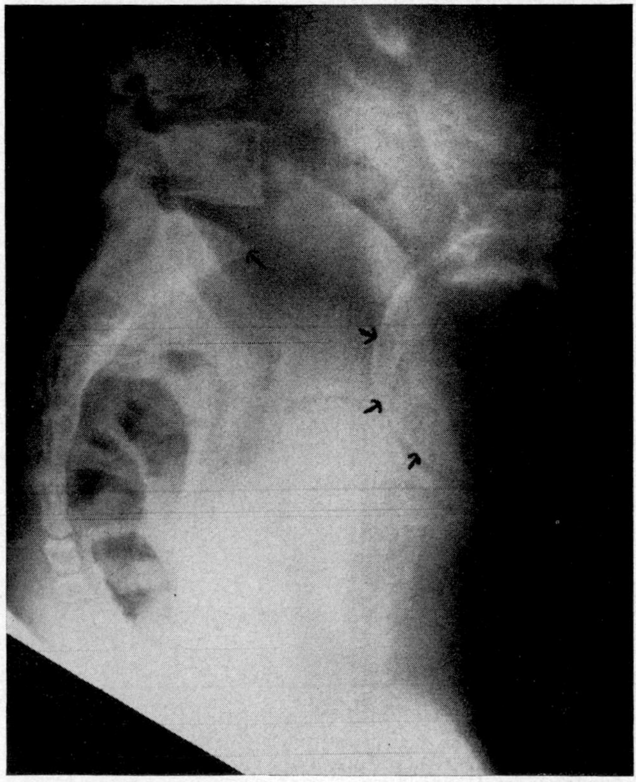

15/FIG. 9.—Erect lateral view. Posterior placenta praevia, grade three. (Fig. 6 shows the semi-inclined view of the same patient.)

could be undertaken. The usual three-hour programme of resuscitative techniques was gone through before life was finally pronounced to be extinct.

Another precaution to bear in mind when one is forced into carrying out an examination under anaesthesia or some vaginal procedure in the acute case with a full stomach, is the danger of passing a stomach tube in a laudable attempt to reduce the hazards of inhaled vomit. The placenta praevia case already bleeding may in fact bleed very much more heavily as a result of gagging with the passage of the

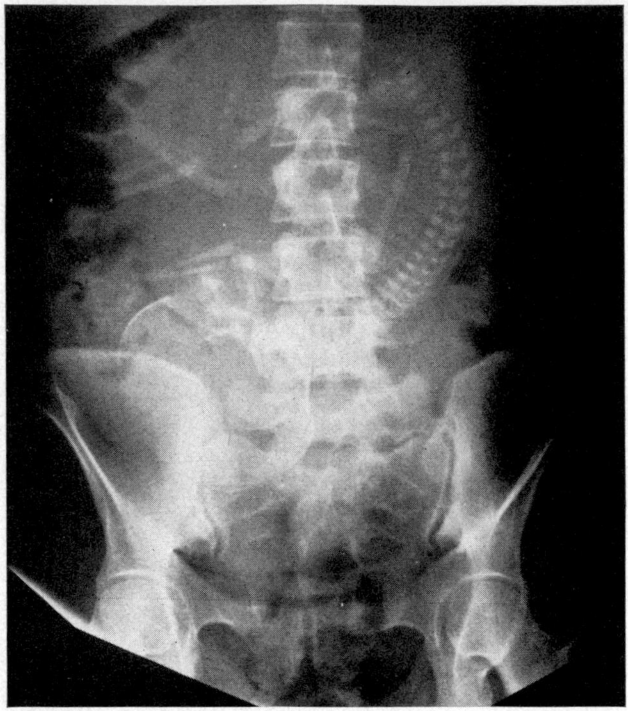

15/Fig. 10 (*a*).—*See opposite.*

tube and it is far safer to induce the anaesthetic with the patient lying on her side and to intubate as soon as she is unconscious. Rapid head-down tilt facilities are, of course, mandatory, as in all modern anaesthesia.

While the most important part of the procedure is the presence of established anaesthesia before starting, the instrument packs for immediate Caesarean section should be at hand. The bladder is drained and the usual aseptic and antiseptic ritual carried out. The vaginal examination is now made.

The head is pressed into the brim, and first of all the fornices are thoroughly explored to see if there is any intervening thickness in the lower uterine segment between finger and the fetal head or presenting part. If the head can be felt clearly through all fornices, one may then proceed to pass a finger through the cervix with increasing confidence. If, on the other hand, a suggestive mass of tissue is felt through the fornices in the lower segment, one should proceed to the rest of the examination with great deliberateness and care. If

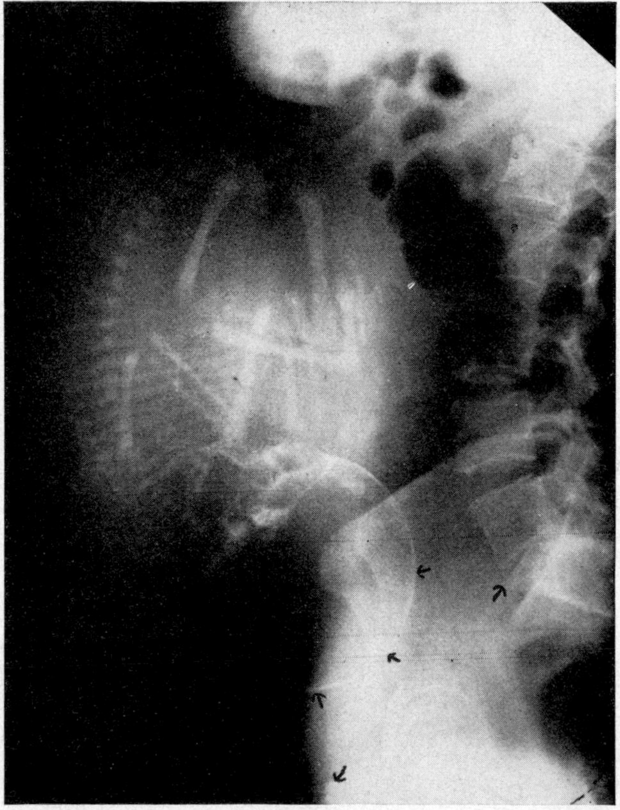

15/FIG. 10 (*b*).

15/FIG. 10.—Left lateral placenta praevia. (*a*) The postero-anterior view shows displacement of the presenting part upwards and to the right. (*b*) The erect lateral view shows displacement of the presenting part away from both the symphysis pubis and the sacral promontory.

the placenta is lying over the internal os, in other words it is of the third or the fourth degree, quite severe bleeding may be provoked at this stage unless one proceeds with great gentleness. The presence of the placenta in this position is not always as easy to diagnose as one would think, and blood clot may easily be mistaken for it. However, on careful palpation the stringiness of the placenta will be observed, which is lacking in the case of blood clot, which feels more friable.

If no placenta is felt over the os, the finger is now passed inside the lower segment and proceeds to explore by sweeping gently in a concentric fashion of ever-widening radius until as much as possible of the region within 3 inches (7·5 cm) of the os has been carefully investigated.

Furious bleeding may occur as a result of detaching the placenta, in which case the examining finger should be kept within the cervix to act as a temporary plug. This haemorrhage has plenty of volume but very little pressure, and it is not difficult to hold it in check with the finger *in situ*, unless the cervix is already more than one finger dilated. Caesarean section must in this case be undertaken at once, and since we have waited patiently until the 38th week the question of prematurity need not further concern us. While waiting for the final preparations for Caesarean section, the finger should be kept *in situ* as long as the bleeding threatens to continue. The gloves are then changed and the operation is begun. Occasionally it is not possible to control the haemorrhage by keeping the finger in the cervix, and in this case roll gauze, 6 inches wide, can be quickly packed into the vagina. If this is not immediately available, one should proceed with the utmost expedition to operate. If the placenta is found over the internal os, but bleeding is not provoked, the occasion still demands Caesarean section forthwith.

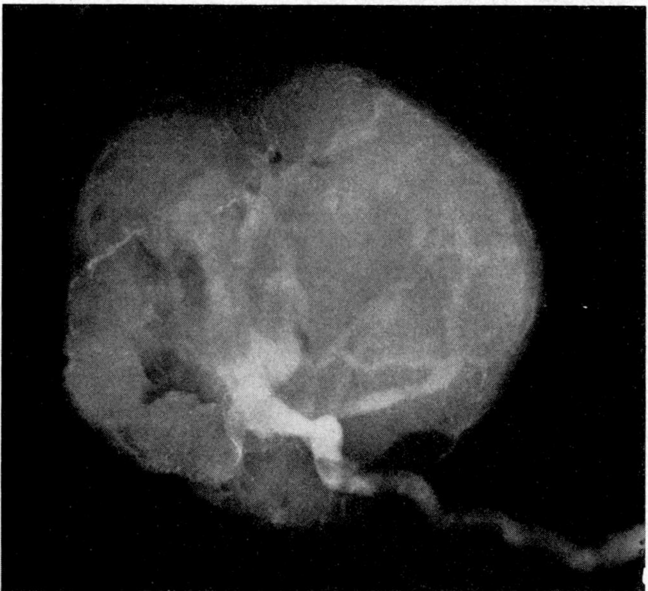

15/FIG. 11.—X-ray of placenta after delivery showing fine granular calcification.

Sometimes bleeding is only slight, usually with the lesser degrees of placenta praevia, and, provided that there are no other obstetrical contra-indications, the forewaters should be ruptured. This will bring the head or the presenting part on to the detached placenta, and should very quickly control further bleeding. The patient should now be watched for about ten minutes, to make sure that bleeding is not going to start again, before she is allowed to come round from her anaesthetic and proceed to vaginal delivery. If, on the other hand, artificial rupture of the forewaters does not control the bleeding and the patient is not already in labour, Caesarean section is undoubtedly the safest course in preference to version, pulling down a leg, or applying Willett's forceps, procedures which belong to a bygone era.

If no placenta praevia is felt and no bleeding is provoked, and the cervix is unfavourable, i.e. like the spout of a teapot, one may decide against rupturing the membranes at this time and return the patient to her bed to await the spontaneous onset of labour.

Treatment of Placenta Praevia

It will have been noted that thus far nothing has been done in the actual treatment of placenta praevia, only a conservative policy of "watch and wait" in the hope of getting past the hazards of prematurity. However, there is an account from Scandinavia[13] of an idea first suggested by Løvset, that an encircling suture of the cervix using thick, grained nylon might be used, as in the Shirodkar operation, to prevent the lower segment of the uterus and the internal os from dilating and allowing further separation of the placenta. The patients so treated were thereafter allowed home. I have no experience of such a technique and am not likely to acquire it, because if the patient did not have a placenta praevia, and it is quite likely I might not yet know, the operation would have been unnecessary; if I knew she had a placenta praevia I would be afraid of triggering off a massive haemorrhage, if one was not already in force demanding evacuation of the uterus in its own right, and even if I succeeded in inserting the suture as suggested I would be terrified to let her home with an established diagnosis of placenta praevia. In fact the dividend of a few weeks' extra shopping in the world outside would hardly seem worth the anxiety entailed.

The outlook in antepartum haemorrhage, in general, has been transformed for the better in recent years, firstly by the ready availability of blood, secondly by the advent of antibiotics, thirdly by the improved methods of anaesthesia, and fourthly, by the increased use of lower-segment Caesarean section. Unfortunately Caesarean section is no guarantee of neonatal survival as babies so delivered in these cases have an increased susceptibility to the respiratory distress syndrome due to hyaline membrane atelectasis.

Most undergraduates have been trained to invoke Caesarean section in their answers as the last resort in treatment, but in this condition it should be the first. This is not to suggest that Caesarean section is always the treatment of choice, and we will presently review the indications for the alternative methods. The advantages of Caesarean section in placenta praevia are that the fetal prospects are good, that maternal mortality is reduced, the cervix is not torn (a danger to which it is exposed by the increased vascularity as a result of placenta praevia) and, in the end, the patient is delivered as a rule with far less loss of blood. In the first two years after opening the Queen Mother's Hospital we lost only one baby in 32 cases of placenta praevia and the section rate was 84 per cent.

Although the lower-segment operation is now almost universally preferred it is as well to beware of two hazards in placenta praevia. Firstly, the placenta, if encountered, should be spared from damage as far as possible because the baby may lose a dangerous amount of blood before the cord is clamped. It is far better to find an edge to the placenta and push it aside in order to extract the baby rather than to cut through it, if this is at all feasible, and in either case because of the danger of fetal haemorrhage the cord should be clamped as soon as possible. Secondly, maternal haemorrhage may be very brisk. The best way of coping with this is to get on with the operation and finish it. Louw recommended packing or ligation of the uterine vessels to control severe bleeding, but fast, determined and accurate suturing of the uterine incision should be adequate in most cases.

Unfortunately the placenta may be morbidly adherent to the lower segment in patches and in the course of trying to separate it haemorrhage may be very profuse. This is not uncommon and the surgeon is torn between the desire to get the uterus sewn up as quickly as possible and at the same time to satisfy himself that the source of the bleeding from within the uterus has been dealt with before it is shut from view. Having closed the abdomen it may now be seen that a patient is bleeding fairly freely per vaginam. Three alternatives have now to be faced; hopeful expectancy, hysterectomy or packing.

Usually the blood transfusion rate is accelerated and the patient is allowed to surface from her anaesthetic, in the hope that with further ergometrine and squeezing the blood out of the uterus all will yet be well, and this is often the case; but sometimes bleeding continues or recurs and in my own experience I have met two such cases of the utmost severity. In the first of these, I saw the patient several hours after her original Caesarean section for placenta praevia and she was now pulseless with a blood pressure of 40/0 mm Hg and receiving her 14th pint of blood. I was put under great pressure to undertake hysterectomy forthwith, but it was fairly obvious that her condition could not stand such a procedure. She was still bleeding, and under a very brisk and light cyclopropane anaesthetic I packed the uterus firmly from top to bottom with a further reinforcement of ergometrine, trusting to my colleague's suturing. The effect was dramatic and with further blood transfusions she rapidly improved and left hospital fourteen days later none the worse for her experience. The pack was removed after twenty-four hours under morphine and this would appear to be the treatment of choice, as in this case she was a young primigravida aged 27.

A more recent case was a grand multipara in her late thirties who continued to bleed furiously after lower-segment Caesarean section for placenta praevia at the hands of a junior but experienced colleague. He called one of his seniors, who, two hours later, removed the

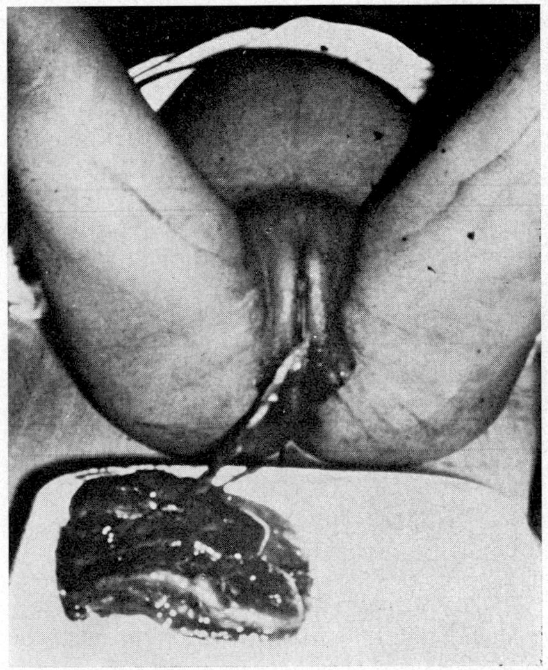

15/Fig. 12.—Case of severe antepartum haemorrhage due to placenta praevia. The patient, para 6-0, was admitted to hospital having had no antenatal care and with a history of 12 hours bleeding and labour pains. During transit from home to hospital she delivered the placenta but retained the baby, as shown above. Spontaneous vertex delivery of a dead baby was achieved 6 hours later following blood transfusion and oxytocin drip. Baby weighed almost 3 kg. Recovered.
(By courtesy, Prof. Majid Memon, Hyderabad.)

uterus. Her condition, nevertheless, continued to deteriorate although there wasn't much visible bleeding from the vagina. Six hours later her condition was truly desperate and intraperitoneal bleeding was strongly suspected. She was curarised, intubated and put onto intermittent positive-pressure inflation, while hypothermia was induced with ice packed round the axillae and neck. In this condition she hovered between life and death for several hours more and I was invited to see her. I might say here that although there were strong grounds for suspecting continued intraperitoneal bleeding in spite of the perfectly routine hysterectomy, with complete confidence about the integrity of the pedicles, the diagnosis was extraordinarily difficult to make in a frozen patient, totally relaxed under curare. The fearful decision had to be made whether to open the abdomen for the third time in eighteen hours in her present very parlous condition. To be mistaken might well prove disastrous. Her circulating blood volume was rapidly estimated by a physicist using a standard dilution technique with radioiodine and he announced what was, to him, the highly improbable result of one litre. Considering the patient's condition I was only too ready to believe this and with the help of one of my ultrasonic machines there could be no doubt that the abdomen was full of fluid, presumably blood. On opening the abdomen there was an enormous quantity of blood everywhere, both retroperitoneal and intraperitoneal, and on examining the pedicles all were perfectly secure, but the raw surface of the bladder and every possible blood vessel in the region of the vaginal vault was streaming blood and it was impossible to overtake the situation by suturing. The condition seemed to be particularly bad on the left side. I therefore ligated the anterior division of the left internal iliac artery, passing an aneurysm needle under it, blind, loaded with strong silk and taking great care not to rupture the underlying internal iliac vein. This did the trick and we had no further trouble. She left hospital seventeen days later with full recovery of her renal function and again apparently none the worse for her terrible experience.

In retrospect I feel that hysterectomy in this case should not have been undertaken and it would have been far better to have packed the uterus firmly and deliberately from top to bottom, but my friend who called me in said that he had had the most tragic experiences from this procedure but, of course, he was referring to the desperate 1930s, when this measure was often undertaken as a last resort in the absence of blood transfusion. This case just described had, in all, 26 pints of blood, which, to date, is my record.

All cases of third- and fourth-degree placenta praevia should be delivered by Caesarean section, not only in the interests of the mother but chiefly in the interests of the child. In deciding the delivery route, the relationship of the presenting part to the brim is of more importance than the nearness of the placenta to the internal os, and an anterior placenta praevia case can be more safely delivered by the vaginal route than cases where the placenta is posterior. If the head can be made to engage in the brim without upsetting the fetal heart, it is an additional indication that the membranes can be ruptured safely. As a general rule, therefore, vaginal delivery is nowadays more and more restricted to those cases of the first and second degree, in which the placenta is anteriorly situated.

Occasionally, a patient's condition may be so moribund from haemorrhage that one may be tempted to defer operation until her condition has been restored by blood transfusion. This procrastination, however, is only permissible if bleeding has already stopped, otherwise matters can only be made worse by every minute's delay. No case is ever so moribund from placenta praevia bleeding as to contra-indicate Caesarean section. In this desperate emergency, rapid classical Caesarean section is indicated. I much regret not having done so in a very acute case who died on the table just after the uterus had been emptied and tragedy might, in fact, have been averted by saving even a few precious seconds involved in carrying out the more formal lower-segment operation. Clearly I had underestimated the gravity of the patient's acute blood loss and encountered the immediate period of primary shock, the signs of which are described in a later chapter as usually appearing about ten minutes too late.

If the patient when first seen is bleeding and already in labour, a vaginal examination should be made, preferably under an anaesthetic, so as to permit the pulling down of a leg if a foot presents and the placenta is not covering the internal os. If the vertex presents, rupture of the forewaters may suffice. This is particularly useful in the case of the multipara. If this simple measure arrests the haemorrhage, nothing further should be done to expedite delivery; in fact, any hurry will be positively dangerous because of the risk of tearing the lower segment and cervix and also of increasing shock. If this does not arrest the haemorrhage it is better to apply gentle traction to the leg brought down or, as the case may be, to the vertex by means of a ventouse cup (vacuum extractor), than to resort to the now discredited Willett's forceps. Slow and very gentle delivery may thus be achieved. This is less traumatic to the maternal tissues in a cervix not yet fully dilated than the ordinary obstetrical forceps. Willett's forceps do far more damage to the baby's scalp and personally I have not used them or seen them used on such a case since before the last war. All the more picturesque and bloody methods of coping with placenta praevia during labour have now gone by the board and one is left fundamentally with the alternative of Caesarean section or artificial rupture of the membranes with spontaneous labour possibly assisted by vacuum extraction. Any unit without facilities for undertaking Caesarean section is not really fit to undertake obstetrics.

General Remarks concerning Vaginal Delivery

Labour must not be hurried. By contrast, the advocates of *accouchement forcé* of a century ago reaped a terrible harvest of disaster, both from increased haemorrhage and shock. All possible steps should be taken to restore the patient's blood volume in order to improve her chances of surmounting the risks of the third stage. Antepartum anaemia, moreover, predisposes the patient to uterine atony. The third stage is full of possible treachery, and a relatively small blood loss now may tip the scales against an already shocked and exsanguinated patient, so that all possible prophylactic steps should be taken, including the use of ergometrine at the completion of the second stage. Not only are the effects of bleeding more marked in placenta praevia delivery, but postpartum haemorrhage is particularly likely to occur for the following reasons. Firstly, part of the placental site is in the lower segment of the uterus and, therefore, in a non-retractile portion. Secondly, the placenta which is praevia is usually larger and thinner than usual and, as a result, the shearing mechanism, whereby the mass of the placenta is detached from the uterine wall in the normal physiology of the third stage, fails to operate effectively, and one is then faced with all the evils of a partially separated yet retained placenta. Morbid adherence, too, is not uncommon. Lastly, because the placental site is generally larger, there is a greater area from which bleeding can occur. The patient cannot be regarded as safely delivered until at least a couple of hours after the placenta has arrived.

Because cervical tears are particularly common, preparations should always be at hand for the proper examination and suturing of the cervix if necessary. The incidence of manual removal of the placenta is somewhat increased, because of morbid adhesion.

Attention to asepsis and antisepsis must be punctilious, because puerperal sepsis is very liable to follow, not from local interference but because the placental site, being both lower in the genital tract and larger than usual, provides a portal of entry which is more quickly reached by ascending infection. Often a certain amount of old blood clot will have been retained in the uterus for a considerable period of time, so that intra-uterine infection may be already established before the completion of labour. The patient, because of her exsanguination, will succumb far more readily to infection in the puerperium than the patient who finds herself after delivery still in possession of nearly all her original blood. All the antibiotics in the world are no substitute for a healthy blood state, and one pint of blood is worth several million units of penicillin.

ABRUPTIO PLACENTAE

There is a dying tendency in the reports from obstetrical departments to classify all cases of antepartum haemorrhage in which evidence of placenta praevia is not established as cases of accidental haemorrhage. Such a classification is too wide, because in at least a quarter of the cases of antepartum haemorrhage an accurate diagnosis of its source cannot be made, and when this is the case such patients should be put in the unclassifiable group.

We are concerned in this section with bleeding from the placental site when it is normally situated wholly within the upper uterine segment. Bleeding can only occur if there is some degree of placental detachment, and for this reason the term "abruptio placentae" is preferred. The process is bound to leave its effect or scar upon the placenta itself, and, unless the clinical evidences before delivery are overwhelming, these placental signs should be looked for and noted after delivery before regarding the case finally as one of abruptio.

The placenta after delivery shows, in a recent case, a depression, usually with a clot firmly attached to it, or, if some time has elapsed between the abruptio and delivery, evidences of a sizeable area of infarction in varying degrees of organisation. Not all cases of abruptio bleed *per vaginam*, and there are minor degrees which end in no more than a retroplacental haematoma, a condition in which the so-called variety of concealed accidental haemorrhage occurs in miniature.

Placenta praevia and "accidental" antepartum haemorrhage have only one thing in common, namely both types bleed as a result of placental separation, but in all other respects they differ totally. In abruptio, the external bleeding is probably the least important feature of the case, and what matters far more is the degree of associated toxaemia, shock, the amount of blood retained *in utero*, and the area of abrupted placenta. In fact, the greater the amount of external, revealed bleeding, the less wide as a rule is the area of placental separation *in utero*, and, conversely, the most severe cases of concealed haemorrhage result in practically total placental separation.

Abruptio placentae, therefore, declares itself as concealed intra-uterine harmorrhage, in which no blood whatsoever appears at the vulva for the time being, or as revealed external haemorrhage, in which practically no blood is retained within the uterine cavity. Most commonly, a mixture of the two varieties obtains. The gravity of the case is directly proportional to the amount of blood retained within the uterus, because herein lies the source of severe degrees of shock. The extent to which bleeding is concealed or revealed is determined far more by the tone of the uterine muscle and its ability to expel the blood to the outside world than by the actual quantity of blood lost. If all the bleeding were revealed, the patient's general condition would vary directly with the amount of blood lost, but in the concealed variety the patient's general condition is grave out of all proportion to the blood lost, even including the quantity apparently retained *in utero*. It is important, therefore, not to be misled into relating the gravity of the condition to the amount of visible haemorrhage. In placenta praevia, on the other hand, haemorrhage is often very much more profuse, and its degree directly accounts for the patient's general condition.

The above categorical statements are almost wholly true but alas not totally so, and the clinical differentiation between unavoidable and accidental haemorrhage, between placenta praevia and abruptio placenta, is not always absolute and there may be an overlap. We have all seen cases due to placenta praevia bleeding who have had a hard, tender uterus with retained blood within it and conversely cases of accidental haemorrhage with surprisingly little pain or uterine hardness that have been due to major degrees of placental abruption.

It is difficult to arrive at a reliable estimate of the incidence of abruptio placentae, and figures should only be accepted from centres in which definite evidences of abruptio are sought and noted, including examination of the placenta after delivery, and to accept the exclusion of placenta praevia as grounds for classifying the case as one of accidental haemorrhage is to rate the incidence too high. True, abruptio is very much less common than placenta praevia—certainly less than half. O'Donel Browne, for example, confining himself to toxaemic antepartum haemorrhage, gave the incidence as 0·6 per cent. In multiparae the incidence is 4 times as high as in primigravidae. To some extent, this is offset by the fact that there are more multiparae and they tend to fall into a slightly older age group, with a consequent general rise in the level of blood pressure, but the incidence increases markedly after the fifth pregnancy, and rapidly repeated childbearing is also a factor. Social factors are undoubtedly important and the frequency of abruptio increases the further down the social scale one searches. Abruptio can occur at any time in late pregnancy, but most commonly does so about the 34th week.

The majority of the genuine cases are of the mixed variety, and the wholly concealed haemorrhage is fortunately an uncommon, though desperate, emergency.

Aetiology of Abruptio

In many instances it is impossible to trace the cause; nevertheless the coincidence of pre-eclamptic toxaemia is by far the most important factor. This however, is only half the truth, for the majority of cases of toxaemia do not suffer abruptio and, in a certain number, the evidences of pre-eclampsia are first seen after the onset of abruptio and not before it. Proteinuria, for example, is frequently found for the first time after shock has supervened. Patients who are already in hospital under observation for pre-eclamptic toxaemia only uncommonly develop abruptio, and there is some doubt in relating pre-eclampsia to abruptio in deciding which is cause and which effect.[19] The number of cases of known pre-eclamptic toxaemia who abrupt is only moderately raised to 1·6 per cent, as against a normal control rate of 1·07 per cent and in the case of hypertension 2·3 per cent.[16, 17] The issue is further fogged by the fact that antecedent hypertension may be masked, when the patient is first seen, by the development of shock, which lowers the blood pressure. Notwithstanding all this, it is generally accepted as one of the entities of the pre-eclamptic state, and it is probable that many more of these cases would actually develop eclampsia were it not for the fact that the blood pressure is reduced first by the shock of concealed haemorrhage.

The theory underlying the association of pre-eclampsia is that there is hypertensive spasm of the vessels supplying the placental site which results in capillary anoxia. When the hypertensive spasm wears off, the damaged capillaries are unable to cope with the vascular engorgement which follows, and bleeding therefore takes place. Both chronic nephritis and hypertension are associated with abruptio and the mechanism here is probably somewhat similar. In many cases of abruptio there is no evidence of toxaemia. In this type of case the antepartum haemorrhage may not only recur during pregnancy but may complicate later pregnancies as well. We are largely in agreement with the view emanating from Liverpool that folic acid deficiency may be a major aetiological factor without overt megaloblastic anaemia being present. Seventy-two out of seventy-three cases of abruptio were found by Hibbard to have this deficiency and we too have found a remarkable reduction in the frequency of abruptio placentae since concentrating upon the early detection of anaemia of all varieties, including folic acid deficiency.

Our own view is that there is a mixed aetiology in this condition partly due to toxaemia, partly to a poor nutritional state, especially associated with high degrees of parity or with nutritional neglect in the case of the unmarried primigravida. The Liverpool view has traditionally been that the main deficiency state which predisposes to abruptio placentae is one which is in fact already operating in the very early stages of pregnancy at the period of early fetal and chorionic development. The finding therefore of folic acid deficiency in mid-pregnancy is thus often too late to be corrected by folic acid supplements which may do no more than prevent the development of megaloblastic anaemia but will not by themselves protect the woman from placental abruption later. All this would fit in with the unhappy phenomenon encountered of recurrent abruption in successive pregnancies and I myself know of one patient who, in spite of hospitalisation and every thinkable precaution, abrupted her placenta for the fourth successive time in one of our own antenatal wards.

As mentioned in Chapter VII the blood of our patients is examined at every antenatal clinic visit and a small but adequate supplementary dose of folic acid is given along with iron therapy, which is reckoned to be about adequate for the Glasgow diet. In fact most of the cases we now see are among the unbooked, and not only those who have had no antenatal care, but perhaps the even more unfortunate who have had inadequate care outside.

There is probably more to the problem than simply folic acid deficiency as an isolated cause and there may indeed be multiple dietetic factors; for example, in Malaysia no increased evidence of megaloblastic erythropoiesis could be found in association with cases of abruptio placentae.[49]

The "supine hypotensive syndrome", a condition in which the inferior vena cava is obstructed by the pressure of the gravid uterus in late pregnancy when the patient lies on her back, is thought to be associated with occasional abruptio, as has been experimentally produced in animals. Certainly recumbency in the dorsal position aggravates shock and hypotension after abruptio has occurred and before the uterus is emptied. These cases should always be nursed in the left lateral position.[28, 56]

In a few cases, the cause can be related to trauma and, in these instances, the bleeding is mainly revealed. The commonest type of trauma likely to cause bleeding is that of external cephalic version, particularly under anaesthesia where the anaesthetic has been used as a misguided excuse for the employment of more than customary force. In hypertensive and pre-eclamptic patients, therefore, because of their increased tendency to abruptio, external version is contra-indicated.

Direct blows to the abdomen may also cause abruptio, although it is remarkable how much violence the average pregnant uterus can withstand without suffering this complication. Coitus is occasionally incriminated, and in a few cases the bleeding appears to follow some great psychological shock, though the mechanism of the latter is obscure.

Occasionally the existence of a short cord has been blamed, but this is only likely to operate as a cause if the patient is in labour with the presenting part advancing. In a few cases, fibroids are held responsible in the same way as they may be regarded as causes of abortion.

Because of the generally accepted influence of multiparity, it has been postulated that subinvolution of the uterus may be a cause. But this, on the whole, is unlikely, because conception in the first place is thereby discouraged. Social factors combined with poor, lifelong dietary habits are often linked with uncontrolled parity.

Lastly, separation of the placenta may follow the sudden release of hydramnios.

PATHOLOGY

The changes in the placenta, as observed after delivery, have already been mentioned, and the freshness of the infarcted area will depend upon the time interval existing since separation.

It has been suggested that in the first place a retroplacental haematoma forms and may build up sufficient pressure to rupture the basal plate, the resulting laceration in which allows a free communication from the intradecidual space of the haematoma into the maternal circulation of the placenta. There now follows a process of what Schneider[44] described as "auto-extraction" of tissue substances including thromboplastin from the decidua directly into the maternal circulation, thereafter to be distributed throughout the general maternal circulation with resulting coagulopathy.

In the full-blown case of concealed haemorrhage the uterus is distended to an appreciably greater size than would apply to the period of gestation, and contains a large retroplacental clot which may have tracked beyond the confines of the placental margin and may even have burst into the amniotic sac. The characteristic Couvelaire uterus shows ecchymoses on its serous surface which may be heavily fissured and from which blood may be oozing. Bleeding may likewise occur between the layers of the broad ligament, and the muscle bundles of the uterine wall are heavily infiltrated with extravasated blood and oedema fluid. It is not certain whether the haemorrhages are entirely due to capillary endothelial damage resulting from hypertension, spasm and anoxia or to the direct effects of some toxin, but it can be easily seen how the uterus itself comes to be atonic, which is one of the features of this condition. In the worst cases of Couvelaire uterus there is usually a blood-clotting defect due to hypofibrinogenaemia. The peritoneal cavity usually contains an appreciable quantity of blood-stained fluid, and occasionally the uterus may actually rupture with profuse intraperitoneal haemorrhage, although this, considering the damage to the uterine wall, is surprisingly rare. The uterine muscle fibres themselves may necrose in patchy areas, yet the case who recovers appears to suffer no residual uterine structural weakness.

The pathological changes of eclampsia may be found in both the liver and the kidneys, even though the onset of eclamptic seizures has been aborted by the shock of the abruptio. Distant organs often show numerous small haemorrhages, for example the ovaries, tubes, liver, suprarenals, heart and meninges, while haematemesis may result from haemorrhages in the gastric mucosa and haematuria may likewise arise from the damaged kidneys. The disturbance, therefore, is by no means confined to the uterus, but is more general (Fig. 13).

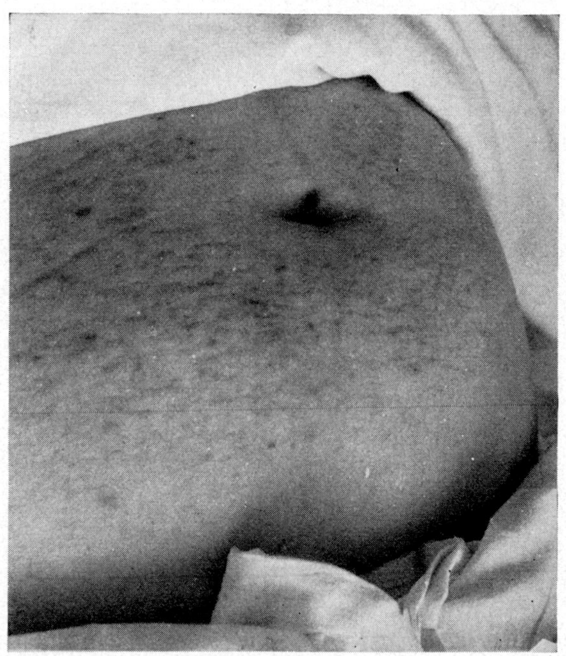

15/FIG. 13.—Purpuric type of rash in a case of abruptio placentae at 34 weeks, with hypofibrinogenaemia, megaloblastic anaemia, thrombocytopenia and twins. She required 4 litres of plasma and 7½ litres of blood. Recovered.

The kidneys are liable to suffer further disaster, either in the form of bilateral cortical necrosis, which is a characteristic sequel of concealed accidental haemorrhage, and is practically always fatal, or a tubular nephrosis may occur as a result of shock. These two causes of suppression of urine and death from uraemia are dealt with more fully in the section on oliguria (Chapter XI).

Sheehan's Syndrome

Some cases manage to survive a severe and prolonged period of shock due to abruptio placentae only to demonstrate later on the signs of anterior pituitary necrosis, namely amenorrhoea, genital atrophy, intolerance to cold, listlessness and premature senility.

Murdoch (1962) followed up 94 patients who had severe postpartum haemorrhage and shock in Glasgow. The follow-up extended up to nine years after the incident and already 11 of them (11·6 per cent) complained of poor health and intolerance to cold although, except for one patient, amenorrhoea (apart from hysterectomy) was not a feature. The severity of the shock would appear to be less important than its duration and the full-blown picture of hypopituitarism may be delayed until the time of the natural menopause. Conversely Murdoch observed that in 54 cases of Sheehan's syndrome the onset of symptoms had first appeared in almost a half of them between the ages of 41 and 50 years (24 cases) and he reckons that the menopause or an earlier pyrexial illness may act as triggers in the case of latent hypopituitarism from obstetrical causes.

Mortality

The condition of abruptio can provide from time to time one of the most desperate situations in obstetrics. What is both surprising and creditable is that nowadays maternal death occurs only very occasionally, thanks to modern treatment of shock, coagulation failure and renal shutdown. For example in a good peripheral unit in a series of 189 cases of placental abruption there was one maternal death.[1] The fetus is of course in great peril and approximately 50 per cent of the babies die. Many might be saved if the case could be got to a well-equipped maternity unit in time since the fetus may survive for an hour or two after quite severe abruption. Nevertheless prematurity is commonly an added cause of fetal death, even if the baby is rescued by prompt Caesarean section. This operation has a somewhat limited role since the patient may be in too severe a state of shock to stand it and it is commonly the case that the pregnancy has not advanced beyond the 34th week of gestation in which case the baby has a poor chance because of the added hazard of prematurity. However it has a definite place when it is clear on examination that labour cannot be induced easily and completed in a very short time, for example, when the cervix is long and very unfavourable. One is particularly encouraged to operate if the baby appears to be of a reasonable size and, of course, alive. Caesarean section is inappropriate when the baby is dead. The quandary is only likely to arise if induction, which is the usual treatment, fails to bring on labour, and in one such case of mine, described later, anuria supervened and clearly I had operated too late.

BLOOD COAGULATION DEFECTS

It might not be out of place to consider here briefly the subject of deficient coagulation as it is particularly one of the complications of abruptio placentae. There are indeed other complications of pregnancy and labour such as amniotic fluid embolism, retained intrauterine dead fetus (especially due to Rh-haemolytic disease) and septic abortion, as will be discussed later, and different mechanisms may operate in producing the ultimate clotting defect according to the causative condition.

The whole subject of blood coagulation has been bedevilled by an inconstant and bewildering terminology, which acts as a "student swamper" and makes the average clinician turn away in frustration and disbelief.

The International Committee for the Nomenclature of Blood Clotting Factors tied up the terminology in accordance with the table below (*Brit. med. J.*, 1962, **1**, 465), since when further modifications have been made and are herewith included.

These factors have a proven separate identity. So far, in obstetrics, we have only to consider a few, but who knows the degree of complexity with which we may yet have to grapple? There are four major stages in coagulation in some of which groups of the above factors may trigger each other off. The process has, in fact, been likened to a cascade or waterfall phenomenon.

Four Stages of Coagulation

1. Formation of activated factor X;
2. Conversion of prothrombin to thrombin;
3. Conversion of fibrinogen to fibrin;
4. Later resolution involving the destruction of fibrin by a process of fibrinolysis in order to restore patency to the clotted vessel.

There is thus a balance between clotting and unclotting known as fibrinolysis and since these are both mechanisms which are controlled by powerful enzyme systems, it can be seen how equilibrium can be lost and the whole situation get out of control.

It will be noted that several of the traditionally accepted numerals have been discarded in the course of characterisation of the purified coagulation factors; for example thromboplastin is no longer known as factor III and calcium is not alluded to by a factor numeral, which would be altogether too pedantic. It will be noted that the existence of factor VI has now been dismissed.

In obstetrics we are mainly concerned with fibrinogen depletion which may be brought about in one of three ways. Firstly, loss of fibrinogen within a retroplacental clot due to abruptio placentae, secondly, intravascular microcoagulation and thirdly, fibrinolysis including fibrinogenolysis.

Hypofibrinogenaemia.—The normal circulating level of fibrinogen in late pregnancy is raised to about 0·45 g per cent and uncontrolled haemorrhage occurs if this level falls below 0·1 g per cent. Many cases of persistent postpartum bleeding in the past were wrongly attributed to the alleged atony of the Couvelaire uterus, when, in fact, they were suffering from hypofibrinogenaemia.

15/TABLE IV

BLOOD CLOTTING FACTORS

Factor I	Fibrinogen.
Factor II	Thrombin.
Factor V	Accelerator globulin, proaccelerin.
Factor VII	Proconvertin, serum prothrombin conversion accelerator (SPCA).
Factor VIII	Antihaemophilic factor.
Factor IX	Christmas factor, antihaemophilic factor B.
Factor X	Stuart-Prower factor.
Factor XI	Plasma thromboplastin antecedent (PTA).
Factor XII	Hageman factor.
Factor XIII	Fibrin stabilising factor.

The association between abruptio placentae and coagulation failure had long been recognised but it was not until Schneider's observations in 1952 that clinicians began to understand the pathology with which they were faced.

At first the generally accepted explanation was that thromboplastins liberated from the retained blood clot or damaged placenta within the uterus, and absorbed into the blood stream, caused widespread microcoagulation throughout the entire vascular tree, too evenly and thinly spread to be clinically noticeable but effectively using up the available supplies of circulating fibrinogen which the liver cannot replace fast enough. It is known that the uterus and the decidua, as well as the lungs, are important sources of tissue thromboplastins when damaged, and this mechanism of microcoagulation may well, in fact, apply in cases of amniotic fluid embolism and retained intra-uterine dead fetus.

In abruptio placentae, however, the observations of Willoughby in this country, Nilsen in Norway and, before these, of Pritchard and Wright in America, have abundantly shown that the loss of fibrinogen from the circulation can, in fact, largely be accounted for by measuring the amount of fibrin within the retroplacental clot. The clot very rapidly retracts, so that its volume at delivery is deceptive simply to naked-eye examination. The fluid components from the clot appear to be absorbed and to dilute further the circulating fibrinogen, haemoglobin and all its other necessary constituents, thereby adding to the patient's anaemia which may become suddenly severe. Coagulation failure is further aggravated. The situation can now be made even worse by the administration of synthetic volume expanders.[55]

It is suggested that quite apart from the factor of fibrinogen dilution by intravenous dextran, the fibrinogen may be precipitated as fibrin or inactivated by forming a fibrinogen-dextran compound.[45] We too have had trouble following dextran infusion in cases of abruptio placentae and have now ceased to use it altogether. After dextran solutions have been used it is more difficult to cross-match the patient's blood for subsequent transfusion—another though less urgent reason for not using them.

Apart from persistent bleeding, often severe, it will be noticed that the blood is slow to clot, sometimes taking over ten minutes to do so and that a clot once formed often liquefies thereafter on incubation. This, the clot observation test described by Weiner, can be done most cleanly at the patient's bedside simply by withdrawing blood from a vein into a dry test tube.

The diagnosis can be confirmed by the thrombin test (Fibrindex or Thrombin (Maw)) on the spot by mixing in a test tube 0·2 ml each of citrated blood and thrombin solution. Clotting should start within 10 seconds in the case of normal blood and the clot should already be formed within a minute. If clotting takes longer than 20 seconds or the clot liquefies after a minute, severe hypofibrinogenaemia is indicated. The Fi-Test (Baxter) claims specificity by using rabbit antibodies to human fibrinogen combined with polystyrene latex. It is only necessary to add one drop of the patient's whole blood diluted in a glycine-saline buffer (provided) to the antibody reagent and clumping should occur within 20 seconds if normal, but low levels of fibrinogen below 0·1 g per cent do not clump. No obstetric unit should be without the means of performing this test which, by indicating the true nature of the patient's peril, may be life saving. It gives only a qualitative rather than a quantitative answer. As soon as possible blood should be sent to the laboratory. Our own practice is to have a stock of labelled tubes containing 1 ml of fresh 3·8 per cent citrate in the freezing compartment of the matched blood refrigerator. Whole blood from the patient is added to this tube up to the 10 ml mark and mixed. It is a good plan to take blood from a normal individual at the same time and in the same way. The fibrinogen level can now be very quickly assayed within about 20 minutes by the Schneider test, in which serial dilutions of the patient's plasma are made up in saline and thrombin is added to each tube. The result is read as the highest dilution at which the fibrin clot becomes visible.[55]

In normal plasma clotting should be observed in all tubes up to a dilution of 1 in 128 and certainly 1 in 64, which corresponds to a concentration of about 200 mg per cent and indicates a safe level of fibrinogen. The clotted tubes are now incubated in order to detect subsequent digestion of fibrin clots. This is one of the main tests which, carried out repeatedly, will indicate whether or not fibrinogen replacement is adequate. A moderate fibrinogen deficiency is revealed at a titre of 1 in 8 to 1 in 32 and severe deficiency may have a titre of 1 in 2, 1 in 4 or no sign of a clot in any of the tubes. A rough-and-ready guide, however, is immediately furnished as to how much fibrinogen to give the patient in order to correct the defect, and it is recommended that titres below 1 in 8 to 1 in 32 require at least 4 g of fibrinogen and titres even lower of than 1 in 8 require 8 g initially. The test should be repeated every hour or two to ensure that a safe level of circulating fibrinogen is being maintained. The actual estimation of fibrinogen level requires a complicated laboratory technique, and takes several hours to complete.

Some years ago I saw a case who was admitted with a severe degree of abruptio and delivered herself shortly thereafter of a stillborn fetus. In spite of a reasonably firm uterus and intravenous ergometrine she continued to bleed after the delivery of the placenta. She required in all one pint of dextrose (at the beginning of the drip), seventeen pints of blood, two of plasma and a further pint of quadruple-strength plasma when the diagnosis of hypofibrinogenaemia became known. Her fibrinogen level was estimated as quickly as possible and found to be at the danger level of 0·1 g per cent. It was the quadruple-strength plasma which saved the day and she left hospital well some days later with a satisfactory urinary output, a haemoglobin level of 10·8 g per cent and a fibrinogen level of 0·35 g per cent, thanks to prompt and massive transfusion (through three drips) which kept just ahead of severe and irreversible shock. Today we would have been a little quicker off the mark in recognising the existence of hypofibrinogenaemia.

Quadruple-strength plasma is viscous and is not used nowadays and the more modern therapy for the treatment of shock associated with hypofibrinogenaemia would be whole blood to replace lost haemoglobin and then a plasma expander. This should consist not of synthetic materials but mainly of fresh frozen plasma, which contains fibrinogen and factors VIII and V as well as the vitamin K-dependent factors II, VII, IX and X. Additionally fibrinogen or cryoprecipitate, which is rich in fibrinogen and factor VIII can be given. A commonly used plasma expander is plasma protein fraction which consists mainly of albumin and this is the most usual plasma expander stocked by the blood transfusion service at present.

In the cases who get over this dire emergency the liver quickly restores the fibrinogen level, often within 48 hours.

The treatment, as soon as the diagnosis is made, is to inject pure fibrinogen 4–8 g intravenously, or the plasma expanders listed above, in preference to double-, triple- or quadruple-strength plasma. Where massive transfusion is necessary, as it often is, the amount of citrate acquired by the patient may be excessive and it is advisable to give calcium gluconate up to 2 g intravenously to counter the citrate effect. Fibrinogen is nowadays readily available and is certainly preferable to plasma because it is possible to correct a deficiency rapidly and by infusion of a smaller volume of fluid.

Some have referred to this as the defibrination syndrome and certainly the loss of fibrinogen is the most important cause of coagulation failure in obstetrics, but other deficiencies must also be looked for as soon as time allows, for example low platelet counts, low levels of factor VIII (antihaemophilic factor), factor IX (Christmas factor), and factor V (proaccelerin). The platelet count is particularly important in cases where hypofibrinogenaemia is due to abnormal fibrinolysis, which is discussed presently. The latter does not lower the platelet count of itself and the loss of platelets is probably due to a severe degree of intravascular clotting, for example, in the pulmonary bed and, in fact, one may be dealing with a case of amniotic fluid embolism whose mechanism differs from that of abruptio placentae.

At one time we held the view that the defibrination syndrome could not be reversed until after the uterus had been evacuated, because it erroneously seemed to us that as long as thromboplastins were being absorbed, any circulating fibrinogen was likely to be deposited further as fibrin; but any persistence of haemorrhage in cases of abruptio in those days was in fact due to inadequate treatment, rather than to the above mechanism.[54] Such a state of affairs may in fact be true with intravascular microcoagulation as may occur after amniotic embolism, but is certainly not true of abruptio placentae where the urgent need is to replace fibrinogen lost within the retroplacental clot, and adequately treated hypofibrinogenaemia can be permanently corrected by an adequate infusion of fibrinogen. In fact, as Willoughby has pointed out, the very fact that such an improvement can be achieved and maintained in circulating fibrinogen levels supports the conclusion that the condition was due to a straight subtraction effect of lost fibrinogen. In the cases he describes, clotting abnormalities were not in fact accentuated by the administration of fibrinogen and furthermore there was no postpartum haemorrhage. The term "consumptive phase" of fibrinogen has been used to signify that the process of fibrinogen depletion is continuing, usually from a different pathology from that found in abruptio placentae, and it is therefore as well to know when giving fibrinogen during this phase is like attempting to rebuild a house that is on fire instead of summoning the Fire Brigade.[46]

It is important to recognise the cause of the hypofibrinogenaemia with which one is faced, because if there is a continuing "consumptive phase" it is likely to be due to the digestion or fibrinolysis of intravascular microcoagulated deposits of fibrin, and stoking up with more fibrinogen will only prolong and aggravate the process. As this hardly happens at all in abruptio placentae, the question of fibrinolysis and antifibrinolytic agents should not therefore feature in the treatment. The situation is altogether different with amniotic embolism and retained dead fetus, and in differentiating the various mechanisms the clinical recognition of the likely cause will be of far more benefit than a whole battery of laboratory tests.

Fibrinolysis can include fibrinogenolysis, and split products of fibrinogen (FDP—fibrinogen degradation products) in themselves may accentuate a clotting defect. Further fibrinogen supplying yet more plasminogen, where activator is still circulating, may magnify and prolong the lytic effect. But more important still perhaps is to recognise that fibrinolysis is a physiological phenomenon designed to restore the patency of the affected blood vessels and as long as the process does not get out of control the effects are entirely beneficial. To reverse them therefore with antifibrinolytic agents may turn a case of incipient recovery into disaster.

I bitterly recall the tragic fate of a patient who represents one of my Caesarean fatalities. She had a bad obstetric history, hydramnios, a high head and an irregular fetal heart without demonstrable radiological abnormality. She was well into her thirties and, for better or for worse—worse as it happened—I sectioned her and delivered a healthy baby without incident except for the massive escape of her excess liquor amnii. She must have got an amniotic fluid embolism, because shortly after an apparently normal recovery from her anaesthetic she collapsed with obvious signs of haemorrhagic shock. On reopening the wound there was total failure of haemostasis at all levels from the skin downwards and complete absence of clotting. The fibrinogen level was apparently nil and huge quantities of triple-strength plasma and fibrinogen were given urgently; in fact, the equivalent of thirteen pints of blood, although haemorrhage itself had not been excessive. The fibrinogen levels were restored to normal within a few hours and there was no further clinical evidence of bleeding, but her condition progressively deteriorated in spite of the treatment and with steadily deepening cyanosis and clinically solid lungs she died in an oxygen tent, within a few hours. At that time epsilon aminocaproic acid (EACA) was new to us and we had tried it although she was not now bleeding, but she died an hour or two later. Looking back, I think the fibrinogen deficiency must have been due to pulmonary intravascular microcoagulation and that the EACA simply prevented the fibrinolysis which might have given her at least a chance. The amniotic embolism was obviously the trigger that set off the whole train of biochemical events, but was not of itself the cause of her deepening cyanosis since the pulmonary signs only developed hours later and after the fibrinogen levels had been restored.

Excessive Fibrinolysis as a Cause of Haemorrhagic State

Normally, if fibrinogen is present in sufficient quantity it is converted under the influence of thrombin to fibrin monomer which then polymerises to fibrin polymer and this in turn gelates to a firm and visible clot. This is the final stage in the complex business of blood clotting. There might, of course, be no end to this process if it once started inside vessels and theoretically the whole vascular tree could become blocked up by continued propagation of clot were it not for the natural anticlotting mechanisms which exist and are due to plasmin, whose function is to prevent excessive clotting and to maintain the patency of the vascular tree throughout the body. Plasmin does not normally exist in a free and active state, but is derived from a normal plasma globulin called plasminogen. This plasminogen has to be activated by an enzyme known as an "activator" in order to be converted to plasmin. These activator enzymes are present in very small quantities in plasma but in large quantities in damaged tissues, particularly lung, uterus, prostate, thyroid and brain. Major trauma to such tissues or any event which causes their liberation into the blood stream in large quantities will therefore cause plasminogen to be converted into this fibrinolytic substance plasmin. This is fairly unlikely to happen in abruptio placentae which is promptly treated by rupture of the membranes, but occurs more readily in amniotic fluid embolism as already stated and in the gradual absorption of thromboplastins which can occur with a retained intra-uterine dead fetus. These activators can also be produced by bacteria, for example, streptokinase and staphylokinase. Such activators, which could theoretically be extremely dangerous in undermining any clotting process, are excreted in the urine as urokinase. It can be seen that plasmin, once liberated, could undermine all clot repair of damaged blood vessels and get completely out of hand were it not for the fact that normal circulating plasma contains antiplasmins which neutralise the fibrinolytic plasmin. The plasmin gets into the clot all right, and helps to digest it by becoming absorbed on to the fibrin molecules, but the antiplasmins do not reach them so easily. In this way the fibrinolytic effect is to some extent restricted to the site of actual clotting. Now the action of plasmin is to digest fibrin into soluble polypeptides and therefore ultimately to destroy clot and restore the patency of the affected blood vessel. This action is to be seen *in vitro* when a patient suffering from a haemorrhagic state due to this cause has blood which, at first, clots in a test tube and then presently the clot dissolves again, a clinical observation of considerable importance. This would make the diagnosis of an abnormal fibrinolytic state of the blood fairly easy were it not for the fact that plasmin also digests fibrinogen and factors V and VIII (antihaemophilic factor) so that an abnormal fibrinolytic state may in certain instances be associated with hypofibrinogenaemia, but not always. This distinction may be important in treatment.

Fibrinolysis may thus be primary or secondary following intravascular clotting. A platelet count and plasminogen assay may help to differentiate between the two because thrombocytopenia indicates intravascular coagulation with secondary fibrinolysis, but marked plasminogen depletion, being due to conversion to plasmin and utilisation as such, is common to both. Unfortunately this assay is a lengthy business and not likely to be of much immediate help to the obstetrician. Theoretically at least if the trouble was primarily one of intravascular coagulation the treatment, paradoxically, would be heparin rather than an antifibrolytic agent. Heparin acts by direct antagonism of thrombin.

As long as the mechanism of a patient's defibrination remains in doubt antifibrinolytic agents should be given with great caution.[11] In deciding the appropriate treatment for such cases, other than abruptio placentae where the issue is direct and clear, it may be of some help to consider which feature of the case is the more worrying, either the haemorrhage or the cardiopulmonary embarrassment. Of the two, the latter is probably the more dangerous in amniotic fluid embolism.

Fibrinolytic inhibitors.—This reaction of converting plasminogen to plasmin under the influence of the liberated activators from damaged tissue can, however, be inhibited by competition from certain natural amino acids, such as lysine, and even more effectively by the less toxic synthetic amino acid known as EACA (epsilon aminocaproic acid). Not only does this substance inhibit the activators of the plasminogen-to-plasmin reaction, but in high concentrations it also directly inhibits plasmin itself in its action upon fibrinogen and fibrin. EACA is excreted in the urine rapidly and is also absorbed to a full extent within two hours of administration by mouth, but in many of the haemorrhagic emergencies in which its use is indicated it is better administered intravenously. A loading dose of 4 to 6 g is first given and then this is followed on the basis of 1 g per hour to replace excretion. It can be given with normal saline, 5·5 per cent glucose, or Ringer's solution, but not with fructose. As a general rule it should not be given in the existing presence of hypofibrinogenaemia until that has been permanently corrected, in which case it may not now be necessary and its use really is confined to cases who demonstrate a continuing clotting defect despite a level of 200 mg per cent of fibrinogen.

A more modern and even less toxic fibrinolytic inhibitor which can be given in smaller dosages is tranexamic acid (Cyclocapron, Kabi).

If fibrinogen levels are not reduced and one is confronted with a haemorrhagic state in obstetrics due to some clotting defect, it will be obvious that to go on pumping fibrinogen into the patient, either in the form of triple-strength plasma or as pure fibrinogen, is only adding fuel to the fire and that what is wanted is something that will inhibit the activators released from the damaged tissues and which are converting plasminogen to plasmin. Emptying of the uterus, of course, removes these activators from further absorption into the circulation, hence the urgent value of the procedure.

Trasylol is another inhibitor of protein-splitting enzymes and thus an antifibrinolytic agent. It is relatively non-toxic apart from occasional urticaria and is rapidly excreted, having a biological half-life of only 150 minutes. It must be given intravenously. Each 5 ml ampoule contains 25,000 units and 2 ampoules may be given straight away and the infusion thereafter maintained. It acts as a competitive inhibitor of plasminogen activator and also of plasmin itself. It has the advantage also of interfering with thromboplastin degeneration thus producing an anticoagulant effect early on in the coagulation process, so it has the advantages of being both anticoagulant and antifibrinolytic. However, it is unwise to use fibrinolytic inhibitors unless the true nature of the coagulation defect is thoroughly understood.

These are powerful and interesting drugs, but the clinician who is not backed by a very competent and advanced haematological service would do well initially to concentrate on the fibrinogen needs of his patient.

Postpartum Haemorrhage

It is commonly said that the incidence of postpartum haemorrhage is no greater than normal after abruptio, but this is misleading, and even a small loss of blood following delivery may be enough to precipitate collapse in a patient whose state was previously parlous. The most torrential postpartum haemorrhage I ever encountered was in a case of severe abruptio placentae, and the story is worth telling as a warning of what may happen if delivery is effected in the presence of complete uterine atony. The patient had a minor degree of pelvic contraction and a large baby weighing approximately 4½ kg. After a normal and fairly rapid first stage, she failed to deliver herself in the second, and the head became arrested in the high mid-cavity of the pelvis. I decided to deliver her with forceps, and the anaesthetist ran into a lot of trouble during the induction. I happened to notice that the patient's finger-nails looked very blanched and asked one of my students to take her pulse. After what seemed a long time he stated that he could not be sure, but that it was certainly over 200. The midwife in attendance felt the uterus and assured me that she was having a "terrific pain" and, fearing the onset of uterine rupture, I made haste to deliver the patient with forceps. At this stage there had been no external bleeding. It proved a difficult delivery and, considering the very powerful contraction of which I was assured, I was surprised that so much traction was necessary to deliver the head. The baby was stillborn on arrival and almost immediately afterwards a large bulge appeared at the vulva, so that I thankfully prepared to receive the placenta. Instead, an enormous clot came out of the vagina, and there followed a haemorrhage the like of which I had read about but had never previously encountered. Nowadays, whenever I see petrol being poured incorrectly from a 2-gallon can, I am reminded of this particular postpartum haemorrhage, which exactly resembled it. Manual removal of the placenta was a matter of seconds, but the haemorrhage continued unabated. Bimanual compression of the uterus was unsatisfactory, because it was so soft that I could not feel what I was compressing, nor was the fundus anywhere to be found. Intravenous ergometrine and pitocin were likewise disappointing, and only a hot intra-uterine douche, coupled no doubt with the patient's extreme hypotension, saved the day. She recovered, and I am thankful that we subsequently had an opportunity to deliver her of a living child by Caesarean section. In retrospect, it is clear that this patient suffered a massive concealed haemorrhage from abruptio, hence the hardness of the uterus mistaken for a uterine contraction, and that I had delivered her in the presence of complete uterine atony.

Another cause of death is suppression of urine, and a very careful watch for diminished urinary output must be maintained before, during and after delivery. Lastly, these cases may easily succumb from puerperal sepsis, not only because of the need which may arise to intervene, but chiefly because the patient's resistance to infection, as a result of blood loss and shock, is greatly diminished.

The Clinical State

Occasionally there are premonitory symptoms, such as cramp-like pains in the abdomen and a small amount of vaginal bleeding, so that the onset of labour may be inferred, but the majority of cases present acutely. The primary symptom is that of abdominal pain to which bleeding is mainly secondary. By contrast, bleeding due to placenta praevia is always painless. In the most severe cases abdominal pain is agonising and shock is profound, but all gradations of severity may be met, depending upon the amount of blood retained and concealed within the uterus. In the less serious cases pain may not be complained of, but palpation of the uterus will always elicit an area of tenderness.

If revealed bleeding is copious and yet the patient has neither pain nor tenderness, it is very unlikely that the case is one of abruptio, and a presumptive diagnosis of placenta praevia will be made.

As already stated, the level of blood pressure may be misleading because the immediately antecedent level may not be known, and a blood pressure which drops precipitately from 190 to 110 mm Hg systolic can be just as much associated with shock as one which has dropped from 110 to 70 mm. Apart from this source of error, however, the usual signs of shock are present in varying degree.

The abdomen is tense and the abdominal wall appears to be very rigid, while the uterus itself has the well-known hard "wooden" consistency, together with great tenderness, so that in severe cases it is quite impossible to identify any fetal parts or to determine the presentation. If the case is seen early enough this wooden hardness may be seen to develop within about half an hour. This hardness of the uterus is a remarkable phenomenon when one considers that it is in a state of acute atony which is by no means due to the mechanical distension of its cavity with blood clot, because the membranes on vaginal examination are not found to be bulging under pressure. In most instances the fetus is already dead, and in any case in which more than one-third of the placenta is abrupted fetal death is inevitable. If the patient is seen almost immediately after the onset of concealed haemorrhage, the fetus may yet be alive, and every now and then can be saved by prompt Caesarean section, but such good fortune is unusual.

Other evidences of pre-eclamptic toxaemia may be present; for example, there may be oedema, but this is variable and is only noteworthy in about half the cases. The bladder should be catheterised and the urine examined, not only for protein, but its quantity, specific gravity, and the presence of casts or blood should be noted. In the majority of cases protein is present, but if associated with a concentrated scanty amount of urine, it may be a shock phenomenon and is not necessarily indicative of pre-eclampsia. Shock proteinuria is probably due to renal anoxia, and can be distinguished from pre-eclampsia by the fact that it usually disappears within 2 days after delivery, whereas pre-eclamptic proteinuria tends to persist for longer.

So great and continuous may be the patient's pain that it is impossible to tell whether or not labour has actually started without resorting to a vaginal examination, and there should be no hesitation in performing this, after adequate sedation with morphia has been achieved, in order to identify the fetal lie and to confirm the prospects of expeditious vaginal delivery.

If signs of cervical dilatation are already present, so much the better, since the patient who is in a state to initiate spontaneous labour has a far more favourable prognosis. The worst cases are those in which pain is severe and haemorrhage slight or absent.

Diagnosis

The diagnosis of abruptio is not usually difficult, and the history of pain associated with bleeding should make one think of it first. The fact that bleeding may be recurrent does not exclude the possibility of abruptio, since the full-blown attack may be preceded by warning haemorrhages. Coexisting signs of pre-eclamptic toxaemia make the diagnosis more likely, although cases of placenta praevia may be incidentally associated with toxaemia. The essential part of the diagnosis depends upon examination of the abdomen for uterine hardness and tenderness, which may be either localised or generalised. The size of the uterus, the height of the fundus and the abdominal girth should all be recorded at the first examination, because an increase in uterine size will accompany, and indicate a deterioration in, the patient's condition due to the accumulation of still further concealed bleeding.

It is less likely that the diagnosis will be missed than that other abdominal catastrophes will be wrongly attributed to concealed haemorrhage, and I have myself made the classic mistake of diagnosing a ruptured appendix in later pregnancy as a case of abruptio. By the time I had changed my mind and decided to operate it was already too late, and the patient died before active measures could be undertaken. The patient in question was a young primipara at about the 30th week of pregnancy, who had been admitted a few days previously with signs of pre-eclamptic toxaemia. She collapsed with acute abdominal pain, had a rigid, board-like, exquisitely tender abdomen, while the fetal heart could not be heard, and it is depressing to reflect that one could easily repeat the same mistake. She was treated with morphia and blood transfusion which availed her nothing, and at necropsy there was generalised peritonitis.

A ruptured uterus may simulate concealed haemorrhage, since both produce severe continuous pain and shock, and in both there is likely to be at least some revealed bleeding *per vaginam*. A history of previous classical Caesarean section complicated by a septic puerperium would, of course, bring this possibility to mind, but uterine rupture can occasionally occur spontaneously in the previously intact organ, especially in grand multiparity. If the patient is fairly obese, it may be very hard to distinguish between the two, but the presence of proteinuria may be of some help in indicating concealed haemorrhage, and a blood pressure higher than the state of shock would suggest may also be a help.

A retroperitoneal haematoma in the broad ligament may simulate a concealed haemorrhage, but, in this instance, the uterus is pushed to one side and is not itself tender nor necessarily hard in consistency, although the area over the haematoma is acutely painful.

A haematoma of the rectus abdominis muscle is by no means rare and may produce the pain, shock and abdominal signs of abruptio, but there is no vaginal bleeding, the fetal heart is not affected, evidences of pre-eclampsia are absent, and the uterus itself is of normal consistency.

Acute hydramnios may have to be considered, but there is no vaginal bleeding and no shock. The fetal heart can usually be heard though sometimes with difficulty, and sonar puts the matter beyond all doubt.

Volvulus of bowel and the rupture of any of the hollow viscera must also be taken into account in the differential diagnosis. These matters are more fully dealt with in the chapter on acute abdominal pain in pregnancy. Rarities, such as a ruptured splenic aneurysm, may enter the diagnostic field about once in a practitioner's lifetime.

Acute pyelitis should not be mistaken for this condition, because it is associated with fever, usually with pyuria, and the pain is situated more to one side than the other. In spite of all that has been said so far in this chapter, placenta praevia may be diagnosed when in fact the case is one of abruptio, even after vaginal examination. The common mistake here is to palpate a boggy mass of clot within the lower uterine segment and, because of the haemorrhage which is likely to accompany the examination, further identification of the mass is forgone, and it is assumed that one is feeling the placenta itself. But even a fairly well organised clot should not be mistaken for the placenta, because the latter is definitely stringy and is not broken up by the examining finger. What makes the differential diagnosis of abruptio placentae so serious a matter is the fact that most of the conditions with which it may be confused call for very definite lines of active treatment, as witness the disastrous case above described, whereas in the majority of cases of abruptio conservatism applies.

Management of Abruptio Placentae

When first seen the patient may be in a state of rapidly advancing shock. Her general condition must be quickly reviewed and then she must be turned into the Sims left lateral position. This is in order to prevent aggravating the hypotension caused by the weight of the gravid uterus on the inferior vena cava. At the same time a suitable sedative such as morphine is given.

A specimen of blood is taken off for haematological investigation, particularly fibrinogen titre for which an answer should be obtainable within less than half an hour. Evidences of a fibrinolytic state should also be sought.

In all but the mildest cases blood transfusion is urgently necessary, at least 4 units being required in the first instance. These patients are severely hypovolaemic at first and their natural response is one of vasoconstriction. Therefore vasoconstrictive drugs are neither necessary nor indicated and the first effort should be directed towards restoring an effective circulating blood volume.

In the clinically severe case, a central venous pressure line at the time[35] provides also a ready route for massive blood transfusion. It is a common mistake to undertransfuse these cases and the aim is to go on transfusing blood until the central venous pressure is raised to 10 cm of water. This is just as important as early delivery.

In the unusual event of being able to estimate effective circulating blood volume in the midst of such a crisis, by either an isotope or dye-dilution technique, it is reckoned that blood volumes below 60 ml per kg of body weight indicate a critical state and below 40 ml presage likely renal failure unless hypovolaemia is urgently corrected within the next two or three hours.[50] I have great distrust of blood substitutes as volume expanders. What the patient needs is blood and plenty of it.

As soon as her general condition starts to rally no time should be lost in inducing labour by artificial rupture of the forewaters. If, however, the baby is alive and the pregnancy of adequate maturity, at least 34 weeks, Caesarean section should be undertaken. In most cases however labour rapidly supervenes after induction, especially if the patient is parous. Because of her extreme pain, which is continuous, it is often difficult to know with certainty when labour has started nor how it is progressing without resort to vaginal examination. But increasing restlessness commonly indicates that labour is well under way. The appearance of blood at the vulva in renewed amount signifies at least that the uterus has started to demonstrate contractile power, otherwise the blood would have remained concealed. At this point it is particularly worth-while making a vaginal examination because the unremitting hardness of the uterus may make it impossible to observe rhythmical labour contractions. It may be found that labour is more advanced than thought and in those cases where the membranes have not already been ruptured this should be undertaken at once.

It is our policy to regard a fibrinogen titre below 1 in 128 as urgently calling for fibrinogen replacement and not to await completion of delivery from the false fear of stoking the fires of fibrinogen depletion. As has been explained, this state is almost always due to a subtraction phenomenon within the rapidly inspissating retroplacental blood clot itself.

The longer the delay between abruptio and delivery, the greater the likelihood of afibrinogenaemia and deepening shock. This is domonstrated by the fact that the characteristic signs of the Couvelaire uterus take a few hours to develop as can be seen when Caesarean section for example is delayed for more than 3 or 4 hours, and with this delay go increasing chances of anuria, and the effects of hypofibrinogenaemia may become more pronounced. The truth of this was brought home to me vividly and tragically shortly after my arrival in Glasgow when I hung on to conservative treatment too long. The patient became anuric 24 hours after admission, although copious blood transfusion appeared to have restored her general condition, thereby encouraging me to hold my hand. She failed to go into labour and with her blood urea rapidly rising I undertook Caesarean section in spite of an absent fetal heart on the third day. She died on the table and necropsy showed complete renal cortical necrosis. At that time we consoled ourselves with the reflection that death would have been inevitable in any case, but I now consider that had I secured delivery earlier on, her kidneys would not have failed.

The use of oxytocin is not usually required and I have had a traditional prejudice most of my life against stimulating a pathological uterus, on the ground that this was akin to flogging a tired horse. The risks, however, of any delay in labour are so much greater than the judicious use of oxytocin that there should be no hesitation in employing it in the unusual cases in which the cervix does not dilate within three hours. Usually the babies are small from prematurity and delivery is easy, but delay in the second stage should be countered by assisted delivery.

We do not favour the use of epidural anaesthesia in these cases since a haematoma, due to a clotting defect, may form in the extradural space and cause local pressure. Even a spinal anaesthetic would be preferable, but is seldom necessary.

Sometimes delivery, when the uterus really "gets going", occurs with quite extraordinary speed. I once examined such a case and found a cervix completely undilated; a few minutes later she went into tumultuous labour and delivered herself precipitately with two almighty heaves, placenta, retroplacental clot and all. The shock which followed was equally dramatic. Fortunately she recovered but the baby was stillborn.

All other forms of treatment are now matters of history and have been discarded. In summary the treatment is as follows:

1. Inject morphine;
2. After rapid assessment turn the patient onto her left side in the Sims position;
3. Transfuse liberally;

4. Set up a central venous pressure line in severe cases;
5. Rupture the forewaters as soon as the hypovolaemic state is being adequately treated by transfusion;
6. Test for afibrinogenaemia and treat accordingly, bearing in mind the possibility of abnormal fibrinolysis;
7. Do not hesitate to employ Caesarean section if the child is alive and not excessively premature;
8. Beware of even minor degrees of postpartum haemorrhage especially if there is any sign of uterine atony. If bleeding continues after emptying of the uterus, bimanual compression may be required as an immediate interim measure, but in really desperate cases I have found a hot intra-uterine sterile saline douche, at a temperature only just bearable to the skin of the operator's forearm, to be lifesaving; but it takes a few minutes to arrange this sort of treatment. At least it is preferable to packing the uterus, which is not likely to be effective. In the unlikely event of bleeding still continuing and with clotting defects already dealt with by fibrinogen replacement etc., hysterectomy may have to be considered. This however is a mutilating step in an already desperate situation which is seldom justified nowadays and it is many years since I have been aware of the need for it.

Decisions are difficult to make in the not so obviously acute case in which, for example, the diagnosis is not in doubt, but response to shock treatment is rapid and the patient appears relatively well and yet labour does not supervene. The question is what to do next. Under these circumstances one is faced with the following choices: firstly, to empty the uterus by abdominal section, which should be avoided if possible if the fetal heart cannot be heard; secondly, to leave the patient strictly alone until she finally goes into labour spontaneously. Occasionally this interval of anxious waiting may be as long as 48 hours or more. However in all previously shocked cases, this is simply asking for anuria, and the patient should be dealt with by oxytocin infusion and a surgical induction.

If, however, deterioration in the patient's general condition appears in spite of *adequate* anti-shock treatment, preparations should be made for Caesarean section. Nevertheless, before undertaking this operation, a vaginal examination should again be made because the apparent deterioration in her condition may merely be due to the fact that labour is now progressing rapidly and the cervix is already dilating well.

Finally, in less severe cases in which the fetal heart persists in spite of the certain diagnosis of a retroplacental haematoma and in which the mother's general condition remains good, it is worth adopting a more conservative line in the hope that pregnancy may safely continue and achieve a more rewarding degree of maturity. In these mild cases of abruptio, with rest in bed and suitable sedation, the pain disappears within a few days and when delivery finally occurs signs of an old crater may be found on the surface of the placenta.

REFERENCES

1. Blair, R. G. (1973). *J. Obstet. Gynaec. Brit. Cwlth*, **80,** 242.
2. Browne, J. C. M. and Veall, N. (1953). *J. Obstet. Gynaec. Brit. Emp.*, **60,** 141.
3. Browne, O'D. (1952). *Proc. roy. Soc. Med.*, **45,** 414.
4. Butler, N. R. and Bonham, D. G. (1963). *Perinatal Mortality*. p. 290. Edinburgh: Livingstone.
5. Crawford, R. M. C., Greig, K. and Sutherland, A. M. (1957). *Scot. med. J.*, **2,** 451.
6. Crawford, R. M. C. and Sutherland, A. M. (1961). *J. Obstet. Gynaec. Brit. Cwlth*, **68,** 545.
7. Donald, I. (1967). *Trans. Coll. Physns. S. Afr.*, **11,** 61.
8. Donald, I. (1976) Mackenzie Davidson Lecture. *Brit. J. Radiol.*, **49,** 306.
9. Donald, I. and Abdulla, U. (1967). *Brit. J. Radiol.*, **40,** 604.
10. Donald, I. and Abdulla, U. (1968). *J. Obstet. Gynaec. Brit. Cwlth*, **75,** 993.
11. Dubber, Anne H. C., McNicol, G. P. and Douglas, A. S. (1967). *Scot. med. J.*, **12,** 138.
12. Fernstrom, I. (1955). *Acta radiol. (Stockh.)*, Suppl. 122.
13. von Friesen, B. (1964). *Acta obstet. gynec. scand.*, **43,** 122.
14. Gottesfeld, K. R., Thomson, H. E., Holmes, J. H. and Taylor, E. S. (1966). *Amer. J. Obstet. Gynec.*, **96,** 538.
15. Hartley, J. B. (1954). *Brit. J. Radiol.*, **27,** 365.
16. Hibbard, B. M. (1962). *Proc. roy. Soc. Med.*, **55,** 640.
17. Hibbard, B. M. (1962). *J. Obstet. Gynaec. Brit. Cwlth*, **69,** 282.
18. Hibbard, B. M. (1964). *J. Obstet. Gynaec. Brit. Cwlth*, **71,** 529.
19. Jeffcoate, T. N. A. (1966). *Proc. roy. Soc. Med.*, **59,** 397.
20. Jeffcoate, T. N. A. (1969). Margaret Orford Memorial Lecture: *Abruptio placentae*. (South Africa).
21. King, D. L. (1973). *Radiology*, **109,** 167.
22. Kobayashi, M., Hellman, L. M. Fillisti, L. and Cromb, E. (1970). *Amer. J. Obstet. Gynec.*, **106,** 279.
23. Louw, J. T. (1956). *S. Afr. med. J.*, **30,** 307.
24. Løvset, J. (1959). *Acta obstet. gynec. scand.*, **38,** 551.
25. Macafee, C. H. G. (1945). *J. Obstet. Gynaec. Brit. Emp.*, **52,** 313.
26. Macafee, C. H. G. (1945). *J. Obstet. Gynaec. Brit. Emp.*, **52,** 786.
27. Macafee, C. H. G. (1960). *Lancet*, **1,** 449.
28. McRoberts, W. A. (1951). *Amer. J. Obstet. Gynec.*, **62,** 627.
29. Millar, K. G. (1966). *Brit. med. J.*, **1,** 1571.
30. Millar, W. G. (1959). *J. Obstet. Gynaec. Brit. Emp.*, **66,** 353.
31. Mitchell, A. P. B., Anderson, G. S. and Russell, J. K. (1957). *Brit. med. J.*, **1,** 611.

32. Moir, J. C. (1944). *Amer. J. Obstet. Gynec.*, **47,** 198.
33. Murdoch, R. (1962). *Lancet*, **1,** 1327.
34. Nilsen, P. A. (1963). *Hypofibrinogenaemia in Premature Separation of the Placenta.* Oslo: Universitetsforlaget.
35. O'Driscoll, K. and McCarthy, J. R. (1966). *J. Obstet. Gynaec. Brit. Cwlth*, **73,** 923.
36. Parks, J. and Barter, R. H. (1963). *Ariz. Med.*, July, 155.
37. Percival, R. (1959). *Proc. roy. Soc. Med.*, **52,** 562.
38. Percival, R. and Murray, S. (1955). *Lancet*, **1,** 1045.
39. Pritchard, J. A. and Wright, M. R. (1959). *New Engl. J. Med.*, **261,** 218.
40. Reed, M. F. (1973). *Brit. J. Radiol.*, **46,** 255.
41. Reid, F. (1951). *Proc. roy. Soc. Med.*, **44,** 703.
42. Reid, F. (1952). *Postgrad. med. J.*, **28,** 445.
43. Russell, J. K. and Warrick, C. K. (1955). *Lancet*, **1,** 785.
44. Schneider, C. L. (1952). *Amer. J. Obstet. Gynec.*, **63,** 1078.
45. Scott, J. S. (1955). *Brit. med. J.*, **2,** 290.
46. Scott, J. S. (1968). *Brit. med. Bull.*, **24,** 32.
47. Seldinger, S. J. (1953). *Acta radiol.* (*Stockh.*), **39,** 368.
48. Stallworthy, J. (1951). *Amer. J. Obstet. Gynec.*, **61,** 720.
49. Thambu, J. and Llewellyn-jones, D. (1966). *J. Obstet. Gynaec. Brit. Cwlth*, **73,** 930.
50. Tovey, G. H. and Lennon, G. G. (1963). *J. Obstet. Gynaec. Brit. Cwlth*, **70,** 749.
51. Watson, H. B., Israelski, M. and Jordan, W. M. (1957). *Brit. med. J.*, **2,** 490.
52. Weiner, A. E., Reid, D. E. and Roby, C. C. (1953), *Amer. J. Obstet. Gynec.*, **66,** 475.
53. Willocks, J. (1971). *J. Obstet. Gynaec. Brit. Cwlth*, **78,** 987.
54. Willocks, J. and MacVicar, J. (1965). *Brit. med. J.*, **2,** 979.
55. Willoughby, M. L. N. (1966). *J. Obstet. Gynaec. Brit. Cwlth*, **73,** 940.
56. Wright, L. (1962). *Brit. med. J.*, **1,** 760.

CHAPTER XVI

INDUCED LABOUR

Dangers of Oxytocin: "Danger of uterus will stand on its top, up-down".

Examination Candidate

An induced labour is one in which pregnancy is terminated artificially any time after the 28th week of gestation by a method that aims to secure delivery *per vias naturales*. Whether or not the intention is fulfilled does not alter the definition, for occasionally, alas, labour may indeed be started only to be concluded by Caesarean section either because some fresh complication arises, as for example uterine inco-ordination, fetal distress, or because the grounds for induction have been inaccurately assessed.

History reveals an understandable reluctance to interfere with the course of labour by hastening its onset, partly because the methods were uncertain, bizarre and often dangerous. The penalties of failure and the hazards of delayed labour have been recognised for centuries and have influenced thinking in obstetrics right up to the present.

The control of infection, however, and the more effective management of uterine behaviour is rapidly modifying our traditionally conservative attitude to what was regarded once as meddlesome midwifery, so that the day cannot be far off when labour of a foreseeable sort and at a predictable time becomes commonplace. In this respect the development of newer and better induction techniques demands less of the so-called art of obstetrics and more of its science; otherwise they are likely to create more problems than they solve. For induction to be safe and effective, fetal assessment and monitoring both before and during labour are essential prerequisites.

Even today no method of induction is both absolutely certain and safe. When something goes wrong it is natural that one should ask oneself whether spontaneous delivery might have occurred had there been no meddling in the first place.

Natural Onset of Labour

The ancient view that labour might be delayed because of perversity and unwillingness of the fetus to emerge into this naughty world we now recognise as not so far wide of the mark. There are many factors, mechanical, maternal, extrinsic, as well as fetal, which contribute to the onset of this extraordinary event. Only recently has the role of the fetal pituitary and adrenal cortex come to be recognised. In sheep, for example, a surge in fetal cortisol level precedes the onset of labour combined with a falling maternal progesterone, and fetal pituitary activity influences the role of fetal ACTH.[28]

Fetal cortisol is also believed to be responsible for the rising levels of lecithin in liquor amnii which are associated with the final maturation of the lung alveoli in preparation for extra-uterine respiration.[26, 38]

The experimental work on sheep has produced some very cut-and-dried results. For example, pregnancy can be prolonged by intra-uterine fetal hypophysectomy.[30] In the human this may explain the tendency of anencephalic pregnancy to go postmature.

Furthermore prostaglandins may increase in the liquor amnii during labour but may not be detectable before that and may be absent in anencephalic postmature labour. One of the experimental difficulties has been that prostaglandins are cleared from the maternal blood by passing only once through the pulmonary circulation. The prostaglandins, particularly E and F have a powerful oxytocic effect locally on the human uterus.

Attempts have been made to simulate this endocrine state of affairs by a single intra-amniotic injection of 20 mg betamethasone.[34] In a small series of cases, already postmature, labour occurred, albeit tardily, in significantly less time than any controlled group injected with normal saline into the amniotic cavity. Interestingly enough one of the failures was that of a woman with an anencephalic pregnancy who was still not in labour even a week later, presumably because the fetus was unable to swallow and absorb the drug. A 20 mg dose of betamethasone given intramuscularly direct into the fetus was more successful.

The use of corticosteroids is not at present an acceptable method of induction because it is too slow, but this work is mentioned to indicate that the fetal as well as the maternal endocrine stage has to be set for the natural onset of labour.

Induction of labour artificially therefore remains one of the most abused procedures in all obstetrics. Attempted before the 36th week, induction is often profitless, dangerous, or both, for mother and fetus.

One should consequently be as ready to defend the indications for induction as for Caesarean section, since it is a good rule in midwifery that any intervention, however apparently trivial, carries with it the responsibilities for the consequences which may be disproportionately severe and which it would be as well to review.

Risks of Induction

Failure to Labour

In a review of over 3000 cases at the Queen Mother's Hospital, MacVicar[32] observed that almost 2 per cent of induced patients required delivery by Caesarean section for no other reason than the failure of the uterus to contract properly howsoever stimulated. Abnormal uterine activity was recognised if full dilatation of the cervix was not achieved in the absence of cephalopelvic disproportion. In addition to these of course there were others who had to be delivered by Caesarean section for reasons not directly related to induction itself. These hard-core cases with inco-ordinate uterine activity are demoralising to all concerned and always raise the question as to whether a more normal type of labour might have ensued if the patient had been left alone. From the patient's point of view her failure to labour may be coupled with the fear that there is something abnormal, particularly with her child. Of all the unspoken fears of pregnancy, this last is probably the most common, and because of its unlikelihood doctors often forget to recognise such mental processes which are after all natural enough to the young, uninformed, lay imagination; hence the very great need for the patient to understand what is being done and why. The effects of anxiety on the labour process are universally acknowledged and the occasional inert labour following induction, whatever the method, is probably due more to this factor than to any other.

Prematurity

Another common risk is that of prematurity due to a mistaken impression of the child's size and an inaccurate history of the menstrual cycle and last period, and induction for "postmaturity" may actually result in premature labour. I once asked all female candidates at an examination how many women were absolutely sure of their dates and the usual answer was "about half". This did not surprise me. When a patient presents herself at a clinic she is often intimidated and anxious not to appear stupid. She therefore produces a date for her last period and after that she "sticks to her story."

In departments properly equipped with sonar and with proper antecedent prenatal care, the risk of unforeseen prematurity is neither acceptable nor excusable.

The best of paediatric units is no substitute for a healthy intrauterine environment up to the time of adequate maturity.

Unforeseen Disproportion

More serious are the clinical mistakes so easily made in assessing relative disproportion. Often, following induction of labour for this reason, the fetal head at delivery shows so little evidence of moulding that one may wonder whether it had ever been necessary to interfere with the course of pregnancy. However, it should be remembered that the premature head, because of its bony pliability, very quickly loses its moulded shape, so that the observation is not quite fair, nor, for that matter, is moulding a desirable occurrence in the premature, even as a vindication of the obstetrician's diagnosis of disproportion. There is no doubt, however, that such cases are often induced unnecessarily early, and babies are just as likely to be lost because of prematurity as saved by preventing a difficult labour at term. In the other direction, a mistaken assessment of disproportion may reveal itself after induction in the course of labour when it becomes clear that the head will not mould through the pelvis. Such disproportion is itself a cause of inert uterine action, so that the trial of labour is no true test at all, and the Caesarean section, now necessary, would have been better left deliberately until term. It is for this reason that many obstetricians hold that trial of labour should be reserved for spontaneous labour only.

Sepsis

With modern methods this risk is negligible, provided that the time interval between induction and delivery does not exceed 24 hours. A long induction/delivery interval (IDI) inevitably invites sepsis, since no procedure conducted through the genital tract can ever be sterile and the presence of detectable amnionitis is certain within 24 to 36 hours.[29] The nature of the infection may be neither foreseen nor controlled by antibiotics. Effects upon the fetus *in utero* are more disastrous than on the mother of today.

So long as the amniotic sac is intact the risks of intra-uterine infection are very much less, but when the forewaters have been ruptured, the chances of infection mount steadily with the passage of time and prejudice the safety of Caesarean section should it become necessary. The baby may not only acquire an active infection before it is born but the infection may be one that remains latent for many weeks after birth yet whose bacteriology incriminates the maternity hospital as its source.

Whatever the precautions taken at amniotomy the presence of pathogenic organisms in the vagina even before surgical interference has been recorded in no less than 38 per cent of the series reported by McCallum and Govan.

Where the fetus is dead *in utero*, surgical methods of induction are so dangerous as to be absolutely contra-indicated. Quite apart from being strictly unnecessary, nothing could be more inviting to gas-forming organisms than the presence of a dead fetus and placenta, and many disasters in the past have occurred with dramatic rapidity.

Placental Site Retraction and Fetal Asphyxia

Nowadays, surgical induction is chiefly limited to methods of tapping the amniotic sac and removing varying amounts of liquor, which reduces the volume of the uterine contents as a whole. The uterus must, therefore, shrink to some extent to compensate for the loss of liquor, and this shrinkage and retraction are mainly confined to the upper uterine segment in which the placenta is normally situated. Some reduction, therefore, of the area of the placental site will occur, but what is more important is that the volume of maternal blood flow through the placenta will be reduced. This may not matter very much for a number of hours, but if, as is occasionally the case, the fetus is already on the verge of asphyxia (and some degree of hypoxia is physiologically present at the end of all pregnancies), then a delayed or protracted labour may tip the scales and result in a stillbirth which is the consequence of prolonged though mild asphyxia.

Partial Placental Detachment and "Bloody Tap"

Where the placenta is sited low in the uterus, surgical induction by hindwater tapping commonly provokes antepartum haemorrhage if placental attachment to the uterine wall is disturbed. Fortunately the bleeding usually stops spontaneously on removal of the catheter, but if prolonged may call for forewater rupture, and if uncontrollable may require delivery at once by Caesarean section.

The other cause of a "bloody tap" is the rupture of vasa praevia or fetal blood vessels encountered in a low-lying placenta. It is clearly a matter of the most urgent importance to decide whose blood is being lost, mother's or baby's. Fetal exsanguination, as an uncommon but serious possibility, has been pointed out by Russell *et al.* (1956) who reported two fetal deaths from this cause following surgical induction by hindwater rupture.

Fortunately it is now possible to identify the blood within little more than ten minutes by the use of the Singer test for fetal haemoglobin, as modified by Anderson. The test depends upon the fact that fetal haemoglobin is more resistant to denaturation by alkali than is adult haemoglobin. The following description of the test is given by Mitchell *et al.* (1957):

Anderson's Modification of Singer Test for Fetal Haemoglobin

Principle.—A sample of blood is allowed to react with an alkali for a set period of time. The reaction is then stopped by an acid solution which also precipitates non-haemoglobin chromogens. The mixture is filtered immediately and the filtrate examined by the naked eye and in a colorimeter.

Reagents.—Alkali: N/12 NaOH or N/12 KOH. Acid-precipitating solution: 800 ml of 50 per cent saturated $(NH_4)_2SO_4$ plus 2 ml of 10

N HCl. Blood: The sample is either pure blood or a mixture of blood and other contaminants issuing from the vagina. It should be collected in a clean heparinised bottle. If collected in an oxalated tube or by means of a siliconed syringe, there is a danger of "fetal" results being obtained from adult blood.

Technique.—The haemoglobin level of the blood sample is first determined. To 2 ml of alkali, 0·1 ml of blood is added and the mixture is shaken. The reaction is allowed to proceed for one minute at room temperature, when 4 ml of acid-precipitating solution is added and the mixture again thoroughly shaken. It is then filtered through a No. 1 Whatman filter paper and the filtrate collected.

The results are usually obvious by naked-eye examination. With adult-type haemoglobin the filtrate is either clear and colourless or a faint brown-amber colour. With fetal-type haemoglobin it varies from a faint pink to a distinct cherry red, depending on the amount of haemoglobin in the sample.

A colorimeter may be used for greater accuracy, especially when both types of blood are mixed and for the elimination of false positive results for fetal haemoglobin which might be obtained by naked-eye inspection.

The timely discovery that the bleeding is of fetal origin may be life-saving if Caesarean section is promptly undertaken within the next hour. A longer period of grace before the fetal heart stops cannot be counted upon.

Accidental Haemorrhage (Abruptio placentae)

Full-blown abruptio placentae may occur following the sudden release of enormous quantities of liquor in cases of hydramnios. For this reason, severe cases should, if possible, be decompressed by "controlled rupture". This is usually attempted with a Drew Smythe catheter before finally rupturing the forewaters. Unfortunately the forewaters in such cases are often ruptured accidentally, thus defeating one's purpose. An alternative is to decompress the uterus by abdominal paracentesis first, with a lumbar-puncture type of needle.

Artificial rupture of the membranes, whether high or low, especially in the case of hydramnios, has other penalties, sometimes unexpected, as, for example, when a very senior Glasgow obstetrician performed this simple operation in the house of a patient with gross hydramnios and complained that the ensuing deluge put the fire out!

Fetal Pneumonia

This is a common penalty of prolonged retention of the fetus *in utero* with ruptured membranes, particularly in association with prolonged labour. The combination of fetal anoxia and the inevitable presence of infected meconium invites deep inspiratory efforts on the baby's part, so that it may be born with an established aspiration bronchopneumonia, which can be fatal. It is customary to give prophylactic antibiotics before delivery in such cases, but although this may protect the mother from the most vicious forms of sepsis, it is less likely to save her child. For one thing the antibiotic must be capable of traversing the placental barrier and reaching the liquor in high concentration and for another the organisms, whose nature is not yet known, should be sensitive to it. So great are the risks, however, that we feel some guesswork is indicated here and for a time it was our practice to give ampicillin prophylactically after 24 hours with artificially ruptured membranes, but we have since switched to cephaloridine.[5]

Cord Prolapse

This should not occur unless either the head fails to engage or there is malpresentation, particularly with oblique or transverse lie, in which case surgical induction is plainly contra-indicated until the lie has been converted to the longitudinal and the presenting part has been made to engage firmly in the pelvis. With a high head, the forewaters should not be ruptured unless the head is first made to engage, but even hindwater rupture with a high head is not devoid of this complicating risk, and a careful examination should always be made at the end of the operation to exclude the presence of a prolapsed cord. If indeed the cord does prolapse at amniotomy, immediate Caesarean section is the only really rational treatment (another reason for carrying out surgical induction of labour only in surgical conditions). We make a rule of carrying out this simple operation in one of our operating theatres and have had reason to be grateful for such strict caution.

Amniotic Embolism

Lastly, amniotic fluid embolism may occur, either at the time of amniotomy or some hours later. It occurs more readily if the uterine contractions are very strong, usually in a multipara, and amniotic fluid is squeezed into a maternal sinus through a hole in the membranes. I know of such an accident which befell a colleague's patient who collapsed immediately following this simple operation and died within a few minutes. In another case on my own unit the patient's doctor had ruptured the membranes on the previous day. She suddenly became very ill, was admitted deeply cyanosed with pyrexia 40·5 °C and gross tachycardia. She died within 45 minutes of delivery by forceps, from amniotic fluid embolism, presumably a sequel to her previous amniotomy. Admittedly these hideous complications are uncommon but their incidence should not exceed nil unless the operation is done for inadequate reasons.

Neonatal Jaundice

In recent years an association between neonatal jaundice and premature induction of labour, especially drug-assisted induction, has been increasingly recognised,[15] so much so that there is now some doubt as to how much hyperbilirubinaemia may be regarded as strictly physiological as previously accepted.

Some degree of transient jaundice, especially in breast-fed babies, has traditionally been accepted. Much depends upon the level of bilirubin in the serum which is regarded as pathological. Few would consider levels below 10 mg/100 ml (171 μmol/l) as significant, but increasing numbers of cases are being recognised in which the bilirubin exceeds 15 mg/100 ml (256 μmol/l).

It is suggested that there is more to this than mere coincidence[14] and that premature interruption of pregnancy may be the main factor, as it occurs anyway in prematurity because of the inability of hepatic enzymes to cope with the bilirubin load which follows birth, due to the haemolysis of excess fetal red cells. It is further suggested[18] that the dose of oxytocin may directly affect the bilirubin levels. It has however been noted that even if labour has been expedited with oxytocin following spontaneous onset, the degree of hyperbilirubinaemia is markedly less than in cases which have been prematurely induced. It is well known[35] that there is a cortisol "spurt" towards the end of pregnancy which may produce a sudden maturation of the various systems which are necessary for survival after birth.[38] These systems include a number of liver enzymes. It is not yet known however at what minimum level brain damage can develop, but the coexistence of hypoxia, hypothermia, acidosis, and a bilirubin level of more than 20 mg/100 ml (342 μmol/l) can together cause brain damage. Liver-enzyme immaturity is the popular explanation at present but undoubtedly stronger oxytocin-induced contractions may lead to hypoxia. Nevertheless pH levels below 7·1 are not necessarily associated with high bilirubin levels. In a search for other possible associated factors the pre-induction medication agents have come under review. It is noteworthy that this increase in neonatal jaundice has more or less coincided with the gradual disappearance of the barbiturates as sedatives in clinical practice, and nitrazepam and bupivacaine have both been incriminated, but unconvincingly.

Meanwhile, whatever the cause of the increasing incidence of neonatal jaundice, the practice of premature induction of labour is growing apace. These findings have been further confirmed in the large survey of more than 10,000 births in Cardiff[15] and actual oxytocin dosage would appear to be a major factor. This appearance of jaundice frequently delayed the mother's and the baby's discharge from hospital although there was no evidence of other harmful effect.

The findings however have been vigorously opposed in a later prospective study of more than 1300 labours[7] where, using the cut-off level of significance as 12 mg or more per 100 ml (205 μmol/l), no difference was noted in the incidence of neonatal hyperbilirubinaemia following spontaneous labour or after labour induced or accelerated by oxytocin. However, the total dose of oxytocin was more significant, particularly when it exceeded 20 units in all as was the case in 12 per cent of induced labours. A further report from Belgium[47] not only exculpated the oxytocin but the prostaglandins as well, up to the third day of neonatal life.

It has been further observed in a large series of over 13,000 term babies born between 1969 and the end of 1974 in Boston that, excluding cases of haematological incompatibility and those weighing less than 2500 g, there was no difference in the number of cases with bilirubin levels exceeding 10 mg/100 ml (171 μmol/l); but what was significant was the manner of the child's delivery, whether spontaneous or instrumental, and it has been suggested that instrumental delivery may cause focal haemorrhages which are not obvious but may nevertheless be manifested by later jaundice[24]; and so the controversy still continues. While some caution must be exercised in not abusing oxytocin administration none can dispute its immense value in the induction and acceleration of labour. In the end the prostaglandins may prove to be the safer in this respect though this is by no means yet established.

In a further similar paper[8] and again using 12 mg/100 ml (205 μmol/l) as the cut-off point no significant association was found in neonatal hyperbilirubinaemia following labour induced or accelerated with prostaglandin E2 as compared with spontaneous labour, nor was there any significant association with the total dose used for induction, unlike the alleged total dose effect of oxytocin. The series was prospective and dealt with more than 400 babies and the results are doubly reassuring.

Fetal Mortality

This is, in most centres, higher than in spontaneous delivery, but considering the very large number of reasons for which labour may be induced it is not really fair to blame the induction without taking into account the indication, which has its own fetal mortality.

History of Induction of Labour

Since antiquity various methods, many bizarre and some frankly dangerous, have been used in an attempt to bring on labour.

Massage of the breasts and uterus are very old but inefficient methods. Something approaching the use of tents dates back to the sixth century, and stretching of the cervix digitally has been long employed. The last century brought with it more ingenuity and at one time electricity was thought of. As far back as 1838 rubber tubing was pushed into the uterus, only to be revived in the form of a stomach tube about ninety years later by Fitzgibbon.

Scanzoni used a hot carbolic acid douche in 1856, and at this time Kraus introduced his bougies, which only since the 1930s have fallen into disuse because of their relative inefficiency, their sepsis rate and the oft-encountered risk of harpooning or detaching placenta.

Kraus' bougies had, however, one virtue over the other foreign-body methods in that they did not displace the presenting part. The writer used them frequently before the last war, and had little serious trouble with them apart from occasionally encountering the placenta, which called for reintroduction of the bougies in another direction and the delay, sometimes of many days, before labour started; it is not safe to leave them in the uterus for more than two days. It is now generally recognised, however, that their use is not justified.

Barnes in 1861 used rubber bags filled with water, but this was only an extension of the more traditional method of using pigs' bladders. It must be remembered that none of these weapons was sterilised in their heyday, and some of the results must have been frightful.

Artificial rupture of the forewaters stands in a class by itself, for it has stood a prolonged test of time, being first used by Denman in 1756 for cases of contracted pelvis, and being known since then as the "English method". It remains to this day the most efficient and most widely used method in spite of the sacrifice of an intact amniotic sac which it entails.

Hindwater rupture with the Drew Smythe catheter was introduced in 1931, but what it gains in safety, in forewater preservation, in reduced amniotic fluid infection and in discouragement of cord prolapse, it loses in efficiency when compared with forewater rupture.

The Unfavourable Cervix

It is the common experience of us all that labour may follow induction expeditiously under the most unfavourable circumstances and conversely the apparently favourable case may be slow to respond. Nevertheless it is as well to make a clinical attempt to assess the likelihood of success when undertaking induction. The nulliparous patient is particularly unpredictable in her behaviour.

The likelihood of success however is indicated by a number of perfectly recognisable findings, namely dilatation of the cervix, its degree of effacement, its consistency and its position within the pelvis, which are all important factors. In addition a fifth factor has to be taken into account, namely the station of the head, whether at, above or below the level of the ischial spines. Bishop introduced a scoring system in 1964 which takes all these factors into account as shown in the accompanying Table. From this Table it will be seen that the maximum possible score would be 13, at which point, of course, delivery would be just about imminent. These signs together indicate, according to Bishop, the proximity to the spontaneous onset of labour, since the total score gradually increases as term is reached.

16/TABLE 1

INDUCIBILITY RATING (BISHOP)
Circle Appropriate Number

Dilatation	0 0	1–2 1	3–4 2	5–6 3
Effacement %	0–40 0	40–60 1	60–80 2	80+ 3
Station	−3 0	−2 1	−1·0 2	+1 +2 3
Consistency	Firm 0	Medium 1	Soft 2	
Position	Posterior 0	Mid 1	Anterior 2	

Total Score...........

0–5 unfavourable
6–13 favourable

He reckoned that elective induction might successfully and safely be performed when the score amounted to 9 or more and in fact in all the cases where he applied it there were no failures and the average duration of labour was less than 4 hours. This clinical examination was recommended at each prenatal visit during the last week of pregnancy. Bishop also recommended it as a method not only of determining the optimum time for elective induction of labour but of deciding the date of elective repeat Caesarean section and it might also thereby forewarn the obstetrician of mistaken prematurity on clinical grounds alone regardless of the patient's menstrual history.

In our own practice we use the Bishop scoring technique on a wide scale and regard totals above 6 as favourable and of good augury for a successful induction whereas totals below 6 are definitely discouraging.

The value of this prelabour estimate of inducibility and the subsequent course of labour has been comprehensively analysed by other workers[23] who noted that as the evaluation score rose, the latent phase became shorter. This is an important matter because the latent phase contributes significantly to a prolonged induction/delivery interval. Of all the factors the degree of cervical dilatation is clearly the most important and this of course is mainly applicable to the multipara. Furthermore a so-called "ripe" cervix does not necessarily correlate to the maturity, nor an "unripe" cervix to prematurity. Although the length of the latent phase in induced labour varies inversely with the prelabour evaluation score and the lower the score the longer will it last, once the active phase of labour supervenes it does not necessarily differ significantly in length or other characteristics from spontaneous labour.[23]

Drug Induction

In modern obstetrics there are now only two classes of drug which are seriously considered in the induction of labour, namely oxytocin, preferably synthetic (Syntocinon), and certain of the prostaglandins. Even so drug induction alone without accompanying amniotomy is seldom regarded as adequate except when dealing with an intra-uterine dead fetus in which all local surgical interference is absolutely contra-indicated.

What is surprising is that the psychiatrists do not yet appear to have tilted at this problem. After all, when one thinks of the effect of air-raids, thunderstorms and emotional stimuli in provoking labour, it would seem that there is scope here, and it is certainly no more ambitious in trying to make labour both brisk and painless.

Oxytocin

The oxytocic factor from the posterior lobe of the pituitary is nowadays prepared in great purity, free of vasopressor substances, and synthetic oxytocin has by now stood the test of many years' reliability. Unfortunately oxytocin is destroyed very rapidly by the enzyme oxytocinase so that intramuscular and subcutaneous injections are either useless or unpredictable in their effects. Admittedly oxytocin can be readily absorbed from the buccal and nasal mucous membranes which for a time made both buccal lozenges containing the drug, and oxytocin snuff, briefly popular. The intravenous dilute drip method however is now practically universal and is an everyday ceremonial in most maternity hospitals, its use being sometimes matched by the degree to which it is abused.

Following a night's sedation, usually with nitrazepam 5 to 10 mg, the drip is set up early on the next morning. The usual procedure is to use the two-bottle method. That is to say in one bottle with a capacity of 1 litre a solution of Plasmalyte 148 is made up in 5 per cent dextrose. In the other bottle, with a capacity of 500 ml, Syntocinon in amount varying from 2 units to 32 units is added to a similar solution from which it passes via a drip-counter through a Y-piece connection close to an indwelling intravenous plastic catheter inserted into an arm vein. The dummy solution is set running first and then the rate of flow of the drip of Syntocinon can be regulated with one of the admirable drip counters of which the Ivac and the Tekmar are our present favourites as they allow only a preset number of drops per minute to pass down the tube by using a photoelectric control mechanism. Failing these luxurious devices, the drip rate can be controlled by plain counting but adjustment is sometimes tedious and in any case one should only handle very dilute solutions of oxytocin in case of a sudden flood of drops with disastrous effects on uterine tone. This is particularly important in the case of the grand multipara in whom the risks of oxytocin infusion even within the first few minutes can be considerable. The importance of having the "Y" connecting piece close to the patient is that it shortens the length of tubing dead-space which may contain residual amounts of oxytocin which it is desired to cut off.

We now insist on reckoning oxytocin dosage only in milliunits per minute and this means referring to the dosage table which is available in all delivery rooms (Table 2).

Clearly where, because of fluid-retaining conditions such as pre-eclampsia, it is desirable to restrict the amount of fluid infused, it is better to start off with stronger solutions of oxytocin provided the above precautions are observed. The discipline of thinking only in terms of milliunits per minute is very necessary if confusion is to be avoided, likewise disastrous mistakes, since the patient's response to dose is very unpredictable at first and demands careful observation and monitoring, preferably throughout the whole procedure but certainly for the first half-hour. Even so, many years ago, we had a disastrous experience in a grand multipara 9 whose reaction right at the beginning of the procedure, and in the presence of an experienced member of staff, caused the uterus to go into titanic spasm and burst. I was summoned hurriedly to the hospital and within twenty minutes had removed the uterus, but the patient was in a state of irreversible shock and died some days later from anuria which we could not manage. This was before the days of dialysis. This experience has made me very cautious ever since.

We are now making increasing use of the "escalation technique" which would horrify Theobald with his long-established doctrine of very dilute physiological dosage, but there are occasions when the uterus continues refractory even to high dosage.

Our usual technique is to set up a solution of two units in 500 ml solution and run it at 20 drops per minute which is equivalent to 5 milliunits/min, then to continue according to the patient's response. This is best monitored by tocography, as is the case now with all our

16/Table 2

Two-bottle Method Regime

	Drops per minute		milliunits per minute
2 units in 500 ml at	10	=	2·66
	20	=	5
	40	=	11
	80	=	21
8 units in 500 ml at	20	=	21
	40	=	43
	80	=	85
32 units in 500 ml at	20	=	85
	40	=	171
	80	=	341

Continue to escalate Syntocinon every 15 minutes until the onset of regular contractions every 2 minutes.

patients, but can be done very competently by experienced clinical observation. The dose is stepped up every 15 minutes until it is running at 80 drops per minute. We then set up the next bottle with 8 units in 500 ml solution and start again at 20 drops per minute, increasing thereafter as before. Except in cases of intra-uterine death, where surgical induction is not allowed, where in any case the danger of uterine rupture is absent, and where there are no fetal interests to consider, one would normally expect to get a reasonable response, i.e. regular contractions every two to three minutes with a dose less than 43 milliunits/min. This is the technique which Turnbull and Anderson very sensibly called "oxytocin titration" and is an important concept inasmuch as it takes account of the individual sensitivity of the patient to the drug. This titration method has been found superior to the infusion of more dilute oxytocin at a slowly increasing rate.[27] The success and safety of titration techniques however depend absolutely upon the availability of staff and proper monitoring facilities; otherwise it would be far safer to stick to the older dilute infusion technique with one unit in a thousand ml of 5 per cent glucose solution and not allowing the drip rate to exceed 40 drops per minute until the patient's sensitivity to the drug had been monitored by observation. In any case whatever infusion method is used and whatever monitoring apparatus is to hand, the patient should not be left unattended throughout the whole process.

We have had considerable experience of variable speed syringe pumps such as the Sage pump[1, 35] and the Rocket pump, in which small quantities of solution, for example 2 units of Syntocinon in 10 ml, can be given very slowly and accurately with instantaneous cut-off if necessary. The speed of the pump is set at the lowest point and gradually increased every five minutes according to the uterine response. By this technique it is not possible to refer to tables such as Table 2 to know exactly what dosage of oxytocin is being given at any time and although the technique may encourage a bolder approach to the use of oxytocin, we nowadays prefer to know exactly what the patient is, in fact, getting.[33]

The danger of uterine rupture is minimal in the case of a nullipara with a normal uterus although it is very real in grand multiparity but in both classes of patient the dangers of asphyxia to the baby in the absence of proper supervision and control are considerable.

One should aim to maintain the lowest possible dosage consistent with regular contractions every two to three minutes and the oxytocin drip should be kept running right through the third stage of labour and preferably for at least an hour thereafter, or two hours following twin delivery, to prevent any atonic third-stage haemorrhage.

The ideal frequency of contractions is about three in ten minutes but what is even more important than the height and intensity of the contraction is the return between contractions to a normal flaccid, resting uterine tone. Apart from cases of intra-uterine death it is now standard practice to combine the setting up of an oxytocin drip with artificial rupture of the membranes at the same time.

The oxytocin drip is at present being used with uncritical abandon on a scale which can hardly be justified on the basis of genuine indications. Wrigley (1962) sounded rather like a voice crying in the wilderness when he concluded, in the large series which he quoted, that it is "questionable whether the oxytocin drip saved the life of a single baby and it is certain that its employment never made labour more normal or more comfortable for the patient". What makes the matter worthy of serious thought is that accidents undoubtedly occur and the procedure cannot be regarded as totally safe. These hazards will be discussed later.

The recommendation to stay with the patient throughout administration is more important in fact for the maintenance of her morale than her physical safety. This last point is more important than commonly realised since a patient left alone, apparently at the mercy of a relentless and pain-producing drug whose administration she can lie back and watch but not control, is very liable to panic.

Uterine spasm should not be allowed to occur even with the hyper-reactive patient. Without the precautions already referred to, it can occasionally be intense and prolonged sometimes for over ten minutes, to the considerable peril of the fetus. In times gone by the teaching was to turn the patient onto her side and administer chloroform speedily by face-mask to alleviate the spasm but the need for this belongs to days of inappropriate dosage and supervision. The patient in any case should be nursed on her side throughout most of her labour.

Contra-indications to Oxytocin Drip

The chief absolute contra-indication is grand multiparity because of the tumultuous precipitate labour which can follow even quite small quantities of dilute oxytocin drip. Even medical supervision at the time may not be sufficient to prevent a sudden disaster of this sort as already described. One such catastrophe alone must wipe out the alleged benefits of many hundreds of other cases so treated.

Because of this danger of uterine rupture I am chary of employing an oxytocin drip in cases of previous Caesarean section, unless, by the opportunity of previous palpation from inside the uterus at a subsequent labour, I can be confident of the integrity of the scar. Previous Caesarean section is not an absolute contra-indication but calls for a slower rate of escalation, commonly approximately half, and of course full vigilance.

Apart from applying the observations involved in Bishop's scoring there are no prelabour methods of determining speed or likelihood of success in labour and we have now dispensed with oxytocin sensitivity tests. After all, if we mean to induce, we induce *and* monitor.

Disproportion, or subclinical varieties of it, are common causes of inert labour and the oxytocin drip is not only likely to fail in such a case but may have damaging effects on both mother and baby. Where hydramnios is present it is resonable to get rid of the overdistension of the uterus by amniotomy first, before using an oxytocin drip. Cases of transverse lie constitute other absolute contra-indications because of the obvious risks of membrane rupture with cord prolapse. We are also opposed to its use in diabetic pregnancy because of the natural hazards to which the fetus is heir in any case and which will not suffer any addition from this extraneous cause. Any pathology of the cervix involving scarring, for example following previous operation or repair, is a further contra-indication because of the risk of splitting.

In cases of multiple pregnancy, there is much to be said for an oxytocin drip being kept running in the course of the second and third stages of labour at a very slow and judicious rate, particularly with triplets and quadruplets where the hazards of uterine inertia and consequent postpartum haemorrhage are very considerable. Such a drip should not be taken down until the uterus is thoroughly well retracted at the end of the whole delivery and an hour or two thereafter.

Because of the misery of an intravenous drip in an otherwise well woman and the forced immobility which it involves, there has always been considerable interest in other possible routes of administration. Oxytocin is destroyed at once in the stomach, which makes the oral route useless and, as already mentioned, intramuscular and subcutaneous injections are futile or dangerous, or both, because of the complete unpredictability of the rate of absorption and destruction; but some of the mucous membranes are capable of absorbing oxytocin at a more even rate. At first the nasal route seemed an attractive alternative using oxytocin snuff, and later a spray, which was found to be as safe as the intravenous route and almost as effective,[11] although it never achieved much popularity in this country. The introduction of buccal oxytocin was immediately accepted, however, and for a time it was hoped that it could replace amniotomy and surgical methods; but it was soon evident that it was no more effective as a medical induction than the old-fashioned methods, including the use of quinine which I remember in the 1930s. Only 67 per cent in one series[45] were successful and of the 33 per cent failures, 22 were successful after artificial rupture of the membranes. The present view is that except for cases of intra-uterine death or as a "trial of induction" in postmaturity (which we do not approve of) the greatest use for buccal oxytocin is following amniotomy for the induction of labour.[41, 42] The maximum dosage as recommended by the makers (Parke-Davis—Buccal Pitocin) is to start with half a scored 200-unit tablet, i.e. 100 units for the first two doses at half-hourly intervals and thereafter to increase hourly with each alternate half-hourly dose until a maximum of 600 units is being given at a time. We ourselves gave up using Buccal Pitocin years ago. The tablets take almost an hour to dissolve when placed correctly between the cheek and the outer border of the upper gums and if an unexpected over-reaction of the uterus occurs they can be spat out and the mouth rinsed. The effect will be abolished within the next fifteen minutes. Some patients have difficulty in not munching the tablets and swallowing them inadvertently and also they tend to accumulate in the mouth to an embarrassing extent, but these minor inconveniences are a small price to pay for the greater comfort and mobility of the patient. All the hazards and precautions necessary with the use of intravenous oxytocin apply with equal force to the buccal route. No advantage whatsoever is gained in safety.

Prostaglandins

The existence of this group of very interesting substances has been known for many years. More than a dozen prostaglandins have been identified in human seminal fluid. Originally prostaglandins were extracted at considerable expense from the vesicular glands of sheep but nowadays, since their chemistry is known, they can be synthesised. They are all derivatives of prostanoic acid and have the property of acting as "local hormones".[17] As such they can be produced in active form in many places and operate near the site of production. In fact prostaglandins are inactivated by a single passage through the pulmonary vascular bed. Of all the varieties of prostaglandin, PGE2 and PGF2α seem to have the most useful potential in initiating and maintaining labour. The other varieties of prostaglandin would appear to have different and apparently contradictory actions on smooth muscle in various parts of the body.

Karim and his colleagues in Uganda had noted that prostaglandin F2α appears in human amniotic fluid during labour and also in the maternal venous blood in variable amounts which prompted the idea that this substance might play a part in the process of parturition. They therefore applied this principle to women at term and successfully induced labour by continuous infusion of 0·5 μg/kg/min of PGF2α in 29 women. An important observation was that the uterine activity was similar to that of normal labour but there was no increase in the resting tone of the uterus. Embrey in Oxford extended the study to include PGE2 and found that, dose for dose, the stimulant properties of PGE2 were very much greater, in fact about five times greater than those of PGF2α. He found that infusion of prostaglandin in the range of 4-8 μg/min at term produced comparable effects to those of oxytocin 5 milliunits/min but the action was slower to occur, with a latent period of 15 to 20 minutes, and the effects were thereafter more prolonged.[21] In a later and larger series[22] he confirmed these satisfactory results in induction by intravenous infusion in a dosage of 0·5–2·0 μg/min using total amounts varying from 100 μg–600 μg without hypertonus or undesirable effects in mother or baby. However he had less success in the induction of abortion since in 3 out of 11 cases the process was not complete and very much greater total dosages were necessary. Roberts and Turnbull however reported hypertonus in some of their cases induced with prostaglandin E2.

It would appear that uterine hypertonus is not only dose-related but patient-related as well and therefore these powerful substances, as with oxytocin, should not be used without adequate monitoring. The technique was introduced in Cardiff of starting the dosage at 0·75 μg/min and doubling the infusion dosage every two hours until a satisfactory level of activity was maintained.

One of the great drawbacks of intravenous prostaglandin administration is the painful phlebitis which results. It clears up very quickly and spontaneously but can be unpleasant while it lasts.

Since prostaglandins come into the class of local hormones, produced locally and with local effects, it was quickly expected that they might prove useful when placed in the vault of the vagina as "do-it-yourself" abortive agents, but it was soon found that not only were large doses necessary but the local irritant effect on rectum and large bowel was unacceptable. As has been described in the chapter on abortion, prostaglandins can only be used satisfactorily within the uterus itself either extra- or intra-amniotically.

The prostaglandins do not appear to be destroyed in the stomach and can be taken by mouth but in the sort of doses needed to induce abortion they will produce intense diarrhoea, nausea and vomiting, far worse than when used by the intravenous route. As a consequence of these observations and experience it is our practice, when having to induce midtrimester abortion on established genetic grounds, to use the extra-amniotic route as already described.

Of the two, prostaglandin E2 appears to be much less toxic in its effects than F2α and we therefore prefer it,[3–6] although in some parts of the world the latter is cheaper and more easily available. PGE2 is marketed as dinoprostone by Upjohn under the trade name of Prostin E2 in different amounts and concentrations according to the purpose, whether for the induction of labour or abortion, and whether or not for intra-uterine, extra-amniotic use. The manufacturers recommend caution in using this drug in patients with glaucoma or raised intra-ocular pressure, or with a history of asthma.

An interesting observation has been made regarding the release of oxytocin as detected in the plasma of women receiving intravenous prostaglandin E2 or F2α intravenously for the induction of labour, the levels being not dissimilar from those found in the late first stage of spontaneous labour.[25] Since oxytocin was found in maternal plasma even when the fetus was dead, and in the plasma of males receiving prostaglandin infusions, it would appear that prostaglandins have a direct effect upon the pituitary gland which may play a part in the oxytocin effects of systemic infusion as distinct from the local effects from intra-uterine administration.

Bearing in mind the high cost of prostaglandin, the sore arm suffered by the patient from intravenous infusion and the long-recognised reliability of synthetic oxytocin, a comparison is necessary for the relative effectiveness of each. This has been undertaken by Craft and his colleagues in the case of patients with intact membranes, using rapid type titration schedules to induce labour in patients near term.[18] The series was a small one but included both primigravid and multigravid patients and the drugs were administered by slow intravenous infusion pump. Their results showed a striking superiority in effect of prostaglandin E2 as compared with oxytocin.

It has been my own personal hope at this time, with my traditional respect for intact membranes, that prostaglandin induction might make amniotomy unnecessary at least until more than half dilatation of the cervix, but there can be no doubt that if an effective and expeditious induction is required, that is to say with an induction/delivery interval preferably within 12 hours, amniotomy has to be combined not only with intravenous oxytocin but with prostaglandin as well. In our own department, in a double-blind trial and restricting the comparison to primigravid patients only, forewater amniotomy was followed by oxytocin intravenously in escalating dosage, and in a comparable series prostaglandin E2 was introduced simultaneously. The cases of course were monitored and it was possible with a combined treatment to use a very much lower dose of oxytocin; in addition the benefits of a shorter labour were also evident.[39]

Bearing in mind that prostaglandins are not destroyed in the stomach it was not long before an assessment was made of oral prostaglandin E2 titration combined with amniotomy.[3–6, 18, 48] The F2α preparation in oral capsules was used at first but produced too much in the way of gastric and intestinal side-effects and was less effective than oral prostaglandin E2 which was given in freshly prepared aqueous solutions. The titration technique was used to control the dose, starting at 0·5 mg in a draught of 50 ml of water, subsequent doses being given at 2-hourly intervals and presently increased if necessary by 0·5 mg increments until uterine activity with contractions occurring every 2 to 3 minutes and lasting 40 to 50 seconds were induced; the maximum dose however did not exceed 3 mg.

The dose of prostaglandin required was related to the prelabour inducibility score and generally the lower the score the greater the dose required and the longer the induction/delivery interval. This was particularly true of primigravidae. In cases with low inducibility scores it would be more logical to use intravenous oxytocin titration because they are likely to have tedious labours anyway and intravenous infusion will be required to combat ketosis. It is consequently the practice in our department to undertake Bishop's scoring and in fact we restrict the use of oral prostaglandins to multiparae[19] with amniotomy. Full monitoring both of fetal heart and tocography was of course maintained throughout. Consequently no cases of hypertonus were observed and side-effects were not severe.

Fortunately Prostin E2 tablets each containing 0·5 mg dinoprostone are now available. An initial test dose of 0·5 mg (1 tablet) may be given. Thereafter we usually give 1 mg (2 tablets) hourly following amniotomy until labour is well established. The dose is then usually adjusted in successive hours between 0·5 and 1·5 mg according to the patient's response. The results in multiparae have been so satisfactory that this is now our preferred technique. An additional advantage is that the patient has more mobility, although this may interfere with monitoring.

There remains the problem of the case with the very unfavourable, unripe cervix with a low Bishop score and here there may well be a place for the extra-amniotic administration of prostaglandins as described by Calder *et al.*[12, 13] A No. 16 French gauge Nelaton urethral catheter is inserted through the cervix into the amniotic space for an optimum distance of 10 to 12 cm beyond the internal os, stiffening the catheter if necessary by inserting the metal stiletto of a Drew Smythe catheter into its lumen. Prostaglandin E2 is made up in normal saline in a concentration of 1·5 μg/ml. Infusion is begun at the rate of 20 μg/hour and increased every 15 minutes by 10 μg until labour is well established. The dose should not exceed 150 μg/hour. The infusion unit is connected by a Y-piece to an intra-uterine pressure manometer. Uterine hypertonus is not a problem and the type of labour is similar to that in cases following amniotomy and with intravenous oxytocin. In Glasgow the technique is favoured for the induction of midtrimester abortion using a Foley catheter with a balloon capacity of 30 to 50 ml and with prostaglandin E2 solution administered by Palmer pump in comparable dosage. By this means the cervix ripens very readily and the catheter is usually extruded at a dilatation of 3 to 4 cm. Then, and not before, amniotomy is deliberately undertaken. Oxytocin infusion intravenously is only added if uterine activity thereafter appeared unsatisfactory as was the case in about 31 per cent of patients with a normal fetus and 3 out of 4 with an anencephalic fetus. The big advantage of these cervical ripening techniques is that amniotomy can be delayed when this is desirable, such as in cases of fetal abnormality or with a high presenting part or where the cervix is particularly unfavourable for amniotomy at the outset.[13, 36] In the series reported by Calder and Embrey, using a balloon catheter, this technique was used amongst others in 7 primigravidae with Bishop scores as low as 0 to 1. Naturally the induction/delivery interval was longer in these very unfavourable cases but all were delivered within 18 hours.

At last the bogey of the really unfavourable cervix as a discouragement to the induction of labour has been coped with. The prostaglandins undoubtedly rival oxytocin in efficacy if not in cost but they also have the additional advantage that they do not cause antidiuresis and this may be most desirable in cases of pregnancy complicated by marked fluid retention as in pre-eclampsia, chronic renal disease or cardiac disease.

Artificial rupture of the forewaters.—This widely used method is not difficult nor is an anaesthetic necessary except in the nervous primigravida. Diazepam 5 mg intravenously usually suffices. Because of the occasional need to employ anaesthesia, however, especially if the cord unexpectedly prolapses, or if acute fetal distress is manifest, or if a "bloody tap" of major degree is encountered, it is a wise plan for the patient not only to have this minor operation in suitable surroundings, such as a proper obstetric theatre where Caesarean section can be carried out, but she should come with an empty stomach. For this reason we aim to carry out all our elective surgical inductions before 12 noon. Quite apart from being safer, it is a lot kinder to the patient.

In the interests of asepsis the patient should be in the lithotomy position, full aseptic and antiseptic ritual must be observed and the bladder must, as usual, be empty.

The introduction of a speculum and gripping the cervix with a sponge forceps is not as a rule necessary, and after passing a finger through the cervix and separating the membranes from the region of the internal os, a long-toothed artery forceps is passed, by touch, alongside the finger in the cervix and the forewaters are "tweaked". A disposable plastic amniohook, resembling a crochet hook is commonly used. Sometimes, because the head is applied closely to the membranes, no gush of liquor occurs, and it may be doubted whether the membranes have, in fact, been ruptured; a few fetal hairs in the tips of the forceps is evidence, of course, but the purpose of the operation is to drain off some liquor. By gently pushing up the head with the finger through the cervix, the operation may often be more successful and intermittent displacement of the head and withdrawal of the finger may produce gushes until the desired amount of liquor has been withdrawn.

If a uterine contraction occurs, so much the better, but care must be taken neither to rupture the membranes nor to displace the head during one in any case where the head is not deeply engaged, for fear of provoking cord prolapse, a disaster which in any event must always be excluded by examination at the end of the operation.

Rarely, it is not possible to pass a finger through the cervix, and blind stabbing with forceps is to be deprecated. Although there are many who would proceed to dilate it forcibly with dilators, the safer view is that the case is not suitable for surgical induction. Sometimes the cervical os is so far back in the sacral position that it is hard to reach even with the longer middle finger. Nevertheless it must be reached and hooked forwards. Often in such cases the fold of endocervix may obtrude below the internal os, which however must be reached and the terminal phalanx of the finger pushed through it if the operation is to be proceeded with. The index finger can sometimes negotiate this potential barrier better, especially after the cervix has been brought forward. The head should be steadied by the other hand on the abdomen. These difficult cases are undoubtedly made more easy by the intravenous injection of 5 mg of valium. If trying to pass two fingers through the internal os, it is easier to pass the index finger through after the middle finger than in the opposite order.

Occasionally some bleeding may occur, usually due to a minor degree of placenta praevia. With the forewaters already ruptured this is almost certain to cease in a minute or two, and only in cases of prolonged and serious bleeding will Caesarean section be indicated. Finally, the fetal heart should be auscultated to ensure that all is well.

Artificial rupture of the hindwaters.—The preliminary steps are the same as for the operation of forewater rupture and the same remarks about anaesthesia apply.

The Drew Smythe catheter is the instrument of choice, and it is introduced with the point of the stilette withdrawn and guided through the cervix by the sense of touch. It is slowly and gently passed between membranes (prevously separated) and uterine wall directly posterior to the presenting part; occasionally a postero-lateral insertion may serve better. On no account is any force to be used, nor is it necessary. When the whole of the distal curve of the instrument has been passed through the cervix the direction of thrust is altered by lowering the handle until the shaft of the instrument is pressing backwards on the perineum. The tip is now safely pointing directly forwards and the stilette is pushed home. A small downward movement of the handle is now made and the moment of membrane puncture can usually be detected. The stilette is now withdrawn and the liquor is collected in a measuring jug (Fig. 1). An alternative instrument is a curved male metal catheter. This is introduced posteriorly or sometimes more laterally and then twisted in its long axis with a flick in order to puncture the amniotic sac. It does not enter the uterus as far as the Drew Smythe catheter and is therefore less likely to encounter placenta but, in my hands at least, it fails more often to rupture the membranes. Removal of about 300 ml of liquor is generally sufficient and often one has to be content with less. As a rule, the success of the induction depends far more upon the period of gestation than the amount withdrawn.

Sometimes, on rupturing the membranes, only a small quantity of meconium-stained liquor is obtained. If the meconium is clearly fresh, i.e. turbid and "particulate" rather than old watery staining, one should be very vigilant for further signs of fetal distress and the fetal heart should thereafter be checked every quarter of an hour if a continuous fetal heart-rate monitor is not available. The fetus is clearly near the end of its tether. These cases come to a high operative delivery rate, either by Caesarean section or forceps, on account of further evidence of fetal distress. There is a higher incidence of fetal abnormality in these cases and an X-ray should be taken while there is yet time, to decide the issue.

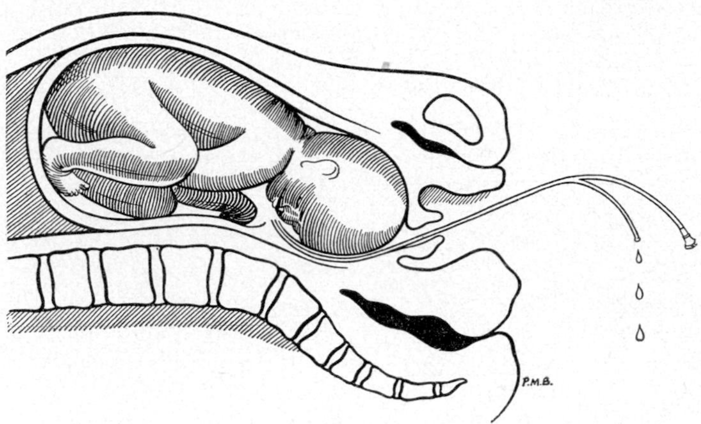

16/FIG. 1.—Hindwater puncture.

Certain troubles may be encountered. The commonest is to be rewarded not by liquor but by frank blood, due either to encountering placenta or vasa praevia; a blood-stained ooze from the decidua is of no moment. When bleeding occurs the Drew Smythe catheter should be withdrawn, and if it does not stop readily, as indeed it usually does, the forewaters should be ruptured. In all such cases the blood passed must be sent forthwith to the laboratory to exclude fetal haemorrhage (see earlier). When the cervix will not admit a finger (a bad omen) and it is decided nevertheless to proceed, it is better to do so under direct vision with the help of a Sims' or Auvard speculum and a sponge forceps applied to the anterior lip of the cervix. With a tight or difficult cervix it is certainly much easier to rupture the hindwaters by passing a Drew Smythe catheter than to rupture the forewaters. An extra-amniotic catheter and prostaglandin administration may be a better choice.

The fetal heart should be auscultated at the end of the operation. Irregularities and slowing of the rate are a warning that the child is not likely to stand the strain of prolonged delay in delivery.

Occasionally a fetal hand may be felt alongside the head during surgical induction. It should be pushed out of reach, and provided the head settles well on to the cervix it is unlikely to give further trouble.

Induction by Intra-amniotic Injections

It has already been mentioned that paracentesis, even with a fine needle, of the amniotic cavity may be followed by labour even when this is not intended. Bengtsson (1962) described the method of inducing therapeutic abortion in women between the 16th and 24th week of pregnancy by injecting hypertonic 20 per cent saline into the amniotic cavity. This injection produced a sharp fall in blood progesterone levels and incidentally he noted that if systemic progesterone was given before the hypertonic saline injection the onset of labour might be delayed for up to two days or more. Bengtsson reckoned that the hypertonic solution destroys placental function and removes the progesterone "block".

Because of the destruction of placental function this method of induction, of course, is reserved for cases of intra-uterine death or gross fetal abnormality, as fetal survival is not involved. The use of hypertonic glucose[50] has now been abandoned after a series of impressive disasters, including clostridial infection of the uterine contents and pressure-induced amniotic fluid embolism. Our own practice is to eschew intra-amniotic injections because of their unacceptable hazards as described in the chapter on abortion.

Indications for Surgical Induction

Whenever there are indications for medical induction, one should as a rule be prepared to acknowledge them for surgical induction as well, and failure of the one method should be followed by an attempt at the other. If one is not prepared to carry out this sequence, one is logically bound to admit that the gounds for interference were in the first place inadequate. To prescribe a medical induction which does not succeed and then to leave the patient to solve the problem for herself is both bad obstetrics and bad psychology, and repeated medical inductions are no better. Such treatment betrays a mind not sufficiently made up or one that has not the courage of its convictions. Intra-uterine fetal death is the only absolute exception to this rule.[37]

For this reason the indications for inducing labour whether by surgical or non-surgical means are grouped together, and are either for maternal or fetal interests or more commonly for a combination of both.

The indications come under two headings:

1. Obstetrical conditions;
2. Certain medical conditions aggravated by pregnancy.

The correct selection of cases in itself presupposes certainty as to the child's maturity. The best paediatric unit in the world is no substitute for a healthy intra-uterine environment up to the time of adequate maturity and there is now no excuse for being in doubt about this, thanks to the precision afforded by modern sonar techniques. The likely danger of neonatal respiratory distress syndrome can be foreseen or eliminated by amniocentesis and estimation of the lecithin: sphingomyelin ratio. Certain phospholipids originate in increasing quantity in fetal lung as it approaches maturity, but after the 35th week of gestation the lecithin component rises very much more markedly than sphingomyelin.[26] The ratio rises from near parity before the 35th week to 8 or more as term is approached. We regard a ratio of 2:1 as borderline and 3:1 as an encouraging sign that respiratory distress syndrome will not afflict the baby after birth.

Obstetric Indications for Induction

1. Pre-eclamptic toxaemia. Both fetal and maternal interests are at stake, but are often not mutually compatible, so that the choice for the moment of induction requires judgement.
2. Eclampsia which is not followed by the onset of spontaneous labour within forty-eight hours demands induction of labour, as the patient is sitting on a volcano.
3. Previous history of large babies. The tendency is for birth weights to increase in successive deliveries. No child is the better for being more than 4·5 kg at delivery and the mother is appreciably worse off.
4. Postmaturity. The risks of this to the baby are generally acknowledged, but mistakes are very frequently made in assessing its degree or significance and the case should be carefully reviewed. Modern sonar techniques now help to eliminate this sort of error. As Wrigley (1958) pointed out, "there is no such thing as an exact date for delivery, any more than there is an exact height or weight for a person", and he took into account, in assessing postmaturity, the amount of liquor relative to the fetal bulk on repeated examination by the same observer.

   The older the patient the more seriously should postmaturity be taken and the more readily should labour, after term, be induced.
5. Recurrent intra-uterine fetal death. This peculiar entity, said to be due to placental insufficiency, may, by the warning history, provide an opportunity to forestall disaster by shrewd or lucky timing.

   Grouped into this class come cases of dysmaturity or the "small for dates" baby. A great deal of interest is focused on this vexing problem and is dealt with in a later chapter, but much effort, and possibly ingenuity, are being devoted to the assessment of intra-uterine well-being, including growth rates as measured by sonar, in order to detect when fetal growth comes to a standstill and thus to determine the optimum moment for elective induction and delivery. An absence of maternal weight gain throughout pregnancy is often a pointer towards the possibility of dysmaturity. That nature is not always the best judge of the optimum time for delivery is evidenced by the phenomenon of macerated stillbirth, or in a less final form in the "small for dates" baby, undernourished, suboxygenated and in all respects dysmature. The baby that is in danger of outrunning its placental reserve, and who would fare better in a healthier extra-uterine environment, is only now beginning to be properly recognised before it is too late. The induction of premature labour is high up on the list of therapeutic alternatives, at least until we can find some method of assisting a child's development while still *in utero*.

6. Cases of mild disproportion. On the whole induction is best reserved for multiparae, in whom the risk of inertia is much less and whose obstetrical prowess can be assessed from the history of previous deliveries. In any case, it is not to be done without full clinical assessment of the pelvis and, if possible, X-ray pelvimetry.
7. Severe hydramnios producing marked pressure symptoms may call for relief. Abdominal paracentesis with a lumbar-puncture type of needle may be tried in the hope of prolonging pregnancy, but the amniotic cavity usually fills up rapidly again if labour is not already provoked and in the end deliberate induction is likely to be indicated. The danger of accidental haemorrhage following artificial rupture of the membranes in these cases has already been described.
8. Monsters. The prolongation of pregnancy is profitless and undesirable. It is better to deliver a small monster than a large one, and, on grounds of humanity as well, pregnancy is better terminated. The back-door escape, however, of Caesarean section is closed should labour subsequently become inert, and it is as well to bear this risk in mind and meet it to some extent by deferring induction until after the 34th week, by which time it is more likely to succeed.
9. Certain cases of placenta praevia in which the placenta is situated clear of the margins of the internal os and in whom a sufficient degree of maturity has been reached to make the risks of prematurity less than those of recurrent bleeding. It need hardly be pointed out that forewater rupture is the only method to consider, as it alone will reduce the chances of further antepartum haemorrhage and the operation should be performed in an operating theatre and under anaesthesia.

10. Rh factor iso-immunisation cases. The degree to which a fetus is affected with haemolytic disease *in utero* can now be determined by amniocentesis and spectrophotometry of the liquor amnii. In moderately or severely affected cases, where pregnancy has already reached the 34th week, induction of labour and delivery of the child in spite of prematurity is safer and more likely to be successful than intra-uterine transfusion, which is reserved for cases that have not yet reached this degree of maturity. The object of the induction is to get the child delivered so that it is available for exchange transfusion after birth and the timing will depend upon the likely severity of the disease.
11. Breech presentation provides a controversial point, particularly with extended legs. With the addition of every half kg to the baby's weight over 3 kg, the fetal mortality begins to climb with increasing steepness, and there is much to be said for inducing labour if the child's size is already reckoned to be approaching that figure. In any case, however, labour should not be induced before the 37th week, as the aftercoming head would be too vulnerable. Naturally, attempts at external version will have been made previously. The choice of method is debatable, but Drew Smythe catheter induction is not only feasible but preferable. Inadvertent tweaking of the testicles has little to commend it! Whichever method of membrane rupture is employed, the risk of cord prolapse is minimal with a deeply engaged presenting breech.
12. Intra-uterine death of the fetus which is radiologically proven is only a relative indication for induction. Spontaneous labour will always start eventually, but the patient can often be spared some very wretched weeks of waiting if labour is induced. Surgical methods, as already stated, cannot be too strongly condemned, but drug induction is both safe and usually efficacious.
13. Hyperemesis with signs of ketosis appearing in late pregnancy, particularly in a multipara, occasionally betokens some acute toxaemic process which is generally ill-understood. Not only should the ketosis be urgently combated with intravenous glucose saline, but labour should be induced forthwith. Many of these cases have hiatus hernia.
14. Icterus gravidarum may be another grave sign of obstetrical toxaemia and has a bad prognosis. Pregnancy must be terminated promptly.

Medical Indications for Induction

1. Chronic nephritis. Pregnancy has no known beneficial effects whatever on the healthy kidney, and where renal function is

already damaged the effects of pregnancy vary between bad and disastrous. If only maternal indications were at stake all such pregnancies should be terminated whenever and as soon as the diagnosis of chronic nephritis is established, and the patient should be sterilised. Mild cases, however, may reach the later months of pregnancy, and in the almost certain knowledge that no future pregnancy is likely to fare better, if as well, it may be justifiable to gamble for a few extra weeks in the baby's interests. Induction has a limited field, however, mainly restricted to the multiparous, and Caesarean section and sterilisation there and then, or subsequently, are generally preferred. Such decisions and the timing of intervention are among the most difficult in midwifery.

2. Hypertension. The effects of pregnancy are, as a rule, harmful here as well, but the position is far less clear cut than in the case of chronic nephritis. Much will depend upon the condition, if known, before pregnancy started, the period of gestation at which hypertension appeared, the rate at which it develops, whether or not other signs of pre-eclamptic toxaemia are superimposed, the age and parity, and many such factors. The risks to the baby of prematurity have to be weighed against those of intra-uterine death, and the longer the hypertension is allowed to operate the more likely is the mother to remain hypertensive for the rest of her life. Induction of labour, therefore, plays a very large part in the management of these cases.
3. Diabetes. Whether or not pre-eclamptic toxaemia is added to this complication, induction of labour is often called for to forestall intra-uterine fetal death, which is a very real risk, and to obviate delivery of an oversized yet premature child of less than usual resilience to the stresses of labour. Wherever possible we try to induce labour by amniotomy between the 36th and 37th weeks of pregnancy since the danger of intra-uterine death rises steeply after this period.
4. Recurrent pyelitis betokens structural alterations in the upper urinary tract which are likely to become permanent if neglected, and the possibility must be borne in mind of more deep-seated urological pathology which prolongation of pregnancy is likely to aggravate.
5. Chorea gravidarum. This complication is sometimes so severe or difficult to control that pregnancy may have to be terminated by Caesarean section. In the later weeks, however, induction of labour may suffice.
6. History of bleeding in earlier pregnancy. As Lennon[29] said, "Placental damage, once sustained, is irreversible and fetal survival depends upon the amount of residual functional

placental tissue and fetal maturity". For this reason (which applies even more commonly to pre-eclamptic toxaemia) we very readily induce cases who have threatened to abort earlier in pregnancy and we are very reluctant to allow them to become postmature for fear of intra-uterine fetal death.

In broad and general principles, however, non-obstetrical diseases are served no better by induction than by awaiting spontaneous delivery at term, for induced labour is, as a rule, no kinder to mother or child and occasionally demands its own price.

Contra-indications to Induction of Labour

Under the following circumstances the induction of labour is absolutely contra-indicated:

1. Disproportion which is more than borderline. It must have been made abundantly clear already that such treatment is little short of wanton folly rewarded with a high failure rate, a prohibitive fetal mortality and the likelihood of maternal morbidity.
2. Where pregnancy has not yet reached the 34th week—except in cases of established eclampsia—firstly, because the onset of labour may be dangerously long in starting and, secondly, because the risks of prematurity are too high; there is, however, one exception in the case of gross fetal abnormality associated with hydramnios which is producing symptoms.
3. Where the lie is other than longitudinal, for obvious reasons.
4. In cases which have previously been subjected to Caesarean section on account of contracted pelvis or who have failed in a previous trial of labour for disproportion.
5. Where a tumour occupies the pelvis.
6. Cases of cardiac disease are exposed to the additional hazards of subacute bacterial endocarditis at the best of times and surgical induction is likely only to increase them, especially if there is subsequent delay in completing delivery, since there is no such thing as an aseptic surgical induction. Usually induction is not necessary in these cases anyway as they tend not to go postmature and spontaneous labour is usually expeditious.
7. Elderly primigravidae with malpresentation are better delivered by Caesarean section without more ado.

Lastly, it is reiterated that surgical induction cannot be too strongly condemned when the fetus is known to be dead.

The above is categorical teaching more or less throughout the world, but it has come to my notice that Professor Townsend of Melbourne, at the 5th World Congress of Gynaecologists and Obstetricians in Sydney (which, for health reasons at the last moment, I could not attend), produced a paper holding the exactly opposite point of view and strongly recommending that the membranes should be ruptured in any case of intra-uterine death after the 20th week of gestation and active steps taken to promote delivery by the use of a determined oxytocin infusion. He produced a series of 40 cases so treated without disaster and claimed that the method eliminated psychological stress for the patient and reduced the hazard of hypofibrinogenaemia,

It is the view of my more conservative colleagues that the chances of developing hypofibrinogenaemia are no more than 25 per cent and that if it does occur the patient may not necessarily bleed but that 8 g of fibrinogen should be at the ready to cope with any bleeding, ante- or postpartum. Delivery itself should prevent recurrence of hypofibrinogenaemia but in the unlikely event of its not ensuing, following blood loss, the further microcoagulation and loss of more fibrinogen can be prevented by heparin. This in turn should be reversed by protamine sulphate within an hour before delivery or before any form of surgery. It is only very rarely necessary to have to go through all these therapeutic steps, which however are trivial compared with a surgical induction which misfires and rewards one with only a few spoonfuls of turbid liquor amnii at amniotomy (Fig. 2).

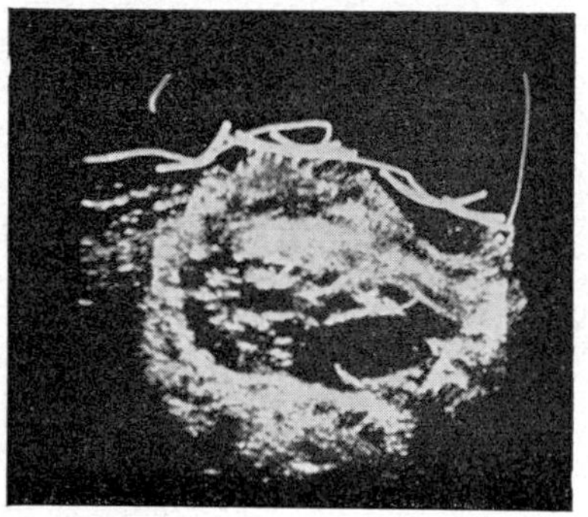

16/Fig. 2.—Ultrasonogram, in longitudinal section, of retained intra-uterine dead fetus due to Rh-haemolytic disease at the 28th week of gestation, the size of uterus being no more than 20 weeks.

Note: Thick Rhesus placenta in the upper part of the picture, i.e. anteriorly, and the relative scanty amounts of liquor (black areas).

The deformed, dead fetal head is partially seen lower right of picture.

Effects of Induction

Even before labour starts, cases of pre-eclamptic toxaemia often show some temporary improvement after rupture of the membranes and the blood pressure tends to drop so that eclampsia may, for a few hours, be less imminent; the respite is, however, only brief, and must not encourage a relaxation in vigilance; nevertheless, it may suffice, particularly in the multipara.

Other immediate effects before the onset of labour are the relief of pressure symptoms from hydramnios and the control, as a rule, of antepartum haemorrhage in cases of minor degrees of placenta praevia.

The penalities are reflected in an increased fetal mortality and maternal morbidity rate, but it is hardly fair to blame induction for these without taking into account the indications for which it is done.

Induction-delivery interval (IDI).—This is now being recorded in an increasing number of maternity reports of various institutions and gives a good indication of the success of induction methods in securing their objective, namely, the onset of labour; what it fails to do, however, is to show up the length of the latent period of waiting before labour ensues, and it is felt that this latent period should be shown in these tables.

It may be considered a paradox that rupture of the forewaters is used as a method of induction on the one hand and yet, on the other, spontaneous early rupture of the membranes often presages a prolonged first stage. The difference in mechanism can be explained in that, in the latter the membranes may have ruptured early because the presenting part does not fit snugly in the lower uterine segment, as, for example, in occipitoposterior positions which, of themselves, cause inertia.

Once the decision to induce labour has been made it is our firm intention that the induction/delivery interval should not exceed 18 hours at most. This we seek to achieve by adequate oxytocin or prostaglandin patient-titration techniques as already described, together with amniotomy. Failure is indicated by refusal of the cervix to dilate over a period of several hours. The risks of intra-uterine infection mount with the duration of labour following amniotomy and after 24 hours the chances of established amnionitis rise to 100 per cent. The baby in such a neglected case suffers even more from such an infection and may be born with an established intranatal pneumonia. If delivery is not achieved within 12 hours of induction the case should be very critically reviewed as to the wisdom of persisting. Monitoring techniques may indicate the onset of fetal distress which may call for delivery by Caesarean section but even in the absence of fetal distress, failure to progress in labour in spite of adequate drug dosage, as like as not by now supported with epidural analgesia, calls for Caesarean section early rather than late.

To perform Caesarean section because induction has failed and because of the threat of intra-amniotic infection is an extreme but perfectly logical point of view, and is the only prudent line to take if the indications for induction were sufficiently pressing in the first place. It is when inductions of convenience are undertaken that trouble, on the rare occasions when it occurs, is particularly galling. I have heard D'Esopo talking of "delivery by appointment" by means of elective induction, but I note that he is careful to restrict the practice to supernormal cases, parous women, with the head well engaged and the cervix already 2 cm dilated.

The idea of elective delivery and induction for reasons of convenience, staffing economics or simple patient comfort has undoubtedly come in the wake of increased safety, improved methods and better fetal and maternal assessment before labour. The incidence of induction has been steadily rising in many obstetric units including our own in the last few years (over 40 per cent) but there has also been a striking reduction in perinatal mortality to just over 15 per 1000, and if corrected for ultrapremature fetuses spontaneously born with birthweights under 1000 g the figure for last year was 13 per 1000 and this included cases of fetal abnormality. Clearly we seem to be heading towards the irreducible minimum, thanks to the fact that all our cases except those in very rapid labour are monitored with the most sophisticated apparatus.

For obvious reasons elective induction is undertaken in the early part of the morning since there is no point in making a patient miserable throughout the night, labouring unnecessarily. This inevitably results in "rush hour" delivery periods in the late afternoon (Fig. 3). This could, in time, affect staffing arrangements in hospital and the maintenance of ancillary services at peak efficiency at times of maximal demand, although full staffing has to be maintained throughout the 24 hours. The policy has come in for a good deal of adverse criticism of an emotive sort at the time of writing. It must not be forgotten that the introduction of anaesthesia into midwifery by Simpson in the last century came in for even more vitriolic abuse from sources both lay and ecclesiastical for interfering with Nature and the God-given pains of childbirth. The hope has been expressed that elective induction of labour, however, might contribute not only to reduction in the perinatal stillbirth rate but also in the number of cases of mature, unexplained stillbirths.[16]

The acid test of this interventionist policy is that the Caesarean section rate should not appreciably rise and the perinatal mortality rate should be reduced. If these results are not achieved the policy should certainly be overhauled. As a counterblast from Dublin, in 1000 consecutive primigravidae, studied prospectively, labour was induced on only 95 occasions, with figures every bit as good as ours on this side of the Irish Sea. The Dublin policy is to accelerate labour after it has spontaneously started rather than expediting its onset for indications which cannot be genuinely sustained.[40]

The situation of "failed induction" as formerly understood must not nowadays be allowed to occur, but at the same time the overall Caesarean section rate should not be wantonly increased or one is forced to the conclusion that there has been bad selection of cases.

As an omen for successful induction, whatever figures may suggest, it is the common experience of all of us that a well-taken-up and effaced cervix, with a thin lower uterine segment and a deeply

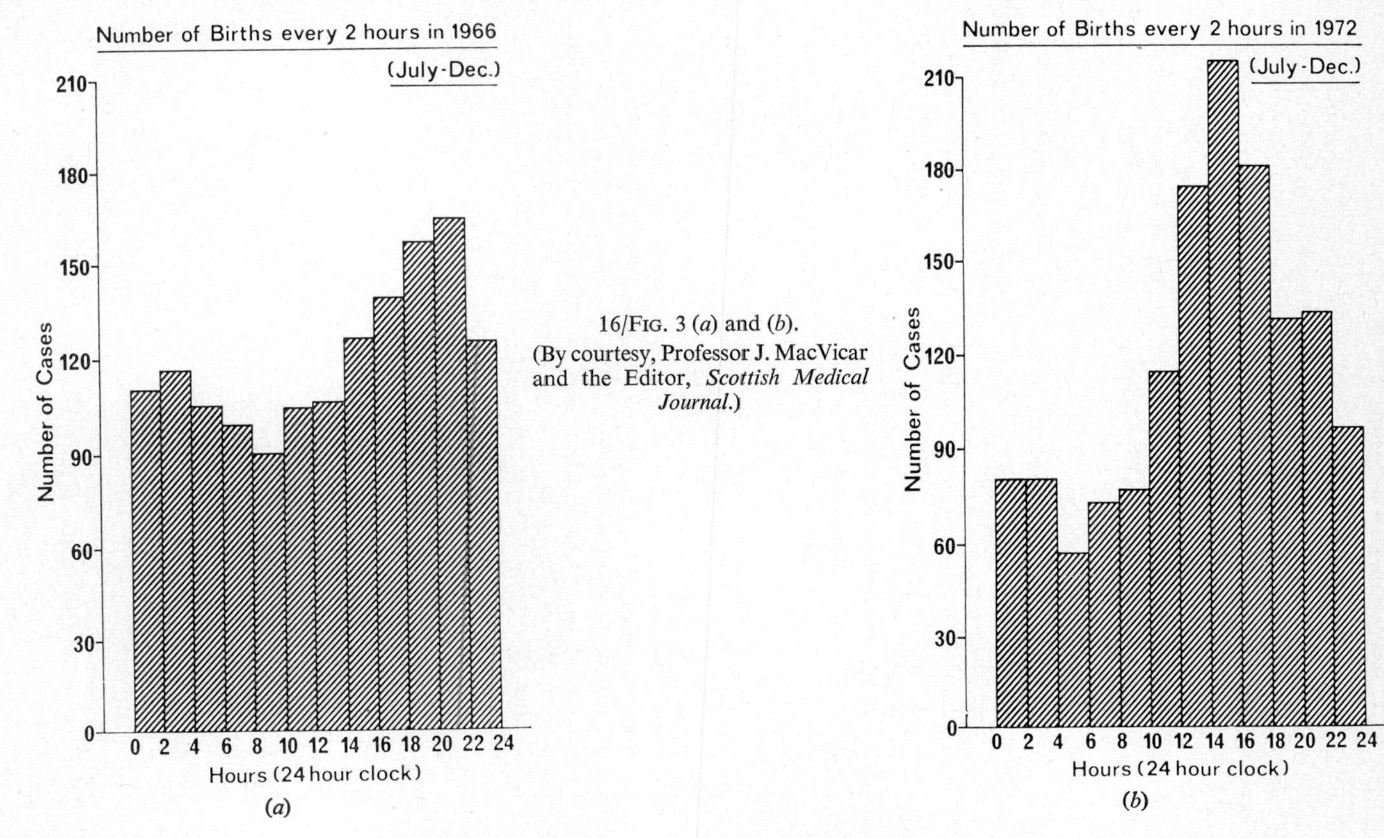

16/Fig. 3 (*a*) and (*b*).
(By courtesy, Professor J. MacVicar and the Editor, *Scottish Medical Journal*.)

engaged vertex, all these, together with a uterus which demonstrates its irritability on palpation, betoken a stage well set for labour and delivery. It is unlikely that the added stimulus of artificial rupture or puncture of the membranes will fail to trigger off the processes of labour.

In conclusion, then, let one's reasons for inducing labour be carefully and honestly weighed, let the circumstances be favourable, and let the Rubicon be crossed with no lingering glances behind.

REFERENCES

1. Bainbridge, M. N., Nixon, W. C. W., Schild, H. D. and Smith, C. B. (1956). *Brit. med. J.*, **1,** 1133.
2. Baird, D. (1957). *Brit. med. J.*, **1,** 1061.
3. Barr, W. (1972). *Proceedings of Symposium at Royal College of Physicians, London, 21 September 1972.* Upjohn.
4. Barr, W. (1973). Personal communication.
5. Barr, W. and Graham, R. (1967). *Postgrad. med. J.* Suppl. **43,** 101.
6. Barr, W. and Naismith, W. C. M. K. (1972). *Brit. med. J.*, **2,** 188.
7. Beazley, J. M. and Alderman, B. (1975). *Brit. J. Obstet. Gynaec.*, **82,** 265.
8. Beazley, J. M. and Weekes, A. R. L. (1976), *Brit. J. Obstet. Gynaec.*, **83,** 62.
9. Bengtsson, L. P. (1962). *Lancet*, **1,** 339.
10. Bishop, E. H. (1964). *Obstet. and Gynec.*, **24,** 266.
11. Borglin, N. E. (1962). *Acta obstet. gynec. scand.*, **41,** 238.
12. Calder, A. A. and Embrey, M. P. (1973). *Lancet*, **2,** 1322.
13. Calder, A. A., Embrey, M. P. and Hillier, K. (1974). *J. Obstet. Gynaec. Brit. Cwlth*, **81,** 91.
14. Calder, A. A., Moar, V. A., Ounstead, M. K. and Turnbull, A. C. (1974). *Lancet*, **2,** 1339.
15. Chalmers, I., Campbell, H. and Turnbull, A. C. (1975). *Brit. med. J.*, **2,** 116.
16. Cole, R. A., Howie, P. W. and MacNaughton, M. C. (1975). *Lancet*, **2,** 767.
17. Collier, H. D. J. (1971). *Proc. roy. Soc. Med.*, **64,** 1.
18. Craft, I. (1972). *Brit. med. J.*, **2,** 191.
19. Davies, D. P., Gomersall, R., Robertson, R., Gray, O. P. and Turnbull, A. C. (1973). *Brit. med. J.*, **3,** 476.
20. D'Esopo, A. (1963). Obstetrical and Gynecological Assembly of Southern California, Los Angeles.
21. Embrey, M. P. (1966). *J. Obstet. Gynaec. Brit. Cwlth*, **76,** 783.
22. Embrey, M. P. (1970). *Brit. med. J.*, **2,** 256, 258.
23. Friedman, E. A., Niswander, K. R., Bayonet-Rivera, N. P. and Sachtleben, M. R. (1966). *Obstet. Gynec.*, **28,** 495.
24. Friedman, E. A. and Sachtleben, M. R. (1976). *Brit. med. J.*, **1,** 198.
25. Gillespie, A., Brummer, H. C. and Chard, T. (1972). *Brit. med. J.*, **1,** 543.

26. GLUCK, L., KULOVICH, M. V., BORER, R. P., BRENNER, P. H., ANDERSON, G. G. and SPELLACY, W. N. (1971). *Amer. J. Obstet. Gynec.*, **109,** 440.
27. HOWIE, P. and MACVICAR, J. (1970). *J. Obstet. Gynaec. Brit. Cwlth,* **77,** 813.
28. KARIM, S. M. M., TRUSSELL, R. R., HILLIER, K. and PATEL, R. C. (1969). *J. Obstet. Gynaec. Brit. Cwlth*, **76,** 769.
29. LENNON, G. G. (1957). *Proc. roy. Soc. Med.*, **50,** 793.
30. LIGGINS, G. C., KENNEDY, P. C. and HOLM, L. W. (1967). *Amer. J. Obstet. Gynec.*, **98,** 1080.
31. MCCALLUM, M. F. and GOVAN, A. D. T. (1963). *J. Obstet. Gynaec. Brit. Cwlth*, **70,** 244.
32. MACVICAR, J. (1971). *J. Obstet. Gynaec. Brit. Cwlth*, **78,** 1007.
33. MACVICAR, J. and HOWIE, P. W. (1967). *Lancet*. **2,** 1339.
34. MATI, J. K. G., HORROBIN, D. F. and BRAMLEY, P. S. (1973). *Brit. med. J.* **2,** 149.
35. MAYES, B. T. and SHEARMAN, R. P. (1956). *J. Obstet. Gynaec. Brit. Emp.*, **63,** 812.
36. MILLER, A. W. F. and MACK, D. S. (1974). *J. Obstet. Gynaec. Brit. Cwlth*, **81,** 706.
37. MITCHELL, A. P. B., ANDERSON, G. S. and RUSSELL, J. K. (1957). *Brit. med. J.*, **1,** 611.
38. MURPHY, B. E. P. (1973). *Amer. J. Obstet. Gynec.*, **115,** 521.
39. NAISMITH, W. C. M. K., BARR, W. and MACVICAR, J. (1972). *Brit. med. J.*, **4,** 461.
40. O'DRISCOLL, K., CARROLL, C. J. and COUGHLAN, M. (1975). *Brit. med. J.*, **4,** 727.
41. RITCHIE, J. M. and BRUDENELL, J. M. (1966). *Brit. med. J.*, **1,** 581.
42. RITCHIE, J. M. and BRUDENELL, J. M. (1967). *ibid.*, **1,** 608.
43. ROBERTS, G. and TURNBULL, A. C. (1971). *Brit. med. J.*, **1,** 702.
44. RUSSELL, J. K., SMITH, D. F. and YULE, R. (1956). *Brit. med. J.*, **2,** 1414.
45. SPENCE, D. N. and CHALMERS, J. A. (1964). *Lancet*. **1,** 633.
46. THEOBALD, G. W., KELSEY, H. A. and MUIRHEAD, J. M. B. (1956). *J. Obstet. Gynaec. Brit. Emp.*, **63,** 641.
47. THIERY, M., DE HEMPTINNE, D., SCHUDDINK, L. and MARTENS, G. (1975). *Lancet*, **1,** 161.
48. TSAKOK, F. H. M., GRUDYINSKAS, J. G., KAVIM, J. M. M. and RATNAUR, S. S. (1975). *Brit. J. Obstet. Gynaec.*, **82,** 894.
49. TURNBULL, A. C. and ANDERSON, A. B. M. (1968). *J. Obstet. Gynaec. Brit. Cwlth*, **75,** 32.
50. WOOD, C., BOOTH, R. T. and PINKERTON, J. H. M. (1962). *Brit. med. J.*, **2,** 706.
51. WRIGLEY, A. J. (1958). *Lancet*, **1,** 1167.
52. WRIGLEY, A. J. (1962). *Lancet*, **1,** 5.

CHAPTER XVII

DISPROPORTION

THE art of obstetrics is more often travestied in the name of disproportion than in any other instance. The prediction that cephalopelvic disproportion will adversely influence labour, as well as the assessment of its extent and the treatment with which the problem is met, are more than matters of mathematical measurement, and demand a skill and experience which no textbook can provide. With modern radiological technique it is possible nowadays to measure up the pelvis in all sorts of planes, and yet the fact that trial of labour is so frequently instituted is acknowledgment enough of the inadequacy of these scientific aids.

The dynamics of labour are more important than the mechanics, and the efficacy of uterine contractions, the capacity of the fetal head to mould and the stamina and the temperamental resilience of the patient contribute more to the outcome of labour in the minor and commoner types of disproportion than the pelvic measurements themselves. An appreciation of the mechanism of labour in disproportion is, therefore, essential.

In this chapter only vertex presentations will be considered, for the delivery of malpresentation with contracted pelvis hardly comes into the realm of good obstetrics. Nevertheless, restricting our consideration to the four vertex positions, it must be acknowledged straight away that occipitoposterior positions have a particularly adverse effect.

Successful delivery will depend in large measure upon good uterine contractions. Unfortunately these are often lacking. To an almost similar extent, an attitude of good flexion on the part of the fetus is essential. Flexion is the essence of normal labour. In flexion, after all, we come into this world and bent up with old age we go in flexion to our graves; flexion is the alpha and the omega—the beginning and the end!

Poor flexion causes poor pains and poor pains aggravate poor flexion. It is altogether a depressing combination. The mechanism of labour has been studied with much detail and ingenuity, and all sorts of models, which are imaginative masterpieces, have been produced to illustrate it. Caldwell, Moloy and D'Esopo have also studied the mechanism of labour by means of radiology but, when all is said and done, difficult labour boils down to an attempt on the part of Nature to force a large foreign body through a somewhat inadequate orifice. The size of the foreign body, that is to say the baby's head, is a major consideration, yet this is one of the more uncertain factors. Sonar, however, is a great help.

In about 1959–60 I noticed that two echo blips were obtainable from the fetal head *in utero* by means of a standard ultrasonic flaw-detector used in industry to reveal deep-seated defects in mental structures. My then ward sister (now matron) was quick to employ it as a means of identifying the presentation in doubtful cases before my grand rounds. The two blips, as shown in the diagram of Fig. 1,

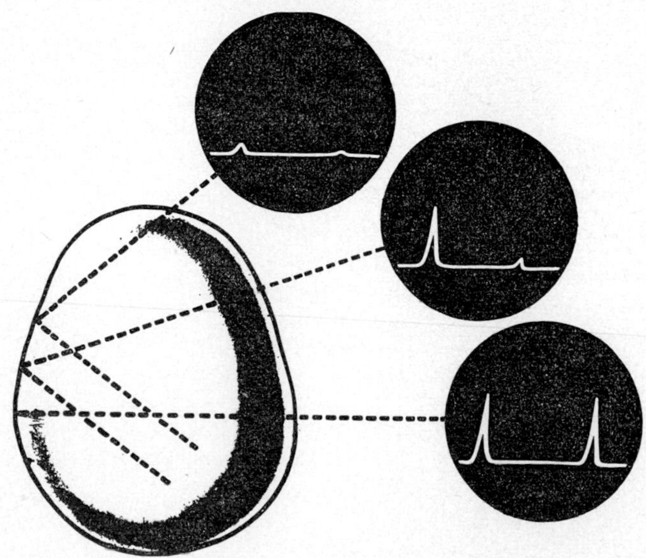

17/FIG. 1.—ULTRASONIC BIPARIETAL CEPHALOMETRY. (Original, 1959–60.)

In the lowest diagram the biparietal diameter is revealed by the simultaneous appearance of two huge echo blips on a cathode ray screen because both reflecting surfaces are at right angles to the beam of ultrasound. In the other two diagrams above these conditions do not apply.

depend upon the fact that the echoes only return to the probe (applied to the abdominal surface through a film of olive oil to secure acoustic coupling) when the incident beam of ultrasound strikes the fetal skull surfaces at right angles.[5] Both sides of the fetal skull can only thus reflect squarely and simultaneously if the beam lies along either the biparietal or the occipitofrontal diameters, i.e. the true diameters of the elliptical fetal skull and not a chord of the ellipse. The biparietal diameter is easily accessible, usually lying anteroposterior, whereas the occipitofrontal is less accessible and anyway is much larger and unlikely to be confused.[6]

The parietal eminence is searched for by palpation and the ultrasonic probe is then applied in this region and rocked about until both blips from the near and far walls of the fetal skull show up simultaneously on a cathode ray screen. It was a logical sequence of this discovery to relate the distance between the two blips to the actual distance between the parietal skull bones, in other words, the biparietal diameter. Willocks and Duggan, of my department, have

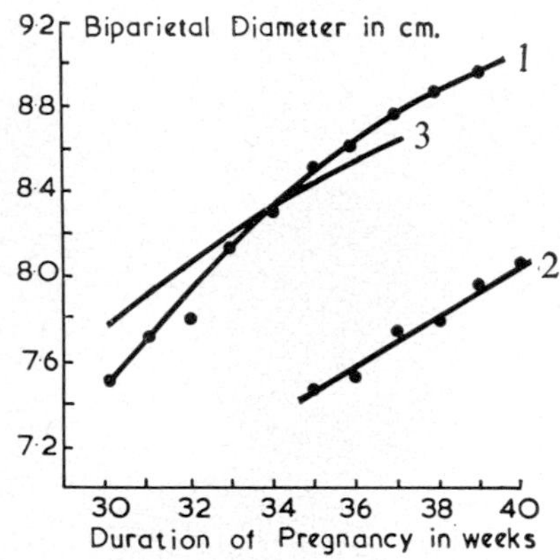

17/FIG. 2.—BIPARIETAL GROWTH CURVES *IN UTERO*.

(1) A normal curve. (2) A case of placental insufficiency. (3) A baby of a diabetic mother with normal growth curve and delivered at 37 weeks.

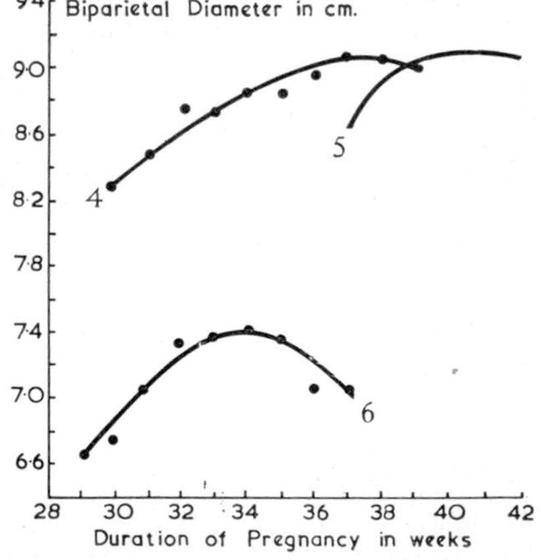

17/FIG. 3.—BIPARIETAL GROWTH CURVES *IN UTERO*.

(4) Demonstrates the reduced growth rate as term is approached. (5) A case of postmaturity. (6) Intra-uterine death resulting in macerated stillbirth (Willocks, 1963).

since developed the technique to a high degree of accuracy, of the order of a millimetre, and have observed the continued rate of growth of the fetal skull in the last weeks of pregnancy (Figs. 2 and

3). This is a very simple technique (from the patient's point of view) and only takes a few minutes without even moving her from her bed.

More recently another one-time member of my department, Stuart Campbell, has refined the technique still further by identifying the fetal head and its exact attitude in two dimensions with sonar, thus identifying the biparietal diameter pictorially beyond all shadow of doubt and usually demonstrating the midline echoes from the falx as well. Then switching the signals from the ultrasonic probe onto A-scan, in one dimension as before, very accurate measurements, often to 0·5 mm, can be made using electronic cursors as devised by Duggan.[20] Ultrasonic biparietal cephalometry is now almost universally undertaken in the more sophisticated departments throughout the world.[9]

That the head enlarges in the last weeks of pregnancy there can be no doubt. There is, therefore, a significant difference in the size of head between the 38th week and the 42nd week of gestation. Now, moulding can reduce the biparietal dimension by a quarter of an inch or more (6–7 mm), but such gross degrees are not compatible with the child's safety and it is not desirable that moulding should cause more than a reduction of 4 mm. In a clear-cut case of disproportion, therefore, it is not fair to the child to rely upon moulding to secure its delivery, except perhaps in the case of the flat pelvis, which demands moulding in only one meridian.

Disproportion at the brim is often partly countered by the mechanism of asynclitism, whereby the lateral rocking of the head presents a slightly diminished diameter, namely, the subparieto-superparietal diameter of $3\frac{1}{2}$ in (9 cm), as compared with the biparietal diameter of $3\frac{3}{4}$ in (9·5 cm). There are two sorts of asynclitism. The commoner is the anterior variety, also known as Naegele's obliquity, whereby the anterior parietal bone presents predominantly so that the sagittal suture lies nearer the sacrum (Fig. 4). This is a favourable mechanism. The other type is the posterior asynclitism, also known as Litzmann's obliquity, in which the posterior parietal bone presents, thereby placing the sagittal suture closer to the pubic symphysis. This is an unfavourable mechanism and augurs very badly for spontaneous delivery if it persists.

Disproportion at the outlet is a definite entity and is dealt with more fully later. One of the most important features here is the width of the subpubic arch and the acuteness of the subpubic angle. A narrow arch and angle cause a great waste in the anteroposterior dimensions of the outlet because the head can only emerge by passing farther back, with detriment to the maternal pelvic floor. Greater forces in delivery are therefore necessary in these cases and outlet difficulties are far more often responsible for extreme moulding and elongation of the head than brim dystocia.

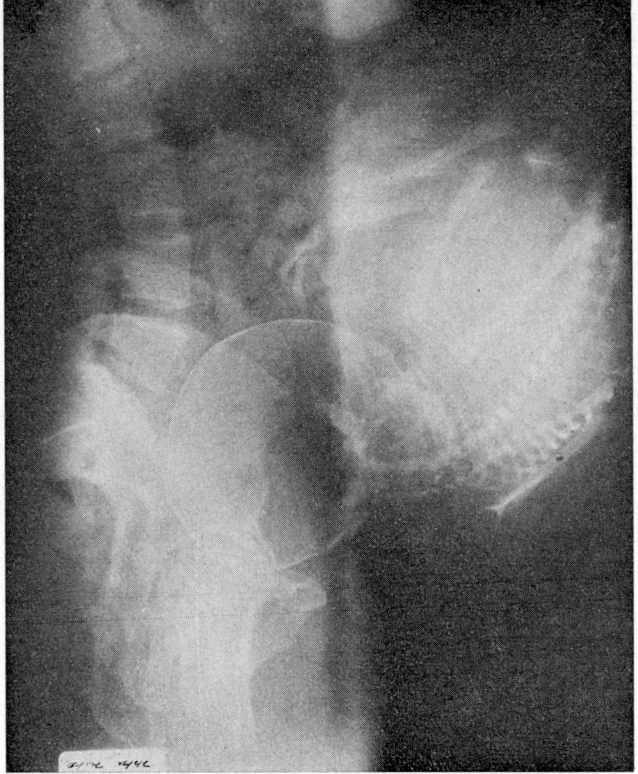

17/Fig. 4.—Anterior parietal presentation.

The mechanism of successful internal rotation of the fetal head may be hampered by the presence of disproportion, but even more commonly is this fault due to uterine inadequacy. The various types of contracted pelvis, however, profoundly influence the mechanism of labour, and these individual aspects will be discussed presently.

When to Suspect Disproportion

It is naturally a part of good antenatal care that major degrees of contracted pelvis should be evaluated long before the patient reaches term. Nowadays, the main problem is confined to the lesser degrees and borderline cases. A fetal head deeply engaged within the pelvis during the last four weeks of pregnancy practically rules disproportion out of court, for there is no finer pelvimeter than the fetal head, but where satisfactory engagement of the head is not present, disproportion is one of the numerous diagnostic possibilities.

Certain general features are worth taking into account in forming an early impression. The stature of the patient is relevant, and although quite small women very often have good obstetrical pelves, any woman whose height is less than 5 feet (1·5 m) should have an accurate assessment of the pelvis made during pregnancy, especially if she is a primigravida. Radiological pelvimetry is, if possible, delayed until after delivery because of increasingly recognised hazard to the fetus. The size of shoe worn also supplies some general indication of bony stature, and contracted pelvis in a woman of medium height or over is rather unlikely if the shoe size is greater than 5. A history or the stigmata of rickets are now rare in this country, but the problem is certainly more common overseas. Deformities of the lower extremities, if congenital or contracted in early youth, should always raise a suspicion of pelvic asymmetry, and spinal deformities are likewise significant. Beware of the primigravida with the pendulous abdomen. This is often due to the inability of the head to find room for itself in the pelvis.

The primigravida is a dark and untried horse, and a proper clinical assessment, at least of the pelvis, should never be omitted during pregnancy. The multipara, however, can supply information of priceless value, and the history should take note not only of the weight of the baby but the duration of labour, the extent of perineal damage, the degree of moulding at birth, the readiness with which the child breathed and the maturity at the onset of labour. A history of previous stillbirth or neonatal death should be very carefully inquired into, as a contracted pelvis might have been responsible. Nevertheless, a successful vaginal delivery in the past does not always guarantee a repetition next time, because successive babies tend to be larger and, in rare instances, the actual capacity of the pelvis may be diminished, especially in high degrees of parity, by partial subluxation forwards of the sacral promontory. The factor of uterine inertia, however, seldom complicates the issue in multiparous labour, although "delayed labour" in a multipara should make one think of the two likely possibilities of unsuspected brow presentation or unsuspected disproportion.

A thorough vaginal examination has remained a vitally important source of information ever since Smellie first measured the diagonal conjugate digitally, and the advent of X-ray pelvimetry in no way dispenses with the need for it. Vaginal examination is often misleading if sought in early pregnancy, and the optimum time for digital assessment is at the 36th week of pregnancy, when the soft tissues are sufficiently dilated to facilitate it. This should be a routine practice in all primigravidae except those already under observation for antepartum haemorrhage.

An appreciation of the mounting hazards of exposure to ionising radiations, which are now known to be genetically cumulative and possibly a factor in malignant disease in childhood (M.R.C. Report 1956 and Stewart *et al.*, 1956), has made nonsense of the statement which once originated across the Atlantic that every bride should have her pelvic measurements inscribed on the inside of her wedding ring! Court Brown *et al.* (1960) however checked the fate of over 39,000 live-born babies of mothers subjected to abdominal or pelvic irradiation in pregnancy between 1946 and 1956 in London and Edinburgh and found only nine to have died of leukaemia by 1958 against an expected natural incidence of more than ten. Lewis (1960) likewise in a smaller series at Queen Charlotte's Hospital actually found more cases of childhood leukaemia among the controls than in those whose mothers had been irradiated antenatally! Nevertheless the average obstetrician of today is reluctant to incur the hazard, however small.

Radiopelvimetry is reserved for cases in which the information sought is vital, for example in forthcoming breech delivery and in which satisfactory measurements may not have been obtainable by clinical methods. Our caution in rationing diagnostic radiology in pregnancy, however, must not be allowed to expose the baby or mother to even greater risks through neglecting to assess mechanical difficulties in labour. In spite of pelvimetry and every conscientious effort to assess disproportion, one is still sufficiently uncertain of the likely outcome to invoke trial of labour to resolve the doubt. Unfortunately, even a trial of labour often fails to answer the question. Gibberd, in the course of his Canadian lecture tour, in a piece of brilliantly analytical criticism, pointed out from a series at Guy's Hospital that, whereas the prediction that the pelvis would prove adequate was wrong in only 1 out of 650 cases, the diagnosis of pelvic inadequacy remained still unproven in about half the cases submitted to trial of labour because for one reason or another the trial could not be carried through to a full and final verdict.

It is to Munro Kerr that modern obstetrics largely owes the direction of its attention to the ability of the foot to fit the shoe or the head to fit into the pelvis, and, whatever other aids to diagnosis we may invoke, above all there remains the cardinal observation—Is the head engaged or is it not, and, if not, can it be made to do so?

The sign of a high head at term in a primigravida is not a welcome finding and calls for investigation as to possible causes. A retrospective study of over 400 unselected primigravidae in London indicated that in the majority the head did not engage spontaneously until after the 38th week of pregnancy.[17] This fact does not however invalidate the desirability of seeing if it can be made to engage by manipulation from the 36th week onwards.

Causes of a High Head at Term

The commonest cause is posterior position of the occiput. This is often associated with some degree of deflexion, which must rank as the second commonest cause. In multiparous pregnancy likewise the head may be late in engaging and in fact may occasionally not do so until labour is well advanced. In all three instances, however, it should be possible to push the head into the pelvis by manipulation. There is a growing tendency, even in Glasgow, to ignore the possible significance of a high head at term in the primigravida and I am constantly deprecating the attitude which, translated in Glaswegian dialect, amounts to "Hoots to a high head." It must, of course, colour one's attitude towards forthcoming labour and how vigorously it is to be pursued, but above all it calls for a thorough clinical assessment—no bad thing!

A full bladder or, it might be added, even a half-full bladder, should never be forgotten as a cause of high head at examination.

Mistaken maturity might be mentioned here as a spurious cause, the head being high simply because the patient is not so far on in pregnancy as her alleged dates would suggest.

A high angle of inclination of the pelvic brim discourages engagement. It occasionally operates singly but is more commonly associated with compensatory lordosis of the spine, and pendulous abdomen, with or without this bony anomaly, may discourage the head from engaging. Sometimes a high head is found which cannot be pushed into the pelvis because that is already occupied by the presenting part of another twin. This mistake is easier to make than one would imagine.

Hydramnios, besides being a cause of unstable presentation, is not uncommonly a cause of high head. The mechanism is obvious. No case, however, associated with hydramnios should be simply dismissed on that account, but should be examined radiologically for fetal abnormality or to exclude multiple pregnancy.

Now, and only now, be it noted, is disproportion mentioned. Naturally disproportion may be due to a contracted pelvis with a normal-sized baby or to an over-sized baby without pelvic contraction. Of the latter, hydrocephalus constitutes an extreme example.

Lastly, there may be an adventitious obstacle to engagement of the head in the form of placenta praevia or the presence of pelvic tumours, such as a fibroid or an ovarian cyst within the pelvis. The above is a large list to consider, and it has been given as far as possible in the order of probability if not of importance. Notwithstanding the above, however, there are some cases, usually fairly muscular girls, in whom no adequate explanation presents itself. It is as though the whole uterus, including the lower uterine segment, tended to ride high. In such cases disproportion is hard to exclude, and only the events of labour will provide evidence in retrospect.

Before proceeding to an account of the assessment of disproportion, mention should be made of a syndrome which, though not common, may, if recognised, give advance warning of difficult labour associated with disproportion. I refer to what is known as the dystocia dystrophia syndrome.

Dystocia Dystrophia Syndrome

These patients are of a definite type which is worth recognising, and Williams (1942) gave a very good account of 62 observed cases. The syndrome was recognised by Horner, but it was De Lee who gave it its clumsy though descriptive name. Characteristically, the patients are of stocky build, somewhat bull-necked with broad shoulders, short thighs and a tendency to obesity. Added to the above attributes there may be a male distribution of hair, and the hands are stubby, with the middle three fingers of approximately the same length. The bony structure of the pelvis tends towards the android type, which often gives rise to deep transverse arrest of the head in the cavity and difficulties at the outlet. The dimensions of the vagina are skimpy, notably in the vaginal vault, and the cervix is small. There may be a family history of dystocia.

It is not surprising that these patients are rather subfertile and often do not conceive until late middle age. Their subfertility may be reflected in irregular menstruation, and spasmodic dysmenorrhoea is common. Having conceived, they have an appreciable tendency to abort. Over half of Williams' cases developed pre-eclamptic toxaemia and the incidence of eclampsia is higher. More than two-thirds of them become postmature.

Labour starts indifferently with the head often high, and in the majority of cases occipitoposterior in position, the membranes rupture early, and labour drags on inertly. The average duration of labour in Williams' cases was over 50 hours and more than two-thirds of his patients had either an occipitoposterior position or a transverse arrest of the occiput at the time of eventual operation. Not one of his cases had a spontaneous delivery. The perineum is rigid, and this, together with the combination of a large postmature baby and an android type of pelvis, often makes rotation and forceps delivery a difficult undertaking.

Their response to induction of labour is usually so unsatisfactory, because of uterine inertia, that it is very doubtful if it is worth performing in these cases. Finally, they complete the unsatisfactory obstetrical picture by lactating very indifferently.

Assessment of Disproportion

Pressing the Head into the Brim

An attempt is first made to push the head into the brim, and many methods are employed to execute this manoeuvre, but because of the resistance of the abdominal muscles and the oblique tilt of the plane of the brim, normally 60° from the horizontal, many of these methods are often unsatisfactory. Sitting the patient up and then palpating is a poor method, because either it is impossible, in this position, for the patient fully to relax her abdominal muscles or the abdominal wall overhangs the area above the symphysis pubis and interferes with the examination. The use of the standing position is little better and increases the angle of pelvic brim tilt, so that it becomes more difficult to push the head into the brim.

My own method is to keep the patient lying on a couch with the knees not fully raised but fairly widely separated, the head being supported by a pillow. Standing on the right of the patient and using the third, fourth and fifth fingers of both hands, the head is gripped at sinciput and occiput. It will be noted that both index fingers and both thumbs are still free. One of the index fingers, usually the left, now reaches over and identifies the position of the top of the symphysis pubis. The thumbs are then pressed backwards against the parietal eminence. A complete grip of the head is thus obtained and its relationship to the symphysis pubis is fully appreciated (Fig. 5). Now, and not before, an assistant applies his hands to the baby's breech and presses the whole child towards the pelvis. At the same time the thumbs which are applied to the parietal eminence press downwards and backwards while the fingers on sinciput and occiput can observe what is happening and the index finger of the left hand is kept as before at the upper margin of the symphysis pubis. If the head is mechanically capable of engagement, it can now be steered into the brim with the thumbs and the whole movement can be fully appreciated. Often the head can be unmistakably pressed well down into the pelvis by this method.

Equivocal terms like "engaging" should never be used. Either a head is engaged or it is free, and if it is free it can either be made to engage or it cannot, and students or candidates who use the term engaging are trying to hedge and get the best of both worlds and deserve no credit. Only one definition of engagement is acceptable, namely that the biparietal diameter has passed the plane of the pelvic inlet or brim.

The term "fixed" is often used as though it were synonymous with "engaged". It should not be used, because this is by no means always the case. A head can be fixed in the brim but still be too large to pass

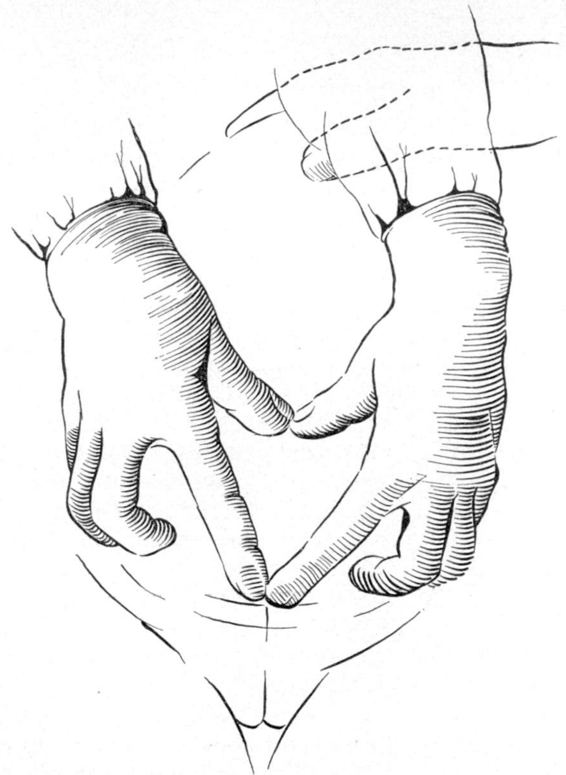

17/FIG. 5.—Testing for engagement. Assistant presses on breech.

through it, or may be deep in the pelvis and so small in relation to pelvic size that it is anything but fixed. A good simile is the case of the egg and the egg-cup. Most eggs will sit fixed in the brim of the egg-cup, but disproportion clearly exists, whereas a bantam's egg is easily engaged within the egg-cup and is not fixed.

If the head cannot thus be pressed into the pelvis a vaginal examination should be performed. After the 36th week, this should be made with proper aseptic and antiseptic ritual. It is true that any pathogenic organisms introduced into the genital canal through careless technique will probably disappear within a few days, but one cannot at this stage of pregnancy be certain that labour might not presently ensue, hence the need for proper precautions.

The Vaginal Examination in Apparent Disproportion

Everything possible must be found out at this examination and nothing should be allowed to interfere with its thoroughness, because it is undesirable to have to repeat it later. To this end it is worth admitting the patient to hospital, at least for the day. She is shaved and properly prepared, an enema is given, and the bladder is emptied. The nervous patient may require an anaesthetic, but usually a powerful sedative is all that is necessary. It is our practice to take her to the Labour Room, and just before the examination to give an injection of up to 100 mg of pethidine with 0·4 mg of scopolamine. Alternatively 5 mg intravenous diazepam can be used.

The patient is now placed in the lithotomy position and after swabbing down and painting is properly draped. The resistance of the pelvic floor is noted and then the presenting part is identified and the state of the cervix observed. The fingers are now gently but firmly pressed onwards until the sacral promontory is reached. In the lithotomy position and under the influence of the drug there should never be any difficulty in reaching the sacral promontory. With the help of sterile callipers, the depth of insertion of the fingers in reaching the promontory is accurately measured. It is a good plan for the operator to know exactly the distance between the tip of his middle finger and the crease of the metacarpophalangeal joint of the index finger. In this way the diagonal conjugate is assessed.

Using the traditional Munro Kerr method and with the help of an assistant pressing upon the fundus of the uterus, an attempt is now made to push the head into the pelvis on top of the fingers lying along the diagonal conjugate. The thumb of the examining hand is swept over the front of the symphysis pubis and feels for overlap. This often needs quite a good manual stretch, as it may be difficult sometimes for the thumb to reach far enough. If the head can be pushed down to the level of the ischial spines, what the Americans call "zero station", brim disproportion can be excluded. If it cannot, the thumb notes the degree of overlap. In first-degree overlap the parietal bone lies flush with the anterior surface of the symphysis pubis (Fig. 6). This amounts to about a quarter of an inch (0·6 cm) of overlap, and, given good contractions and a favourable position, the chances are that the head will go through. If, however, the head is felt by the thumb to overhang the symphysis pubis, second-degree overlap is diagnosed. The outlook then for vaginal delivery is very poor.

Unfortunately, the assessment is not as simple or cut and dried as most descriptions, including the above, would infer, and there are certain snags, the chief of which is that although the pelvis seems large, the diagonal conjugate above reproach and the head of no more than reasonable size, yet it is still impossible to push the head down to the level of the ischial spines. One may rightly feel certain that there is no question of disproportion, although the Munro Kerr test has failed, and in all honesty it has to be admitted that one sometimes comes away from the examination with doubts far from resolved.

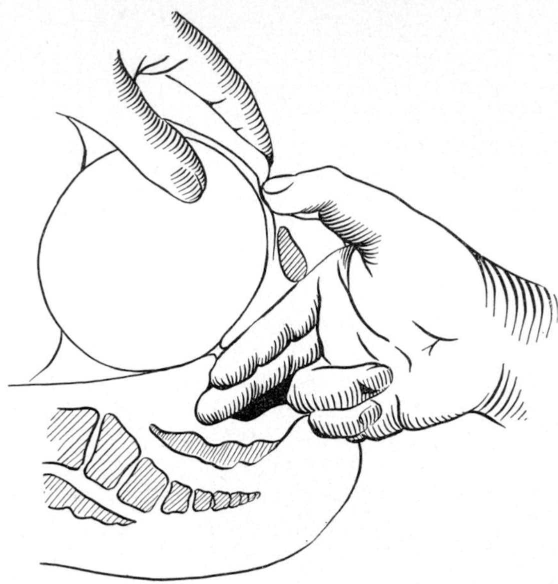

17/Fig. 6.—Testing for overlap. (Munro Kerr method.)

In the normal pelvis the diagonal conjugate should measure not less than $4\frac{3}{4}$ in (12 cm), but this measurement alone is not enough. The examination is not complete without further observations. The finger should be swept round the inside of the pelvic brim and an estimate made of its shape, particularly the fullness of curvature of the anterior portion. Any tendency to "beaking" suggests an android type and diminishes the *effective* lengths of the antero-posterior diameters. The length of the symphysis pubis should also be noted. An unfavourable sign is the impression of great pelvic depth which one gets with the android pelvis and with cases of high assimilation. The angle of inclination of the pelvic brim is also noted; the steeper the angle the less favourable the prognosis. The fingers are now swept around the side walls of the pelvic cavity in order to detect any tendency to convergence. The prominence of the ischial spines and the depth or width of the sacrosciatic notches can be easily assessed, and the finger is now swept down the anterior surface of the sacrum, noting any false promontories, irregularities, straightness, angulation and general roominess of the sacral bay. The sacro-coccygeal joint is tested for mobility and finally completion of the examination involves an estimate of the outlet. The subpubic arch should comfortably accommodate the backs of two fingers. It should be in the shape of the Norman arch rather than the Gothic.

The length of the descending pubic rami is also observed and, using the fingers of both hands, an estimate of the subpubic angle is made. The normal angle is somewhere between 80° and 85°. It will be noted that we distinguish between subpubic arch and subpubic angle, although as a general rule an acute angle tends to go with a narrow arch and vice versa. Lastly, with the patient still in the lithotomy position, the intertuberous diameter can be very satisfactorily assessed with the knuckles. Obstetricians should know the width of their four knuckles. Depending on the size of one's hand, either the knuckles of the first interphalangeal joints can be used or the knuckles of the clenched fist, which appears to be a more stable measurement. The examination thus conducted is of priceless value, and properly carried out with a co-operative patient can yield almost as much information as a whole set of X-rays. It is an examination which calls for good patient handling. Gentleness is essential as the patient is likely to be frightened by the general ritual of the labour theatre. A running commentary must, therefore, be kept up with the patient throughout and there must be no hesitation in explaining what is going on and reassuring her on every good point noted. This is very important, because if the patient once suspects that she is mechanically incapable of delivering herself the subsequent outcome of labour is prejudiced from the first.

Measurements of the Normal Pelvis

A consideration of the pelvic diameters in three planes will suffice, namely the plane of the brim, the cavity, and the outlet. There are one or two observations to be made before giving the traditional list. Firstly, the true conjugate may be of less relevance than the obstetric conjugate. The latter is measured from the inner margin of the upper part of the symphysis pubis to the nearest point of the sacrum, which often lies below the actual promontory. In certain cases the difference may be as great as 0·5 cm and since the head must negotiate this smaller diameter it should, in such cases, be separately noted. The transverse diameter of the brim is usually taken as the widest measurement, but, particularly in the android type of pelvis, this diameter lies rather closer to the sacral promontory and is not fully available in labour. It is, therefore, worth noting what is known as the available transverse diameter. This latter measurement is made transversely at mid-distance between fore and hind pelvis.

Traditionally the normal true conjugate has been given as 4¼ in or 10·8 cm, but it is now generally recognised that the correct figure should be 4½ in (11·43 cm).

The average value of the obstetric conjugate varies from 11·2 to

11·8 cm. The transverse diameter of the brim varies from 12·6 to 12·9 cm (5–5⅛ in) (Chassar Moir). The interspinous diameter is 10–10·8 cm (4–4¼ in).

One cannot draw a hard and fast line of demarcation at which contracted pelvis is categorically diagnosed. The shape of the pelvis and the angle of inclination must also be taken into account. Disproportion, however, in a given pregnancy occurs when delivery cannot be safely accomplished because of a reduction in one or more measurements of the bony pelvis. The average biparietal diameter is 3¾ in or 9·5 cm. A diameter of 9·6 cm represents a fairly large head. If any of the diameters in any of the three planes measures less than 4 in (10·5 cm) one can fairly safely state that contracted pelvis exists. The decision as to the method of delivery is discussed later. A true conjugate, however, of 3½ in (8·9 cm) or less represents gross pelvic contraction, and a baby small enough to negotiate such straits is often too fragile to do so in safety.

Clinical examination of the pelvis will only produce an estimate of the true conjugate by inference from measuring the diagonal conjugate. This is generally accepted as being half an inch greater than the true conjugate; in other words, in normal cases, practically 5 in (12·6 cm) but this difference is by no means standard, and in order to obtain really accurate measurements one has to resort to radiology. Intravaginal measurements taken with callipers have not even been discussed; they are difficult to make, uncomfortable to the patient and too inaccurate to be of much use. Sonar is too imprecise.

Radiology, in the case of the maternal pelvis, has brought to obstetrics almost as much as it has to orthopaedic science. The fact that it may be abused is no reflection upon radiology but rather upon the clinician who lacks sufficient common sense and clinical judgment to make intelligent use of it. Chassar Moir dismissed the fear that more radiology would lead to unnecessary intervention by saying that this will only occur when bad radiology is combined with bad obstetrics. Proper clinical examination of the pelvis, however, must never be omitted simply because X-rays are available. Both sources of information should be studied, for one is complementary to the other. We will now review what radiology has to offer in the study of disproportion. A fuller description of the technical aspects of radiological pelvimetry by Dr Ellis Barnett will be found at the end of this chapter.

X-RAY PELVIMETRY

Not only can the pelvis be very accurately measured by modern techniques, but the general shape and type of the pelvis are revealed, and this is almost as important as actual measurements. The relationship of the head to the pelvis can also be studied and, in certain cases, progress of labour can be observed. To some extent bony dystocia can also be forecast at certain levels other than the brim and this knowledge may be helpful in modifying the conduct of a difficult labour.

Of all the available views, a lateral X-ray taken in the erect position is unquestionably the most valuable. The following is a list of the points to be observed and the information which can be obtained from a lateral X-ray:

1. The relation of the head to the pelvic brim.
2. The angle of inclination of the pelvic brim.
3. Posterior position of the occiput.
4. Angulation of the fetal neck; this is likely to occur when occipitoposterior position is combined with a high angle of pelvic inclination. It is an unfavourable sign because it indicates some misdirection of the uterine thrust, the components of whose force tend to be directed in front of the symphysis pubis instead of downwards into the cavity of the pelvis (Fig. 7).
5. The measurement of the true conjugate.
6. A false promontory, if present.
7. The measurement of the obstetrical conjugate if different from the true conjugate.
8. The shape of the sacrum and the fullness of the sacral bay. A straight sacrum or one with a reverse curve is unfavourable.
9. Measurement of the sacral angle. This is the angle subtended by the true conjugate and the anterior surface of the first two pieces of the sacrum (Fig. 8). It is an observation of the greatest importance and is not sufficiently stressed in current teaching. The angle is normally greater than 90°, in which case it can be confidently predicted that a head which has once negotiated the brim will find its passage easier thereafter. On the other hand, a sacral angle of less than 90° suggests funnelling, and labour is likely to become more difficult as it proceeds.
10. The number of pieces in the sacrum, indicating the possible presence of an assimilation pelvis. High assimilation, i.e. incorporation of the fifth lumbar vertebra in the sacral body, is an unfavourable sign.
11. The width and depth of the sacrosciatic notch. The notch should be wide and fairly shallow in the good pelvis.
12. The anteroposterior measurement of the outlet.
13. The relationship of the sacral attitude to the pubis and descending rami. The latter should be nearly parallel to a line joining the sacral promontory and the sacral tip. Convergence in a downward direction is an unfavourable sign.

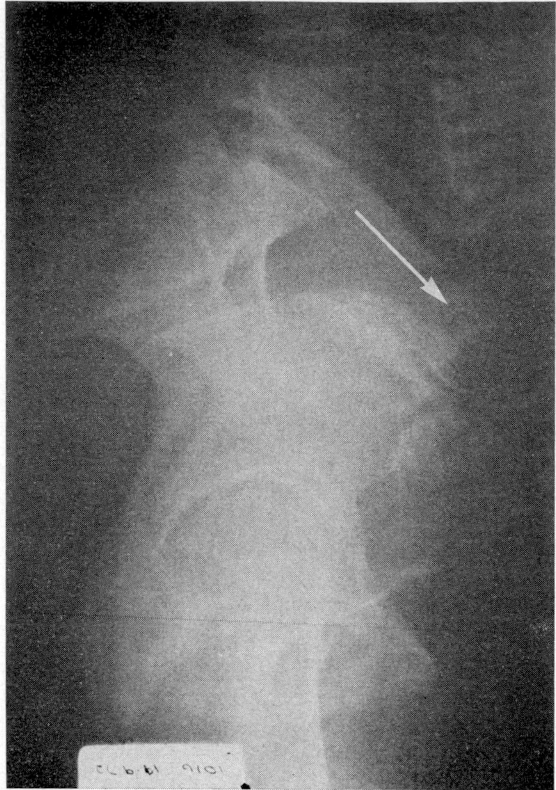

17/FIG. 7.—Angulation of fetal neck, associated with occipitoposterior position. An unfavourable sign. Minor degree of disproportion. Failure to progress after 9 hours. Caesarean section.

To obtain all the above information the picture must be very well taken and properly centred. The heads of the two femora and the acetabular margins should be superimposed upon each other or at least very nearly so.

The brim view is also valuable because, apart from the actual measurements, anteroposterior, oblique and transverse, which it furnishes, its shape largely indicates the type of pelvis. Unfortunately, as pointed out by Dr Ellis Barnett later, this involves a much higher exposure to radiation. A discussion of the features and influences upon labour of the various genetic types will follow presently. The outlet view is on the whole somewhat less important, as much of the information can be obtained by clinical means.

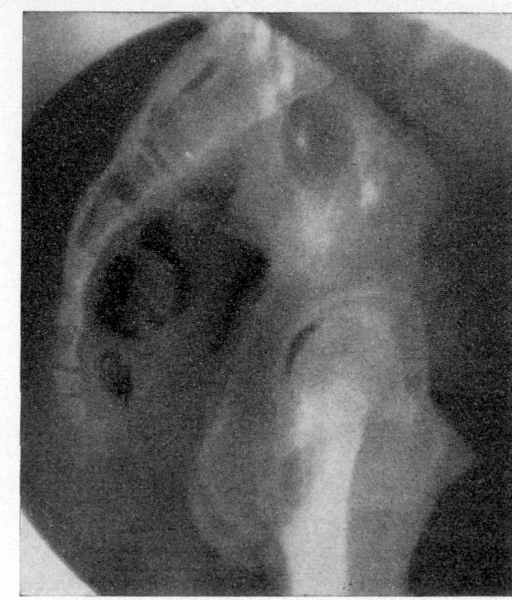

17/Fig. 8 (*a*).—Acute sacral angle.

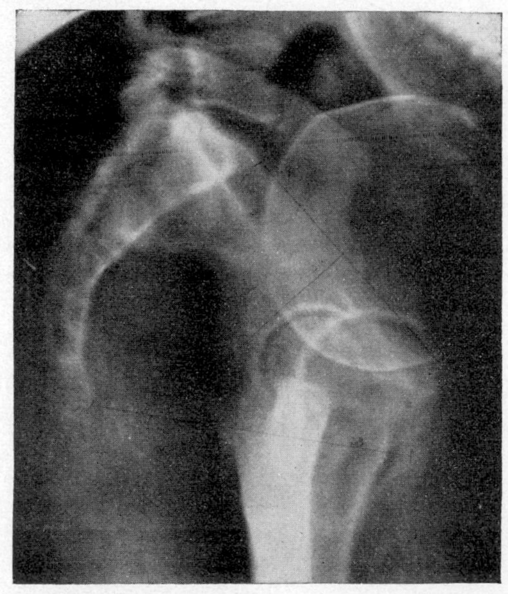

17/Fig. 8 (*b*).—Obtuse sacral angle.
(By courtesy of Dr J. W. McLaren.)

Types of Contracted Pelvis and their Influence on Labour

Attempts have been made, notably by Caldwell and Moloy, to classify the types of female pelvis, whether or not contraction is present. Their classification is now more generally accepted than that of Thom. The pelvic type becomes much more important when contraction in any of the diameters is present. Caldwell and Moloy may be out of fashion now but at least they defined four generic, parent types applicable, more or less, to the majority of women. In rough figures the type frequency is as follows: gynaecoid 50 per cent, android 18 per cent, anthropoid 26 per cent, platypelloid 5 per cent. None of these types is pathological unless any of the diameters are substantially reduced below average. The following are the characteristics of each (Fig. 9).

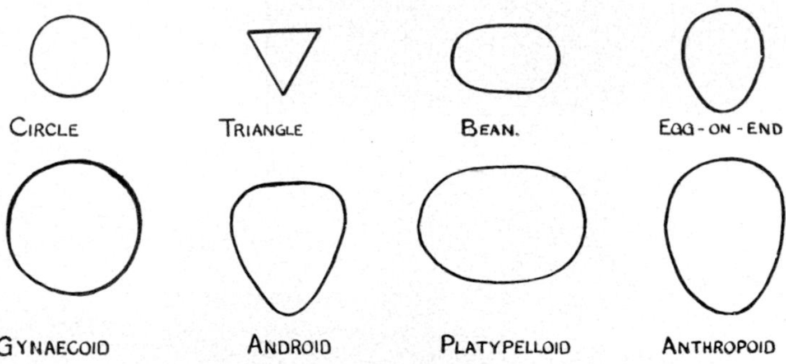

17/Fig. 9.—Diagrams of Caldwell-Moloy types.

Gynaecoid.—The brim is well rounded and there is a good, full curvature of the fore pelvis. The maximum transverse diameter does not lie far behind the mid-point of the true conjugate, with the result that the area of the hind pelvis is only somewhat less than that of the fore pelvis (Fig. 10*a*). The cavity of the pelvis is almost the segment of a sphere and there is no convergence of the side walls. The ischial spines are not prominent and the sacrosciatic notches are relatively wide and shallow in a vertical diameter. The sacral bay has a full and even curve. The subpubic arch is normal in shape and the subpubic angle is not less than 85°, while the descending pubic rami are short and slender. The sacral angle exceeds 90°.

Android.—This is more like a triangle with the base towards the sacrum. The fore pelvis is beaked rather like the bows of a ship, and

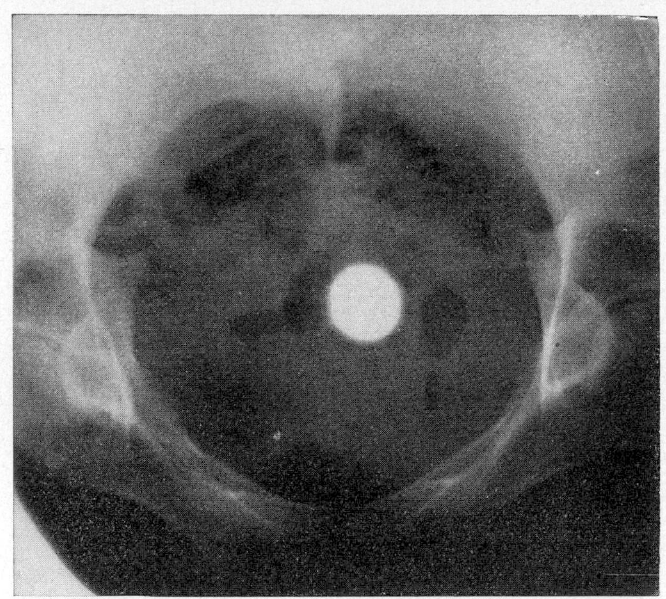

17/Fig. 10 (*a*).—Gynaecoid pelvis.

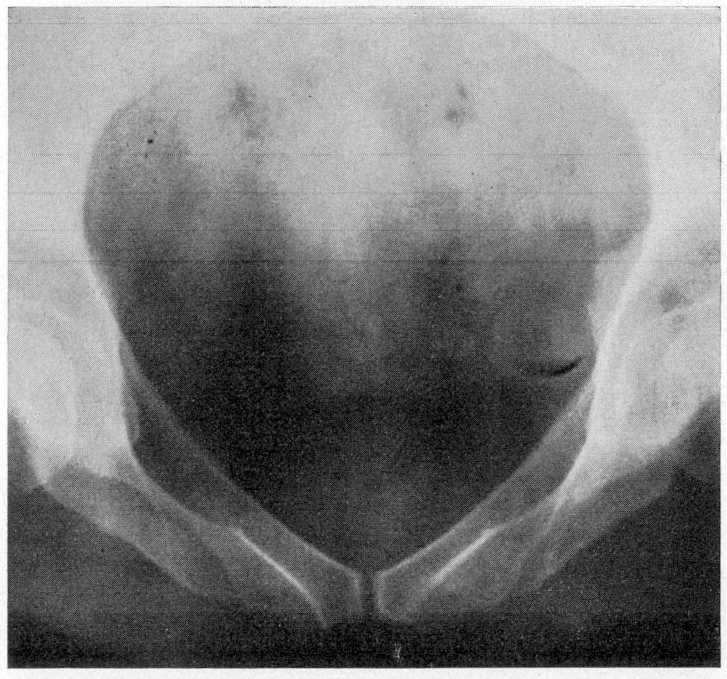

17/Fig. 10 (*b*).—Android pelvis.

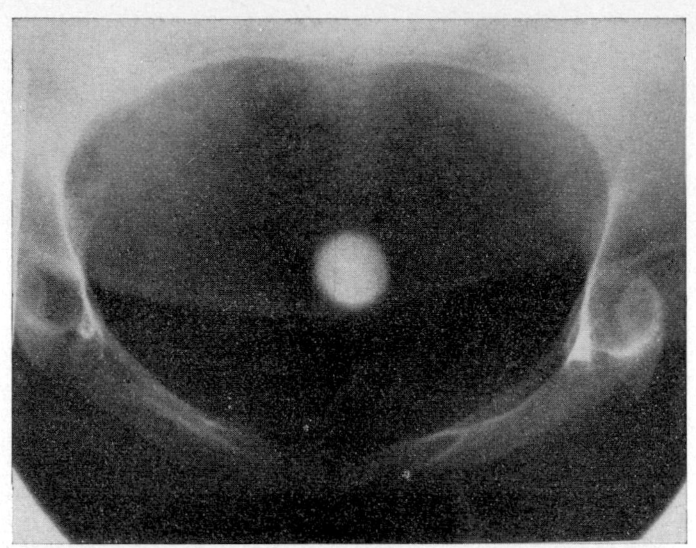

17/FIG. 10 (*c*).—Platypelloid pelvis.

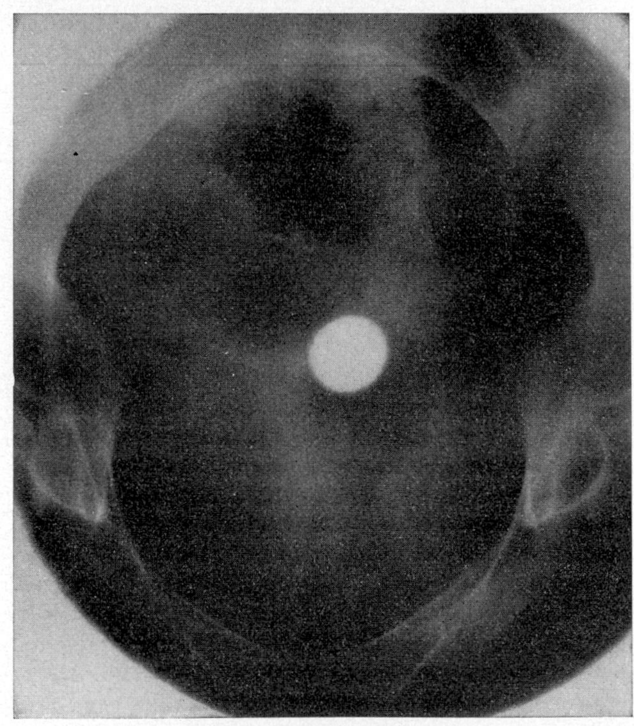

17/FIG. 10 (*d*).—Anthropoid pelvis.
(Figs *a*, *b*, *c* and *d* by courtesy of Dr J. W. McLaren.)

the maximum transverse diameter of the brim intersects the true conjugate very close to the sacrum so that the area of the hind pelvis is only a fraction of that of the fore pelvis (Fig. 10*b*). Because of the beaking of the latter the fetal head is unable to make use of much of the fore-pelvis area and has to pass at some distance posterior to the symphysis pubis. The side walls of the pelvis tend to converge downwards, the ischial spines are often prominent and the sacrosciatic notches are narrow and deep in a vertical direction. The length of the symphysis pubis is greater than usual, the subpubic arch tends towards the Gothic, the subpubic angle is definitely acute and the descending pubic rami are long and thick. The head in its passage to the outlet is not able to make use of much of the subpubic space, and therefore has to emerge farther back. The angle of brim inclination is steep and the sacral angle is less than 90°.

Platypelloid.—This is the flat type of pelvis. The transverse diameter is very much larger than the anteroposterior diameter and the sacral promontory tends to encroach upon the area of the hind pelvis (Fig. 10*c*). The cavity tends to be more roomy than usual, the side walls of the pelvis diverge downwards, the sacral angle is greater than 90°, the sacrum may be somewhat flattened in its upper portions with a rather sharp curve forwards near its tip. The sacrosciatic notches are very wide and shallow in a vertical direction and the ischial spines are not prominent. The symphysis pubis is not deep, the subpubic arch is wide and the subpubic angle is in excess of 90°. The outlet diameters are consequently increased.

Anthropoid.—In this type the brim has an anteroposterior diameter which exceeds the transverse, giving it an oval appearance. The maximum transverse diameter may intersect the true conjugate fairly near its mid-point, providing a reasonable ratio between the areas of fore pelvis and hind pelvis, but the normal engagement of the head in the occipitotransverse position is discouraged (Fig. 10*d*). The cavity and outlet have no gross distinguishing characteristics.

The pelvic types are not as pure as the above description would suggest, and there are all manner of subdivisions, for instance a woman may have a gynaecoid hind pelvis and an android fore pelvis and all sorts of combinations may occur in the different straits. When contraction is present, however, the pelvic type may materially influence the mechanics of labour. The small gynaecoid pelvis, which used to be called the small round or justo minor pelvis, provides a tight fit the whole way. The mechanics are those of normal labour calling for increased expulsive forces if delivery is to be achieved, and extreme degrees of flexion of the fetal head will be required. The android type of contracted pelvis is one of the most treacherous and may easily be missed on clinical examination alone. What makes it more dangerous is that the clinical estimate of the diagonal conjugate may show no reduction, and indeed the true conjugate may be normal but, as already hinted, much of this length is wasted in the narrowness of the fore pelvis. Even when the head has safely negotiated the brim it meets increasing difficulties in the cavity because of funnelling, so that labour may come to an obstructed halt at a later stage with the head tightly wedged, unable to rotate and incapable of advancing. When it reaches the outlet the head meets even greater trouble. Extreme moulding may cause it to appear at the vulva long before the main bulk of the skull vault has properly reached the pelvic floor. Because of the need to pass farther back from the symphysis, the perineum and other maternal soft tissues are subjected to increased stress and damage may be extensive. There is only one compensation in difficult labour with a contracted android pelvis, namely that the narrowness of the fore pelvis provides a protective arch for the bladder neck and its supports, so that damage in the form of subsequent stress incontinence or pressure necrosis of the bladder neck, resulting in vesicovaginal fistula, is less likely to occur in this type of disproportion than in other types.

The anthropoid type of pelvis, when contracted, discourages transverse engagement of the head, so that it engages either occipitoanterior or occipitoposterior. Should the latter occur, long internal rotation is not likely to take place and a persistent occipitoposterior position results. Under these circumstances it may be unwise to attempt to rotate the head to the occipitoanterior position in order to deliver with the forceps, and these cases are better delivered in the unreduced position, namely, face to pubis.

The contracted platypelloid type of pelvis influences labour in a manner similar to the rickety flat pelvis. Here the difficulties are mainly confined to the brim, where most of the pressures of engagement are borne on the sacral promontory and on the back of the symphysis pubis, to the great detriment of the bladder neck, which lies between two bony millstones. If there is uterine obliquity and the occiput happens to lie on the same side as the obliquity, the parietal eminences may get held up on the brim and cause the head to become deflexed, even resulting in a secondary face presentation. Indentation of the cranial bones by the sacral promontory may occur, and even a depressed fracture may in rare instances be caused. Asynclitism is often a necessary mechanism, as has been explained earlier. Chassar Moir has shown by means of a simple model, consisting of a wire hoop and child's balloon, that, for a given circumference, a head will more easily negotiate a contracted flat pelvis than a small round brim.

Once the head has passed the brim, all is relatively plain sailing, although internal rotation may occur late because of the usually flattened sacrum. Outlet dystocia is most unlikely.

Classes of Pelvic Deformity

Firstly, there are those which are due to diseases affecting the skeletal system as a whole. Of these, rickets is the principal offender. Not only may it produce stunting in growth, with general contraction, but the characteristic deformity is flattening of a type which exaggerates the worst features of the platypelloid pelvis, inasmuch as the sacral promontory may bulge so far forward as to give the brim a reniform shape (Fig. 10*e*).

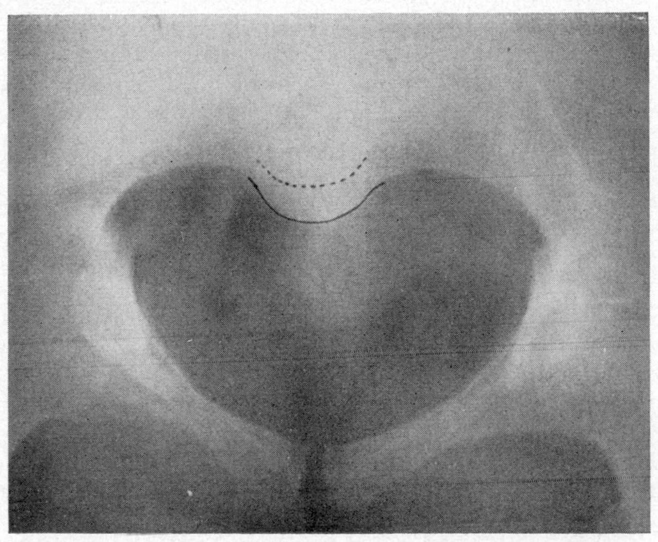

17/Fig. 10 (*e*).—Flat pelvis with marked encroachment of the sacral promontory. Probably due to rickets.
(By courtesy of Dr Ellis Barnett.)

Secondly, the pelvis may be deformed as a result of disease in one of the lower limbs, contracted in childhood or of congenital origin. Examples are poliomyelitis, congenital dislocation of the hip, tuberculous arthritis of the hip, serious injuries, and talipes. The woman who comes into the antenatal clinic with a severe limp requires a careful investigation of her pelvis.

Thirdly, there may be abnormalities of the spine. Scoliosis is often associated with disease affecting the lower extremities, and in these cases there may be pelvic asymmetry.

Kyphosis is important, particularly in relation to its site. A high dorsal kyphosis is usually offset by a compensatory lordosis, so that the pelvis is not altered in shape, although one must mention other obstetric considerations, such as the reduced distance between xiphisternum and symphysis pubis which may make a transverse lie inevitable for want of room in the abdominal cavity. A kyphosis situated low down in the spinal column may, for like reason, encourage a pendulous belly. The outlet tends to be contracted in the latter instance, but these cases often go into premature labour so that the baby may be small enough to be delivered by the vaginal route.

There are two types of assimilation pelvis, the high and the low (Fig. 11*a* and *b*). In the former, the last lumbar vertebra is incorporated in the body of the sacrum, thus not only increasing the sacral length but placing the sacral promontory at a higher level than normal. This has the effect of steepening the angle of pelvic inclination and reducing the sacral angle well below 90°. It may be a potent cause of dystocia (Fig. 11*a*). In the low assimilation pelvis only four pieces comprise the body of the sacrum and there are no obstetrical disadvantages (Fig. 11*b*),

Every undergraduate student remembers the freak pelves of Naegele and Robert. They are mainly of museum interest and only a very few cases of the latter have been recorded. In the Naegele pelvis one sacral ala is not properly developed, resulting in profound asymmetry (Fig. 12). In the Robert pelvis the condition is bilateral.

Spondylolisthesis, too, is rare, though less so. The lumbar spine is subluxated forward on the sacrum, thus reducing the anteroposterior diameter of the brim. In grand multiparity something akin to this process may occur.

Osteomalacia, very rare in this country, produces a three-cornered-hat type of pelvis.

Lastly, to complete the list, deformities of obstetrical significance may result from pelvic fractures, chondroma and osteoma.

Outlet Contraction

There are those who do not believe in the existence of outlet contraction as an entity. They state categorically that if a head can be got through the brim it can be got through the outlet. I agree, as far as my own experience goes, but I have seen cases in the hands of very able colleagues where this has not been so. The above sweeping statement is technically true, but the price paid for vaginal delivery may be very high indeed. Unfortunately, the price is paid by the baby, who may suffer considerable cerebral damage, and the mother, whose soft parts may never be the same again. The amount of traumatic force which may have to be employed in delivering such cases with forceps can reduce the art of obstetrics to brutish barbarism.

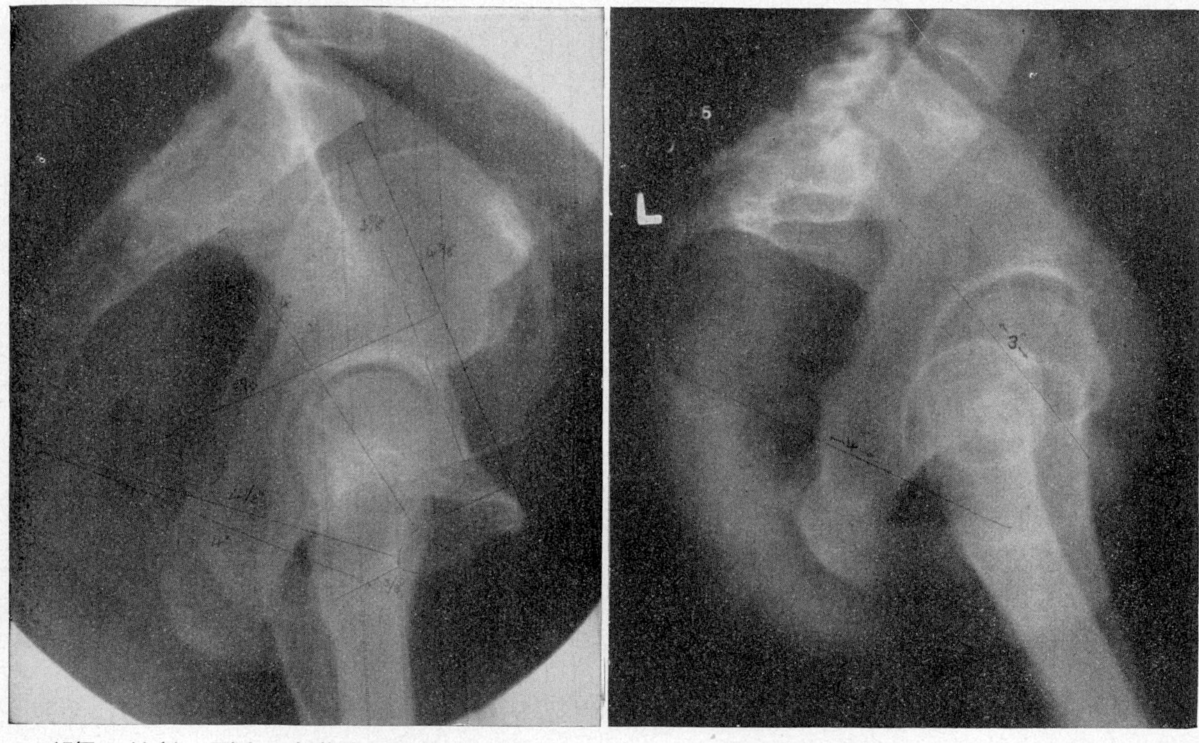

17/FIG. 11 (*a*).—High assimilation, android pelvis. 17/FIG. 11 (*b*).—Low assimilation, flat pelvis.
(By courtesy of Dr J. W. McLaren.)

The diagnosis of contracted outlet is often wantonly made in order to explain difficulties encountered in forceps delivery, which are more often due to faulty technique or a tight pelvic floor, and this diagnosis is one of the commonest with which patients are admitted to hospital after a failed attempt at forceps delivery. (In the majority of such cases the cervix is found to be not fully dilated, hence the difficulty.) Nevertheless, the condition undoubtedly occurs, although it is uncommon. The contracted android pelvis is likely to provide more instances than any other.

An examination of the outlet is a part of the routine assessment of the pelvis during the antenatal period. Firstly, the distance between the ischial tuberosities is estimated with the knuckles and it will often be found that in early pregnancy this transverse diameter is apparently contracted. In the majority of cases, however, the loosening up of the pelvic joints during pregnancy causes some widening before term. The importance of the subpubic arch and subpubic angle has already been mentioned. The anteroposterior diameter of the outlet

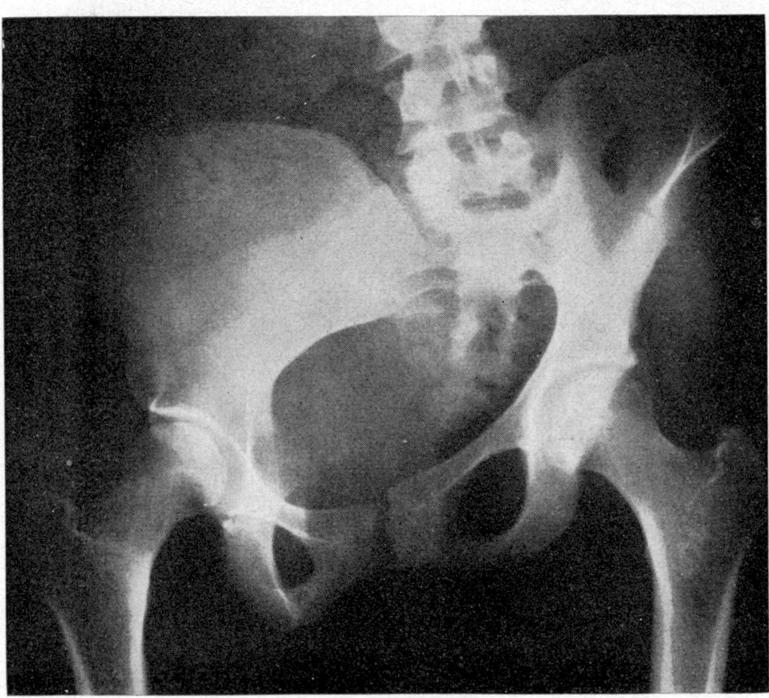

17/FIG. 12.—Naegele pelvis.
(By courtesy of the late Dr G. W. Garland.)

is measured from the bottom of the symphysis pubis to the tip of the sacrum. If this measurement is found to be less than 4 in (10 cm), outlet contraction can be accepted as definite on clinical grounds. It is not difficult to make accurate measurements of the pelvic outlet without X-ray pelvimetry, but outlet views are well worth obtaining if there is any doubt. The information may be of vital importance to the conduct of labour. For instance, trial of labour is not applicable if the pelvic outlet is in doubt, because the true state of disproportion will not be apparent until very late in labour.

One may be reluctant to plan abdominal delivery simply because X-ray pelvimetry indicates a contracted outlet. It is in these cases that, having made a very full vaginal examination, preferably under anaesthesia, there is something to be said for allowing the patient to proceed in labour. If all seems well and the second stage of labour is reached fairly easily, one may proceed to what is now referred to as a trial of forceps should further progress come to a halt. If it now appears that forceps delivery will be difficult and hazardous, it is far better to resort to Caesarean section at this stage than to blunder on, doing irreparable damage. Injudicious force, besides injuring the baby, may even dislocate a sacroiliac joint or disrupt the symphysis pubis.

The other alternative when faced with outlet obstruction is to resort to symphysiotomy. Needless to say, if the baby is unquestionably dead, perforation is the treatment of choice rather than a strenuous forceps delivery with the fetal head intact. Perforation makes a surprising difference to the ease with which the head can be delivered. Only in rare instances should it be necessary to resort to more destructive procedures, for only the gross types of contraction justify them and should have been noted long ago.

In remote parts of the world where antenatal care is not available, gross degrees of contraction may first be encountered late in labour, and cephalotripsy and cranioclasm still have their place in the neglected and seriously infected case. There are, nowadays, few obstetricians in this country who have much experience of these ghastly operations, and, considering the good conditions under which they work, the patient is probably better off with a lower segment Caesarean section than to be shocked, exsanguinated, lacerated and bruised by the prolonged piecemeal delivery of a dead and infected child's body. Things should never have been allowed to come to this pass.

Hydrocephalus

The commonest indication for craniotomy these days is hydrocephalus. Since the hydrocephalic fetus commonly presents by the breech, the treatment is straightforward, because the aftercoming

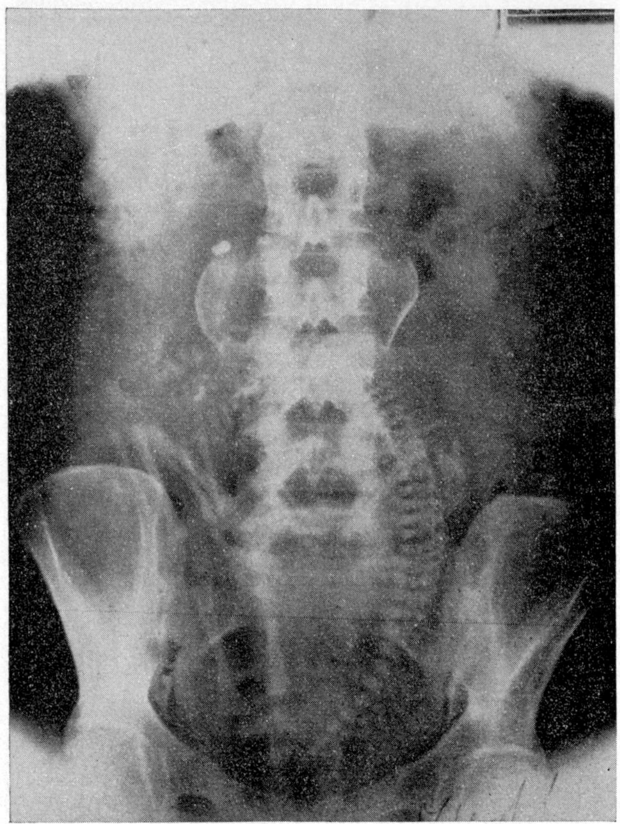

17/Fig. 13 (*a*).—Extended breech presentation, not apparently abnormal.

head is easy to tap. By pulling downwards on the neck, the head is safely stabilised and perforation in the suboccipital region is simple. Alternatively, a metal cannula can be pushed up the spinal canal from below in order to draw off the cerebrospinal fluid. This is an even easier matter when there is associated myelocele, but otherwise the method has no advantage over perforation.

When the hydrocephalic fetus presents by the head (as occurred in 68 per cent of Feeney and Barry's 304 cases), treatment is less simple; for one thing, the head is above the brim and, for another, it is often difficult to stabilise its position; the cervix may not dilate very readily, thus increasing the hazards of perforation, and great care has to be taken in inserting the perforator that the points do not slip off at glancing incidence and damage maternal tissues. The

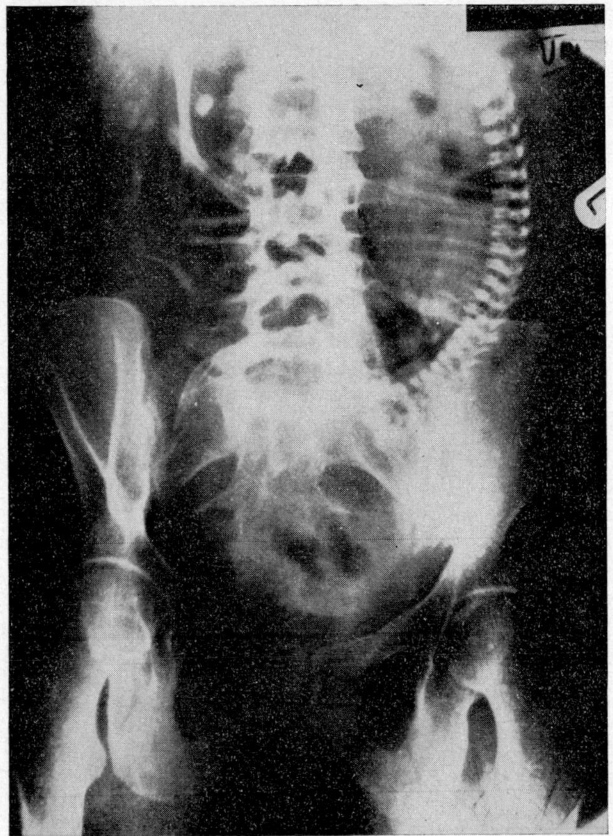

17/Fig. 13 (*b*).—Same case as Fig. 13*a* 5 weeks later. Gross hydrocephalus has developed, although the vertex now presents.
(Fig. 13 *a* and *b* by courtesy of Miss Lois Hurter.)

head can also be slowly decompressed from below by inserting a lumbar puncture needle through a fontanelle. This does not kill the baby. There is an alternative method of tapping the hydrocephalic head through the anterior abdominal wall, after catheterising the bladder, but this is not without its risks and free bleeding may be started up if one is unlucky enough to strike a large blood vessel. The catheter itself may become blocked.

TREATMENT OF DISPROPORTION

We have already considered the plight of the patient and her doctor when disproportion is diagnosed only late in labour. It is part of the essence of modern obstetrics that the diagnosis should have been gone into before labour ever starts. Under these circumstances one has the choice of three methods: elective Caesarean section, trial of labour, and induction of premature labour.

Elective Caesarean Section

This is the method of choice for all cases in which the degree of pelvic contraction is gross. In fact, there is no reasonable alternative. Any pelvis with a true conjugate of less than $3\frac{1}{2}$ in (9 cm) is severely contracted, and a normal-sized baby cannot be reasonably expected to negotiate the diameters in safety. True, some women with such pelves, especially of the flat variety, are capable of delivering themselves vaginally, but the amount of moulding called for constitutes a serious risk. A small and premature infant might theoretically fare better, but the softness of the skull and the well-known liability to intracranial haemorrhage in premature infants more than offset the advantage of reduced size.

If borderline disproportion is present in the elderly primigravida, the only prudent thing to do is to deliver her by Caesarean section. Her obstetrical future is too short to justify doing otherwise.

All malpresentations which cannot be corrected by external version, if associated with contracted pelvis, indicate elective Caesarean section. There can be no trial of labour, for example, in a breech presentation. The verdict would come too late.

Major degrees of contraction of the outlet also call for Caesarean section, for reasons above stated.

Induction of Premature Labour

Theoretically this would be an ideal method of meeting the problem if only one could be completely certain of the degree of disproportion, if one could guarantee effective uterine action, if any method of surgical induction were both certain and safe, and if there were no penalties to prematurity. Alas, it is just on these very matters that this solution may let us down. In the cases in which this line of treatment appears to have been successful it has to be admitted that the absence of moulding of the fetal skull seriously questions the original need for intervention. In other words, in the cases in which it succeeds it is hard to be certain that it was necessary and in the cases where it fails the results may be disastrous. The penalties of a long induction-delivery interval have already been dealt with in the chapter on induced labour, and one's hand is often forced in these cases into performing Caesarean section, an operation which is prejudiced in advance in spite of antibiotics. Moreover, there must always remain the suspicion in these cases that if the patient had been left strictly alone and not induced she might have delivered herself spontaneously.

The indications, therefore, for induction must be very clear cut, and primigravidae are as a rule unsuitable because, obstetrically speaking, they are unknown quantities and the fetal mortality may be as high as 20 per cent in the presence of disproportion.

The only cases generally accepted as suitable for induction are those in whom disproportion is no more than borderline and in whom a history of a previous delivery is available on which to assess the patient's obstetrical prowess. In the fit multigravida, therefore, who has had, for example, difficulty in delivering herself of an 8-pound (3·6 kg) baby because of disproportion, there is a very strong case for inducing labour prematurely next time.

One might well be tempted to try to get the best of both possible worlds by surgically inducing the patient near term when the disproportion is only of a very minor degree, in the hope of securing vaginal delivery before further enlargement of the fetal head renders it difficult. In doing so one makes also the mental reservation that a trial of labour will be conducted and resorts to Caesarean section at the first sign of trouble or arrest of progress. This procedure is undoubtedly becoming more popular but is questionable. It smacks of meddlesome interference, and labour is sufficiently likely to be in need of stimulation as a result of the induction to prevent the subsequent trial from being a fair one.

TRIAL OF LABOUR

Trial of labour dates from about 1925. Because we cannot yet foretell how well a patient with disproportion will surmount her difficulties, a wait-and-see policy is adopted. This is not as casual as it sounds, for these labours are conducted with great vigilance and with full facilities in the background for the safe performance of Caesarean section. It goes without saying that a patient should not be aware of one's mental processes and above all that the trial should be conducted without ceremony.

This practice has conferred many benefits to date. Firstly, it has reduced the rate of Caesarean sections electively decided upon. Secondly, it has eliminated an enormous amount of unwarranted and injudicious induction, and thirdly, a successful trial of labour practically guarantees a woman's obstetrical future. It is not without its disadvantages, however, chief of which is that it often proves nothing and, as Gibberd pointed out, trial of labour may become a test not of disproportion but of readiness of the cervix to dilate, and in half the failures disproportion remains unproven because Caesarean section had to be undertaken on account of uterine inertia or fetal distress. In Gibberd's series the cervix was less than half dilated at the time when Caesarean section was performed in nearly 70 per cent of these cases at Guy's between 1934 and 1950. In other words, more trials fail because of ineffectual contractions than because of proven disproportion. Good contractions, after all, are worth half an inch of true conjugate.

Another disadvantage is that the fetal mortality is higher than would be the case with elective Caesarean section, and death from intracranial haemorrhage after trial of labour serves only to condemn it in retrospect. The maternal morbidity rate is also raised, but nowadays this is a less serious consideration. Not the least of the disadvantages is the fact that when a woman fails in a trial of labour she has now to face a major surgical operation, demoralised, disappointed, dehydrated, frightened and, at least potentially, infected.

Trial of labour is definitely not applicable to quite a large number of cases, as follows:

1. The elderly primigravida.
2. Cases of malpresentation.
3. Where there is outlet contraction.
4. In the presence of pre-eclamptic toxaemia or hypertensive disease.
5. Where any cardiac or pulmonary lesion or other relevant medical disease complicates pregnancy.
6. If the true conjugate is less than 3½ in (9 cm), because in such cases the prospects of success are too remote.
7. If a genuine previous trial of labour has failed.

Trial of labour should on no account be conducted outside a hospital which is not only well equipped but, and this is more important, is properly staffed so that the case can be adequately watched.

Conduct of the Trial of Labour

For the trial to have maximum validity the onset of labour should be spontaneous and not induced. Everything should be done to preserve the membranes intact for as long as possible. In respect of duration, the trial only commences from the time of membrane rupture. Up to this point the mother and baby are hardly at risk, but from now on the condition of both must be frequently observed and the rate of progress estimated. As long as the head remains not engaged the patient should be nursed in bed, and no enema should be given once labour has started for fear of provoking rupture of the membranes.

As soon as the membranes rupture, the patient must be examined to exclude prolapse of the cord. Often the head will now be found to have engaged in the pelvic brim and this is a good moment to assess its position. A fluid-balance chart should be maintained, bearing in mind that the longer dehydration can be staved off, the later will maternal distress appear.

There are two criteria of progress:

1. The progressive descent of the presenting part.
2. The progressive dilatation of the cervix.

Either, singly or together, denotes progress.

Nowadays the tendency is to shorten trials of labour in order to reduce the risks to the fetus. It is useless to set an arbitrary time limit to the duration of the trial after the membranes have ruptured. Various authorities have recommended periods ranging from two to seven hours, but the case should be judged on its own merits and account taken of the rate of progress, the general condition, the patient's fortitude and the state of dilatation of the cervix so far achieved. The onset of fetal distress calls from prompt intervention. There should be no hesitation in using intrapartum radiography in the case that is not going well. A lateral view, erect if possible, is particularly important, but features to note are any evidence of fetal abnormality as this will discourage the employment of Caesarean section, signs of moulding of the fetal head (Fig. 14), the level of the head and its attitude, e.g. occipitoposterior, and unfavourable factors such as inclination of the head on the neck. The decision to operate is better taken early rather than late.

The conduct of labour with disproportion in the case of the African woman presents an altogether different set of problems. For one thing the African pelvis is extraordinarily shallow so that the head may bulge at the vulva before the biparietal diameter has yet passed the brim and uterine inertia is very unusual. The chances of having to face a really difficult forceps operation are usually prevented either by spontaneous delivery due to tumultuous pains and a more or less physiological type of autosymphysiotomy, or the clamant need for a Caesarean section with the established threat of obstructed labour. In the European woman the position is far less clear cut.

In many ways the most difficult cases are those in which a mid-cavity forceps operation becomes necessary after a long and difficult first stage. Having gone so far one is reluctant to turn back, but vaginal delivery may be secured at too high a price, especially to the baby, and a difficult forceps operation of this nature may be almost as dangerous to the baby as internal version and breech extraction. This is a task for the skilled obstetrician only and, if the forceps delivery threatens to prove very difficult, Caesarean section, even at this late stage, may be the wiser course. In such cases forceps delivery should only be attempted on an operating table in an operating theatre equipped for Caesarean section so that there need be no hesitation in proceeding to abdominal delivery. If in doubt, section is safer than savagery with forceps.

One cannot afford to be so impressed by survival statistics that one ignores the patient's subjective experiences, and to many women a long and unsuccessful labour evokes the firm resolution "never again".

The institution of trial of labour may easily encourage slovenly clinical assessment of the patient, on the argument that there is time

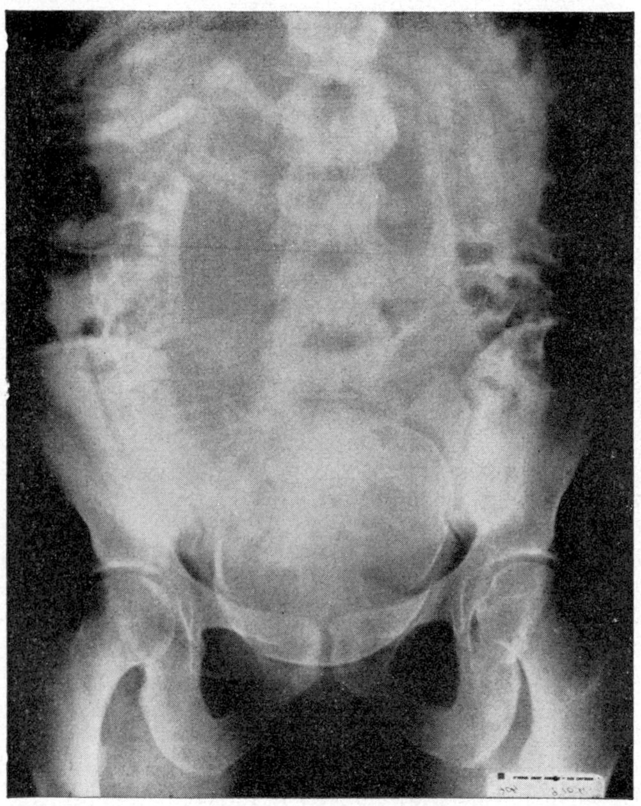

17/FIG. 14.—Moulding of the fetal head in labour with disproportion. An intrapartum X-ray taken after 18 hours with the membranes ruptured, with strong contractions and without advance during the last 12 hours. Maternal height 4 ft 11 in (1·47 m). Cervix 4 cm dilated. Delivered by lower segment Caesarean section. Birth weight 9 lb 6 oz (4·3 kg). Postnatal pelvimetry indicated a true conjugate of 10 cm with a small gynaecoid pelvis with contracted outlet.

enough to start worrying when the patient fails to make progress in her delivery. Nothing could be more deprecated than to subject a woman wantonly to an ordeal which has no reasonable prospect of rewarding success. It is not only bad science, it is bad doctoring. Furthermore, one's attitude to the labour itself should take into account every available feature, including the capacity of the cavity and the outlet. If one were only concerned with the problem of brim dystocia, as in the rickety flat pelvis, one could afford to be less punctilious in the safe knowledge that once the true conjugate was negotiated all would be well.

Trial of labour, therefore, just as much as induction of premature labour for disproportion, calls for scrupulous attention to every detail and the employment and intelligent use of every diagnostic aid. There is, after all, little credit in seeing the head negotiate the brim only, thereafter, to wreck the outcome in the course of a difficult forceps delivery. With foreknowledge of the lower pelvic straits one may well be influenced to curtail a trial of labour which at an earlier stage is not promising well.

Trial of labour may be the best that we can do under the circumstances, but it should never be allowed to degenerate into trial by ordeal.

Pelvic Osteoarthropathy

This interesting condition though not normally associated with disproportion had best be described here. As a result of the hormones of pregnancy, particularly "relaxin or progesterone," the joints of the pelvic girdle loosen up resulting sometimes in an abnormal separation and mobility at the symphysis pubis. The patient begins to feel considerable pain in her back and tenderness over the symphysis in the last month of pregnancy and the gap between the two halves of the pubis can sometimes be so wide as to be easily palpable. Because of pain in the pubic region I have seen such cases diagnosed as having a urinary infection. The diagnosis is not difficult to make provided it is thought of and can be confirmed by getting the patient to stand out of bed, first on one leg and then on the other, while the examiner's fingers palpate the symphysis pubis. The level of the two halves of the symphysis will be found to alter in relation to each other as the patient shifts her weight from side to side and the diagnosis can be further confirmed by X-ray (Fig. 15). The treatment is to put the patient to bed on a mattress with a hard board underneath it, which will greatly relieve her discomfort. She has, after all, a more or less physiological symphysiotomy and labour is not usually complicated, but the condition may persist for some weeks after the puerperium and great care should be taken not to subject the pelvic girdle to undue strain by encouraging too early ambulation, particularly without

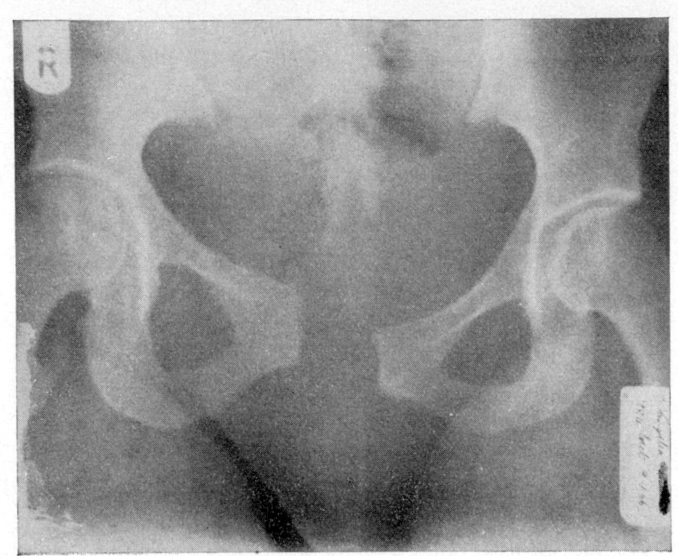

17/FIG. 15 (*a*)

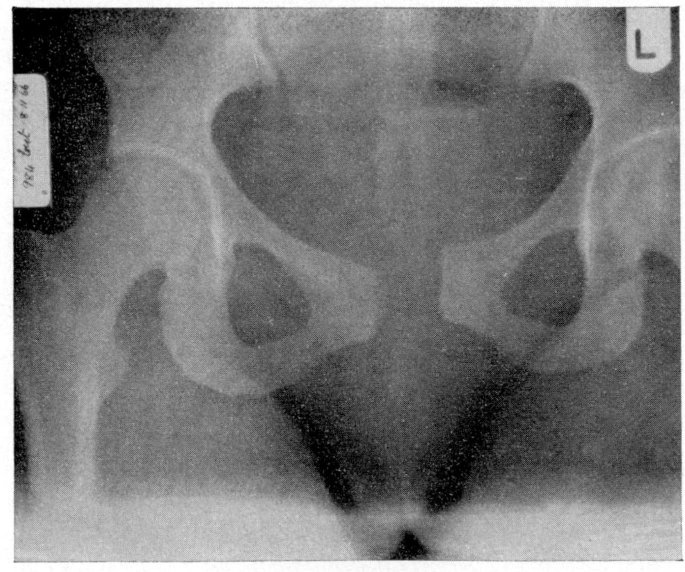

17/FIG. 15 (*b*)

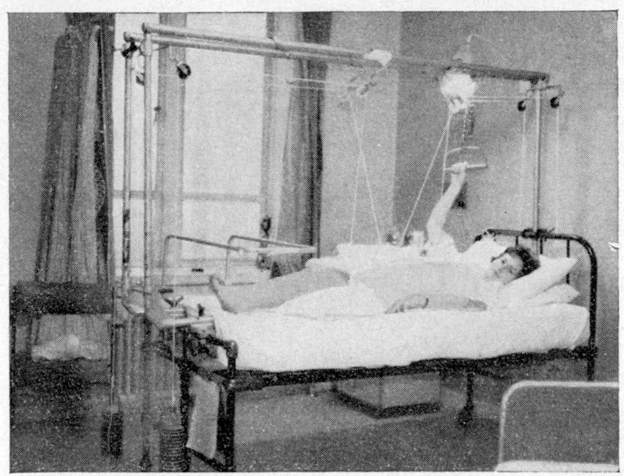

17/FIG. 15 (*c*)

17/FIG. 15.—Pelvic osteoarthopathy.
(*a*) Patient standing on right leg.
(*b*) Patient standing on left leg.
(*c*) Pelvic girdle maintained in a felt sling support during puerperium.

adequate support from strapping and binders. In extreme cases it is best to make a felt sling for the whole pelvis suspended by pulleys and weights from a Balkan beam (Fig. 15*c*). In the case shown here this had to be maintained for three weeks before the patient could be comfortably got out of bed. Fortunately in the postnatal weeks the pelvic girdle becomes more stable.

SAFETY ASPECTS OF RADIOLOGICAL PELVIMETRY

by ELLIS BARNETT, F.F.R., D.M.R.D.
Radiologist, Royal Maternity and Women's Hospital, Glasgow

The possible radiation hazard in obstetrics is still regarded as a major consideration in the selection of cases for radiological pelvimetry. Radiologists are acutely aware of the dangers of excessive radiation, and since the initial report by Stewart *et al.* in 1956, radiological techniques generally have been analysed with reference to radiation protection and reduction of dosage to the patient. In this respect also, further attention has been paid to X-ray apparatus and emphasis placed upon accurate coning down of the X-ray beam to cover only the essential area, the use of faster films and X-ray screens, and the application of various protective shields. In addition, increased filtration of the X-ray beam ensures that only the hard (that is, more penetrating) radiation reaches the patient.

The report of the Adrian Committee (*Radiological Hazards to Patients*, H.M. Stationery Office, 1960) summarises the present attitude and makes certain recommendations. In view of the great importance of this subject not only in obstetrics but in medicine generally, the reader is strongly recommended to study this report. However, several extracts relevant to obstetrics are recorded below for general guidance.

"Our survey has shown that in the present circumstances, the dose to the gonads from any X-ray examination is small in comparison with that considered by the Medical Research Council to be acceptable to the individual, without causing any undue concern on behalf of himself or his offspring."

"Pregnant women should be subjected to pelvimetry only after thorough clinical examination by an experienced obstetrician. The full radiological examination is necessary for only a small proportion of primigravidae, and very few multigravidae, but once decided upon, the examination should be very thorough. Of the four projections in common use—erect lateral, anteroposterior, subpubic arch and outlet, and superoinferior or inlet—the last named presents by far the highest dosage to both the maternal ovaries and the foetal gonads, and should be omitted whenever possible." In support of this are the figures recorded for the average gonad doses in milliroentgens per exposure to the fetal gonads and maternal ovaries during radiological pelvimetry, as listed below.

PROJECTION	DOSE	
	Maternal Ovary	*Fetal Gonads*
Anteroposterior	460	630
Lateral	577	535
Subpubic arch and pelvic outlet	670	140
Superoinferior pelvic inlet or Thom's	992	2242

Most radiologists agree that the superoinferior or Thom's view (Fig. 16) should now be avoided wherever possible, in view of the greater dose particularly to the fetal gonads. The anteroposterior view of the pelvis is an acceptable alternative to the Thom's view, although the shape of the pelvic brim cannot be as readily appreciated due to foreshortening. There is evidence to show that using the anteroposterior view with very accurate coning of the X-ray beam by means of triple lead diaphragms, the dose to the fetal gonads is reduced to a negligible level (Fig. 17). Should the Thom's brim view be deemed necessary in a particular case, the radiation to the fetal and maternal gonads can be reduced by placing a lead disc of suitable size in the path of the primary beam and close to the X-ray tube. The resultant film will show only the bony pelvis, the pelvic cavity being obscured (Fig. 18).

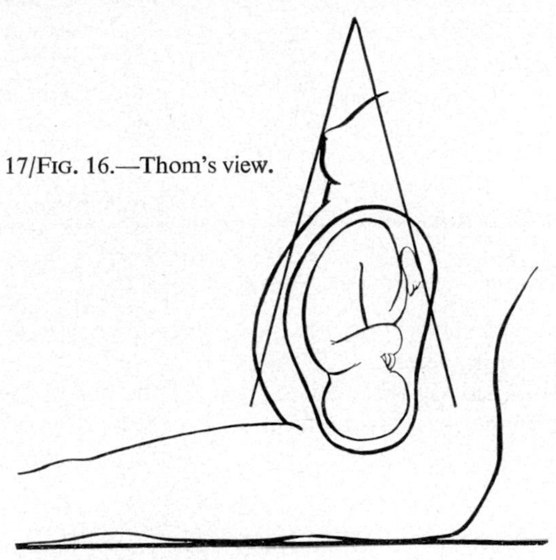

17/FIG. 16.—Thom's view.

THE TECHNIQUE OF X-RAY PELVIMETRY

It must be emphasised at the outset that in radiological pelvimetry the consideration of pelvic shape is just as important as the calculation of certain linear measurements. Pelvic shape is discussed earlier.

The basic views of the maternal pelvis used for the purpose of pelvimetry are:

1. Erect lateral view (Fig. 19).
2. Outlet view (Fig. 20).
3. Anteroposterior view (Fig. 21).
4. Thom's brim view. For the reasons already stated this view should be avoided wherever possible.

In the X-ray department of The Royal Maternity Hospital, Glasgow, the first three views indicated above are used when a full pelvic assessment is desired. But the erect lateral film is without a doubt the most important, and if only a limited examination is necessary this is the view of choice, for very often cephalopelvic disproportion can be appreciated or excluded, as far as the inlet and mid-pelvis are concerned, by examination of this film even without measurements.

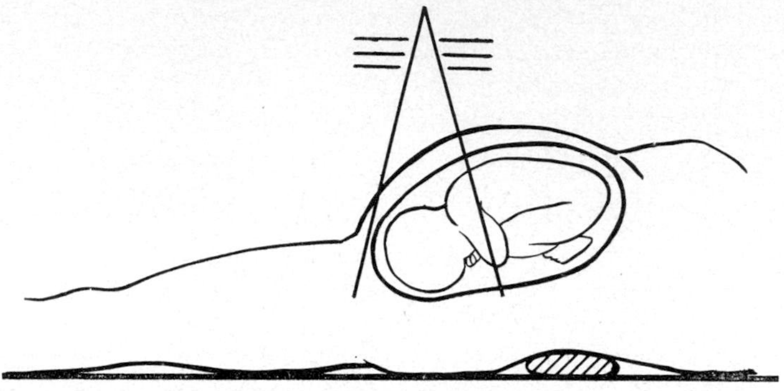

17/FIG. 17.—Reducing X-ray dosage of fetal gonads.

Nevertheless, whenever possible, we prefer to evaluate the pelvic capacity more completely.

Having obtained the three basic views of the pelvis, certain pelvic diameters are measured on the films and corrected for magnification

17/FIG. 18.—Thom's brim view with masking off of fetus by means of a lead disc.

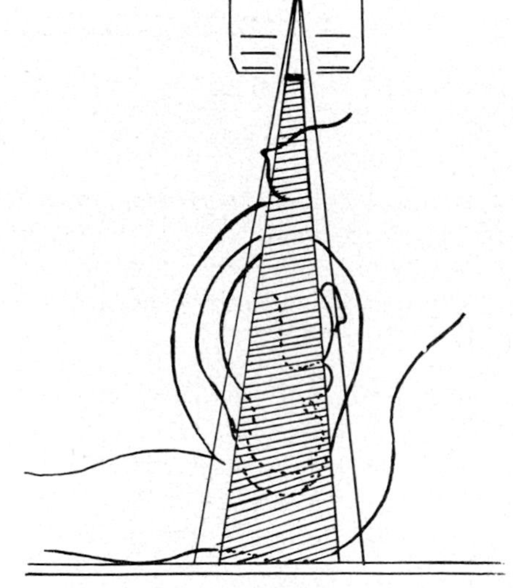

by the simple geometric problem of comparison of similar triangles as shown in Fig. 22. The thickness of the X-ray table (HB) is fixed, and the distance of the X-ray tube from the table (AH) is also kept constant. Thus the only variable is the distance of the diameter in question (EF) from the table top, that is, the distance GH, and this will of course vary with the thickness of the patient. For the lateral view, we measure the distance between the natal cleft and the top of the X-ray table, whereas for the anteroposterior view the pubis-to-table-top distance is determined. The outlet film is taken in such a position

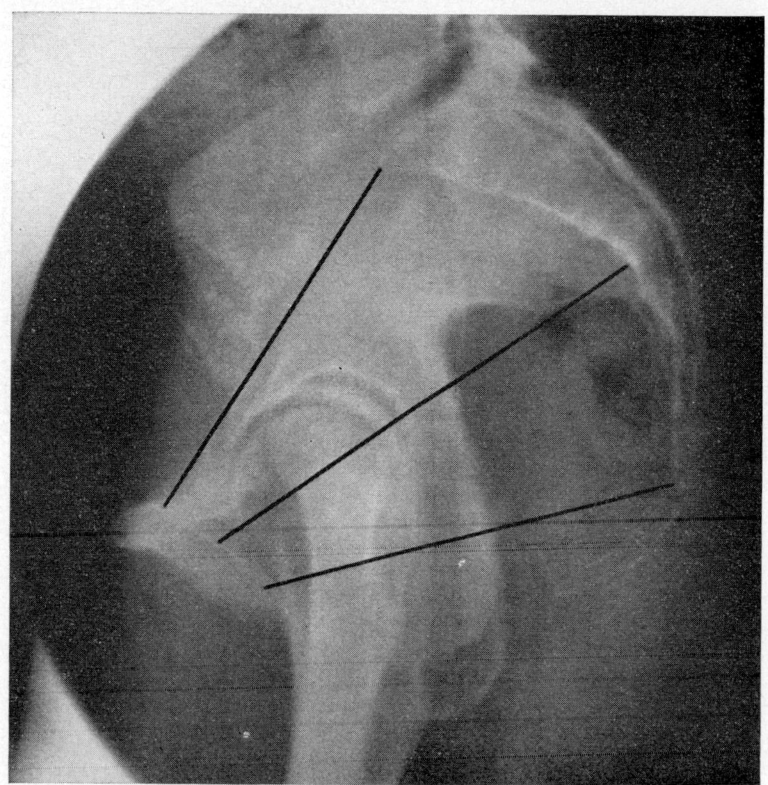

17/FIG. 19.—Erect lateral view.

that no measurement on the patient is necessary, as will be discussed.

Various authorities utilise different pelvic diameters. We use the following combination of pelvic diameters (Figs. 19, 20 and 21).

From the lateral film:

1. The available (obstetric) conjugate diameter of the inlet, which is a line joining the upper limit of the posterior wall of the symphysis pubis just where it starts to curve forwards, to the nearest point on the sacrum. The posterior extremity often, but not necessarily, coincides with the sacral promontory.

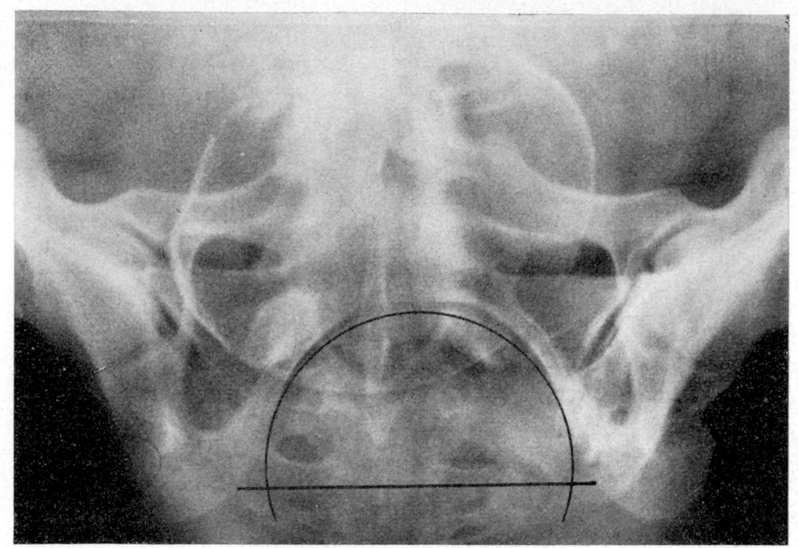

17/Fig. 20.—Outlet view.

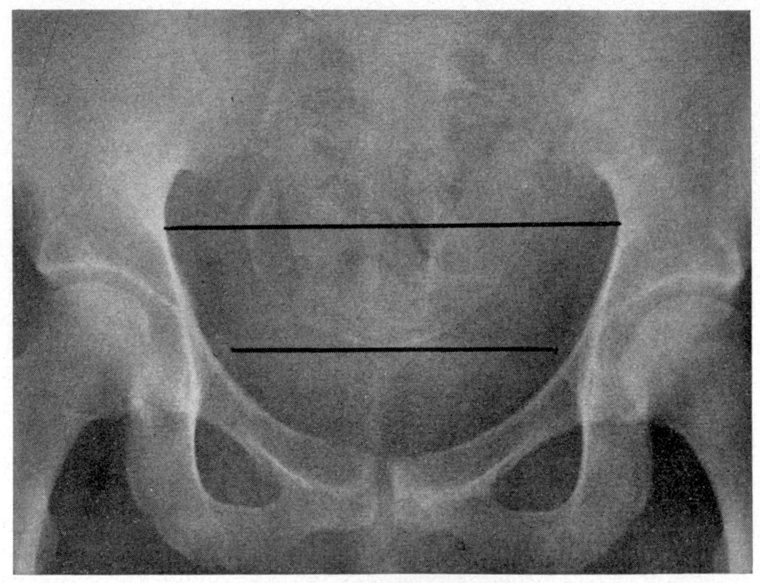

17/Fig. 21.—Anteroposterior view.

2. The anteroposterior diameter of the mid-pelvic cavity, which is taken as a line joining the middle of the posterior wall of the symphysis pubis to the middle of the anterior surface of the third piece of the sacrum.

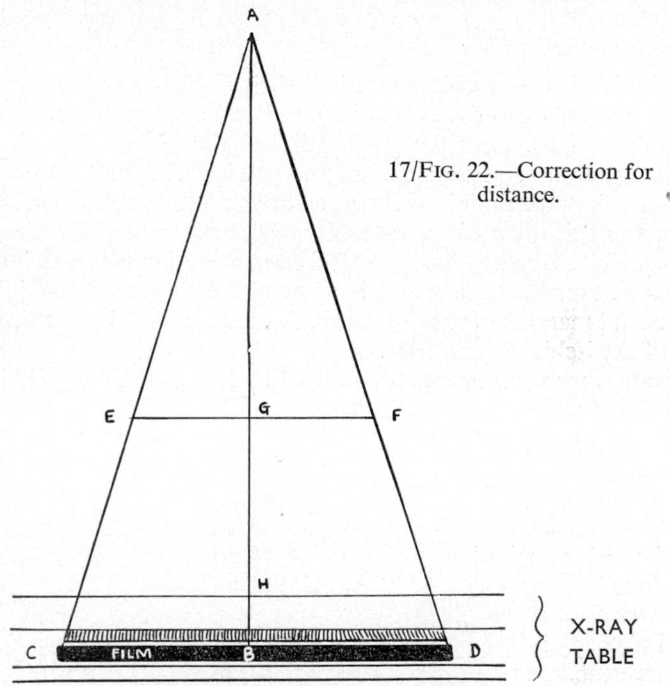

17/Fig. 22.—Correction for distance.

3. The anteroposterior diameter of the lower strait. (This diameter is often referred to as the anteroposterior diameter of the outlet, but strictly speaking it is not in the plane of the outlet, therefore the term lower strait is recommended.) This is a line joining the lower limit of the posterior wall of the symphysis pubis just where it starts to curve forwards, to the first sacro-coccygeal joint, thus taking into account the occurrence of partial or complete fusion of the coccyx to the sacrum.
4. The sacral angle (see Fig. 8).

From the anteroposterior film:

1. The transverse diameter of the inlet, which is taken at the widest transverse diameter that can be measured on the film.
2. The bispinous diameter, which is a line joining the tips of the ischial spines.

Blair Hartley has shown that the transverse diameter of the inlet and the bispinous diameter lie respectively $\frac{2}{3}$ and $\frac{1}{3}$ of the distance of the symphysis pubic from the table top, with the patient supine. Thus, having measured the pubis-to-table-top distance on the patient, the correction factors for these diameters can be readily calculated.

From the outlet film:

This view is taken with the patient sitting directly on the film, and bending as far forwards as possible, the abdomen lying between the separated thighs. Thus the positioning of the patient for this view brings the transverse diameter of the pelvic outlet and also the inferiŏr ischiopubic rami into close relationship to the film. Therefore, using a sufficiently great tube-to-film distance, the magnification will be negligible. To allow for the soft tissues overlying the ischial tuberosities we take the transverse diameter of the outlet as a line joining the medial margins of the descending rami at a level 1 cm above the tips of the ischial tuberosities.

The average measurements recorded by Ince and Young (1940) in a survey of 509 cases are as follows:

INLET		
True Conjugate	=	11·83 cm
Transverse	=	13·06 cm
Posterior Sagittal	=	4·87 cm
Area	=	121·30 cm^2
LOWER STRAIT		
Pubosacral	=	11·97 cm
Intertuberous	=	10·90 cm
Ischial bispinous	=	9·95 cm.

The subpubic angle can be measured by joining the two extremities of the transverse diameter of the outlet to a point at the lower border of the pubic symphysis, but we feel that this angle is of little practical value, as it does not allow for the curvature of the descending ischiopubic rami. It is much more important to assess the capacity of the subpubic arch and to determine the extent to which the average fetal head can utilise the space available. This is done by determining the waste space of Morris. A circle 9·3 cm in diameter is applied to the outlet film between the descending rami. This will give a practical indication of the extent to which the average fetal head can utilise the arch. Morris (1947) considers that the head, moulded in the attitude of flexion, approximates closely to a cylinder with the biparietal, suboccipitobregmatic, and occipitofrontal diameters more or less equal. The diameter of this cylinder at term may be taken as 9·3 cm.

Normally the distance between the lower border of the symphysis and the circumference of the circle is not more than 1 cm and the coronal diameter of the circle should be at least 1 cm in front of the ischial tuberosities. Obviously if the waste space is large the anteroposterior diameter of the lower pelvic strait as measured on the lateral

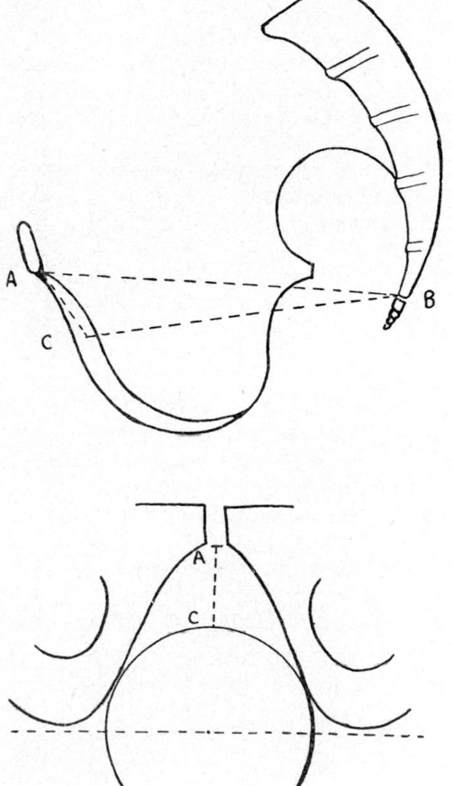

17/FIG. 23.—Available anteroposterior diameter of lower strait.

AB = Anteroposterior diameter of lower strait.

AC = Waste space of Morris.

CB = Available anteroposterior diameter of lower strait.

film is false for practical purposes, as the head cannot fully utilise the whole of this diameter, which must therefore be adjusted and the *available* anteroposterior diameter of the lower strait be determined as shown in Fig. 23. The only measurement of the fetal head which is thought to be measurable with sufficient accuracy on routine views is the biparietal diameter as measured on the erect lateral film when the head is presenting in the occipitotransverse position, and is not deviated to either side in the anteroposterior view.

REFERENCES

1. CALDWELL, W. E. and MOLOY, H. C. (1939). *Amer. J. Roentgenol.*, **41,** 305, 505, 719.
2. CALDWELL, W. E., MOLOY, H. C. and D'ESOPO, D. A. (1935). *Amer. J. Obstet. Gynec.*, **30,** 763.
3. CAMPBELL, S. (1968). *J. Obstet. Gynaec. Brit. Cwlth*, **75,** 568.
4. COURT BROWN, W. M., DOLL, R. and HILL, A. B. (1960). *Brit. med. J.*, **2,** 1539.
5. DONALD, I. and BROWN, T. G. (1961). *Brit. J. Radiol.*, **34,** 539.
6. DONALD, I., MACVICAR, J. and WILLOCKS, J. (1962). *Proc. roy. Soc. Med.*, **55,** 637.
7. FEENEY, J. K. and BARRY, A. P. (1954). *J. Obstet. Gynaec. Brit. Emp.*, **61,** 652.
8. GIBBERD, G. F. (1952). Eighth Annual Meeting of Society of Obstetricians and Gynaecologists of Canada, June 6th.
9. GOLDBERG, B. B., ISARD, H. J., GERSHON-COHEN, J and OSTRUM, B. J. (1966). *Radiology*, **87,** 328.
10. HARTLEY, J. B. and FISHER, A. S. (1955). *A Plan for Radiography in Obstetrics*, 2nd edit. Manchester: United Manchester Hospitals.
11. INCE, J. C. H. and YOUNG, M. (1940). *J. Obstet. Gynaec. Brit. Emp.*, **47,** 130.
12. LEWIS, T. L. T. (1960). *Brit. med. J.*, **2,** 1551.
13. MOIR, J. C. (1947). *J. Obstet. Gynaec. Brit. Emp.*, **54,** 20.
14. MORRIS, W. I. C. (1947). *Edinb. med. J.*, **54,** 90.
15. M.R.C. Report (1956). *The Hazards to Man of Nuclear and Allied Radiations.* London: H.M. Stationery Office.
16. STEWART, A., WEBB, J., TILES, D. and HEWITT, D. (1956). *Lancet*, **2,** 447.
17. WEEKES, A. R. L. and FLYNN, M. J. (1975). *Brit. J. Obstet. Gynaec.*, **82,** 7.
18. WILLIAMS, B. (1942). *J. Obstet. Gynaec. Brit. Emp.*, **49,** 412.
19. WILLOCKS, J. (1963). M.D. Thesis, Univ. Glasgow.
20. WILLOCKS, J., DONALD, I., DUGGAN, T. C. and DAY, N. (1964). *J. Obstet. Gynaec. Brit. Cwlth*, **71,** 11.
21. WILLOCKS, J,, DONALD, I., CAMPBELL, S. and DUNSMORE, I. R. (1967). *J. Obstet. Gynaec. Brit. Cwlth*, **74,** 639.

CHAPTER XVIII

MANAGEMENT OF LABOUR

O, that a man might know
The end of this day's business ere it come!
But it sufficeth that the day will end,
And then the end is known.
SHAKESPEARE, *Julius Caesar*, Act V, Sc. 1.

A LABOUR which is unduly prolonged is likely to give rise to one or more of three types of distress, namely maternal, fetal or "obstetricians' distress". Of the three the last may be easily the most dangerous! These cases tax clinical judgment, often to the limit, and then a second opinion, come freshly on the scene, is worth a lot. In hospital practice this is usually automatic, but in domiciliary work importuning relatives may easily distract judgment already wavering in the cause of plain humanity, with the result that intervention is often prematurely, ill-advisedly or unnecessarily undertaken.

Dawn should not rise twice upon the same labour. Nowadays we would regard any labour lasting more than 24 hours as pathological and, in the case of the multiparous patient, positively sinister. All such cases need the facilities of a properly staffed and equipped obstetrical unit.

We have come a long way since the days in the 1930s when my first obstetrical case laboured for five days (and I too!) and although she delivered herself spontaneously in the end, she became acutely psychotic a few days later and was removed to a mental institution where, so I learned, she did not do well. These were days when we were more concerned with maternal survival than fetal wellbeing, Caesarean section, usually classical, carried a mortality of not less than 5 per cent and the philosophy of those days was that the first baby at least was always expendable in the interests of the mother's obstetrical future. I first came into obstetrics towards the end of a truly horrific period of maternal hazard and suffering and my memory is more deeply engraved with the disasters of those days than it is with any subsequent successes.

UTERINE FUNCTION

An adequate study of this cannot be made by observation and palpation alone, and various tocographic techniques have been used which fall into two main classes: (*a*) external, (*b*) internal.

An example of the former is the guard-ring tocograph (Fig. 1) devised by Smyth (Nixon and Smyth, 1957). A flat perspex plate is applied to the abdominal wall, turning the area covered into a flat surface. In the middle of this plate there is a hole about one inch in diameter through which a "button plunger" projects from a fairly stiff leaf-type spring. Two strain-gauges are bonded to the leaf spring, one above and one below and form two of the resistances of a Wheatstone bridge circuit. Any change of pressure within the uterus

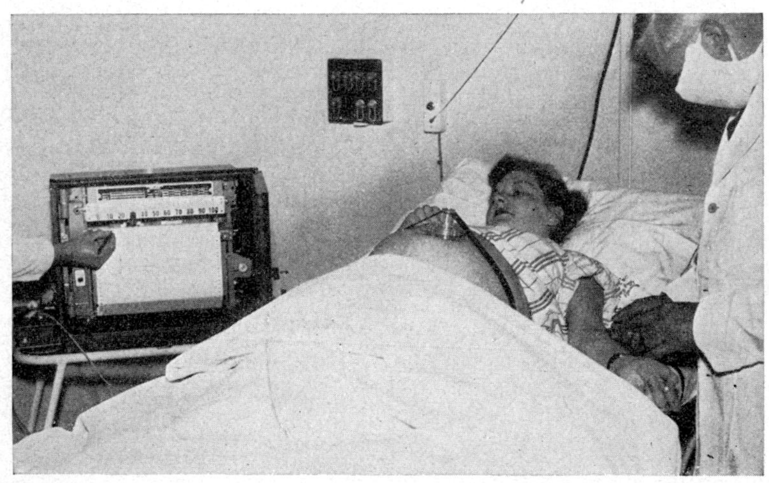

18/Fig. 1.—Guard-ring tocodynamometer.
(By courtesy of Dr C. N. Smyth.)

is transmitted to the button plunger moving in the central hole of the perspex plate and thus the leaf spring is subjected to stress which increases the tension on one strain-gauge and at the same time relaxes it on the other, thus altering their electrical resistances in opposite directions. This unbalances the Wheatstone bridge, the electrical imbalance so induced being proportional to the distorting mechanical force. By suitable amplification very stable (i.e. free from drift) records can be made.[47, 48]

Good records of the patterns of uterine activity can thus be obtained, as indeed they also can by careful clinical palpation, but it is less certain that absolute intra-uterine pressure measurements can be made by this means as there is some evidence that the figures given are affected by the pressure with which the apparatus is applied to the abdominal wall, and the thickness and natural resistances of this wall presumably play a part too.[19] The method, however, has the great advantage that it subjects the patient neither to risk of infection nor to discomfort.

The disadvantages of internal methods are of course the risks of sepsis due to the presence of a foreign body. The method is to insert a fairly large polythene tube into the amniotic sac by means of a Drew Smythe catheter introduced at the same time as performing induction of labour by hindwater rupture or through a flexible plastic tube to encourage the catheter tip to get above the presenting part. The polythene tube is connected to an electromanometer.

The internal method described above only gives a picture of uterine activity as a whole with the resultant pressures achieved, and Caldeyro and his colleagues (1950) made interesting observations by combining external and internal methods. They have shown that in normal labour there is good synchronisation of activity and have also detected asynchronism and other anomalies in abnormal labour.

The pacemakers of the uterus are believed to be situated in the region of the tubal ostia, from which waves of activity spread synchronously downwards. In the colicky type of uterus there may be ectopic pacemakers. The above workers have found the following characteristics of satisfactory uterine action:

1. There are large rises in intra-amniotic pressure exceeding 24 mm Hg;
2. There is fundal dominance as compared with the strength of mid-zone activity and the lower segment shows minimal action;
3. There is good synchronisation;
4. The wave pattern is regular;
5. There is good relaxation of the uterus between contractions as demonstrated by a satisfactory resting baseline of intra-amniotic pressure. In normal labour this amounts to no more than 5–6 mm Hg but in hypertonic and colicky types of uterine action the "resting" pressures may exceed 15–20 mm Hg and in fact may remain dangerously above the pain-threshold level.

This last observation is of particular importance, because of the need for uteroplacental circulation to recover its volume between contractions. The interference with effective uterine blood flow caused by uterine activity has been well demonstrated by the clearance rates of radiosodium injected into the myometrium. It was found that whereas the blood flow was normal in nearly all cases early in the first stage of labour, more than half showed a significant reduction towards full dilatation. Those cases showing signs of fetal distress demonstrated a great reduction in effective uterine blood flow. The mechanism of fetal asphyxia in prolonged and difficult labour is thus well illustrated.

Studies of this nature throw a great deal of light on the behaviour of the uterus, especially in cases of inco-ordinate action. However, the lower segment is not entirely passive, as is commonly taught, but undergoes contraction, relaxation and retraction, though in lesser degree. This can be observed at Caesarean section, and were it not true every case of placenta praevia would die of postpartum haemorrhage.

Pain

Attempts have been made to study pain and an individual's threshold to it by various methods of dolorimetry, but there is still much that modern science has not yet evaluated concerning the sensation of pain in childbirth. Pain is believed to be capable of reaching the potential maximum at the end of the second stage of labour, but the pains of the first stage, by a process of exhausting repetition, can be just as serious a matter and far more demoralising to the patient. Leaving aside the question of individual threshold, it is important to consider why one type of first stage should be so much more painful than another. The critical level of pain production in the human uterus is believed to be a pressure exceeding 25 mm of mercury. The pain produced may be due either to the stretching of the structures adjacent to the uterus, including neighbouring ganglia, or may be in the nature of an ischaemic cramp. The latter is probably the more important. Certainly after-pains cannot be attributed to stretching. The lower segment of the uterus is probably far more sensitive to pain than the upper segment, and pain due to stretching thereof is mainly referred to the back, whereas the upper segment refers pain to the hypogastric area. The less backache, therefore, in labour as a rule the more efficient the uterus and, conversely, the worse the backache the more does it signify inco-ordinate action, since it suggests that the lower segment and cervix are providing abnormal resistance to the expulsive efforts of the upper segment.

Functions of the Membranes

The older doctrine of the sanctity of the membranes was more or less built in with the bricks in my obstetrical philosophy. No labour is so pleasing and satisfactory to mother and child as when intact membranes are maintained right up to full dilatation at which point a gush of clear, clean liquor amnii flushes out the genital tract, followed, not so many minutes later, by the delivery of a clean, healthy, screaming baby. This is Nature at her best and I never cease to marvel at such normality. It is a safe doctrine which can only be dispensed with in the presence of full monitoring facilities. It would be a pity otherwise if the old lessons had to be relearned by younger generations the hard way.

The evil significance of prolonged labour is directly proportional to the time which has elapsed since rupture of the membranes. This is the most important landmark in the first stage. With very few exceptions, intact membranes mean an intact mother and an intact baby.

I was once dilating upon the virtues of intact membranes to my students and remarked frivolously that if I were much of a poet I would write an ode to their graces, whereupon one of my audience, J. McMullan by name, who was then an undergraduate student, went home and produced the following sonnet which was duly published in the *St. Thomas's Hospital Gazette*:

Shall I compare thee to de Ribes's bags
Thou art more natural and more temperate:
Rough pains come but still the labour lags
And Voorhee's lease hath all too short a date.
Often the obstetrician finds
Early rupture runs a tedious course:
Sometime too strong the muscle binds
And harms the fetus by untempered force.
But thy eternal safety shall not fade
Nor bring infection to that fair thou hast
Nor shall death come to mother nor to babe
When intact to the second stage thou last.
So long preserve thy precious charm,
And keep mother, child and all from harm.

The following, then, are the advantages of intact membranes:

1. The maintenance of even hydrostatic pressure equally applied to the whole fetal surface;
2. The chances of intra-uterine infection are enormously reduced during prolonged labour;
3. Constriction ring does not occur;
4. Rupture of the uterus is very rare except in the presence of pre-existing pathology of the uterine wall;
5. Fetal asphyxia is less likely, because an intact amniotic sac discourages major degrees of retraction at the placental site with its consequent reduction in uteroplacental circulation;
6. Rotation of the body of the child in cases of occipitoposterior position is not discouraged as is the case with a dry labour;
7. The cord may present, but until the membranes rupture it cannot prolapse;
8. The fetus is very unlikely to contract intranatal pneumonia.

It will be noted that the dilating power of the bag of forewaters has not been mentioned in the above list. This property is nowadays discounted. The incidence of inertia and prolonged labour is not significantly altered by the fact of early rupture of the membranes, but the effects of delay are magnified, in particular fetal distress and maternal infection.

Types of Anomalous Uterine Action

The old division of inertia into primary and secondary types is now obsolete. The former term simply indicated that uterine contractions had been ineffectual from the start of labour, while the second is far better described as "uterine exhaustion". It is more important, when labour is extended by faulty uterine activity, to define, as far as possible, the nature of that fault in one's diagnostic terminology, because there are marked differences in prognosis and treatment. The following are the varieties of inefficient uterine action with which we are concerned.

1. Hypotonic inertia;
2. Hypertonic inertia:
   (*a*) Defective polarity;
   (*b*) Colicky uterus;
   (*c*) Constriction ring;
3. Asymmetrical uterine activity;
4. Cervical dystocia.

Hypotonic inertia.—This is the least serious of the above varieties, although labour may be more prolonged than in the case of any of the others. It comes nearest to true primary inertia, but is not always primary in respect of time, as it may supervene in a labour which has previously been proceeding at a normal pace. The patient and her baby are in no immediate danger. The contractions come fairly regularly but infrequently, and relaxation in between is complete, so that the uteroplacental circulation is not unduly interfered with and the patient does not readily develop signs of maternal distress. The prognosis on the whole is fairly good. Labour after all is simply proceeding in a lower gear and is at any time capable of spontaneous acceleration. Reassurance and a good night's sleep are all that is usually required, and these patients often appreciate some homely simile such as being likened to a "slow oven". The condition is easily recognised by observing a few contractions. As in normal labour, the uterus can be felt to harden under the examining hand before the patient experiences any pain, and likewise the contraction outlives the duration of the discomfort. The uterus between contractions is perfectly soft and is not tender, and palpation of the fetus easy.

Hypertonic states.—The outlook here is altogether less favourable. In all of them the intra-uterine pressures are liable to exceed the critical pain threshold level of 25 mm Hg, even between contractions. Because of this increased pressure during the so-called resting phase the uteroplacental circulation is impeded and fetal asphyxia may develop, in some cases even while the membranes remain intact. Often a type of reversed polarity would appear to be at work whereby the lower segment offers resistance because of its hypertonicity to the relatively ineffectual contractions of the upper segment. This is a state of affairs which can be reproduced experimentally in monkeys by stimulation of the hypogastric nerves and, because of the overactivity of the lower segment and the stresses to which it thereby becomes subjected, severe pain may be referred to the back, a symptom which helps to distinguish the case from one of hypotonic interia. There is often rectal and colonic spasm in sympathy while the stomach and bladder become distended, so that vomiting and retention of urine or at least failure to empty the bladder spontaneously are troublesome features which make matters worse. These last are probably sympathetic effects of hyperactivity.

The patient suffers much and enjoys little respite from her pains. To the examining hand the uterus is not only tender but reacts to quite gentle manipulation by painfully contracting, so that palpation of the fetus is often hampered. Another cardinal feature is the presence of pain which both precedes and outlives a palpable uterine contraction.

The term "colicky uterus" largely explains itself. There is a lack of normal polarity and the uterus appears to be suffering from a continual crop of extrasystoles without any co-ordination to give them effect.

Constriction rings in the first and second stage of labour only occur with ruptured membranes. They resemble the "hug-me-tight" uterus in many aetiological respects, but represent areas of intense local hyperactivity. The ring usually forms round some indentation in the fetal surface, most commonly round the neck, and the junction of the upper and lower segments is one of the more usual sites. A constriction ring can seldom be diagnosed by abdominal examination and is only found when the hand is inserted to ascertain the cause of delay or at Caesarean section. We prefer the term constriction ring to contraction ring, although the two are synonymous and in no way to be confused with the retraction ring of Bandl, of which more anon under "obstructed labour". Because polarity is deranged the lower segment is not thinned out nor stretched in cases of constriction ring and there is no danger of uterine rupture from labour obstructed due to this cause. Attempts to deliver the fetus forcibly past the ring only make it clamp down the more viciously. Fortunately, the condition is reversible, but only with the lapse of time, generous sedation or epidural anaesthesia.

Cervical dystocia.—This not very common condition comes into a subcategory of its own. Occasionally it results from some structural abnormality of the cervix of acquired origin, as a result, for example, of fibrosis and scarring following cervical cautery, trachelorrhaphy or amputation. In other instances the cervix may be poorly developed and incapable of ready dilatation or there may be an excess of fibrous tissue within its substance. In labour, cervical dystocia may also represent another variety of inco-ordinate uterine action. In any case, a mechanical obstruction is offered to delivery. This is situated at the external os, which presents to the examining finger an unquestionably hard, leathery and undilatable rim. The presenting part is well applied to the cervix, and the other forces of labour have usually driven it low into the pelvis. In these cases full dilatation of the cervix can only be achieved at the expense of tearing, and occasionally annular detachment of the cervix results. It is an important condition to recognise in labour, because not only does it account for the delay in the first stage and for the patient's pain, which may be very great, but also because of the likelihood of extensive damage.

A somewhat similar condition occasionally occurs in which the os becomes displaced upwards and behind the leading surface of the presenting part so that there is a tendency for the anterior wall of the lower segment to sacculate, since the cervical canal is out of the line of thrust (sacral os). If the bony fit of the pelvis is a tight one, necrosis may occur, and the presenting part may side-track the cervix and burst its way through the lower segment into the vagina. A similar mechanism may occur posterior to the cervical canal, and as a rule the rent above the external os does not subsequently heal and can be found at later examinations. I had one such case with a large posterior aperture into the uterine cavity who, presumably as a result of it, suffered subsequently a series of very bloody abortions.

False labour.—Normally a patient is not painfully aware of uterine activity until the commencement of labour, but this is not invariably so. Before being certain that labour has started, the cervix, too, should show at least some sign of dilating. I once had a patient who had apparently agonising uterine contractions throughout the last eight weeks of pregnancy. She repeatedly turned up at a nursing home where she was booked for her confinement, but there was no sign whatever of cervical dilatation until she reached term, whereupon she delivered herself spontaneously and without trouble. Subjectively at least she had been in the first stage of labour for two months.

Cases of postmaturity have often demonstrated a short period of false labour round about term, and such a history may be of help in deciding if a case is in fact postmature. It is often difficult to decide whether a patient is in true or false labour and overnight observation is usually necessary.

Maternal and Fetal Mortality

Nature and time are unreliable allies (Jeffcoate, 1961). Thirty years ago the incidence of prolonged labour lasting more than 48 hours was over 3 per cent. Under these dreadful circumstances the mortality rate for both mother and baby was roughly quadrupled, the fetal death rate rising with the duration of the first stage of labour and the time which had elapsed since the membranes ruptured, the last factor being particularly important.

Sepsis and haemorrhage took their toll of maternal life while the chief causes of fetal death were intra-uterine asphyxia, tentorial damage and intracranial haemorrhage, and intranatal pulmonary infection in which the baby is born with an already established pneumonia. This last hazard, alas, occurs too often even today, especially in the case of the premature.

Aetiology

Many cases of prolonged labour are not due purely to uterine functional faults, so that catastrophe may, for example, arise from underlying causes, such as overlooked disproportion, undiagnosed malpresentation, particularly brow, or accidents following the treatment adopted for those conditions—either a difficult instrumental delivery with all its attendant risks, or a Caesarean section undertaken too late.

The extent of morbidity cannot easily be assessed. Apart from puerperal pyrexia in the mother, the cervix, pelvic floor and bladder sphincter mechanisms may suffer much residual disability, nor should one overlook the late psychological sequelae which affect both the mother as well as her husband in their attitude towards further childbearing. Fetal morbidity is even more serious especially as regards the central nervous system and the child's subsequent intellectual capacity. I well recall one of my old teachers, the late Kenneth Bowes, speculating on how much prolonged uterine activity it took to damage a child.

Today with modern treatment prolonged labour is scarcely permitted. For example the National Maternity Hospital in Dublin in the year 1975 had only three cases in which labour exceeded 24 hours in over 2000 primigravid labours, an incidence of 0·05 per cent. The cause of delay in each case was disproportion. Two of the patients had already been in labour for 24 hours or more when admitted and the fundamental mistake was the failure to recognise the simple fact that the lack of progress in labour, in spite of efficient uterine action, was due to disproportion. The height of all three cases was less than 160 cm and one of them was postmature. Looking back on our own practice I cannot recall a labour in recent years lasting longer than 24 hours in any of our patients, nor can my colleagues whom I have consulted and I would have to search the records too far back to find one.

Primiparity is the most important constant factor in disordered uterine activity. The multiparous uterus, faced with mechanical difficulty, sometimes fights it and ruptures in the process. The primiparous uterus nearly always responds by becoming inert in the first instance and then inco-ordinate. Such a case neglected would become septic as a matter of course. The influence of age, though somewhat overrated in the past, is additionally important however, because the effects of prolonged labour are increasingly significant.

Overdistension of the uterus, either from twins or polyhydramnios, is a traditionally accepted cause of inert labour, but it is more than 20 years since I personally have seen a case of labour lasting more than 48 hours with twins. Hydramnios benefits from the drawing off of excessive quantities of liquor, preferably by amniocentesis if gross, to allow slow decompression and to discourage prolapse of the cord or placental abruption.

Grand multiparity is dangerously accepted by some as a cause, the supposition being that much of the uterine wall is infiltrated with fibrous and elastic tissue. It is a safe rule, however, to regard all cases of delayed labour in multiparae as being possibly due to an undiagnosed brow presentation, until this has been excluded by very thorough vaginal examination. Fibroids, too, are blamed for inertia, but the majority of cases thus complicated encounter no such difficulties, at least in the first stage of labour, and it is possible that the attendant's interest in the patient's fibroids may contribute much to her anxiety. Uterine hypoplasia is also quoted as a cause by people who are more ready to guess than to think. This is obviously nonsense: how else could the uterus have carried a pregnancy right up to term, and if anybody can diagnose uterine hypoplasia at 40 weeks' gestation he must be either a magician or a poet. Hormonal imbalance has also been postulated, but only in a nebulous and as yet unsubstantiated way.

Of all the malpresentations and malpositions the occipitoposterior position is the most important in prolonging labour, though there is here some admixture of cause and effect, since a lively uterus will soon deal with poor rotation of the occiput. The other malpresentations, save the extended breech, operate as obvious causes in prolonging labour and demand recognition and treatment in their own right. Beware particularly of undiagnosed brow presentation and minor degrees of hydrocephalus.

Any cause of badly fitting presenting part in the lower uterine segment deprives labour of one of its most important mechanical stimuli. Placenta praevia must be included under this heading. Congenital abnormalities in the uterus very occasionally cause inertia, but in many cases labour runs a perfectly normal course, so that the condition is not even suspected.

There are certain general types of patient who tend to labour badly and the dystrophia dystocia syndrome is an extreme case in point. This has been dealt with more fully in the chapter on disproportion. The association of obesity and inert labour is common experience, and in these cases there is often also a family history of prolonged labour, so that it would appear that the endocrine make-up of the patient is important in a general sense.

Postmaturity is not infrequently associated with long and difficult labour. At least a part of the reason for this is mechanical because of the hardness and slightly increased size of the fetal head. Cause and effect here are mixed together since postmaturity besides discouraging brisk labour may, itself, be the result of disordered uterine activity. The older the patient the more sinister does the combination become.

The injudicious use of powerful drugs can often be rightly blamed for holding up labour. Nobody would expect a patient who was kept continuously under a deep anaesthetic to deliver herself smartly, and to a lesser extent the same argument must apply to the too early administration of "knock-out" drugs.

Let us never forget the full bladder and the full rectum, particularly the former. Not only are uterine contractions reflexly inhibited, but it is quite astonishing how even a moderately filled bladder can discourage deep engagement of the presenting part.

The question of inertia following induction of labour has been dealt with in the chapter on induced labour. It is a matter of some importance and readily incriminates injudicious interference of this sort.

Anxiety and fear have been so largely accepted as causes that the science of obstetrics has become cluttered up with much speculative theory and it is difficult to sort out the wheat from the enormous quantity of chaff. All women facing labour do so with some degree of fear, some reacting more outwardly than others; but a patient can be frightened into labour just as well as she may be reputedly frightened out of it. Thunderstorms are terrifying to many people and in most induce a state of some sort of excitement, but midwives are usually extra busy at these times. A woman who has previously had a horrifying labour has extra reason to fear the next. Many, in fact, from fear decline to embark on further pregnancies. On this basis inertia ought to be more common amongst multiparae than in primigravid patients. But the reverse is the case. It might be argued, however, that the fear of the unknown is more potent than fear of the known, but the professional torturers of history do not appear to have worked on this principle, and they should know! Surely the explanation of the differences in suffering and the length of labour between the primigravida and multipara lies in the fact that anatomically the two women differ. The multipara has had her cervix stretched in a previous labour, and it is suggested that, since this stretching is always accompanied by some degree of structural damage to the cervix, some type of modified local sympathectomy has been achieved by nature.

Much specious argument has been expended in explaining prolonged labour in terms of psychological aberrations and, as a result, all manner of therapy has come into vogue ranging from hypnosis to simple reassurance, the latter being obviously desirable without invoking scientific justification. Patients who can be bothered and who have the time can, according to taste, sit around relaxing, breathe Yoga fashion, or romp about in the gymnasium of a department of physiotherapy training their muscles. The cardiac case, who does not get this training, is seldom inert. All this huge and varied fabrication is based on the observation that the course of labour can be modified by the patient's mental state. This is too obvious to need further elaboration, but the methods of dealing with the matter have often little basis in science and are probably less effective than frank witchcraft and certainly less picturesque. A patient's reactions to her condition are on the whole more important than the condition itself, and if these reactions can be modified, as it is agreed they indeed can, so much the better. The patient who trusts her doctor and has healthy insight into the processes through which she is going, co-operates in her labour in the comforting knowledge that she will not be asked to bear more than is reasonably necessary and no scheme of antenatal preparation for labour, however elaborate or grotesque, can be accepted as a substitute for confidence between the doctor and his charge.

Management of Prolonged Labour

The optimum duration of labour is now generally regarded as between 6 and 12 hours, the primiparous patient usually taking a few hours longer than the multipara. Ideally the cervix should dilate roughly 1 cm to the hour. Precipitate labour due to tumultuous pains is hazardous to the baby from the point of view of intracranial damage and the occasional delivery of a baby rapidly and spontaneously into a lavatory basin has nothing to commend it. We have all had experience, however, of the case who goes through the first stage of labour painlessly and I remember a colleague's wife, admitted to hospital for observation because of mild hypertension, who rang for the midwife because she quite suddenly found the baby in bed beside her, the baby showing no signs of wear and tear.

Alas, Nature left to her own devices often fails to achieve the pattern and duration of labour which we now accept as normal. The objective now therefore is to recognise the case in which prolonged labour is threatened and to prevent it from developing. Unfortunately throughout the world only a minority of obstetric units have the staff or the equipment for safely extending the rapidly growing practice of accelerating labour, so much of what follows is directed towards these less fortunate units as well as the better equipped.

General care.—Everything should be done to stave off, for as long as possible, the onset of maternal distress in the hope of delivery being completed before one's hand is forced into operating. Now, the signs of maternal distress are chiefly those of dehydration and ketosis. The lower the fluid intake, therefore, the sooner will labour dehydrate the patient. It was once taught that no opportunity should be lost of encouraging the patient to drink adequate quantities of fluid such as sweetened drinks flavoured with fruit juices. Unfortunately the very patient most in need of fluid and carbohydrate is also the one least likely to benefit from such treatment. At best she will vomit most of it and at worst she will merely accumulate it by the pint, unabsorbed, in her hypotonic stomach and upper intestine, where it lies treacherously in wait to be vomited back if, and when, a general anaesthetic has to be given. She will then be lucky indeed if she does not aspirate some of this deadly and copious vomit. We now regard fluids by mouth as dangerous in prolonged labour because of this risk, and unhesitatingly prefer the intravenous route to combat dehydration and ketosis. We ourselves use Plasmalyte 148 (Baxter FKB 25 83), which contains 5 per cent dextrose. Laevulose 20 per cent in water (Baxter FKB 042, or Laevuflex—Geistlich) can also be given, 500 ml to 2 litres every 24 hours, by intravenous infusion. Laevulose can be given when there is a primary need to correct ketosis. It is now our practice to forbid all food and drink by mouth during labour and we only allow our patients to suck ice cubes. This, together with 4-hourly attention to oral hygiene by the nursing staff, suffices to keep the patient's mouth and throat comfortable nowadays when labour is measured in hours rather than days.

The signs of maternal distress are a dry tongue, a rising pulse above 100, later a rising temperature and in advanced cases a hot, dry vagina, with possibly some purulent secretion. The urine becomes increasingly concentrated and scanty, and presently, if the patient is vomiting and has achieved only a very unsatisfactory carbohydrate intake, acetone, albumin and sometimes red blood corpuscles appear. Acetone in the urine, in any appreciable quantity, is an indication for the setting up of an intravenous drip. The customary solution for infusion is 5 per cent glucose, but in our own practice, where only the best is still not quite good enough, we have gone over to the use of laevulose which can be given in any desired concentration, up to 50 per cent even, without damaging the vein walls and causing thrombosis. There is no point, however, in giving such high concentrations in a patient who is already dehydrated and therefore needs fluid as well, although the only disadvantage of giving too much is that there is urinary spillage before this carbohydrate can be properly made use of. An infusion rate of 0·75 g of laevulose per kg body weight per hour up to 2 g per kg body weight can be given over prolonged periods. Alternating with the laevulose solution, an infusion of Ringer's solution is much to be preferred to the traditional normal saline because the former contains a far more representative set of much-needed electrolytes, including potassium. Two litres of such intravenous therapy can make a most astonishing difference to a patient's well-being and often to the progress of her labour. The treatment of maternal distress, apart from the treatment of the cause, is not surgery but judicious intravenous therapy.

If there is any doubt about the patient's ability to empty her bladder completely, there should be no hesitation in catheterising, since it often takes very little urine in the bladder to hold up labour. The modern objections to catheterisation, on the gound that the urinary tract may be infected thereby, are less pressing in maternity units than in gynaecological or general wards where the bacterial population is much more dangerous.[18]

Until fairly recently we used to instil 50 ml of pure 1:5000 solution of chlorhexidine and leave it in the bladder at the end of catheterisation, as is the practice in our gynaecological wards, but a fairly prolonged and controlled trial of results as regards urinary infection showed no difference and we have since abandoned the practice. What really matters is that the aseptic technique should be above reproach and sterile gloves for catheterisation should always be worn. Wet, slimy hands are a bacteriological insult to any bladder. The volume of all the urine passed must be measured and charted and each specimen must be tested for specific gravity, protein and acetone. It is always surprising to me how rapidly ketonuria can develop in a woman in hard labour.

Provided the head is engaged an enema may be given, but is preferably withheld if the head is above the brim after the onset of labour, because of the danger of the membranes rupturing and the cord prolapsing unless the presenting part is well applied to the lower uterine segment. Today in fact we prescribe very few enemas and then only usually because the rectum is obviously heavily loaded with material which may soil the second stage.

The patient in normal labour can be up and about during the day, provided the head is engaged, but she should remain in bed if malpresentation is present because of the risk of cord prolapse. She should not be allowed to the toilet unaccompanied once labour is established and the door should never be locked.

Vulval pads are preferably only worn if needed for the sake of comfort because of a very copious discharge of liquor amnii. Otherwise they merely encourage infection. She can be assisted to a shower in early labour or sponged down twice daily as required.

Mobility is highly desirable until the point of labour at which analgesia is required.

A pelvic examination is made at least once every three hours, my own preference being for rectal examinations undertaken in the left lateral position to assess the station of the head and progressive dilatation of the cervix.

Preferably, the woman in labour should not find herself alone from beginning to end, and this is where the company of her husband can be so very useful. He can be taught to massage the small of her back when labour begins to get really uncomfortable towards the end of the first stage. The point to teach is that there should be no friction on the skin itself, otherwise it would become red and sore, but that the flat of the hand should be pressed firmly over the sacro-iliac joints and a slow rotatory movement made of the subcutaneous tissues against the underlying bone. The secret of the art is to observe the onset of a contraction but not to start this form of massage until the patient asks for it. The pain wears off as the massage is being continued and presently the patient attributes the natural relief of her pain with the subsidence of the contraction to the efficacy of the massage. I used to think this was quite a good confidence trick on both husband and wife until I came to appreciate the tremendous benefit from a very skilled midwife who massaged my own back when in hospital following one of my three heart operations, when I developed a really horrifying degree of faecal impaction due to the simultaneous administration of diuretics and pain-relieving drugs of the codeine variety. I can testify, though a mere male, to the reflex relaxant effect it has upon the pelvic floor.

In all cases where labour is not expeditious a high vaginal swab should be taken for bacteriological culture. The use of prophylactic antibiotics without first demonstrating the bacteriological need for them is to be deprecated, except in the case of patients with cardiac lesions who are very liable to acquire subacute bacterial endocarditis at this time. Cephaloridine is particularly suitable given intramuscularly in half- to one-gram doses twice a day. Some such antibiotic should also be given in all cases where there is even a minor degree of maternal pyrexia, when the membranes have been ruptured for some time previously, where there is established evidence of genital infection, of course, and in cases of diabetes who are additionally susceptible.[1, 2]

Most Gram-positive and many of the Gram-negative organisms encountered in prolonged labour are sensitive to cephaloridine. Sensitive organisms include staphylococci, streptococci, including *Str. viridans*, the clostridia, coliforms and *Proteus*. This drug is capable also of crossing the placental barrier in an effective concentration and will remain in the baby's serum for many hours, thus helping to protect it from infection. The drug works its way round to the liquor amnii in adequate concentration in two or three hours after administration.

We are now using a standard partogram chart for all cases in labour (see end paper). This is marked out for all of 24 hours. Where full, continuous monitoring facilities are not available the fetal heart should be recorded at least every half hour, preferably quarter-hourly, throughout the first stage, and noted immediately after every contraction in the second stage. On this chart are also recorded details of amniotic fluid and any tests of pH of fetal scalp blood. The station of the head is recorded at each pelvic examination whether rectal or vaginal; the figure zero station representing the level of the presenting part at the ischial spines, with minus 1, 2 or 3 cm for levels above and plus 1 and 2 for levels below. At station 0 +2 the head is well on the pelvic floor and visible at the vulva. The position of the head as regards sagittal suture and fontanelles is recorded at the same time, also the effacement of the cervix and the degree of dilatation from 0 to 10 cm which latter represents full dilatation. Its effacement is also recorded. The contractions (frequency, strength and duration) are likewise charted and the concentration or dosage of Syntocinon or prostaglandin are recorded in milliunits per minute or milligrammes respectively. On the same partogram analgesics and their timing are also recorded, also epidural anaesthesia and all amounts used for topping up. There is a space for remarks, and fluid amounts, for example from vomitus, are also recorded. The blood pressure and pulse and also details of the urine complete a really comprehensive chart which gives a total bird's-eye view of any given labour without the necessity for thumbing through dangerously thick folders of notes. Furthermore, having to complete this partogram ensures the correct discipline of supervision.

In addition to all the above it need hardly be reiterated that a pelvic examination should be undertaken as soon as possible after the membranes rupture, if they have not been ruptured earlier. This is principally to exclude prolapse of the cord at this time and to take note of the state of the cervix and how well the presenting part settles on the lower uterine segment.

In the second stage of labour the patient must never be left even for a brief moment and she should not be encouraged in active pushing until the head is clearly visible at the vulva and beginning to distend the pelvic floor. At this time the anus will appear to open and the anterior wall of the rectal canal can be seen. Gone are the days when we used to exhort the patient to take a deep breath, hold it and push, and many is the subconjunctival haemorrhage I have seen in the past following labour of this slave-driven type. It is only ineffective and encourages subsequent prolapse, not only in the patient but sometimes, I feel, in the case of sympathetic bystanders as well. The patient will push soon enough involuntarily when the head gets sufficiently low on the pelvic floor and encouragement to push should be reserved until then. Until this stage the patient should make full use of self-administered analgesia such as Entonox nitrous oxide and oxygen mixture, so that her plasma becomes progressively saturated and its effect is more immediately available following the onset of subsequent contractions.

Our midwives are instructed to ensure the presence of a doctor if delivery is not evidently imminent after 20 minutes in the second stage, or if organised pushing for this period appears to be ineffective. An early decision can therefore be made as to the desirability of episiotomy and possibly low forceps or ventouse assistance. In the old days medical help was only sought after two hours of ineffectual pushing by which time the state of both mother and child was considerably worse.

A doctor must also be present in all cases where third-stage problems are anticipated such as when there has been a history of postpartum haemorrhage or of retained placenta in a previous labour, in all cases of grand multiparity (para 5 and over) and where labour has been stimulated or accelerated by the administration of oxytocic drugs.

Throughout the second stage the fetal heart should be noted as soon as possible after each contraction has worn off. It is here particularly that anomalies of fetal heart rate can be missed without continuous monitoring by electronic means.

In common with many modern and well equipped up-to-date obstetric units we are in the happy position of being able to monitor every case in labour, except those cases who are already well advanced in obviously progressing and satisfactory labour. In other less extravagantly equipped units monitoring facilities have to be reserved for problem cases, but further clinical observation and recordings as described on a proper partogram chart go most of the way towards meeting the problems of fetal and maternal distress. The emphasis is on the standard of thoroughness.

The staff of the labour suite should notify the Paediatric Department in the following categories of cases, firstly during labour, so that an incubator can be in readiness and secondly when delivery is imminent, so that a member of the paediatric staff can be in attendance to receive the baby:

1. Pre-term labour (37 weeks gestation or under);
2. Fetal distress;
3. Breech delivery;
4. Caesarean section;
5. Twin delivery;
6. Diabetic mother;
7. Where morphine or Omnopon have been given within 4 or 5 hours, or intravenous pethidine within the previous hour;
8. Rh iso-immunisation cases;
9. Forceps deliveries;
10. Ventouse deliveries;
11. Antepartum haemorrhage of all varieties;
12. Severe pre-eclampsia or eclampsia;
13. Polyhydramnios;
14. Previous siblings with a known congenital defect.

The justification for routine continuous intrapartum fetal monitoring is rapidly becoming more clear to those of us employing it. The perinatal mortality is significantly reduced primarily by the elimination of intrapartum stillbirths which, except for gross degrees of fetal abnormality, are usually preventable, and with it there is a significant lowering of neonatal mortality from injuries, stresses and infections inflicted during labour. This has been achieved without an increase in the incidence of Caesarean section; in fact the reverse is true[21] because more discrimination can be employed in estimating the significance of clinical signs of apparent fetal distress. The result is that Caesarean section, when indicated, is more readily undertaken before damage is done; on the other hand fewer cases are unnecessarily delivered abdominally, with a baby full of vigorous protest and obviously not in need of such intervention. This double benefit of lowered perinatal mortality combined with lowered incidence of Caesarean section is an irrefutable vindication of an apparently extravagant technique.

FETAL DISTRESS

The term Fetal Distress covers a number of ugly realities of which hypoxia is only one, albeit the chief one. Other contributory factors in fetal distress are antecedent subnutrition in the uterus due to placental inadequacy from a very large variety of causes, including partial separation, mechanical stresses in labour, intra-uterine infection and the action of drugs. Our methods of assessing the baby's well-being, or the reverse, before birth are extremely crude and depend mainly on observation of the fetal heart rate and the passage of meconium. A combination of slowing and irregularity is the most serious, while slowing alone to below 120 beats a minute is significant, and below 100 a minute more sinister. Fetal tachycardia above 160 may provide an earlier warning of trouble to come.

Alterations in the fetal heart rate are therefore not necessarily due to hypoxia but to other causes and so-called fetal distress does not necessarily mean fetal hypoxia. It is often thought that unexpected death before delivery is due to inadequate fetal heart monitoring, but this is not necessarily so. Nevertheless one has to recognise three mains classes of cause in fetal bradycardia. One results from head compression and the slowing is related to the contractions both in timing and severity. The second variety involves cord compression which is more variable in its relationship to the contractions and may produce a type of vasovagal response in the baby. Both these classes affect the bowel by vagal stimulation and consequently meconium is passed. It is not true however to say "no death without defaecation." Stillbirth can indeed occasionally occur without the passage of meconium and conversely, as is explained further on, some babies can be delivered coated with meconium and yet be fighting fit at delivery. In the third and more difficult class of uteroplacental insufficiency, which may be aggravated by oxytocin, there is sometimes a more delayed type of slowing in relation to the uterine contractions.

The clinical observations leading up to the diagnosis of fetal distress do not sufficiently distinguish between the three types mentioned above, of which the last is probably the most treacherous because fetal death may occur with less warning.

Continuous fetal monitoring.—The value of this is established beyond all doubt. It involves a simultaneous study of alterations in fetal heart rate and uterine contractile activity. It is almost impossible to achieve this in any meaningful way without resorting to specialised electronic apparatus. The clinical signs of fetal distress are: significant alterations in fetal heart rate, irregularity in rhythm, slowness to recover a normal rate after decelerating as a result of uterine contraction, meconium in the liquor amnii and excessive or tumultuous fetal movements. By the time these clinical signs are fully recognised it may be already too late and the baby may be either severely hypoxic or sometimes damaged beyond recovery. Most of us now agree with Beard and his colleagues in the course of the last ten years that what is wanted is an early-warning system which can detect the threat of fetal asphyxia and acidosis in advance. This is in fact now available by simultaneous recording for which a variety of quite expensive but excellent pieces of apparatus are commercially available.

It was Hon however who in the late '50s pioneered the study of continuous fetal heart rate changes but in those days was handicapped by having to apply electrodes to the abdominal wall by means of suction cups.[23] The fetal ECG was invariably overshadowed by maternal electrocardiographic patterns and deciphering the traces was, as I well remember, very difficult in spite of all sorts of filtration techniques. The initial objective was to detect early fetal life from 16 weeks onwards, and it was claimed that the technique might also be helpful in diagnosing twins. Since those early pioneering days, which also included attempts at phonocardiography, which was never really satisfactory because of interference and fetal movements, the technique has been enormously simplified by the use of the ultrasonic Doppler effect and even more reliably still by the application of electrodes direct to the fetal scalp.

There is no excuse however for neglecting to obtain continuous records of the fetal heart for want of expensive apparatus. This can be done even in poorly equipped units by using a simple fetal heart rate detector working on the ultrasonic Doppler principle, applying the transducer to the abdominal wall and counting the number of beats for each ten seconds. With such a detector, fetal heart sounds can be observed right throughout a contraction and uterine contractions are recorded at the same time by abdominal palpation. Carefully performed, results are thoroughly worthwhile and match up almost to those obtained by the most sophisticated monitoring techniques.[49]

The normal combined monitoring trace is illustrated in Fig. 2, in which the rate does not vary outside the limits of 120 to 160 beats per minute and any alterations, mainly decelerations, occur synchronously with the uterine contractions and, even then, by not more than about 30 beats per minute. At the same time the uterine tocographic trace should show good relaxation between contractions which allows time for the restoration of placental circulation. Such variations were classed by Kubli *et al.*[25] as minor and therefore innocuous. They also regarded absence of minor beat-to-beat variation as an unfavourable sign. Early dips in fetal heart rate can be caused by fetal head compression, for example while passing through the brim, or later in the second stage, but provided they are not excessive and do not lag behind the peak of uterine contraction do not signify immediate fetal danger. These are commonly referred to as Type I Caldeyro-Barcia dips. Really ominous are the Type II dips or as they are better described "late decelerations" with slow recovery as in Fig. 3. Such a record indicates the establishment of severe fetal hypoxia and distress. Baseline tachycardia and bradycardia outside the above limits are mainly significant if alterations in the fetal heart rate are provoked by uterine contraction. Any lag-phase in deceleration, i.e. one extending into the period between uterine contractions and recovering slowly, increases the importance of abnormal baseline figures.

A loss of beat-to-beat variation is defined as variations of five or less beats per minute. One must take into account however that the previous administration of diazepam reduces beat-to-beat variation. Baseline bradycardia is more serious than tachycardia, but in either case it is the timing and depth of the dips which is significant. Between these two extremes are a number of variable patterns and attempts are often made to distinguish between cord compression and uteroplacental insufficiency. The greater the deceleration, the worse the fetal asphyxia and with later deceleration the situation is worse still. An extreme example is shown in Fig. 4 in which it can be seen that there is a hypertonic type of uterine activity with very poor

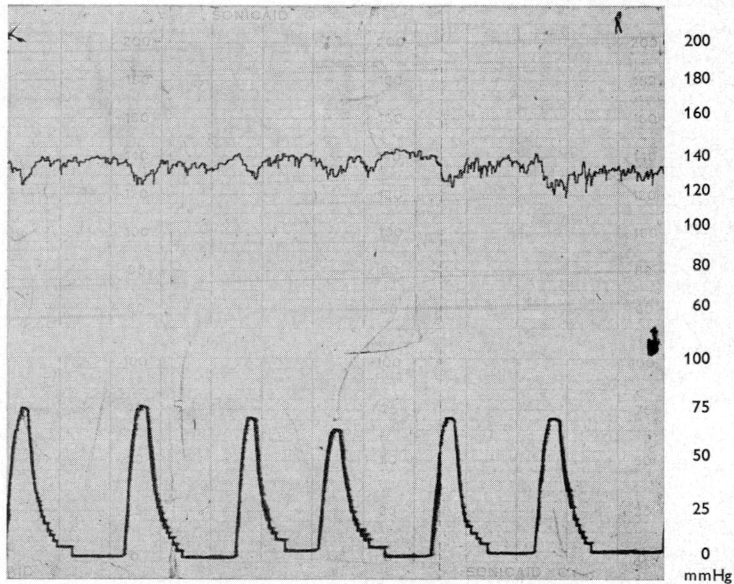

18/Fig. 2.—Normal combined monitoring trace. Upper line records the fetal heart rate and shows good beat-to-beat variation and decelerations of less than 20 beats per minute, mostly synchronous with uterine contractions. Lower line is a tocographic record of normal uterine action, with well-timed co-ordinated pressure rises and good relaxation between contractions. Spontaneous delivery.

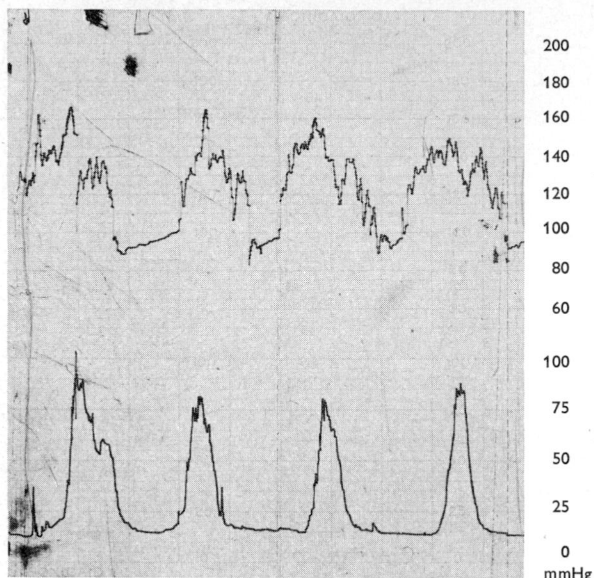

18/Fig. 3.—Late deceleration in fetal heart rate with considerable lag-time following uterine contractions. Recovery is also slow. The patient, though para 5, had not been pregnant in 7 years and because of fetal distress shortly thereafter required delivery by mid-cavity forceps. The baby weighed 3·43 kg and became hypoglycaemic.

relaxation. This is accompanied by a steadily rising baseline tachycardia and then finally a drop to below recordable levels. In this figure the scribbled word "TRUE" indicates the authenticity of this record. Delivery with such a pattern is urgent.

More usually however the early warning signs provided by continuous monitoring provide an indication for fetal blood sampling as described below and, if heeded early enough, time is usually available to determine the fetal blood pH and therefore the degree of acidosis which finally indicates the asphyxial state or otherwise of the baby.

Cord accidents such as compression from tight winding round the fetal neck or knotting (Fig. 5) cannot be foreseen clinically but warning of danger may be provided by an abnormal monitoring trace. At the first sign of trouble one must make sure to keep the patient turned off her back and if an oxytocin drip is running it should be slowed down or stopped until the fetus shows signs of recovery. Apart from degrees of fetal abnormality incompatible with survival, fresh stillbirth on such a regime should be regarded as an avoidable tragedy.

Before membrane rupture one has to resort to the ultrasonic

Doppler method but this may require frequent readjustment of the position of the transducer head. A really accurate method of fetal heart rate monitoring depends upon scalp electrodes. These are of several types and all require partial dilatation of the cervix for their application and of course membranes already ruptured. The first of these was the clip electrode applied with a special forceps but even

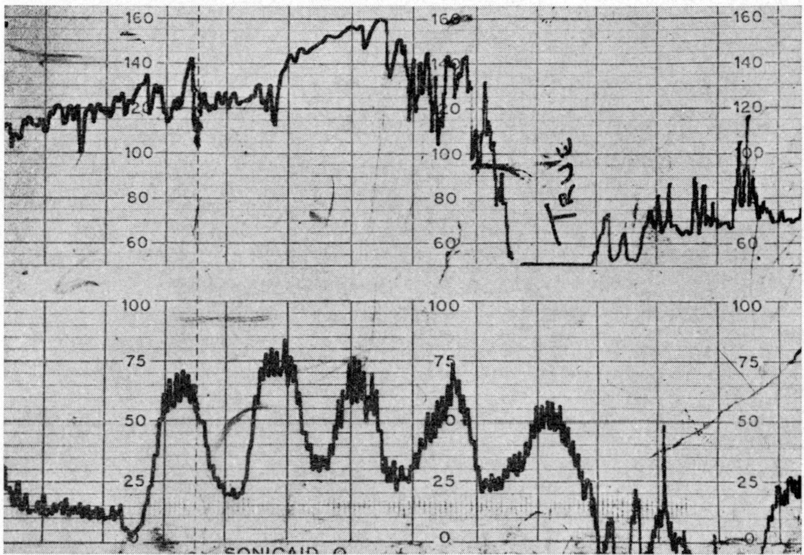

18/Fig. 4.—Effects of overstimulation by oxytocin. Note the uterine hypertonus with failure to relax properly. The effect on the fetus was a rising tachycardia initially, then a catastrophic deceleration to below recordable level. There was some recovery after turning off the oxytocin infusion but delivery by Caesarean section was necessary.

simpler was the hook-type electrode which can be home-made, using a bit of insulated armature wire from which the insulation has been removed for the last half-centimetre. This is passed through a 23-gauge disposable needle so that the half-centimetre of exposed electrode tip protrudes. This exposed tip is now bent over like a fish-hook but parallel to the shaft of the needle. The needle itself is bent to an angle of about 30° to facilitate application through the cervix and after suitable sterile precautions the needle can be driven tangentially into the scalp either through an amnioscope under direct vision, or by direct digital manipulation, taking care not to puncture the glove which is all too easy. The syringe needle is now slid back over the wire, the other end of which is connected up to the recording apparatus, along with a neutral electrode from maternal abdomen or thigh. Better still, though more expensive, is the spiral screw type electrode which is pressed directly against the fetal scalp and twisted clockwise until the screw is truly home and unlikely to be dislodged.

I am not satisfied in my own mind that the desire to apply a scalp electrode in itself justifies amniotomy sooner than need be since, with trouble and care, ultrasonic records, especially with multi-head transducers can be very satisfactory.

Whenever any labour, induced or spontaneous, is being urged on with oxytocin administration, particular note should be taken of the uterine tocographic trace since excessive dosage may produce an abnormal pattern; either excessive tone, too frequent contractions, or variable colicky types.

Ideally contractions should come about three in every ten minutes with full relaxation between. Peak pressures of 75 mm Hg are normal. In the second stage, of course, the addition of maternal expulsive

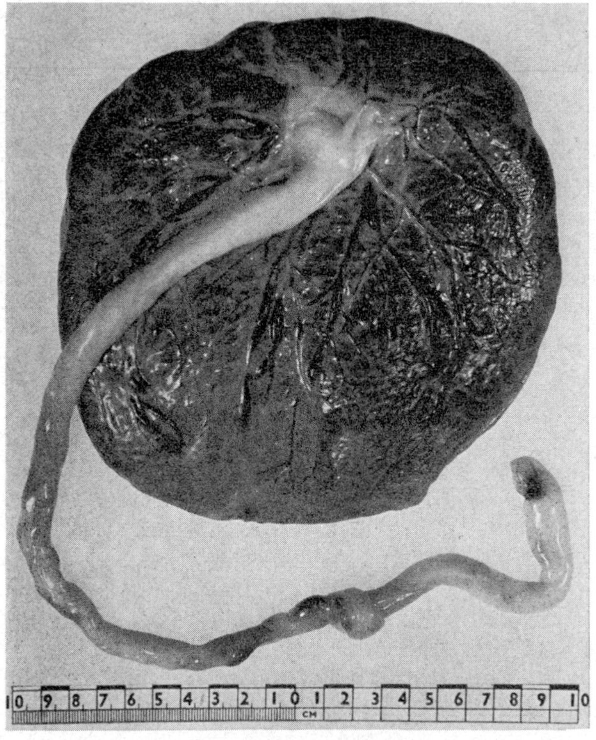

18/FIG. 5.—A true knot in the cord. It resulted in the baby being freshly stillborn.

effort enormously increases the overall pressure applied to well over 100 mm Hg.

Fetal acidosis.—An interest in the biochemistry of fetal distress may contribute more both to the understanding and treatment.[55] Fetal acidosis in labour may be of two types, namely, metabolic and respiratory, of which the metabolic is the commoner and more serious and it is to some extent related to maternal acidosis which usually appears during the last two hours of labour.[44] Measurements of base excess, the metabolic component of the acid base balance, may indeed indicate fetal acidosis and imminent fetal distress and it is possible to reduce both maternal and fetal acidosis by the administration of sodium bicarbonate in standard solution of 155 mEq per litre. Running the infusion rate at about 2·5 ml per minute up to 6 ml per minute is the recommended dosage.[44] In the assessment of fetal distress, the only accurate method is to look at the fetal blood itself and herein lies the importance of Saling's work.[45, 46]

One of the amazing compensatory factors in fetal physiology at birth is the ability of the central nervous system, and in fact the baby as a whole, to survive quite prolonged periods of hypoxia by resorting to anaerobic metabolism which is many times less efficient than standard aerobic metabolism of carbohydrates but adequate to sustain life. Anaerobic metabolism depends upon an adequate supply of glycogen, an increasing amount of which is laid down in the tissues, notably the liver and myocardium, as term and the stresses of labour approach. The brain stores no glycogen and is dependent upon an active circulation of glucose derived from glycogen to keep it alive. Tissue glycogen is broken down first to lactic acid and then in the presence of oxygen converted to pyruvic acid. When anaerobic metabolism occurs because of the lack of oxygen, the lactic acid is not thus converted and an assessment of the lactic/pyruvic acid ratio gives an index of anaerobic metabolism. It will be seen therefore that a prolonged period of hypoxia will use up glycogen to a more deadly degree than a brief episode of fetal distress late in the second stage. This accounts for the ready response of the latter type of case to resuscitation at birth even though the baby is coated with thick, fresh meconium, whereas the baby who has been chronically deprived of oxygen, and therefore in the ultimate stages of glycogen depletion (without which there is no life), may die with far less dramatic warning.

Amnioscopy

No death without defaecation. This would appear to be the basis of Saling's theorem that the threat to fetal life can be foreseen by observing meconium in the liquor amnii. Although this is not invariably the case, nevertheless the association of meconium and asphyxia, or perhaps in the more important negative sense of fetal health and clear liquor, is sufficiently common to make observation in the liquor thoroughly worth while. I have frequently been infuriated by juniors who rupture the membranes in the course of vaginal examination in labour and give as their excuse that they wanted to see if there was any meconium in the liquor. There is now no such excuse for this mischievous habit because the liquor can be viewed through the intact bag of forewaters by means of one of Saling's conical amnioscopes.

The sight of clear liquor with flakes of white vernix floating within it is certainly reassuring that all for the moment is well. As long as a finger can be got through the cervix it is possible to introduce one of these amnioscope specula which are conical and have an obturator rather like that in a proctoscope. The sight of clear liquor may encourage one to hold off inducing labour because of suspected placental inadequacy, particularly in association with postmaturity for example. I have found that the use of the lithotomy position is by no means invariably necessary; in fact in the apprehensive patient and particularly in the case of one not already in labour, the full left lateral Sims' position is much less distressing. Whichever position is used it is important to protect the sensitive lower anterior vaginal wall from pressure. Therefore it is recommended that after inserting two fingers in the vagina to protect the subpubic region and turning the palmar surfaces of the fingers backwards, the amnioscope should be introduced with the pressure directed onto the perineum. In this way the point can be guided into the cervical canal with very little discomfort. If the liquor looks meconium-loaded it is a simple matter to rupture the membranes there and then under direct vision. The use of a mattress wedge to tilt the patient 10 to 15 degrees to one side when in the lithotomy position obviates the additional hazard of inferior vena caval occlusion and is now our general practice.

Fetal blood sampling.—This can be undertaken at any stage of labour after the membranes are ruptured; again my own preference is for the left lateral position, although the lithotomy position is more commonly employed. The technique has been fully described by Morris and Beard.[36] The speculum is applied to the fetal caput which is wiped clean with small swabs, for which purpose dental swabs are admirable, and the area under review is then sprayed with ethyl chloride in order to make it hyperaemic and to "arteriolise" the capillary blood as far as possible. The skin is painted with a little silicone jelly to encourage the formation of a proper globule of blood on puncturing it, and then a stab is made with a guarded knife whose blade projects beyond the holder no more than 2 mm. Very often one fails to draw blood adequately and an attempt to make a small linear incision is defeated by the scalp moving with the knife. The lower the head in labour, the easier is this manoeuvre to carry out. Once a drop of blood forms at the puncture site it is aspirated carefully into a heparinised capillary tube. It is important to obtain an unbroken column of blood within this tube especially if it is proposed to undertake P_{CO_2} measurements. Sometimes bleeding is embarrassingly persistent from the scalp and the only method of stopping it is to apply continued pressure. The blood sample should be examined as soon as possible, preferably within a matter of minutes and the first observation is the fetal pH. Admittedly a low figure may not be abnormal if much of this is due to maternal acidosis.[3] On the other hand a pH above 7·25 indicates that the baby is not in severe fetal distress even before undertaking further micro-Astrup measurements of fetal acid-base status. Sometimes there is difficulty in applying the rim of the amnioscope satisfactorily to the fetal scalp and liquor amnii or maternal blood may leak under its margins and thus contaminate the sample. Also the site of puncture may be lost by fetal or maternal movement. In these cases a suction amnioscope can be used, i.e. one with a suction rim round its margins and connected to a ventouse vacuum pump so that fixation by suction can be rapidly obtained at approximately 0·5 kg/cm^2. The results of the blood sample correlate perfectly well with those obtained by using the standard amnioscope.[6, 7]

A very extensive experience has been obtained in Queen Charlotte's Hospital which the rest of us throughout the country are now belatedly following up, because it is quite clear to all that far too many Caesarean sections are being unnecessarily undertaken for a diagnosis of fetal distress, which the baby refutes by crying lustily at birth. There was indeed a reduction straightaway in the Caesarean section rate, purely for fetal distress, at Queen Charlotte's Hospital, from 49 cases in 1964 to 26 in 1965, and it is unusual to perform the operation for clinical signs of fetal distress if the pH is within normal limits.[4, 5] However, where the fetal pH is low and particularly if it is less than 7·2, the evidence of fetal asphyxia must be regarded as overwhelming. A level of 7·1 represents greater danger and 6·9 is practically incompatible with fetal survival. In the first few minutes after birth acidosis is likely to be even worse and the possible association of severe and prolonged degrees with subsequent neurological damage is worth bearing in mind.

Pain-relieving Drugs

The majority of mortals faced with the ordeal of severe pain need, and therefore deserve, drugs of one sort or another to make it tolerable. If psychoprophylactic methods could eliminate the need for pain relief by drugs, labour itself would undoubtedly benefit and the baby would be spared the depressant effects upon its centres, which all such drugs, in some degree, are bound to inflict. The performance of the uterus throughout labour and particularly in the third stage would likewise be more physiological. Everything, unfortunately, has its price and nothing in this world can be got for nothing. Drugs are no exception, since none is wholly without penalty and no drug yet devised can ever be both harmless and effective at the same time.

As far as possible, however, such drugs should conform to the following criteria:

(*a*) They should effectively relieve pain;
(*b*) They should not cause fetal respiratory depression;
(*c*) The course of labour should not be adversely affected and in particular the ability of the uterus to maintain retraction should in no way be undermined;
(*d*) Elimination should be rapid in order to prevent accumulation;
(*e*) The safety margin should be wide and there should be no undesirable side-effects.

All the above is asking too much.

Sedatives

The best that can be said for sedatives is that they are harmless. They may, in the very early stages of labour, encourage the patient to have a ration of sleep before labour really gets under way and this is useful in the nervous patient, who then has a chance to wake up some hours later with labour convincingly established. Nitrazepam 5 to 10 mg by mouth is our present favourite.

Hypnotics

These, of which the barbiturates form the most important group, have no effect in raising the pain threshold but allay anxiety and may promote sleep. Only the short-acting drugs of this class should be employed, such as Seconal (quinalbarbitone) or Amytal (amylobarbitone) or Nembutal (pentobarbitone) in doses of up to 0·2 g. The longer-acting barbiturates may seriously depress the fetus at birth. Unfortunately the baby's respiratory centres are extremely susceptible to barbiturates, particularly in prematurity and unfortunately these undesirable effects may persist for quite a few days after birth, the baby remaining sleepy with sluggish reflexes, disinclination to feed and with a fall in body temperature. As for labour itself, the woman becomes unco-operative and is the more likely to require assistance in the second stage on that account. These drugs have the further effect of depressing maternal respiration as well which is undesirable, particularly in a patient who may subsequently require general anaesthesia.

Basal Narcotics

These are more potent and the safest is undoubtedly paraldehyde, since it does not cause much respiratory or circulatory depression. Between 70 to 80 per cent of the drug is destroyed within the body and the remainder is excreted through the lungs, so that all within range suffer the smell which, to the majority of people, is most unpleasant. It is much too hateful to take by mouth, but it used to be traditional practice to give it per rectum, in doses of freshly prepared 10 per cent solution, 5 ml per kg of body weight up to a maximum of 300 ml. This route is messy and uncertain, especially as the patient is liable to return some of it before it is all absorbed leaving one in doubt about how much she has retained. The best way to give paraldehyde is by deep intramuscular injection (although some give it intravenously in eclampsia). The dose by intramuscular injection is from 5 to 10 ml and the injection must be deep or considerable pain and, later, an abscess may be caused. If it were not for its smell this drug would undoubtedly be used more, since it does not interfere with uterine action and produces considerable lethargy and quite a deep sleep. Unfortunately its action is not very prolonged and the patient may be clamouring for further relief at the end of three hours.

Narcotics

Pethidine (Demerol) is 1-methyl-4-phenyl piperidine-4-carboxylic acid ester hydrochloride and is every bit as effective as morphine in relieving pain. There is probably no drug which can produce addiction quite so fast as pethidine, it is said even within twenty-four hours, and it is for this reason that its use is almost wholly restricted to relieving the pain of dying or of child-bearing, neither of which can be described as constantly recurring conditions or providing the setting for addiction. Pharmacologically pethidine is analgesic, sedative and antispasmodic. One hundred mg of pethidine should be reckoned as the equivalent of 10 mg of morphine and therefore the usual 100 mg dose is too small to alleviate the pains of strong labour. Even when given in larger doses, and one can safely go up to 200 mg, pain relief is likely to be much more satisfactory if hyoscine is given at the same time.[22] By using hyoscine the dosage of pethidine can be reduced.

Pethidine would appear to be less likely to cause third-stage uterine atony than morphine but its effects on the fetal respiratory centre are just as bad. Some patients vomit repeatedly after morphine whereas pethidine seldom produces this undesirable side-effect.

Labour should be well established before pethidine is given in order to allow one the opportunity to assess a patient's likely analgesic needs and to avoid "shooting one's bolt" too soon. Certainly the os should be showing signs of dilatation, preferably over two fingersbreadth in a primigravida and up to this amount in a multipara. Normally one would expect to have to give the second dose at about three-quarters dilatation of the cervix and 150 mg of pethidine alone at this point may suffice. One has to remember that the effect should preferably have worn off by the end of the second stage so that the baby will not require special resuscitation. The primigravida is likely to need at least two injections of pethidine unless labour is very expeditious. If it is prolonged she will need many more, but it is better to give repeated doses than doses which are too large.

What usually happens in our practice nowadays is to go straight ahead with an epidural anaesthetic if one dose of pethidine does not last long enough or is ineffective.

Pethidine can be given intravenously, but in reduced dosage and very slowly over a few minutes, because of the sudden respiratory depression which intravenous injections produce. I once, and only once, gave 200 mg of pethidine intravenously and the apnoea which followed quite horrified me! This route should be reserved for acute cases such as the multipara who insists on bearing down before full dilatation. The intravenous dose of pethidine should not exceed 50 mg and hyoscine 0·4 mg may, with advantage, be added, but less may suffice. Apart from sudden repiratory depression, rapid intravenous injection may produce dizziness, nausea and vomiting of a very unpleasant degree, hence the need to give the injection slowly, preferably diluted in at least 10 ml of saline.

A study of respiratory minute volumes in newborn infants was made by Roberts and Please (1958) and Roberts *et al.* (1957), using a trip spirometer (Donald and Lord, 1953), and they found that pethidine, even in average doses, is capable of reducing these volumes, particularly during the first few hours of life. Fortunately we have antagonist drugs in the form of nor-allylnormorphine (nalorphine) and levallorphan. If 1 mg of such an antagonist is combined with 100 mg of pethidine the analgesic effect is considered to be little if at all diminished and the respiratory depression of the infant is very markedly reduced.

Levallorphan is available combined with pethidine in suitable dosage as indicated above and marketed as Pethilorfan. Where this precaution has not been taken earlier in labour, nalorphine can be administered to the mother during the second stage to counteract the narcotic effect on the baby's respiratory centre and the dose intravenously for this purpose is 5 to 10 mg. Most of us, however, prefer to await the arrival of the baby to see if nalorphine is even necessary. Given intravenously into the umbilical vein in a dose of 0·2 to 0·5 mg it will immediately correct the depressant effects of not only pethidine but morphine, Omnopon, heroin and the other drugs of this class, but it is useless against other pain-relieving drugs and, if given either unnecessarily or in excessive dosage, may of itself produce excessive cerebral stimulation of the baby or more likely a severe respiratory depression which may be very hard to counteract. Naloxone (Narcan) is an alternative and has now been cleared by the Committee on Safety of Medicines. It has the advantage of being purely an antagonist to morphine, pethidine and also pentazocine.

Our own practice is to use morphine or Omnopon or heroin very seldom late in labour, but we rely upon pethidine and counteract its effects upon the baby, if necessary, with nalorphine. Pentazocine (Fortral) is reputed to have a pethidine type of action as regards pain relief because less crosses the placenta into the fetal circulation and it is less addictive. Its effect however is rather brief.

Morphine will always have a place in the relief of pain in labour, although it has been largely replaced by pethidine. Of its power to elevate the pain threshold there can be no doubt, producing relaxation, apathy, lethargy and sleep. The patients often wake up from it without any appreciation of the hours of suffering which they have been spared and I can recall my singular lack of gratitude for it in periods of great pain in my own life. Morphine, of course, in common with drugs of this class and power, besides depressing the respiratory centres of the baby, has the characteristic disadvantages of encouraging uterine atony, which in the third stage can be positively dangerous, and occasionally of inducing vomiting in the patient; nevertheless, many labours, inert because of anxiety and tension on the part of the patient, are paradoxically hastened by the mental apathy which morphine induces.

Heroin, like morphine, is a useful drug with similar applications. The dose can be varied between 10 mg and 2·5 mg. The usual dose is 5 mg. Like morphine it depresses respiration in the mother as well, but its analgesic action is both rapid and profound, and in prolonged difficult and colicky labours the drug is unquestionably of very great value.

Tranquillisers

These have more to offer in the control of pain in labour than would at first have been expected. Amongst their many pharmacological properties, which have been described as vagolytic, sympatholytic, sedative and anti-emetic, their greatest use in labour is their undoubted power of potentiating the activity of a number of drugs acting upon the central nervous system, i.e. anaesthetics, hypnotics and analgesics. The common tranquillisers used in obstetrics are chlorpromazine (Largactil) and promazine (Sparine). An example of the use of this synergistic action is provided by Lacomme *et al.* (1952) who devised a "lytic cocktail" which consisted of an infusion of 500 ml of pyrogen-free glucose saline containing 50 mg of chlorpromazine and 100 mg of pethidine, the drip being run fairly rapidly until the patient showed signs of pain relief when the drip rate was cut back to 30–50 drops per minute and subsequently adjusted according to her needs. Another method of administering tranquillising drugs is the injection of a combination of:

Pethidine	100 mg
Chlorpromazine	50 mg
Promethazine	50 mg
Distilled water to 20 ml	

Of this solution 2 to 3 ml may be given intravenously when labour is established and repeated as necessary intramuscularly.

In our own practice we prefer promazine to chlorpromazine, having had one very troublesome case of jaundice which was attributed to the latter. The danger of agranulocytosis has also to be borne in mind. Promazine (Sparine), on the other hand, has proved of the greatest value and would appear to have a very high safety factor. Given slowly by intravenous injection in the form of promazine 50 mg, pethidine 50 mg, and hyoscine 0·4 mg even the most hysterical and colicky type of patient "keels over" in a few seconds and may sleep for several hours without apparent respiratory depression and may thereafter be found to be at full dilatation of the cervix or nearly so within that time. Nevertheless, behaviour may be unpredictable and the patient should be constantly supervised after such treatment. The hyoscine is most likely to be responsible for this and more often nowadays we inject 50 mg of promazine intravenously first, observe the effect, and reinforce it, if necessary, within half an hour with 100 mg of pethidine intramuscularly. The combination is certainly most useful.

Promazine hydrochloride is a member of the phenothiazine group of drugs and is regarded as one of the least toxic members of this family. Besides its useful anti-emetic effects it reduces the amount of pethidine required by potentiating the latter's analgesic effect and although inducing relaxation and even sleep between injections, does not interfere with the physiological course of labour. It is also safe even in premature labour, since there is no fetal respiratory or circulatory depression.

Thrombophlebitis is a very rare complication after intravenous injection, but is most easily avoided by diluting the Sparine with saline and avoiding concentrations higher than 25 mg per ml. Such an injection should also be made very slowly.

Promazine is believed to be safer than chlorpromazine as far as the fetus is concerned since the phenothiazine which has been detected in the urine of babies whose mothers have been given the latter, has not been found in either fetal blood or urine after promazine, even though it has been given intravenously and Pollock *et al.* (1960) doubt if Sparine crosses the placental barrier in significant amounts. Experiences in our own unit with this drug have been reviewed by MacVicar and Murray (1960) and our favourable view of the drug continues to this day.

Tachycardia sometimes occurs but would appear to be the only noteworthy side-effect from Sparine. The course of labour is not slowed up, but rather the reverse. So far we have not observed any untoward effect on the baby, nor upon its respiratory centre at birth. The happy property of this drug would appear to be its ability to induce a state in the patient of unawareness of her present miseries, a sort of "medical leucotomy". In our view Sparine is one of the most important drugs to have been introduced into obstetrics since the discovery of pethidine.

On the whole we tend to distrust polypharmacy in labour and combinations of drugs should be used sparingly. However, not only may Sparine potentiate the analgesic properties of pethidine but Phenergan (25 mg by injection) is also useful.

One should always bear in mind the possible effects of any drugs used on subsequent general anaesthesia. Although Sparine is unlikely to produce a hypotensive effect in the customary thiopentone/relaxant/nitrous-oxide/oxygen technique, a severe fall in blood pressure may occur if halothane is used; in any case an unpopular anaesthetic because of its encouragement of atonic postpartum haemorrhage. Promazine however should not be used if spinal or epidural anaesthesia is in the offing.[15, 20] Our steadily increasing use of epidural anaesthesia is now pushing this medication into the background. A reminder here could profitably be given that anaesthetists should always be informed of all drugs administered before his advent, so that he may be on the lookout for rare cases of untoward interaction between the drugs and subsequent anaesthetic agents.

Sedatives and analgesic drugs should be used very sparingly in cases of hypotonic inertia and mainly reserved to ensure, if necessary, a good night's sleep, but in the hypertonic types these drugs can be used far more liberally, where, by allaying the patient's anxiety and fear, quite apart from relieving her pain, they may have the paradoxical effect of accelerating the course of labour.

Inhalation Analgesics (Self-administered)

These all have the advantage of rapidity of effect and reversibility on discontinuing the administration. Ever since Queen Victoria had the pains of childbirth relieved by intermittent whiffs of chloroform (*narcose à la reine*) this method of analgesia has never lost ground.

Chloroform may be dead but it will not lie down. In all the years of anaesthetic history nothing has yet been found quite so handy, unobjectionable and effective in domiciliary practice. Unfortunately coroners take a very hard view of its use in spite of the great skill and safety achieved with it by an older generation of obstetricians. Its free vaporisation in a Junker inhaler greatly increases the safety of administration as compared with the drop-on mask technique, as dangerous concentrations are avoided thereby and it takes quite a lot of hard bag-squeezing to produce real anaesthesia with a Junker machine.

Chloroform becomes dangerous when there is much adrenaline being secreted by the patient, where administration is prolonged, when induction is repeated several times, and when the patient has a period of apnoea and a dangerously high concentration is allowed to accumulate under the mask for the patient suddenly to inspire, but these objections cannot apply to self-administration techniques. Chloroform undoubtedly depresses uterine activity and may increase the incidence of postpartum haemorrhage and since it crosses the placenta it may seriously depress the fetus. Its powerful and untoward effects on the heart in a small fraction of cases, however, are nowadays thought to cancel out its advantages, namely smooth and rapid action, convenience and efficacy. The great tragedy is that nothing, as yet, has fully taken its place in domiciliary practice.

Ether

This is much too slow and certainly too hateful to a conscious patient to be used for analgesia, although the admixture of chloroform, 1 part in 8, will take a great deal of the nastiness out of ether.

Nitrous Oxide and Air

The natural death of this type of analgesia is long overdue. The Minnitt apparatus which had a very long innings since well before the last war, gives an unreliable mixture which in any case is bad but, even worse, has been found to give the lowest oxygen concentrations at low respiratory minute volumes so that patients already suffering from respiratory depression are likely to be rendered even more hypoxic.[32] It delivers a 50/50 mixture of nitrous oxide and air. This means that the amount of oxygen administered is likewise cut by half, producing a state of mild hypoxia in the mother and even worse in the baby. Fetal distress due to hypoxia can be seriously aggravated by such an oxygen-impoverished mixture. The maternal contra-indications to its use are (1) marked cardiac disease; (2) pulmonary diseases; (3) hypertensive states; and (4) anaemia.

Nitrous Oxide and Oxygen

This is easily the most satisfactory of the inhalant analgesics since the full effect from nitrous oxide can be obtained by increasing the concentration up to between 70 and 80 per cent while the mother still obtains a normal supply of oxygen or even better. A commonly used apparatus in this country has been the Lucy Baldwin machine, which unfortunately is both expensive and heavy, thus somewhat offsetting its other obvious advantages. The use of the machine should, however, be supervised and care taken to see that the oxygen cylinders do not run out.

Undoubtedly the handiest method of administering nitrous oxide and oxygen analgesic mixtures is to use premixed gas cylinders with the Entonox delivery apparatus which supplies a 50/50 nitrous oxide and oxygen mixture. With us this has become the standard method. This, however, has one hazard which might be encountered if the cylinder is left out of doors and subjected to freezing, so that a phase separation may occur, as the two gases will vaporise again at different temperatures. The danger is mainly confined to cylinders which are not completely full, but even a temperature no lower than −8 °C in the case of a half-full cylinder may cause phase separation. Our senior anaesthetist, Moir, has recommended certain safety precautions such as that the cylinders must never be stored in open or unheated buildings and before use they should be inverted or rolled on the floor two or three times to make sure that the nitrous oxide and oxygen are truly mixed, and that if the cylinders have been allowed to get cold outside, below freezing point, they should be stood for five minutes in warm water not above 35 °C and then inverted at least three times. So portable and handy has this method of self-administered anaesthesia become that it is likely to supplant all others very soon.

Trichloroethylene (Trilene), CCl_2CHCl

This is really a colourless fluid smelling somewhat like chloroform, but for safety it has been coloured with waxilline blue. It has great value as an analgesic as compared with other volatile anaesthetic drugs, since the patient can obtain relief without actually losing consciousness and where unconsciousness is induced it is of only very brief duration. Unfortunately the drug passes freely across the placenta and accumulates in the fetal tissues (just as it does in the maternal tissues), and can produce apnoea in the baby which, fortunately, is short-lived.[17] Because of this possibility of accumulation it is as well to reserve Trilene for the latter part of the first stage and the second stage, unless labour is obviously being very expeditious. For use by midwives there are very suitable inhalers constructed to give the mother concentrations of 0·35 to 0·5 per cent Trilene vapour in air. They are proof against being heated and therefore of giving dangerously high concentrations and cannot be misused in this way. Examples are the Emotril and the Tecota inhalers. For doctors who wish to vary the Trilene vapour concentration the Cyprane inhaler is a beautiful little machine, extremely portable and effective and well worth the small space it occupies in the bag for domiciliary use. Although designed for self-administration the patient should not be left alone with it. One minor disadvantage of Trilene is that it can produce tachycardia both in mother and fetus, a point worth remembering.

Conduction Analgesia during Labour

Where the primary purpose is to relieve pain in labour, mainly the first stage thereof as distinct from the need to provide anaesthesia for operative delivery itself, methods of conduction analgesia have not yet gained wide acceptance in this country because of the technical difficulties of administering them, the supervision which they entail and the unpredictable period of time over which they may have to be maintained before delivery is completed. Where labour cannot be concluded before the effects have worn off, the technique must be capable of being safely and easily repeated. While local analgesic agents eliminate the dangers associated with general anaesthesia, the drugs employed nevertheless carry special hazards of their own and alarming idiosyncrasies are occasionally encountered, especially where the drug is accidentally injected either into the general circulation or misplaced in the case of epidural or caudal blocks. If circulatory collapse occurs, oxygen and circulatory stimulants must be given at once and, in severe cases of collapse, cardiac massage, nowadays by the external method, may be required. Where the reaction to the analgesic drug takes the form of convulsions, intravenous thiopentone in 2½ per cent solution may be required to control them, starting with an initial dose of 3 to 4 ml followed by intermittent, single-ml doses as required.

To a large extent the older paravertebral block and paravertebral lumbar sympathetic block techniques[41] have been replaced by caudal and epidural analgesia. Uterine tone and activity are not directly affected and the period of anaesthesia depends on the type of analgesic fluid used.

Paracervical Nerve Block

Using the correct apparatus this is a very simple technique. Its only disadvantage is the rather short duration of effect which is seldom much more than an hour although newer anaesthetic agents such as bupivacaine 0·5 per cent with adrenaline 1:200,000[13] may act for longer. With regard to apparatus, all that is really wanted is a specially constructed guard tube with a bulbous end with which to probe the lateral vaginal fornices and a needle which protrudes no more than 7 mm beyond its tip. Both guard tube and needle must be of an adequate length to reach as far up as the lateral fornices, in practice at least 14 cm in length. The patient is placed in the dorsal position (the lithotomy position is not necessary) and after the usual antiseptic precautions the guard tube is introduced and pressed firmly into the lateral fornix, if anything slightly posteriorly, and then the needle is passed through the guard tube. With a syringe attached, a preliminary aspiration is carried out to make sure that a blood vessel has not been entered and then 10 ml of the anaesthetic solution is injected on each side into the loose paracervical tissues.[12] This technique is particularly useful towards the end of the first stage in the case of the patient who tends to bear down prematurely before dilatation of the cervix is completed. The two hazards are firstly, of course, inadvertent intravenous injection, as with all local anaesthetic techniques, in which case the patient may become rapidly pale, dyspnoeic and distressed. The other hazard is that of fetal bradycardia. Although this is said not to matter and to wear off fairly quickly, I have been driven to carry out emergency Caesarean section on a doctor's wife in whom the bradycardia persisted for over an hour. The baby, fortunately, was well. It is important not to exceed the recommended dose.

Because of the very short-lived effect and the rapid demoralisation in a patient who, once relieved, wakes up again to the full horror of labour, there has been shown considerable interest in a continuous form of administration.[50] Here, using a combination of special guard tubes, puncture needles and stilettes, the paracervical tissues are reached as before and a curved Teflon catheter is inserted into the pelvic cellular tissue on each side. The catheters are designed to have a built-in, curled tip, rather like a pig's tail, which coils up within the loose cellular tissues and maintains them in position for the duration of the rest of labour. The operation is facilitated by injecting 3 ml of anaesthetic solution through the puncture needles before inserting the catheters in order to distend the area of lodgment and allow more room for their curled tips to take up position. After removal of the various inserting tubes and the stilette, an additional anaesthetic agent is added according to the patient's needs, in 5 ml amounts on each side. As before, the effect wears off in about an hour and repeat injections are necessary. A warning here must be given against the use of prilocaine (Citanest) for this purpose. If more than 400 mg of this drug are given, there is a danger of methaemoglobinaemia and I had one such patient who went very blue from this cause and had some circulatory collapse. The treatment of this unusual complication is the intravenous injection of methylene blue (1–4 mg/kg body weight of 1 per cent solution) which reduces the methaemoglobinaemia and clears the cyanosis.

These cases require just as much minute-to-minute supervision as those under caudal and epidural anaesthesia and therefore there is now a greater preference for these methods than the use of paracervical block which does not produce the same widespread relief from pain.

Low Spinal (Saddleblock) Anaesthesia

This is carried out as a one-shot procedure for forceps delivery. An anaesthetic solution made up in 6 per cent glucose to ensure that its specific gravity is greater than that of CSF is introduced by lumbar puncture in the lumbar region with the patient sitting vertically, thus allowing the heavy solution to produce a suitable low anaesthetic. It is however more likely to produce postoperative headache than other forms of regional anaesthesia due to leakage of cerebrospinal fluid through the puncture hole, and also hypotension may be profound. It is more popular in the United States of America than it is in this country with the steadily increasing use of epidural anaesthesia.

Epidural Anaesthesia

The motto here is sooner rather than later and before the patient's morale is undermined. It is much to be preferred to caudal analgesia which is rapidly falling into disuse throughout the country. It is also safer than the caudal which is not only more difficult but the approach to the epidural space through the sacrococcygeal hiatus is dirtier, harder, and fails more often. The volume of anaesthetic solution moreover has to be much larger in caudal analgesia and the risks of accidental dural tap are just as great, according to Moir. In the caudal approach, a soft, malleable needle is used to approach the epidural space and through it is passed a fine nylon catheter further in. Occasionally the malleable needle can get in some strange places and I remember one case many years ago who did not walk properly for three months.

Better by far is our present practice of continuous epidural analgesia, in which the space outside the dura mater is approached through the lumbar region of the back as in lumbar puncture, but care is taken not to penetrate the dura. The epidural space is identified by the "loss-of-resistance technique". A blunt-tipped plastic catheter is then advanced into the epidural space, the needle is withdrawn and the catheter is connected to a sterile syringe filled with 0·5 per cent bupivacaine. This is now regarded as the drug of choice in preference to a formerly popular 2 per cent lignocaine with 1:200,000 adrenaline added. The main advantage is that the duration of effect is considerably longer and even the addition of adrenaline only marginally prolongs the effect.[33, 34, 35] This syringe is sealed inside a transparent polythene bag and strapped to the abdominal wall so that further injections can be given without the need to scrub up or endangering asepsis. Bupivacaine preferentially selects the sensory roots before the motor roots and by careful attention to dosage the effect can be predominantly a sensory one so that complete paralysis is not achieved. The initial dose is in the region of 7 to 8 ml followed by similar top-up doses when the reappearance of pain necessitates them, at intervals of 2 to 4 hours.

There are certain hazards which have to be recognised and are sufficient to indicate the need for an anaesthetist skilled in the technique to be in charge. The do-it-yourself obstetrician who undertakes his own epidurals already has his hands far too full to cope with complications in which action has to be very prompt and recognition swift and sure. The practice of epidural analgesia is therefore necessarily confined to units who can supply 24-hour anaesthetist cover. The common risk is that of accidental dural tap. If this is not recognised and the anaesthetic is introduced, a dangerously high spinal anaesthetic may result with a catastrophic lowering in blood pressure and even perhaps respiratory paralysis. The introducing needle is usually of Tuohy type through which the epidural catheter is threaded, and this makes quite an appreciable hole in the dura mater. If this happens an epidural anaesthetic should immediately be achieved through another segment. By doing so, not only will the initial objective be achieved but the epidural anaesthetic solution will help to maintain the extradural pressure and prevent the leak of CSF through the puncture previously inflicted. Even so, the rest of the labour should be conducted somewhat differently with the patient being discouraged from pushing or causing any rise in cerebrospinal fluid pressure. For the same reason delivery must be delayed until electively achieved with the forceps. After delivery the extradural pressure must be maintained with a final epidural injection of 50 ml of saline. Thereafter the patient should be nursed prone as much as is practicable for the next 24 hours.

To minimise headache from loss of CSF through a dural puncture hole, CSF production should be maintained with a high fluid intake of 3 litres per 24 hours for the next two days. If in spite of these precautions headache develops the procedure is to perform what is called a "blood patch". This consists in taking 10 ml of the patient's own venous blood in a sterile and non-heparinised syringe and injecting it into the epidural space. This stops the headache within ten minutes and the procedure should be repeated if it fails. The patient in any case should be nursed flat.

Another serious complication is hypotension which can occasionally be very severe. It is most likely to come on within about a quarter of an hour of the administration of the anaesthetic (as the latter begins to take effect). It should therefore be watched for very closely. It is undoubtedly aggravated by the supine position in which the patient may be lying and she must be immediately turned onto her side and her head must be lowered. It is also necessary to counter the hypotensive effect of sympathetic blockade by administering at least 500 ml of any crystalloid substance, for example, saline, or Ringer lactate solution, to compensate for the dilatation of blood vessels. If this fails to restore the pressure above 100 mm Hg ephedrine should be given intravenously as a vasoconstrictor and also to increase cardiac output. It is this latter factor, so important in the maintenance of placental circulation, which makes ephedrine the drug of choice as compared with pure vasoconstrictors. Further intravenous therapy can be continued with Plasmalyte which contains glucose.

Another complication of epidural analgesia is retention of urine because of the insensitivity of the bladder; this must be watched for and where necessary dealt with by catheterisation.

Occasionally the technique fails to produce analgesia in one particular segment, usually L1, because one or more nerves, especially on the right side, escape blockade. Pain in the groin region results. This is best dealt with by topping up the injection with the patient lying on the affected side, so that the solution, which tends to sink in tissue fluids will pick them off.

Another complication is the puncture of an epidural vein, which of course must be recognised before the injection is proceeded with.

Tachyphylaxis is a curious phenomenon occasionally encountered especially with carbonated lignocaine. It is manifested by an ever decreasing duration of effect, even from repeated doses given as often as half-hourly. We have had much less trouble from this source since using bupivacaine which also has the advantage that less gets across the placenta into the fetus, 95 per cent becoming locked to maternal plasma proteins. The risk of toxicity is also less. For similar reasons prilocaine should not be used because, as already stated, an accumulation may cause methaemoglobinaemia.

An accidentally given spinal anaesthetic may not only produce severe hypotension but respiratory and cardiac arrest as well, with far more dramatic speed than is ever likely with an epidural injection. For this reason facilities for intubation and a respirator, and for cardiac resuscitation, should always be available. I know of one case in another city who has lived for many years as a vegetable because of such a catastrophe.

The diagnosis of full dilatation is only likely to be made by vaginal examination as the patient is unlikely to want to bear down and for this reason too over 90 per cent of cases have to be delivered by either forceps or ventouse. When full dilatation of the cervix is diagnosed, and not before, and if all else is well, the patient can be partially let out of her epidural analgesia and switched over progressively to Entonox analgesia in good time so that she is more likely to achieve spontaneous delivery by her own expulsive efforts, or at least delivery may be completed with the ventouse or low forceps.

There are certain precautions which must be observed. For example, we prefer not to start an epidural anaesthetic in patients whose labour is being induced with oxytocin until uterine response to oxytocin has been studied for about two or three hours and the dosage stabilised. In cases who have had a previous Caesarean section there is a very natural fear that an epidural anaesthetic may mask the physical signs of uterine rupture; of local tenderness there may be none and to wait for signs of a rising pulse or bleeding *per vaginam* is to wait too long. Uterine contractions however are more likely to cease and further progress in labour is not likely to be achieved. Selwyn Crawford states that in the case of a properly administered epidural anaesthetic the pain of uterine rupture, if present, will "get past" an epidural sieve.

Many of the troubles attributed to epidural anaesthesia are due to inferior vena caval compression because of the patient's lying in the supine position, and with blood pooling in the lower body and limbs.[33] Even during delivery with forceps she should be tilted to one side with a wedge mattress. The incidence of deep venous thrombosis in the legs is less likely if caval compression is at all times avoided. Crawford does not regard twins as a contra-indication to epidural analgesia provided these precautions are observed.[14] Regarding my own personal, disastrous case referred to in the chapter on twins, Crawford and Moir, in discussing the case, both agreed that the tachyphylaxis demonstrated was probably due to lignocaine and the severe hypotension to inferior vena caval compression. The resulting hypotension is much more serious in any case with twins whose placental circulatory demands are correspondingly greater. Another reputed disadvantage of epidural analgesia in twin delivery is possible difficulty with the delivery of the second because of a uterus which is overactive and may clamp down too soon after delivery of the first.

Notwithstanding all this, epidural anaesthesia has a most important part to play in the management of inco-ordinate uterine action, quite apart from its great uses as a single-shot anaesthetic for difficult instrumental deliveries. The relief of the patient is quite astonishing to witness. She more or less grins her way through labour and we are always prepared to consider the advisability of this type of analgesia after six hours of labour in primigravidae, provided the case is otherwise obstetrically normal. One has plenty of time now to correct maternal acidosis and to give the cervix every chance to dilate; another advantage to be reaped is the excellence of uterine retraction in the third stage so that blood lost from the episiotomy usually exceeds that from the placental site.

Once the patient has been given the treat of epidural analgesia, however, her attendants are absolutely committed to complete delivery during the course of that anaesthetic, because the patients take it very hard to be exposed to the unaccustomed pain of the late first stage of labour if the anaesthetic is allowed to wear off too much. There is obviously a limit to the desirable length of time for maintaining epidural analgesia and we are certainly reluctant to allow the business to go on for more than 18 hours and usually much less. It follows that one must be prepared to deliver either by forceps or by Caesarean section within that time according to the degree of dilatation achieved.

This account is full of cautionary remarks which are reason enough for not using this type of analgesia indiscriminately; in fact with careful selection combined with enthusiasm for the method the incidence of epidural analgesia at the Queen Mother's Hospital, Glasgow, is now 25 per cent and rising all the time.

Counter irritation and distraction.—An interesting method of which we have a limited experience is the use of what is called "white sound". This is a curious noise involving a wide spectrum of frequencies producing a resultant sound rather like the continuous noise of a wave breaking upon a beach made up of fine pebbles. This weird continuous noise is mixed up with good music, such as a Schubert quartet. The first time I used this instrument the expensive part of it, namely the Hi-Fi recording of the quartet, was not available, only the curious noise, so we abandoned culture for the moment and supplied the more practical element via headphones to a patient who was making very heavy weather of her first stage and suffering uncontrollably with each contraction. For hours thereafter she grinned her way through each contraction and said it was "smashing" but she still came to Caesarean section that evening for total lack of progress. I do not think the Schubert would have made much difference. Dentists are known to find this method helpful, especially with children who take less kindly than most of us to assaults in the dental chair, but I doubt if we are yet in a position to say that the same beneficial effects cannot be more simply produced by the judicious use of pain-relieving drugs.

Psychoprophylaxis.—The late Grantly Dick-Read developed almost a cult for the easing of childbirth's miseries by mental as well as physical relaxation. By now generations of labouring women have acknowledged benefit from this type of brain-washing which was more readily accepted in the United States than in this country. In somewhat similar fashion a psychoprophylactic preparation for childbirth is more popular and acknowledged on the other side of the English Channel. At a meeting of the Natural Childbirth Trust in London in March, 1961, Dr Pierre Vellay of Paris described his methods of psychoprophylactic preparation, continuing the work of Lamaze who is said to have derived his technique from Russian methods. He claimed that 35 per cent of all deliveries by this method are completely painless, in 63 per cent there is tolerable pain and in only about 5 per cent is there a total failure. Dr Vellay attributes painless childbirth so achieved to a combination of the correct conditioned reflexes, adequate training exercises and successful human relations. Where psychiatric probing reveals disturbance, the services of a "psychosomatician" are called in, but to judge by the report of this meeting, in 80 per cent of cases pregnancy and labour are sufficiently normal for obstetrician and midwife to suffice and this should make those of us who practice this branch of medicine feel a little better! He said that 30 per cent of all women in France are delivered by this method of psychoprophylaxis. The fees charged for the course, which consists of some lectures, a visit to the obstetrical unit and a film, etc., are refunded by the Securité Sociale. He claims that it is possible to deliver a woman with forceps without any need for anaesthesia. At this same meeting the late Dr Lee Buxton, after a study of thirty-three obstetrical units in Europe and the United States, found more than twenty different methods of psychological preparation for childbirth and he suggested that if we were to look for a common denominator in all these methods it might be the personality or enthusiasm of the person conducting the labour, or even the kindness, competent humanity and care given by someone trained to give it. I wonder if this is not just part of the essence of good doctoring and whether it might not be as well to abandon some of the grandiloquent phrases which tend to suggest that doctors hitherto have not known how to understand, succour and comfort their patients. The subject is an emotive one and a large number of women have been so greatly helped by modern psychoprophylaxis that it deserves a better account than I can give. Accordingly Dr Alan Giles of Stobhill Hospital, Glasgow, who has great experience of it has kindly supplied an essay on psychoprophylaxis at the end of this chapter.

Acceleration of labour.—Throughout this chapter there has been the underlying theme that a labour lasting longer than 18 hours is undesirable and therefore in modern practice to be avoided. I wholeheartedly agree with our Irish colleagues, notably O'Driscoll *et al.*[38] who pointed out that we are too much preoccupied with the mechanical aspects of difficult and prolonged labour and too often we invoke disproportion as a cause. For nearly quarter of a century I have preached myself that good contractions are worth half an inch of true conjugate. Furthermore good uterine activity discourages unsatisfactory attitudes such as deflexion and occipitoposterior and persistent transverse attitudes of fetal head.

While it is vital not to overlook even minor degrees of disproportion, one recognises that nature left to her own devices frequently fails to produce an expeditious and safe delivery, as in the past, because of poor uterine behaviour. This can now be accurately and safely overcome by judicious oxytocin stimulation and O'Driscoll and his colleagues in Dublin, in a remarkable series of 1000 consecutive primigravidae, adopting an aggressive approach to the control of uterine activity, were able to whittle down the admission of disproportion in these cases to less than one per cent; in fact where trial of labour fails the diagnosis of disproportion can only be entertained if uterine activity has been genuinely adequate.[38]

There is a subtle difference between the terms "acceleration" and "augmentation" of labour. O'Driscoll quite firmly prefers the former. Many others of us have with considerable success augmented and incidentally accelerated labour where it has already been induced by escalating doses of oxytocin.[30, 31] The important point about the Dublin attitude is that acceleration is only applicable to labour once it has spontaneously started and that induction simply prolongs the period of stress to the mother. In fact the incidence of induction at the National Maternity Hospital in Dublin is only 6 per cent and their results fully justify this philosophy. There, the policy is that the patient admits herself to the labour unit when she thinks herself in labour because of painful contractions or because of show, or spontaneous rupture of the membranes. The first three hours after this self-admission to hospital are crucial and in that time an assessment can be made as to whether or not she is really in labour and if so a partogram chart is initiated. Counting of the duration of the labour only starts from when the cervix begins to show dilatation at the rate of about 1 cm an hour and the diagnosis of labour is disqualified unless the cervix is dilated. If in spite of painful uterine contractions there is no progress as evidenced solely by dilatation of the cervix, descent of the presenting part being regarded as less important, after the lapse of two hours the forewaters are ruptured and labour accelerated with oxytocin. The assessment therefore in the first three hours really dictates the management of the case. This principle of acceleration therefore should only be applied to a case who has already started labour. Furthermore the assurance that she is likely to be delivered within the next twelve hours makes her more ready to thole the pain of labour, and the use of analgesic drugs, commonly restricted to 50 mg of pethidine, would be regarded by many of us as stingy.

An important point in the Dublin management is that a given midwife is allocated to each individual case throughout the whole of her labour and everything is done to allay apprehension and to produce a truly physiological pattern of uterine behaviour. As a result operative intervention can be delayed until the head is sufficiently low for a simple forceps delivery if necessary and, in fact, mid-cavity forceps deliveries and all types of difficult instrumentation are regarded as anathema. This must be a midwife's paradise! On this side of the Irish Sea, where labour is commonly induced on a much more extravagant scale, uterine activity is again secured by intravenous oxytocin medication in steadily increasing dosage.[30, 31]

The sensitivity of each individual uterus to oxytocin dosage varies enormously and Turnbull and the rest of us use the phrase "oxytocin titration" which means progressively increasing the dosage until satisfactory uterine behaviour is obtained.[51, 54] This can, of course, be done by using a dilute solution and increasing the rate of the drip but water-intoxication may result and in any case large quantities of fluid may not be desirable. We therefore have considerable experience of delivery pumps, such as the Rocket pump and the Sage pump and other pumps which deliver carefully controlled doses of the drug. Most now operate by accurately counting the number of drops passing a photo-electric cell and thereby controlling the feed to a set speed. In this way quite high concentrations of oxytocin can be given accurately in relatively small quantities of fluid. For instance with the Rocket pump, 4 units of Syntocinon are mixed with 20 ml of sterile water giving a strength of 1 unit of Syntocinon in 5 ml. The charged syringe is attached to the manometer tubing and flushed through with the solution and then attached to the giving set. The dial on the pump is increased by one figure every fifteen minutes until it reaches the figure 10 or until good uterine contractions are felt every two minutes and lasting about 40 seconds. If there is still an inadequate response a new solution is made up by increasing the strength of the solution fivefold and reducing the dial to one-fifth of the previous setting and continuing the escalation exactly as before.

The procedure with the Sage pump is similar. Starting with a strength of one unit of Syntocinon in five ml, the settings on the dial are increased initially every five minutes until the figure 1·0 is reached and thereafter by 0·5 increments every fifteen minutes. If there is still no effect the strength of the solution is, as before, increased five times and the rate of infusion set back to one-fifth of its previous rate. The rate of escalation thereafter is somewhat slower but applied every 15 minutes. For the drip technique there are many comparable machines on the market, such as the Ivac and the Tekmar which we commonly use, and which are all capable of giving a very accurately controlled dose of Syntocinon. They can be switched off instantly and of course they should be slowed down as soon as adequate oxytocin titration has been achieved.[8]

The unwelcome part of this procedure is the latent period of oxytocin titration between amniotomy and the commencement of cervical dilatation which may vary from minutes to hours. Full monitoring of uterine activity by an external or, better still, by an internal catheter-fed tocograph, combined with fetal heart recording we regard as an essential precaution; but good clinical observation as described earlier, provided it is continuous and thorough, can be equally safe.

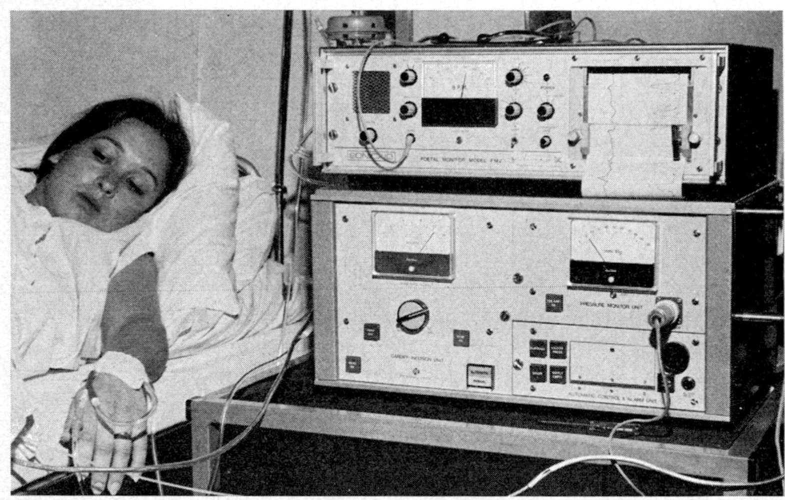

18/Fig. 6.—Combined use of Cardiff oxytocin infusion pump and FM2 Sonicaid fetal heart rate monitor above. A satisfactory, well-controlled induced labour resulting in spontaneous delivery of a healthy baby.

It is important however to be aware of the dosage rate of oxytocin being given and this should always be recorded in milliunits per minute. The Cardiff infusion pump is an admirable piece of apparatus which guarantees safety of administration by controlling its own rate according to the pressures recorded by intra-uterine catheter, and in any case the rate cannot be driven over 32 milliunits per minute (Fig. 6). It has every conceivable type of safety feature built in so that labour can be not only safely augmented but accelerated as well. The FM2 Sonicaid fetal heart monitor fits neatly on top of it.

Uterine hypertonus must never be allowed to occur and provided this is avoided and the uterus is allowed to relax well between contractions, the technique is very safe. The primigravid uterus is practically immune from rupture from being over-driven unless it is actually pathological. More caution is necessary in the case of the grand multipara and I have the gravest reservations about allowing the dose of oxytocin administration to exceed 8 milliunits per minute in such a case.

As soon as a stable pattern of uterine behaviour is achieved labour can thereafter be maintained without further escalation. For example 7 milliunits of oxytocin per minute is a likely level of dosage required and there is nothing to be gained by running excessive maintenance levels.[8]

Having thus artificially overcome uterine atony it is important to maintain the drip for at least an hour after completion of the third stage in case of reaction with postpartum haemorrhage.

The Dublin technique, without a large array of sophisticated electronic apparatus, has at the time of writing been boiled down to a fairly standard procedure in which 10 units of Syntocinon are added to 1 litre of 5 per cent dextrose and the infusion rate started at 10 drops to the minute, with slowly progressive increase thereafter to a maximum if necessary of 60 drops per minute, which works out at 40 milliunits. Only in the presence of a dead fetus is it regarded as wise or safe to go much above this level although we occasionally, in a refractory case, have to go up to 64 milliunits per minute. In missed abortion, of course, as previously described, very much higher doses can safely be used and may, in fact, be necessary.

As in Dublin, Valium may be used occasionally to enhance the action of pethidine but their usage of epidural analgesia is very much lower than ours.

In conclusion this drug-controlled active management of labour although a form of pharmacological *accouchement forcé* stands fully justified in modern obstetric practice by eliminating most of the horrors and hazards of unnecessarily prolonged labour.

Alas, even with all these modern techniques and safety precautions, success cannot be counted upon and one's hand may be forced into operative intervention at the onset of fetal distress, refractory behaviour and lack of progress and, of course, the hazards associated with malpresentation to which the technique of accelerated labour is not properly applicable.

Operative treatment.—Decisions here may be very difficult particularly if the patient is near to full dilatation and one has to make up one's mind whether to assist in securing vaginal delivery or to undertake vaginal bypass by Caesarean section. In years gone by I have applied the obstetric forceps through a cervix only three-quarters dilated and accelerated labour with continuous light-weight traction, an admirable ladder of ascending infection being thereby supplied. This line of treatment is only of historical interest.

The ventouse (vacuum extractor) comes into a different category and may resolve a lingering first stage most satisfactorily. To use it, as I have, in a case of labour lasting more than four days because of indolent hypotonic inertia with the cervix still only four fingersbreadth dilated and to have the patient quietly and successfully delivered without haemorrhage or other mischief within the next half hour, is an experience sufficient to convince the most stubborn.

Where the cervix is more than three-quarters dilated and the pelvis is roomy, it is often possible by digital manipulation to push the cervix above the maximum diameters of the presenting part and to deliver with forceps. This is an operation calling for considerable skill, but is certainly preferable to applying the forceps without first stretching the cervix over the fetal head and relying upon brute force to deliver, a procedure which is shocking both physically and aesthetically. The ventouse nowadays makes a better and safer delivery of this sort.

Often, after reaching full dilatation at last the patient may be too exhausted by her first stage to achieve spontaneous delivery in the second, and operative delivery with forceps or a ventouse is likely to be required. The risk of postpartum haemorrhage in the neglected and exhausted case is bound to be high as well. It will be seen, therefore, that there are certain hazards to vaginal delivery "at any price".

Though largely replaced by the ventouse, incision of the cervix is worth considering but only in a very few cases, and this procedure should be reserved for the rare instances of cervical dystocia with the head low within the pelvic cavity. Duhrssen's incisions consist of a series of short nibbles round the posterior margin of the cervix, but it is often more effective to make a frank cut. O'Sullivan recommended cutting the cervix to a depth of half an inch on each side at nine o'clock and three o'clock, but it is probably safer to keep away from the mid-lateral area and incise at eight o'clock, six o'clock and four o'clock. There is one technical snag about this, namely each cut should be completed in one bite, because the V-shaped gap in the cervix which it makes is immediately flattened out and cannot again be identified, so that a second bite taken in the same region is unlikely to coincide with the original cut. The cervix must now be pushed up over the head, especially in front. O'Sullivan performed this operation with only analgesia instead of anaesthesia, and the patient could sometimes now be left to proceed to spontaneous delivery. Where, however, a general anaesthetic has been used, one is more or less obliged to proceed to forceps delivery rather than face the prospect of having to induce a second anaesthetic should spontaneous delivery not occur.

Provided the head is very well applied to the cervix there is usually surprisingly little bleeding from incising it, but the cases must be very carefully selected and the following conditions must be present:

1. The head must be very deep, preferably on the pelvic floor;
2. The cervix must be at least 3 fingersbreadth dilated;
3. There must be no suspicion of contraction of the bony outlet;
4. The cervix must be tightly and thinly stretched over the head;
5. Contractions, though weak, must be regular in nature.

It will be seen, therefore, that the operation is quite unsuited to the colicky type of uterus. In any case very profound shock may be caused, mainly because of the traction which is felt upon the imperfectly prepared lower uterine segment before full dilatation and only exceptionally can this be regarded as the operation of choice.

There are two criteria of progress in labour, namely progressive dilatation of the cervix and progressive descent of the presenting part. As long as either is present labour can be said to be progressing, but if neither criterion is satisfied in the course of 6 hours if not sooner, the question of Caesarean section arises. The universal use of the lower-segment operation together with the exhibition of antibiotic drugs, where indicated, has made this outcome of labour a far preferable method to brutish delivery before the completion of the first stage. While deploring the indiscriminate use of abdominal delivery in these cases, the plea is here made for Caesarean section a little too early rather than too late.

Complications

It is not enough nowadays to confine one's view of results merely to maternal and fetal survival. Such a narrow view will soon come to be condemned as neo-Georgian. The maternal morbidity rate rises according to the duration of labour, particularly from the time the membranes rupture. Apart from the genital tract, urinary infection increases with the need for repeated catherisation. One of the greatest risks of operative delivery, whatever its nature, lies in the anaesthetic. These patients are sometimes in poor shape, often dehydrated, ketosis may be marked and their stomachs are treacherously full, so that vomiting easily complicates the induction of anaesthesia.

Among the sequelae one must consider the prospects for future labours and the attitude of the patient towards embarking upon further pregnancies. Jeffcoate pointed out the significant fact that, of those who were ultimately delivered by Caesarean section after a prolonged and difficult labour, almost half avoided further pregnancies, and of those who were delivered by forceps the percentage who remained voluntarily sterile was only a little less. This is a point of no mean importance. The outlook for future labours is usually satisfactory provided on the previous occasion vaginal delivery was achieved, whether by forceps or not, but the repeat Caesarean section rate remains very high, especially if the cervix did not reach more than half dilatation.

Neonatal complications and morbidity are if anything even more serious. Birth asphyxia can do the child nothing but harm which is even more related to its duration than its extent and neurological damage may be severe, even more so if the baby is dysmature. Sepsis of many varieties may be incurred during the process of birth, the first and most obvious manifestation of which is neonatal pneumonia, umbilical sepsis and occasionally fulminating generalised septicaemia. Sometimes infection contracted in the process of birth may manifest itself weeks later in the form of meningitis or osteomyelitis, for example. Not least amongst the sources of neonatal morbidity are the iatrogenic causes: the ill-advised, the over-drugging and the frankly traumatic. It is not for nothing that one talks of the Valley of the Shadow of Birth.

OCCIPITOPOSTERIOR POSITION

Occipitoposterior positions, because of their frequent adverse effect upon the length of labour, deserve consideration here on their own. About 10 per cent of all vertex presentations occupy posterior positions at the onset of labour, but in about four-fifths of these labour is not much affected. The other 20 per cent, in rough figures, require some form of intervention.

On average, labour is prolonged about 3½ hours in primigravidae and about 1¾ hours in multiparae.

The occipitoposterior position, though common, cannot truly be regarded as normal. There are many reasons for the normal occipito-anterior position, among which are the respective curvatures of the maternal lumbar and fetal spines. Clearly it is more suitable for these curvatures to lie in parallel than with their convexities opposed, and if, as happens in occipitoposterior positions, these curvatures are opposed, it is easy to see how a deflexed attitude of the fetus results. Furthermore, in the erect posture there is more room anteriorly for the curvature of the fetal back. A lesser factor is the position of the placenta, since the fetus tends to face it *in utero*, and it is known that the placenta is more commonly sited on the posterior wall than on the anterior, though the difference is not great enough to account for the frequency of occipito-anterior positions.

Most cases of O.P. malposition are usually unexplained.

If the head should engage in an anthropoid type of brim with the occiput posterior in the first instance there is, of course, reason enough for its unwillingness to negotiate the relatively narrower transverse strait by long internal rotation, and these cases often prefer the shorter rotation into the hollow of the sacrum.

The well-known military attitude so often seen in a tight uterus signifies a state of deflexion, but it would be hard to say whether this was a cause or effect of occipitoposterior position.

A flat pelvis, with uterine obliquity towards the same side as the occiput, encourages deflexion of the head after the manner of producing a secondary face presentation (which constitutes an extreme example), and this may be a minor aetiological factor. Lastly, some cases are attributed to primary brachycephaly which shortens the lengths of the lever from the frontal region to the atlanto-occipital

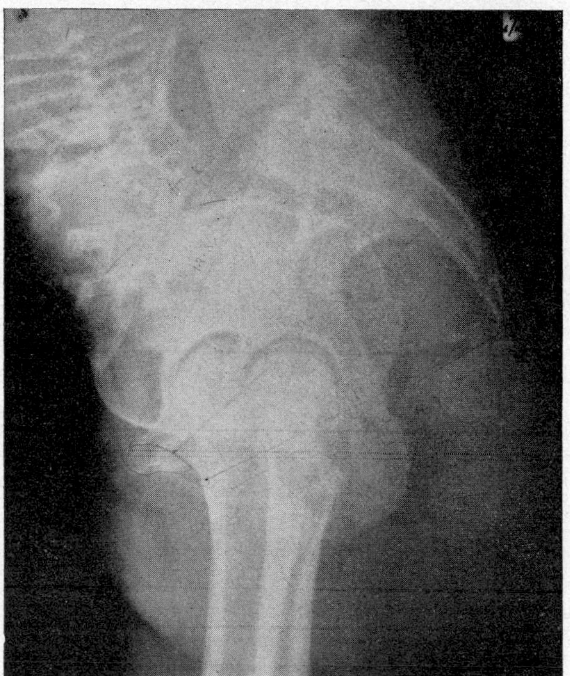

18/FIG. 7.—Persistent occipitoposterior position, two hours in second stage of labour after 26 hours in the first stage. Note moulding and extension of head. Delivered by Caesarean section. Birth-weight 4 kg.

(By courtesy of Dr R. A. Tennent.)

joint and therefore reduces its effective moment in flexing the head.

Quite apart from the generally accepted need for long internal rotation of the occiput through three-eighths of a circle (which will depend both on really adequate uterine contractions and pelvic roominess), the mechanism of labour is adversely affected in many other ways. The axis of uterine thrust, for one thing, transmitted from the fundus through the fetal vertebral column tends to operate at a mechanical disadvantage, because it is out of alignment and not at right angles to the pelvic inlet (Fig. 7). The steeper, therefore, the angle of inclination of the pelvic brim the more serious does this factor

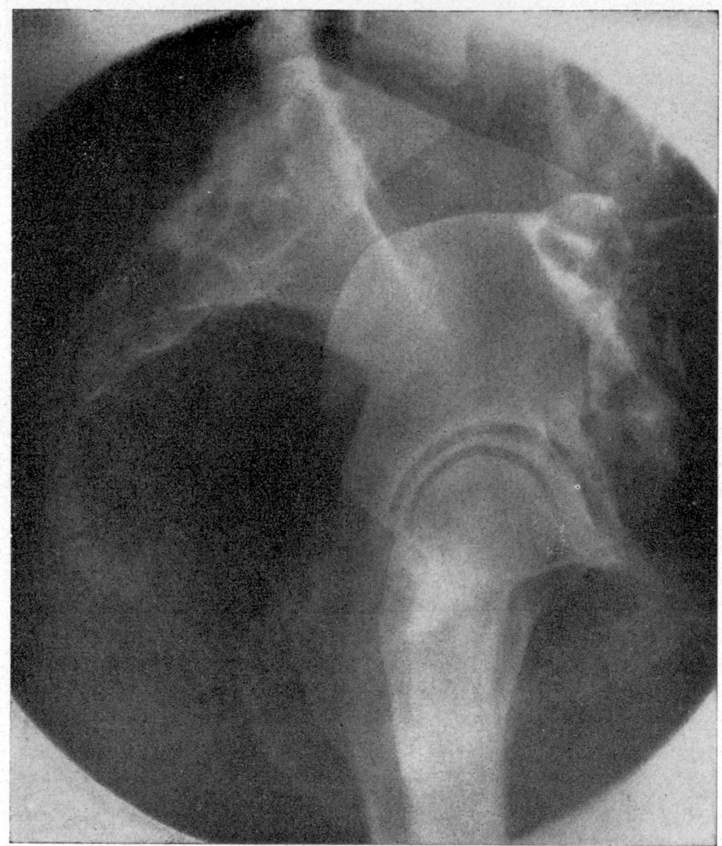

18/Fig. 8.—Angulation of neck.

become, so that on taking a radiograph there will often be observed a marked lateral angulation of the fetal neck (Fig. 8). The forces necessary to drive the head deeply into the pelvis are often misdirected and therefore misspent.

Now, in the multipara with her more lax abdominal wall the uterine body sags farther forward, so that the direction of uterine thrust through the fetal spine more nearly approaches the direction of engagement. This partly explains why occipitoposterior positions seldom inconvenience the labouring multipara.

The deflexed head presents an ovoid rather than a sphere to the lower segment and therefore tends to fit badly, so that poor pains result from inefficient stimulation. The forewaters are not plugged off efficiently by the presenting part during uterine contraction and the membranes rupture early so that rotation is somewhat discouraged as a result.

If deflexion is marked, the occipitofrontal diameter of 11·3 cm (4½ inches) may present instead of the suboccipitobregmatic, and mild cases of deflexion present with the suboccipitofrontal measuring 10·25 cm (4 inches). This is a common cause of high head at term. If both fontanelles remain at the same level, in what is called by some authorities the median vertex position, the head, in its descent through the pelvis, inadequately presents the vertex to the gutter mechanism of the pelvic floor, which is therefore unable to choose which variety of internal rotation to encourage. Transverse arrest of the head then results. As long as transverse arrest remains uncorrected, the patient is incapable of delivering herself, and the head usually sticks in the mid-cavity at a level at which about two pennyworth of scalp or caput can be seen on separating the labia.

Occasionally the posterior fetal shoulder may get caught on the wrong side of the maternal vertebral column and this, too, discourages internal rotation.

When the occiput remains posterior, its mechanical pressure backwards towards the rectum is very liable to give the patient the desire to bear down and push before full dilatation, and it is very common indeed for the onset of the second stage to be prematurely diagnosed by the attendant. As a result, the patient may be urged to push with her pains, all to no purpose, so that, after the lapse of a statutory period, delay in the second stage is diagnosed and preparations are made for forceps delivery which might not have been necessary if the patient had not been encouraged to exhaust herself with fruitless efforts prematurely.

If labour proceeds to face-to-pubis delivery, it is obvious that greater diameters must ultimately distend the vulval outlet. Maternal lacerations are therefore more common and the narrower the subpubic angle happens to be the worse will be the damage to the pelvic floor.

A narrow subpubic angle presents a less attractive escape gap to the presenting part, so that, particularly in the android type of pelvis, the condition of deep transverse arrest of the head persists. Similarly, a poor sacral bay favours transverse arrest.

It is not surprising, therefore, that the operative delivery rate is high. Of those cases who start labour with the occiput posterior, approximately 63 per cent deliver themselves spontaneously with the occiput anterior, about 14 per cent have spontaneous face-to-pubis deliveries and the remaining 23 per cent require operative delivery. The frequent need for episiotomy is obvious, and the technique and pitfalls of manual rotation of the occiput and forceps delivery are described in the chapter on forceps.

Because of the increased length of labour and the greater need for operative intervention maternal morbidity is naturally higher. The fetal mortality is higher in cases requiring rotation and forceps. The jam-pot type of moulding which is characteristic of the persistent occipitoposterior presentation is particularly unfavourable from the point of view of tentorial damage because of the extreme elevation of the falx cerebri which it entails.

It would not be an exaggeration to say that occipitoposterior positions and transverse arrest of the head account for more second-stage trouble than all the rest put together.

OBSTRUCTED LABOUR

This should never be encountered in modern obstetric practice, for it can only result from woeful neglect. Only the briefest summary will therefore be given. Its causes include disproportion, brow presentation, persistent mentoposterior position, shoulder presentation and impacted breech. One of two possible sequences of events must now take place. Either the uterus will give up the unequal struggle and become inert from exhaustion, the patient ultimately dying of sepsis, or, more commonly, the contractions come more fast and furious until the uterus relaxes not at all between pains. This tetanic condition of the uterus is called tonic contraction. The upper segment has retracted fully at the expense of the lower segment which is stretched to the limit and beyond. The junction between the two segments is represented by a ridge, Bandl's ring, which rises higher in the abdomen usually at an oblique angle. The patient's condition is desperate. Pain is continuous and very severe, the uterus is hard and so tender that palpation of the fetus is impossible. The maternal pulse is rapid, usually over 120 per minute, and may be thready. The temperature is raised and all the signs of dehydration are present, including a dry, dirty tongue, a hot, dry vagina, and highly concentrated, scanty urine containing albumin, acetone, blood and casts. Uterine rupture is imminent, and most commonly occurs through the posterior wall of the thinned-out lower segment. The baby is of course already dead from asphyxia, and unless very prompt and skilful treatment is immediately available the mother, too, is well on her way to the next world. Of all obstetric deaths it is probably one of the most terrible, and in underdeveloped countries often made worse by attempts outside to bring about delivery.

PSYCHOPROPHYLAXIS

by ALAN M. GILES,
B.Sc., M.B., Ch.B., D.P.H., F.R.C.O.G., F.R.C.S.(Glas.)
Stobhill General Hospital, Glasgow

Psychoprophylaxis is a psychological method of antenatal preparation designed to prevent or at least to minimise pain and difficulty during labour. The pregnant woman is taught how to use her natural brain processes to her advantage.

The psychoprophylactic method of preparation is based on the following principles described by Pavlov. (1) Man is constantly being conditioned by experience and environment. (2) Conditioned reflexes can be established by the use of speech. (3) Old reflexes can become weak and new reflexes can be established. (4) The effect of one group of stimuli on the brain can be diminished by the inhibitory effect of other stimuli. (5) By a process of selection and concentration on stimuli from one source, stimuli from another source can be made secondary. (6) Inhibition of stimuli can be conditioned.

Applying the principles of his experiments, the Russian obstetricians Platonov, Velvosky and Nicolaiev evolved the method at the same time as Dr Grantly Dick-Read was developing his ideas on "natural childbirth". Read stated that fear produced tension and tension produced pain. He advised relaxation during a contraction. The Russians did not agree with Read. On the contrary, they advocated activity both mental and physical during labour. In 1951 Dr Lamaze, a French obstetrician, visited Russia and saw women, trained in psychoprophylaxis, deliver without pain. On his return to Paris he and Dr Vellay adapted the Russian method for use in the Western world. The method has now spread to some forty-four countries.

Childbirth is surely the greatest physical act performed by women. It can also be a great emotional experience. The physical and psychological aspects cannot be separated. For most women labour is a time of apprehension, of fear and agony. This need not be so. As a result of suitable antenatal preparation the majority of women can have labour that is easy and painless, or almost painless, and can actually enjoy the labour and experience a sense of fulfilment. It can be postulated that the basic sensations from the contracting uterus are those of tightness and that these sensations are interpreted by the brain as pain only when there are added factors due to emotion or to previous conditioning. The Russian obstetrician Nicolaiev states that it is necessary to reshape the mind of the woman who has come to believe that pain in labour is inevitable. Nicolaiev reshaped the woman's mind by a process of deconditioning and reconditioning. To this method of antenatal preparation was given the name psychoprophylaxis—prevention by use of the mind.

The Conditioned Reflex

The conditioning probably begins at puberty. The attitude of the girl's mother to menstruation, dysmenorrhoea and childbirth may produce either a favourable or an unfavourable impression. The mother may thus start the formation of an adverse conditioned reflex.

In the years between puberty and pregnancy the girl gathers information from many sources: from her schoolmates, from her older sisters. She overhears gossip about pregnancies and births. She reads about the subject in newspapers and magazines. She watches television. The information is absorbed by her brain and creates a conditioned reflex. The information may be favourable—descriptions of happy and normal births, but on the other hand it may be of tragedies, of sickness in pregnancy, of long difficult labours, of stillbirths and deaths and fetal abnormalities, and above all of pain. Some of the expressions used to describe the birth process are unfortunate. The word "labour" itself conveys an impression of unpleasantness, and many still use the word "pain" when they should say "uterine contraction".

As a result of her experience and environment during the years before her pregnancy, during the antenatal period, and even during her labour, a patient is conditioned favourably or unfavourably. If unfavourably, the reflex will be—signal: contraction of the uterus, result: pain and difficulty. If the patient has pain in labour then fear, apprehension and tension appear. A defence mechanism may be called into play. Release of adrenaline may cause ischaemia and spasm of the uterus, and result in even more intense pain. The patient may attempt to reject the cause of the pain, i.e. the contractions of the uterus, and so may prevent the normal increase in tempo of the labour and the normal increase in strength of the contractions. The result is often a long and painful labour.

During training in psychoprophylaxis the patient is deconditioned and reconditioned by the use of speech and by detailed education. Again and again it is stressed that the uterus is a muscle similar to that of the bowel and that when a skeletal muscle or smooth muscle contracts pain is not usually felt. The sensation should be that of tightness. But, if the muscle is in spasm, as during indigestion, pain will be felt. The woman is asked to feel her own painless Braxton Hicks contractions. In the last few weeks of pregnancy she proves to herself that the uterus can contract without pain. A patient who has had a painless labour is introduced to the class and asked to describe her experience. By persuasion and constant repetition the woman is made to accept that the uterus can contract painlessly. A new conditioned reflex is produced: contraction of uterus = tightness.

Furthermore, the woman is taught that the contractions of the uterus dilate the cervix and that the quicker the cervix dilates the shorter will be the labour. She is persuaded to welcome the onset of the next contraction and to hope that it will be strong. A new conditioned reflex is built up; signal: contraction of uterus, result: welcome tightness. The conditioned reflexes at play during labour are even more complex than those described above.

Concentration and Selection

Another neurophysiological principle was described by Pavlov. Arriving at the brain are large numbers of stimuli. Some process of selection is necessary to prevent mental chaos. If man did not have a power of concentration and selection he would not be able to carry out any continuous action but would be frequently diverted by the arrival of new stimuli at the brain. In everyday life man selects certain stimuli and rejects others, e.g., the husband reading the sports page does not hear his wife speak. The use of a counter irritant may relieve pain.

It is possible to use this principle during labour. A woman's active participation in her labour can inhibit stimuli from the uterus, can eliminate pain. In psychoprophylaxis the woman is required to be active, both mentally and physically. By this alertness and activity the patient's brain is flooded with stimuli which tend to crowd out, to minimise the stimuli from the uterus. The sensation of tightness is therefore lessened and any tendency for the tightness to become pain is reduced and delayed. In an attempt to make the stimuli from the uterus secondary, the patient is instructed to select and concentrate on some extraneous activity during the contraction. An untrained patient, feeling pain during the contractions, tends to concentrate on the sensations from the uterus. She will be relaxing on her bed. During the contraction she will close her eyes, unfortunately stopping all light stimuli, and she will hold her breath, reducing stimuli from her chest. She concentrates on the painful contraction of the uterus making it seem more intense. The trained woman is taught to concentrate on her breathing, on knitting, reading or watching television. By this concentration the woman makes the stimuli from the uterus secondary and so reduces their effect.

Pavlov states that an inhibition can be conditioned. That is, a signal can be made to cause inhibition or suppression of a previously expected effect. In psychoprophylaxis the woman is taught to breathe in a definite manner and is told that this will prevent any sensation of pain.

Training

Education is detailed. The Birth Atlas is used in teaching the anatomy and physiology of pregnancy and labour. Much time is spent in discussing in detail everything that happens, from admission procedures and conduct of the first stage, to the actual delivery. The patient is told exactly what each procedure will be and the reasons. A tour of the labour room and introduction to the labour room staff is arranged. Fear of the unknown is as far as possible removed. The patient develops faith in the method, confidence in the staff and, most important, faith in her own ability. Psychoprophylaxis is made a discipline.

In the training programme described by Vellay of Paris, the main emphasis is placed on the lectures which are really a form of psychotherapy. Throughout the lecture course there is constant repetition of the general principles, thus deconditioning and reconditioning the woman's mind. The Pavlovian principles involved are described using many simple examples which the patient can understand. An appeal is made to her intelligence. Intelligence is not synonymous with education or culture. The less intelligent patient may prove easy to train because she has absorbed less adverse information and because she may develop faith more easily.

The exercises described by Vellay of Paris are few and are simple, and are used mainly as a vehicle for the psychotherapy. The main exercise is the practice of the shallow breathing which will be carried out during the contractions of the first stage of labour. This breathing drill acts in several ways. As the patient is required to practise it every day she has therefore to think about the method daily. During the actual uterine contractions in labour this breathing acts as a distraction on which the patient concentrates. During the training period the practice of the shallow breathing affects the conditioning on an inhibition. The patient comes to believe that by breathing during the contraction she will not feel pain. And lastly, instead of holding her breath, as do many women during a contraction, the trained woman ensures a continuous absorption of oxygen from her lungs during labour.

The degree of success of the method is dependent on many factors. There is the ability and willingness of the patient herself to learn and carry out the detailed practice. The quality of the teaching is of great importance. The teacher should be someone with a full knowledge and experience of midwifery. Order of preference would be doctor, midwife, physiotherapist. Probably a team of all three would be ideal. The personality and teaching ability of the individual would obviously influence the choice of personnel. There is no place for lay teachers, even although their enthusiasm and motives are beyond question.

The conduct of the staff during the patient's labour is another important factor which can contribute greatly to the chance of success. The staff must understand psychoprophylaxis. They must supervise the patient's breathing, they must encourage her to be mentally and, up to a point, physically active. The labour lounge should be specially designed to provide interest and distraction. Sleep should be discouraged and hypnotics should not be given routinely. If the patient's brain is sleepy the stimuli from the uterus will become primary. The atmosphere in the labour room should not be that of a busy casualty department. The staff should be kindly and firm but not sympathetic, and there should be no suggestion of preparing the patient for an ordeal to come. The patient who is going to have an easy labour does not require sympathy. The patient's faith may be lightly held and can easily be upset by sceptical doctors and midwives. If the patient does experience pain she should be given an analgesic. The patient herself is the best judge of her need and should be consulted. She should not be given drugs routinely because she is in strong labour. It is obvious that the presence of untrained patients having pain will lessen the trained patient's chances of success.

If the patient fails, she is naturally disappointed but at Stobhill Hospital there has not been a case who was psychologically upset. On the contrary, most of these women study the method more intensely during their next pregnancy and often succeed then. If the method was practised universally the population as a whole would lose its fear of childbirth and come to accept that labour can be a painless process. In this Utopia new generations will be favourably conditioned and the need for antenatal training will be less.

There are many forms of antenatal preparation. The simplest is the reassurance given by the doctor or obstetrician at the patient's routine antenatal visits. Many of the methods place the main emphasis on complicated exercises. The choice of words used by the teachers is more important than the actual exercises, accounting for differing success rates found throughout the country. Many of the "relaxation class" teachers have absorbed some of the principles of psychoprophylaxis but do not feel competent to discuss brain function and conditioning in detail. They still concentrate on exercises. Whatever the method used, the most important factor is the "psychotherapy" and the ability of the teacher to get it over to the patient.

Parisian psychoprophylaxis is a definite discipline combining the necessary psychological conditioning and simple exercises, the meaning and purpose of which can be readily understood by patients, physiotherapists, midwives and doctors.

REFERENCES

1. Barr, W. and Graham, R. (1967). *Postgrad. med. J.*, Suppl. **43,** 101.
2. Barr, W. and Graham, R. (1967). *J. Obstet. Gynaec. Brit. Cwlth,* **74,** 739.
3. Beard, R. W. and Morris, E. D. (1965). *J. Obstet. Gynaec. Brit. Cwlth,* **72,** 496.
4. Beard, R. W., Morris, E. D. and Clayton, S. G. (1966). *J. Obstet. Gynaec. Brit. Cwlth,* **73,** 562.
5. Beard, R. W., Morris, E. D. and Clayton, S. G. (1967). *J. Obstet. Gynaec. Brit. Cwlth,* **74,** 812.

6. BEARD, R. W., FILSHIE, G. M., KNIGHT, C. A. and ROBERTS, G. M. (1971). *R.C.O.G. 2nd College Study Group to Consider Methods for Monitoring the Fetus in Pregnancy and Labour.*
7. BEARD, R. W., BAIN, G., JOHNSON, D. A. N. and BENTALL, R. H. C. (1970). *Lancet*, **1**, 330.
8. BEAZLEY, J. M., BANOVIC, I. and FELD, M. S. (1975). *Brit. med. J.*, **2**, 248.
9. BONSTEIN, I. (1958). *Psychoprophylactic Preparation for Painless Childbirth.* London: Wm. Heinemann Med. Bks.
10. CALDEYRO, R., ALVAREZ, H. and REYNOLDS, S. R. M. (1950). *Surg. Gynec. Obstet.*, **91**, 641.
11. CHERTOK, L. (1959). *Psychosomatic Method in Painless Childbirth.* Oxford: Pergamon Press.
12. COOPER, K. and MOIR, J. C. (1963). *Brit. med. J.*, **1**, 1372.
13. COOPER, K., GILROY, K. J. and HURRY, D. J. (1968). *J. Obstet. Gynaec. Brit. Cwlth*, **75**, 863.
14. CRAWFORD, J. S. (1975). *Brit. J. Obstet. Gynaec.*, **82**, 929.
15. DOBKIN, A. B., KEIL, A. N. and WONG, G. (1961). *Anaesthesia*, **16**, 160.
16. DONALD, I. and LORD, J. (1953). *Lancet*, **1**, 9.
17. DONALD, I., KERR, M. M. and MACDONALD, I. R. (1958). *Scot. med. J.*, **3**, 151.
18. DONALD, I., BARR, W. and MCGARRY, J. A. (1962). *J. Obstet. Gynaec. Brit. Cwlth*, **69**, 837.
19. DUGGAN, T. C., LAUGHLAND, A. W. and MACGREGOR, J. (1966). *Lancet*, **1**, 488.
20. DUNDEE, J. W. and MOORE, J. (1962). *Brit. J. Anaesth.*, **34**, 247.
21. EDINGTON, P. T., SIBANDA, J. and BEARD, R. W. (1975). *Brit. med. J.*, **3**, 341.
22. HINGSON, R. A. and HELLMAN, L. M. (1956). *Anesthesia for Obstetrics.* Philadelphia: J. B. Lippincott Co.
23. HON, E. H. and HESS, O. W. (1960). *Amer. J. Obstet. Gynec.*, **79**, 1012.
24. JEFFCOATE, T. N. A. (1961). *Lancet*. **2**, 61.
25. KUBLI, E. W., HON, E. H., KHAZIN, A. F. and TAKEMURA, H. (1969). *Amer. J. Obstet. Gynec.*, **104**, 1190.
26. LACOMME, M., LABORIT, A., LE LORIER, G. and POMMIER, M. (1952). *Gynéc. et Obstét.*, **4**, No. 3, bis.
27. LAMAZE, F. (1958). *Painless Childbirth. A Psychoprophylactic Method.* London: Burke Publishing Co.
28. LANCET (1961). Report: Training for Childbirth. **1**, 765.
29. MACVICAR, J. and MURRAY, M. H. (1960). *Brit. med. J.*, **1**, 595.
30. MACVICAR, J. and HOWIE, P. (1967). *Lancet*. **2**, 1339.
31. MACVICAR, J. and HOWIE, P. (1970). *J. Obstet. Gynaec. Brit. Cwlth*, **77**, 817.
32. MOIR, D. D. and BISSET, W. I. K. (1965). *J. Obstet. Gynaec. Brit. Cwlth*, **72**, 264.
33. MOIR, D. D. (1973). *Pain Relief in Labour*, pp. 102–119. Edinburgh: Churchill Livingstone.
34. MOIR, D. D. (1975). *Scot. med. J.*, **20**, 167.
35. MOIR, D. D., SLATER, P. J., THORBURN, J., MCLAREN, R. and MOODIE, J. (1976). *Brit. J. Anaesth.*, **48**, 129.

36. Morris, E. D. and Beard, R. W. (1965). *J. Obstet. Gynaec. Brit. Cwlth*, **72,** 489.
37. Nixon, W. C. W. and Smyth, C. N. (1957). *J. Obstet. Gynaec. Brit. Emp.*, **64,** 35.
38. O'Driscoll, K., Jackson, R. J. A. and Gallagher, J. T. (1970). *J. Obstet. Gynaec. Brit. Cwlth*, **77,** 385.
39. O'Sullivan, J. V. (1948). *Proc. roy. Soc. Med.*, **41,** 312.
40. Pollock, G. B., Spitzel, J. J. and Mason, D. J. (1960). *Obstet. and Gynec.*, **15,** 504.
41. Reich, A. M. (1951). *Amer. J. Obstet. Gynec.*, **61,** 1263.
42. Roberts, H., Kane, K. M., Percival, N., Snow, P. and Please, N. W. (1957). *Lancet*, **1,** 128.
43. Roberts, H. and Please, N. W. (1958). *J. Obstet. Gynaec. Brit. Emp.*, **65,** 33.
44. Rooth, G. (1964). *Lancet*, **1,** 290.
45. Saling, E. (1962). *Arch. Gynäk.*, **197,** 108.
46. Saling, E. (1964). *Geburtsh. u. Frauenheilk.*, **24,** 464.
47. Smyth, C. N. (1957). *J. Physiol. (London).*, **137,** 3P.
48. Smyth, C. N. and Wolff, H. S. (1960). *Lancet*, **2,** 412.
49. Steer, P. J. and Beard, R. W. (1970). *J. Obstet. Gynaec. Brit. Cwlth*, **77,** 908.
50. Tafeen, C. H., Freedman, H. L. and Harris, H. (1966). *Amer. J. Obstet. Gynec.*, **94,** 854.
51. Turnbull, A. C. and Anderson, A. B. M. (1968). *J. Obstet. Gynaec. Brit. Cwlth*, **75,** 32.
52. Vellay, P. (1959). *Childbirth without Pain.* London: Hutchinson & Co.
53. Velvovsky, I. *et al.* (1960). *Painless Childbirth Through Psychoprophylaxis.* Moscow: Foreign Languages Publishing House.
54. Weaver, J. B., Pearson, J. F. and Turnbull, A. C. (1974). *J. Obstet. Gynaec. Brit. Cwlth*, **81,** 297.
55. Wood, C., Newman, W., Lumley, J. and Hammond, J. (1969). *Amer. J. Obstet. Gynec.*, **105,** 942.
56. Wright, H. P., Morris, N., Osborn, S. B. and Hart, A. (1958). *Amer. J. Obstet. Gynec.*, **75,** 3.

CHAPTER XIX

TECHNIQUE AND PITFALLS OF INSTRUMENTAL DELIVERY

THE development of the obstetric forceps dates from the innovation made by one of the members of the Chamberlen family around A.D. 1600, since when innumerable modifications and improvements have been made right up to our own time. The fascinating history of this aid to delivery is well dealt with in certain of the larger text-books, such as that of Greenhill-DeLee, and Munro Kerr and Chassar Moir's *Operative Obstetrics*. It will not be discussed at length here; suffice it to mention a few of the landmarks of major importance.

The original forceps had no pelvic curve, and this introduction is attributed to Levret in Paris during the first half of the eighteenth century. This was a major advance. It was Smellie who first used the forceps for the aftercoming head in breech delivery. Even the introduction of the pelvic curve only partially obviated the difficulties of high forceps application, and in 1877 Tarnier conceived the idea of axis traction employing a principle not far dissimilar from that of the modern Milne Murray forceps. The principle of axis traction at once made possible a more satisfactory pull in conformity with the curvature of the birth canal with an associated decrease in the amount of force necessary, thus sparing the maternal tissues, to say nothing of the fetal head, because it is consequently possible to resolve the forces of traction into their more appropriate components and to pull in the correct direction. In the case of a brim or high-cavity application the only alternative to axis traction is the use of Pajot's manoeuvre, in which the same resultant effect is attempted by pressing downwards on the shanks of the blades at the same time as traction is exerted (Fig. 1). This manoeuvre, incidentally, was introduced before the discovery of the principle of axis traction and is far cruder. Nowadays the importance of axis traction is dwindling, as the high forceps operation is only rarely performed in sound obstetric practice.

Neither axis traction nor the use of Pajot's manoeuvre, however, dealt adequately with the usually associated problem of the malrotated head, and to Kielland must go the honour of making the greatest single advance in forceps design, since when little of major importance has come on the scene.

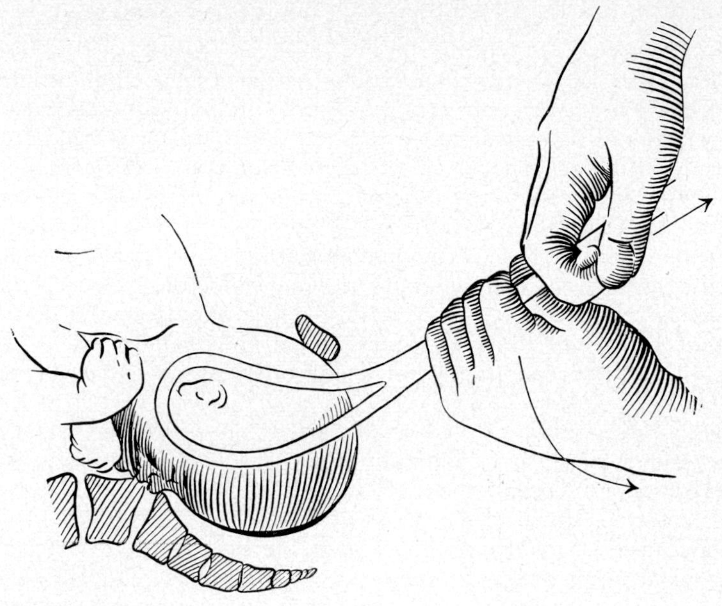

19/FIG. 1.—Pajot's manoeuvre.

FUNCTIONS OF THE OBSTETRIC FORCEPS

The chief of these is to supply traction in cases in which the unaided expulsive efforts of the mother are insufficient to effect a safe delivery in time. The second function is that of rotation, and this can only be guardedly mentioned, for, with the exception of Kielland's forceps, which are designed and eminently suitable for the purpose, rotation of the fetal head with forceps, whether by Scanzoni's manoeuvre or any other diabolical practice, is very questionable. The third function of the forceps is to provide a protective cage for the head from the pressure of the maternal parts, an advantage which is most noticeable in the case of the aftercoming head in breech delivery. In the latter case the forceps properly handled can prevent uncontrolled and too rapid delivery of the head with all its dangers of sudden decompression.

Lastly, the forceps to some extent decreases the transverse diameter of the head by compression, but in so doing increases the vertical diameter. Only where a perfect cephalic application has been achieved is this hypothetical function an advantage, and compression achieved between face and occiput, for example in a thoroughly bad application, is likely to be nothing less than lethal.

Types of Forceps

Time was when many obstetricians, as part of the climb to fame, designed a new type of obstetric forceps to suit their fad or fancy, and space will not be wasted here in enumerating them. Quite apart from variety in design, Rhodes (1958) drew attention to the not inconsiderable discrepancies by different manufacturers in the measurements of allegedly the same design of forceps. A certain haphazard development, too, has led to no very clear idea of what the measurements should be, and amongst other recommendations Rhodes suggests that the distance apart of the tips should be 3·0 cm the widest distance between the blades 9·0 cm, the blade length 16·0 cm and the radii of cephalic and pelvic curves 11·25 and 17·5 cm respectively.

Only three main types will be considered (Figs. 2, 3 and 4). Of all the varieties of axis traction forceps that of the Milne Murray type is one of the best, because the traction rods are applied to the bases of the fenestrae, which is the point at which the traction should be applied and where the hinging is most necessary. There is also the further advantage that the degree of flexion of the head can be independently controlled by the main handles of the instrument. There are innumerable varieties of long curved forceps, such as those which can be used with and without their axis traction attachments, and individual preference and training must determine the choice.

The second main group consists of the short curved forceps, such as the Wrigley pattern, which by their lightness and generous cephalic curve are ideal when the head is on the perineum. These beautiful little instruments are worth their weight in gold and can be applied with delicate ease and with the minimum of anaesthesia; they are kindness itself to both the baby's head and maternal soft parts.

The third main class is Kielland's forceps or some variation on this basic type which, with their sliding lock and peculiar shape, can, in practised hands, make wizardry of a difficult forceps delivery of the badly rotated head. I would be content to go through the rest of my obstetrical career with no forceps other than a pair of Kielland's and a pair of Wrigley's.

Conditions which must Obtain for Forceps Delivery

A legitimate indication must be present. This is mentioned first, because many of the troubles in obstetrics are due to interference which is either unwarranted or premature or both. The further indications will be dealt with presently.

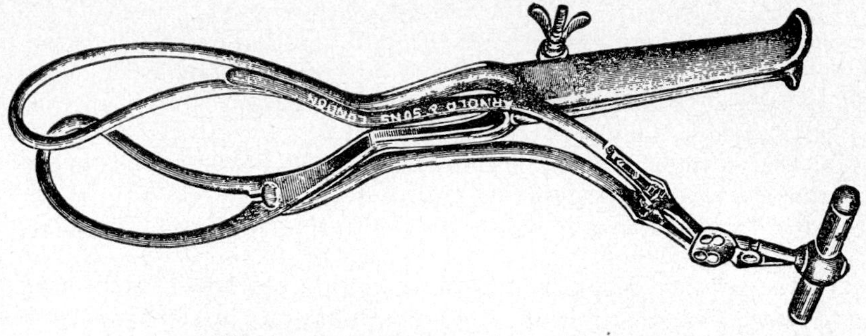

19/Fig. 2.—Milne Murray axis traction forceps.

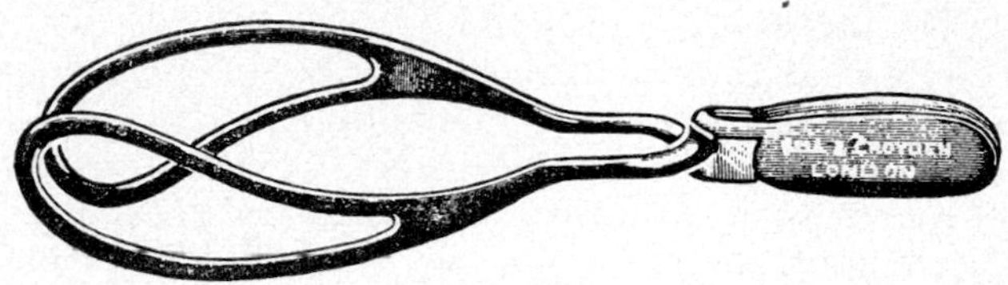

19/Fig. 3.—Wrigley's forceps.

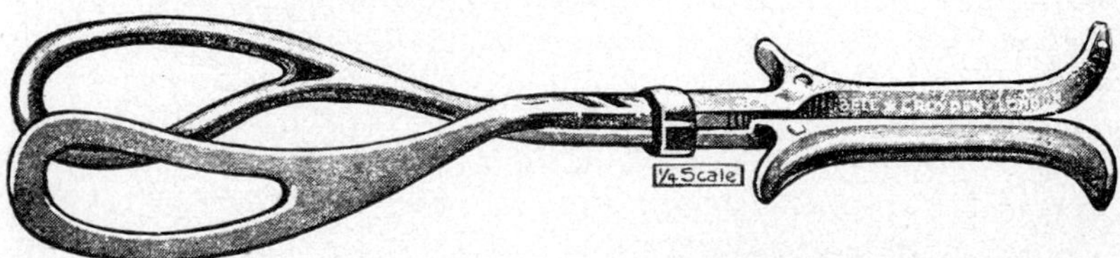

19/Fig. 4.—Kielland's forceps.

(Figs. 2, 3 and 4 by courtesy of John Bell and Croyden.)

Delivery must be mechanically feasible. By this is meant that there should be no insuperable bar to delivery because of disproportion. While one can arrive at a very reasonable estimate of the size of the patient's pelvis, the same cannot be said about the size of the baby's, head without very specialised techniques, but if it is deeply engaged in the pelvis then, clearly, its diameters must be less, at least, than those of the brim and mid pelvic straits. This does not necessarily mean that in every case no further mechanical difficulty may be encountered, although outlet contraction with a good sized brim is very uncommon. As a general rule, vaginal delivery can be completed in any case in which the head passes satisfactorily through the brim, but occasionally it may be achieved only at a severe price. Estimates of the true conjugate are a guide, but no more, to the feasibility of forceps delivery, because the strength of uterine contractions and the capacity of the head to mould cannot be forecast. Nevertheless, in any case in which the true conjugate is less than 3¾ inches (9·5 cm), the prospects of safe vaginal delivery must be carefully questioned.

The presentation must be suitable. The only presentations applicable are vertex presentations, face presentations where the chin is anterior, never when it is posterior, and the after-coming head in breech delivery.

The position of the head must be known, not only in respect of its level, but the degree of rotation and flexion must be accurately assessed before the forceps is applied. To apply the forceps blindly to a malrotated head, particularly one arrested in the transverse position, can play havoc with the baby.

The cervix must be fully dilated. The words "or nearly so" are often added, but have given rise to more trouble in forceps delivery than all the other difficulties put together. Often on examining the patient before applying the forceps a fringe of cervix can be felt, and it may appear that the cervix is so near to full dilatation that the head may be eased past it. Now there is all the difference in the world between a cervix which is fully dilated and one which is not quite so, and it is easy to be deceived about the practicability of forceps delivery there and then. Even though it appears that the cervical rim can be pushed over the maximum diameters, traction on the forceps can only mean traction on the lower uterine segment with its neighbouring rich nerve supply in the bases of the broad ligaments. A profound degree of shock is the not uncommon reward, and the cervix is almost bound to suffer more damage, in the form of a lateral split, than is usually foreseen. This state of affairs is commonly encountered in occipitoposterior positions where the patient shows, to all outward appearances, the signs of being fully dilated and is therefore encouraged to bear down. No advance of the head occurs, however, and after the lapse of an hour or two signs of maternal distress may develop and preparations are made for forceps delivery. The situation presently develops all the ingredients of a shambles. With the patient now anaesthetised, one is faced with the unwelcome alternatives of either delivering her through an incompletely dilated cervix, with all its attendant risks, or of calling off the anaesthetic and leaving her to continue her labour until she is unquestionably in the second stage. If at this point fetal distress is already established, one may have to choose the former alternative or perform Caesarean section. In other respects the latter is by far the safer course, although at the time it may appear the less humane. The original mistake, of course, was in diagnosing full dilatation prematurely. True, a rectal or a vaginal examination without an anaesthetic may have been made originally, but the mis-diagnosis may be made because the cervix was not reached by the examining finger. This is a sequence of events which is so often encountered that there is a strong case for not interesting oneself in the moment of full dilatation until the head is on the pelvic floor and the patient is bearing down of her own compulsive volition. If this rule were more frequently followed, the premature application of the forceps before full dilatation would be very much less common and disasters thereby avoided.

To add the obstetrical crime of forceps delivery before full dilatation, simply because one has been mistaken about the cervix in the first place, is seldom justifiable; nevertheless, from time to time circumstances arise in which the risks of such a delivery have to be taken advisedly. This is a task only for the experienced operator. In the majority of cases the situation should not have been allowed to arise. The application of the ventouse before full cervical dilatation is much less of a crime, and may have to be undertaken deliberately.

The patient must be suitably anaesthetised. The modern preference is for local analgesia whenever practicable, i.e. in the vast majority of cases (see later). Obstetrical anaesthesia is an art in its own right and is full of treachery, especially as the patient's stomach is often full. Induction should be smooth and quick, so that the patient is steered past the risk of asphyxia which is even more damaging to the baby than to the patient herself. Thereafter a light plane of anaesthesia should be maintained. The first plane of the third stage is the ideal level, as uterine activity is thereby less likely to be affected.

The bladder and rectum must be empty. The former is the more important of the two; nevertheless, either of them, when not empty, can reflexly hold up progress in labour and attention to them may often remove the apparent indications for forceps. Even more important is the danger to which a full bladder is exposed in forceps delivery. An empty bladder is very much less vulnerable. The passage of a catheter, therefore, before applying the forceps is a routine necessity. Because the head is jammed tightly against the symphysis pubis it may often be difficult to insert a catheter. This demands not the use of greater force but a slight elevation of the head to overcome the obstruction of the urethra. The catheter should be passed a fair distance inside and if no urine is at first withdrawn it may be necessary to pass in half of its length. This is because the lower part of the bladder may be empty due to compression by the fetal head. Suprapubic pressure should be applied not only in the midline but on both sides of it in order to tap every available drop of urine.

Uterine contractions should be present. Not only do they indicate the likelihood of the uterus retracting suitably after the extraction of the child, but any contribution to expulsive force which the uterus can supply reduces by that amount the traction force necessary with the forceps. In most cases a contraction is reflexly stimulated as soon as the forceps is pulled upon. To deliver in the presence of complete uterine atony is to invite one of the worst-known varieties of postpartum haemorrhage.

Lastly, the membranes should have been already ruptured. This is less important, because delivery is perfectly possible with intact membranes, but the point is that this very fact alone may be the cause of delay and their deliberate rupture may remove the apparent indication for forceps.

Local Analgesia versus General Anaesthesia for Forceps Delivery

There can be few greater therapeutic insults offered to a woman in labour than inexpertly administered anaesthesia. A formidable collection of unhappy reminiscences has convinced me that obstetrical anaesthesia is no job for the occasional anaesthetist and unsupervised junior house officers. The only reason why chloroform once enjoyed a peculiar reputation for safety in parturient women was its relative rapidity of induction before vomiting occurred and the fact that general practitioners used it with the patient lying on her side for forceps delivery in the left lateral position, thus incidentally reducing the risks of inhaled vomit.

It would be an exaggeration to say that anaesthetists, today, kill more mothers in labour, and babies, than do obstetricians, but careful reading between the lines of maternal mortality reports will far more often implicate anaesthetic accidents than the statistics would suggest. Parker[32, 33] long ago reckoned that aspiration of inhaled vomit was responsible for 4 per cent of maternal deaths occurring in Birmingham and this may be an understatement as post-mortem proof is often lacking. It is not the large chunks of solid matter that may be aspirated that cause the trouble as a rule, though they can be dangerous enough, but the highly irritant brown fluid, often made more deadly with glucose, copiously regurgitated and sucked deeply down the bronchial tree, far beyond the reach of even bronchoscopic suction, which is not only lethal but may leave little trace unless the patient survives for more than a day and long enough for the bronchiolar reaction to be demonstrable at necropsy.

Mendelson (1946) differentiated two types of case following aspiration of vomit: the obstructive group due to solid particles of food and the "asthmatic" type which is the commoner danger in obstetrics and whose importance is now better recognised. At the time of induction or recovery from inhalation anaesthesia vomiting occurs, but it is often not realised at the time that foreign matter has been aspirated. For a variable period up to a few hours the patient's condition may at first appear to be satisfactory but presently cyanosis, dyspnoea and marked tachycardia with hypotension develop. A type of pulmonary oedema sets in together with bronchospasm sometimes and progressive collapse usually. Death may occur within 12 hours in the worst cases or sometimes in 4 or 5 days if an aspiration bronchopneumonia supervenes.

Fortunately, in the majority who survive and whose perilous adventures do not find their way into maternity reports, recovery would appear to be complete. Treatment consists of oxygen and antibiotics. Digoxin is often given but usually fails to control the tachycardia.

Intravenous aminophylline (250 mg) may be tried if bronchospasm is evident. Bronchoscopic suction is usually disappointing and one feels remarkably helpless when faced with this clinical picture. I have seen a patient die within a few hours, chattering and excited to within an hour or two of death, with deep cyanosis which an oxygen tent affected not at all, and an uncontrollable tachycardia. There had been no haemorrhage but the antecedent labour had been prolonged.

It was suggested by Hausmann and Lunt (1955) that the underlying pathology is an acute adrenal failure and they appear to have had some success with intravenous hydrocortisone started immediately (100 mg given within 4 hours in a 5 per cent glucose drip). If hypotension is very severe, noradrenaline should be added to the drip (e.g. Levophed 2–4 mg to the half-litre) and the drip regulated around 10–20 drops per minute according to very frequent blood-pressure readings.

Clearly, this is an ugly complication of operative delivery which it is worth going to great lengths to prevent. The patients, after all, are unpremedicated and often in poor metabolic shape before anaesthesia, quite apart from their full stomachs. Some anaesthetists empty the stomach first by passing a stomach tube—probably the safest course, but by no means wholly effective. For a brief while the intravenous injection of apomorphine to induce vomiting to be followed with atropine enjoyed a short vogue. To be really safe a cuffed endotracheal tube is necessary but with inexperienced anaesthetists the damage may be done before the tube is passed or, let it not be forgotten, after it has been prematurely withdrawn.

The problem is further aggravated by the fact that few labour ward beds can be rapidly tilted into the head-down position should vomiting occur and far too many labour wards are without efficient mechanical suction instantly available. In order to minimise the hazard of acid aspiration we make it an invariable rule now to give 14 ml of standard magnesium trisilicate mixture by mouth immediately before all general anaesthetics and when there is abdominal distension in prolonged labour we pass a stomach tube as well. The effects of the magnesium trisilicate mixture last for up to two hours by way of neutralising the gastric contents.

Quite apart from the more dramatic risks of obstetric anaesthesia enumerated above, there must also be remembered the effects upon the baby in addition to those of accidental asphyxia.

All anaesthetics not only put the mother to sleep, but the baby and the uterus to some extent as well.

Finally, if one counts up all the anxious time one has spent awaiting the arrival of a suitable anaesthetist, it is small wonder that modern local analgesia has been welcomed on an increasing scale.

It is now the practice in my unit to use local analgesia, if possible, in all forceps deliveries in which the vertex presents, the only absolute contra-indications being eclampsia and cases for trial of forceps (see later), in which the possibility of Caesarean section as an alternative is being considered. Even the "hysterical" patient can usually be talked into co-operation, if necessary with the help of intravenous promazine (Sparine) 50 mg or 5 mg of diazepam. Furthermore, we now prefer to train our junior residents in the techniques of forceps delivery having first effected local analgesia, since a bad or rough application cannot be made without protest from the patient and less traction effort is required because of the contribution which the patient and her uterus can be encouraged to make in delivering the head. In fact, forceps delivery under local analgesia is not only safer for the mother, but the lively condition of the unanaesthetised babies proclaims it as the method of choice. The popularity of low spinal or saddle-block anaesthesia, which is so widespread in the U.S.A. is less widely shared in the United Kingdom. Our own reasons for preferring pudendal nerve block are its simplicity, its great safety and, not least, the fact that the patient retains her expulsive reflexes and is able to contribute to the delivery and reduce the traction effort with forceps. Often the patient is already under the influence of an epidural anaesthetic because of first-stage difficulty and this will then suffice but a one-shot epidural anaesthetic is often used.

Technique of Local Analgesia

Lignocaine hydrochloride (Xylocaine 1 per cent) or, as an alternative, prilocaine (Citanest 1 per cent) have proved, in our experience, the most useful agents yet tried. They are remarkably non-toxic and complications are rare, and are only likely to follow accidental intravenous injection or frank overdosage. Allergy has not been reported, but dizziness and collapse may occur if a large quantity of the drug rapidly enters the circulation. Hypotension may require a pressor drug such as ephedrine intravenously (dose 10–15 mg) during the immediate emergency and if it persists 100 mg of hydrocortisone should be given by drip infusion. The commonest cause of hypotension however results from inferior vena caval compression and it is now our standard practice, even with the patient in the lithotomy position, to impart a tilt of approximately 10° to one side by means of a wedge mattress. Convulsions may be controlled by intravenous thiopentone. Such accidents are very unlikely in standard dosage which gives a good duration of analgesia sufficient for most forceps operations and repair of episiotomy thereafter. Its spreading power is so great that the use of hyaluronidase is unnecessary; in fact, by increasing the rate of diffusion, hyaluronidase proves a nuisance by shortening the duration of anaesthetic effect.

In a study of 100 primigravidae, prospectively half of whom were delivered under epidural block and the other half by forceps under pudendal block with perineal infiltration, no difference was found in postpartum headache, disorders of micturition or backache between the two groups.[30]

Perineal Infiltration

Local infiltration of the perineum is all that may be necessary for the performance of episiotomy and very low outlet forceps or the application of the ventouse at the end of the second stage. Indeed, if the fetal head is very low it may be impossible to reach the ischial spines for the purpose of pudendal nerve block without hurting the patient. It is also sufficient for most perineal repairs. The technique is very simple. Using a long, fine needle, on a 20-ml syringe, 10–20 ml of 1 per cent lignocaine is injected fanwise, from a point in the midline at the fourchette. If possible it is as well to insert a couple of fingers into the vagina first to put the perineal tissues on a slight stretch.

Premedication—for delivery under local analgesia.—The best premedication of all is a thoughtful and careful explanation to the patient of what one is about to do, explaining the help that is about to be offered for her baby's sake as well as her own and securing her intelligent co-operation. A conversational patter maintained throughout with the patient will often suffice for even apparently hysterical patients. It is here particularly that the rapport established between doctor and patient in the course of good antenatal care begins to reap its dividends. However, the situation on the psychological front may have been allowed to get out of control before operative intervention is contemplated. In these cases we have found intravenous injection of Sparine or diazepam, as described in the previous chapter, of great help. There are all manner of variants on this theme. The medication is given about 10 minutes before the patient is placed in the lithotomy position and draped.

Pudendal Nerve Block

The only apparatus required is a 20-ml syringe and a fine needle at least five inches in length. The aim of the injection is to place the solution around the internal pudendal nerve as it passes into the ischiorectal fossa adjacent to the ischial spine. In actual practice the spread of effect of lignocaine makes up for indifferent technique to a most comforting extent. It will be remembered that this nerve leaves the pelvic cavity above the pelvic diaphragm through the lower border of the sacrosciatic foramen and, in company with the pudendal artery, winds round the outer surface of the ischial spine and then enters the ischiorectal fossa below it. At any distance thereafter it may give off inferior haemorrhoidal and perineal branches before it goes on to reach the clitoris. Quite a small quantity of local anaesthetic, therefore, placed in the strategic position near the inferior and outer border of the ischial spine will achieve a wide field of anaesthesia.

There are two methods of placing this injection and for both a one per cent solution of lignocaine or prilocaine without adrenaline or hyaluronidase is recommended. The older and now dying method is to inject via the ischiorectal fossa. For this purpose a weal is first raised on either side at a point midway between the ischial tuberosity and the anus. A finger is then placed in the vagina and the ischial spine identified. The ischial spine is aimed for with the needle and the finger in the vagina helps to guide it just below its inferior border. The plunger is withdrawn to make sure that a vessel has not been entered and a solution of 10 ml of lignocaine is injected on each side. A further 5 ml can be placed just medial to the ischial tuberosity in order to block an aberrant inferior haemorrhoidal nerve and finally 5 to 10 ml can be injected under the greater part of the length of skin covering each labium majus, in order to block any filaments from the ileo-inguinal nerve. In actual fact this latter procedure is seldom necessary. It will be noticed that the total dose now given does not exceed 40 to 50 ml of one per cent lignocaine which is well within the safety limit. It used to be my practice to infiltrate the perineum first with about 15 ml in order to make the examination and the palpation of the ischial spines more comfortable for the patient and also to cover up any deficiencies in technique. Such is the spreading power of lignocaine, however, that even a reasonably approximate approach to the ischial spine on the point of emergence of the pudendal nerve is sufficient to produce an efficient block and the extra dosage in the perineum is not usually necessary. The makers of lignocaine advise restricting the total volume administered to no more than 50 ml of one per cent solution, although I have often exceeded this dose. The anatomical details of the technique have been well illustrated by Gate and Dutton (1955). If one is less confident of this technique and wishes to fall back on larger quantities of solution it is better to use a half per cent strength, which is also quite effective, rather than increase the dose.

The second method of achieving pudendal nerve block, and one which we increasingly favour, is by the transvaginal route as graphically described by Kobak *et al.* (1956) and by Huntingford (1959). This technique provides the shortest possible route to the nerve and would seem to be the last step in the evolution of pudendal nerve block. A six-inch, seventeen-gauge spinal needle is recommended, together with a 20-ml syringe. The index and middle fingers of one hand, held in apposition, reach for the ischial spine. If there is difficulty in palpating it because it is not prominent, the sacrospinous ligament can be felt as a ridge converging on it. The shaft of the needle can be placed in the groove between the two fingers and the needle and is thus made to penetrate the vaginal skin just below the ischial spine. The direction of the needle is now altered so that it is parallel with the table on which the patient is lying. This will take the point of the needle slightly behind the spine and, after aspiration to ensure that a blood vessel has not been entered, a very accurately placed injection is possible. If blood is aspirated it is better to withdraw the needle and reinsert it slightly more to the midline to avoid the vessels.

This technique involves the intravaginal use of two fingers and it is very easy to puncture the glove with the needle tip.

The method which Huntingford recommends is slightly different and involves guiding the needle to the tip of the ischial spine by the index finger of one hand with the thumb of the same hand flexed on the shaft of the needle. When the needle point is at the tip of the ischial spine, it is advanced about 0·5 cm to bring it over the sacrospinous ligament, then, by bending the point of the needle by firm pressure with the index finger against the resistance of the thumb on the shaft the sacrospinous ligament is penetrated and following aspiration for blood, as before, the injection is made deep to the sacrospinous ligament.

At this point mention should be made of the Iowa trumpet. I was introduced to this delightful instrument by Dr Edwin McDaniel of Thailand and I am very grateful to Dr Dan S. Egbert of Fort Dodge, Iowa, for sending me one for my own use. It consists of a guide for a 5-in needle which can only project a few millimetres beyond a blunt, bulbous tip. At the proximal end of the guide is a ring for the thumb, while the finger can be placed over the bulbous tip which is guided onto the lower tip of the ischial spine before the long needle is passed through it and inserted in the usual fashion.[8] The use of this instrument makes child's play of pudendal block anaesthesia and secures an accurate placing of the solution and therefore anaesthesia is almost immediate. This can be verified by asking the patient to draw in the anus which she should now be unable to do because of levator paralysis, also needleprick in the region of the anus produces no response from the external sphincter. The pelvic floor becomes very much more slack after pudendal block has been achieved, thereby facilitating operative procedures and examination even before episiotomy. The duration of anaesthesia is seldom less than thirty minutes, sometimes more, and can easily be extended by further injection later when it wears off, but it is adequate in most cases for the subsequent repair of an episiotomy and for many cases of manual removal of the placenta, if a general anaesthetic for this operation is not immediately available. My own enthusiasm for pudendal block using the Iowa trumpet may to some extent be conditioned by the fact that I usually put in some local perineal infiltration as well and there are some who have suggested that the efficacy of pudendal block simply depends upon the perineal infiltration alone.[36] This I do not believe, because the forceps operation under perineal infiltration alone is seldom a painless affair.

One of the arguments against using adrenaline with lignocaine, apart from the fact that it is unnecessary, is that there is danger of sudden ventricular fibrillation if the patient at the same time has trichloroethylene, for example, from a self-administering inhaler.[23] If any form of self-administered inhalation anaesthetic is required because of a partially unsuccessful pudendal block, then the 50/50 nitrous oxide and oxygen mixture as delivered by the Entonox apparatus would be the most suitable.

The ensuing operation calls for great finesse. By careful reassurance of the patient, careful timing of movement, slow and deliberate gentleness and attention to the direction of pull, it is possible to slip on the forceps blades and deliver the head with less pain and discomfort for the patient than a normal spontaneous delivery in a primipara. Smellie must have worked with such delicate touch on far less suitable but unanaesthetised patients in his day and we would do well to remember his example.

Not least of the advantages of a well-conducted delivery under pudendal block analgesia is the lively interest and co-operation of the patient in what is her greatest hour.

To exploit the technique of this method to the full one must become familiar with the use of Kielland's forceps, since rotation of the head is best done with this beautiful instrument. Manual rotation requiring the half hand, or more often the whole hand in the vagina, may require general anaesthesia.

Local analgesia was successful in 94 per cent of all types of forceps delivery in Scott and Gadd's series (1957) and in 84 per cent of all cases of delivery by Kielland's forceps, although a supplementary injection of chlorpromazine ($12\frac{1}{2}$ mg) and pethidine (100 mg) was necessary in a minority of cases (where we would use promazine).

Scott uses a proper operating table with the patient's buttocks overhanging the edge, in order to facilitate the application of the anterior blade of Kielland's forceps in the direct method of application (see later). These workers have shown the traction forces applied by the use of a dynamometer attached to the handles of the Kielland's forceps, and they class as moderate traction forces of from 35 to 50 lb (16 to 23 kg), and 70 lb (32 kg) as severe, above which level damage to the baby's head is likely.

Epidural Anaesthesia

Well-executed pudendal nerve block is so efficient that the fuller type of anaesthesia produced by the epidural route is seldom called for in the case of operative vaginal deliveries. Nevertheless, where it is necessary to remove pain completely or in cases where the possibility of proceeding to Caesarean section is being considered in the event of failure to deliver by the vaginal route, there is much to be said for inducing epidural anaesthesia in the first place. Continuous epidural anaesthesia has already been discussed at some length in the previous chapter. The disadvantage is that the patient can contribute nothing, or practically nothing, to her own delivery by voluntary bearing down efforts because of her temporary paraplegia, and most of the forces to achieve delivery have to be applied through the instrument used. Nevertheless, this technique enjoys very great popularity in the United States, and deservedly so. In competent hands it provides a most excellent and safe anaesthetic, particularly from the baby's point of view. The technique is as follows: the patient lies on her left side with the legs moderately flexed and the shoulders parallel. There should be no attempt to flex the spine unduly since this stretches the dura and also reduces the capacity of the peridural space. After infiltration of the skin in the midline between either the 2nd and 3rd or 3rd and 4th lumbar vertebrae, a fairly large-bore needle with a sharp stilette (similar to a 16-gauge Tuohy needle) is inserted, keeping constantly in the midline, and advanced until the tough ligamentum flavum is encountered. The latter is the important structure which indicates the correct progress of the needle, and as the needle goes beyond this tough medium there is a definite sense of release conveyed through the needle to the operator. Attempts to inject fluid or air whilst the point of the needle is still in the ligament result in a rebound of the piston, whereas, when the point is in the peridural space the syringe empties easily. The hanging-drop technique may be employed to estimate the progress of the needle. It is essential to appreciate the dangers of inadvertent intrathecal injection, since the introduction of a large volume of fluid into the subarachnoid space would cause a high spinal anaesthetic, high enough to produce respiratory paralysis, a state of affairs which must, be instantly recognised and dealt with by artificial respiration. Furthermore there is likely to be a severe drop in blood pressure. Therefore, after ascertaining the inability to withdraw cerebrospinal fluid, a test dose of 2 ml is advisable, followed by a pause of about 5 minutes to check for the development of somatic anaesthesia. If the test proves negative, it should be followed by a further injection of about 20 ml. A fairly large pillow beneath the head and shoulders of the patient will ensure that the analgesic fluid will extend caudad and thus include the sacral nerves so essential in vaginal deliveries. The solutions used are the same as in caudal blocks, again preferring lignocaine or prilocaine, 1 per cent, or 1·5 per cent without adrenaline. Slow injection is desirable, as this minimises the likelihood of hypotension. Bupivacaine 0·5 per cent produces a longer effect although this is not likely to be needed.

It is interesting to compare the blood loss at forceps delivery carried out under different types of anaesthesia and this has been investigated at the Queen Mother's Hospital by Moir and Wallace (1967) in 214 consecutive and unselected mid-cavity forceps deliveries in which episiotomy was performed at the same time. The estimation was carried out by the haemoglobin extraction dilution technique using the Perdometer apparatus into which were fed all gowns, gloves, swabs and in fact almost every drop of blood lost at delivery. It is a sort of washing machine containing a solution which extracted the haemoglobin and passed the washing fluid of known volume through a photoelectric mechanism, adjustment having been previously made for the patient's known haemoglobin. The amount lost was very much greater than expected whatever the anaesthetic, a fact which no longer surprises me; but the mean loss was found to be 518 ml under general anaesthesia, 412 ml under pudendal block and only 276 under epidural analgesia, much of the latter coming from the episiotomy wound.

Indications for Forceps Delivery

It has for long been customary to think of the indications in terms of faults in forces, passages and passenger, but this generalisation needs qualifying. Agreed the forces may be inadequate; nevertheless they should be present. With regard to faults in the passages, the only genuine indication in this class is undue resistance to delivery by maternal soft tissue. Bony disproportion is not a proper indication; in fact it may be a positive contra-indication. Faults in the passenger are more usually due to malrotation and deflexion than anything else, and it will be seen that this classification of indications is far too incomplete and misleading to be any longer acceptable. It is, therefore, better to class the indications for forceps as maternal, or fetal or both.

Physical maternal distress is indicated by a dry tongue, a rising pulse, a variable degree of pyrexia, and in extreme cases by hotness and dryness of the vagina. Of these the dry tongue is the most important. No woman in the second stage of labour with a clean moist tongue can be genuinely regarded as physically distressed however heavily she appears to be weathering her labour. In other words, dehydration is a part of the mechanism of maternal distress; the urine likewise shows increasing specific gravity and in advanced cases may contain appreciable quantities of albumin and acetone.

In certain general maternal conditions the threat of maternal distress becomes an indication for forceps delivery and its frank development cannot be tolerated, for example, in cases with cardiac lesions, pulmonary tuberculosis, and thyroid disease associated with dyspnoea. Likewise in eclampsia, at full dilatation, forceps delivery is indicated in both maternal and fetal interests. The fetal indications are mainly those of asphyxia or the threat thereof. Unfortunately the signs of fetal distress are only clinically apparent when fetal asphyxia in already advanced and irreparable damage may already have been done. The subject of fetal distress has been dealt with in the previous chapter, and in the second stage of labour calls for delivery forthwith.

There are additional fetal indications in which the threat of fetal asphyxia is so definite as to constitute an immediate indication for delivery. Instances of such are prolapse of the cord at full dilatation and eclamptic seizures in the mother. A very significant sign of fetal asphyxia is the appearance of violent convulsive movements of the baby indicating that it is literally in its death throes.

Of course, to apply the forceps to the head of a distressed fetus is to increase its distress somewhat further. Nevertheless, it is safer to deliver it forthwith than to leave the original conditions of asphyxia still in full operation. A baby *in utero* will not withstand genuine distress for very long. In such a delivery everything possible must be done to spare further trauma to the baby's head and an episiotomy is obligatory.

Failure to advance is an accepted indication, but it must be qualified in the light of the nature of the uterine contractions. Although a duration of the second stage of 2 hours is regarded as a more than adequate maximum, midwifery cannot be run according to the clock, and in some cases of hypotonic uterine inertia the patient may be regarded simply as performing a perfectly normal delivery but in a slower gear. In these cases, in the absence of fetal and maternal distress, labour can safely be allowed to continue normally.

More commonly, however, it is apparent that the patient's own expulsive forces are not enough of themselves to effect delivery and in these cases failure to advance becomes a genuine reason for operating long before the elapse of two hours; in fact lack of progress in spite of good contractions for an hour calls for action. In any case of doubt a vaginal examination should be made and the reason for the delay may then become more apparent. An occipitoposterior position or a head which is not rotated from the transverse position will in many such cases be found to be the real cause.

Incidence of Forceps Delivery

This varies very widely from one institution to another and from one obstetrician to another, even though the maternal morbidity and fetal mortality figures may not vary much, which suggests that the use of forceps might be overdone.

The incidence in hospital practice is naturally much higher than outside mainly because of selection and the greater availability of services. Our own incidence of instrumental delivery, predominantly forceps, was 24 per cent in 1975. Approximately three-quarters are in primigravid patients. The indications in the order of numerical importance are as follows:

Fetal distress;
Delay or the threat of delay in 2nd stage;
Deep transverse arrest of head;
Persistent occipitoposterior position;
Maternal indications.

In a few cases, about half a dozen each year, the ventouse may be used to pull the head down to a lower station but delivery thereafter is completed with forceps because of detachment of the cup. It is interesting to note that ten years ago there was a neonatal loss of 11 cases (1·7 per cent) of which congenital malformations were responsible for five of the six neonatal deaths, the remaining neonatal death being due to meconium aspiration. Of the five stillbirths, four were delivered after 41 weeks gestation with cessation of the fetal heart during the first stage of labour. These fresh stillbirths are capable of practically being eliminated thanks to the increased use of monitoring during labour and provided, of course, that a severe fetal abnormality does not prejudice the issue.

In short, one is reminded that the indications for which forceps may be deemed necessary may, in themselves, be more dangerous to fetal life than the operation itself which should not be attempted in the face of mechanical difficulty.

Technique of Forceps Application

The patient is placed in the lithotomy position on a wedge mattress to tilt her laterally 10 to 15 degrees in order to prevent caval compression and resulting hypotension. The old-fashioned method of using the left lateral position has now been abandoned. Not only does the lithotomy position facilitate aseptic technique, but by improving accessibility a correct orientation of the position of the baby's head is easier.

The vulva and surrounding skin are liberally sponged with antiseptic, the bladder is catheterised and the patient draped in sterile towels. A pudendal block anaesthetic is administered and a thorough vaginal examination may now be made. This entails inserting at least the half hand, and in any case where there is the slightest doubt there should be no hesitation in using the whole hand. It is often worth patiently ironing out the perineum with the fingers of both hands in order to facilitate this examination.

Having noted the depth of engagement of the head, a digital assessment of the size and shape of the pelvis should be made to ensure that vaginal delivery is possible and safe. In the course of this one should be satisfied that the cervix is, in fact, fully dilated, in which case its existence is barely palpable and no rim, or gutter caused by the fornices, can be felt, since at full dilatation the vagina, cervix and uterine cavity should form one continuous tube. By inserting the fingers where there is most room and by the use of patient gentleness it should be possible in most cases to avoid seriously displacing the fetal head upwards. Occasionally, in the case of a tight fit, the bones of the fetal vault may be felt to go in momentarily like a ping-pong ball when pressed. This disconcerting sign is fortunately of little significance. An attempt is now made to identify the sutures, which can be very difficult in the presence of a large caput. The sagittal suture by its length and straightness can usually be identified without too much difficulty, but it is often hard to distinguish between the two fontanelles. Theoretically this should be easy because, in the case of the anterior, four suture lines radiate from it and in the case of the posterior only three, in which the sutures join in the shape of a Y. Nevertheless, within the cramped space of the vagina, it is terribly easy to be mistaken by counting sutures. If the finger is slowly and deliberately swept round the fontanelle, counting each suture in turn, it is often impossible to be sure whether a fourth suture felt is in fact the first one felt for the second time. Even an assessment of the angles at which they diverge from each other can be difficult. A better method is to place the index and ring finger of the examining hand on two of the sutures which seem farthest apart and then to palpate with the middle finger to identify whether one or two intervening sutures remain (Fig. 5). In certain instances, especially if the head is high, this too may be difficult because of the awkward position for the examining hand. There should be no hesitation in using either right or left hand according to whichever is most convenient. Another method of fontanelle identification which is sometimes useful depends upon the fact that the parietal bones often overlap the frontal bones, whereas overlapping does not usually occur at the frontal suture, so that a finger placed on each frontal bone is able to depress first one and then the other relative to its partner. Often, the frontal suture is hard to feel, but the cranial bones near the anterior fontanelle feel softer than those farther back near the posterior fontanelle. Notwithstanding all the above, doubt may still remain about the exact position of the head,

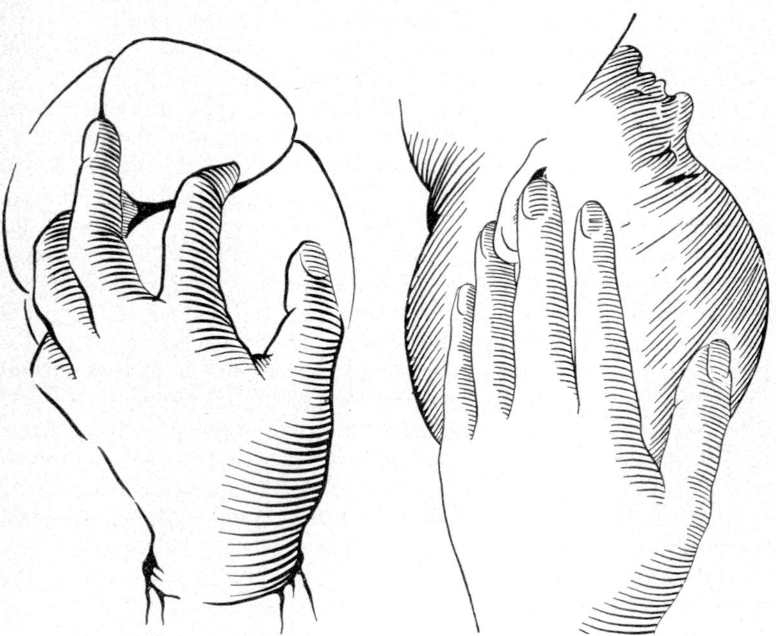

19/Fig. 5.—Suture counting.

19/Fig. 6.—Feeling for and identifying an ear.

and in these circumstances it is necessary to identify an ear. For this purpose the fingers have to be pushed much farther in and often the use of the half hand will not suffice. It is usually easier to reach an ear by the posterior than by the anterior approach, and care should be taken to dislodge the head upwards as little as possible, if necessary steadying it by suprapubic pressure. To reach the flange of the ear is not enough, because the ear is often bent over on itself so that the pinna points in the wrong direction. To obviate this mistake the finger should identify the external auditory meatus so that the pinna can be straightened out. An ear properly felt resolves all doubt (Fig. 6). An alternative method is to pass the hand farther up alongside the head to identify the nape of the neck.

The correct orientation of the position of the head is the most important part of the operation, because a proper cephalic application of the blades is a necessary condition for safe delivery. The use of Kielland's forceps will be discussed later, but for the usual types of instrument the occiput must always first be rotated to the anterior position except when the head is very low and the occiput dead posterior, when a deliberate face-to-pubis delivery with the help of an episiotomy is usually to be preferred.

Applying the Blades

Having rotated the occiput to a suitable position, there are two standard methods of applying the blades of the usual long curved forceps. The method preferred by the writer is to insert the right hand laterally alongside the head and, holding the left blade of the forceps between finger and thumb of the left hand, lightly to steer it directly alongside the baby's head. In this manoeuvre the handle of the forceps blade starts above the symphysis pubis and parallel to the right inguinal ligament on the patient's right and swings down in an arc towards her left (Fig. 7). The left half hand is now inserted alongside the baby's head and the manoeuvre repeated with the other blade held as before but in the right hand. Correctly applied, the locks should come easily together and the handles should be very little separated. The other standard method is to insert the left hand into the vagina in front of the hollow of the sacrum and to introduce each blade in turn posteriorly first, then manipulating it round to the side of the baby's head. The blades should lock comfortably and easily as before.

Difficulty may be experienced in applying the blades. This is no indication for the use of more force, which should, anyway, never exceed the power which three fingers can apply, and it indicates rather the need for re-examination. If the cervix is not fully dilated, one may fail to apply the forceps simply because the point of the blades is being pushed into one of the vaginal fornices. The most common source of difficulty, however, is due to the fact that the head has not been properly rotated with the occiput anterior. Under these circumstances the locks may fail to come together or the handles may appear to be widely separated. This assuredly denotes a faulty application and demands re-examination, correction of the malposition and applying the blades again. Cramming the forceps

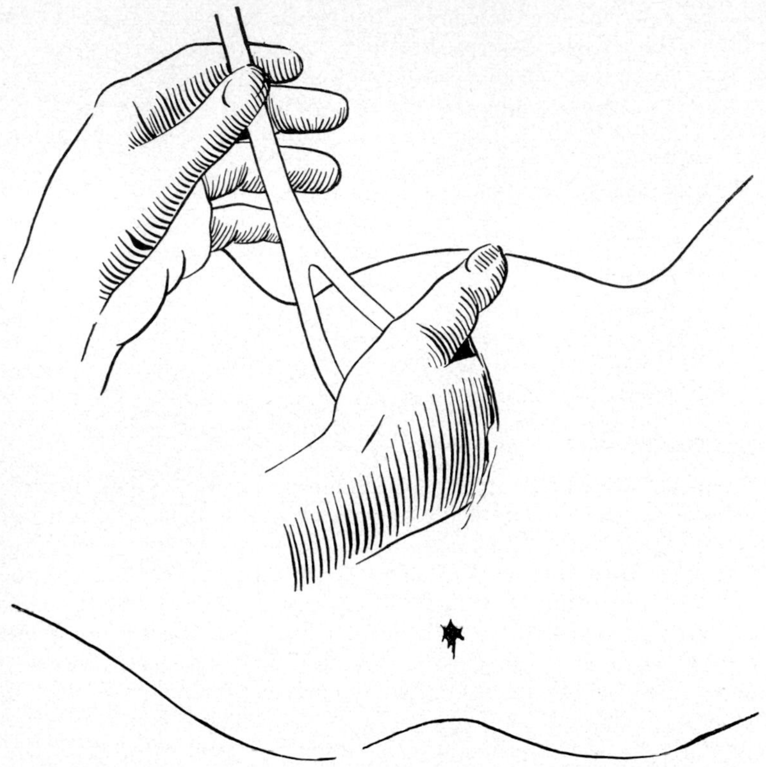

19/FIG. 7.—Inserting left forceps blade.

together by brute force is only to be deplored. Sometimes failure to lock the blades is due to the fact that they have not been introduced far enough, and it is a common mistake for beginners to hold the handles too far forward, which prevents the proper insertion of the blades. A correct cephalic application advertises itself by the ease with which the handles come together. In this position the blades lie along a line joining the chin and junction of the posterior and middle thirds of a line joining the anterior and posterior fontanelles.

Manual Rotation of the Occiput

This is a very necessary part of the forceps operation in which the occiput is not already anterior. It requires a certain amount of knack and at times can be very difficult. During its performance two objectives must not be forgotten, namely to maintain as far as possible a good degree of flexion and to avoid undue displacement upwards of the head. If the head escapes above the brim it may be reluctant to engage again in its new position, so that one is faced with the alternatives of a high forceps application, an internal version and breech extraction (very hazardous) or Caesarean section. Some upward displacement is inevitable in order to facilitate manual rotation, but its degree should, as far as possible, be controlled. In the case of ROP and ROL positions, it is usual to use the left hand and vice versa so that the movement of forearm and wrist is one of pronation (Fig. 8). The rotation of the head should be accompanied by rotation of the trunk by manipulation of the baby's anterior shoulder *per abdomen*, and one should not be content with less than overcorrection to a few degrees on the opposite side of the midline in order to ensure against the malposition recurring. Beware of using too much lubricant as it will make the grip too slippery. One of the great advantages of the use of Kielland's forceps is that rotation can be completed with the minimum of displacement of the fetal head and these forceps prevent the malposition from recurring. Often, too, the head is more easily rotated at a lower level in the pelvis than can be achieved by the hand. This will be discussed more fully later.

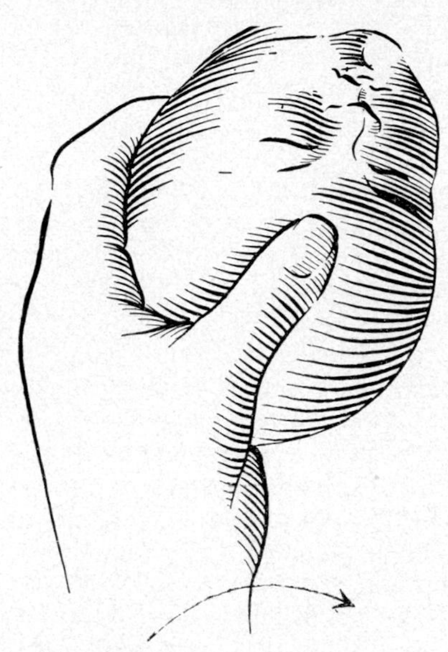

19/FIG. 8.—Manual rotation of head in ROP position.

An alternative method of manual rotation is to pass the fingers up over the baby's face, thus improving flexion, and to rotate by supinating the arm, using the right hand in ROP positions and the left hand for LOP positions. Sometimes it suffices to reach up no further than the anterior fontanelle, using the pressure of the ulnar border of a finger on the fontanelle margin to achieve rotation. The sacral promontory sometimes prevents full rotation by getting in the way of the sinciput. The remedy is to displace the head a little farther upwards, but a hand must, at the same time, be applied to the abdomen to control the displacement and to push the head down into the pelvis again when the sinciput can be negotiated into the opposite parasacral bay.

The deliberate employment of manual rotation of the head before full dilatation of the cervix, in order to expedite a first stage which is dragging on from three-quarters dilatation, is usually a waste of time since delivery cannot yet be completed with forceps and the malposition is likely to recur. It occasionally happens, however, that one may be examining a patient under anaesthesia in order to determine the cause of delay, in which case an attempt at manual rotation is justifiable. Under these circumstances the ventouse may prove the most suitable instrument, being less likely to damage the cervix.

Traction Difficulties

The difficult forceps operation must presently become as much of an anachronism as cranioclasm and cephalotripsy. A mother's pelvic tissues, may, with luck, recover. A child's brain may not. The amount of force which can be justified in pulling on the forceps should not exceed that which can be applied by the forearms alone.

Whether the standing or the sitting position is employed is a matter of personal taste, but, on the whole, better control is obtained with the latter. In either event there are few things more distressing to mother, baby and onlookers than a powerful man applying his weight, aided by the pressure of his feet up against the bed, to extract the child. Such force is clearly misapplied and therefore both unnecessary and harmful. One has only to compare the bearing down pressures which the patient in normal labour exerts to deliver herself (pressures which amount to not much more than 200 millimetres of mercury), and the immense force which is sometimes injudiciously employed. Clearly in such instances something is wrong. Either the case is not suitable for forceps delivery or a proper cephalic application of the forceps is lacking. Thirdly, the case may be one of undiagnosed persistent occipitoposterior position, or brow presentation, or perhaps traction is being made in the wrong direction, usually too far forwards, so that the back of the maternal symphysis is taking the brunt of the operator's effort, to the lasting detriment of intervening structures, particularly the bladder neck and its supports. The direction of the birth canal should be remembered in relation to the station of the baby's head, so that in high mid-cavity positions the direction of pull is somewhat downwards and backwards, gradually levelling out as the head descends and finally turning upwards and forwards as the occiput stems round the symphysis pubis (Fig. 9).

If, therefore, with reasonable traction no advance is made, attention should be directed to the possibility that traction is being exerted in the wrong direction or that the occiput is directed posteriorly or, again, that the cephalic application of the blade may be faulty. Only when one has considered these possibilities should one consider the less likely diagnosis of contracted outlet. In all the above instances, except the first, re-examination is called for after removing the blades. This is far better than pressing on to the very death (of the baby)!

Another disconcerting accident associated with forceps traction is the slipping off of the blades. This is most injurious to both mother and child. The commonest cause of this is the undiagnosed persistent occipitoposterior position, in which instance the forceps obtain

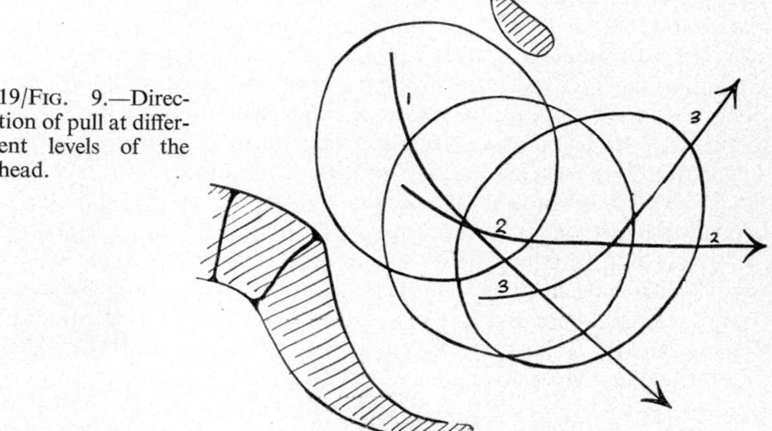

19/Fig. 9.—Direction of pull at different levels of the head.

a far less secure grip of the head. The other cause of the blades slipping off is an oblique or anteroposterior application over the baby's occiput and face.

Lastly, an appreciable degree of vaginal bleeding may appear at this stage of the operation, which can be very worrying, especially since, delivery not being completed, it is not possible to find its source and deal with it. It usually originates from a split in the vaginal wall or an internal tear of the perineum and usually ceases as delivery proceeds.

If traction is made in association with a uterine contraction, the amount of force necessary is by that much reduced. Fortunately, as soon as pulling starts, a reflex contraction is usually evoked. Steady but intermittent and convincing pulls should be made, and the locks should be eased open a little between whiles, in order to relieve the baby's head from continuous compression. As soon as the resistance of the pelvic floor is met it is customary nowadays to perform episiotomy, and there is much from the baby's point of view to commend this practice, inasmuch as it reduces the wear and tear upon the baby's head.

Towards the final point of forceps delivery, traction is being made more or less directly upwards, and care should be taken to control the force used in order to minimise the extent of perineal damage. As soon as the head is crowned, the forceps should be removed, whereupon the delivery of the head can be slowly completed by extension as in the conduct of a normal second stage.

Vaginal bypass in the form of Caesarean section is infinitely preferable for the baby and often for the mother too, rather than difficult forceps delivery, and evidence of cerebral damage has been noted in 18·7 per cent of quite a large series of cases in which difficulty was experienced in the course of mid-cavity forceps delivery.[39] This is sufficient to condemn difficult forceps delivery in retrospect. In this series the main factors appear to have been some degree of contracted pelvis, especially with a flat sacrum and restriction of the cavity associated with transverse arrest or posterior position of the occiput. This naturally raises the question of trial of forceps. By this is meant the application of forceps with the mental reservation that should the operation prove difficult there should be no hesitation in removing the blades and resorting forthwith to Caesarean section, for which preparations have been fully made in advance. To undertake a proper trial of forceps, therefore, it is mandatory that the operation not only finishes but starts in a properly equipped operating theatre. It is our practice at the Queen Mother's Hospital to carry out all obstetrical operations, even the simplest, under full surgical conditions in an operating theatre, but very few units are thus generously equipped and if a patient happens, as is likely, to be in what is euphemistically called a forceps delivery room, the business of removing her into an operating theatre, commonly on a different floor (and even in one place where I worked, across a snow-covered courtyard) is so daunting as to discourage one from resorting to Caesarean section and trying yet again another good hard pull. This is certainly not trial of forceps. I have done enough "bathroom obstetrics" in my life to know that the best judgments are only made under the best conditions, and preparedness in every physical and geographical sense for Caesarean section is an indispensable ingredient of a true trial. Successful trial of forceps indeed is most rewarding, but an unsuccessful trial terminating in Caesarean section is an unpleasant business for mother, baby and obstetrician. All the more need therefore for a full pre-operative assessment. Trial of forceps is like lion taming; it is not the sort of exercise one would willingly undertake in expectation of failure.

Face-to-pubis Delivery with Forceps

Unwittingly performed, because of missed diagnosis about the position of the child's head (and we have all from time to time made this mistake), the head is liable to pop out suddenly with extensive damage to the perineum, unless prophylactic episiotomy has been performed. This, too, is one of the cardinal causes of a third-degree tear. Nevertheless, in certain cases it is preferable to deliver in the unreduced POP position deliberately, provided care is taken to prevent the forceps from slipping off or the head from suddenly popping out. With a generous episiotomy, made in advance, this method is preferable to manual rotation under the following circumstances:

1. If the head is already bulging the perineum and the patient has only failed to deliver herself spontaneously face-to-pubis at the last stage of the head's descent.
2. In cases of marked anthropoid shape of the pelvis. In this instance the rotation of the head would involve negotiating the narrower transverse diameter so that it becomes neither necessary nor wise.
3. In cases of prolonged and dry labour, in which the uterus is so closely applied to the baby's body that it is impossible to rotate it in conformity with the rotation of the head.

It can be argued with some justification that in cases in which the occiput lies directly posterior one should accept this as an indication for proceeding with face-to-pubis delivery, since the pelvis in such cases must be either anthropoid in type or roomy enough to have allowed the head to have rotated into this position so there is now no indication for turning it. Furthermore, the mechanics of moulding are better left undisturbed at this late stage.

The position is altogether different in the more commonly met cases of transverse arrest of the head or where the occiput lies obliquely posterior. These cases must be rotated.

Incidentally, the jam-pot moulding in occipitoposterior position so often described in textbooks is rather uncommon. More often a lop-sided oblique moulding occurs in conformity with the oblique or transverse position of the baby's head, and even in the full face-to-pubis position one more often sees the moulding of extreme flexion which exaggerates to a depressing degree the apparent vertical length of the baby's forehead, before the eyebrows can be made to appear from under the symphysis pubis.

Forceps to the Aftercoming Head

It is a mistake to regard the use of forceps as the last resort in dealing with the difficult delivery of the head in a breech delivery, because, by now, it may be too late. The forceps should be sterilised and available in advance especially in the case of primiparous breech delivery, so that there need be no delay in applying. In the first place, the head should be brought as low down as possible by hanging the body of the child downwards until the occiput lies up against the back of the symphysis pubis. An assistant then raises the legs of the child so as to lift the body out of the way. The forceps blades are applied on either side of the baby's head from underneath its body, that is to say on its ventral aspect (13/Fig. 2). An episiotomy should, of course, have been made already. A great advantage of the forceps in these cases is that the head can be gently extracted and its rate of delivery accurately controlled. Unfortunately, it is not possible to perform this operation without the help of a second pair of hands to lift the body of the child.

Forceps in Face Presentation

It is essential that the chin be already fully rotated to the front before the forceps is applied, except, of course, in the case of the Kielland's forceps which may be used for the rotation of the face. An episiotomy is absolutely essential in these cases, and traction should at first be continued somewhat downwards and backwards in order to maintain the fullest possible extension of the head until the chin unquestionably clears the bottom of the symphysis pubis. Thereafter, the head is delivered by flexion. In this sort of delivery the forceps blades should be applied with the handles rather farther forward than in the case of the vertex deliveries, so that when traction is made in the correct direction, as above, any attempt by the head to become flexed will be thereby discouraged.

Failed Forceps

In recent years the emphasis upon certain causes of failure to deliver with forceps, notably cases of disproportion, has shifted, largely as a result of antenatal care. Miller in 1927 found that there was an incidence of 17·6 per cent of cases of failed forceps amongst a series of 500 emergency admissions to hospital, and of these the cause of failure was disproportion in no less than 40 per cent, of which 7 cases had outlet contraction. In 1928 he published a series of 558 cases of failed forceps collected from Edinburgh, Glasgow and Manchester. The causes were listed as follows:

Disproportion with flat pelvis predominating	221	(outlet contraction 14)
Constriction ring	6	
Occipitoposterior positions	161	
Face presentation	12	(5 persistent mento-posterior)
Brow presentation	8	
Hydrocephalus	8	
Breech	2	
Shoulder	2	
Ovarian tumour	2	
Locked twins	1	

Furthermore, in no fewer than 151 cases there was no evidence of disproportion and the head was in normal position, and it was probable that the failure was due to premature intervention originally.

A very different state of affairs was described many years later by Freeth (1950), who enumerated 100 cases of failed forceps between the years 1941–48 from the Birmingham Maternity Hospital. Three-quarters of these cases were primigravidae, and persistent occipitoposterior position and transverse arrest of the head accounted for no less than 50 per cent, while the cervix was not fully dilated in 20 per cent. There were 5 cases of contracted outlet, 4 of hydrocephalus, and odd cases of face and brow presentation, constriction ring, ovarian cyst and septate vagina made up the remainder. Freeth also made the interesting observation that 29 per cent of the cases were apparently more than two weeks overdue.

The difference between Miller's figures and those of Freeth is very striking in the much smaller importance of disproportion as a cause in more modern times. It will be noted that in both series hydrocephalus was by no means a minor factor, and slight degrees of this abnormality constitute a serious pitfall. Without a previous X-ray, such as diagnosis is not always easy to make, especially when the characteristic separation of the sutures has been obliterated by the forces of labour. When a case is sent in from outside by a doctor who has failed to deliver a patient with forceps, he usually attributes his difficulty to a contracted outlet, but in a significant majority of cases the patient, on being examined in hospital, is found either to be not fully dilated or to have a fetus in a malrotated position. With regard to the former diagnosis I often suspect that the doctor outside has been unjustly blamed for applying the forceps before full dilatation of the cervix; sometimes the cervix, I am sure, shuts down after a failed attempt, much as a constriction ring may form. It is inconceivable that the doctor could have inserted the blades without accepting this hypothesis in cases where the cervix is found to be only half dilated or less.

We once received an interesting call from a general practitioner to take over a case of failed forceps and he explained on the telephone that this case was rather different inasmuch as the main difficulty had not been in putting the forceps on but in getting them off. On inquiry as to where the forceps were at the moment he replied that they were still inside the patient and that the patient was already in a waiting ambulance. He then requested, with some urgency, that we return his forceps after recovery, a point on which we quickly reassured him that this was indeed our invariable practice. A few minutes later, however, he rang again in a much more cheerful voice to state that he had had a brainwave and had given the patient an injection of 10 units intramuscularly of oxytocin and that the patient had promptly delivered herself of baby, forceps and all. He apologised for having troubled us but stated with some satisfaction that he had got his forceps back.

There is a special type of failed forceps which is not uncommon in hospital practice and follows what has been apparently a successful manual rotation of the occiput. In these cases the head has escaped above the brim and has become deflexed. It is also less likely to re-enter the brim in the anteroposterior position unless the pelvis is of gynaecoid or anthropoid shape or of huge diameters, in which case it should not have been necessary to displace the head so far in the first place. When this accident occurs, a high forceps application is far more dangerous, and also less likely to succeed, than performing internal version forthwith, with its equally serious dangers of fetal death and uterine rupture. The other alternative of proceeding straightway to Caesarean section is better employed in the interests of the child.

Parry Jones (1952) summarised the causes of difficulty in forceps delivery under the headings of maternal and fetal. He listed the maternal causes as follows:

1. Cervix not fully dilated;
2. Disproportion;
3. Generalised tonic contraction of the uterus;
4. Constriction ring;
5. Non-dilatability of the paravaginal tissues.

Fetal causes he listed as follows:

1. Malposition;
2. Deflexion;
3. Large baby;
4. Shoulders impacted at the brim.

In spite of all these lists which various writers have produced, there is no doubt that premature intervention with forceps is responsible for a far larger number than the figures indicate. A patient is often diagnosed as being fully dilated because of her desire to bear down and because the cervix is not palpable on rectal examination or vaginal examination without an anaesthetic. This is common, particularly in occipitoposterior positions. Then, after two hours of ineffectual pushing, it is decided to apply the forceps because of failure of the head to advance. Now, at any time during this last two hours the patient may, in fact, have become fully dilated and the second stage has not lasted anything like as long as estimated. The result is that less moulding can have occurred and intervention is undertaken far sooner than one would have contemplated had the time of full dilatation not been mistaken. It is a mistake to interest oneself in the duration of the second stage as measured by the clock, and a patient should be encouraged to use her best efforts only when the head is actually seen to be on the pelvic floor. In this way much premature maternal distress will be avoided and there will be fewer cases of unnecessary or too early application of the forceps, with resulting failure in a proportion of cases.

Mortality and the Risks of Failed Forceps

Earlier reports, such as those of Miller and Feeney, show a thoroughly depressing mortality rate both for mothers and babies. The principal causes of death are shock, sepsis, uterine rupture and postpartum haemorrhage, while the persistent ill-health which may follow cannot even be approximately assessed. Miller long ago reckoned that 50 per cent suffered from impaired health and quoted a maternal mortality of 10 per cent (54 cases), of which 37 died as the result of sepsis. In a different series he reported 17 deaths out of 88, a mortality of 19 per cent. Feeney (1947), in reporting 121 cases of failed forceps in Dublin, and adding a further 225 cases from the literature, found a maternal mortality of 11 per cent, but only the complicated cases were included in these figures, so that the maternal mortality was correspondingly exaggerated.

The institution of the Flying Squad and the more effective use of chemotherapy and antibiotics, together with the present availability of blood for transfusion, has enormously improved this depressing picture, and Freeth (1950) found a maternal mortality of 2 per cent. Caesarean section after a failed forceps delivery is now nothing like so hazardous as formerly.

The improvement in fetal mortality is nowhere near so satisfactory. In Miller's series fetal mortality was 64 per cent and in Freeth's series in 1950 it was still as high as 34 per cent, excluding cases of hydrocephalus. Three major factors contribute towards these bad results both for mother and child. Firstly, the condition which originally caused the failure to deliver with the forceps, secondly, the repeated intervention to which the patients were inevitably subjected, with its attendant risks of sepsis and shock, and thirdly the need which was often present for the repeated induction of anaesthesia. In this last respect chloroform was especially dangerous, and even the pre-operative use of a 10 per cent glucose infusion did not provide adequate protection.

Undoubtedly a certain percentage of cases of failed forceps never needed the operation in the first place, and it is therefore interesting to review the outcome. Miller, for instance, reported that in 78 cases in the disproportion group, subsequent spontaneous delivery or low forceps delivery finally occurred, indicating that intervention, even although there was disproportion, had been premature. In Freeth's cases 62 per cent were delivered with the forceps, no less than 17 per cent had a spontaneous delivery, 8 per cent had internal version and 6 per cent were delivered by Caesarean section, while craniotomy and breech delivery made up the remainder. The lesson to be learned from all this history is that one should never ignore or transgress the indications for forceps delivery nor flout the conditions which must be present before attempting it. To be wrong in the selection of one's cases is bad enough, and to fail, having put one's hand to the plough, only makes matters many times worse.

Trial of forceps, advisedly undertaken, however, comes into a completely different class. Here, one recognises all the difficulties in advance and has made due preparations for them. Such an operation must be undertaken on an operating table, in a properly equipped operating theatre with an anaesthetist in attendance. The decision to abandon the forceps and to proceed to Caesarean section must not be regarded as a matter of "failed forceps" but as an enlightened step in recognition of the hazards, particularly to the baby, of persisting with vaginal delivery.

Kielland's Forceps

This really wonderful instrument makes possible a true cephalic application, regardless of the station of the head, which is impossible with the usual long curved forceps types without prior rotation. The Kielland forceps achieves this objective by interrupting the pelvic curve at the commencement of the shanks, which are bent backwards at a slight angle with the blades. The other important feature is the sliding lock which caters for varying degrees of asynclitism. The Scanzoni manoeuvre in the case of the malrotated head is so crude by comparison with a rotation with Kielland's forceps that it does not really merit description.

Those who have once mastered the technique of using Kielland's forceps are enthusiastic, and most of the criticism comes from ignorant or prejudiced sources. The argument has even been advanced in one major undergraduate teaching hospital that Kielland's should never be used because the students might get the wrong idea and be encouraged later on to try using it themselves when they entered practice. If this argument had anything in it, students who were destined for general practice ought never to see a hysterectomy or any other major surgical procedure. This is not to deny the instrument is tricky and is not for the occasional obstetrician. House surgeons should be taught carefully how to handle it, preferably with local analgesia (see earlier), by seniors who are well practised, for, in inexperienced hands, there are undoubtedly pitfalls which we will now review. This is an argument for learning to use the instrument correctly rather than for condemning it out of hand.

Risks of Kielland's Forceps

Because of the sliding and therefore unstable lock, considerable damage can be done to vagina and cervix and occasionally lower uterine segment if the blades are not correctly applied in the first place. Under these circumstances the points tend to rise away from the baby's head and, in the course of rotation, can lacerate the maternal tissues. A tight skimpy vagina is particularly vulnerable. The bladder may thus be injured and give rise to a vesicovaginal fistula from direct laceration or from pressure necrosis. Spiral tears of the vagina are reported in addition to tears of the cervix, and the lower uterine segment can be ruptured especially in the classical method of applying the anterior blade. Parry Jones mentioned other risks, which, however, are not peculiar to Kielland's, but may occur with any forceps delivery, for example, dislocation of a sacro-iliac joint, fracture of the terminal part of the sacrum, separation of the symphysis pubis and injury to the nerve trunks of the sacral plexus.

Risks to the baby are considerably reduced by the use of Kielland's forceps, because far less compression to the fetal skull can be achieved across the fulcrum of the sliding lock than with the usual forceps. Moreover, the ability to obtain an accurate cephalic application enormously lessens the strain upon the tentorium cerebelli. Facial abrasions and depressed fractures of the skull are no more likely with this than with any other forceps. One risk, however, must be mentioned, and that is the trapping of the cord or possibly the baby's hand if the classical method of application of the anterior blade is used. Prolapse of the cord is regarded as one of the risks, but it is considerably less than with high upward displacement of the head in order to achieve manual rotation.

There is undoubtedly a tendency to cause more damage to the perineum with Kielland's forceps, mainly because of the angle of the shanks, but this can be minimised by an episiotomy which in any case should always be carried out in conjunction with Kielland's forceps delivery because the perineum is very liable to get in the way of the shanks and may prevent the proper application of the blades.

Method of applying Kielland's Forceps

It is best to perform episiotomy first since this facilitates the application of the blades. There are three methods—classical, wandering and direct. The classical method was mainly introduced for the high forceps operation with the head not properly engaged, and has now been largely discarded because of the modern abandonment of this operation. However, it merits description. The anterior blade is applied first between the baby's head and the symphysis pubis with the concavity of the cephalic curve directed upwards. In order to decide which of the blades is the anterior one it is a good rule to assemble the forceps in front of the patient before applying them, so as to obtain the correct orientation of the position which they will occupy once they have been inserted. Needless to say, in this assembly, the concavity of the pelvic curve is directed towards the child's occiput, whose position is already known following proper examination. The anterior blade is then slipped in "butter side upwards". It is essential to use only finger-light force, and no attempt must be made to rotate it butter side downwards until it has been pushed in far enough. It is not until the more or less rounded junction of blade and shank is lying between the baby's head and the symphysis that it will be safe or even possible, without force, to rotate it (Fig. 10).

When the blade has been pushed in far enough, it will be found that the shank is pressing against the posterior vaginal wall. With

KIELLAND CLASSICAL METHOD

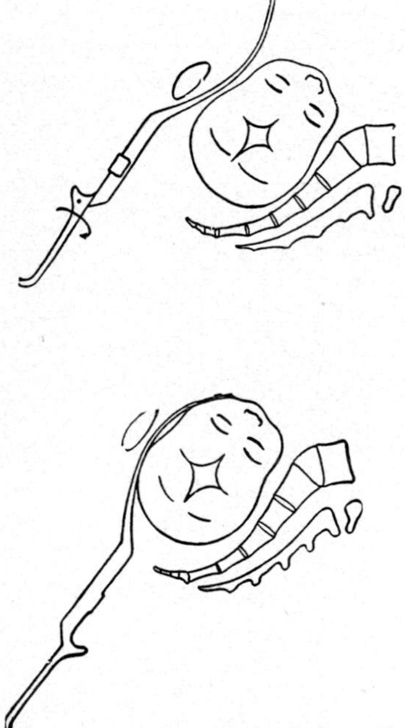

19/Fig. 10 (*a*).—The position of the blade before rotation (*A*); the position of the blade after rotation (*B*).

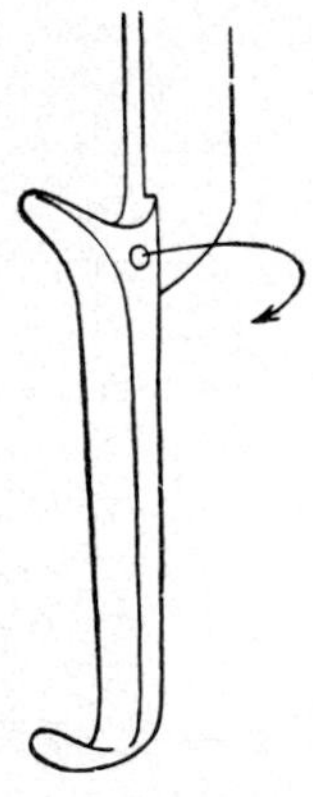

19/Fig. 10 (*b*).—The direction knob lies on the same side as the pelvic curve. Rotation of the blade is carried out towards the same side.

very gentle and careful manipulation the blade is now turned through 180° on its long axis, so that the pelvic concavity is turned against the convexity of the fetal skull, and to make matters simpler there is a small knob on the handles which points in the direction in which the blade should be turned. Some difficulty may be encountered in this manoeuvre, the commonest being due to the tight application of the fetal head against the top of the symphysis pubis. Now it goes without saying that unless a finger can be inserted between the head and the symphysis pubis, a blind attempt to force the forceps blade in this area is not justified and another method of application is to be preferred. The higher the head, however, the less likely is this difficulty to operate and the more applicable the classical method.

Another common cause of failure is that the blade has not been inserted far enough, in which case the fault will be advertised by the fact that the handle instead of sloping downwards towards the perineum is more horizontal than it should be.

Occasionally a constriction ring may prevent the insertion and proper rotation of the blade, and lastly the child's anterior shoulder may get in the way. If difficulty is encountered, force must on no account be used to overcome it, but as a rule it is surprising how easily the blade slips round. It is at this point that there is always the chance that a loop of cord may get caught as the blade is pulled back home to engage upon the head.

With the head in the transverse position and the blade correctly applied, the handle should be sloping somewhat downwards and a little to the side of the midline on the opposite side to the baby's occiput. If an assistant can now steady it at this point so much the better. The posterior blade is now applied, and in many ways it is the more difficult of the two, because the point of the blade often bumps up against the sacrum and it appears impossible to negotiate the sacral promontory. The secret is not to use more force, but to depress the handle which is usually being prevented by the perineum. It is this fact which makes an initial episiotomy so valuable in order to assist one in drawing the perineum backward and out of the way. If, in spite of drawing the perineum well back and depressing the handle, the obstruction of the sacrum is still felt against the tip of the blade, more room may be found slightly to one or other side of the midline.

The wandering method is the one most generally applicable. It is usually recommended that the anterior blade be applied first, but this is optional, and personally I prefer to start with the posterior blade. The same technique with the posterior blade is followed, but in this case it is easier because the other blade is not now taking up room nor is it in the way. Again, it is a common mistake not to slide the blade in far enough. When correctly applied (and it is a good plan to aim for the baby's ear), the handle is sloping somewhat downwards towards the floor and a little towards the opposite side to which the occiput lies. The anterior blade is now applied laterally directly over the baby's face guided by two fingers. By very careful manipulation of the handle and with two guiding fingers, the blade is gently "jilled" through a quarter of a circle around the periphery of the pelvic cavity, until it matches up with the posterior blade (Fig. 11). Carried out this way it will now be found, in the case of the right occipito-lateral position, that the handles will have to be crossed on each other for the locks to meet, but this can always be easily and gently done. With the occiput to the left the handles do not have to be crossed over. As the locks engage the shanks should, of course, be in line with each other, and it will now be noticed that one blade is farther in than the other. In other words, the head is nearly always in a position of some degree of asynclitism. This is gently corrected by the sliding lock.

The direct method of application is used when the head is very low or very small, since there is not enough room otherwise to apply both blades directly without one of the above manoeuvres.

Above all, always remember to keep the handles well down. Failure to observe this is responsible for more difficulties with Kielland's forceps than any other fault.

Rotation of the Head

Having corrected any asynclitism with the help of the sliding lock, the mobility of the head within the pelvis is cautiously assessed with the forceps and a gentle attempt is made to rotate it. Only finger force should be used. If it appears that the head cannot be rotated in its present position, it is a good plan to draw the head down a little in the uncorrected position and to try again, and if this fails to push it up slightly and repeat the attempt at a slightly higher level. In this manner, by carefully feeling one's way and always keeping the handles well down, the safest level at which to rotate the head can be determined, the safest being that at which least force is necessary. The sense of control of the head has to be experienced to be believed. Lastly, it is a wise precaution to desist from attempts to rotate the head while a contraction is in force.

Traction with Kielland's Forceps

The direction of pull is largely determined by the direction in which the handles are pointing. This is somewhat downwards (more so than with ordinary forceps) until the occiput appears behind the symphysis. On no account must the handles be raised, even so far as

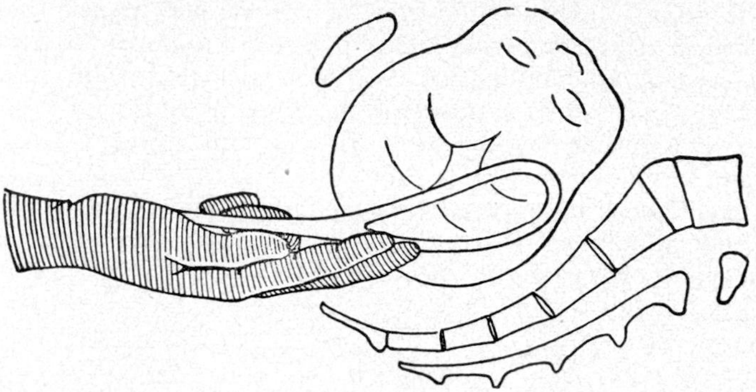

19/FIG. 11 (*a*).—Second movement of wandering. The internal fingers rest behind the fenestration, ready to push the blade anteriorly.

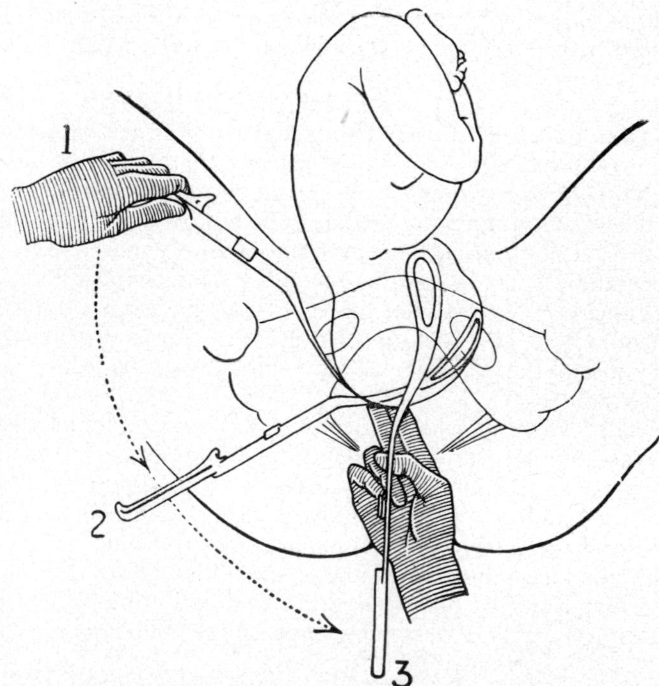

19/FIG. 11 (*b*).—The three main movements of wandering.
(Figs. 10 and 11 from *Kielland's Forceps* by courtesy of Dr E. Parry Jones and Butterworth & Co.)

the horizontal, until this point is reached. At no time do the handles rise so high as in the case of the ordinary long curved forceps.

As soon as the now rotated head is pulled well down on to the pelvic floor, a light, low forceps of the Wrigley pattern may be applied in the place of the Kielland forceps, in order to spare the perineum additional damage, but this is a refinement which is hardly necessary, and with care in the direction of pull at the outlet the operation can be completed with Kielland forceps with great finesse.

There can be few operations in all midwifery so satisfying as a correctly performed delivery with the Kielland forceps, especially under local analgesia only. See Figs. 12–18.

Bony Contraction of the Pelvic Outlet

Sometimes contraction of the outlet is not discovered until in the course of a forceps operation. This is a regrettable but nevertheless occasional fact. The subject is dealt with more fully in the chapter on disproportion, but we must consider here the steps to be taken when, having applied the forceps, it is clear that a serious degree of bony obstruction exists.

There are three alternatives now before us: the most commonly practised is to deliver the child with forceps by brute force. This is highly deplorable. It has been said that in practically every case the head that will pass through the brim can be got through the outlet. True, but at a fearful price sometimes which is borne both by mother and baby. It is in these cases that symphysiotomy comes into its own. The operation is not difficult and makes a tremendous difference to outlet difficulties. Few people in their senses, who had foreknowledge of outlet contraction, would plan to deliver the case by forceps and symphysiotomy as an elective decision, and Caesarean section would be preferred.

The third alternative is to remove the forceps and proceed to Caesarean section forthwith. Craniotomy is only to be considered if the baby is unquestionably dead. There is no doubt that either Caesarean section or symphysiotomy is vastly preferable to the first method of brute force, in which not only may the child be seriously damaged or killed, but the mother's sacro-iliac joints may be dislocated, her bladder and its supports traumatised, and her pelvic floor damaged beyond reasonable hope of adequate repair.

19/Fig. 12 (*see opposite*).—Applying the posterior blade of Kielland's forceps in a case of transverse arrest with the occiput to the right.

19/Fig. 13 (*see opposite*).—The posterior blade of Kielland's forceps when properly placed points the handle somewhat downwards and laterally.

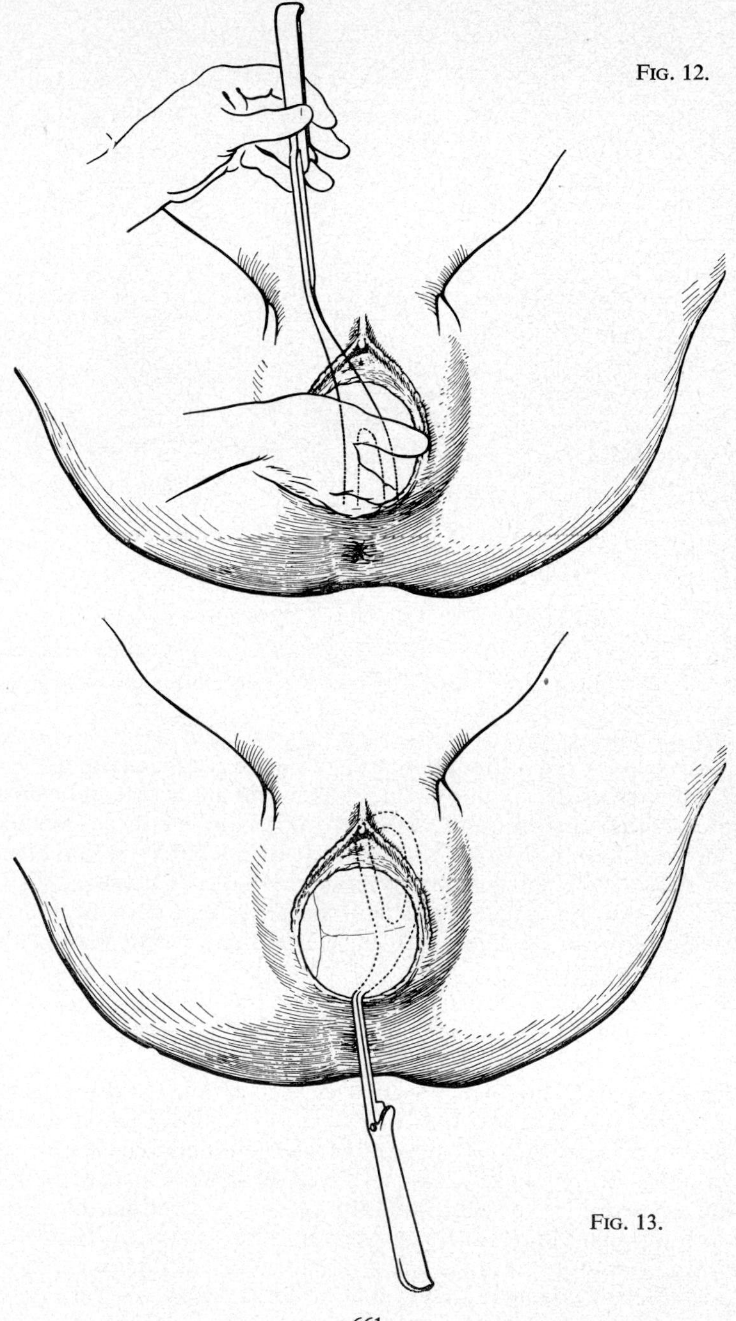

Fig. 12.

Fig. 13.

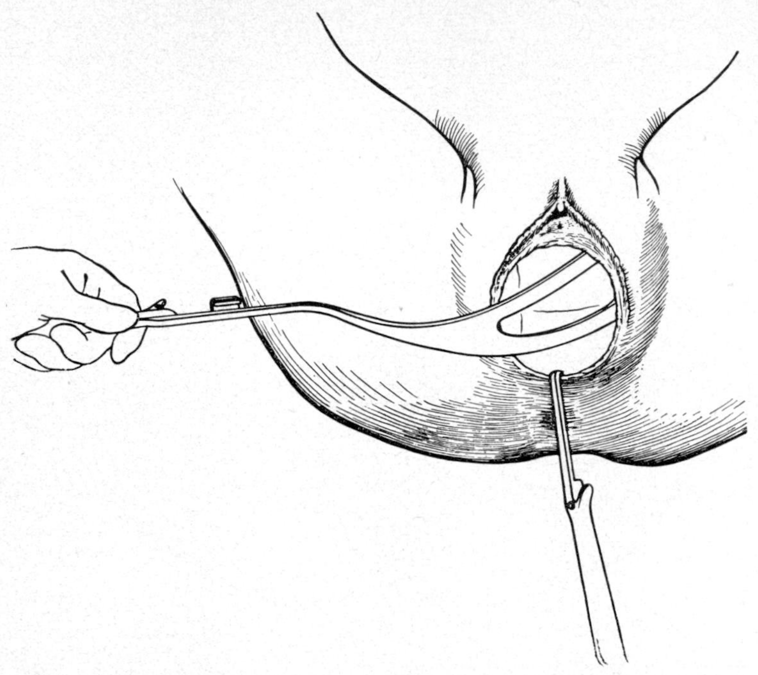

19/Fig. 14.—Inserting the anterior blade of Kielland's forceps over the face.

If the baby is unquestionably dead and there is difficulty in delivering with forceps (and this is most likely in the case of a hydrocephalic head) perforation, of itself, may make all the difference. Although I have occasionally in the past used the Winter combined cranioclast and cephalotribe without getting into trouble, it is a heavy, brutish instrument and, if available, several pairs of Morris bone forceps can be applied to the perforated area to extract the head more elegantly.

Symphysiotomy

This is an operation which has never been popular in this country nor in the United States. It is by no means new, and has had brief vogue from time to time during the last few hundred years. The alternative of pubiotomy has been if anything consistently less popular. Much of the unpopularity of these operations has been earned through faulty selection of cases. As a method of treatment of brim disproportion it is quite unsuitable, and its only indications are in cases of outlet disproportion late in labour or in the case of

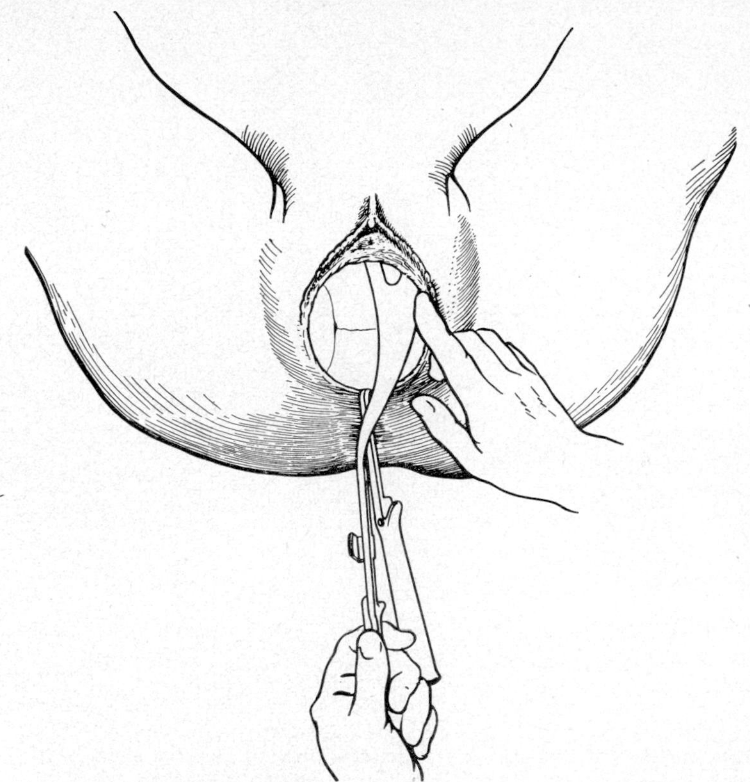

19/Fig. 15.—"Wandering" the anterior blade into position. Note how the handles will have to be crossed over in ROT positions for the lock to engage.

immovable malposition of a deeply placed fetal head. The cases, therefore, for which it is considered are usually those of android, funnel-shaped pelvis.

In primitive communities, as Seedat and Crichton (1962) have shown, there is still a place for symphysiotomy since many patients disappear into the bush and insist on being delivered at home next time and the theory is that a patient who has had a symphysiotomy will fare better and more safely in a subsequent delivery than one who has had a previous Caesarean section. From the point of view of uterine rupture and catastrophic death a long distance from medical aid this may be true, but in other respects the matter may be regarded as open to some argument. A further reason given is that the high infant mortality rate makes repeated delivery by Caesarean section hardly worth while. This too is debatable by civilised standards, but Seedat and Crichton had a large series of 505 cases in

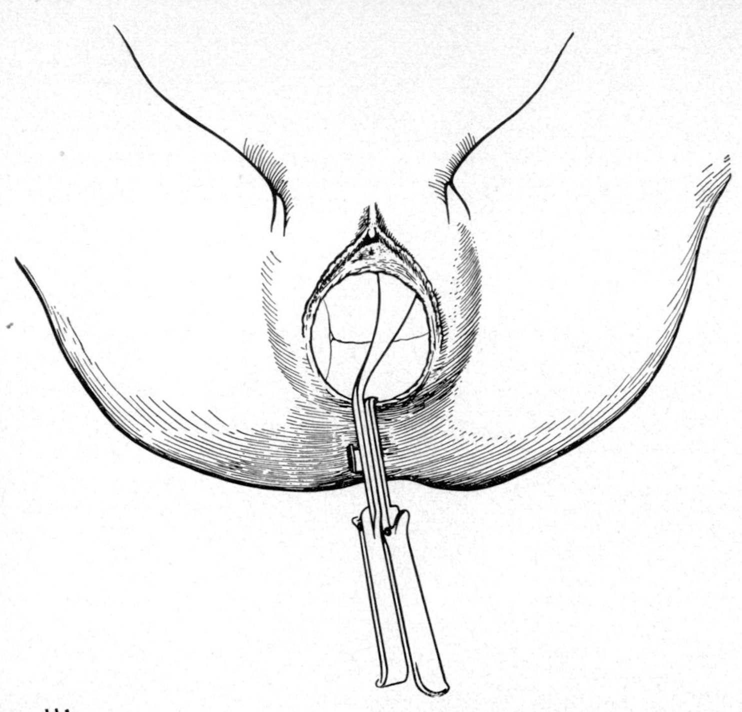

19/FIG. 16 (*above*).—The Kielland's forceps immediately after application and before correction of asynclitism. Note the position of the handles, sloping somewhat downwards and laterally to the side away from the occiput.

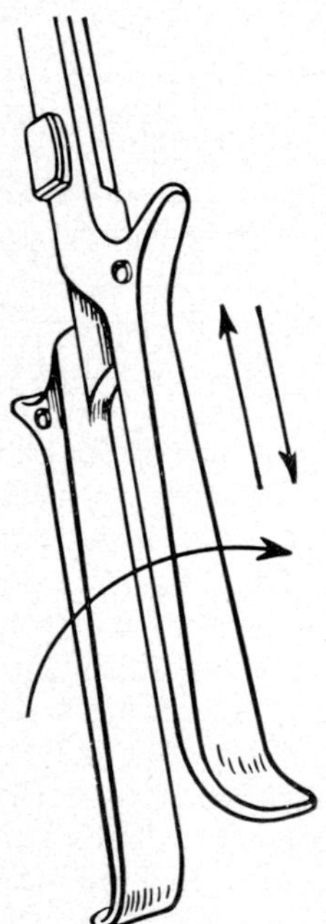

19/FIG. 17.—Correcting asynclitism and rotating from occipitotransverse to occipitoanterior position.

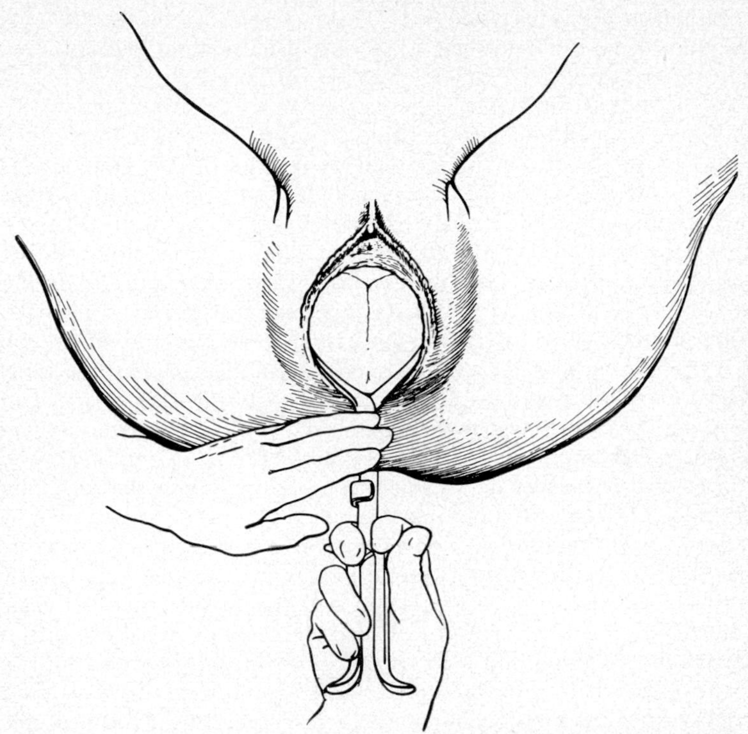

19/FIG. 18.—Traction and Pajot's manoeuvre applied to the Kielland's forceps.

Bantu women without maternal mortality and with only ambulatory difficulties in 16 cases and stress incontinence in a further 5, a truly remarkable record. In the following year (Crichton and Seedat, 1963) they published details of 1200 cases in Natal with 4 instances of vesicovaginal fistula and 12 of vestibular together with sometimes urethral tears, all of which were successfully repaired and for which the antecedent pressure necrosis was more of a factor than the operation itself. The situation is very similar in Nigeria where symphysiotomy is commonly employed in the management of disproportion.[6] Since so large a proportion of the world's population live under conditions which these workers describe it would be wrong for those of us who practise in more fortunate communities to dismiss the importance of this operation.

Pubiotomy is usually performed by inserting a Gigli saw behind the pubis to one side of the midline and severing the bone. It is on the whole a more traumatic and vascular procedure than symphysiotomy. It is more than forty years since I last saw this operation.

Technique of symphysiotomy.—There are two methods, the open and the closed, the latter being the more usually described, although the former has had a vogue in Dublin.

In the closed method a subcutaneous approach is made with a long solid scalpel, the incision being placed just above the symphysis pubis. The blade of the knife is then inserted on the flat close against the front of the symphysis pubis and then turned through a right-angle so that the cutting edge faces backwards. A finger is kept in the vagina so as to get a better idea of what is happening; and the symphysis is divided from before backwards through the greater part, but not all, of its thickness. The legs are removed from the lithotomy poles and held by assistants who, by pressing on the trochanters and abducting the thighs, produce a distractive force which slowly tears the remaining fibres of the posterior part of the symphysis pubis. The finger in the vagina is able to appreciate this, and a separation of no more than 1 to $1\frac{1}{2}$ inches ($2\frac{1}{2}$ to $3\frac{1}{4}$ cm) is allowed. The transverse diameters of the outlet are immediately increased and thereafter delivery is facilitated.

It is a good plan always to insert a fairly stiff catheter into the bladder before starting the operation and to use the finger in the vagina to displace both the urethra and the bladder neck laterally well to one side of the symphysis before cutting it. An alternative to the above closed method is to work from behind forwards and from above downwards, introducing the knife behind the symphysis pubis at its upper border and keeping strictly to the midline. Probing with a needle may occasionally be necessary to identify the joint. Unless spontaneous delivery follows quickly it is becoming increasingly common now to complete the delivery with the ventouse.

The open method is favoured by Barry in Dublin. Here the mons is incised vertically in the midline, bleeding points are secured and the front of the symphysis pubis is exposed to direct vision. The linea alba is incised, and a finger is inserted from above behind the symphysis pubis together with a narrow-bladed scalpel whose cutting edge is directed forwards so that the symphysis is severed from behind forwards. The same precautions are taken about holding the legs and controlling the amount of separation achieved. The operation tends to convert the dimensions of the outlet into a transverse oval, so that if Kielland's forceps is now applied to a transversely arrested head, it is often better to extract it in the unreduced position.

Fibrous union always occurs and the pelvic girdle nearly always regains its former stability, so that locomotion is not interfered with. During the puerperium the pelvis is supported by strapping or binders and the legs are usually bandaged together, but for the first few days there is often considerable oedema which may provide some nursing trouble, especially in catheterisation. The patients seem to suffer remarkably little pain. Nursing the patient on her side is also recommended.

It is true that the bladder or its supports may be injured in such cases, but this is not the direct result of operative technique, more often being due to the delivery which follows after the protective bony arch supporting the bladder has been robbed of its supporting properties as a result of severance. At the completion of the operation a large speculum is inserted and a very careful search made for any signs of splitting or tearing of the anterior vaginal wall. It goes without saying, therefore, that the manipulation with the forceps after symphysiotomy must be carried out with extra care. One of the very great advantages of symphysiotomy is that the pelvis remains permanently enlarged, so that subsequent deliveries are likely to be much easier. In a city like Dublin, where high degrees of parity are common, this is a factor of some importance, as it helps to eliminate the need for repetitive Caesarean section with all its penalties.

In Figs 19*a*, *b* and *c* will be seen pelvimetry radiographs taken before and after symphysiotomy in a case which Barry demonstrated personally to me on a visit to Dublin. Although there is a small permanent increase in the transverse measurements, much of the benefit likely to appear in subsequent labours will be due to the ease with which the symphysis pubis will "open up" for the occasion.

On this side of the Irish Sea, however, obstetricians are inclined to prefer repeated Caesarean section for contracted pelvis, since they prefer to inflict a soft tissue injury on abdominal wall and uterus than a skeletal injury on the pelvic girdle, a prejudice perhaps but a natural one!

THE VENTOUSE (Vacuum Extractor)

The idea of delivering a baby's head with the aid of suction is by no means new but it is generally accepted that Sir James Young Simpson in Edinburgh was the first to produce an apparatus which actually worked and successfully achieved delivery. Malmström's modern vacuum extractor differs only in detail and refinement from Simpson's suction tractor of 1849, of which Simpson produced a number of variants. The idea had doubtless arisen from the old practice of cupping. Chalmers (1963) in his historical review recounts the pithy phrase of Neil Arnott, another Scot, who envisaged such a machine and observed that the tractor seemed "peculiarly adapted to a purpose of obstetric surgery, namely as a substitute for steel forceps in the hands of men who are deficient in manual dexterity whether from inexperience or natural ineptitude." Such an attitude of prejudice reinforced by the less efficient materials of the last century have possibly been responsible for the delay of over a century before the true merits of vacuum extraction came to be accepted in Europe. Interest certainly waned in the method until Malmström, with very much better design and materials, produced the present ventouse which is now gaining a much more rapid acceptance.[24, 25, 26] The most violent criticism of the ventouse nearly always comes from people who have the least experience in using it, commonly none at all.

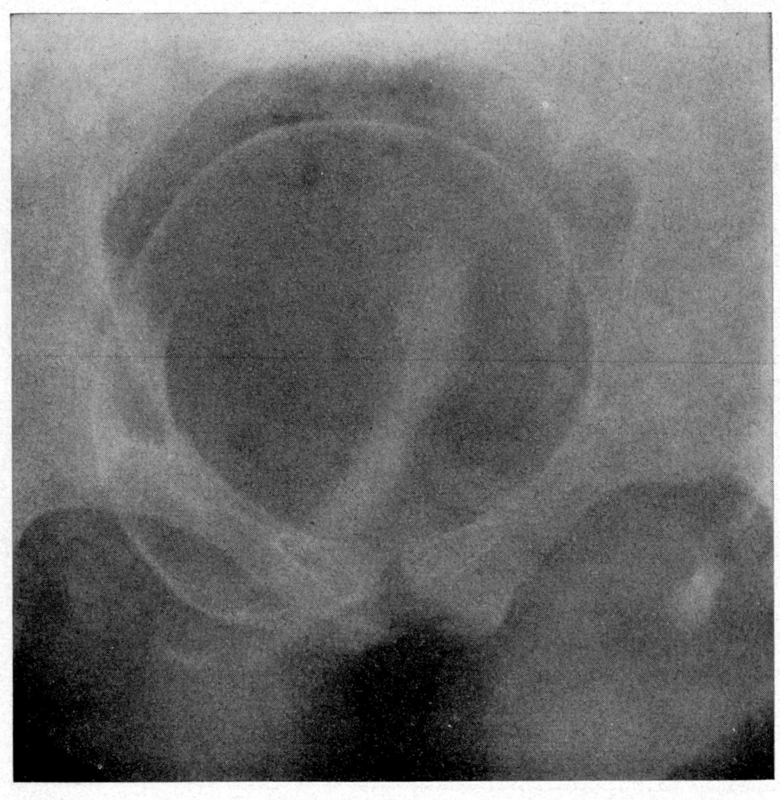

(*a*)

19/Fig. 19.

(*a*) Contracted pelvis before symphysiotomy. True conjugate 10·8 cm, transverse 11·5 cm.

(*b*) (*opposite*). Outlet view before symphysiotomy.

(*c*) (*opposite*). Same case after symphysiotomy and delivery of healthy baby weighing 7 lb 12 oz (3·5 kg) delivered in the unreduced transverse position with Kielland's forceps. Transverse diameter 11·8 cm. Separation at symphysis pubis 1·6 cm.

(Fig. 19 *a*, *b* and *c* by courtesy of Dr A. P. Barry.)

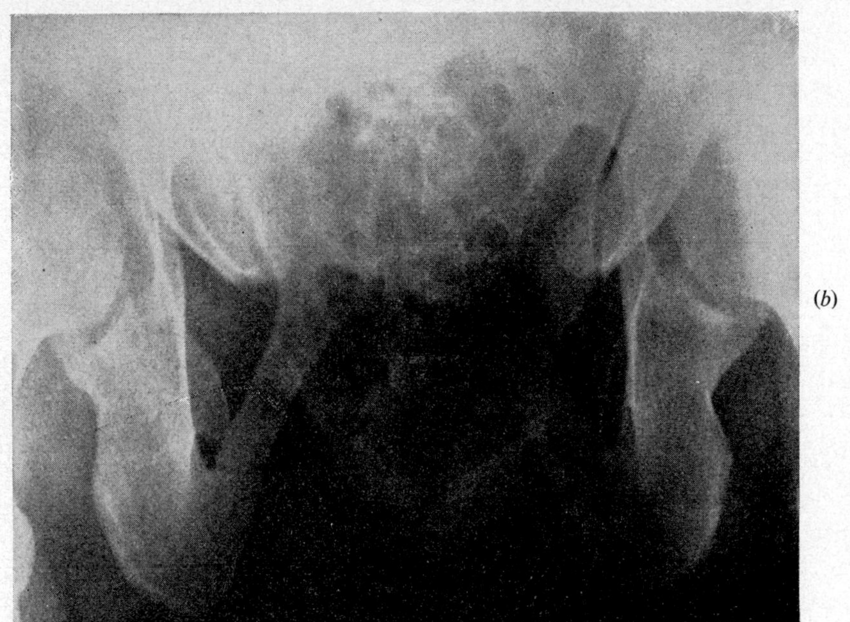

(b)

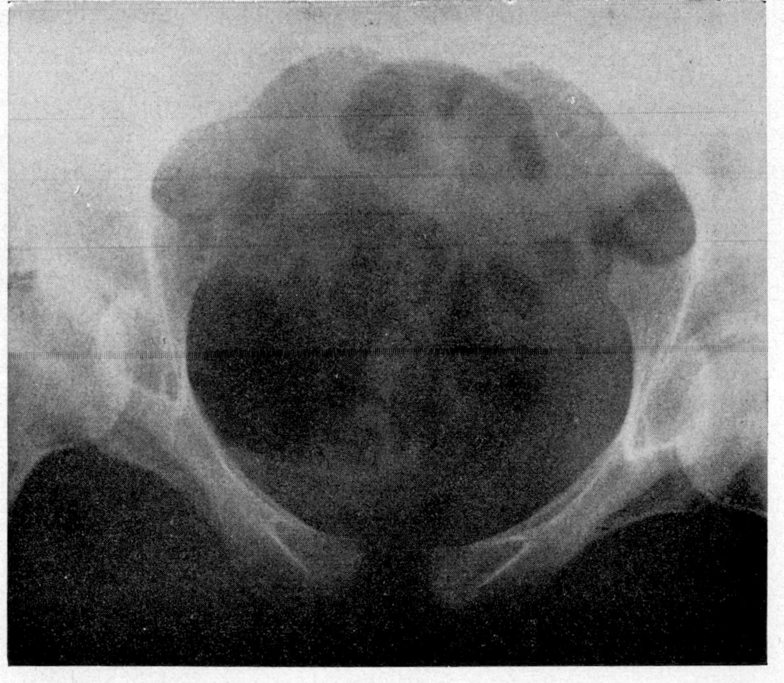

(c)

Simpson's cup with its incorporated piston and barrel must have been difficult to apply to a head not well down in the pelvis and was probably ineffective for pulls of more than a few kilograms, but the Malmström cup (Fig. 20) does not rely upon leather or rubber contact with the scalp but from the interesting shape of the metal cup and its flange which, following on the gentle building up of the vacuum by means of a very well made pump, allows the skin of the scalp and the induced caput succedaneum to "unfold" inside the cavity of the cup practically obliterating the potential space within it and forming the well-recognised "chignon" (Fig. 21). This secures an extremely satisfactory and atraumatic grip of the scalp without affecting the underlying structure of skull bones and brain.

Malmström's modern instrument has gained popularity throughout Western Europe and, in fact, in Professor Snoeck's department in Brussels, which I visited in 1961, I observed that this instrument had completely replaced the obstetric forceps since 1958, without any increase in the Caesarean section rate. It was first taken up in this country on a large scale by Chalmers and Fothergill who reported very favourably upon it in a series of 100 cases, and since then have gone from strength to strength, with a progressive incidence of vacuum extraction and fall in overall fetal mortality.[4, 5]

We ourselves have now acquired a considerable experience with it and our present use amounts to about 20 per cent of instrumenlal deliveries. Naturally the most comprehensive evaluation of indications and results comes from Sweden—its country of origin.[26]

Description of instrument.—A self-explanatory diagram is shown in Fig. 20. The most important part, of course, is the interestingly shaped cup already mentioned. Traction on this is achieved not through the rubber tubing which maintains the vacuum, but through a plate attached inside the cup to a chain that lies inside the lumen of the tubing and is fixed by a pin which is part of the assembly of the traction bar. A suction bottle with accurate vacuum gauge and a very well made pump, together with a bracket for hanging on the side of the bed, complete this fundamentally simple equipment. There is also an efficient vacuum-release valve. Vacuum pressures are recorded in kilograms per square centimetre, a designation which my much-forgotten arithmetic is incapable of translating into pounds per square inch, millimetres of mercury, or any of the better-recognised terms of measurement. Below is a table designed to provide an idea of the suction used.

The more recent types of ventouse apparatus have a traction chain attached to the centre of the cup independently of the vacuum-raising nozzle which is placed eccentrically. This facilitates application especially when it has to be made far back and also gives one a wider freedom of directional pull.

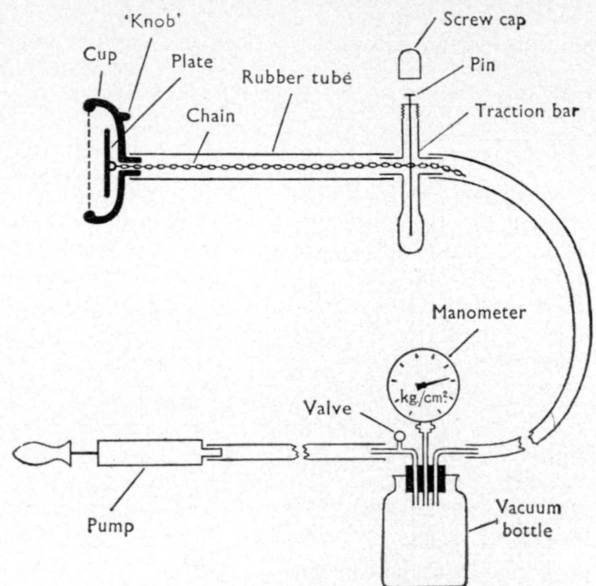

19/FIG. 20.—The Malmström cup.

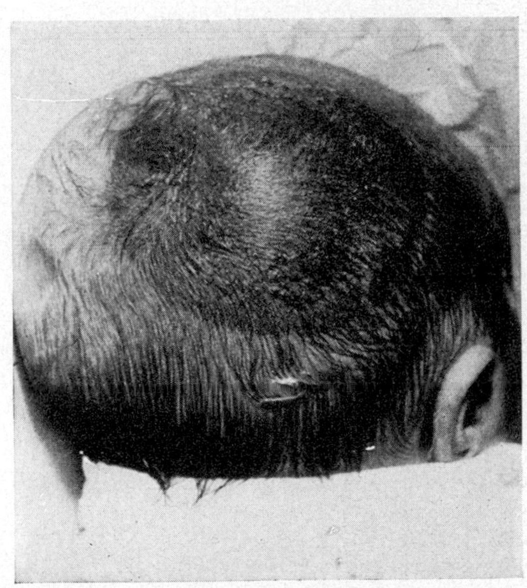

19/FIG. 21.—"Chignon" caused by the ventouse. It has usually disappeared within a few hours and leaves a discoloured mark which fades within a week. (By courtesy of Dr R. J. Fothergill, Dr J. A. Chalmers and the Editor, *Practitioner*.)

Glasgow Royal Maternity Hospital. First 132 cases

19/TABLE 1

ANAESTHESIA FOR VACUUM EXTRACTOR

	Percentage
General anaesthetic	15 (11·4)
Pudendal block	102 (77·3)
Local infiltration of perineum	8 (6·1)
Inhalational analgesia	4 (3·0)
No anaesthetic	3 (2·2)
	132

19/TABLE 2

FAILURES WITH VACUUM EXTRACTOR

Total 26 (19·7%)

Delivered by Caesarean section	2
Delivered by forceps	24
V.E. produced full dilatation of cervix in	7
Failure due to faulty technique in	9
Failure due to unsuitable case in	10

19/TABLE 3

INDICATIONS FOR VACUUM EXTRACTOR

	Percentage
Prolonged first stage	15 (11·4)
Fetal distress in first stage	15 (11·4)
Accidental haemorrhage in first stage	1 (0·75)
Prolonged second stage	65 (49·2)
Fetal distress in second stage	20 (15·1)
Severe pre-eclampsia in second stage	4 (3·0)
Cardiac disease in second stage	6 (4·5)
Brow presentation in second stage	1 (0·75)
Brow and prolapsed cord in second stage	1 (0·75)
Compound presentation (hand and head) in second stage	1 (0·75)
Breech presentation in second stage	1 (0·75)
Twins in second stage	2 (1·5)
	132

Technique of use.—There are certain rules which should be followed if the best results are to be obtained. The first of these is to use the largest possible cup. There are four sizes and if the cervix is fully dilated, or anywhere near so, the largest cup can nearly always be applied. If the head is already bulging the perineum, local infiltration only with 1 per cent lignocaine will suffice, but usually we employ pudendal block, the technique of which has been described

19/Table 4
Pressure Conversion

kg/cm^2	lb/in^2	mm Hg
0·1	1·422	73·56
0·2	2·844	147·11
0·3	4·266	220·67
0·4	5·688	294·22
0·5	7·110	367·78
0·6	8·532	441·34
0·7	9·954	514·89
0·8	11·376	588·45
0·9	12·798	662·00
1·0	14·220	735·56

earlier. General anaesthesia may be used but, on the whole, it is not favoured because the function of the ventouse is simply to lead the head out with the help of the patient's own expulsive efforts and her active co-operation is much to be desired. I would liken the operation to leading a horse through a gate; one steers the animal out by its head but the major propulsive power is supplied by its own muscles. This differs very much from the principle of forceps delivery under general anaesthesia, where much greater tractive efforts have to be applied.

Having induced pudendal nerve block the perineum is retracted with two fingers of one hand and the cup inserted with the knob, for reference, pointing towards the baby's occiput. The cup is pressed up against the baby's scalp and it is said to be best if it can be placed as near to the lambda as possible, but my own practice is to apply it to the most dependent and accessible part of the scalp, even over the parietal eminence in cases of transverse arrest of the head. This can be quite useful as will be seen later. One should at this stage ascertain, as far as possible, that no vagina or cervix has been included within the rim of the cup and an assistant is now asked to work the pump for a few strokes until a vacuum of 0·2 kilograms per square centimetre is registered on the gauge. Now is the time to make a proper check to ensure that no cervix or vagina has been included because there is just enough suction to maintain the cup in position. It is surprising how easy it is to include a bit of cervix and I have done so twice. Very careful palpation right round the rim of the cup is necessary to exclude this. If cervix or vagina is included in the cup it is difficult to achieve a stable vacuum and a hissing leak will almost at once be heard when traction is applied; also no advance whatever will occur, so the mistake will be very readily recognised on further examination or on the cup pulling off. The crescent of included cervix looks a little dusky as a result of being included but I have not seen any harm result from it. With the cup properly applied, the longer one can take in building up the vacuum the more satisfactory will the artificial caput inside the cup become. If one is in a great hurry, because of fetal distress for example, the vacuum can be built up in two or three minutes, but a much less satisfactory grip of the head is obtained and with all the patience in the world we prefer to spend at least eight minutes in building up the vacuum of 0·8 kilograms per square centimetre, which is what we usually employ. During this period the patient can be kept in intelligent conversation and full time is allowed for the pudendal block to take effect.

I have deliberately sought to measure the traction forces which can be applied before the cup pulls away from the scalp. For this purpose I waited, and had to wait a long time, for a fresh stillbirth which occurred in a case of hydrops late one Saturday afternoon. I hurriedly made in my workshop a sort of miniature lavatory seat to fit the baby's head exactly, wedged the head into this "brim" and applied the ventouse in the standard manner. I then rigged the whole thing up in the mortuary so that weights could be applied directly to the ventouse in increasing amounts and at 23 lb (10 kg) the vacuum broke and the cup came off. This is a very much smaller force than is usually applied with forceps as has been described earlier and constitutes one of the great safety factors in this operation.

As soon as the vacuum has been built up properly traction can begin, preferably synchronously with a uterine contraction, although as soon as pulling starts, of course, the uterus contracts in sympathy. Malmström recommended and indeed it is the usual practice to pull at right angles to the plane of the cup, but in order to do this the perineum has to be pulled well back with two fingers of the other hand in the vagina, but I have found it useful, especially in cases of malrotated head, to pull in different directions about 10 degrees off this perpendicular axis, watching the cup and any of the head that is visible to see if movement or rocking or any type of rotation looks like taking place. It will be appreciated that in cases of transverse arrest of the head the cup, if applied to the most dependent and accessible part of the scalp, may be over the anterior parietal eminence, or partly so, in which case the slight pulling off axis may swing the head most impressively and rotate it into the occipito-anterior position. Sometimes this does not occur until the head has come further down on the pelvic floor, but this technique demonstrates most beautifully the mechanics of spontaneous labour which has simply failed because the expulsive efforts of the uterus and patient have been inadequate hitherto to achieve what the assistance of the ventouse now brings about so easily. It is certainly most interesting to see an occipitoposterior rotate with the help of the ventouse almost spontaneously under the influence of the gutter mechanism of the pelvic floor. This operation involves no displacement of the head and is the nearest thing to physiological normal delivery that can be achieved. The forceps, after all, tends to fix and determine the position of the head at the will of the operator. The ventouse allows the head to come the way it wants to, even sometimes face to pubis, and this is one of the most delightful features of the operation.

The warning hiss that the vacuum is about to break and the cup come off can usually be taken as an indication either that one is pulling too hard (and to one who has been used to forceps it takes a lot of discipline to restrict one's tractive efforts to what is suitable for the ventouse), or else it is because maternal soft parts have been included within the rim, thus calling for re-examination. If the cup does come off no great harm is done. One of my patient's commented, "What was that?" The cup can be immediately reapplied over the same chignon as before, but it is a bad thing to do so more than once and one should consider alternative methods of delivery. There is a temptation to use the cup for screwing the head round, but this is not to be recommended as it tends to abrade the scalp. Less than half a dozen pulls with contractions will indicate the likelihood of success and one should be able to have a fair idea within twenty minutes whether to persist or not.

Our own failure rate, Table 2, was depressingly high at first. The 132 cases quoted in these tables date to the beginning of 1963, since when, of course, our experience has considerably enlarged. Unfamiliarity with the instrument was mainly responsible and, to some extent, bad selection of cases.

The direction of pull is largely determined by what looks most rewarding and since adopting this principle the success rate has improved enormously.

The vacuum is released as soon as the head is crowned and delivery is then completed in the normal way. The indications for the use of the ventouse are listed in Table 3. The great indication, of course, is for the hypotonic case in the absence of mechanical disproportion who hangs fire at about four fingers' dilatation. We do not like applying the instrument at less than this degree of dilatation, not only because it is more difficult but for fear of damaging the cervix, although others are more bold in this respect. To deliver a woman within half an hour, after many days of tedious and unrewarding labour, is a very satisfying experience and much to be preferred to Caesarean section or forceps. Willocks (1962) who, in my department, has used the apparatus more extensively than any of us, has listed the following major indications:

1. To deliver some cases of fetal distress occurring late in the first stage of labour.
2. To complete delivery in some cases of uterine inertia late in the first stage.
3. As an alternative to trial of forceps in some multiparae in whom second-stage delay is associated with deflexion and malposition of the fetal head at the pelvic brim or high in the pelvic cavity.
4. To rotate and deliver the head in many cases of occipito-transverse and posterior positions.

He also adds that the ventouse may be used instead of forceps in the second stage and I agree that it makes a very pleasant alternative to the simple low forceps operation. I had the gratifying experience of delivering one of my own staff midwives with the ventouse after an hour and a half of profitless second staging and her comment after delivery was, "I am so glad I managed it all myself". She did not even know at the time that she had been delivered with the ventouse. I wonder if one could say the same even for the easiest of low forceps operations and I felt this was tribute indeed to the gentleness of the method.

One talks of trial of forceps with all preparations in the foreground rather than in the background for Caesarean section if the trial fails. The same principle can be applied, particularly before full dilatation, in the case of the ventouse and we call it the "Ventouse-Caesarean section sequence". In actual fact, as our Tables show, the ventouse nearly always succeeds and the need for Caesarean section does not, therefore, arise, but one of my colleagues in Glasgow has referred to it in derisory terms as "the suck it and see". I would agree however with the statement[10] that very high vacuum extraction must initially be regarded more or less as a trial of ventouse, which, if failure occurs, should be followed immediately by Caesarean section. There is a natural temptation to follow a failed vacuum extraction, with suspected disproportion, by the application of forceps, but if these two fail, the baby and the mother are now in poor shape and whenever I have gone through the whole miserable sequence of failed ventouse, failed forceps, and ultimate Caesarean section I have much regretted not having gone straight to section without an intervening attempt at forceps. The cumulative effect of all three methods is something which I do not wish to encounter again.

Hazards.—The literature is already replete with grisly accounts of sloughing scalps, intracranial haemorrhages, cephalhaematomata, depressed fractures of the skull, death and destruction, which accord ill with our own experience and that of colleagues of mine in other centres who have acquired a proper experience of the instrument. All this has helped to fan the prejudice of reactionary obstetricians, some of whom have argued fiercely with me and with apparent intelligence and then finally confessed that they had never even seen the instrument used or had certainly not attempted to use it themselves. Tradition dies hard and midwives of both sexes are often remarkable for their conservatism. Huntingford (1961) produced a very depressing account but on an extremely small series of cases and by our standards would appear to have made much more prolonged and possibly determined efforts to deliver than we would have attempted. Our own rule is to review the suitability of the case for delivery by this method if success does not appear to be likely within twenty minutes and certainly the delivery must be completed within about forty-five minutes of the application of the cup. Otherwise one is obviously asking for trouble. Nowadays one would think very seriously before tugging away at a baby's head with forceps for more than threequarters of an hour and might be justified in considering Caesarean section as a less traumatic method of delivery, particularly from the baby's point of view, and the same philosophy should apply to the ventouse. We do not now talk about brute force in obstetrics but we still practice "brute forceps". Fortunately one cannot employ force with the ventouse because it simply pulls adrift from the scalp. Theoretical objections have been raised that the vacuum applied to the scalp increases the incidence of intracranial haemorrhage, but by what mechanism is not clear. Snoeck, in fact, worked out that intracranial stress and the risk of haemorrhage were much less with vacuum extraction than with forceps delivery. After all, this is simply a form of skin traction as employed in orthopaedic surgery and the point of application of force is at the point of attachment of the scalp in the region of the base of the skull.

We have become much interested in the occasional phenomenon of scalp haematoma which may be so serious as to require neonatal blood transfusion.

A serious kind of bleeding in the baby at or shortly after birth is a subaponeurotic haemorrhage following ventouse delivery. It differs from cephalhaematoma in that it is not limited to the sutures and is not subperiosteal. In a three year period up to the end of 1967, in 232 out of 6,439 deliveries a ventouse was used and of these 232 cases, 9 had subaponeurotic haemorrhage; two of them were fatal—one at least being due to a failure to recognise the need for blood transfusion earlier.

The characteristic clinical finding is diffuse pitting oedema of the scalp and occasionally fluctuation. Later, bruising may appear. The signs of haemorrhage may not be evident for $1\frac{1}{2}$ to 48 hours after delivery. Much later there may be hyperbilirubinaemia. Certainly the danger of this complication should be recognised if the thrombotest is below 10 per cent. The trouble is that the action of phytomenadione is not sufficiently rapid to deal with the acute hypoprothrombinaemic case who is bleeding. Therefore carrying out thrombotesting is always desirable and if the levels are pathologically low transfusion is indicated before waiting for signs of its immediate effects. The transfusion of fresh frozen plasma 10 ml/kg if given at an early stage is admirable. This precaution is particularly valuable in low-birth-weight infants with low thrombotest levels.[1]

Willoughby, our haematologist, reckons that the thrombotest is very low in 10 per cent of all babies, but that no harm results from this unless some haemostatic insult is inflicted, in this case, the ventouse. We therefore do thrombotest examinations on all cases of ventouse delivery except those at very inconvenient hours of the night when we give vitamin K_1 (intramuscular phytomenadione) prophylactically (5 mg) and of course this drug is also given in cases of recognised hypoprothrombinaemia.

Our own perinatal mortality in the first 132 cases is 3 per cent and corrected for intra-uterine death, gross prematurity and fetal abnormality the figure works out at 0·9 per cent, which can hardly justify condemning the operation as a lethal procedure. Lange (1961) in Denmark has compared a series of 480 cases of vacuum extraction delivery with 376 cases of forceps delivery and has concluded that the former involves less danger for the mother and infant than forceps, with a perinatal mortality of about half. He, too, considers the method more physiological.

Reference has already been made to the use of the ventouse to complete delivery after symphysiotomy. The African pelvis is very shallow compared with the European and it is not uncommon for part of the head and caput succedaneum to be visible at the vulva, with the biparietal diameter still nowhere near negotiating the pelvic brim. I am much impressed with the combined effects of symphysiotomy and ventouse extraction from witnessing the procedure in Uganda, carried out under local anaesthesia with the whole matter finished and done with within a quarter of an hour. Since about a quarter of instances of uterine rupture in underdeveloped countries are in previous uterine Caesarean scars, this would appear to be a thoroughly worth-while alternative in treatment.[14] Nevertheless symphysiotomy is only permissible if no more than two-fifths of the head is still above the brim regardless of moulding as observed *per vaginam* at the vulva.

As might be expected, those who have used the instrument most are the most enthusiastic and even allowing for slight admixture of cause and effect I think the advent of the ventouse should be regarded as a major advance in operative obstetrics. Delivery can be achieve with extreme gentleness and finesse and with a minimum of anaesthesia.

Let us never forget there is no such thing as a minor anaesthetic.

REFERENCES

1. AHUJA, G. L., WILLOUGHBY, M. L. N., KERR, M. M. and HUTCHISON, J. H. (1969). *Brit. med. J.*, **2**, 743.
2. BARRY, A. P. (1952). Personal communication.
3. CHALMERS, J. A. (1963). *J. Obstet. Gynaec. Brit. Cwlth*, **70**, 94.
4. CHALMERS, J. A. and FOTHERGILL, R. J. (1960). *Brit. med. J.*, **1**, 1684.
5. CHALMERS, J. A. (1964). *Brit. med. J.*, **1**, 1216.
6. COX, M. L. (1966). *J. Obstet. Gynaec. Brit. Cwlth*, **73**, 237.
7. CRICHTON, D. and SEEDAT, E. K. (1963). *S. Afr. med. J.*, **37**, 227.
8. EGBERT, D. S., KEETTEL, W. C. and LEE, J. G. (1960). *J. Iowa St. med. Soc.*, Aug., 499.
9. FEENEY, J. K. (1947). *Irish J. med. Sci.*, **1**, 190.
10. FJÄLLBRANT, B. (1964). *Gynécologie*, **157**, 161.
11. FOTHERGILL, R. J. and CHALMERS, J. A. (1961). *Practitioner*, **186**, 559.
12. FREETH, D. H. (1950). *Brit. med. J.*, **2**, 18.
13. GATE, J. M. and DUTTON, W. A. W. (1955). *Brit. med. J.*, **2**, 99.
14. GEBBIE, D. A. M. (1966). *Brit. med. J.*, **2**, 1490.
15. HAUSMANN, W. and LUNT, R. L. (1955). *J. Obstet. Gynaec. Brit. Emp.*, **62**, 509.
16. HUNTINGFORD, P. J. (1961). *Lancet*, **2**, 1054.
17. HUNTINGFORD, P. J. (1959). *J. Obstet. Gynaec. Brit. Emp.*, **62**, 26.
18. JONES, E. P. (1952). *Kielland's Forceps.* London: Butterworth & Co.
19. KERR, J. M. M. and MOIR, J. C. (1956). *Operative Obstetrics*, 6th edit. London: Baillière, Tindall & Cox.
20. KOBAK, A. J., EVANS, E. F. and JOHNSON, E. R. (1956). *Amer. J. Obstet. Gynec.*, **71**, 981.
21. LANGE, P. (1961). *Dan. med. Bull.*, **8**, 11.
22. MCDANIEL, E. B. (1963). Personal communication.
23. MACGREGOR, W. G. (1966). *Lancet.* **1**, 147.
24. MALMSTRÖM, T. (1954). *Acta obstet. gynec. scand.*, **33**, Suppl. 4.
25. MALMSTRÖM, T. (1957). *Acta obstet. gynec. scand.*, **36**, Suppl. 3.
26. MALMSTRÖM, T. and LANGE, P. (1964). *Acta obstet. gynec. scand.*, **43**, Suppl. 1.
27. MENDELSON, C. L. (1946). *Amer. J. Obstet. Gynec.*, **52**, 191.
28. MILLER, D. (1927). *Brit. med. J.*, **2**, 685.
29. MILLER, D. (1928). *Brit. med. J.*, **2**, 183.
30. MOIR, D. D. and DAVIDSON, S. (1972). *Brit. J. Anaesth.*, **44**, 1197.

31. Moir, D. D. and Wallace, G. (1967). *J. Obstet. Gynaec. Brit. Cwlth*, **74**, 424.
32. Parker, R. B. (1954). *Brit. med. J.*, **2**, 65.
33. Parker, R. B. (1956). *Brit. med. J.*, **2**, 16.
34. Rhodes, P. (1958). *J. Obstet. Gynaec. Brit. Emp.*, **65**, 353.
35. Scott, J. S. and Gadd, R. L. (1957). *Brit. med. J.*, **1**, 971.
36. Scudamore, J. H. and Yates, M. J. (1966). *Lancet*. **1**, 23.
37. Seedat, E. K. and Crichton, D. (1962). *Lancet*. **1**, 554.
38. Snoeck, J. (1960). *Proc. roy. Soc. Med.*, **53**, 749.
39. Tennent, R. A. (1965). *J. Obstet. Gynaec. Brit. Cwlth*, **72**, 872.
40. Willocks, J. (1962). *J. Obstet. Gynaec. Brit. Cwlth*, **69**, 266.

CHAPTER XX

RESUSCITATION OF THE NEWBORN

To breathe or not to breathe—that is the question.

The term asphyxia neonatorum explains itself, but behind this outward manifestation of inability to breathe lies a whole sea of troubles, much of which has not yet been properly fathomed and is now engaging much interesting modern research.

Perinatal mortality embraces all stillbirths, whether macerated or fresh, and all neonatal deaths within the first week of extra-uterine existence and when one looks through tables of such statistics, whether national or local, it is readily appreciated that one is confronted with a very wide range of reasons for a baby's refusal to breathe at birth or successfully to maintain respiration thereafter. One has to review the whole subject and efficacy of resuscitation of the newborn against this wide pathological background and in the past failure to do so has been responsible for the rapidly changing fashions in resuscitative techniques, which have varied through the years from the bizarre to the picturesque and only a few have been based upon sound scientific fact. The reasons for respiratory failure at birth, in fact, differ so widely and it is so difficult in the crisis of such an emergency to make a satisfactory differential diagnosis that it is not surprising that no set order of procedure has yet proved satisfactory, and treatment has to fall back upon the general lines of maintaining oxygenation of the heart and vital brain centres by one means or another until a more definitive diagnosis and treatment can be instituted.

Important though the business of resuscitation must be, it has to be recognised that one is often dealing with overwhelming pathology and that the clinician is often presented with a hopeless case from adverse factors which have been operating already before birth and against which his resuscitative techniques can only have a marginal value in reducing perinatal loss. Any major improvement in fetal survival chances will come, not through radical changes in methods of resuscitation, but in the better control of the complications of pregnancy and labour and above all in the elimination of prematurity. Abnormal labour may indeed be bad for the fetus but abnormal pregnancy may be even worse.

The national perinatal mortality rate has been steadily dropping but continues to vary from region to region, from below 20 per 1000 in the rural and less socially deprived areas of the country and approaching 30 per 1000 in the less favoured. In the less developed countries of the world the perinatal mortality may be more or less treble these figures and undoubtedly socio-economic factors are if anything more important than the degree of obstetrical skill locally available. In all areas of the world however the figures are consistently improving. Intra-uterine asphyxia of all varieties ranks highest on the list of causes.

Congenital malformations occupy an increasingly important role in the incidence both of stillbirth and neonatal death. Cerebral birth trauma is fortunately a dwindling factor in modern obstetrical practice but asphyxia during labour whether due to placental inadequacy or to cord accidents, in spite of the increased use of intrapartum monitoring, is still an important cause of perinatal death. Prematurity, especially if complicated by infection during labour or by the respiratory distress syndrome after delivery is still a potent cause of neonatal death.

Over the last 20 years there has been a progressive decline in the perinatal mortality figures of our own hospital practice from about 75 per 1000 to under 16 per 1000 live births (Table 1).

20/TABLE 1

THE QUEEN MOTHER'S HOSPITAL

	Percentage
Section Rate	9·6
Instrumental delivery rate (overall)	24·0
Epidural rate (overall)	25·0
Induction rate (induced, *not* in labour)	46·0 (6 months figs.)
Vaginal breech rate (overall, including twins)	0·8
	per 1000
Stillbirth rate	7·8
Perinatal mortality rate	15·3
Perinatal mortality rate (corrected to exclude infants weighing less than 1000 g)	13·0
Total deliveries: 2672	

In considering stillbirth, or for that matter any perinatal death, it is often possible and indeed advisable to consider it under two headings, namely, the pathology that caused the death, and the obstetrical factor. For example, in a case of maternal antepartum haemorrhage a baby may die because of asphyxia, but the obstetrical cause might be placenta praevia, or abruptio placentae.

Apart from the contribution made to disaster by gross fetal abnormality, the dice is often loaded against the baby in advance by pre-eclamptic toxaemia, abruptio placentae, intra-uterine growth retardation and other types of as yet unexplained placental insufficiency, and the employment of even very skilled resuscitative techniques may have only a marginal value in cases thus prejudiced from the first. Where however the baby's poor condition at birth is due to more immediate adverse effects in labour itself much more can be expected of resuscitation. It is now our view that all fresh stillbirths are, theoretically at least, preventable and call for detailed inquiry. This even includes cord accidents where, with adequate monitoring and vigilance, timely intervention might have saved the baby's life.

All modern, well-equipped maternity hospitals have good Paediatric Departments, with the anomalous result that many cases of what are really previable abortions have to appear in the neonatal death list because of temporarily successful resuscitation. If however babies weighing less than 1000 g are excluded from the tables a more encouraging figure can be claimed, as in Table 1.

The situation over most of the country has been rapidly improving with a declining birth rate in the city; in fact it looks as though "The Pill" is now beginning to work in our area and certainly degrees of parity are nothing like what I remember even in the 1950s. Many new maternity beds have been opened up, including the Queen Mother's Hospital (114 beds). This hospital opened in January 1964 and in the first 5000 births the perinatal mortality rate was 38 per 1000, and 8 per cent of the patients were unbooked. Improvement towards the present figure has been progressive, although it has been achieved at an ever mounting rate of operative intervention, including induction of labour.

If a baby fails to breathe satisfactorily at birth, it will be appreciated that there is usually a very good reason for it and that the greatest hope for the future lies in prevention in the form of more successful antenatal and intranatal management. For a baby to be able to initiate respiration it must be fit enough to do so and undoubtedly the achievement of a flying start is vitally important.

A baby's first breath is a remarkable phenomenon, and it clearly calls for a very great and intricately co-ordinated effort. We have sought to measure these efforts by recording the pressure swings within the chest at birth (Donald *et al.*, 1958). Our technique has involved passing a fine plastic catheter half-way down the oesophagus through one of the nostrils and connecting it to a very sensitive electromanometer. In a number of cases the catheter can be inserted after the delivery of the head but before the birth of the shoulders, and our results indicate that the first respiratory efforts are commonly in the region of 40 cm of water pressure. With the onset of crying some seconds later, the swings of pressure, above and below zero, amount to 90 cm and over, a figure comparable to what an adult can deliberately achieve by attempting forced respiration against a closed glottis or hand placed over nose and mouth.

This is what happens in the healthy mature baby and these respiratory efforts not only open up the lung alveoli directly but, perhaps even more important, they draw blood into the pulmonary vascular system causing a diversion from its former right-to-left shunts through the foramen ovale and ductus arteriosus, as had obtained before birth.

In fact, for the first hour or two of life, the blood flow through the ductus is reversed from left to right, thus sending blood newly returned from the lungs back through the pulmonary artery for a second helping of oxygen. This mechanism improves oxygenation while the lungs are still relatively inefficient, but as soon as the oxygen saturation of the blood exceeds 90 per cent the ductus arteriosus closes functionally and the adult type of circulation through the heart and great vessels is established (Dawes *et al.*, 1953; Born *et al.*, 1954).

The proper filling of the pulmonary vascular bed achieves, in addition to oxygenation, two other very important effects. Firstly, inspired fluid can be rapidly absorbed from the alveoli and, secondly, the pulmonary capillaries have erectile properties and so help in establishing and maintaining the architectural patency of the alveoli (Carter, 1957; Jaykka, 1957). In fact no important circulatory changes have been observed before the first breath and from a study of the structural appearance of lungs of fetuses that have died perinatally Jaykka (1958) has found that the capillary bed is not patent in areas of atelectasis within the lungs and that a non-patent capillary bed implies that there has been no erection of the capillary network and may, in fact, be one cause of atelectasis since it is believed that capillary erection is a prerequisite of normal expansion of the lung. Furthermore, the entrance of air into a lung in which the capillary bed has not been opened up will result in abnormal expansion. In the opinion of Karlberg (1960) half the adaptive changes concerning lung function and pulmonary circulation are instituted within the first two minutes of the onset of respiration and thereafter the rate of adaptation is more evenly spread over the next few days.

The resistances to initial aeration of the lungs are caused firstly by the moist cohesion of the alveolar walls, secondly, by inelasticity of lung parenchyma before the phenomenon of capillary erection by diversion of blood flow has taken place and, thirdly, interference with alveolar duct patency by liquor amnii and meconium, etc. Karlberg, too, reckons that no appreciable lung inflation is possible with anything less than the exercise of pressures of 20 to 40 cm of water, which are considerably greater than those used in normal respiratory effort. From cineradiographic study it would appear that the lower and posterior parts of the lungs are aerated first.

The inspiratory volume of the first breath is reckoned to be between 20 and 75 ml as compared with the usual 15 to 20 ml of resting tidal volumes later on in a normal baby. Crying may raise the figure to 130 to 160 ml.

The resistance of the lungs to expansion, that is to say the lung compliance, consequently improves so that there is a progressive and rapid fall in the amount of effort needed on the part of the baby to maintain respiration. This is very important when one compares the satisfactory aeration achieved within a few minutes by a healthy vigorous baby with the respiratory difficulties associated with atelectasis and prematurity.

We have repeatedly demonstrated the reduction in respiratory effort required which accompanies progressive pulmonary expansion and have made simultaneous recordings of the increasing tidal airs which indicate a bigger ventilatory reward at the same time.

In order to establish this physiological train of events a flying start to respiration is very necessary. Even a premature baby, if it achieves this flying start, can expand its lungs to full radiological clarity within 2 hours and is thereafter most unlikely to develop the pulmonary syndrome of the newborn (Donald, 1954).

The causes of the onset of respiration are usually a combination of factors.

Firstly, the child finds itself in a state of acute anoxia due to the cutting off of the oxygen supply from the mother. In normal labour this occurs as soon as the head is born, at which time the placenta has probably started to separate and the placental site will have already undergone some retraction in any case. The head and face turn a livid blue at this stage, which is an encouraging indication of the state of the baby provided further delivery is not delayed beyond a minute or two, and, if the chest is not too tightly wedged within the pelvic cavity, the baby will often cry forthwith.

As soon as it is born, the stimulus of anoxia is reinforced by innumerable afferent stimuli which crowd in on the baby's central nervous system from skin, muscles and joints. The process of birth must come as a rude and painful shock. In certain animals, the fetus falls on to its snout, which acts as a very efficient receptor for such afferent stimuli (Barcroft, 1946).

The carotid sinus plays an important part. Its response depends upon both chemical and pressor receptors. A rise in blood pressure stimulates respiration in a manner not seen in animals in which the carotid sinuses have been denervated experimentally, and these sinuses are important chemical receptor organs in oxygen lack. This sensitivity may exceed that of the respiratory centre itself.

In like manner breathing is markedly depressed by sinus denervation in animals. The accumulation of carbon dioxide also stimulates the respiratory mechanism, but only if it is functionally healthy and not handicapped or depressed by antecedent anoxia, immaturity or cerebral compression.

Aetiology of Asphyxia Neonatorum

In the first place, the baby may lack the necessary equipment to start or to maintain respiration. This is particularly the case in very premature infants where alveolar development may not be sufficiently advanced. Such infants, for a time, may be able to oxygenate their blood by breathing with their bronchioli which are capable of respiratory distension, but they often die within a day or two from pulmonary atelectasis.

Secondly, the respiratory centre may not be sufficiently sensitive to normal stimuli because of immaturity, or it may be depressed by any condition causing a rise in intracranial pressure, by drugs and anaesthetics, and it may be damaged by previous anoxia so that a rising carbon dioxide level may reach lethal proportions before it can stimulate it.

Thirdly, blood circulation may be so reduced as a result of fetal shock that the supply of oxygenated blood, even if available, is unable to reach the respiratory centre in sufficient quantity to revive it.

Lastly, mechanical factors may prevent blood oxygenation, as, for example, where the respiratory passages are blocked by the aspiration of foreign material, or when there is delay in delivering the aftercoming head in breech presentation or serious difficulty in delivering the shoulders of a large baby.

Asphyxia before Delivery as a Cause of Asphyxia at Birth

This is perhaps the most important class of causes.

Anything which interferes with placental circulation may damage the vital centres and their responsiveness following delivery.

Separation of the placenta, whether normally situated or praevia, may be insufficient to kill the fetus straightaway, but often causes either premature inspiration *in utero* or results in unresponsiveness at birth. The placenta which is praevia has the further risk of being compressed during labour by the presenting part.

Pre-eclamptic toxaemia, and especially eclampsia, subject the child to varying degrees of anoxia which may damage it beyond recall, and placental infarction, particularly the diffuse variety, may operate in like fashion.

Prolonged labour with the membranes ruptured exposes the child to mounting anoxia due to the progressive retraction of the placental site, in addition to intranatal pneumonia.

Cord accidents such as compression or tight winding round the neck and, more unusually, true knotting, are still fairly common in labour.

Any condition which precipitately lowers the maternal blood pressure reduces placental oxygenation, as for example in shock, or in antepartum haemorrhage in which the effects of hypotension may be added to those of placental separation.

A fairly common predisposing cause is maternal asphyxia in the course of inducing anaesthesia, and the ideal general anaesthetic which is free from this risk has yet to be discovered. Vomiting often complicates induction of anaesthesia, especially in the labouring woman whose stomach has been liberally plied with fluids in the course of labour, and the effects of such asphyxia can be as disastrous to fetus as to mother. Long after the latter appears well oxygenated following "induction asphyxia", the uterus, with its slow but plentiful circulation, remains a dusky colour, as can be seen at Caesarean section after a stormy passage through the lighter planes of anaesthesia.

The signs of fetal distress during labour are usually those of asphyxia *in utero* and resuscitation after birth is consequently prejudiced.

Of all the drugs which depress respiration at birth, morphia and its allied derivatives are the chief offenders and for that reason should not be given in the last four hours before delivery. In the case of premature deliveries the safety interval is even longer. Pethidine is less dangerous in this respect, but is best withheld during the second stage. Roberts *et al.* (1957) found that pethidine given to the mother during labour reduced the minute volume of respiratory activity in the baby by 10–15 per cent for some hours after birth. Fortunately nalorphine can counteract respiratory depression due to morphia and pethidine.

Even better as an antidote to respiratory depressants is a newer drug, naloxone (Narcan Neonatal) 0·01 mg/kg body weight intravenously. This drug is designed to antagonise the narcotic drugs including pentazocine without other respiratory depressant effects as may occur with nalorphine given in injudicious dosage.

The mother may have been given Pethilorfan which contains pethidine combined with levallorphan and is more potent than nalorphine. This drug has enjoyed popularity for many years as a safe narcotic for the mother without penalty of depressing the fetal respiratory centre. The standard maternal dose is 2 ml containing 100 mg of pethidine and 1·25 mg of levallorphan. During labour it can be administered to the mother more than once as necessary.

The barbiturates also contribute to neonatal asphyxia and a study of the concentration levels of phenobarbitone in maternal serum and umbilical cord serum has shown that the levels are within 5 per cent of each other and that the rate of elimination from the blood of the newborn is slower than or equal to that in adults. The baby therefore suffers just as much of a hangover as its mother and may well be in less of a condition to have to face it. Paraldehyde still remains one of the safest drugs in this respect.

All general anaesthetics have some influence on neonatal breathing, depending more upon the depth of maternal narcosis than on the particular agent; Trilene, however, is reasonably safe though often inadequate as an anaesthetic. Nitrous oxide and air analgesia lowers the percentage oxygen saturation of the maternal blood and should not be continued in the presence of established fetal distress

Every acute attack of anoxia depletes the fetal glycogen reserves and chronic hypoxia depletes them chronically.

This anaerobic type of metabolism is extravagant and about seven times less efficient than ordinary glucose metabolism and results in fetal or neonatal acidosis due to lactic acidaemia. Though inefficient it nevertheless enables the baby at the time of birth to withstand quite astonishing levels of hypoxia.

There is very little glycogen in the liver early in pregnancy, but the stores increase rapidly and according to Shelley (1961) having reached at term double the level of the adult liver these hepatic glycogen reserves fall, after birth, very rapidly to about one-tenth of their former value within three hours, thereafter rising gradually to adult levels within the next two to three weeks. The fetal brain stores very little glycogen but uses glucose, if necessary by anaerobic metabolism, although it does require an active circulation to supply it with glucose carried in the blood, and this depends upon an active myocardium (Mott, 1961). The myocardium, to maintain efficiency and therefore an effective circulation to the brain, depends upon its own glycogen reserves and these too are depleted in hypoxia. This is one of the reasons for the feeble, slow heart beat of the severely distressed baby at birth. The resistance of the brain of the newborn to anoxia is due to its ability to metabolise glucose anaerobically and this in turn is furnished by the glycolysis of the liver stores, but survival will depend upon how well the stores of glycogen in the myocardium last out (Stafford and Weatherall, 1960). Experiments on newborn animals in an atmosphere of nitrogen show that survival depends on myocardial glycogen and when this is finally depleted circulatory failure ensues. A compensatory mechanism may put off the evil moment here since no animal can maintain its body temperature in the presence of anoxia, and cooling may prolong survival possibly by retarding the utilisation of cardiac glycogen, hence the case for hypothermia as a therapeutic measure, but if oxygen is supplied and reaches the circulation an attempt may be made to maintain temperature by using up the glycogen reserves and death may follow. It is known that a baby, if warm, can survive without food for many days, but if it is allowed to get too cold it may use up its reserves of carbohydrate in an attempt to maintain body temperature and may then die in a state of hypoglycaemia (Mann and Elliott, 1957).

The state of the glycogen stores within the body, and particularly within the myocardium, therefore greatly influence a baby's ability to withstand anoxia and, since it takes many hours for myocardial reserves of glycogen to be built up again, it can be seen that chronic deprivation or repeated shortages of oxygen are far more deadly than the dramatically acute fetal distress which may occur late in the second stage and from which the baby in this latter instance may make a much more dramatic recovery regardless of the technique employed (Donald, 1963). The importance will, therefore, be appreciated of those factors capable of reducing stores of fetal glycogen before or during birth and, therefore, the chances of survival, such as maternal malnutrition, placental insufficiency, especially pre-eclamptic toxaemia and intra-uterine hypoxia of all varieties.

The concept of "placental insufficiency" is frequently invoked to explain intra-uterine anoxia and the mechanism and extent are by no means predictable or discernible in a large proportion of cases, but when perinatal mortality occurs as a direct result of asphyxia during labour the cause is usually much more obvious. Dawkins and colleagues (1961), in analysing one hundred such deaths, found that only two had no recognisable aetiological factor and they noted that the major causes of intrapartum asphyxia were complicated vaginal delivery, premature separation of placenta and inadequate placental reserve, more than half the deaths occurring in association with maternal toxaemia. In fact when toxaemia was combined with postmaturity or difficult labour the hazards were greatly increased, but postmaturity in otherwise uncomplicated cases rarely caused fetal death during labour.

Fetal Conditions as Causes of Asphyxia at Birth

The presence of mucus, often tenacious, and thick meconium in the upper air passages is rightly often blamed, and although post-mortem examination does not, as a rule, reveal such foreign matter in significant amounts, it would appear imprudent at least not to take the simple steps of clearing it out. Liquor which is not thickened with meconium is probably innocuous, for respiratory movements of the baby normally occur for some time before the onset of labour, although they are not deep. In any case normal liquor is readily eliminated from the tract or absorbed. Mucus regurgitated from the stomach is an additional source of trouble and gastric aspiration is increasingly practised.

Intracranial haemorrhage, howsoever caused, whether by the mechanical trauma of labour or by asphyxia, operates differently, and the baby's asphyxia is only one of the several manifestations of fetal shock. Even in the absence of significant intracranial bleeding, cerebral oedema may act in the same fashion.

In prolonged and infected labour with the membranes ruptured, intranatal bronchopneumonia is not uncommon. Clinically, these cases are often hard to distinguish from classical hyaline membrane disease, although radiologically the distinction can be made.

Very rarely, congenital abnormalities such as laryngeal atresia may prevent the onset of respiration.

Above all, if labour is complicated by asphyxia, then any mucus, meconium or blood which may be aspirated as a result is bound to increase the handicaps of a respiratory centre already depressed.

Pathology

The immediate effects of asphyxia are those of venous engorgement, especially in the brain where the vessels have already endured much in the course of labour and whose walls may finally give way. If the tentorium cerebelli is torn the brain is at once flooded with blood, but moulding, by dragging the apex of the tentorium upwards, may sufficiently restrict venous flow to raise back-pressure to the point at which smaller tributary vessels rupture, even though the tentorium is not actually torn. Cerebral oedema also occurs.

Apart from the brain, venous engorgement and capillary haemorrhages are likely to occur throughout the body, especially in the liver and under its capsule, in the lungs, suprarenals and heart muscle, where petechiae (Tardieu's spots) are characteristically seen. There is arteriolar constriction and the circulation is reduced, particularly to the brain with its vital centres, including not only the respiratory but the vasomotor centre as well, which are soon paralysed so that the signs of shock are manifested.

In cases of asphyxia developing after birth Edith Potter and Rosenbaum described an accumulation of cerebrospinal fluid which may not be noticed at autopsy unless the skull is opened carefully. This is more likely to occur after Caesarean section and in premature infants. It is associated with atelectasis which may be secondary, and although it may be due to mechanical causes, such as the sudden removal of the child from intra-uterine pressure, it is more likely to be the result of anoxia. The increase in fluid and the resulting pressure from it is then likely to aggravate the child's respiratory difficulties.

The vicious circle is easily completed. Asphyxia begets vasomotor and respiratory depression, which in their turn cause further asphyxia until irreversible changes end in the child's death.

The Clinical Stages of Asphyxia Neonatorum

In the past it has been customary to describe two types, namely the blue and the white, but the former may merge into the latter, which is a stage of decompensation and failure; on the other hand, white or pallid asphyxia may present from the first, in which case it comes as an outward manifestation of profound fetal shock, however caused.

Cases of white asphyxia would be more accurately described as grey. The point at issue, however, in the difference in colour of the two types, is the state of the peripheral circulation. In both, asphyxia may be profound, but good circulation in the skin is necessary for lividity to show itself, and the better prognosis in the blue variety lies in the better circulatory state.

The signs of early asphyxia, then, are a full and powerful heart beat which is also slower than usual, a mechanism whereby oxygen may be to some degree conserved, and the skin is a dusky blue.

Later these signs give place to grey pallor, a weak apex beat and flaccidity. The worse the child's condition, the slower the heart beat and the first sign of recovery is its acceleration, which precedes improvement in skin colour. The lips have a dirty purple colour, the anal sphincter is toneless, the tongue tends to fall backwards and the jaw is relaxed. The vocal cords lie separated from each other in the paralysed position, so that intubation is not usually difficult, for the reflex tone of the glottis, in common with the other reflexes, has gone.

Respiration is for a time very shallow, punctuated with occasional gasps, but soon becomes very infrequent and finally stops altogether.

Within ten to fifteen minutes the changes are irreversible, and the longer it takes to oxygenate the baby and restore its failing circulation, the greater will be the damage to the brain cells, and it is only possible to speculate on the extent to which its intellect, for example, may be impaired, not to mention the grosser evidences of neurological injury which may originate in the hazards of delivery.

In cases of intracranial bleeding vasomotor tone is poor from the very beginning; the mechanism is different here and there is no livid stage. The prognosis is correspondingly less favourable.

A baby that has suffered a recent severe blood loss, for example from ruptured vasa praevia, is pale but active and has normal muscle tone.

Even though the immediate response to resuscitation may be satisfactory, there are cases which relapse some hours later and develop respiratory distress. Apart from cerebral irritation, oedema or compression, which is the commonest cause, a few of such cases must be attributed to the aspiration of foreign material. Now, the aspiration of liquor amnii at birth, although admittedly common, would not account for secondary atelectasis some hours later; it is therefore probable that regurgitation of mucus from the stomach occurs and, chiefly in the case of the weak or premature infant, some of this mucus may find its way into the respiratory tract. The observations of Gellis, Priscilla White and Pfeffer with regard to the stomach contents at birth, particularly after Caesarean section, will be referred to later.

In classifying asphyxia neonatorum, it is now more commonly the practice to grade it according to its severity rather than the baby's colour. Attempts to evaluate and compare different treatments and to assess subsequent progress are usually defeated for want of an objective standard which can be employed by a number of observers at birth. The scoring system, however, originally devised by Virginia Apgar (1953) deserves note. In this method the condition is assessed exactly one minute after birth in respect of five features, namely heart rate, respiratory effort, reflex irritability, muscle tone and colour, allowing a maximum score of two for each, as shown in Table II. The advantages of such a system are its ease of application, the reduced chances of observer error and non-interference with, nor modification by, resuscitative techniques since the assessment has strictly to be made at a given age, in our practice at 120 seconds.

The Evaluation of the Newborn Infant (Apgar) Method of Scoring

I have noticed with irritation when I am operating, that paediatricians often "take one off for colour". My taunt that in at least one instance the mother was an African is by now apocryphal.

Sixty seconds, or more commonly nowadays 120 seconds, after the *complete* birth of the infant (disregarding the cord and placenta) the following five objective signs are evaluated and each given a score of 0, 1 or 2. A score of 10 indicates an infant in the best possible condition.

Treatment of Neonatal Asphyxia

In these days of demarcation disputes it might be debated whose job it was to resuscitate the newborn. This, however, is a crisis which brooks no argument and the answer is quite simply "anyone present who is competent to cope". The need, therefore, to train obstetri-

Sign	0	1	2
Heart rate	Absent	Slow (Below 100)	Over 100
Respiratory effort	Absent	Slow Irregular	Good Crying
Muscle tone	Limp	Some flexion of extremities	Active motion
Response to catheter in nostril (tested after oropharynx is clear)	No response	Grimace	Cough or sneeze
Colour	Blue Pale	Body pink Extremities blue	Completely pink

cians, anaesthetists and paediatricians in standard resuscitative techniques, including particularly tracheal intubation, is obvious. It is only in larger units that all three categories of individual are likely to be present at the same time and only then in the more complicated cases. There is, therefore, some need to try and predict the type of cases where skilled resuscitation will be needed. Prediction is important in order to indicate that a doctor who can give undivided attention to the infant should be present at the delivery of all these high-risk patients (Corner, 1962). Ideally these would include all operative deliveries, all cases of malpresentation, fetal distress, twins, premature labour and in cases where the mothers appeared clinically to be "small for dates". The importance of obtaining a flying start to respiration has already been mentioned and, in fact, about three-quarters of all cases of respiratory distress have Apgar scores below six (see later) and some trouble at birth is nearly always present in the majority of cases who subsequently develop hyaline membrane disease. A baby apparently well at birth can, within two and a half minutes of complete apnoea, drop its percentage oxygen saturation dangerously and with it follows the inevitable acidosis, so that the pH of the blood falls at the rate of about 0·1 per minute.

The history of neonatal resuscitation reflects little enough credit on the knowledge or imagination of those practising it, and the baby has often had to demonstrate a will to survive capable of defeating the most determined assaults of its wellwishers. In the Old Testament the prophet Elisha had some success with mouth-to-mouth insufflation, but perhaps he was ahead of his time.

To William Smellie, Scottish obstetrician of the eighteenth century, the matter was simple enough. To make the baby cry it should be well whipped and have its nose rubbed with onions. I once came across an account from an eighteenth century combined textbook of Theology and Midwifery which recommended inflating the intestine with tobacco smoke, with clysters. A converted non-smoker, like myself, can only heartily endorse the suggested use of this insanitary and expensive habit. In the last century Schultze's method of swinging the baby above the head and causing it to jack-knife, so as to compress its chest, enjoyed a certain vogue and a very eminent obstetrician in Northern Ireland claims to have survived this form of resuscitation at his own birth. Buist in 1895 described his use of it to the Edinburgh Obstetrical Society in the following words, "Standing in a space cleared in the midst of a small room, whose other denizens were withdrawn into the corners, my feet planted well apart and arms extended I taught the neonatus to perform a series of grand circles, while the meconium distributed itself in trajectories for which the room and its inmates, including the physicians, formed a comprehensive recording surface." Just before the turn of the century subcutaneous injection of tincture of belladonna and whiskey was recommended, provided that it was Irish whiskey. Even when I was a student we were taught the value of rubbing the baby's gums with brandy, which the midwives were reputed to have flavoured with meconium in order to discourage inroads by a thirsty student body.

A list of the methods of artificial respiration which were taught even in my own day relied on the principle of elastic recoil of the chest wall as in adults but, of course, this phenomenon is not to be found in the shocked baby with unaerated lungs. Now these techniques have given way to airway clearance and positive pressure lung inflation in a baby too ill to make its own respiratory efforts.

As Gibberd has long pointed out, three conditions must be satisfied:

1. The air passages must be patent;
2. A suitable atmosphere must be available;
3. Respiratory movements must be adequate.

One might add a fourth condition, namely blood circulation must be adequate to revive the vital centres with oxygenated blood. Nevertheless we must face the sober truth that if a baby has even half a chance to breathe it will take it and its ultimate fate, whether to live or whether to die, is largely determined before resuscitation even starts.

Clearance of airway.—If possible, before the first gasp is taken, the mouth, pharynx and nostrils should be cleared by suction.

The traditional mucus catheter is totally inadequate for the purpose. Quite apart from its inefficiency, it is a septic weapon, and the sight of a midwife pulling down her mask, holding the other end between her teeth and blowing down it to clear it before reinsertion makes a mockery of all the other aseptic precautions. However, any mucus extractor is better than none. In hospital practice suction should, of course, be mechanical, either by connecting to a water suction pump attached to a nearby tap, which is both simple and efficient, or in the case of modern units, to the suction pipes which have been built into all labour wards and nurseries. The end of the sucker must be of soft rubber to avoid damaging the pharyngeal mucous membrane. The end of the sucker tube should also be cut off square so as to discourage sucking in the mucous membrane and so destroying the effect.

It is particularly important to clear the pharynx as soon as the mouth is born in the case of the aftercoming head in breech delivery, or as soon as the head is delivered in Caesarean section, or in forceps deliveries. The ceremonial wiping of the eyelids can well wait until this far more necessary step has been taken.

As soon as the child is completely delivered it should be held up by the ankles with its back steadied against the front of the operator's chest. This leaves him a free hand with which to direct the end of the sucker. The suction pressure should not exceed 50 mm Hg (Figs 1. and 2).

It is recommended that the baby should not be held by its heels above the level of the placenta, as this may deprive it of 50 to 100 ml of its own blood. This provides yet another reason why I personally, being tall, prefer the sitting position for undertaking forceps delivery.

Now, and not before, the cord may be divided and the child may be handed to the midwife in the happy knowledge that the most important steps have already been taken.

The child is now laid, slightly turned to one side with the head downwards, in a warmed cot or tray inclined at about 30 degrees from the horizontal. The purpose of the head-down slope is to facilitate drainage of secretions and fluids and to discourage their aspiration, but once the pharynx and stomach have been properly emptied by mechanical suction the baby will be the better off from being propped up and relieved of the embarrassing weight of the liver on its diaphragm.

Resuscitation trays can be improvised in which the portion supporting the head can be easily lowered to facilitate intubation, should it be necessary. The usual type of cot is not satisfactory, because the side at the head end gets in the way if a laryngoscope has to be used.

Should the child not show signs of spontaneous breathing within

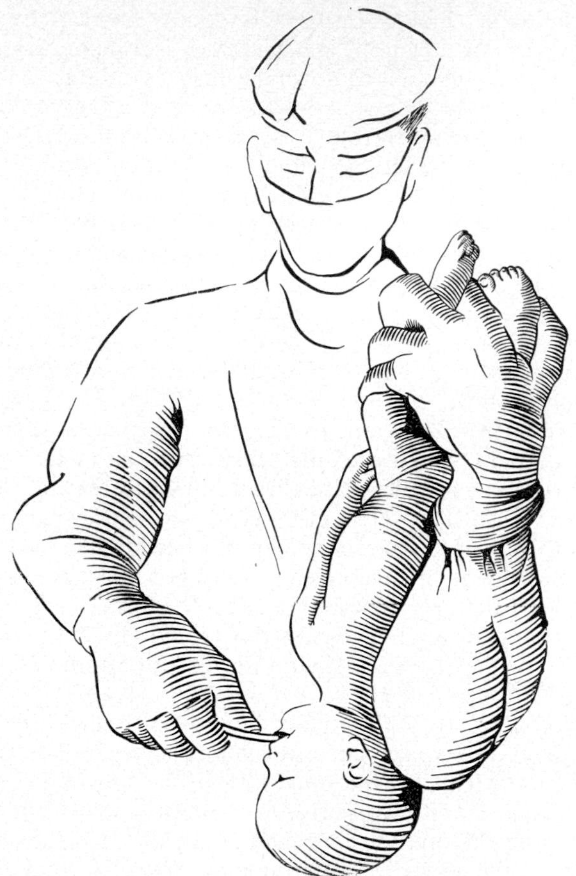

20/FIG. 1.—Method of holding baby immediately after delivery, and sucking out pharynx.

three minutes there should be no hesitation in clearing the glottis with the help of an infant's laryngoscope. Unfortunately, too many obstetricians are reluctant to familiarise themselves with the use of this instrument and tend to put off using it until the situation has become desperate and is made yet more desperate by unskilled hands.

If the glottic reflex is not present, the trachea should be intubated forthwith with a small, curved, soft plastic tube made specially for the purpose, for example close-fitting plastic laryngeal tubes such as Warne's neonatal catheters. The point to remember is that if the child is in any state to resent this manoeuvre there is no need for it, and in the circumstances which call for it there is no difficulty in carrying it out gently and quickly.

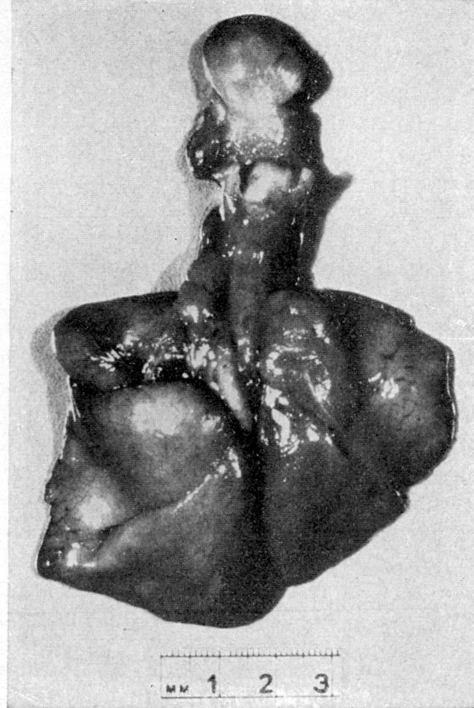

20/Fig. 2.—Mucus blocking glottis.

Any mucus in the trachea can be sucked out now, and intermittent positive pressures of oxygen up to 35 cm of water can be applied with the help of a manually operated rubber bag or some such device. The purpose of this is not to inflate the alveoli as might be expected, for in any case far higher pressures than this would be necessary, but the bronchial tree is thereby flooded with oxygen, some of which is directly absorbed; should the child take even a small breath, it can be certain of receiving a good concentration of oxygen of which it is in serious need. Should no improvement occur in a further few minutes, the outlook is grave indeed.

The value of intubation and the supply of oxygen by endotracheal catheter under positive pressure is now no longer questioned. It is only regretted that so few who attend women in labour are sufficiently trained to employ it, and those in need of practice should use every opportunity afforded by fresh stillborn or dead babies. Unskilled attempts may do more harm than good. The technique has been minutely described by Barrie (1963) and the following is a summary:

Tracheal intubation.—A nurse steadies the baby on its back on a resuscitation shelf or tray. The head is held in a lightly extended position. It is a great mistake to hyperextend the head. Holding the laryngoscope in the left hand the blade is passed over the back of the tongue until the epiglottis is seen. Now comes the slightly more difficult part of locating the glottis. If there is any mucus or debris lying about, it should be aspirated now. The laryngoscope is then passed down further, beyond and behind the epiglottis. Except in extreme degrees of flaccidity the expected triangular opening will not be seen but rather a dimple in the middle of a pinkish-coloured mound, which may open during a gasp. To get a good view, the tip of the laryngoscope blade has to hook under the epiglottis and lift it up against the root of the tongue. Barrie reckons it easier to use the tip of the blade advanced into the space between the root of the tongue and the epiglottis (the vallecula) and to raise the whole instrument so as to lift both structures forwards and thereby to obtain a view. The risk of damaging the epiglottis is thereby reduced. The position of the baby's head may have to be altered to achieve this. Suction is now applied to clear the airway and using the right hand an endotracheal tube is passed for 2 cm into the trachea, or until the shoulder of the tube, if present, impacts in the glottis. Care must be taken not to displace the tube on removing the laryngoscope. A bronchial catheter should suck clear secretions lodged further down and now, in the absence of an oxygen bag and manometer, an attempt is made to inflate the lungs using cheek pressure only. If the operator does his own puffing he will experience a characteristic resistance described by Barrie as like inflating a balloon. Oxygen by a side tube introduced into the operator's mouth is a helpful idea. If the catheter has been introduced too far only one side of the chest will expand, usually the right, and the tube should be withdrawn. If the abdomen bulges instead of the chest, clearly one has introduced the catheter into the oesophagus instead of the trachea. A fine suction catheter should remove any mucus secretions lying about and the treatment thereafter is continued with short, sharp puffs of oxygen using the manometer as a safeguard to limit pressures to no more than 35 cm of water for as long as the child's colour can be maintained and the heart continues to beat. This period may exceed an hour and may still be followed by complete recovery. Pressures less than 30 cm of water are unlikely to produce much visible chest expansion but higher pressures than this, if lasting more than a fraction of a second, may rupture alveoli, producing emphysema and areas of haemorrhage in the lungs, or even pneumothrax (Fig. 3). This treatment, originally introduced by Gibberd and Blaikley in 1935, has stood the test of time better than most others, but clearly is not without its own dangers. Although a gasp is induced very frequently and the benefits of the immediately available oxygen within the bronchiolar system are dramatic, Cross *et al.* (1960) have also noted a marked apnoeic response to lung inflation. As long, however, as the heart rate continues to accelerate or to maintain itself above one hundred beats per minute this method of artificial respiration will maintain efficient oxygenation for the vital centres. It is doubtful, however, if the alveoli are properly opened up without the presence of spontaneous inspiratory efforts which are necessary to bring about the circulatory readjustments already referred to within the pulmonary vascular tree, but the immediate benefit of endotracheal insufflation lies in oxygen absorption from the bronchi and bronchioles and a guarantee of an effective airway.

Difficulties of intubation are more often the result of faulty positioning of the child's head and lack of confidence on the part of the operator than anything else and certainly the manoeuvre can be made easier by pushing back on the cricoid. This helps to close the oesophagus and is also useful in the course of mouth-to-mouth insufflation. Where for one reason or another endotracheal intubation cannot be carried out, an attractive idea has been suggested of using a rubber rat-tailed ear syringe and applying it, after clearance of the air passages, to one nostril while blocking the other and the mouth. Since the bulb has a capacity of about 60 ml it is very suitable as a safe method of trying to inflate the air passages of the newborn. Again the trachea should be pushed backwards to help obliterate the oesophageal lumen and prevent the diversion of most of the air from the syringe bulb into the stomach (Lerman, 1967).

Since it so often happens that adequate skilled attention is not available at delivery, it is necessary to consider alternatives.

The old-fashioned method of standing in front of the fire, dangling the child by its ankles, may assist fluid to drain from its air passages and keep it warm, but to hold the child in this attitude for any length of time must greatly engorge the cerebral veins; moreover, the weight of the liver on the flaccid diaphragm discourages any inspiratory attempt.

Another method securing an airway is to draw the tongue forwards with a tongue forceps. It used to be thought that intermittent tongue traction reflexly stimulated breathing but, apart from acting as an unpleasant afferent stimulus, no such anatomical reflex in fact exists.

There are now some very useful baby-size airways on the market and these may be used to deal with the sagging tongue.

A fine rubber catheter passed into the nasopharynx via a nostril, through which oxygen is slowly run, is a safe and moderately effective method. Better still, is intermittent positive-pressure ventilation (IPPV) with bag, mask and oral airway, sixty times a minute, using pressures up to 30 cm of water.

Whatever method is used, gentleness of handling is the first essential. The child is in no need of afferent stimuli—its arrival into the outer world supplies these in plenty and its inability to respond

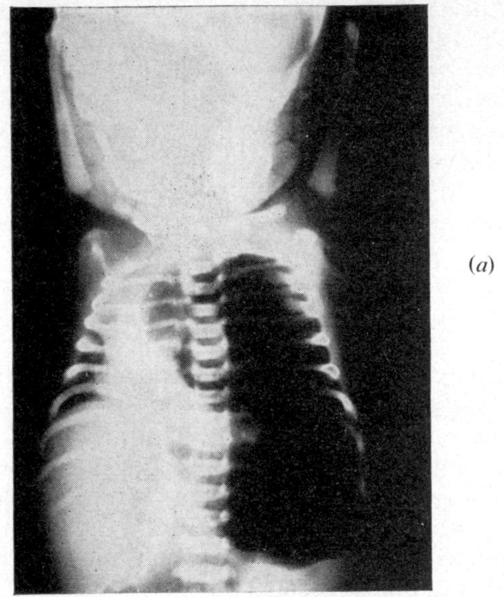

(a)

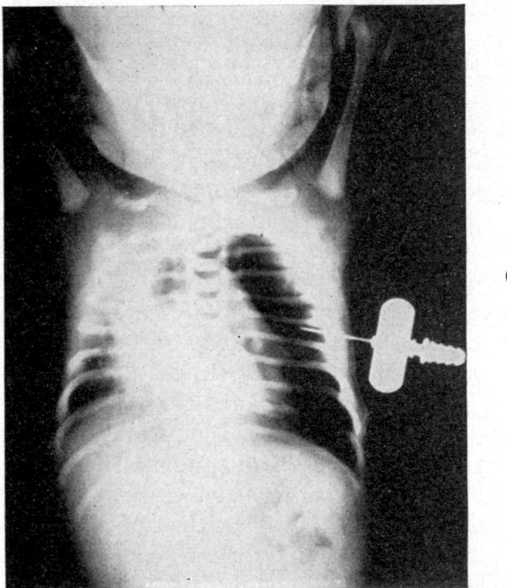

(b)

20/Fig. 3.—(a) Traumatic pneumothorax from intubation and positive-pressure ventilation. (b) Pneumothorax relieved by prompt aspiration. Baby survived.

to them is due to something pathological. Slapping, pinching, spraying with ethyl chloride, anal dilatation and other such measures can only be regarded as primitive as well as futile.

In spite of what has been said above, the practice of bastinado, i.e. torturing the soles of the baby's feet by slapping and flicking, still goes on all over the country and not so long ago was even demonstrated in a dismally bad B.B.C. television programme!

As soon as possible, the child should be either wrapped up in a warm blanket or placed in a warmed oxygen cot and in either case left in peace.

Immersion in a tub of warm water has now gone out of fashion because no one has yet devised a satisfactory method of doing so with the head tilted downwards!

A suitable atmosphere.—The asphyxiated baby's first need is for oxygen to revive the vital centres. Of carbon dioxide it already has a gross excess. The fatuity, therefore, of blowing carbon dioxide at its face must be obvious, and yet it is surprising how long it has taken for this practice to die out. Any alleged response was due more to the stimulus of the cold gas than to its composition, and it might as well be noted again that if the child was well enough to respond to such a stimulus it was well enough not to need it. Undoubtedly the portability of the very small carbon dioxide cylinders for a long time commended their use.

To supply mixtures of 95 per cent oxygen and 5 per cent carbon dioxide is also pointless, at least during the first hour of life. Later on such a mixture may be given intermittently, when anoxia has been remedied, in the hope of encouraging alveolar expansion.

Now, pure oxygen is a pulmonary irritant if used over a long period of time but this is of no present concern when coping with an asphyxiated baby. The risks of inducing retrolental fibroplasia in premature infants do not arise before at least two or three hours of excessive oxygen treatment.

In the emergency of frank asphyxia, the need for oxygen is so urgent that it should be given neat—even delivery through a glass funnel over the face is better than nothing. A polythene funnel is in fact better still as it can be moulded to a better fit round the child's face. Once breathing has become established the percentage of oxygen in the atmosphere to be breathed should be planned deliberately, ideally with the help of an oxygen analyser; percentages varying from 25 to 35, according to the maturity of the child and its general condition, should, if possible, be maintained in the incubator. Unfortunately, in most units the concentration of oxygen achieved depends more upon guesswork and the leaks in the apparatus than upon intelligent management, a matter to which cases of retrolental fibroplasia bear tragic testimony.

Aspiration of gastric contents.—As already mentioned, small quantities of gastric fluids, swallowed or indigenous, may be regurgitated and, in the very sick child, may either produce laryngeal spasm by being aspirated, giving rise to characteristic cyanotic attacks, or their inhalation may be even deeper. Gellis, White and Pfeffer found that the amount of fluid aspirated from the stomach was much greater after Caesarean section (average 14 ml), and where the mother had diabetes in addition the average amount was 20 ml, whereas after low forceps delivery the average was only 2 ml. These workers further observed that those babies whose stomachs were not aspirated at birth and subsequently as necessary, developed respiratory embarrassment following Caesarean section four times more commonly than those so treated. This is a very important observation and confirms our own practice. In fact, where resuscitative measures have to be taken with the child at Caesarean section, gastric aspiration should be one of the routine procedures. Suction can be applied through a number four French rubber catheter passed down the oesophagus and aided by gentle manual pressure on the abdomen. The end of the catheter should be cut off square. This practically eliminates the risk of sucking mucous membrane into the lumen and damaging it.

The fluid aspirated contains the solid constituents of liquor amnii which has been swallowed in the natural course of events but which remains in the stomach for want of the pressures supplied by the process of vaginal delivery. This is a matter which goes far towards explaining why Caesarean section babies sometimes fail to do well.

With the vigorous baby, who is in no need of resuscitation, such measures are not necessary, since it is well able to deal with its own secretions.

Drugs used in resuscitation.—There is not much choice here. Lobeline and nikethamide are not without their dangers as the margin between stimulation and convulsions is none too wide. In fact analeptic drugs are looked upon with increasing disfavour as they may do more harm than good.

Intravenous injection into the umbilical cord can sometimes be difficult if the vein is empty and collapsed, and accidental injection into an umbilical artery can be dangerous and produce necrosis over the buttock. Holmes (1961) recommended overcoming this difficulty by applying a sponge holder on the cord 10 cm from the umbilicus and leaving a 15-cm length of isolated umbilical vein remaining engorged proximal to the clamp and ligature at the point of separation of the baby. Drugs are now injected into the distended vein, the sponge holder is removed and a column of blood containing the drug is milked into the general circulation.

The use of adrenaline, often injected directly into the heart, is no more than a ritual performance, and I have never seen any good come of it, although I have often used it as a last resort. External cardiac massage is more likely to succeed if anything can. On the whole analeptic drugs have fallen out of favour.

Where failure to breathe has been aggravated or provoked by the administration of morphine or its derivatives or of pethidine during the last few hours of labour, an antidote to the depressant effects on the baby of these drugs exists in N-allylnormophine (nalorphine). Given in dosage of 0·5 mg into the umbilical vein, the effect is often dramatic, but this substance is useless against other sedatives such as the barbiturates. Naloxone (Narcan) 0·01 mg/kg is now regarded as better still.

Babies suffering from asphyxia at birth are intensely acidotic and, in fact, the worse their condition the lower the pH. Levels of pH 7·2 are common in early primary apnoea and as the child's condition worsens the pH may fall to 7·0. At a pH of about 6·8 the child's condition is frankly desperate. An immediate infusion is necessary of 10 ml of 8·4 per cent sodium bicarbonate, followed by 10 ml of 10 per cent glucose, repeated if necessary. The buffer substance TRIS (trishydroxyaminomethylamine) should be considered, but time is usually against one and nothing should be allowed to deflect those in attendance from the urgent necessity to oxygenate the baby, best of all by endotracheal intubation.

Methods of artificial respiration.—The old traditional methods of artificial respiration have now gone by the board, and rightly so, for three very good reasons. In the first place, they cannot be carried out without considerable exposure and handling, which is likely to be more vigorous as the child's condition appears more desperate, when in fact, bearing in mind its shocked condition, it really needs warmth and peace. Secondly, these methods, as a rule, rely on compression of the thoracic cage followed by natural recoil, in the hope that air will be drawn into the lungs. Since the baby is in a state of shock, and therefore toneless, there can hardly be much recoil. Thirdly, chest compression is supposed to drive air out of the alveoli which is then replaced by fresh air on recoil; although this may be the case in adults whose alveoli were previously expanded, the principle cannot apply to the newborn whose alveoli are still collapsed so that there is no air to express in the first place.

These methods are, therefore, not only a waste of time but also harmful.

Mouth-to-mouth insufflation has been practised since antiquity. More recently a layer of gauze over the child's mouth has been added as a refinement for the benefit of the midwife in order to reduce her intake of vernix and meconium. The operator's mouth should include both the baby's nose and mouth. Any air insufflated finds its way, of course, not into the lungs but into the stomach, from which there can be little benefit and the risks of sepsis are considerable.

Intratracheal insufflation, already described, still holds pride of place among resuscitative techniques.

Bearing in mind the Queckenstedt phenomenon, any rise in intrathoracic pressure is immediately matched by a rise in intracranial pressure via the great veins draining the skull cavity, which are without effective valves. Our pilot experiments on cats have shown a rise and fall in pressures within the skull which closely follow the pressure changes within the chest. It may follow, therefore, that anything which grossly increases thoracic pressure may have harmful effects on the brain. Now, where the skull bones are reasonably mature, and therefore firm, any rise in the intravenous pressure in the skull would be offset by the resistance of the skull to expansion. If this were not so, coughing and crying would be dangerous activities. With the very premature child, however, this protection is much less, and it may account for the high incidence of intracranial bleeding which occurs in the premature, however delivered. In the past this has been blamed on abnormal fragility of the blood vessels in prematurity, but I doubt whether this is really so and whether the mechanism has not hitherto been misunderstood.

Augmented respiration.—This is the principle underlying the author's method of artificial respiration (Donald and Lord, 1953). Fundamentally it involves synchronising the action of the respirator with any spontaneous respiratory efforts which the baby may be making. We have repeatedly demonstrated the mechanical load which a sick, shocked, narcotised or premature baby may have to shoulder in initially expanding its lungs, diverting the blood flow into the pulmonary vascular bed and overcoming the moist cohesion of its alveolar walls. Indeed, in such cases the respiratory effort required may be too much for it and it therefore fails to make that very important flying start to respiration, which we believe to be vital.

In our earliest respirator experiments we soon found that mechanical devices which operated on a pre-set and arbitrary rhythm and without regard to the baby's breathing attempts were not only ineffectual but often did more harm than good by actually working, from time to time, in direct opposition, or anti-phase, to the child's own respiration—if any, and often provoked what we termed "protest apnoea" (Donald and Young, 1952).

As a result of this I came to experiment with the principle of augmented respiration, in which a variety of respirators were produced, all of which were triggered by a photoelectric mechanism that detected the onset of each spontaneous inspiratory attempt and immediately set the apparatus into an inspiratory phase to assist the baby's breathing. The baby thus automatically controlled its own respirator according to its needs. In the total absence of spontaneous respiration a pre-set rate of operation cut in, until the next inspiratory effort by the baby triggered the mechanism once more in step with the baby.

We are convinced that if there is any virtue in artificial respiration, and we believe there is and there appears to be a renewed interest in the subject, it must operate in accordance with this simple and rather obvious physiological principle.

The case for effective artificial respiration is further strengthened by the observations of Dawes *et al.* (1953) who found that artificial positive-pressure ventilation immediately increases the rate of pulmonary arterial blood flow which is accompanied by (or indeed may be due to) a fall of nine-tenths of the pre-existing pulmonary vascular resistance. Jaykka (1957, 1958) also observed that the effects of artificial respiration and the erectile expansion of the lung capillaries are additive in effecting lung aeration.

Rocking methods.—Eve's rocking method is a very useful addition to treatment. By rocking the baby in its longitudinal axis the weight of the liver and abdominal viscera causes downward and upward displacements of the diaphragm, thereby encouraging the passage of air in and out of the lungs. There is, however, as Eve points out, the important advantage that circulation is first improved by increasing venous return, particularly from the head; this helps to remove carbon dioxide from the brain and vital centres; in other words "Restore the circulation and the brain restores itself".

Rocking can be done quite simply by holding the baby's body across one's chest and swaying from side to side through an arc of 40 to 70 degrees, performing about ten cycles a minute, the only disadvantage being that it is not easy to administer oxygen at the same time.

Phrenic-nerve stimulation.—A phrenic-nerve stimulator on the lines of the Sarnoff apparatus aroused a brief interest some years ago but like other mechanical and electrical pieces of apparatus it never caught on widely. In fact the storerooms of obstetric units are littered with discarded machines which no one can bring himself to throw out because of their admirable ingenuity and so they continue as dust-collecting, space-occupying nuisances. Our own department is no exception.

Administration of gastric oxygen.—Some years ago Yllpo drew attention to the fact that an oxygen bubble in the stomach of a baby disappeared, on radiological examination, within ten minutes.

This was followed up by the introduction of intragastric oxygen as a means of resuscitation by Akerren and Furstenberg and within a very few years the treatment was widely hailed and accepted throughout the whole world—as dramatically, in fact, as it has now been rejected by almost the same people who originally acclaimed it. After such a glorious innings it has now been thoroughly debunked from various quarters (Cooper *et al.*, 1960, Coxon, 1960).

The really disturbing thing about this story is how far we are removed from being able to assess the value of any particular treatment and that the so-called scientific world in this respect is still subject to fashion and guesswork. There is no doubt, however, that the newborn baby very rapidly fills its intestinal tract with swallowed air and this would appear to depend on respiratory activity, including crying, so that these X-ray evidences furnish a good index of vigour at birth. It is now very much doubted that the phenomenon in any way assists the baby's oxygenation (Fig. 4).

Cardiac massage.—This is clearly only applicable where a baby dies at the moment of birth or thereafter when the institution of this treatment can be immediate and before irrevocable brain damage is done. Open cardiac massage by thoracotomy, with all its entailed hazards, has been replaced by closed chest cardiac massage which is further facilitated by the softness of a baby's thoracic cage. Pressure is made downwards with two fingers just to the left of the sternum, towards the vertebral column, depressing the chest wall for about 2 cm, 80 to 100 times per minute. Needless to say pulmonary ventilation must be maintained at the same time and the single-handed operator will, therefore, have to employ mouth-to-mouth breathing as well (Gallagher and Neligan, 1962). If someone is present to maintain pulmonary ventilation by endotracheal oxygen so much the better, but it is important that both procedures should be combined. A good rule of thumb is "3 thumps and 1 puff" rhythm. It is best to lay the baby on a hard surface such as a trolley top and although the heart may readily restart, inflation must be maintained until spontaneous respiration is satisfactorily re-established. A number of reports of success from this prompt line of treatment are now coming in, but clearly it is rather limited. In the case of stillbirths death has seldom occurred so recently before access can be obtained to institute cardiac massage and even if success could be won, it would only be rewarded by the tragedy of permanent cerebral damage. The neonatal babies who suffer from cardiac arrest usually do so for some gross reason which is already defying treatment. Nevertheless, if opportunities are not to be lost one must be mentally alert at the time of the crisis in order not to lose precious seconds.

Hyperbaric oxygen treatment.—In recent years for a while there was hope that the use of a high-pressure oxygen caisson, into which the baby could simply be put and in which pressure could rapidly be built up to four atmospheres, might meet the asphyxiated baby's oxygen need by absorption through exposed mucous membranes.

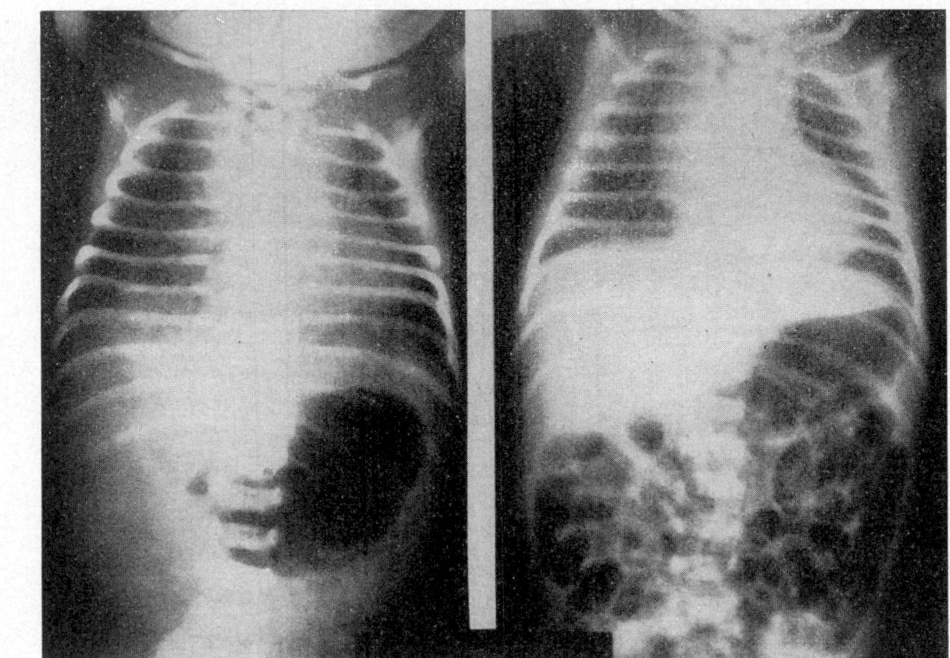

20/FIG. 4.—Premature infant. Note appearance in lungs of hyaline membrane atelectasis (see Chapter XXVIII). Child recovered. (*a*) Age 2 hours. "Aerogastrie"; (*b*) Age 9 hours. "Aerocolie."

(By courtesy of Professor R. E. Steiner.)

One of the merits claimed for the technique was that it might spare the baby the hazards of pulmonary damage such as pneumothorax from positive-pressure inflation techniques (Hutchison *et al.*, 1962). Another advantage claimed was that it might reduce the need for trained staff, skilled in intubation. The apparatus itself is expensive and any unit in a position to purchase it should be also in a position to supply the necessary trained staff, and there has been a general reluctance to accept any method which might delay tracheal intubation and oxygenation in the baby who was really in need of it. This only goes to emphasise the need for training more junior staff whether paediatric or obstetric, as well of course as anaesthetists, in the art of intubation.

It is always difficult to evaluate any new treatment of asphyxia neonatorum, which may be due to so many different causes in babies of such differing weights and maturity as are likely to present one with the emergency. However, an attempt at a controlled trial of hyperbaric oxygen versus intubation and intermittent positive-pressure with oxygen, as a method of resuscitation in babies, has been carried out jointly at the Queen Mother's Hospital and the Royal Maternity Hospital, Glasgow, selecting the patients by a system of cluster and random sampling (Hutchison *et al.*, 1966). The trial was carried out over many months and covered a sufficiently large group of cases to be able to infer from its results that there was practically no significant difference between the two methods, whether the babies were mature or premature.

Nobody denies the value of endotracheal intubation and positive-pressure assistance to the asphyxiated baby's breathing. Experiments on asphyxiated animals at birth have very little relevance in assessing this sort of treatment. They are not strictly comparable to the case of the baby whose myocardial glycogen reserves may have been undergoing prolonged depletion before the moment of birth. Although Cross and his colleagues (1964) observed that in such a deliberate experiment of asphyxiating mature fetal rabbits at birth beyond "the last gasp", 10 of 12 treated by intermittent positive-pressure ventilation recovered whereas none of all the 17 which received hyperbaric oxygen survived. Gupta and Tizard (1967) have pointed out the difference between babies in primary apnoea and those terminal cases asphyxiated beyond the "last gasp", a matter which can only be decided retrospectively, and they suggest that the efficacy of any new method of resuscitation should only be judged in the case of babies in terminal apnoea. It is as well that terminal cases of apnoea are so relatively uncommon compared with the others or one might indeed find oneself constantly trying to salvage cases with a questionable long-term prognosis.

Ideally every baby at its birth should have in attendance somebody capable of safe, atraumatic endotracheal intubation, whereupon the controversy would be quelled. Today there is no generally accepted alternative.

Prophylaxis.—One may well ask, in view of the frequent occurrence of the emergency of neonatal asphyxia, whether something cannot be done to reduce this hazard. Unfortunately, there is no specific prophylactic measure, for much of the whole art and science of obstetrics is challenged, and there is not a great deal of credit in delivering a baby barely alive as a result of its almost catastrophic entry into the world.

Good antenatal supervision should forestall many of the possible difficulties of labour, will prevent the greater part of eclampsia, and will play at least some part in mitigating the prematurity risk, to mention only a few examples.

In labour itself the early detection of fetal distress is important, the choice of drugs and their timing should be judicious, episiotomy will often spare a baby the last lethal straw and skilful use of the obstetric forceps may make all the difference between intracranial haemorrhage and survival. The use of pudendal block local anaesthesia, whenever possible, in forceps delivery makes an impressive difference to the incidence of neonatal asphyxia.

Late prognosis.—Obstetricians often lose sight of the infant they have delivered, and reports assessing the part which asphyxia at birth may have played in causing subsequent disability are not numerous. A later low Apgar score, for example at 10 minutes, has, on the whole, a worse long-term prognosis than an immediate low score.

Schreiber, in an analysis of 900 mental defectives, found that there was evidence of some birth asphyxia in 70 per cent. Although one of the editorials of the *British Medical Journal* (1952) rather played down the late damaging effects, one is inclined to the view that anoxia never did anyone any good, even a baby, and although it is no more than conjecture, it is more than likely that ten minutes' asphyxia will at least reduce a sixth-form intelligence to that of the lower fourth. In Aberdeen, however, Fraser and Wilks (1959) have given a somewhat less depressing picture having followed up 100 children who had suffered delay in the onset of satisfactory respiration at birth. In 40 of the cases asphyxia had been severe. Nevertheless, neurological examination at the age of seven and a half years showed major abnormality in surprisingly few, but minor disorders of personality and perception as compared with the control group were noted. Likewise in Aberdeen, Fairweather and Illsley (1960) investigating mentally handicapped children came to the conclusion that social and genetic factors were more responsible than obstetric complications for the development of the disabilities.

A study of school performance at the age of 11 has been undertaken in the case of 50,000 children whose birth records were known (Barker and Edwards, 1967). It was interesting to note that they found impaired performance mainly associated with only 5 of the obstetric complications studied, namely, prematurity, post-maturity, toxaemia, occipitoposterior position and delivery in an ambulance. This last-mentioned type of event was a little difficult to explain even on the basis of social grading of the mothers.

The nearest that I personally have come to making a controlled observation was in the case of uniovular twins with serious delay and very difficult delivery of the second twin through a cervix which had already to some extent shut down. There was also a marked deflexion of the fetal head. For many days thereafter this unfortunate child showed all the classic signs of cerebral irritation. In spite of my request to the mother to keep in touch with me I lost track of her until one night, seventeen years later, she 'phoned me up from a neighbouring hotel and invited me to see the children. I hurried round miserably expecting to see one perfectly normal child and one spastic and grossly handicapped. To my intense relief both boys chattered excitedly about their studies and when challenged to identify which was which I had to admit that I could not tell the difference.

Any luck which I have had in this subject has, as usual, been undeserved.

Mention has already been made in Chapter I of "at risk registers" in order that the fate of children may be followed up by casting the observation net as wide as possible, but the value of this has been challenged by Richards and Roberts who maintain that such registers have led "to a situation in which an undefined population is being screened for undefined conditions by people who, for the most part, are untrained to detect the conditions for which they are looking," and rightly claiming that there is no alternative to sound clinical examination of all infants in the neonatal period and appropriate screening thereafter; but this is a counsel of perfection. In the words of Know, "The only sensible action to be taken with respect to at risk registers is to abandon them".

The most severe cases which manage to survive may suffer cerebral diplegia. Cerebral palsy may not only be attributable to genetic factors, to maternal infection in early pregnancy or to toxaemia, but may be due to damage through anoxia or intracranial bleeding in the course of labour. Multiple pregnancy and prematurity and likewise kernicterus are also believed to be important causes. The significance of convulsions is particularly ominous and Craig (1960) noted that, apart from the high mortality following them (42 per cent), in the survivors who are followed up for the next three years the incidence of mental or physical handicap was nearly three times (8 per cent) as compared with those who had had postnatal asphyxia without convulsions. Fits within the first 48 hours have the poorest prognosis both as regards neonatal death and subsequent neurological or intellectual defect and in fact the earlier the fits occur, the more likely are they to be associated with cerebral birth injury. Hypoglycaemia and later hypocalcaemia may also be early causes of fits in the newborn. As can be imagined the differential diagnosis in the case of the latter two types is of great importance. The immediate control of the fits, in addition to treating the predisposing cause if applicable, is to induce sedation with phenobarbitone or diazepam.

The degree to which subsequent epilepsy may be caused by brain damage at birth has not yet been fully determined, but long ago Earle *et al.* in necropsy studies of 157 cases of temporal lobe epileptiform seizures found that in 63 per cent there was evidence of compression or damage at birth to the temporal lobes believed to be caused by a temporary herniation, under pressure of the skull at birth, through the incisura of the tentorium cerebelli involving particularly one or both hippocampal gyri. In the intellectual field all gradations from mental backwardness to personality disorders and epilepsy may originate from life's first critical quarter of an hour, and it is as well to assume that in resuscitating the newborn one is fighting not only for the child's life but for its very wits.

In summary, resuscitation procedure is usually carried out in the following order

1. Clear the pharynx, mouth and nostrils by suction.
2. Lay child, head sloped downwards, in warm cot—until aspiration of stomach completed and then prop up to assist breathing.
3. Supply oxygen either by tent or face mask, but only if cyanosed and breathing.
4. If child is limp, insert an airway to deal with sagging tongue.
5. If no improvement, rocking may be employed.
6. If still no improvement after a few minutes, the trachea is intubated under direct vision and positive-pressure lung inflation employed. *N.B.*—If the child is born in marked white asphyxia, this is done earlier.
7. If respiratory depression can be attributed to morphine or pethidine given to the mother, inject 0·5 mg N-allylnormorphine into umbilical vein.
8. Inject 10 ml (mEq) of 8·4 per cent sodium bicarbonate intravenously.
9. External cardiac massage, combined with continuing pulmonary ventilation.

Fortunately, most cases revive before the whole of the above ritual has to be gone through, and those that do not are by now irretrievably dead.

Further Treatment—Cerebral Irritation

Once the immediate emergency of asphyxia in the labour ward has been overcome the baby may, nevertheless, continue in some jeopardy for the next 48 hours, particularly if fetal shock was severe in the first place. It may demonstrate signs of cerebral irritation, of which the following are the more significant:

1. Liability to apnoeic, grey or blue attacks;
2. Twitching and convulsions;
3. Hyperexcitability on switching on a light in the room or making a sharp noise;
4. High-pitched shrill cry;
5. Restlessness and wakefulness;
6. Grunting respirations;
7. Rapid, shallow or irregular respiration;
8. Blue lips;
9. Rolling eyes;
10. Neck rigidity;
11. Bulging anterior fontanelle;
12. Temperature instability;
13. Occasionally hypo-activity.

The differential diagnosis is often a matter of great clinical difficulty. Atelectasis, especially with hyaline membrane, pneumonia, intraventricular haemorrhage in premature babies and subdural haemorrhage in the more mature, can be very difficult to distinguish without special tests, but radiology of the chest (Donald and Steiner, 1953) and spirometry may be of assistance. The treatment of cerebral irritation demands minimum handling, sufficient oxygen concentration in the atmosphere to maintain a good colour but no more than is strictly needed, warmth and repeated aspiration of pharynx and stomach by suction at the first sign of a blue attack. Because of the dangers of regurgitation it is necessary to withhold all fluid or feeding, for 48 hours often, except for the administration of sedatives, for example, phenobarbitone 8 mg/kg/day or chloral 100 mg/kg/day in syrup, which may be repeatedly required to afford the child sorely needed rest.

Congenital Malformations Requiring Emergency Surgery

Certain conditions are immediately obvious at birth or shortly thereafter and any hope of survival depends upon the availability of immediate surgery. These include meningomyelocele which must be covered and kept moist with a sterile, wet dressing during transportation, and exomphalos which likewise must be handled with great care to prevent exposure and rupture of the translucent sac containing intestinal contents in the region of the umbilicus.

Retrognathia is immediately recognised by the small underslung jaw and there is immediate danger of suffocation due to respiratory obstruction from falling back of the tongue.

Oesophageal atresia is especially to be expected in cases of hydramnios. It is frequently associated with a tracheo-oesophageal fistula and in any case the contents of the blind pouch are liable to overspill into the lungs so that the child will drown. The condition is recognised by the failure to pass a rubber catheter down the mouth into the stomach.

Diaphragmatic hernia, most commonly on the left side of the diaphragm, is a source of severe respiratory distress due to displacement of the mediastinal contents and compression of the lung on the opposite side.

Intestinal obstruction, both high and low, is associated with early serious vomiting, the early onset of which depends upon the height of the level of obstruction. Quite apart from the dangers of regurgitation and inhalation there is rapid dehydration and electrolyte imbalance. Likewise distension will depend upon the level of obstruction and will be the greater the lower the level of obstruction. The intra-abdominal pressure rapidly interferes with respiratory movement.

Vomiting may be projectile.

Absent anus or anal atresia should be recognised at once and the degree of defect can be estimated by X-ray of the baby in the inverted position when the level of gas in the bowel is readily seen.

In the ideal situation, as in our case, full paediatric operating facilities are available on the spot but usually the baby requires immediate transportation to a hospital. During transportation it must be kept warm and at all costs the respiratory passages must be kept clear by aspiration of the mouth, pharynx and, if possible, the stomach, using a mucus aspirator. The baby must be nursed prone or at least on its side to prevent aspiration into the air passages of vomitus or mucus dribbling from the mouth. Aspiration of stomach contents may be necessary every few minutes during the journey. In cases of micrognathia and retrognathia the baby must be actually nursed prone to keep the tongue forwards. Wet, sterile dressings are applied to meningomyelocele or exomphalos, and must be kept moist with sterile saline.

Obviously the baby must be accompanied by a doctor or experienced nurse. It should not be overheated but certainly not allowed to cool and a portable incubator should be available with a supply of oxygen. Cases of gross diaphragmatic hernia producing severe respiratory embarrassment may require intermittent positive-pressure respiration, bearing in mind the danger of traumatic pneumothorax which is easily induced. To meet this danger, should it occur, sterile needles and syringes should be at hand to decompress the pneumothorax even in the course of a journey and, in such cases, an anaesthetist should be in attendance.

The availability of immediate radiography at birth does much to help the initial diagnosis, for example, the discovery of fluid levels and levels of gas within the abdomen. Even meconium peritonitis may be diagnosed sometimes if calcification is visible within the distended abdomen. The matter thereafter is one of paediatric surgery and the results can often be surprisingly rewarding. I have even seen a case of very gross exomphalos in an early primigravida, in whom operation was thought not to be feasible in the hospital where I was then working, in which complete success was obtained in a highly specialised paediatric centre to which the child was immediately transferred.

The operability and success of treating meningomyocele depends essentially upon the speed with which the case can be dealt with. Minutes rather than hours count and provided there is no associated handicap such as Down's syndrome or mental defect the results can be gratifyingly good (Rickham, 1971).

Finally, choanal atresia, though rare, provides a surgical emergency because the baby can only breathe through its mouth and attempts to feed may suffocate it.

REFERENCES

AKERREN, Y. and FURSTENBERG, N. (1950). *J. Obstet. Gynaec. Brit. Emp.*, **57,** 705.

APGAR, V. (1953). *Curr. Res. Anesth.*, **32,** 260–267.

BARCROFT, J. (1946). *Researches on Prenatal Life.* Oxford: Blackwell Scientific Publications.

BARKER, D. J. P. and EDWARDS, J. H. (1967). *Brit. med. J.*, **2,** 695.

BARRIE, H. (1963). *Lancet*, **1,** 650.

BORN, G. V. R., DAWES, G. S., MOTT, J. C. and WIDDICOMBE, J. G. (1954). *Cold Spr. Harb. Symp. quant. Biol.*, **19,** 102.

CARTER, R. E. B. (1957). *Lancet.* **1,** 1292.

COOPER, F. A., SMITH, H. and PASK, E. A. (1960). *Anaesthesia*, **15,** 211.

CORNER, B. (1962). *Proc. roy. Soc. Med.*, **55,** 1005.

COXON, R. V. (1960). *Lancet*, **1,** 1315.

CRAIG, W. S. (1960). *Arch. Dis. Childh.*, **35,** 336.

CROSS, K. W., DAWES, G. S., HYMAN, A. and MOTT, JOAN C. (1964). *Lancet*, **2,** 560.

CROSS, K. W., KLAUS, M., TOOLEY, W. H. and WEISSER, K. (1960). *J. Physiol.* (*Lond.*), **151,** 551.

DAWES, G. S., MOTT, J. C., WIDDICOMBE, J. G. and WYATT, D. G. (1953). *J. Physiol.* (*Lond.*), **121,** 141.

DAWKINS, M. J. R., MARTIN, J. D. and SPECTOR, W. E. (1961). *J. Obstet. Gynaec. Brit. Cwlth.*, **68,** 604.

DONALD, I. (1954). *J. Obstet. Gynaec. Brit. Emp.*, **61,** 725.

DONALD, I. (1963). "Asphyxia neonatorum", in *The Obstetrician, Anaesthetist and Pediatrician.* Oxford: Pergamon Press.

DONALD, I., KERR, M. M. and MACDONALD, I. R., (1958). *Scot. med. J.* **3,** 151.

DONALD, I. and LORD, J. (1953). *Lancet*, **1,** 9.

DONALD, I. and STEINER, R. E. (1953). *Lancet*, **2,** 846.

DONALD, I. and YOUNG, I. M. (1952). *J. Physiol.* (*Lond.*), **116,** 41P.

EARLE, K. M., BALDWIN, M. and PENFIELD, W. (1953). *Arch. Neurol. Psychiat.* (*Chic.*), **69,** 27.

EVE, F. C. and FORSYTH, N. C. (1948). *Lancet*, **2,** 554.

FAIRWEATHER, D. V. I. and ILLSLEY, R. (1960). *Brit. J. prev. soc. Med.* **14,** 149.

FLAGG, P. J. (1931). *Amer. J. Obstet. Gynec.*, **21,** 537.

FRASER, M. S. and WILKS, J. (1959). *J. Obstet. Gynaec. Brit. Emp.*, **66,** 748.

GALLAGHER, B. and NELIGAN, G. (1962). *Brit. med. J.*, **1,** 400.

GELLIS, S. S., WHITE, P. and PFEFFER, W. (1949). *New Engl. J. Med.*, **240,** 533.

GIBBERD, G. F. and BLAIKLEY, J. B. (1935). *Lancet*, **1,** 138.

GUPTA, J. M. and TIZARD, J. P. M. (1967). *Lancet*, **2,** 55.

HOLMES, J. M. (1961). *Brit. med. J.*, **1,** 1317.

HUTCHISON, J. H., KERR, MARGARET M., INALL, J. A. and SHANKS, R. A. (1966). *Lancet*, **1,** 935.

HITCHISON, J. H., KERR, M. M., MCPHAIL, M. F., DOUGLAS, T. A., SMITH, G., NORMAN, J. N. and BATES, F. A. (1962). *Lancet*, **2,** 465.

JAYKKA, S. (1957). *Acta. paediat.* (*Uppsala*), **46,** Suppl. 112.

JAYKKA, S. (1958). *Acta. paediat.* (*Uppsala*), **47,** 484.

KARLBERG, P. (1960). *J. Pediat.*, **56,** 585.

KNOW, E. G. (1970). *Arch. Dis. Childh.*, **45,** 634.

LERMAN, S. I. (1967). *Lancet*, **2,** 265.

MANN, T. P. and ELLIOTT, R. I. K. (1957). *Lancet*, **1,** 229.

MOTT, J. C. (1961). *Brit. med. Bull.*, **17,** 146.

POTTER, E. L. and ROSENBAUM, W. (1943). *Amer. J. Obstet. Gynec.* **45,** 822.

RICHARDS, I. D. G. and ROBERTS, C. J. (1967). *Lancet*, **2,** 711.

RICKAM, P. P. (1971). *Brit. med. J.*, **4,** 286.

ROBERTS, H., KANE, K. M., PERCIVAL, N., SNOW, P. and PLEASE, N. W. (1957). *Lancet*, **1,** 128.

SCHREIBER, F. (1938). *J. Amer. med. Ass.*, **3,** 1263.

SHELLEY, H. J. (1961). *Brit. med. Bull.*, **17,** 137.

STAFFORD, A. and WEATHERALL, J. A. C. (1960). *J. Physiol.* (*Lond.*), **153,** 457.

YLLPO, A. (1935). *Acta paediat.* (*Uppsala*). **17,** Suppl. 1, 122.

CHAPTER XXI

POSTPARTUM COLLAPSE

In an emergency it is strange, but nevertheless true, that the more desperate the patient's condition the more difficult may accurate diagnosis become. If the delivery has been a difficult one, the attendant's powers of judgment may be undermined by temporary loss of morale, and reactions vary widely according to temperament from that of "Put her legs down, wrap her up, she will probably be all right presently," to gloomy speculations about the extent of hidden injuries inflicted, and only experience will counter the highly individual variations in outlook.

It is true, however, that in the absence of active bleeding, time and nature are on one's side, and it is generally wise to remember that if in doubt about what to do one should do nothing, apart from obvious routine resuscitative measures, until that doubt is clearly resolved.

Only a small minority of cases of collapse after delivery occur without haemorrhage. Bleeding brooks no delay, both in stopping it and replacing quantitatively that which is lost; but from time to time it will appear that the deterioration in the patient's condition is out of all proportion to the amount of blood which she has lost, and it is the assessment of this factor, the factor of coincident or superimposed shock, which is the theme of this chapter, and an attempt is made to present the problem from the viewpoint of the doctor who finds himself confronted with such a worrying situation.

It is obvious that messy delivery, in which blood is allowed to run to waste on to sheets and bedding and into the bucket and which cannot, therefore, be even approximately measured, is going to deny the opportunity of relating the woman's condition to haemorrhage alone, and the habit of tidy work is just as important as in other branches of surgery. As far as possible all blood lost should be carefully collected for measuring. Even an unsutured episiotomy can surreptitiously cost a patient half a litre of blood and the slow but steady trickle may pass, for a time, unnoticed.

The importance of "blood accountancy" can, therefore, be stressed *ad infinitum* but never *ad nauseam.*

Where it can be reasonably certain that a patient has lost, for example, no more than half to three-quarters of a litre and yet is collapsed, two groups of conditions must be quickly reviewed:

(*a*) Blood is being lost but not externally;
(*b*) Other shock-producing factors are operative.

Since the conditions in the first group demand the promptest treatment, a search in this direction should first be undertaken, and the most likely sites are within the body of the uterus itself, the peritoneal cavity and the retroperitoneal spaces.

A uterus which is slowly filling with blood may often be fairly hard, and only the increase of its overall size may reveal what is happening; the impression of size on palpation is more important than actual height of fundus.

Quite large quantities of blood can lie in the peritoneal cavity without producing many physical signs locally, although general signs of shock are obvious; pain is often much less than would be expected, of abdominal rigidity there is of course none, tenderness may be very indefinite, and the most noticeable features may be bulging of the flanks, dullness to percussion and the patient's clear dislike of lying down flat and thereby allowing blood to run up under the diaphragm.

Many haemorrhages into the retroperitoneal tissue spaces and between the layers of the broad ligament are overlooked if not large, but they too add to the patient's shock over and above the amount of blood lost to circulation.

The following is a table classifying the various causes of post-partum collapse, bearing in mind always that shock and haemorrhage are interlocked in a sort of synergism.

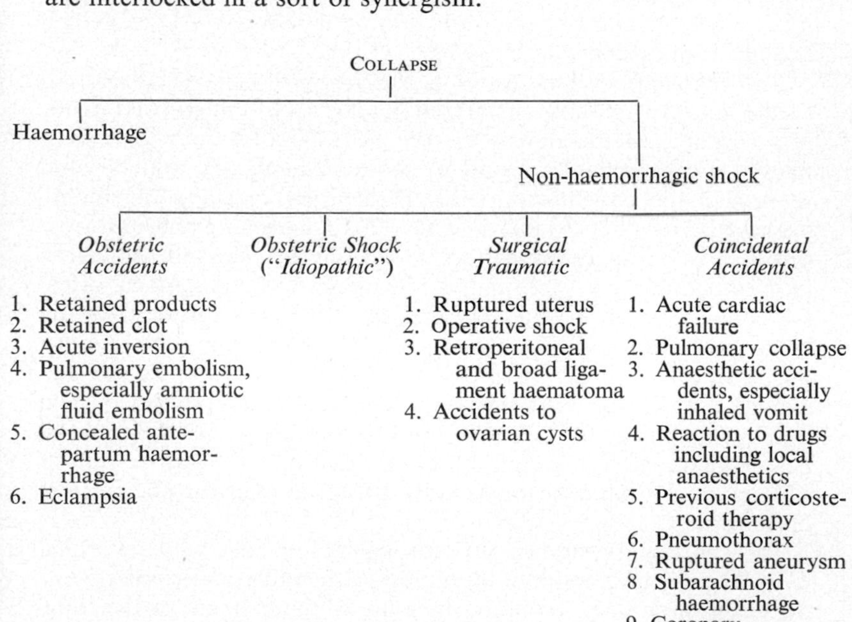

COLLAPSE
Haemorrhage
Non-haemorrhagic shock
Obstetric Accidents
Obstetric Shock ("Idiopathic")
Surgical Traumatic
Coincidental Accidents
1. Retained products
2. Retained clot
3. Acute inversion
4. Pulmonary embolism, especially amniotic fluid embolism
5. Concealed ante-partum haemorrhage
6. Eclampsia
1. Ruptured uterus
2. Operative shock
3. Retroperitoneal and broad ligament haematoma
4. Accidents to ovarian cysts
1. Acute cardiac failure
2. Pulmonary collapse
3. Anaesthetic accidents, especially inhaled vomit
4. Reaction to drugs including local anaesthetics
5. Previous corticosteroid therapy
6. Pneumothorax
7. Ruptured aneurysm
8 Subarachnoid haemorrhage
9. Coronary thrombosis

Published data on postpartum shock deal only with cases that end in death, and innumerable cases of profound shock occur in practice which never find their way into print because they recover and the reason for the shock cannot always be accurately attributed.

HAEMORRHAGE

In the haemorrhage group, patients vary widely in their reaction to blood loss and the amount of collapse thereby suffered. The highly multiparous patient, besides being more liable to bleed on that account alone, stands haemorrhage worse than the primigravid patient quite apart from the question of age; the stresses, moreover, of previous child-bearing and child-rearing may tell their tale. Antenatal health is therefore of very great importance. There is nothing like anaemia to beget anaemia, and the positive health measures of good antenatal care go a long way towards fortifying the patient against the vicissitudes of labour. A woman approaching labour with a haemoglobin of 65 per cent (9·6 g) or less faces it with some peril, and all antenatal conditions producing fatigue exaggerate the effects of labour itself. Where some complication of pregnancy has occurred such as antepartum haemorrhage, be it due to placenta praevia or accidental placental separation, only a relatively small postpartum loss is necessary to tip the scales towards a state of collapse.

A lengthy, exhausting and dehydrating labour likewise magnifies the effects of postpartum bleeding.

It is, therefore, difficult to relate the degree of collapse absolutely to quantitative blood loss without taking such antecedent factors into account. At the end of the second stage of labour there is a physiological mechanism, akin to shock in miniature, which helps to protect the patient from haemorrhage by reducing the blood pressure. Any shock factors which may develop or be already operative are superimposed upon this mechanism but with this important difference—their clinical manifestations are delayed, often by as many as ten minutes, so that by the time a further drop in blood pressure is recorded as the result, for example, of bleeding, one is already so many minutes out of date in assessing the general condition. To recognise this is to improve one's choice of the optimum moment for active intervention in ridding the patient of her placenta with the minimum of additional operative shock. This point is dealt with more fully in the chapter on postpartum haemorrhage.

The general appearance of the patient, coupled with an exact knowledge of the amount of blood lost is, therefore, more objectively important even than the blood pressure at the moment or the state of the pulse.

NON-HAEMORRHAGIC SHOCK

This does not differ in its manifestations from shock encountered in other fields of medicine.

Sheehan (1948) fully described his findings at autopsy in a large number of obstetrical disasters and made interesting observations.

Blood flow is greatly reduced, but not evenly throughout the body, since the processes of vasoconstriction spare the brain with its vital centres as far as possible. Blood flow through the skin is greatly reduced, hence the impression of pallor and coldness. Such circulation as persists in the skin is sluggish, and the damage done by a hot-water bottle, which a healthy person would regard as no more than very warm, can be very extensive because the heat is not carried away and dispersed and any toxic products from local overheating are not rapidly diluted in the circulation.

Muscle blood flow and all visceral blood flow is reduced, so that stagnation and pooling are general, except in the brain as aforesaid.

All renal filtration usually stops at systolic blood pressures of less than 80 mm Hg, so that anuria results. The duration of uncorrected shock will determine in large measure the recovery of renal function.

The heart is operating under grave handicaps, the venous return is reduced and atrial filling is poor, so that cardiac output falls, and even acceleration of the heart cannot compensate for the deficiency because of a stroke output which may be as low as 20 ml.

These effects, namely vasoconstriction and tachycardia, are the result of sympathetic activity, and as Sheehan pointed out, are highly protective in cases of haemorrhage by mitigating further blood loss and maintaining blood supply to the vital centres, but where shock without blood loss occurs, this mechanism may be harmful by embarrassing the heart's action through poor venous return and thus precipitating cardiac failure.

The need is therefore to judge how much the patient's state is due to bleeding and how much to shock factors.

The latent period of delay in falling blood pressure has already been mentioned. There are two stages in the process. Initially, there is a fall in pulse pressure because the diastolic pressure is first increased due to vasoconstriction and the systolic pressure is for a time maintained; then, as the condition worsens, vasoconstriction begins to fail, the heart meanwhile becoming more inefficient, and both systolic and diastolic pressures fall together. The awareness of pain is for some unknown reason dulled.

Other autonomic effects are to be found in dilatation of the stomach, the ascending colon and the proximal half of the transverse colon, corresponding to the predominant sympathetic nerve supply of the intestinal tract.

The liver is liable to suffer central necrosis in the lobules due to vasoconstriction and reduced blood pressure, a state of affairs made worse[3] if there is also pre-eclamptic toxaemia or if further vasoconstricting drugs are given, and these changes in the liver may have something to do with irreversibility in shock.

Postpartum Pituitary Necrosis

The anterior lobe of the pituitary is very susceptible to damage, and as a result of thrombosis in the vessels supplying it, suffers necrosis to greater or lesser degree. The immediate effects are less noticeable and serious than the remote. There is initially a tendency towards hypoglycaemia and lactation is never established. Later the signs of hypopituitarism are manifested (Simmonds' disease), a condition which used to be called superinvolution, and in which there is a degree of genital atrophy with amenorrhoea and usually sterility.[13] The term Sheehan's syndrome is now used when referring to this type of hypopituitarism dating from haemorrhage and shock at delivery. Murdoch (1962) analysed 57 cases admitted to Glasgow hospitals with this diagnosis since 1950. The commonest reasons for admission being lassitude, nausea and breathlessness of increasing severity. Of these patients, 10 were already dead at the time of review and it would appear that pyrexial illnesses are particularly dangerous in precipitating hypopituitary coma. Any disease associated with vomiting has likewise a bad effect. There may be some delay in the development of the full-blown Sheehan's syndrome and in any case in which there has been severe haemorrhage or shock at delivery and in whom lactation does not subsequently occur, damage sustained by the anterior pituitary should be watched for in the course of the next year, declaring itself in amenorrhea, intolerance to cold, lassitude and general debility. Microcytic anaemia often adds to the patient's wretched state and does not respond readily to iron therapy, but may be helped by the addition of testosterone.

The patients may be subjectively much improved by treating with thyroid extract and cortisone 25 mg daily.

General listlessness, apathy and intolerance of cold will remain with the patient for the rest of her prematurely senile life, perhaps another thirty years, until, with increasing tendency to myxoedematous changes and a persistent anaemia, some intercurrent infection closes the tragic chapter. The fact that this disease is not more commonly seen is due to the number of candidates for it who die before it has a chance to reveal itself, and in the future the more prompt treatment of postpartum collapse, which is now more generally available, should lessen the incidence still further, for the duration of a state of shock is more damaging in the long run than the degree. Up to the present only the stimulus of another pregnancy, itself an unlikely event, will restore youthful health by bringing about a hypertrophy of such glandular tissue in the anterior pituitary as has escaped ischaemic necrosis.

Anuria

Another grave sequel of protracted shock is acute renal tubular necrosis, dealt with more fully elsewhere. It has already been stated that renal filtration ceases with systolic blood pressures below 80 mm Hg, and, within the course of a very few hours of uncorrected shock, sufficient renal damage is sustained to stop the secretion of urine completely or reduce it to a few turbid ounces. Any case of severe shock ought, therefore, to be very carefully watched for several days for signs of urinary suppression.

The Factor of Prolonged Labour

Of Sheehan's 147 cases which he examined post-mortem, it was found that, leaving aside cases of uterine rupture, the fatal cases resulting from a strenuous delivery had in no instance laboured for less than two days, and it is clear that resistance to shock depends very much upon the condition in which the first as well as the second stage of labour leaves a patient. Fatigue, dehydration and acidosis are thus powerful contributory factors.

Turning now to the table previously given, some of the causes of collapse require some discussion.

Obstetric Accidents

Retained Placenta without Bleeding

There is no creature more treacherous than a woman who retains her placenta after delivery of her child. Not only may she start a severe haemorrhage at any unpredictable moment, and cannot therefore be left unattended, but as time goes on her general condition is very liable to deteriorate, though the mechanism of this phenomenon is not yet understood. Of Sheehan's 147 fatal cases, no fewer than 35 had retention of the placenta for over two hours, and even though manual removal might be very difficult, the shock thereof as a cause of death is very unlikely if undertaken within the first two hours of the third stage. Where haemorrhage has occurred it is, therefore, obviously desirable that the patient's condition should be restored sufficiently to allow manual removal of the placenta to be undertaken within that time interval, and, as is discussed in the chapter on postpartum haemorrhage, this opportunity may be missed through neglect of very prompt restorative measures as soon as the primary blood loss occurs, so that by the time manual removal is decided upon the patient is sinking for the second time and cannot surface anything like so quickly. This is a thoroughly dangerous situation, in which the shock of the operation in an exsanguinated and hypotensive patient has to be weighed against the shock induced by longer retention of the placenta and the long time it may take for the blood transfusion to bring her to a safe level for operation.

If a placenta does not separate within two hours of delivery of the child, the chances of a safe and spontaneous separation are becoming too slender to count upon and there is, therefore, nothing to be gained by waiting. One knows of cases in which the placenta has been left in the uterus for several days without harm to the patient, but such sang-froid on the part of the attendant is little better than recklessness, and one wonders how thorough was the watch kept upon her throughout this time.

Authorities vary in the time limit they set; most of us take steps to deliver the placenta after one hour of waiting, and anything up to about four hours is probably safe though pointless, and two hours can be taken as a sensible maximum. At the end of the second stage the patient is naturally tired and in need of a good sleep, thus it is impossible to observe a protracted third stage and at the same time keep her both warm, dry and comfortable.

Retained Clot

To a lesser extent much of what has been said above applies here. Quite apart from the fact that clot will encourage further bleeding, such a patient often "perks up" very noticeably after the uterus has been emptied by a judicious squeeze which every midwife administers before turning her back on the patient. This sound and simple practice is often neglected at the end of a Caesarean section while the patient is still anaesthetised and therefore in no state to object, and it is certain that it makes a great difference to the immediate postoperative condition on return to the ward.

Acute Inversion

This is dealt with fully elsewhere, but as a cause of collapse it must be very quickly excluded or treated, and should be one of the first possibilities to cross the obstetrician's mind. Cord pulling is now more fashionable, but it is well to remember that about 15 per cent of cases of acute inversion occur spontaneously and for no apparent reason. In three-quarters of such cases the placenta is inserted at the fundus, the least common site of all, and there is no means of foreseeing this possibility except by incidental knowledge from previous sonar placentography antenatally.

The complete inversion of the third degree is the rarest variety, and it is where the inverted mass does not protrude into view that such a cause of collapse may be overlooked. Abdominal palpation should be made at once to determine the whereabouts and the shape of the uterine fundus, and where this is in doubt, for example in a case of gross obesity, a vaginal examination may have to be made.

Pulmonary Embolism

This rare complication of labour has been noted from time to time, and the embolus may consist of air, thrombus or liquor amnii with its ingredients of meconium, vernix caseosa, etc. (Steiner and Lushbaugh).

For an air embolus to enter the circulation, part at least of the placental site must be exposed which in the normal third stage is unlikely before its completion and delivery of the membranes. Nevertheless, it would appear to be a wise precaution to keep the patient's knees together and to wait for the uterus to harden before changing her position, for example from left lateral to dorsal.

An air embolus may be introduced in the course of intra-uterine manipulation which has been preceded by some placental separation. Attempts to hurry up blood transfusion by increasing the pressure of air within a transfusion bottle, usually by means of a Higginson's syringe, for example, may end in sudden catastrophe and I have had one such case in my own experience. I had just finished operating on her for a severe and haemorrhagic vault laceration and left instructions for the remainder of the almost full bottle of blood which she was then receiving to be given. Leaving the department, I got no further than the hospital gate when I was recalled to find that the patient, who only a few minutes before had been making a good recovery, was now dead, yet only about half the bottle of blood had been given. In fact blood clot had formed well up the filter inside the bottle and the pressure had been built up inside the bottle with a Higginson's syringe in order to complete the transfusion hurriedly and quite unnecessarily. A truly massive air embolus had been instantly fatal. Modern transfusion-giving sets are far safer in this respect than the older patterns, but, even so, a watch must be kept to see that the bottle does not empty and that only blood and not air is being driven down the tubing. The effects of embolism are immediate and shock will have to be treated at once. Intravenous morphia 15 mg with oxygen therapy are the two most useful emergency measures. Transfusion and infusion are both contra-indicated if there is no blood loss to replace, inasmuch as they aggravate the pulmonary oedema which, in any case, is bound to develop. When cardiac arrest occurs because of an air embolus, cardiac massage is only likely to make matters even worse, because air will be driven into the pulmonary circulation. The correct treatment is aspiration of the air out of the right ventricle with a wide-bore needle. Unfortunately there is seldom time for effective treatment which in any case is only likely to benefit the borderline case. A useful, immediate first-aid procedure is to place the patient in the head-down, left lateral position in the hope of displacing the bolus of air towards the apex of the right ventricle. In the case of smaller volumes of air now in the right side of the heart it may be possible for pulmonary circulation to continue until the air bubble is gradually passed piecemeal and less dramatically into the pulmonary system.

Amniotic fluid embolism is more common than is recognised and Steiner and Lushbaugh who originally described it reckoned that it was the commonest cause of obstetric death during labour or in the first ten hours of the puerperium. It produces profound shock, dyspnoea, tachycardia, cyanosis and, if not immediately fatal, hyperpyrexia. The worst case of this sort which I have encountered was admitted in strong labour after artificial hindwater rupture to induce labour two days earlier. On admission she was obviously dyspnoeic, grossly cyanosed, her temperature was 105°F (41°C), the fetal heart was absent and her condition was indeed desperate. There had been no vomiting. As the cervix was almost fully dilated she was delivered with forceps without difficulty, but died without haemorrhage in spite of oxygen and restorative measures 45 minutes later. Necropsy revealed massive amniotic fluid embolism but the site of entry of the liquor amnii into the circulation could not be demonstrated. Presumably the previous surgical induction, coupled with powerful uterine action, had established an entry track.

The emboli consist of particulate constituents of liquor amnii, namely epithelial squames, fat, lanugo hairs and meconium and can be demonstrated in the pulmonary arterioles and alveolar capillaries (Figs. 1 and 2).

Of all the causes of sudden disaster in labour, amniotic fluid embolism ranks high and, in fact, over a third of sudden deaths in a series reported from Liverpool[17] would appear to have been due to this cause. The diagnosis can only definitely be established in the case of maternal death as a necropsy finding, and even so the evidences may have disappeared because of autolysis if there is much delay in carrying out the examination, as is often the case owing to inquest procedure; but the presumptive diagnosis is justified on clinical grounds when there is sudden collapse with tachycardia, tachypnoea, cyanosis and hypotension. The two other conditions which produce an almost identical picture are acute pulmonary oedema due to

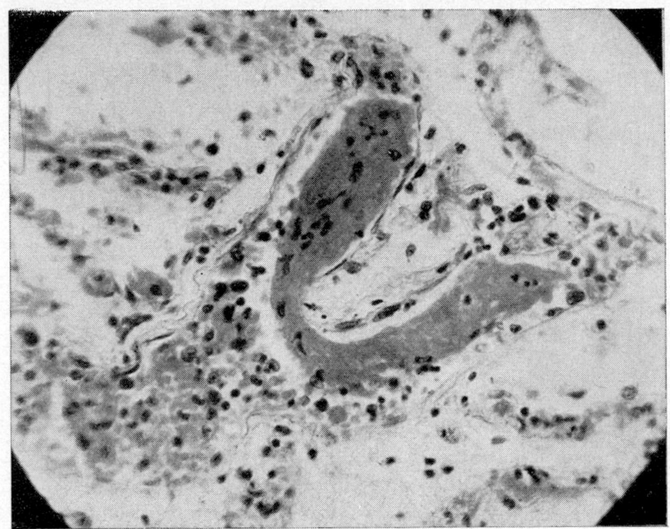

21/FIG. 1.—The section of lung capillary showing embolic mass of vernix material. The capillary is greatly distended and there is a leucocytic reaction in the vessel and in the capillaries of adjacent alveoli. (H. and E. × 500.)

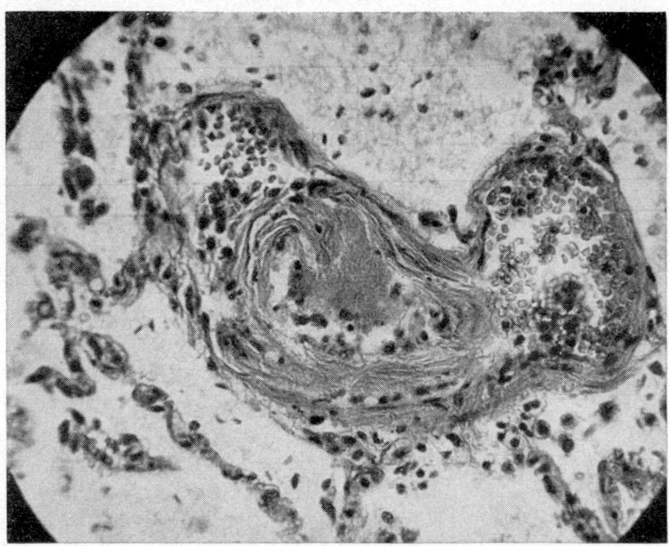

21/FIG. 2.—Dilated pulmonary vessel containing an embolic mass. The embolus consists of vernix material surrounded by bundles of squames. (H. and E. × 500.)

(Figs. 1 and 2 by courtesy of Dr A. D. T. Govan.)

mitral stenosis and the inhaled vomit syndrome presently to be described.

In by no means all cases, however, is death from amniotic fluid embolism immediate, and clotting defects may develop within the course of the next hour or two due to intravascular microcoagulation involving particularly the pulmonary tree, thereby aggravating cyanosis. Blood coagulation failure from this variety of hypofibrinogenaemia may, in fact, be the first evidence that amniotic fluid embolism has occurred (see Chapter XV). Although I have encountered serious haemorrhage in such a case, this can be controlled by fibrinogen replacement. The lethal factor is the vascular obstruction to the pulmonary circulation. The very worst thing to do at this point is to prevent fibrinolysis by the use of antifibrinolytic agents and it is far preferable, almost paradoxically, to use heparin intravenously to prevent further vascular occlusion, using a loading dose of 5000 units intravenously immediately, followed by a drip administering 1000 units per hour. No more fibrinogen should be given than is strictly necessary for the control of bleeding. The patient's danger is more immediate from her lungs than from her anaemic state. The diagnosis can to some extent be assisted by immediate X-ray, taken usually with a portable X-ray machine, because of the gravity of the patient's condition, but provided the patient does not die within the first few hours from the amniotic fluid embolus itself or, more likely, from injudicious treatment, resolution is rapid, presumably due to natural fibrinolysis of the widely scattered microthrombi (Fig. 3). If this variety of embolism, however, presents with pulmonary signs first, without signs of haemorrhage, then heparin must be given courageously and without hesitation before the patient's lungs "solidify".

Figure 3 illustrates one of our own cases.[19] The embolism occurred during the patient's third Caesarean section and was associated with considerable blood loss. Pulmonary signs of cyanosis together with shock appeared during the operation which was carried out under endotracheal anaesthesia and not following it, as might have been expected, in the vomit aspiration syndrome. Ventilation was with difficulty adequately maintained with intermittent positive-pressure using 100 per cent oxygen; at the same time attempts were made to maintain a degree of positive pressure during expiration to discourage increasing pulmonary oedema. Repeated tracheal aspiration was necessary to remove fluid from the lungs and aminophylline was administered. The base excess of –5 mEq/l was quickly apparent and the pH of the blood rapidly fell to 7·28. This was corrected with 100 mEq of sodium bicarbonate and low-molecular-weight dextran was given in the hope of increasing the pulmonary blood flow. Frusemide was also given intravenously (20 mg) to reduce pulmonary oedema

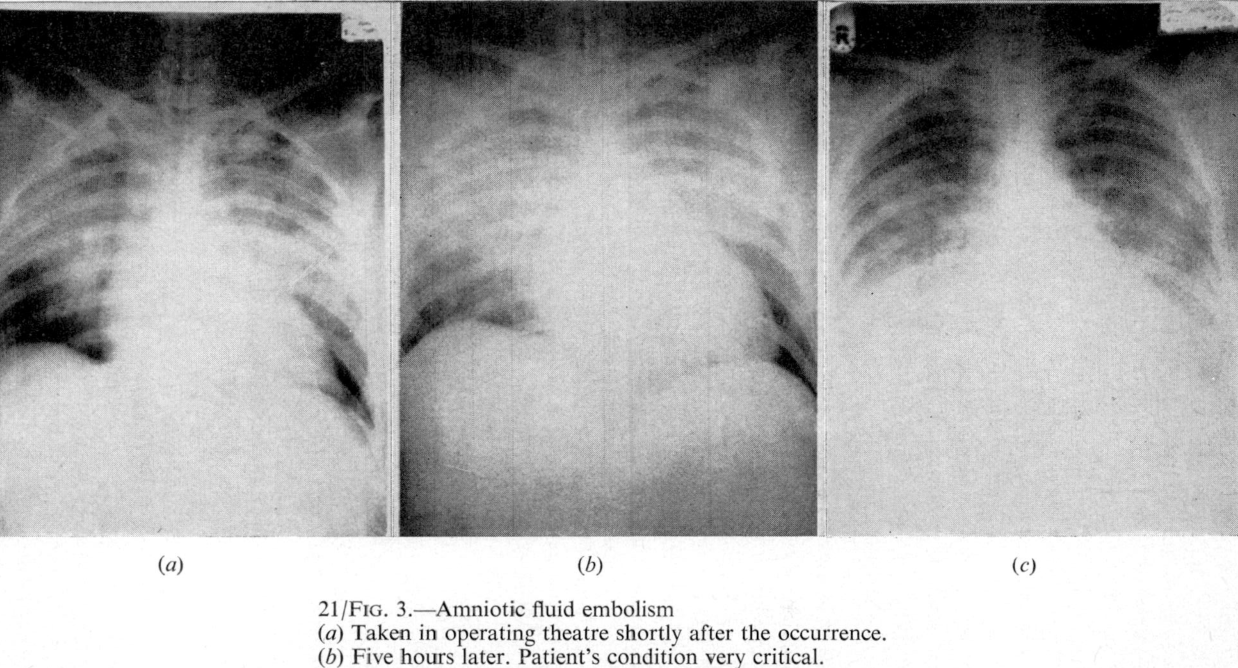

(*a*) (*b*) (*c*)

21/FIG. 3.—Amniotic fluid embolism
(*a*) Taken in operating theatre shortly after the occurrence.
(*b*) Five hours later. Patient's condition very critical.
(*c*) The following day nearly 24 hours after the onset.

Note the very rapid alteration in radiological appearances.

and digoxin 0·5 mg together with intravenous hydrocortisone to maintain the circulation. It will be noted that fibrinogen was not given in spite of the haemorrhage attending the operation. The blood loss was simply replaced. This case was much debated among us and we reckoned that the intermittent positive-pressure ventilation helped to reduce the pulmonary oedema, and at least we did not fall into the trap of aggravating the condition by giving the wrong treatment; the prompt correction of biochemical imbalance in the form of metabolic acidosis doubtless contributed to the recovery. These cases are sufficiently rare to leave one in considerable doubt as to how to cope with the emergency which is often completely unexpected and the above outline of treatment was unanimously agreed by all of us at the time.

Concealed Antepartum Haemorrhage (Abruptio Placentae)

The patient who has weathered this grave emergency to the point of delivery has little in reserve to withstand even minor third-stage difficulties. Attempts, therefore, to hurry delivery before recovery both of uterine tone and general condition are fraught with more than usual danger, and no less than 25 of Sheehan's cases died after delivery as a result of shock following concealed antepartum haemorrhage. Precipitate labour following abruptio placentae can lead to very profound shock, even in the absence of further haemorrhage.

Surgical-Traumatic

Ruptured Uterus (see Chapter XXIII)

The fact that a woman has managed to deliver herself by no means rules out a diagnosis of uterine rupture, and where delivery has followed operative intervention, such a possibility is even more prominent.

I have known spontaneous rupture to occur both at the end of a straightforward delivery and during the apparently normal delivery of the second of twins.

It is a condition which carries a very high mortality if neglected through failure to diagnose it, and even when treated still remains one of the worst hazards of childbearing. A previous Caesarean section scar, particularly of the classical variety, should prime one's suspicions of uterine rupture in cases of collapse. Lower-segment scars may rupture rather insidiously. Internal version, difficult forceps operations, especially those involving rotation of the fetal head and, in fact, any major manipulative measure, all carry the obvious risks of inflicting rupture which may only be appreciated after extraction of the child. The diagnosis is by no means easy, particularly in incomplete rupture, but where shock persists in spite of adequate blood transfusion to replace blood lost, this possibility should come readily to mind and the diagnosis promptly established by digital exploration of the uterus.

Operative Shock

Apart from any gross injury, the obstetric patient has no peculiar immunity from traumatic shock any more than the surgical case. It is nevertheless surprising how much sheer force the parturient woman will stand, provided that such force is not misapplied either in nature, timing or direction. However, the case is quite different if, for example, the cervix is not fully dilated and forcible delivery of the head, even though successful and without lacerating the cervix, is absolutely certain to produce some degree of shock, often very great. In such a case the lower segment of the uterus is pulled upon together with the attached ligaments with their rich supply of nerve fibres, and this fact, together with the light plane of anaesthesia usually employed, provides an adequate reason for shock; this complication is probably the commonest cause of all.

Antepartum haemorrhage of any variety predisposes the patient to traumatic shock. Another all-too-frequent source of shock in the past has been the repeated use of Credé's method of attempting to deliver the placenta, and there are many obstetricians who have been so impressed by the damage thereby inflicted that they feel it is a manoeuvre which should be abandoned; it has now disappeared from our own practice.

Innumerable such instances of misapplied force could be given; what makes matters so difficult is the uncertainty at the time whether or not some serious injury has been caused which calls for courageous surgery in a situation which is already grave.

Retroperitoneal and Broad-Ligament Haematoma

These cases are usually due to incomplete uterine rupture, though occasionally there may be a traumatic rupture of the utero-ovarian venous system without tearing of the uterine wall. The source of the trouble is often not immediately obvious; the swelling may at first be very soft and boggy and only very careful examination may discover it.

Accidents to Ovarian Cysts

Torsion may occur in labour, and very occasionally a cyst finds itself in the path of the presenting part, and whether it ruptures or not shock is certain to occur.

Coincidental Accidents

The patient with a cardiac lesion may collapse and die within the first 24 hours. Here one is forewarned but not necessarily forearmed, and even the most careful treatment (see Chapter V) will not prevent every such disaster.

A case of eclampsia may suddenly show a most precipitate fall in blood pressure, a very serious sign, usually betokening a major vascular accident, often multiple. In some cases acute suprarenal failure is the likely mechanism.

Inhaled vomitus in anaesthesia is now becoming one of the more prominent hazards of midwifery as others are reduced or eliminated, in spite of the increased attention which is being given to this branch of anaesthetics. There is probably no obstetrician alive who has not, more than once, been frightened almost out of his wits by his anaesthetist.

The combination of inexperienced anaesthetist, Boyle's anaesthetic machine and Clauson's harness in a labour room without mechanical suction devices instantly available and without labour ward beds capable of immediate head-down tilt, has provided most obstetricians of my vintage with their full share of alarms. The calamitous effects of inhaled vomit are often even more lethal to the unborn baby.

Inhaled Vomit Syndrome

This is nowadays recognised much more readily as a clinical entity. There are two main varieties. The first, due to inhalation of solid material which blocks off a main branch of the bronchial tree, is an obvious and well-known matter. Lung collapse, pneumonia and lung abscess follow in the case inadequately treated by bronchoscopy. But this sort of accident is relatively uncommon in obstetric practice. More common and treacherous is the type of accident to which Mendelson (1946) drew attention. Here, liquid and highly irritant gastric contents are deeply inhaled and result in an asthmatic type of behaviour in a patient whose condition progressively deteriorates after apparent recovery from the anaesthetic. Clinically there is cyanosis, tachycardia, wheezing from pulmonary oedema and deepening shock. It is by no means always obvious that vomit has in fact been aspirated and the differential diagnosis between amniotic fluid embolism, acute pulmonary oedema due to mitral stenosis and cardiac failure, and this syndrome may be difficult. More than half the deaths attributable to general anaesthesia are associated with inhaled acid vomit.

In reviewing seven cases Parker attributed the development of this "acid-aspiration" syndrome to progressive and generalised bronchospasm, thereby explaining the interval which usually elapses between the end of the anaesthetic and the onset of serious symptoms. Anoxia, cardiac failure and massive pulmonary oedema are the immediate causes of death, often within a dozen hours and sometimes a day or two later when pneumonia is usually superadded.

Treatment is a matter of urgency. The head should be turned to one side and the pharynx immediately emptied by mechanical suction. The patient should be tilted head downwards (and in how many labour wards is this possible?) and if there is any cyanosis a laryngoscope should be passed and any accessible solid foreign material removed. It will probably be necessary thereafter to proceed with the anaesthetic and operation, but if respiratory difficulties of any sort appear following the cessation of the anaesthetic, the likelihood of acid aspiration should be recognised. With the help of a bronchoscope, under renewed anaesthesia, the bronchial tree should be sucked clear as thoroughly as possible. Oxygen should be given and aminophylline (250 mg) injected intravenously to relieve bronchial spasm. It is doubtful if the spontaneous breathing of 100 per cent oxygen is adequate when artificial ventilation with oxygen through an endotracheal tube is not only more efficient but reduces the tendency to pulmonary oedema.[7] Hydrocortisone, 200 to 300 mg, should be given intravenously followed by 100 mg six-hourly intramuscularly, or maintained in an intravenous drip if one is being used, the dose being gradually tapered in the course of the ensuing four or five days. As hydrocortisone prevents the normal response to secondary bacterial invasion, broad-spectrum antibiotics should be employed. There has been debate whether lavage of the lungs with large volumes of bicarbonate or saline might be of use to neutralise the aspirated acid, but the general opinion is that this may only spread the trouble and in fact prove dangerous.

This is one of the big hazards of modern operative obstetrics and for this reason forceps deliveries are being increasingly performed under pudendal block local anaesthesia which is adequate for four out of five cases. Where, however, an inhalational anaesthetic has to be given, the stomach may have first to be emptied by stomach tube. Cases of prolonged labour also demonstrate gastric inertia and usually have treacherously full stomachs. Glucose drinks coaxed into them during the first stage of labour lie unabsorbed within the stomach to be regurgitated when anaesthesia is induced. Intravenous fluids are, therefore, not only more effective but very much safer from this point of view. Even the precaution of passing a stomach tube may not be enough to empty the stomach adequately, quite apart from its unpleasantness in a demoralised patient. Even though all fluids have been restricted since labour became fully established it is now our standard practice, as advocated by Taylor and Pryse-Davies (1966), to administer prophylactic antacid by mouth and for this purpose 14 ml of magnesium trisilicate, B.P.C., are given shortly before anaesthesia is induced. This is sufficient to neutralise 140 ml of gastric contents. Magnesium trisilicate is superior to half-strength aluminium hydroxide which tends to be more viscous and therefore less beneficial if it should be aspirated. The aim should be to raise the pH of the gastric contents to above the critical level of 2·50, below which human lungs would appear to be particularly vulnerable, quite apart from the mechanical dangers of aspiration.

Chloroform is now generally agreed to be a dangerous anaesthetic in spite of its traditional place in midwifery, and it is a pity that what it saves in producing a smooth induction it loses in the direction of ventricular fibrillation and liver damage, for there is no handier agent in domiciliary practice. It is the frequently repeated induction of anaesthesia which multiplies the risks particularly.

Previous corticosteroid therapy produces a hazard of increasing importance. It is now generally agreed that the adrenals may require as much as two years to recover fully from the suppressive effects of corticosteroids and during this period the patient may be incapable of mustering the normal physiological responses to stress, particularly of trauma and operation. Admittedly there is some compensation in the stimulus which pregnancy provides to the maternal adrenals and this may be enough for weathering a normal pregnancy and labour, but when pregnancy or delivery are complicated by vomiting, infection, blood loss, operation or any stressful complication, the patient faces the risk of sudden acute collapse and death unless additional supportive therapy equivalent to 200 mg of cortisone acetate intramuscularly is supplied during each 24 hours, preferably for one day before the emergency, in so far as it can be foreseen, and for at least two or three days thereafter depending upon her general condition. In a real emergency it is wise to administer the corticosteroid in a glucose saline intravenous infusion, controlling the dosage by blood pressure readings. If the clinician is confronted with sudden collapse due to this cause of suprarenal inadequacy the intravenous route should certainly be chosen, as the rate of absorption from intramuscular injection is too slow and unpredictable. The need, therefore, to be aware of previous corticosteriod therapy is very real and in my own unit cardiac arrest occurred in a patient whose doctor at home had been treating her many months earlier with cortisone for "rheumatism" and of which we had no knowledge. Information of this sort is even more urgent than knowing the patient's blood group.

Another cause of sudden and unpredictable collapse is drug sensitivity. This may occur even in the case of local anaesthetic agents used, for example, in pudendal block. Fortunately lignocaine has a very good record in this respect but accidental intravenous injection may produce some degree of collapse. There is probably no such thing as a drug to which some patient somewhere in the world is not sensitive and this possibility should be borne in mind in attempting a diagnosis of the cause.

Spontaneous pneumothorax is an uncommon complication but it becomes particularly dangerous if it goes on to tension pneumothorax, and we have indeed had such a case in a woman who smoked so heavily that she benefited the Chancellor of the Exchequer to the tune of 60 cigarettes a day. The state of her lungs can be imagined and she presumably managed to rupture a subpleural emphysematous bulla as a result of her coughing and chronic respiratory disease. Unfortunately, because of a complicating antepartum haemorrhage, she had to have a general anaesthetic for vaginal examination, halothane in oxygen being chosen and positive-pressure ventilation being avoided. In the course of the ensuing labour epidural anaesthesia was given to avoid the need for respiratory depressant drugs and directly after the injection of the main epidural dose she collapsed with acute dyspnoea, bronchospasm and cyanosis. Naturally the immediate reaction was to blame the epidural anaesthetic but in fact it was fortunately noticed that there was tracheal deviation to the left. The patient was now *in extremis* but prompt relief of the intrapleural pressure, by the insertion of a needle in the seventh intercostal space, dramatically saved her life.[18] This story serves to remind one of how quickly one has both to think and act in a case such as this where faulty observation, or the institution of routine antishock methods, would have been rewarded only be certain death of the patient.

Pulmonary collapse completes the list of commoner causes. The remainder are more in the nature of curiosities: anaphylactic phenomena, paroxysmal tachycardia, subarachnoid haemorrhage, coronary thrombosis, ruptured heart valves and ruptured aneurysm, splenic, renal or mesenteric, to mention a few, and in doing so for the sake of completeness it must again be stressed that the commonest things most commonly occur and should be looked for first.

Idiopathic Obstetric Shock

The more carefully the case is considered and examined the less often will this diagnosis be made; in fact, there are many who deny that it exists. This is an overstatement. Every now and then a patient inexplicably collapses and dies, and at autopsy, usually by the coroner's pathologist, no causative lesion whatsoever can be discovered. Then, and then only, may the diagnosis of idiopathic obstetric shock be made, for there is no alternative.

One can only speculate on the mechanism by which it is produced and at the same time marvel that it does not occur more often when one considers that to some women, labour, even uncomplicated labour, is the greatest ordeal they have ever had to undergo. Stretching of the parts may be a factor in susceptible individuals, just as stretching of the anal orifice may produce surgical shock. Pain, bruising, dehydration and frank terror may all play their part, but it is very difficult to say how often such shock occurs without being certain of the thoroughness of post-mortem examination in a large number of obstetric disasters. Sheehan found no such case in his 147 cases. In the *Report on Maternal Morbidity and Mortality in Scotland*, 1929–33, in 100 fatal cases quoted by Munro Kerr and Chassar Moir rapid labour was listed in two, and in seven cases the cause of death was undetermined, but it is not certain how far all other possible causes were excluded. The diagnosis of idiopathic shock, therefore, can only be made by a complete process of elimination which is impossible until after death and particularly in the case of amniotic fluid embolism post-mortem autolysis very rapidly destroys the evidence.

Prophylaxis against Postpartum Collapse

The first essential is to save blood loss at all times and in all places. There is no greater obstetrical commandment than this, and the second is never to overestimate a woman's powers of endurance.

Antenatal care should eliminate as far as possible and wherever possible the handicaps likely to operate during labour, particularly anaemia, and, where they cannot be eliminated, to mitigate their effects, for example by securing a week or two of maximum rest for the damaged heart.

In labour itself good supervision not only delays the onset of maternal distress, but also goes far towards preventing postpartum collapse by combating dehydration, discouraging ketosis by the timely use of an intravenous glucose drip and encouraging the maximum amount of rest and relaxation by the judicious use of sedatives.

THE FLYING SQUAD

Since Farquhar Murray established the first flying squad in Newcastle-on-Tyne in 1935 no fewer than 172 maternity hospitals in England and Wales have developed this service. About 3000 such calls are dealt with annually (about 1 per cent of all domiciliary deliveries). This in itself might be regarded as a condemnation of domiciliary midwifery, but in areas where there are shortages of maternity beds the flying squad has a very vital role.

The original squad in Newcastle dealt with 353 cases in its first twelve years of operation and Stabler (1947) gave an account of this pioneer work which is likely to be of historical importance as, apart from its other intrinsic interest, it covers the period before and after the institution of blood banks. Before 1940 intravenous saline was the main restorative, since stored blood was not then available.

Twenty-seven cases of acute haemorrhage or shock were transferred to hospital but nine of these died and Stabler blamed the journey. This was certainly true before the availability of adequate blood transfusion in the patient's home, but would not be the case nowadays. For this reason Stabler reckoned that the squad should be capable of, and equipped for, anything and everything on the spot. He therefore recommended not only staffing with an experienced obstetrician, assistants and anaesthetist, but six items of baggage as follows:

1. Large box for drugs, anaesthetics, syringes, bowls, instruments and intravenous giving sets;
2. Small box for gowns, drapes, dressings and gloves;
3. Small box sufficient for abdominal surgery;
4. Crate of dried plasma, saline and 3–4 pints of group O Rhesus negative blood;
5. Bundle of blankets and hot-water bottles;
6. Oxygen cylinders and B.L.B. mask and fittings.

Today we would also insist on a portable anaesthetic apparatus for the administration of nitrous oxide, oxygen and a volatile anaesthetic agent and intermittent positive-pressure ventilation. Intubation equipment and an efficient suction machine, usually foot-operated, are also essential. Neonatal resuscitation equipment and an incubator for transporting the baby to hospital must also be immediately available.

It is quite clear that many of the cases whose deaths are described should never, by present-day standards, have been booked for domiciliary delivery, for example, cases of previous Caesarean section, diabetes, fibroids, previous postpartum haemorrhage, cardiac disease and toxic goitre, and the existence of flying squads should not encourage this type of practice.

There are two ways of regarding the function of a flying squad. The area covered, the state of the roads and transport facilities will to some extent determine the choice although these are rapidly becoming more uniform, especially with the addition of helicopter ambulances for island communities.

The Stabler point of view envisages a squad capable and ready to perform Caesarean hysterectomy, for example, on the kitchen table, on the ground that delay and transfer to hospital may be more dangerous than operating in primitive conditions. The other point of view, to which we subscribe, is that the function of the squad is to resuscitate the patient and to make her fit for the journey to hospital. With adequate transfusion this is nearly always possible.

The main difficulty about desperate surgery in desperate circumstances is the safety of anaesthesia and if the condition is not all that desperate the patient is far better off dealt with in hospital. On the other hand if her condition is truly desperate she is not in need of surgery but of resuscitation. The so-called minor anaesthetic can all too easily end in major catastrophe. There is no such thing as a minor anaesthetic. In both 1960 and 1961, 188 flying squad calls were answered from our hospital (376 cases). Postpartum haemorrhage, as might be expected, was the commonest reason, followed by retained placenta with or without bleeding. Antepartum haemorrhage came third, with abortion and eclampsia further down the list. Today antepatum haemorrhage is the commonest reason for sending out the squad. The number of calls is higher than ever before, mainly because of increased use made of the service by doctors outside. The results of applying the principle of full resuscitation and then removal of the patient to hospital accompanied by the squad and in the case of third-stage complications coverage with ergometrine, and in all cases, where indicated, by continuing blood transfusion would appear to justify this policy. There were no maternal deaths over many years and full aftercare of the patient is made possible. In our part of the world there is a shortage of anaesthetists and unless full and competent anaesthetic facilities can be provided, including mechanical suction and head-down tilting facilities, we feel that more lives are likely to be lost from anaesthetic accidents than will be saved by being operated on in the home. With our practice in a very crowded area, the distances are short and the ambulance service first-class. A different state of affairs exists, for example, in Lanarkshire where calls have to be answered from as far away as 20 miles. Liang (1963) has given a full account of the flying squad service of the Bellshill Maternity Hospital in this country. This squad is equipped with an ambulance with major resuscitating facilities, including the ability to tip the head down on a stretcher (Leslie, 1963). Even so it is felt by this squad that manual removal of the retained placenta is the only operative treatment that a flying squad team should perform in the home, or possibly the rapid extraction of a baby in a case of prolapse of the cord when the state of the cervix is suitable. Certainly our own policy is to remove the placenta, if possible, by the Brandt-Andrews technique or simple expression if it is already separated, rather than admit the patient unnecessarily to hospital, but we are not alone in our policy of regarding the squad as primarily a resuscitation team. Fraser and Tatford (1961) describe a similar set-up from St. James's Hospital in South London, where it is agreed this type of practice is suited to the urban type of service. Again in this service, if signs of placental separation are present the placenta is delivered by maternal effort, by simple fundal pressure, or by the Brandt-Andrews technique. If signs of separation are doubtful the patient is catheterised and if the placenta does not separate, an intravenous drip is set up and the patient is removed to hospital. She is not removed until her blood pressure has been restored to 100 mm systolic and is always kept in hospital under observation for 48 hours, and with this practice we would heartily agree. When manual removal was necessary, again it was performed in hospital. The patient is transferred, with an infusion running, in all cases in which the placenta fails to respond to one attempt at simple expression in the home or when postpartum haemorrhage exceeds a litre or in all patients in whom the blood pressure has at any time before or after the arrival of the squad fallen as low as 100 mm Hg. As in our case the patients are strictly supervised on the journey into hospital.

When a patient fails to recover her blood pressure in spite of resuscitative treatment a difficult diagnostic problem is, of course, posed, and uterine rupture looms large amongst the possibilities. All the more need, therefore, to get the patient into hospital where more efficient treatment can be given.

Alas, there is no safe and effective anaesthetic yet discovered for emergency operations by the flying squad in the home. Chloroform induction may be disapproved of by coroners, but is still much beloved of clinicians. A 1 in 8 mixture of chloroform in ether is a safe anaesthetic on a Schimmelbusch mask, but does not provide such a quick and smooth induction as open chloroform. For a very brief anaesthetic, such as for a manual removal of the placenta, intravenous thiopentone is probably the most widely used, but laryngeal spasm, and in all general anaesthetics the danger of inhaled vomit even after the passage of a stomach tube, occasionally provide a situation with all the ingredients of a shambles in the home. I, personally, will not undergo a general anaesthetic in a dental chair. I have yet to meet the dentist who has personal experience of external cardiac massage, let alone thoracotomy and I have yet to see the dental surgery with adequate bronchoscopic suction facilities. A woman emerging from a dangerous labour is in a much more dangerous situation and the same rules should apply.

There remains now the question of staffing. A junior house surgeon does not constitute a "squad". A very good composition is that of the Cape Town Obstetric Flying Squad (Hagberg, 1956), namely Obstetric Registrar and House Surgeon, Trained Sister and pupil midwife, and two medical students. He might have added an anaesthetist, since the anaesthetic is often the the most hazardous part of the venture.

Apropos the above remarks on the flying squad I received the following counterblast from the late Frank Stabler in a personal letter, which well deserves quoting:

> "With regard to the Flying Squad I remain unrepentant. It is transport that kills these women and the length of the journey is not important. It is the lifting out of bed on to a stretcher and at the other end, from a stretcher on to another bed. To transport a woman who is still bleeding or who has the placenta still *in utero* seems to me nonsense.
>
> I think the squad should be capable of facing anything and I think the talk of primitive conditions is just the delusion of hospital-minded people. What matters in coping with a patient is the man and his hands, not the site at which he is working. It is easier and more economical to do things in hospital but it is not safer.
>
> I once coped with a gamekeeper's daughter and to reach the house we drove a couple of miles over a moorland track and walked the last half mile over the heather. She had a central placenta praevia. In all she lived 45 miles from the nearest hospital. I doubt very much whether she would be alive today if we had resuscitated her and then transported her.
>
> I like your sentence, 'The main difficulty about desperate surgery in desperate circumstances is the safety of anaesthesia and if the condition is not all that desperate the patient is far better off dealt with in hospital.' One can transport an anaesthetist and his apparatus to the patient and we do so. You then say 'if she is not all that desperate she can be dealt with in hospital' but what if she *is* all that desperate, and lastly, the patient is no better off dealt with in hospital, only the surgeon is."

Treatment of Collapse

The following, in summary, is given as a practical guide in the steps to be taken, and the suggested order thereof:

1. Arrest haemorrhage, if any.
2. Ensure patient's airway.
3. Set up an intravenous drip of saline or plasma pending the arrival and cross-matching of blood. The decision to use blood and in what quantity to give it can be made presently. Do not give artificial plasma volume expanders, certainly not before grouping and blood cross-matching, with which they may interfere.
4. Give oxygen. Give morphia 15 mg.

Now start thinking carefully:

5. Find the fundus and note its size, shape, consistency and position.

6. If fundus satisfactory and bleeding controlled, wrap patient warmly, using hot-water bottles no hotter than warm and well covered.
7. Raise foot of bed.
8. Start serial blood pressure and pulse recordings.
9. Have the placenta examined for completeness.
10. Attend to transfusion rate of drip as appropriate: one unit of blood can be given safely in any case, for no labour is completely dry. If the drip is running too slowly because of vessel spasms, it can be encouraged by the addition of 3 ml of 0·2 per cent procaine to the drip.

A drip introduced by needle is always preferable to a "cut-down" since the flow already present in the vein helps to prevent spasm, but sometimes one has no choice.

Noradrenaline is now preferable to methedrine in profound shock and can be given 2–4 ml of Levophed 1 mg/ml diluted in a half-litre of saline. Another very potent vasopressor drug with a prolonged duration of action which we have found very useful is metaraminol bitartrate (Aramine) 1 per cent. This drug is supplied in 1 ml and 10 ml ampoules, each ml containing 10 mg. It is best to set up 15 to 100 mg in 500 ml of normal saline or 5 per cent glucose and to administer it as an intravenous infusion controlling the drip rate according to the response. In very severe emergencies, however, where an immediate effect is urgently required it is permissible to give from 0·5 mg to 5 mg (0·05 ml to 0·5 ml) by direct intravenous injection. The effect lasts from 20 minutes to one hour. The drip method is safer and to be preferred.

By now, the diagnostic field will have been narrowed. If in spite of the above measures the patient's condition still deteriorates or fails to rally, look for signs of internal bleeding. In arriving at a diagnosis remember that these are the conditions which must first be excluded:

(*a*) Uterus is not empty;
(*b*) Uterus is ruptured;
(*c*) Uterus is inverted.

Having got thus far, the other possibilities can be more quietly reviewed in the knowledge that for the moment all essential and prudent steps have been taken.

CARDIAC ARREST

There are two main types of cardiac arrest, namely, cardiac asystole and ventricular fibrillation. It is impossible to differentiate between the two except by electrocardiography or inspection of the heart after opening the pericardium, but in fact there is no pressing need to distinguish them because both require, with equal urgency, immediate cardiac massage if permanent brain damage is not to be inflicted. It is not even safe to count on the three or four minutes' grace said to be allowable after cardiac arrest, because the observation of arrest may not have been made immediately and in any case many valuable seconds can be lost with stethoscopes and sphygmomanometers in a futile attempt to satisfy oneself that the heart has in fact stopped. Meanwhile cerebral anoxia mounts.

Before stopping to think about the aetiology, the pathology and biochemistry associated with stoppage of the heart we must first consider the emergency action to be taken. Absence of bleeding, changes in heart rate and rhythm, especially bradycardia and cyanosis should already have alerted one to the possible diagnosis. To wait for the pupils to dilate is to wait too long. Palpation of the femoral or the carotid arteries or, if the abdomen is already open, of the abdominal aorta is the only diagnostic luxury one should allow oneself however.

The first thing to do is to give the patient a sound blow over the lower sternum, in fact a punch or two may start the heart again, and to secure an immediate airway. A Brook airway is admirable for the purpose. The head should be lowered into a head-down position and the legs should be held upright in order to increase the blood pressure in the cerebral vessels and to improve the venous return to the heart. No time should be lost at this stage in trying to make injections into the heart cavities and the first step after securing an airway by lowering the head and fully extending the neck is to start external cardiac massage, which requires only two strong hands and plenty of determination. If the patient is on a soft bed cardiac massage will not be effective and she should be dragged straight onto the hard floor. The object of external cardiac massage is not to restart the heart but to pump an adequate supply of oxygenated blood to the brain.

External Cardiac Massage

The heel of one hand is placed over the lower end of the sternum (not the xiphisternum) and the other is applied over it; the full weight of the operator's body from the waist upwards should be used to produce sharp depressions of the sternum at least 3 or 4 cm towards the vertebral column. This sharp compression should be completely released between each stroke. The number of compressions should be between 70 and 80 to the minute and especially in older patients the sternum or ribs may in fact be fractured, but this to Coroner's pathologists occasions no surprise nor criticism.

If single-handed this cardiac massage will have to be interrupted every minute or less to inflate the patient's lungs with three or four breaths, as when the prophet Elisha gave mouth-to-mouth respiration to the son of the Shunammite woman (II Kings, 4:34–35). The pharynx is cleared out with a swab wrapped round the finger, or by handkerchief, and the head is tilted right back to open up the airway and this, in fact, is more efficient than trying to lift forward the angles of the jaw. The nostrils are pinched closed, or the nose is closed off by pushing it sideways with the operator's cheek whilst he applies forceful exhalation pressure directly into the patient's mouth, or, if the mouth is kept closed, directly into her nose.

To discourage air going down the oesophagus into the stomach it may be a help to apply pressure to the epigastrium and to press backwards on the cricoid, but, above all, the head must be held tilted back in full extension. Gastric distension may easily provoke regurgitation of gastric contents straight into the operator's own face and mouth, and I can recall my own sense of shame and dismay at the disgust which I personally experienced on such an occasion. If an endotracheal tube is already in place and an anaesthetist present, ideal pulmonary ventilation can be properly maintained. Various double-ended airways are also often available amongst first-aid equipment.

The single-handed operator is at an enormous disadvantage without any equipment or help and the best he can do is to adopt an alternating pattern of activity of about two or three breaths of exhaled air for every dozen or less compressions of the heart. Help should, of course, be sent for but as Milstein has remarked "should not be waited for."

External cardiac massage by the closed method described above is not as efficient as internal cardiac massage following thoracotomy, but the difference is not all that great. Both types of cardiac massage produce a cardiac output of about one-sixth of what might be expected with a normally functioning heart. Nevertheless life can be effectively maintained for half an hour or so by the efficient use of it, while preparations to restart the heart are undertaken. Unfortunately, and this applies particularly to obstetrics, external cardiac massage is even less effective than internal when there has been massive haemorrhage, because the heart fills very poorly; hence the need to avail oneself of every possible drop of blood by raising the legs vertically. This unfortunately requires another pair of hands which one may not be able to spare. Obviously if there has been massive haemorrhage little will be gained by massaging an empty heart and massive transfusion will be required to fill it. Some favour intra-arterial transfusion, or, if the chest is already open, direct infusion into the cavity of the left ventricle via the apex. Normally there is no time for such refinements.

Air embolism as already discussed may produce a type of cardiac arrest which will not respond to cardiac massage; in fact the situation may be aggravated unless the air can be evacuated from the right side of the heart at once.

At the earliest possible moment the trachea should be intubated so that effective positive-pressure ventilation can be maintained regardless of cardiac massage, although it is preferable for the anaesthetist to regulate his ventilation of the lungs usually by manual bag-squeezing, so as not to coincide with the acts of sternal compression.

Internal Cardiac Massage

If external cardiac massage is to have any hope of success it must be capable of producing a palpable carotid or femoral pulse; in fact quite reasonable perfusion pressures can be achieved by this method, but, particularly after haemorrhage, this objective may not be achieved.

It should be possible to make up one's mind within the first minute or two whether external massage is being effective and if in any doubt to proceed at once to internal massage by thoracotomy. The first time I ever carried this out I made the mistake of remaining on the right hand side of the patient with the result that I had poor control of the extent of my incision or its depth and, in my haste, cut the underlying lung because of failure to wait the fraction of a second necessary for the lung to fall away from the parietal pleura with the opening of the cavity and I also accidentally incised part of the ventricular muscle wall of the heart, so that a few valuable seconds were lost in suturing, as well as yet more blood.

The incision should extend from the left edge of the sternum along the fourth, fifth or sixth intercostal space, right back, if possible, to the posterior axillary line, or as far as the hardness of the operating table will allow. Too small an incision makes the insertion of one or both hands very difficult. The time for care in making the incision is in opening the parietal pleura, as already suggested. If possible the internal mammary artery should be avoided at the anterior end of the incision but at the moment this hardly matters since it will not be bleeding anyway and can be ligated later before closing the chest. Asepsis though desirable is immaterial in such an emergency.

Having made the incision, extending as far back as possible, the ribs are retracted using both hands at first in order to insert one hand into the chest cavity, usually the left hand, if one is standing, as one should, on the left hand side of the patient. The use of a rib retractor will prevent a great deal of wrist discomfort and chafing. The hand should be passed right behind the heart and then a compression towards the deep surface of the sternum carried out. The other hand can supply counterpressure over the front of the sternum.

The heart may start beating on its own after the first few compressions, but if it does not there should be no hesitation in slitting open the pericardium, making first a small incision to allow the entry of air as in opening the peritoneal cavity in ordinary abdominal surgery and then extending the incision from the apex to the base of the heart anterior to the phrenic nerve which should be avoided. The incision can be enlarged towards the right at its lower end. Now it is possible to work with both hands, and very efficiently too, and the palms and thenar eminences should be used in preference to the points of the fingers which may damage the myocardium.

What is particularly discouraging is when the heart appears not to fill adequately between each compression and this is very likely to be experienced where massive haemorrhage has been one of the precipitating causes of the cardiac arrest. It is a mistake however which I have made in the past of waiting for cardiac filling as felt by the hands, which may reduce the massage rate to less than 50 a minute, and one should proceed at a rate of 80 whether the heart is filling or not, while awaiting the proper restoration of blood volume. If bleeding now begins to appear from the incision one has reason for congratulation, as there must be some sort of a circulation established. The bleeding points can now be secured.

The patient after half an hour begins to lose heat to a dangerous extent and it will not be easy to restore the heart beat below a temperature of 30 to 31 °C. Warm Ringer's solution poured into the chest may help to raise the heart temperature but this should be done with caution.

Once efficient cardiac massage, either internal or external, has been established the immediate emergency is over and some thought can be given to the cause of the cardiac arrest, its type and the method of restoring the heart beat. It is now important to distinguish between the two main types, namely cardiac asystole and ventricular fibrillation. An electrocardiograph machine will by now have been attached to the patient. The trace in the case of asystole simply shows a straight line whereas ventricular fibrillation shows a random and irregular electrical wave pattern. If the pericardium is already open the differential diagnosis can be made by looking at the heart. Coarse fibrillation is a more welcome sign than very feeble fibrillation which may escape notice. The former is said to feel like a "bag of worms".

In asystole the heart is soft, relaxed and motionless and as hypoxia is one of the commonest causes the coronary veins may look almost black. Ventricular fibrillation is revealed as an irregular twitching or unco-ordinated writhing.

The damaging effects of hypoxia on the heart must be realised and the need to counter it by adequate pulmonary ventilation at the same time must be met before one can hope to restart the heart. Hypoxia will of course, be aggravated by haemorrhage resulting in an inadequate circulating blood volume, by hypercapnia and anaesthetic drugs and the effects of a high level of serum potassium are particularly damaging. The conducting mechanism within the heart is sharply reduced by hypoxia. Hyperkalaemia can in fact be associated with either asystole or ventricular fibrillation, and potassium is released from all the tissues of the body under the influence of anoxia and can be still further raised by the transfusion of stored blood. A high potassium level causes a loss of conductivity within the heart whereas calcium ions increase the contractility and prolong systole and shorten diastole. The ratio of potassium to calcium ions is therefore important and must presently be corrected by the injection of calcium gluconate. In addition to this if, as is likely, a large transfusion is being given, the calcium ions will be necessary to combat the citrate effect of stored blood and it is our own practice after the first two units of blood to give 1 g usually as 10 ml of a 10 per cent solution of calcium gluconate for every two units of blood given after the first couple.

Quite apart from the damaging hydrodynamic effects of hypovolaemia, haemorrhage causes a release of large quantities of adrenaline into the circulation, one of the effects of which is to stimulate the liberation of potassium from the liver, so that hyperkalaemia may itself be an immediate precipitating cause of cardiac arrest. The avoidance therefore of haemorrhagic hypotension by prompt correction of blood volume deficiencies is an important prophylactic measure. To some extent intravenous digoxin may help to counter the effects of potassium intoxication of the heart, which is now suffering from diminished myocardial contractility.

The importance of distinguishing between asystole and ventricular fibrillation at this stage lies in the fact that there are certain differences in treatment, although asystole can turn to ventricular fibrillation and vice versa. If cardiac massage restores the heart beat the point is academic and this may suffice in cases suffering from an overdosage of the cocaine class of drugs, but if the heart beat does not recover following massage and the diagnosis of ventricular fibrillation is made, electrical defibrillation is most clearly called for. This procedure is bound to fail unless full oxygenation of the myocardium can first be obtained by cardiac massage and forced pulmonary ventilation. It is easier to defibrillate a heart which is in coarse ventricular fibrillation than in feeble, but massage may help to coarsen the variety of fibrillation in the first place. If not, the injection of adrenaline may help. Defibrillation can be carried out either externally or by direct application of electrodes to the front and back of the heart, preferably covered with lint made wet with

Ringer's solution in order to distribute the area of electrical shock. All assistants should stand well clear because voltages of some hundreds are used. Defibrillation may be followed by asystole and one should wait for at least a quarter of a minute in the hope of a spontaneous contraction starting up. Failing this, the heart must again be massaged. Most defibrillators work with alternating current. My own personal experience of high voltage (2000 volt) direct current defibrillation on each occasion has been while I was under an anaesthetic. I understand the jump on the table is impressive but I am glad not to have witnessed it in myself! Most units now have electrical defibrillators to hand, but in their absence one may have to resort to the use of procaine which diminishes myocardial irritability and helps to control fibrillation. It is not, however, an effective alternative to electrical defibrillation, although adrenaline may improve its efficacy. If procaine hydrochloride has to be used the dose is from 50 to 200 mg. If, however, it merely produces reduced tone in the myocardium and the defibrillation fails, 5 to 10 ml of 1 in 10,000 adrenaline should be given intravenously to restore a more vigorous type of fibrillation before making another attempt (Milstein).

Treatment of asystole.—As before, the first treatment is cardiac massage and forced pulmonary ventilation with 100 per cent oxygen. Five to ten ml of a 1 per cent solution of calcium chloride should be given at once, either intravenously or directly into an exposed heart chamber. A 10 per cent solution of this dosage has been recommended but is caustic and may cause necrosis if it misses its target. Adrenaline, 5 to 10 ml of a 1 in 10,000 solution, may also be effective in starting up a heart in asystole but may precipitate ventricular fibrillation which, however, can be electrically reversed. Again it must reach the coronary circulation to be effective locally and therefore active cardiac massage must be maintained in order to obtain an effect.

The direct intracardiac injection of drugs like calcium chloride or adrenaline in the case with the closed chest who has been maintained with external cardiac massage, is best made by inserting a long needle about 10 cm vertically through the fourth left space close to the sternum. If the heart is exposed the injection should be made into the left ventricle entering via the apex and taking care to aspirate blood to ensure that the point of the needle is within the ventricular cavity.

There is still hope as long as the myocardium shows signs of responding to massage, drugs or electrical defibrillation, even though repeated attempts to restart the heart may have to be made. Indeed coarse fibrillation is a far more encouraging sign than complete asystole or very fine and feeble fibrillation. Once the heart has been started the chest should not be closed for at least half an hour because of its liability to stop again, and mechanical respiration through an endotracheal tube should be maintained for hours, although if spontaneous respiration does not reappear within 12 hours the outlook is very gloomy.

Acidosis in cardiac arrest.—The damaging effects of hyperkalaemia have already been mentioned and these can be to some extent countered by improving the potassium/calcium ionic ratio by the intravenous injection of calcium gluconate, but it must not be forgotten that very severe metabolic acidosis comes on in a matter of minutes of cardiac arrest even though cardiac massage is promptly instituted. Our own rule-of-thumb method is to give 200 mEq of sodium bicarbonate, i.e. 200 ml of 8·4 per cent solution, as an immediate measure once other more pressing matters have been attended to and the following formula is recommended:

$$\text{Dose of sodium bicarbonate in mEq} = \text{weight of the patient in kg} \times \text{the duration of cardiac arrest in minutes} \times \tfrac{1}{10}$$

The immediate availability of micro-Astrup biochemical control of the blood chemistry is a great help.

Further care.—After half-an-hour's observation to see that cardiac activity is maintained, the pericardium may be closed. This should only be partial and designed to prevent the apex of the heart from herniating outwards, and water-tight closure may embarrass the heart's action or may cause tamponade from haemopericardium. Milstein recommends the use of interrupted sutures at intervals of 2 cm along the lowest 5 to 6 cm of the percardial incision, the upper two-thirds being left open. The mammary artery must be secured preferably by under-running sutures as its ends retract easily and after dealing with any other bleeding points a spray of Polybactrin may be squirted into the wound, or some other antibiotic powder, and the ribs should be approximated with a few pericostal sutures of strong catgut. The intercostal muscles are then sutured with continuous catgut as much as possible and a separate suture layer for the pectoral muscles. The incision must be made airtight to enable the patient to breathe and a drainage tube of wide bore should be inserted into the pleural space in the lateral chest wall well below the original incision and sutured to the skin. The free end is connected to an underwater seal. A mechanical suction pump applied to the drainage bottle may assist pulmonary expansion and pleural cavity drainage.

At the earliest safe opportunity the patient should be moved into an intensive care unit for follow-up treatment, which may include hypothermia for suspected brain damage and supervision for anuria, assisted respiration and biochemical control.

Summary of Immediate Emergency Steps

1. Don't waste time—it only wastes life.
2. Head down and tilted back.
3. Two or three precordial punches.
4. Clear airway and inflate lungs for three or four breaths.
5. External cardiac massage—if necessary on hard floor.
6. If ineffective, perform thoracotomy without wasting time on asepsis.
7. Internal cardiac massage.
8. Continue pulmonary ventilation.
9. Transfuse as necessary.
10. If internal cardiac massage ineffective open pericardium and massage heart.

Total permissible elapsed time to date—3 minutes.

From now on, treatment can be more planned and deliberate with the help of assistants.

There is no longer any such thing in maternity hospitals as acceptable sudden death. A harrowing three-hour ritual lies ahead before the diagnosis of maternal death is likely to be acknowledged and all hope finally abandoned.

REFERENCES

1. *British Medical Journal* (1957). Editorial, **1,** 453.
2. Fraser, A. C. and Tatford, E. P. W. (1961). *Lancet*, **2,** 126.
3. Govan, A. D. T. and McGillivray, I. (1950). *J. Obstet. Gynaec. Brit. Emp.*, **57,** 233.
4. Hagberg, C. J. (1956), *S. Afr. med. J.*, **30,** 1140.
5. Leslie, D. W. (1963). *J. Obstet. Gynaec. Brit. Cwlth.*, **70,** 291.
6. Liang, D. Y. S. (1963). *J. Obstet. Gynaec. Brit. Cwlth.*, **70,** 83.
7. McCormick, P. W. (1966). *Proc. roy. Soc. Med.*, **59,** 66.
8. Mendelson, C. L. (1946). *Amer. J. Obstet. Gynec.*, **52,** 191.
9. Milstein, B. B. (1963). *Cardiac Arrest and Resuscitation.* London: Lloyd-Luke (Medical Books).
10. Murdoch, R. (1962). *Lancet*, **1,** 1327.
11. Parker, R. B. (1954). *Brit. med. J.*, **2,** 65.
12. Sheehan, H. L. (1948). *Lancet*, **1,** 1.
13. Sheehan, H. L. and Murdoch, R. (1938). *J. Obstet. Gynaec. Brit. Emp.*, **45,** 456.
14. Stabler, F. (1947). *Brit. med. J.*, **2,** 878.
15. Steiner, P. E. and Lushbaugh, C. C. (1941). *J. Amer. med. Ass.*, **117,** 1245 and 1340.
16. Taylor, G. and Pryse-Davies, J. (1966). *Lancet*, **1,** 288.
17. Tindall, V. R. (1965). *Proc. roy. Soc. Med.*, **59,** 63.
18. Vance, J. P. (1968). *Anaesthesia*, **23,** 94.
19. Willocks, J., Mone, J. G. and Thomson, W. J. (1966). *Brit. med. J.*, **2,** 1181.

CHAPTER XXII

POSTPARTUM HAEMORRHAGE

"If you can fill the unforgiving minute with sixty seconds worth of distance run."—KIPLING.

THIS is indeed the unforgiving stage of labour, and in it there lurks more unheralded treachery than in both the other stages of labour combined. The normal case can, within a minute, become abnormal and successful delivery can turn swiftly to disaster. The obstetrician's judgment must be sure and swift, and errors of commission carry with them penalties as great, or greater, than those of omission. Increasing experience serves only to sharpen one's alertness during this stage, and there is no room for complacency in any case, however normal, until the placenta has been delivered for at least half an hour, with the uterus well retracted and with minimal bleeding.

It is far more important to understand the physiology of this stage of labour than to know the mechanisms of the second stage and the only safe management is one based upon this knowledge.

PHYSIOLOGY OF THE THIRD STAGE

An excellent opportunity is afforded at Caesarean section to observe the process of placental separation and uterine retraction, for both the inside and the outside of the uterus can be watched at the same time. The shrinkage of the uterus which occurs after the delivery of the baby is not a rapid phenomenon as in the case of skeletal muscle contraction, but occurs almost surreptitiously. It is after a few minutes that the pallor of the uterus and the wrinkling of its surface bear witness to the immense degree of retraction which has been taking place. As seen at operation this shrinkage would appear to be a gradual and progressive phenomenon, and this fact alone should stress the importance of never hurrying the third stage.

Intermittent contractions are of course superimposed, but as a rule they are not usually noticeable to the hand palpating through the abdominal wall for at least ten minutes; it would appear that the contractile activity of the uterus is, for a short while, somewhat in abeyance after the effort of delivering the fetus, although retraction continues progressively. In twin delivery the uterus appears to take a similar rest after the delivery of the first child.

The method of placental separation can also be witnessed profitably at Caesarean section. The commonest mechanism is that associated with the name of Schultze, in which the central portion separates first, followed by a concentrically enlarging area so that the placenta bulges into view with the centre of the fetal surface presenting. For a long time it was thought that this mechanism was caused by the collection of blood behind the centre of the placenta which spread towards its margin, thus completing separation, but this retroplacental haematoma is now regarded as a result of separation rather than a cause.

The other method is that described by Matthews Duncan in which the placenta as a whole is sheared off the uterine wall and presents with its inferior margin first. It is very much less common and is probably more often associated with difficulties in spontaneous delivery of the placenta. The membranes, moreover, are more easily torn instead of being peeled off progressively as in Schultze's method.

The reason for placental separation is almost certainly the mechanical effect of shearing, for the area of the placental site is reduced to a diameter of 10 cm or less, to which the bulk of the placenta cannot readily accommodate itself. In normal cases there is not much resistance in the decidua at the plane of cleavage. The membranes, however, are often very adherent and, having no appreciable bulk, are not sheared off the uterine wall by the reduction in area to which they are attached. This phenomenon, too, can be demonstrated at Caesarean section. The placental mass progressively peels off the membranes, but it is not uncommon for the latter to delay for a time the spontaneous delivery of the placenta. It is at this stage that fundus fiddling becomes particularly dangerous as, thereby, retroplacental blood may be forced to track towards the outside world between the membranes and the uterine wall. Once this track has been formed, blood can trickle away continually while the placental mass, by its retention *in utero*, discourages uterine retraction. Further bleeding can now go on to the point of exsanguination. A failed attempt at Credé's expression often demonstrates this, but in more serious degree.

The presence of blood clot, or placenta, or both within the uterine body may stimulate contractions, but inevitably interferes with retraction, and only the latter will safeguard the patient against postpartum haemorrhage.

The greater part of the uterine musculature is composed of the intermediate criss-cross layer of muscle fibres which are arranged trellis fashion, and through the interstices of which the maternal blood vessels supplying the placental site run a tortuous course. Closing the gaps in this trellis by retraction shuts off the supply of blood to the placental site, and for this reason these fibres are known as "the living ligatures of the uterus".

More often than not the placenta is separated from its attachment to the uterine wall with the contraction which completes the delivery of the baby's body, provided this is not hurried, and only the adherence of the membranes, the temporary cessation of further uterine contractions and the rest from bearing down efforts which the patient takes, delay the immediate delivery of the placenta.

A marked change overtakes the patient as a whole immediately following the birth of her child. Whereas she was hot, she now feels cold and starts to shiver, and often the maternal blood pressure undergoes a temporary fall following the exertions of the second stage. This may contribute some protection against the risks of postpartum haemorrhage. There does not, hitherto, appear to have been much study of the immediate behaviour of the blood pressure in the first few minutes following delivery, but the hypotension is only transitory. There is some rise in blood pressure during the uterine contractions of the second stage.

It is popular nowadays to refer to a fourth stage of labour and its dangers, but this seems to be unnecessary, for the patient who bleeds half an hour after the delivery of her placenta is, in fact, a case of third-stage haemorrhage, inasmuch as it is due to inadequate retraction of the uterus which is part of the essential mechanism of the third stage.

Management of the Third Stage

More tuition is concentrated upon this matter in the training of undergraduates and midwives that on any other part of the subject, yet faulty management remains one of the commonest sources of trouble. It is customary to conduct this stage with the patient in the dorsal position, mainly for two reasons: firstly, the abdomen can be more easily examined, and secondly, the exact amount of blood lost can be collected in a dish, the edge of which is kept pressed against the perineum. A very suitable dish for the purpose and one which we use in preference to the usual kidney dish has been designed and described by Murdoch (1958). The importance of blood accountancy is dealt with fully in the chapter on postpartum collapse; suffice it to mention here that it is impossible to relate a patient's general state to the factor of haemorrhage without knowing exactly the extent of the loss involved. Blood allowed to run over the sheets or into a bucket is blood left out of the reckoning and the amount is usually a great deal more than appearances would suggest.

On the vexed subject of early or late clamping of the cord and its influence on the amount of blood "transfused" from placenta to baby, the strength of uterine contraction at the very end of the second stage, or the very beginning of the third stage, is what really determines the quantity rather than the time interval before clamping. In the healthy baby the transfusion is partly completed by the end of one minute and fully at three minutes. Oxytocic drugs accelerate the process so that one minute suffices to complete it.[11] Respiration does not appear to affect placental transfusion.

In this country many patients complete the second stage of labour in the left lateral position, it being believed, perhaps wrongly, that the perineum can be more easily saved from "damage". The great disadvantage, however, is the need to turn the patient over on to her back in the third stage, and this is always one of the more anxious moments. Many times I have witnessed a brisk gush of blood accompanying the shift of position, and it occurs at a time when one is relatively more disorganised. For those, therefore, who conduct normal delivery in the left lateral position, certain precautions should be taken in turning the patient on to her back, the most important of which is to ensure that the fundus of the uterus is hard and well contracted before starting and the knees should be kept together while moving. This will keep the labia in apposition and discourage the possibility, admittedly remote, of air embolism through the placental site should placental separation have occurred already.

During the ensuing period of waiting the patient is cold and acutely conscious of the wetness round her buttocks, and it is difficult to keep her warm because of the need to keep the abdomen uncovered for examination and inspection. The only safe coverings for the thighs at this time are sterile drapes which are not always available, although they certainly should be. While waiting for the signs of placental separation to appear, the time can profitably be passed by allowing the patient to handle her child and, wherever feasible, to put it to the breast. This has a remarkable effect on uterine activity.

Signs of placental separation.—There are only two of really convincing value. The first of these, namely feeling the placenta by vaginal examination, is commonly frowned upon, although I have no hesitation in surreptitiously making such an examination after a forceps delivery because already enough intravaginal interference has occurred to make further cautious vaginal examination of no moment. The other convincing sign is that of lengthening of the cord, and when observed there is never any doubt about it, for it is never less than several inches and often as many as six or more (15 cm). This invaluable sign is all too often missed and usually unnecessarily so. In separating the baby from its mother the very first step should be to apply a clamp to the cord as close as possible to the vulva after gently lifting up any slack which may be in the vagina. The other clamp can then be applied towards the fetal end of the cord, as usual, and the cord severed.

Now, for some reason which I have never been able to fathom, tutors in midwifery persist in the ridiculous ritual of making the clumsy-fingered student tie bits of twisted string neatly, and about half an inch apart, at the chosen point of cord division. A little piece of wool is then applied to collect the small drop of blood which appears on cutting the cord with scissors, as if such finesse mattered at all in the face of the general messiness of labour! What matters, of course, is that during all this misguided activity cord-lengthening passes unobserved, whereas a clamp applied at the vulva as aforesaid will leave one in no doubt. A very senior midwife once told me that it would not be safe to teach the method of applying the proximal clamp close to the vulva for fear of the adventitious structures which might be included by the flustered pupil. Horrid thought!

The other signs of separation are less conclusive. The fundus of the uterus becomes globular, like a cricket ball, instead of pyriform and somewhat flattened. This is because the placenta has left the upper uterine segment which is now empty and well retracted. Unfortunately, especially in well-covered patients, mistakes in interpretation are made every hour of every day. The uterus is said to become more mobile, as is indeed the case when the bulk of the placenta is sitting in the vaginal vault, but the elicitation of this sign savours of fundus fiddling. The level of the fundus rises after expulsion of the placenta from the upper segment, but this is also true of the uterus which is filled with blood and is too unreliable a sign. A bulge is sometimes visible above the symphysis pubis, but this too may be misinterpreted and may be due to the presence of urine in the bladder. Lastly, a test of placental separation frequently employed must be mentioned only to condemn it in unequivocal terms: it consists in drawing the uterus upwards by manipulation through the abdominal wall and observing if any length of cord is dragged into the vagina from its previous position over the fourchette and perineum. This is hardly good asepsis. Such a test is both unreliable and meddlesome.

Very often, as if to satisfy curiosity, the fundus is seized and pushed downwards to see if this effects delivery of the placenta and, times without number, this hit-or-miss type of diagnosis is the signal for a train of events which starts with a trickle of blood and a protest from the patient and ends in near disaster. Many books still refer to the small gush of blood as being one of the signs of placental separation. This is bad teaching and true only in so far that bleeding could not occur at all unless there was some degree of separation.

Unfortunately, this sign gives no indication of whether or not the separation is complete. It does, however, indicate that blood collecting behind the placenta has now found a vent to the outside world and that the former restrictions on handling of the fundus now no longer apply.

"Controlling the fundus."—A hand is gently laid upon the abdominal wall over the fundus to observe it, but in some institutions the fear is so great that the fundus will be kneaded, pummelled, pushed about and generally fiddled with that this practice is forbidden and reliance is placed upon visual observation of its contour, looking tangentially across the abdominal wall. Anyone, however, who cannot be taught to keep his hand on the fundus absolutely still should be strongly advised not to take up midwifery. It is commonly thought that the hand in this position can control the fundus from rising and from filling up with blood. This of course is nonsense, because an atonic uterus will fill up with blood wherever one's hand is placed. One might well ask, then, what is the purpose in applying the hand to the abdominal wall at all. It is undoubtedly valuable and superior to visual observation: firstly, the state of uterine activity can be observed as the uterus hardens and softens with the return of uterine contractions; secondly, the subsidiary signs of placental separation can be observed, and thirdly, and perhaps this is the most important reason, the fundus does not get lost. Without a hand constantly aware of the exact position of the fundus one may, in the presence of a sudden brisk haemorrhage, be in doubt at first as to whether the fundus is under the costal margin or inverted into the vagina, and some valuable seconds may be lost in the search.

Throughout the period of waiting the right hand is kept immersed in a bowl of antiseptic, not so much in order that a manual removal of the placenta may be immediately undertaken as to keep the hand sterile for the subsequent examination of the perineum. "With the patient's welfare in mind, an impatient obstetrician is far better off doing gynaecology."[24]

Since the third stage is always a time of anxiety which no obstetrician every wholly outlives, there is a very natural tendency to wish to get it over, but in cases in which oxytocic drugs have not been given at the end of the second stage it is a valuable rule to regard a minimum period of twenty minutes as essential for the safe delivery of the placenta, even though one may be reasonably satisfied that the signs of placental separation have already occurred. Now this may seem an extreme view, and one might argue that it is pointless to wait after the placenta has left the upper uterine segment. Mistakes, however, are so often made that it is a pity to grudge the few extra precautionary minutes. In almost all cases this patience will be rewarded by the uterus completing its physiological functions fully, and there are only three admissible reasons for ignoring this simple practice: firstly, haemorrhage, which of course demands treatment in its own right; secondly, in cases in which the patient is already under an anaesthetic and there may be very good reasons for terminating the operation; and thirdly, after the intravenous use of oxytocic drugs. As a student I attended for a fortnight a hospital where this twenty-minute rule was in force, and although the rule was not always intelligently applied, inasmuch as attempts were often made to secure the delivery of the placenta whether signs of separation had occurred or not, nevertheless these injudicious attempts were made with impunity, because sufficient time had been allowed for the uterus to assume full control of the situation. Only if the patient voluntarily expels her own placenta should the third stage be shortened in the normal case.

Delivery of the placenta.—After the lapse of a measured twenty minutes and with the evidences of separation present, it is infinitely preferable to get the patient to expel her own placenta than to resort to pressure upon the fundus. The routine use of the uterus as a piston to drive out the placenta is usually unnecessary and probably damaging to the uterine supports, and to many patients, in retrospect, this is accounted the most unpleasant part of labour. The patient's co-operation should in all cases be sought and encouraged. With the uterus well retracted and hard, like a cricket ball, she is exhorted to bear down. Support to the flabby abdominal wall with the flat of the hand is often a great help.

Cord traction.—This has been traditionally denounced as a dangerous practice. To be honest, we all do it. It is, of course, particularly humiliating if the cord breaks off, and it makes a surprising amount of mess too. There is little harm in the practice provided the placenta is wholly out of the upper uterine segment, in which case there is less need for it. Counter-control through the abdominal wall should always be applied on the body of the uterus with the other hand, otherwise the cervix, and perhaps more, may easily appear at the vulva. The position is altogether different when the placenta is still within the upper segment, and inversion of the uterus is only as uncommon as it is thanks to the fact that fundal insertion of the placenta is unusual, and to the fact that most people respect the rules! To exert cord traction with the fundus of the uterus anything but firmly contracted is certainly asking for trouble.

The use of one hand, with the palmar surfaces of the fingers applied to the anterior surface of the uterus at the level of the junction of upper and lower segments, thus drawing the uterus upwards, is an important part of the cord traction manoeuvre. This method of delivering the placenta is now usually known as the Brandt-Andrews method of delivery, after the two men who described and practised it independently.[5, 1] It is also known as controlled cord traction.[15]

The important feature of the manoeuvre is not the pulling on the cord, as has been witnessed in apes at delivery, but the dragging upwards at the same time of the uterus towards the umbilicus. The direction in which the cord is pulled is also important. This should be somewhat downwards and backwards. The attendant stands on the patient's right and with the flat of the left hand facing towards the patient's head the uterus is pushed upwards and backwards while the right hand draws the cord downwards and backwards. This has the effect of straightening out the genital canal in line with the pull on the placenta. To those formerly used to delivering the placenta by pushing on the fundus as a piston, the temptation to pull on the cord and at the same time press downwards on the fundus is very natural, but this defeats the whole object of the exercise because it curls the uterus over in anteversion, re-forming the right angled bend of the genital canal and making the traction on the cord totally ineffective unless the placenta is already in the vagina. Another common mistake is to pull the cord too far forwards and upwards.

Cords vary enormously in their tensile strength and with firm and steadily increasing tension a tearing sensation may easily be felt. Clearly the cord is now going to break and it may be necessary to desist and wait for further descent of the placenta spontaneously. The patient can greatly reduce the amount of tractive effort necessary on the cord by bearing down herself at the same time.

These attempts can be repeated every two or three minutes only synchronously with complete hardening of the uterus of course, but if delivery of the placenta is not achieved within twenty minutes by this technique one should be ready to recognise the need for manual removal of the placenta.

Controlled cord traction, following the use of intravenous ergometrine given with the delivery of the anterior shoulder, is recommended as a routine procedure in normal cases by Spencer (1962), who considered the method safe and a desirable alternative to Credé's expression. In a thousand of her cases the umbilical cord broke in twenty-six but no harm came of this. She believes that if the placenta is still attached to the uterine wall, controlled cord traction will not succeed and this is certainly true wherever there is morbid adherence of the placenta, but in such cases nothing short of manual removal is likely to succeed. It is claimed for the method that the third stage is appreciably shortened and the total amount of blood lost much reduced even in normal cases. The manual removal rate is not increased as a result of using this technique. A constriction ring, or a cervix that has closed down, may prevent the delivery of the placenta, and sometimes the inhalation of amyl nitrite works like a charm, one capsule being broken under a mask over the patient's nose. The treatment may be repeated if necessary, but failure or continued bleeding calls for manual removal of the placenta forthwith.[15]

There is one possible disadvantage of controlled cord traction as a routine method of shortening the third stage and that is, in my experience, the somewhat increased tendency of the uterus to relax and fill with blood about ten minutes or so later, but this has to be offset against the frequent occurrence of slow filling of the uterus with blood before delivery of the placenta in cases of unhurried spontaneous third stage.

The practice in my own unit is to give an intramuscular injection of Syntometrine (1 ml containing 0·5 mg ergometrine and 5 units of synthetic oxytocin) at the end of the second stage and not to use other routine methods of accelerating the third stage. Where the intravenous route is used, usually as a prophylaxis against haemorrhage following instrumental delivery especially under epidural anaesthesia, oxytocin (5 units) has been found to be as effective as ergometrine and far less likely to provoke vomiting. Oxytocin is also preferred, because of fewer cardiovascular side-effects in cases of hypertension and cardiac disease.[21]

Where labour is completely normal and there is no bleeding we teach our students to wait and to watch for signs of spontaneous placental separation, to keep a hand on the fundus only when it cannot be clearly seen through the abdominal wall in order to avoid losing it and, after the lapse of adequate time for full spontaneous placental separation, to get the patient to deliver the placenta by her own expulsive efforts. This is undoubtedly the right approach for pupil midwives and undergraduate students. Any third-stage difficulty calls for more qualified intervention, as is described later.

Retained membranes.—The weight of the placenta after delivery should always be supported so that it does not wholly drag upon the membranes and tear them. Suspending the placenta by the cord and twisting the membranes into a rope is quite good practice but, above all, the complete delivery of the membranes depends upon gentleness, patience and care. The fundus of the uterus should be massaged vigorously during the procedure, and this helps to loosen the membranes from the uterine wall by ensuring full uterine retraction. Should a portion of chorion break away and not be delivered, it is no very serious matter and certainly does not justify exploring the uterine cavity.

Retention of placental tissue.—The placenta should be examined as soon as possible, and if it is found that a cotyledon or a succenturiate lobe is missing, the only safe thing to do is to anaesthetise the patient and explore the uterine cavity with the gloved finger forthwith. To yield to the temptation of hoping that all will be well and that the administration of ergometrine will suffice is to take a serious risk. One may be tempted to adopt this foolish, optimistic attitude either because the patient has had a perfectly normal delivery and one is, therefore, reluctant to take radical measures once everything is apparently over, or because the patient has had a dangerous delivery and one is reluctant to add to her trials by yet further operative procedures. It can only be answered that, in the first instance, the patient is easily well enough to stand it, and in the second, she may be too ill to withstand the far more serious risk of the inevitable secondary postpartum haemorrhage.

It is customary to examine the placenta for missing cotyledons by cupping it, concave, in the palms of two hands, but this method easily conceals any missing gaps and it is better to examine the placenta convex over the backs of both hands to reproduce its attitude *in utero*. In nearly all cases of secondary haemorrhage from whom quite sizeable amounts of placental tissue have subsequently been removed on uterine exploration, reference to the notes indicates that there was no sign of any missing cotyledons, which shows the inadequacy of the traditional method. The possibility of a retained succenturiate lobe will be indicated by the appearance of torn vessels running up to the edge of the rent in the membranes.

In exploring the uterus one may be dismayed by the impression of roughness of the placental site to the examining finger, but careful examination will reveal whether or not placental tissue is still within the uterine cavity.

Leaving the patient.—The patient should not be left unattended as long as the placenta is still within the genital tract, nor should she be left until a full hour after delivery is completed. The so-called fourth stage has already been referred to and is a period commonly marred by haemorrhage. Apart from retained placental tissue, already mentioned, the chief cause of bleeding is the gradual collection of a large clot of blood within the uterine cavity. Nothing begets haemorrhage so much as haemorrhage, and the presence of a clot *in utero* interferes with uterine retraction and encourages atony.

Before leaving the patient, therefore, the fundus should be examined, firm contraction secured by kneading, and the body of the uterus should then be squeezed to make quite sure that the uterus is empty. The amount of blood appearing at the vulva which is permissible should be no more than sufficient to soil a pad in the course of an hour or two. Any bleeding in excess of this amount demands treatment.

Ergometrine in the Third Stage of Labour

This life-saving drug has made all the difference to the safety of labour. Formerly its use was taboo until after the delivery of the placenta because, it was preached, a constriction ring with hour-glass retention of the placenta would occur. This theory, in common with so much traditional teaching, is not true, and the use of ergometrine as a prophylaxis against haemorrhage before placental separation has everything to recommend it, provided that the uterus is not subjected to handling. Anything is better than the loss of blood—even a constriction ring, should it occur.

It is now known that the incidence of hour-glass contraction is not increased by the use of oxytocic drugs at the beginning of the third stage, and that in those cases in which this complication occurred a history of abortive attempts at Credé's expression could nearly always be elicited. In the past, accidents from pituitary preparations were not uncommon and were occasionally associated with profound shock. Modern commercial preparations of oxytocin are better purified and safer than before, nevertheless there seems to be no good reason for preferring even these to ergometrine, which is known to be both safe and reliable. The combination of both in one preparation such as Syntometrine (Sandoz) appears to be ideal.

In many hospitals throughout the country an intramuscular injection of 0·5 mg of ergometrine has become routine as soon as the head is delivered or alternatively at the very beginning of the third stage. The injection can be simply given by the midwife, and within a few minutes the uterus demonstrates a very healthy tone. Workers in these institutions are usually emphatic about the benefits, and although the actual incidence of postpartum haemorrhage is only to some extent lowered, the significant fact is that the size of the haemorrhage, when it does occur, is very much less. In other words, there may be almost as many blood losses of over 500 ml but there are many fewer cases of blood losses of over a litre, and it is this second factor which matters most.

It might be as well to ask if there are any drawbacks. There is certainly one serious risk, namely the case of the undiagnosed twin. To give ergometrine while the second twin has still to be delivered is certainly a serious matter, made even worse should the lie not be longitudinal, and the child must be very expeditiously delivered if it is to survive the uterine spasm which occurs as a result of ergometrine.

If ergometrine is given intravenously as a prophylactic measure against haemorrhage, the timing of the injection is important if the best results are to be obtained. Its administration should coincide with the crowning of the head or with the delivery of the anterior shoulder. Thereafter, the delivery of the body should await the contractile response of the uterus. By this means satisfactory separation of the placenta is encouraged.

An effect which is almost as rapid can be obtained by the intramuscular injection of ergometrine coupled with hyaluronidase and Kimbell[14] in comparing 1700 cases so treated at the moment of crowning, with 700 untreated controls, found that the incidence of haemorrhage was nine times as high in the latter and that the manual removal rate was not increased as a result of ergometrine so given. He, too, inclined to the view that retention of the placenta may be encouraged if the drug is given too late, for example, after the delivery of the child's body.

With the help of tocographic studies Embrey and his colleagues at Oxford have explored the advantages of using a combination of oxytocin for its speed of action and ergometrine for its duration of effect (Syntometrine). They confirmed tocographically that hyaluronidase accelerated the action of intramuscular ergometrine by about two minutes. Having found that the full effect after intramuscular injection of ergometrine alone was as slow as seven minutes this, in their opinion, was a rather disappointing improvement, and the addition, of oxytocin was found to speed up the response of the uterus.[10, 11, 12] The observations of the Oxford workers have been abundantly confirmed by others using Syntometrine in Worcester, Manchester and by ourselves and it would appear that intramuscular Syntometrine makes as good a substitute as can be obtained for intravenous ergometrine under circumstances in which such an intravenous injection cannot be given. There remains the one debatable point, having given Syntometrine, whether to adopt a highly active policy and secure delivery of the placenta forthwith by fundal pressure or controlled cord traction, or to wait for signs of placental separation. Our own view at the moment is that after giving Syntometrine, and provided there is no bleeding, there is nothing to be lost by waiting a few minutes and allowing time for the placenta to descend at least some distance down the genital canal, peeling off the membranes behind it.

The oxytocic response of intravenous ergometrine is fully established within forty-one seconds (average time) as against nearly five minutes with intramuscular ergometrine plus hyaluronidase, and seven minutes with ergometrine alone intramuscularly, but Syntometrine is effective within two and a half minutes.[12]

Definition of postpartum haemorrhage.—The definition of postpartum haemorrhage is arbitrary. Blood losses of over half a litre are almost universally accepted as indicating postpartum haemorrhage, whether it comes from the placental site or from laceration of the genital tract. This standard is not wholly satisfactory, for the danger of postpartum haemorrhage depends more upon the rate at which blood is lost than upon its actual amount, and the patient's ability to withstand haemorrhage has also to be taken into account. However, for statistical purposes, it serves well enough. The usual time-limit set for the application of this definition is up to 24 hours after delivery. Thereafter bleeding is designated "secondary postpartum haemorrhage" (see later).

Causes of Postpartum Haemorrhage

Apart from lacerations, uterine inversion and clotting defects (which are dealt with elsewhere), there is only one cardinal cause of postpartum haemorrhage, namely anything which interferes with retraction of the uterus as a whole and of the placental site in particular. In the majority of instances this is because the uterus is, for various reasons, atonic. Less commonly mechanical factors may play a part, such as the presence of fibroids or a partial pathological adherence of the placenta to the uterine wall preventing emptying, however good the uterine tone. Inversion is dealt with elsewhere, but it must be remembered that it may be accompanied by severe haemorrhage. It will be seen, therefore, that the majority of cases are due to imperfect retraction as a result of uterine atony, and the remarks just made about the routine use of ergometrine apply in this direction. It is therefore necessary to seek for the factors which predispose to uterine atony. The retention of the placenta may be the cause of imperfect retraction because of morbid adherence, but is far more commonly the effect, since morbid adherence is rather unusual and certainly not as common as operators describe in recounting their experiences in manual removal.

Factors which predispose to uterine atony in the third stage.—High degrees of multiparity probably constitute the commonest cause, and this fact has never been wholly satisfactorily explained, for the grand multipara usually goes through the first and second stages of labour exhibiting the very reverse of sluggish uterine action. It may well be that, in her case, uterine contractions occur with a vigour out of all proportion to the ability of the uterus to retract, a fact which comes fully to light only in the third stage. After the first four or five deliveries each successive labour carries a somewhat greater risk of postpartum haemorrhage, and since these women, often as a result of rapidly repeated childbirth, overwork, poverty, malnutrition and chronic iron-deficiency anaemia, are in a poorer condition to withstand even a moderate postpartum haemorrhage, it will be seen that the effects are far more serious.

The next most important predisposing factor is that of multiple pregnancy. In cases of twins (and hydramnios too) the uterus, because of over-distension, may be lacking in retractile power; but even more important is the fact that in twins the double placenta is a relatively large structure, which is less readily delivered, and the area of the placental site is greatly increased so that bleeding, when it does occur, is doubly profuse. Added to all this there is the possibility that some of the large placental site area has overlapped on to the lower uterine segment where retractile power is poor.

Placenta praevia itself, besides causing inevitable antepartum haemorrhage, is often a cause of postpartum haemorrhage, the effects of which are aggravated by the antecedent bleeding, and it is a strange paradox that one of the commonest causes of death in APH should be PPH. The same obtains in cases of accidental haemorrhage, and the most terrible haemorrhage I have ever witnessed followed delivery of a woman with abruptio placentae.

Uterine exhaustion following a prolonged, inert labour is often classed as one of the principal causes of postpartum haemorrhage, though this has not been my experience. It is certain that when haemorrhage does occur its effects are more pronounced because the patient is already dehydrated as a result of her labour. It is the loss of available circulating fluid rather than the number of available red cells which accounts for the immediate evidences of shock in postpartum haemorrhage. With regard to prolonged labour it must be remembered that many of these cases have been fairly heavily narcotised and the uterine atony in the third stage is often due to drugs and anaesthetics.

Precipitate labour is quite often followed by postpartum haemorrhage which is not necessarily due to grand multiparity. It is probable that in these cases the placenta is detached at the end of a precipitate second stage, and the uterus, which in any case requires a few minutes to achieve retraction, is unable immediately to follow up its sudden emptying with suitably maintained shrinkage.

Anaesthetics produce atony more as a result of the depth of general narcosis achieved than because of individual drug propensities, and for this reason chloroform and ether are reputedly dangerous in high dosage. Nevertheless, certain drugs seem to affect the uterus less adversely than others, notably cyclopropane, the use of which I always welcome during Caesarean section, not only for this reason, but also because of the high oxygenation rate with which it is given. Relaxant drugs of the curare class do not interfere with uterine contraction, nor do the lighter anaesthetics like nitrous oxide or Trilene. General debilitating diseases predispose the patient to some extent to postpartum haemorrhage, but their chief contribution lies in magnifying its effect.

Most people are agreed that a patient with a previous history of retained placenta runs an appreciably greater risk of the same misfortune in subsequent deliveries. It would seem only prudent, therefor, to deliver such a case in an institution. Dewhurst and Dutton (1957) in a review of 132 labours in which there had been a previous history of abnormal third stage found that in 23 per cent this stage was again abnormal and that even one or more intervening labours without trouble did not eliminate the dangers of recurrent mishaps in the third stage of the next labour. A woman, therefore, who has once had third-stage trouble, be it haemorrhage, placental retention or manual removal, should be suspected of being capable of a repeat performance.

They recommend in such cases the routine prophylactic use of intravenous ergometrine at the delivery of the anterior shoulder. Yet even this precaution did not prevent serious haemorrhage in all cases —a sobering thought. The availability of suitable cross-matched blood for transfusion is clearly essential in the patient with a bad third-stage history and hospital confinement indicated absolutely.

Fibroids undoubtedly increase the likelihood of third-stage bleeding, not only because they may mechanically interfere with uterine retraction, but also because when they impinge upon the inner surface of the uterus the decidual reaction in this region is sometimes less complete. Should the placenta happen to be sited here, some degree of morbid adhesion may be encountered. This is a matter which cannot be foreseen in a case complicated by fibroids except by sonar, and it is as well to bear the risk in mind. Fortunately, bleeding usually ceases once the uterus is empty, even though fibroids may be present in marked size or number. Should bleeding continue after the uterus has been proved empty by exploration, it may be necessary, in rare instances, to resort to hysterectomy.

Lastly, as already stated, one of the most common, if not the most trivial, causes of postpartum haemorrhage is the presence of clots in the uterus. Their very presence seems to paralyse the uterus from further retractile activity and they are all too often overlooked. Their effect can hardly be wholly mechanical, because it is such a simple matter to squeeze them out.

Estimates of blood actually lost at delivery vary from guesswork to near mendacity, according to temperament, but the amount is nearly always greater than reckoned. Using a haemodilution technique (Perdometer) in which we have collected all blood, swabs, soiled towels and gloves in a sort of washing machine with a known volume of haemolysing detergent, it is possible, after correcting for the patient's known haemoglobin level, to calculate the blood loss accurately.

For years it has always bothered me that haemoglobin levels in patients 3 days after Caesarean section were so often a couple of grams per cent lower than the estimated blood loss would account for until this investigation produced the likely explanation. In a study of over 500 cases[27] it was found that the average blood loss at Caesarean section was nearly one litre (!) and at forceps delivery just over 400 ml. Spontaneous vaginal delivery, as might be expected, cost the patient least blood of all (less than 300 ml in 83 per cent of cases to which episiotomy added a further 130 ml). It is quite clear therefore that one can safely double a colleague's estimate of blood actually lost, and in some cases treble it, without fear of exaggeration.

Prophylaxis

The first important step is to spot the losers, or rather the blood losers, and arrange for their delivery in an institution which is capable of supplying immediate anaesthesia, resident skilled obstetric cover and full laboratory services, including those necessary for massive transfusion. General practitioner obstetric units do not normally fulfil these requirements. Patients in the following categories should have blood cross-matched on admission to the labour suite:

History of postpartum haemorrhage;
Antepartum haemorrhage;
Previous Caesarean section;
Haemoglobin under 10 g/100 ml;
Intra-uterine death;
Fetal distress.

In general, whenever there is a possibility of Caesarean section or excessive haemorrhage, blood should be cross-matched.[29] In the first chapter of this book the indications for hospital booking are fully given. Many of them are concerned with the risk of haemorrhage and, of these, all cases of grand multiparity, multiple pregnancy, antepartum haemorrhage of any variety and a past history of third-stage troubles constitute the most important groups. The incidence of postpartum haemorrhage is also higher in women under the age of twenty years, whatever their parity, and in those over the age of forty.

Vigilance during the third stage there must always be, but it would be well to consider more specific measures. Of these the most important is to be ready with ergometrine. Valuable minutes may easily be lost in procuring a syringe and opening an ampoule, and the syringe should always be charged with 0·5 mg of ergometrine or Syntometrine some time during the second stage and kept in readiness in some standard position. In domiciliary practice the mantelpiece is suggested. The drug will in any case not be wasted, for it can be given before leaving the house should its use not have been previously necessary.

Antenatal supervision, in so far as anaemia is routinely diagnosed and corrected during pregnancy, is also an important measure to insure the patient against the possible effects of haemorrhage.

The chances of postpartum haemorrhage can be reduced by good management. Even one's management of the second stage of labour is of importance. Only an irresponsible person would deliver a woman with forceps in the complete absence of uterine contractions, and anyone sufficiently ignorant to commit this crime could be expected to be incompetent to cope with the inevitable haemorrhage rewarding his folly. Even in normal delivery, however, it is important to deliver the baby's trunk slowly in order to allow a little time for uterine retraction to follow up the egress of the baby's body. This rule applies particularly after the intravenous use of ergometrine if the full benefits of this treatment are to be enjoyed.

Once bleeding starts, even though the amount is not initially serious, it is far better to act too soon that too late. A common and treacherous situation is one in which very small gushes repeatedly occur, none of them, by themselves, at all alarming, but whose effect is cumulative. It is important here not only to measure very accurately how much the loss is adding up to, but to be quite clear about what is happening inside the uterus. At a time when one of these little gushes is taking place, it will usually be found that the uterus is hard. The gush then stops and, for a time, it is thought that all is well, yet when it recurs the uterus is again found to be firm and well contracted. What is happening of course is that during the periods of arrested external bleeding the uterus is relaxing and filling itself with blood and the gush which occurs with the observed hardness of the uterus represents blood actually lost a minute or so earlier. Once this sequence of events is established, it becomes less and less likely that the placenta will be spontaneously delivered, and although the case may be nowhere near classification as one of postpartum haemorrhage, it is far better to take note of the warning before it is too late.

One is often reluctant to intervene because, for the time being, the patient's general condition seems so satisfactory but, as explained in the chapter on postpartum collapse, the signs of a rising pulse and a falling blood pressure are usually ten minutes out of date, so that intervention, when it comes as a result of these indications, comes too late.

One's only defence, therefore, is to start thinking alertly when the 250 ml mark is reached and to be prepared to act when the loss reaches 450 ml. If one waits until the statutory half-litre has been lost, intervention will only have to be undertaken under conditions far less favourable. Beware therefore of inertia not only in the uterus but in the attendant!

The patient's own blood is more precious than any that a blood bank can provide and a surer defence against puerperal sepsis than all the antibiotics in the world. It would be better to carry out manual removal of the placenta with imperfectly sterilised hands, while the patient still remains in possession of most of her own circulating blood volume, than to carry out the same operation with the most rigid asepsis in a patient already dangerously exsanguinated.

Treatment of Postpartum Haemorrhage

The uterus must be emptied of its contents whether they be blood clots, placenta, or both. This is the first principle of treatment, and the order in which the various measures are employed differs in some respects, depending upon whether the placenta has already been delivered and upon the briskness or persistence of the haemorrhage.

Bleeding after Delivery of the Placenta

The fundus of the uterus should at once be sought and kneaded by brisk massage through the abdominal wall until the uterus hardens with a contraction. Then, and not before, it is firmly squeezed to expel the blood clots which are almost certainly present within its cavity. This alone may suffice.

In carrying out this simple measure it is important to avoid pressing the uterus down into the pelvic cavity, which is not only useless but may be harmful, because venous drainage is to some extent obstructed and haemorrhage is, therefore, likely to be increased. While squeezing with one hand, the other hand should steady the uterine body from below, being placed on the abdominal wall just above the symphysis pubis. Quickness of movement is more useful than sheer brute force, from which the patient cannot protect herself by contraction of her very lax abdominal wall.

At the earliest opportunity the placenta should be examined to make sure that it is complete and that there is no evidence, in the form of torn vessels at the edge of the chorionic rent, to suggest that a succenturiate lobe has been left behind. If either a cotyledon or a lobe is missing, exploration of the uterine cavity will, of course, be necessary.

Ergometrine should be injected as soon as possible,[19, 20] and the choice of the intravenous or the intramuscular route will depend on the urgency of the haemorrhage. For this reason a sterile syringe already loaded with ergometrine and kept in a standard position in readiness for the injection will often prove a great standby. The intravenous route is to be preferred where seconds rather than minutes count and an almost certain effect is assured within forty seconds. The intravenous dose favoured is 0·25 mg of ergometrine. This is twice the dose recommended by Chassar Moir, but the margin of safety is wide. It is not necessary to exceed this dose intravenously, as some patients may exhibit side-effects, such as dizziness, vomiting and weakness of the limbs. Intramuscular injection of ergometrine will usually produce its effect within seven minutes and often less, the standard dose in this instance being 0·5 mg. Syntometrine, already described, is even better, and acts more quickly.

If the uterus refuses to harden up with the initial rubbing, and this is rather uncommon, no time should be lost in injecting one of these drugs. Massage of the uterus will now be effective.

A uterus which keeps softening and losing successive little trickles of blood, especially after twin delivery, may be kept in a better state of activity by maintaining an oxytocin drip infusion for an hour or two.

If bleeding still continues, a laceration of the cervix or vagina should be suspected, as discussed later, but one should not forget as a possible cause of prolonged trickling after a complete delivery of the placenta and with no evidence of a tear of cervix or vagina and where there is no clotting defect, that the cause may, in fact, be due to a minor degree of uterine inversion. Bimanual compression of the uterus is very seldom called for in such cases and hot intra-uterine douches even less frequently.

The uterus can often be compressed very efficiently through the abdominal wall, without resorting to vaginal manipulations, by raising it out of the pelvis with the right hand and passing the left hand behind the fundus. This hand now presses the uterus forward over the right hand and, moreover, the lower part of the uterus can be compressed against the sacral promontory.

Bleeding before Delivery of the Placenta

One's immediate reactions will depend upon whether or not the patient is under an anaesthetic, because if she is already anaesthetised, for example for forceps delivery, manual removal of the placenta can be undertaken more readily. In these cases intravenous ergometrine should already have been injected as soon as the anterior shoulder was born (see chapter on Forceps) and one is now working at a considerable advantage.

When a patient is not under a general anaesthetic, decisions are usually harder to make. It is true that manual removal of the placenta can be undertaken without a general anaesthetic; in fact I have done so myself with the help of self-administered Trilene, but except in grave emergency or when the placenta is obviously loose in the lower uterine segment and controlled cord traction has just failed to deliver it, such a practice is not to be recommended. I was once rash enough to give a talk to the Mothers' Union of our Church on "what to do about a woman upstairs unexpectedly having a baby", but the meeting soon degenerated into a series of personal obstetrical reminiscences by the various members of my audience. One of these included a description in graphic terms of having one's placenta removed without anaesthesia, which electrified the audience. It made the evening!

The first thing to do, of course, is to massage the fundus of the uterus vigorously until it hardens, and, whether or not this is successful in temporarily arresting the bleeding, no time should be lost in injecting ergometrine intravenously or intramuscularly, according to the rapidity of the blood loss. This is far better treatment within the first minute than resorting to possibly fruitless and damaging attempts at Credé's expression of the placenta in the unanaesthetised patient.

The importance of not fiddling with the fundus during the conduct of the third stage has already been dealt with at length, and one's actions now are in strange contrast to this previous inactivity. Once blood has started to appear at the vulva the arguments for keeping hands off the fundus of the uterus no longer apply, and so-called fiddling, to the extent of purposive massage, is now called for. Rubbing up a contraction in any case produces no more than a temporary respite from bleeding. This is bound to recur until the placenta has been safely delivered.

Credé's Method of Expression of the Placenta

This is a subject on which strong views are held by some authorities in opposing directions. That it is resorted to more often than necessary there can be no doubt, and it is equally certain that it can produce or aggravate shock. Consequently many obstetricians think that there is no justification whatsoever for its use. Controlled cord traction or the Brandt-Andrews technique may make Credé's expression unnecessary in many cases and should be tried first. On the other hand, by its judicious use it is possible to save many a patient from the need for manual removal of the placenta, and most of us now take a middle view, permitting one attempt at Credé's expression before the patient has received an anaesthetic, a further attempt once anaesthesia has been induced, to be immediately followed by manual removal of the placenta should this second attempt fail. (If possible, the bladder should be emptied first by catheterisation provided time allows.)

Unless one is possessed of a very powerful masculine hand it will usually be found that two hands are required. A common method is to pass the fingers behind the body of the uterus and to squeeze the front wall with the opposed thumbs. Alternatively, in a thin woman, it may be possible to squeeze the uterus between the palms of the two hands. The upper part of the uterus should be squeezed first, and in doing so the uterus should not be driven down into the depths of the pelvis, which is both shocking and ineffectual.

On no account should Credé's expression ever be attempted unless the uterus has first been made to contract either by brisk massage or by the injection of ergometrine. If the uterus cannot be made to harden up, then Credé's method of expression is absolutely contraindicated, for not only will it fail but acute inversion of the uterus is likely to result.

If a large clot has already collected in the uterus, it is necessary to maintain the pressure in order to secure the delivery of the placenta. This is a method which calls more for knack than for force. Much of the latter is often grossly misapplied by the novice. As soon as the placenta has been expelled, it is necessary to rub the uterus again to maintain a good state of contraction until bleeding ceases. The effect can be reinforced by the injection of more ergometrine.

The amount of ergometrine given in the repeated injections should not exceed 1·0 mg. If, as often happens, the attempt fails, and one is simply rewarded by further bleeding, it may be necessary to give a further injection of ergometrine while anaesthesia is being induced.

Stock should at all times be taken of the patient's general condition. Fortunately, where shock is profound, bleeding will usually greatly diminish, if not stop altogether, and this temporary respite should be made use of to set up an intravenous infusion. If cross-matched blood is already available, so much the better, but usually there will be some delay in obtaining it and, in the meantime, normal saline may be given. The patient's most urgent need is for an adequate circulating blood volume. The decision when to proceed to deliver the placenta under anaesthesia will depend upon the state of the patient's blood pressure. If the systolic pressure is less than 100 mm Hg there are considerable risks in proceeding further until the state of shock and exsanguination has been to some extent corrected, and in the chapter on postpartum collapse details are given of how to choose the best moment for operative intervention.

Until the patient's condition warrants an anaesthetic, ergometrine, blood transfusion and oxygen are one's main standby. During this anxious period, the blood pressure must be repeatedly observed, and no time must be lost, as soon as the systolic pressure exceeds 100 mm Hg, in proceeding to the removal of the placenta. If there is delay now, the patient will assuredly bleed again, and shock this time will be less easily corrected.

In making the second attempt at Credé's expression under an anaesthetic, all preparations should be at hand for proceeding to manual removal should the attempt fail and an intravenous drip should already be in action. These circumstances demand the presence of another practitioner, and in domiciliary practice one would be well advised not to proceed further single-handed.

In most large population centres there are, nowadays, flying squads who will come readily to one's aid. While waiting for the arrival of help the bladder should be catheterised, the patient should be given morphia and, if available, oxygen. She should be kept warm, for shock is greatly aggravated by cold, and one has to rely on the ergometrine already given to protect the patient from further bleeding.

Every obstetrician should carry in his bag some fluid suitable for intravenous use. Even saline is better than nothing. Where no fluid suitable for intravenous use is to hand, ordinary tap water, run slowly into the rectum, will help to restore the patient from a state of complete pulselessness. Dextran is not without drawbacks. In the first place it must not be given until a specimen of the patient's blood has been taken for grouping and cross-matching as its presence in the patient's circulating blood may interfere with the test. Secondly, it may interfere with the mechanism of blood coagulation.[25]

It is far better to rely upon these measures than to resort to further traumatic attempts at Credé's expression, pending the arrival of help. Before the days of flying squads one had only the choice of transferring the patient to hospital, in a condition already precarious, or of coping with the situation on the spot with the help of a partner. The more desperate the patient's condition the more likely was the second of these alternatives to be the safer procedure, unless transport to a nearby hospital was readily available. The advantages of transferring the patient to hospital, however, are that really massive transfusion becomes possible and expert anaesthesia is available. Local circumstances, therefore, must decide the choice.

The institution of the flying squad, with its ready supply of Rh-negative Group O blood, has simplified the dilemma and has been responsible for the saving of many lives. We always keep a fresh stock of four units of Rh-negative, Kell negative, Lewis A-negative, Group O blood, screened for Anti-A haemolysins at the ready for immediate transfusion to any recipient in urgent need, and have on occasion used all of it too.

Let us now assume that the patient's general condition is fit for anaesthesia, that an attempt at Credé's expression or, preferably, controlled cord traction has already failed, the placenta still remaining *in utero*, and that all preparations are to hand.

The patient is anaesthetised with some quick-acting anaesthetic, of which thiopentone is one of the most useful, and during the induction the obstetrician dons sterile gloves. It is a regrettable fact that the shortage of skilled anaesthetists may, in many instances, deny otherwise up-to-date maternity units the immediately available service they should have. Rather than wait for expert anaesthetic help, manual removal of the placenta under a sort of "hypoanaesthesia", using a combination of pethidine (Demerol) 50 mg intravenously, pudendal block and trichloroethylene, has proved a useful expedient[9] which, however, is to be deplored since it might encourage Health Authority Staffing Committees to view full anaesthetic cover with less urgency. After drenching the vulva with antiseptic solution a catheter must be passed, for, if there is time for anaesthesia there is also time for catheterisation. The abdomen must be covered with a sterile towel. Through the towel the second attempt at Credé's expression may be made, again having assured oneself that the uterus is well contracted. If this attempt fails or if it cannot be undertaken because the uterus cannot be made to contract satisfactorily, one is now ready to proceed in a matter of seconds to manual removal of the placenta. The above precautions of asepsis are always worth while before attempting expression, in order to obviate delays if manual removal is necessary.

The patient should not be put in the lithotomy position without the consent of the anaesthetist because of the danger of vomiting.

Manual Removal of the Placenta

To quote Bruce Mayes, "The really difficult part about manual removal is the decision to undertake it." Under the procedure outlined above, this decision will have already been taken and there will now be no hesitation.

The vulva has already been cleansed with antiseptic lotion and the bladder has been emptied. The cord should be cut off short at the vulva. One hand in the shape of a cone is insinuated into the vagina. Time should not be wasted removing perineal sutures. If necessary they can be replaced later. The cord is followed until the placenta is found.

The other hand is just as important as the hand inside the uterus. There is a very natural tendency to forget about the existence of this second hand whose function is to steady the fundus of the uterus and prevent it from being pushed up towards the costal margin. During manual removal of the placenta the uterus is very inclined to relax, with the result that the internal hand has to be introduced almost to the entire length of the forearm if this precaution is not taken.

Using the external hand correctly, it should not be necessary to introduce the other hand farther than two or three inches above the level of the wrist, the fundus being guided on to the fingers inside by external manipulation. If, through faulty technique, the fundus of the uterus is allowed to drift into the upper abdomen, the placental sinuses are opened up and haemorrhage becomes profuse. The risk of perforation of the uterine wall is also considerably increased.

Finding the placenta is not usually difficult and can be facilitated by keeping the cord taut while inserting the hand. It now has to be remembered that no retreat is permissible until the placenta has been completely detached.

Having reached the insertion of the cord in the placenta the periphery is sought. Some now proceed to separation by working from above downwards, but in actual fact it is easier to work by starting from the already detached portion. This is usually the inferior margin, and a plane of cleavage is here already demonstrated.

As far as possible the fingers should be kept together, working in the manner of an egg slice removing an egg from a frying-pan, at all times remembering the functions of the external hand pressing through the abdominal wall.

If a fold of the membranes can be kept in front of the advancing fingers, so much the better. Frenzied clawing with the individual fingers is to be deprecated, because the placenta will be torn to ribbons and much of it will be left behind. In few operations is there a greater need for patient determination.

Working from the detached margin upwards, the placenta will have been completely detached by the time the upper margin is reached, but it should not be removed from the uterus until one's fingers have reached above this margin.

Having now satisfied oneself that the whole placental mass is free within the uterine cavity, it is best delivered by traction on the cord, retaining the hand inside the uterus for a final exploration of its cavity.

Carried out deliberately and carefully, this operation can sometimes be remarkably bloodless but, in any case, bleeding must not undermine resolve. A failed attempt at manual removal is nothing short of disastrous.

The operation is not usually difficult, but there are certain points which are worth discussing. Occasionally there may be difficulty in reaching the placenta because of the presence of an hour-glass constriction ring. This is dealt with later. The other main difficulty is when an area of morbid adherence of the placenta is encountered. There is no doubt that this is far more often diagnosed than is actually the case, and I have now noted that right-handed operators tend to attribute morbid adhesion in the region of the right cornu of the uterus, whereas left-handed operators seem to diagnose this trouble in the left cornu, and it is suggested that this finding is occasionally more subjective than objective. When, however, this pathological condition is encountered, the difficulty may be very great, and it is almost impossible to remove the placenta without leaving shreds of tissue behind. Under these circumstances one has to be content with the best that one can do.

Having successfully completed manual removal of the placenta, most cases will usually stop bleeding. Occasionally, when there is gross uterine atony, haemorrhage continues unabated. Intravenous ergometrine is more likely to be successful than any other measure, but sometimes one may have to resort to bimanual compression of the uterus forthwith.

Bimanual Compression of the Uterus

The clenched fist is placed in the anterior fornix and the body of the uterus is compressed against it by a hand placed behind the uterus through the abdominal wall. Considerable haemostatic pressure can be applied in this way, but it cannot be maintained for more than two or three minutes because of fatigue. During this time, however, the uterus usually contracts and arrests haemorrhage.

There is one great pitfall about this procedure, namely that the case most urgently in need of it often has a uterus so atonic that it cannot be felt and therefore cannot be convincingly compressed. When the uterus is too soft to be palpable, one may even doubt whether the clenched fist is in the anterior fornix. In such cases it may be necessary to resort to a hot intra-uterine douche.

Intra-uterine douche.—A hot intra-uterine douche is a very certain method of stimulating an atonic uterus to contract. It is not without its obvious dangers, and should only be used when other measures fail to control the bleeding. It is customary to put some antiseptic lotion in the douche, but it is the heat which matters rather than the constituents. To be effective, therefore, the temperature should be not less than 118°F (47·8°C) in the douche can. Temperatures greater than this carry with them the risk of producing a sloughing of the vagina, especially in a patient who is severely shocked, under an anaesthetic, and in whom the blood circulation rate is very slow.

All air should be driven out of the piping before the douche nozzle is inserted into the uterus, because of the risk of air embolism. The can should be held not more than 2 feet above the level of the uterus, because greater pressures may force fluid along the Fallopian tubes. The risk of sepsis is, of course, increased by using an intra-uterine douche, but the dangers of present haemorrhage are far more pressing. This procedure is nowadays only known to members of my generation but its rediscovery is more than likely. [13]

Uterine tamponade.—This is a desperate measure and is very seldom employed in this country, although it is more popular in the United States. Enormous quantities of sterile roll gauze have to be used, each length being knotted to the previous one.

The gauze is best introduced by a hand passed well into the uterus with the other hand steadying the fundus from outside through the abdominal wall. It is most important to pack the upper portion of the uterus thoroughly, and a common mistake is to introduce some half-hearted packing only into the lower part of the uterus, leaving a large cavity above, which of course just fills with blood.

The packing is more likely to exert its effect by stimulating the uterus to contract rather than by direct pressure upon the placental sinuses. If, however, the uterus relaxes above the pack instead of contracting, as it may well do, matters are made very much worse.

It is impossible to pack the uterus properly without an anaesthetic, and the operation is both dangerous and useless unless done with great thoroughness.

I have only used this method of controlling haemorrhage once, and that was in a case who had been delivered by a colleague by classical Caesarean section for placenta praevia. A large portion of the placenta was found to be accreta and the placenta could only be removed piecemeal. Much of it was left behind, and haemorrhage during the operation was torrential. I first saw the patient some hours after operation, and she was then receiving her eleventh unit of blood. Her bed had been changed twice because of soiling with blood, she had air hunger and was pulseless. Her blood pressure was less than 50 mm Hg systolic. She was far too ill for hysterectomy and was moreover still bleeding. In this case I explored the uterus, removed a large quantity of retained blood clot and as much remaining placental tissue as I could, and packed the uterus firmly with gauze. The effect was dramatic and the patient rallied, leaving the hospital a fortnight later none the worse for her experience and with her uterus still *in situ*. The pack was very slowly removed under morphine premedication 24 hours later.

It is in cases of placenta praevia which continue to bleed postpartum that packing is likely to be more useful than at any other time. This is because the placental site is situated in a non-retractile portion of the uterus and, rarely, packing alone may control the haemorrhage.

On the whole it is not an operation to be lightly considered, and the case well enough to stand it in safety is likely not to need it, and other measures should suffice. Oxidised cellulose gauze has been used by some obstetricians, but Titus reports that he found its use unsatisfactory, because he had to remove large portions of partially dissolved material piecemeal at a later date.

Attention to the Patient's General Condition

So long as the patient is actively losing blood no general resuscitative measure can ever hope to keep pace with the deterioration so caused. Therefore, the first step must always be to arrest acute haemorrhage. Many cases, however, will subside into a condition of uncorrected shock unless prompt resuscitative measures are taken. Of these, blood transfusion is by far the most important, and no time should be lost in setting one up, as already mentioned. Pending the arrival of cross-matched blood, plasma or even normal saline may be given, but the sooner the patient receives whole blood the better, for this is what she is losing. The use of whole blood is regarded as shotgun prescription by Blood Transfusion services, because it is wasteful and could be more rationally replaced by "Blood Component Therapy." The blood components currently available are red blood cell suspensions, platelet concentrates, Christmas concentrate, fibrinogen, fresh frozen plasma, cryoglobulin precipitate, human AHF concentrate, human normal immunoglobulin, a variety of human specific immunoglobulins, dried plasma, salt-poor albumin and plasma protein solution, superconcentrate of factor VIII and another of factor IX.[28] The choice in fact compares with the extravagant menu of an expensive restaurant. It is not surprising if the half-demented clinician coping with desperate haemorrhage weakly asks simply for blood.

It is very easy to waste time by busying oneself with minor and less effectual measures to restore the patient's general condition when one's whole concentration should be directed towards the intravenous drip.

If the veins are collapsed it may be difficult to make the drip run at more than a drop every second or two. Nikethamide 0·25 ml injected into the drip tubing sometimes encourages it to speed up and warming of the limb occasionally helps. Rapid transfusion can be given under positive pressure with one of the rotary roller-type pumps now on the market (Fig. 1) and no maternity unit should be without some such device. On no account should positive pressure without the blood bottle be generated by means of a Higginson syringe attached to the vent tube, once a common but terribly dangerous practice. I have seen a patient killed within a few seconds by a massive air embolus which forced its way into the delivery pipe.

Most patients are undertransfused rather than overtransfused since the blood loss is usually greater than reckoned and the effective blood contents of the standard bottle amount only to 400 ml since the remainder is made up of citrate.

Pulse and blood-pressure records may not reveal the full degree of exsanguination and the adequacy of blood replacement, because a circulating blood volume as low as 70 per cent of normal may fail to cause variations in pulse rate or blood-pressure level.[16] Usually, therefore, the amount of blood transfused depends upon guesswork, but the measurement of central venous pressures provides the readiest guide in an emergency. The method is not only simpler but more useful than estimating blood volumes by dye or isotope dilution techniques.

To measure central venous pressure a plastic catheter of previously

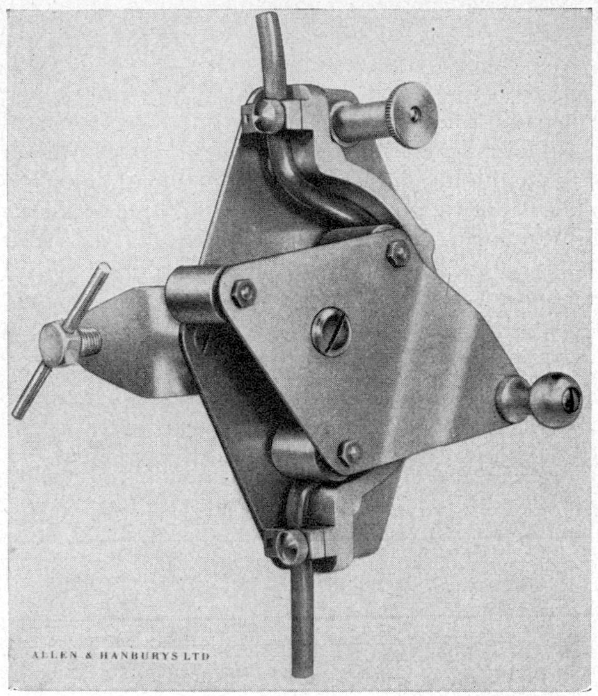

22/FIG. 1.—Martin Transfusion Pump.
(By courtesy of Allan & Hanburys, Ltd.)

estimated length is passed into the superior vena cava through a No. 14 gauge needle, either via a jugular vein or from an arm vein, which we prefer. It is connected both to drip infusion and to a water manometer by a three-way tap and the column of water height is measured above the manubriosternal junction which is 5 cm above the level of the superior vena cava with the patient in the dorsal position. Using the manubriosternal junction as a reference point the normal range of central venous pressures is from 5 to 12 centimetres of water. Transfusion should be maintained until this range is achieved and pulmonary congestion due to overtransfusion will not occur unless the upper limit is exceeded. The most uncertain feature in measuring central venous pressure is determining the exact level of the reference point on the patient (usually the manubriosternal angle) in relation to the manometer scale. This difficulty is readily solved by using a partially fluid-filled loop which can be spread between patient and manometer and, by raising or lowering the whole loop, the exact level of the reference point can be applied to the manometer scale.[23]

The foot of the bed is raised, morphia is given to allay restlessness and the patient is wrapped up in dry, warm bedding. The blood pressure and pulse are recorded every quarter of an hour and a watch is kept for renewed bleeding. One should aim, so far as possible, at replacing quantitatively the measured amount of blood lost. Where there is difficulty in maintaining a reasonable blood pressure Aramine is a useful addition to the drip, or hydrocortisone (see Chapter XXI).

The longer a patient remains in uncorrected exsanguination and shock, the longer will it take for the above resuscitative measures to succeed, and if they are instituted with the minimum delay, one is usually rewarded by a remarkable recovery in the patient within three hours.

Notes on Transfusion

The following notes are extracted from an admirable pamphlet on the subject issued by the Ministry of Health, in association with the Department of Health for Scotland, for the National Blood Transfusion Service, 1958, and, more recently, the Revised Notes on Transfusion (1973) issued by the DHSS.[6]

Banked blood should not be used unless there is a clear line of demarcation between the sedimented cells and the supernatant plasma, which should be straw coloured and free from visible signs of haemolysis. The latter may be indicated by a reddish-purple discoloration in the supernatant plasma spreading upwards. The blood should have been stored at 4°C and should not be time-expired. At no time should the blood have been allowed to freeze, as frozen and thawed blood may be lethal and blood which has been out of a refrigerator for more than 30 minutes should not be used.

Packed cells, made by discarding the plasma and adding the cells of one or more other bottles should only be prepared from blood less than a fortnight old and should be used within twelve hours of preparation.

Plasma is supplied with 400 ml of pyrogen-free distilled water in which it is dissolved after 5 minutes shaking. Failure to dissolve within 10 minutes indicates rejection. Reconstituted plasma should be used within 3 hours.

In a previously healthy patient in urgent need of blood following haemorrhage a transfusion rate of 100 ml minute until the systolic blood pressure reaches 100 mm Hg is well tolerated, but the rate should thereafter be cut back according to the state of the blood pressure.

In correcting chronic anaemia and in patients suffering chronic debilitating disorders, especially cases of cardiac disease, the rate of administration should not exceed 20–40 drops/minute for fear of embarrassing the heart. Signs of overload are jugular-vein filling and moist sounds from pulmonary oedema at the lung bases.

The clinician administering the blood is responsible for ensuring that grouping and compatibility testing have been adequately carried out—preferably under proper laboratory conditions, and only in the gravest emergency should Group O Rh-negative blood be used blindly since even this may contain anti-A or anti-B antibodies and uncommon immunisation against even Rh-negative antigens is possible.

Samples of the patient's serum for testing should always be taken before any dextran-like substance has been infused. 5–10 ml is collected with a dry, sterile syringe and placed in a dry, sterile tube after removing the needle (to avoid the damage caused by squirting).

Full compatibility testing and grouping takes a few hours but laboratories can carry out modified compatibility tests within about half an hour in emergencies, which are preferable to the crude prewar methods we used to employ of mixing a drop of the blood to be given on the back of a saucer with a drop of the patient's serum, obtained from the lumen of a broken-off capillary pipette end, and watching for signs of agglutination. Proper testing therefore means a 24-hour laboratory technician service.

Blood should not be warmed after removal from the refrigerator except in cases of exchange transfusion in babies.

Venepuncture is far preferable to cut down and cannulation, and a number of ingenious needle mechanisms are now available for introducing polythene catheters into veins.

In setting up the transfusion bottle and giving set, a clip should be closed on the tubing just proximal to the needle. After the air vent to the bottle has been opened the afferent tubing should be hung down and the clip near the end opened over a dish until blood runs out. The clip is then closed and the distal end, lifted in a U until it is at the same level as the bottom of the drip chamber. The clip can then be slowly opened until all air has been expelled from the tube. This avoids flooding the drip chamber.

The patient should be carefully watched for the first 30 minutes to stabilise the drip rate and to observe any unfavourable reactions.

All urine should be kept, measured and tested for albumin. The samples should not be discarded for 24 hours in case of any haemoglobinuria or subsequent signs of transfusion reaction develop.

Treatment of Transfusion Reactions

In the event of a severe transfusion reaction occurring due to the giving of incompatible blood, the following treatment is suggested in order to lessen the risk of anuria:

500 ml 10 per cent Rheomacrodex in dextrose (or approx. 1 g/Kg) to be given as soon and as quickly as possible, followed by a further similar quantity given over the next hour.

The decision that incompatible blood has been given may be made on the basis of:

1. The severity of reaction, or
2. A comparison of the group shown on the bottle with that given in the patient's case notes, or
3. Subsequent verification in the laboratory that either the patient's alleged group or that of the bottle was erroneous.

It would not necessarily be justifiable to delay treatment until laboratory confirmation was obtained.[29]

Complications of Blood Transfusion

1. *Febrile Reaction.* Grade 1.—Temperature to 37·8°C. Grade 2. —Temperature above 37·8°C, with sensation of chill but no shivering. Grade 3.—Rigor.
2. *Circulatory Overload and Pulmonary Oedema.*
3. *Haemolytic Reaction.* This follows the giving of incompatible blood or blood already partly haemolysed by freezing, heating, infection or prolonged storage.

   The symptoms are often of rapid onset and include fever, dyspnoea, headache, constricting sensation of chest and intense lumbar pain.

   Haemoglobinuria and jaundice develop subsequently, the former in a few hours and the latter within a few days.

   Death, when it occurs, is usually due to acute cardiac failure or suppression of urine.
4. *Air Embolism* is another dangerous complication usually due to connecting a Higginson's syringe to the transfusion bottle to speed up the drip, but it can also occur from faulty apparatus, even after puncturing the tubing to inject substances into the blood being given. This last hazard is reduced if the puncture is made at the distal end of the tube nearest the needle.

   Air embolism should be promptly treated by clamping off the source, turning the patient on to her left side for two hours and giving oxygen.
5. *Allergic Reactions* such as urticaria, rashes and angioneurotic oedema.
6. Transfusion of already infected blood may produce symptoms at first indistinguishable from those of a haemolytic reaction, except that there is extreme hypotension with warm extremities.

There may also be vomiting, diarrhoea and abdominal pain. Antibiotics and vasopressor agents will be required.

7. *Homologous Serum Jaundice* may follow transfusion with blood or plasma, although all dried plasma in this country is prepared from pools from not more than 10 donors nowadays, all of whom are screened for Australia antigen. The condition is clinically indistinguishable from infective hepatitis but the incubation period is from 40–150 days.

Coagulation Defects Postpartum

This subject has been very thoroughly reviewed by three experts in this field, namely Bonnar, McNicol and Douglas,[2, 3, 4] who have given a comprehensive summary of the history of recognising coagulation defects as causes of postpartum haemorrhage dating back to the observations of de Lee in 1901. A brief account is also given in Chapter XV in this book.

Of the numerous defects, hypofibrinogenaemia was the first to be recognised in association with abruptio placentae. Later it was noted as a complication of amniotic fluid embolism, retention of a dead fetus *in utero*, initially from Rh-haemolytic disease, and also in cases of retained placental tissue and septic abortion.

In addition to low or absent circulating fibrinogen, additional deficiencies are now recognised in the form of thrombocytopenia together with reduced levels of factors V, VIII and IX.

In obstetrics although the dominant factor in a haemorrhagic diathesis is lack of fibrinogen, other mechanisms frequently operate and the matter is important because particular deficiencies can now be recognised and treated properly by replacement.

The list of factors involved in final coagulation (which depends upon the conversion of fibrinogen to fibrin) is given in Chapter XV.

The normal clotting mechanisms could go on indefinitely to produce total coagulation of blood were it not for the compensatory fibrinolytic enzyme systems which are invoked in response to what would otherwise be an impossible situation. The role of the enzyme plasmin, which is directly responsible for fibrinolysis, has already been described. Fortunately for the clotting process it exists in an inactive form, namely plasminogen, and its conversion to plasmin has to be positively activated, otherwise it would digest not only fibrin but fibrinogen, prothrombin, factor V and factor VIII as well. This plasmin activator would in itself wreck the whole process of blood coagulation by fibrinolysis were it not for the fact that it has first to overwhelm its inhibitors known as antiplasmins. Normally these inhibitors are present both in serum and platelets in sufficient amounts to hold the process in check; but activator levels converting plasminogen to plasmin rise very sharply in response to trauma and various other stimuli such as adrenalin.

Normally plasminogen is included in a fibrin-forming clot but activators diffuse gradually into the thrombus and trigger off the process of fibrinolysis, that is to say digestion of fibrin and dispersal of the clot. Were this not so, no vessel would ever regain patency once a clot had formed.

The digestion of fibrinogen and fibrin results in the appearance of fibrin degradation products (FDP) which can be readily detected.

The finding of raised levels of fibrin degradation products is no more specific than the finding of a raised erythrocyte sedimentation rate. It merely draws attention to the existence of a problem without identifying it. The normal FDP level is 5 micrograms per ml. The determination of a low platelet count is of far more diagnostic significance than finding a raised FDP level.

When plasmin activity reaches pathological proportions however, not only is fibrinogen depleted but also the coagulation factors prothrombin, factor V and factor VIII. The blood clotting time is enormously prolonged and such viable clots as are formed are very readily digested.

There is thus a state of dynamic equilibrium in health which can readily be upset in disease and this applies to a number of complications in pregnancy as well.

Most of the coagulation factors, particularly fibrinogen, are progressively increased during the second and third trimesters of pregnancy, right up to labour, and this in itself is a protective mechanism against uncontrollable haemorrhage. But the extent to which the competing fibrinolytic system is enhanced has not yet been completely demonstrated.

As already mentioned, abruptio placentae with a massive retroplacental blood clot in itself mechanically subtracts very large quantities of fibrinogen from the circulating blood volume and the effect is further aggravated by haemodilution, but the coagulopathic mechanisms are more complicated in such conditions as intra-uterine fetal death. Here it is suggested that the enhanced ability to coagulate reverts to normal levels thus robbing the patient of this protective hypercoagulability and furthermore fibrinolytic activity may be increased. This process takes time, usually about a month after intra-uterine death has occurred.

In summary, coagulation defects in pregnancy are likely to occur under four main conditions:

1. Abruptio placentae;
2. Missed abortion and intra-uterine death;
3. Amniotic fluid embolism;
4. Septic abortion.

Abruptio Placentae

Although the subtraction of fibrinogen within the retroplacental clot is undoubtedly the main factor, there is also an associated diffuse intravascular coagulation particularly involving the pulmonary vascular bed. The latter is precipitated by the liberation of tissue thromboplastins for which the placenta and decidua form a generous source. The local damage within the uterus following abruption is surely enough to trigger off this mechanism. The intravascular fibrin formation also involves the small vessels of the kidney and the pituitary gland, but fibrinolysis may operate in time to prevent irreversible damage. Needless to say fibrin degradation products can be plentifully demonstrated in the blood of such cases.

The process of fibrinolysis now enters on the scene and may incidentally destroy the haemostatic plasma factors already enumerated and may interfere with fibrinogen polymerisation and therefore make protective blood-clotting unstable. It is important therefore, when confronted with a coagulation defect, to recognise as early as possible which mechanism is primarily responsible since the use of fibrinolytic inhibitors in certain defibrination syndromes, particularly affecting the lungs, may practically turn the vascular bed solid. It would be all very well if their effect could be localised as is reckoned to be possible in cases of menorrhagia for example, but where disseminated intravascular coagulation is involving the lungs, as in amniotic fluid embolism, the use of these inhibitors, such as EACA may be dangerous in the extreme. I have in a previous chapter described my own personal catastrophic experience in this respect.

In abruptio placentae the most serious deficiency to correct therapeutically is that of fibrinogen, since in this condition this is the dominant feature. The use of fibrinogen itself or of concentrated plasma may in the majority of cases suffice, but better and more specific results may be obtained by the use of cryoprecipitate preparations of plasma which are particularly rich in the other clotting factors such as factor VIII. This kind of *in vitro* titration can of course only be undertaken in centres where advanced haematological services are available.

Intra-uterine death

Here the depletion of coagulation factors is gradual and can be observed in the course of awaiting delivery. The fall in fibrinogen levels becomes noticeable after three weeks. Fortunately the majority of cases go into spontaneous labour before this unwelcome lapse of time. The associated disseminated intravascular coagulation which occurs as the result of the gradual liberation of thromboplastins progressively consumes fibrinogen, factor VIII and platelets. The reduction in the last-named is particularly significant and easily assessed. Naturally the process of fibrinolysis starts up in response to the intravascular coagulation and this causes a rapid release of fibrin degradation products which themselves contribute to faulty conversion of fibrinogen to fibrin. The process of progessive defibrination will continue until the uterus is empty and paradoxically this can best be corrected meanwhile by intravenous heparin. This is, in fact, logical since it arrests the process of disseminated intravascular coagulation which results in consumption of not only fibrinogen but factor VIII in particular and the other clotting factors as well.

What has been said above about intra-uterine death applies to a lesser extent in cases of missed abortion in the second trimester, although I have had a patient who hung on to her dead pregnancy for nearly two years in spite of attempts to shift it with intravenous oxytocin; she was apparently none the worse for it. The pregnancy was too far advanced to encourage us in evacuating the uterus surgically.

Amniotic Fluid Embolism

The main pathology here is undoubtedly in the lungs following the initial phase of profound shock. The haemorrhagic state does not usually develop at once but occurs within the next few hours. The condition is probably fairly common though only those that are fatal are fully recognised. Unexplained shock and postpartum haemorrhage should alert one to the diagnosis, especially if shock and cyanosis are out of all proportion to the amount of blood lost. Cases of Caesarean section associated with antepartum haemorrhage from placental separation of whatever variety are particularly vulnerable, and the differential diagnosis of the nature of clotting defect is a matter of urgency.

The levels of fibrinogen, platelets and factors V and VIII rapidly fall in cases of disseminated intravascular coagulation. Stoking the patient with fibrinogen tends to increase the conflagration. The finding of a low platelet count particularly should reveal what is happening.

In a very short time increased fibrinolytic activity is invoked which further aggravates the coagulation defect.

Provided these patients survive the initial primary shock, which may indeed require blood transfusion, the correct treatment on recognising the nature of the coagulopathy is to stop the disseminated intravascular coagulation by the use of heparin, which may be life-saving. These patients may die from the *coup de grace* administered by fibrinolytic inhibitors such as EACA, with solid lungs and deepening cyanosis. A chest X-ray will give warning of this dangerous pulmonary state (see Chapter XXI).

Septic Abortion

The mechanism of coagulation defect here is similar and the method by which the abortion has been procured is highly relevant. I have encountered cases brought near to the point of death by the use of soap detergent douches administered under pressure, and the X-ray appearances in the lungs are not dissimilar from those seen in cases of disseminated intravascular coagulation from other causes. I encountered one such case in the United States which was presented to me as one of recurrent pyaemic emboli (in spite of negative bacteriology) on whom my colleagues had, foolishly, as I pointed out, ligated the inferior vena cava, which was totally irrelevant treatment. My comment that the patient had barely survived, not thanks to their surgical treatment but in spite of it, was received with characteristic American generosity. We have seen identical cases in our own country in which intra-uterine detergent was undoubtedly the precipitating factor. One of our cases ended up with a quadriplegia, having survived her anuria and ultimately the other hazards of her precarious state. On this memorable occasion she made a dying deposition to the sheriff and his officers denouncing the abortionist but, since she ultimately survived, the evidence became invalid.

Recognition

In addition to intractable bleeding from an obvious site such as the uterus, the cervix or vagina, which cannot be controlled by standard treatment, there may be more general signs of coagulation failure such as bruising, prolonged bleeding after venepuncture and haemorrhages in skin, especially in the neighbourhood of a sphygmomanometer cuff and from suture sites and intramuscular injections. A specimen of blood should be firmly clotted within five minutes and should remain firm without subsequent lysis for the next quarter of an hour. But this is only a crude test. More specific tests are described in Chapter XV. The quickest methods of estimating fibrinogen depletion are those which estimate what we call the fibrinogen titre. Kits for this are available for bedside use. By now the full services of an up-to-date haematological department should be in action whatever the hour of day or night.

Management

Apart from cases which gradually develop clotting defects, for example, an intra-uterine death, the situation is usually one of extreme urgency and there may not be sufficient time for spontaneous recovery of clotting ability to occur. Blood transfusion is of course the first immediate necessity but stored blood is often poor in platelet content and factors V and VIII, and the fresher the blood transfused the better. Fresh blood naturally is ideal.

Fibrinogen concentrates (4 to 8g) are preferable even to fresh frozen plasma, which itself is more effective than triple- or quadruple-strength plasma which, because of its viscosity, cannot be given rapidly, and anyway such plasma infusions have a high potassium content which may cause cardiac arrest.

The fibrinolytic inhibitors such as epsilon-aminocaproic acid (EACA) have little place in the management of obstetrical haemorrhage for reasons already given. In fact they may be positively dangerous where there is disseminated intravascular coagulation.

Our attitude towards Trasylol is similar.

Intravenous heparin is the only anticoagulant which is applicable in obstetrical defibrination syndromes. An intravenous drip or constant infusion pump should deliver, 1500 units per hour.

If the patient is not already delivered as for example in cases of abruptio placentae, the sooner she can be made safe for delivery and the delivery accomplished the better. While preparations are being made for delivery, the nature of the clotting defect must be investigated. Usually fibrinogen depletion will have to be corrected, but if there is marked thrombocytopenia, fresh blood containing viable platelets, or a platelet transfusion, is highly desirable. Cryoprecipitate preparations may also be of great value.

When fibrinogen concentrates are given 6 g can be dissolved in 300 ml of distilled water and infused over a period of a quarter to half an hour. This is likely to be far more effective than whole bank blood by itself, although this too is required for oligaemia.

In the absence of fibrinogen concentrate a litre of fresh frozen plasma should be given which will supply 3 g of fibrinogen and factors V and VIII, the circulating volume being made up with transfused whole blood. My distrust of synthetic plasma expanders continues to this day and, in my experience at least, they aggravate haemorrhage.

In cases of intra-uterine death, coagulation studies are performed at weekly intervals from the first fortnight onwards. An oxytocin infusion, in high dosage if necessary, should be employed to expedite delivery and forestall the development of a haemorrhagic state.

Fibrinogen may have to be given to stave off haemorrhage from hypofibrinogenaemia, but if this does not restore normal clotting, intravenous heparin, as outlined above, will be necessary to arrest disseminated intravascular coagulation. Delivery must then be determinedly sought as soon as the fibrinogen level is restored to over 200 mg per 100 ml and before a further consumption of fibrinogen is allowed to take place.

In cases of amniotic fluid embolism immediate treatment of shock with blood, and of cyanosis with oxygen, must be followed as soon as possible by treatment appropriate to the coagulation defect. Once the immediate emergency is under control the patient is more likely to die of hypoxia than blood loss.

It is the common experience of us all that when the patient has required a very large transfusion, for example of 5 litres or more, generalised bleeding is likely to persist. This is because banked blood is deficient in viable platelets and to some extent in factors V and VIII. These have to be replaced either by fresh blood or by cryoprecipitate preparations. Citrate intoxication is also to be feared in truly massive transfusion of several litres of citrate blood given rapidly. This can be countered by 10 ml of a 10 per cent solution of calcium gluconate per litre of citrated blood already transfused in excess of 2 litres. Fortunately the healthy liver is able to detoxicate citrate rapidly.

A number of haematological disorders, such as the varieties of thrombocytopenia, require appropriate management in collaboration with the haematological department. In idiopathic thrombocytopenic purpura, for example, steroid treatment if already in force will require an increase of dose to cover the stress of delivery by whatever means. Nevertheless fresh blood or fresh platelet-enriched plasma should be available in the unlikely event of a haemorrhagic accident in the course of delivery.

Von Willebrand's disease is a genetic condition in which bleeding time is increased and factor VIII is diminished. Fortunately there is usually foreknowledge of the condition before delivery and if there is trouble the factor VIII level in the blood can be raised by the infusion of cryoprecipitate covering the period of labour and the first few days of the puerperium.

Patient Already on Anticoagulant Therapy

The hazards from drugs such as warfarin, have come in for a good deal of speculation because their low molecular weight enables them to cross the placenta and possibly cause a fetal haemorrhagic diathesis. Prolonged treatment with heparin, however, of a patient requiring anticoagulation during pregnancy is hardly practicable and our own preference is to convert to heparin a fortnight before delivery or, if a more urgent situation develops before that, to reverse the warfarin with 20 to 50 mg of vitamin K_1 intravenously. The effect of heparin during delivery can be quickly eliminated by stopping the drug temporarily and recourse to reversing its effect with protamine sulphate is seldom necessary.

Risks of Postpartum Haemorrhage, Immediate and Remote

Postpartum haemorrhage in 1945 accounted for 9·4 per cent of all maternal deaths (Registrar-General). It has now dropped to third place but it is doubtful, however, whether figures from this source give a true picture, and many patients who do not die as a result of their haemorrhages remain handicapped for many years to come with indifferent health and chronic anaemia.

If the patient escapes immediate death from haemorrhage, she still remains very liable to develop puerperal sepsis, for nothing so predisposes the patient to infection as the loss of blood. The saving of blood at all times and in all places is far more important than the most rigid aseptic technique, and no chemotherapy, however advanced, can guarantee the mastery of infection in the case of the seriously anaemic patient.

Gibberd once quoted a mortality for manual removal of the placenta of between 5 and 15 per cent, but it is usually the severity of the haemorrhage indicating the manual removal which is lethal, rather than the operation itself. Nowadays, when manual removal is much more readily undertaken, the mortality has shrunk to low proportions.

The operation of manual removal is, however, easily fatal if undertaken in a patient whose blood pressure at the time is below 80 mm Hg systolic, and, if possible, it is preferable to secure a blood pressure of over 100 before undertaking it.

The choice of anaesthetic makes an appreciable difference, nitrous oxide being particularly dangerous because of anoxia in a patient already anaemic.

If the systolic blood pressure remains below 80 mm Hg for more than a very few hours, the patient is liable to develop anuria due to tubular nephrosis. All renal filtration ceases when the blood pressure reaches these low levels, and these cases should be watched carefully for signs of oliguria during the next few days.

After a severe postpartum haemorrhage it is common for a patient to be unable to establish lactation, and chronic subinvolution may undermine her gynaecological health for years to come.

Anterior pituitary necrosis (Sheehan's syndrome), though fortunately uncommon, is a very serious risk in a patient who remains shocked and acutely anaemic for any length of time. This is discussed more fully in the chapter on postpartum collapse.

A chronic iron-deficiency anaemia may remain as a permanent sequel to postpartum haemorrhage unless steps are taken to correct it during the puerperium. The haemoglobin should, as a matter of routine, be estimated 48 hours after delivery, and it will often be found that the patient has lost far more blood than was thought likely at the time. Blood transfusion, especially of packed cells, greatly expedites convalescence, but in less severe cases intensive iron therapy very often suffices, and it should be one's aim to restore a normal blood picture to the patient within the first six postnatal weeks.

Extra-placental Bleeding

If a patient continues to bleed although it is known that the uterus is empty and, by its hardness on palpation, it appears to be well retracted, the source of the haemorrhage must be sought in the cervix, vaginal vault, vaginal walls or perineum.

An episiotomy usually bleeds far more than a second-degree tear, and efficient suture will deal effectively with it. The worst haemorrhage from the vulva usually occurs from tears in the neighbourhood of the clitoris. This can be controlled by underrunning a mattress suture.

More commonly the continued loss of bright blood usually indicates a laceration of the cervix. As a source of postpartum bleeding this is not common following normal delivery, but after forceps delivery or breech extraction it is a relatively frequent complication. One is often tempted to temporise in the hope that the bleeding will cease spontaneously, which admittedly often occurs, but it is not wise to procrastinate for more than a minute or two. During this time the necessary instruments should be mustered for obtaining a proper view of the whole extent of the cervical perimeter. These instruments are: (1) a large Sim's speculum (2) three pairs of sponge forceps—they are far more satisfactory than vulsella, which tend to tear the cervix; (3) a liberal supply of gauze swabs; (4) a good light.

The cervix is often oedematous and bruised, and its lips may be very much distorted at the end of delivery, so that it is not always an easy matter to identify a laceration and the bleeding point at its base. Digital palpation from inside is not satisfactory, and it is far better to obtain a proper view by dragging each successive portion of the cervix well into sight, with the help of the speculum and the sponge forceps. One obtains a hold of any accessible portion of the cervix with the sponge forceps, and then, with the help of a second pair, works round the margin of the cervix towards the lateral edges. By pulling the speculum laterally and the sponge forceps medially a good view of the lateral fornices can be obtained.

Arterial bleeding from the cervix will be seen coming usually from the depth of the cleft caused by the laceration. As a temporary measure this bleeding region can be grasped with the third pair of sponge forceps while sutures are prepared.

The main indication for suture of a cervical laceration is to control haemorrhage. It is very doubtful whether it is worth sewing up a laceration which is not causing bleeding because, for some reason, these lacerations never heal well however carefully sutured, and the cosmetic effect at postnatal examination is almost invariably disappointing.

It is often easier to put the first suture in, not at the base of the laceration, but at the corners of its most distal margin. A finger can then be passed inside the cervix deep to the tear, and by gentle traction on the first suture the remaining sutures can be inserted very accurately (Fig. 2).

Occasionally, and this applies particularly to vault lacerations as well as cervical, it may be possible to control haemorrhage by applying sponge-holding forceps to the rent edges but impossible to replace them with haemostatic sutures because of cutting out, or inaccessibility combined with a parlous state of the patient. In such cases the safest course may be to leave the clamps in place for 24–48 hours, strapping them together. To prevent the patient dislodging them with her thighs one foot should be bandaged to the knee of the opposite leg (Fig. 3).

Hour-glass Constriction Ring (Contraction Ring)

The incidence of this troublesome complication to some extent varies with the amount of meddlesome interference which is undertaken during this stage of labour. The old fear that the use of oxytocic drugs before the delivery of the placenta would evoke it has not been borne out by experience since the routine use of these drugs in this manner was introduced. In almost all cases in which constriction ring occurs after the use of an oxytocic drug, some evidence can be found that the body of the uterus has been irritated by

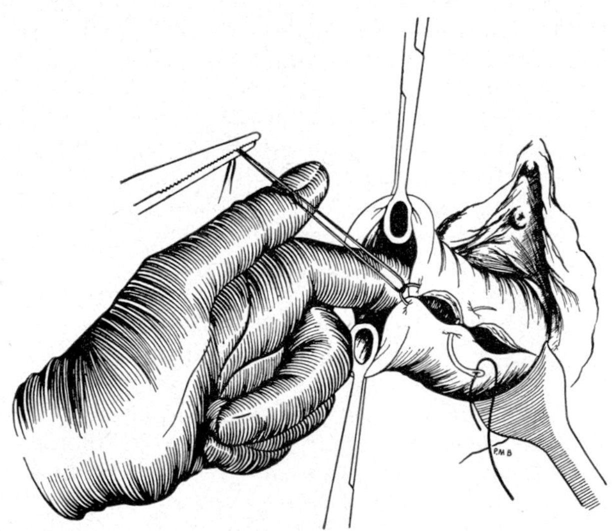

22/Fig. 2.—Cervical suture.

attempts at Credé's expression or by general mishandling. Intra-uterine manipulations during the second stage of labour to some extent make the uterus irritable and such a ring may develop during the third stage.

The diagnosis can only be made, of course, by inserting, or attempting to insert, a hand into the uterus, and in the course of manual removal of a placenta the development of such a ring may be noticed. Fortunately, its onset is fairly gradual, and it is often possible to complete the removal before the ring has closed down too tightly.

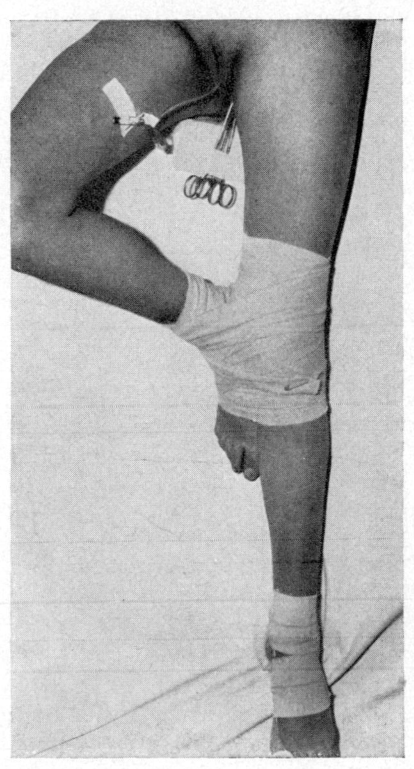

22/FIG. 3.—Method of preventing dislodgement of haemostatic clamps.

In extent, a contraction ring varies from a complete constriction, making the upper portions of the uterus totally inaccessible, to minor degrees of ridging. In the former instance, if the hand is introduced in order to remove the placenta, the cord will be found to disappear through the vault of a smooth dome which represents the part of the uterine cavity below the ring. The placenta is thus completely out of reach. These cases, because of the very tightness of the ring, are incapable of bleeding for the time being. This ring cannot be penetrated, and as the patient is not bleeding, time can safely be allowed for it to wear off. The patient should be given morphia 15 mg, and within four hours it will be found that the ring has relaxed and the placenta can now be removed. During this period the patient should, of course, be kept under careful observation and the appearance of bleeding during this period will indicate, firstly, that the ring is relaxing, and secondly, that the placenta is endeavouring to separate and intervention should thereupon be undertaken.

The less extreme varieties of ring will allow the passage of two or more fingers, and in such cases the constriction will often yield to passive dilatation. Deep general anaesthesia encourages relaxation of the ring and in many cases amyl nitrite works like a charm. This drug is made up in small capsules and is highly volatile. The capsules are surrounded by little cotton bags to prevent the scatter of glass splinters. They are broken and immediately placed underneath the anaesthetic mask. However quickly one does this, much of the vapour will escape, and it is usually advisable to use two capsules. Often within a few seconds a ring which has appeared impassable seems to vanish, and the examining hand finds itself within the main cavity of the uterus without further difficulty. As soon as the placenta has been removed it matters not at all whether a ring reforms.

Retention of the Placenta without Bleeding

This is by no means uncommon and because of the concern which it is likely to cause it is hard to remember that as long as the patient is not bleeding she is in no immediate danger. A scrupulous vigilance of the third stage must be maintained throughout the period of waiting, and it is particularly important to satisfy oneself that the uterus is not slowly and silently filling with blood behind the placenta. This will be indicated not only by a rise in the level of the fundus, which may be very gradual, but by a very definite impression of an increase in size of the uterus as a whole. These signs point to the fact that bleeding is occurring and supply the indications to interfere.

In other cases the uterus seems merely to be inert and no signs of placental separation appear. One soon begins to wonder how long it is profitable to continue the wearisome observation of the third stage. While waiting, however, it is as well to remember that the apparent uterine inertia may be due to a full bladder, and a catheter should always be passed. It is common to find that 200 ml or more of clear, pale urine have surreptitiously collected in the bladder since the delivery of the child. One was originally assured by catheterisation that the bladder was empty at the end of the second stage and this apparent diuresis in the third stage may come as a surprise. Much of this urine has probably been dammed back within the dilated ureters and renal pelves by the mechanical pressure of the child's head during the second stage.

After passing a catheter the uterus often appears to wake up and the signs of placental separation then follow.

If the placenta does not separate within an hour it is rather unlikely to do so spontaneously for a long time and most obstetricians are prepared to intervene before two hours have elapsed.

There are certain good reasons for discouraging an unduly prolonged retention of the placenta. Firstly, as long as the placenta remains undelivered, the patient is liable to start bleeding at any time. Secondly, supervision cannot be relaxed throughout this period. Thirdly, the patient cannot be left undisturbed in her own warm bed where she would be only too glad to have a sleep after the exertions of her recent labour. Fourthly, there is the occasional risk that the patient may develop a variety of postpartum collapse due to retention of the placenta alone. Finally, the longer the placenta is left in the uterus the greater are the chances of puerperal sepsis.

Every now and then an enthusiast for conservative methods decides to leave a placenta *in situ* for an indefinite period, in the hope that it will safely autolyse and ultimately be discharged, just like in cattle, and we have all heard of cases in which the placenta has been left in for several days without apparent ill effects. If the attendant prescribing this treatment were prepared to remain with the patient throughout this time and not to relax vigilance, we would have more respect for his attitude, but in many of these cases the placenta is removed by his house surgeon as soon as his back is turned.

If, after catheterisation and waiting, the placenta is still retained, preparations should be made for its removal, if necessary under anaesthesia. Although this may sound pessimistic, it is far better to be prepared for every eventuality before starting to rub up a contraction and squeezing the uterus, because, if anything goes wrong and bleeding starts, delays in completing delivery of the placenta may now be serious.

If the patient has not already received some ergometrine, 0·5 mg should be injected intramuscularly. This alone may do the trick, but in any case it is far better than pushing on the fundus of the uterus to see what happens, a mistake that is often rewarded by the onset of bleeding which one may not be able to arrest immediately.

An anaesthetist should now be summoned, sterile drapes should be at hand and preparations made for the possibility of having to proceed to manual removal of the placenta if simpler measures fail.

Causes of retention of the placenta.—There are four main causes of retention of the placenta:

1. *Inertia.* This can often be countered by the injection of ergometrine which is preferable to uterine massage.
2. *Adherence of the membranes to the uterine wall.* This is a common cause, and one in which treatment by Credé's expression is most likely to succeed, or as an alternative, cord traction (see earlier).
3. *The presence of a constriction ring.* This has already been dealt with.
4. *The placenta may be totally morbidly adherent* (*placenta accreta*).

This last condition will not be diagnosed until an attempt at manual removal has to be made. In a study of 14 cases of placenta accreta in

Glasgow, Millar (1959) noted the greatly increased incidence of placenta praevia as an aetiological factor, a point which my own experience confirms. The cause is thought to be primarily the result of a defective decidual reaction, probably hormonal in origin, rather than the result of previous trauma such as manual removal and curettage which themselves are required because of it. The association with uterine inversion is also recognised.

Treatment for this rare and ugly condition (which, be it remembered, may be encountered by those undertaking manual removal of the placenta in domiciliary conditions) consists of "grubbing out" the placenta as best one can and controlling the haemorrhage as far as possible by bimanual compression, blood transfusion and even by uterine packing. Finally, severe degrees of placenta accreta may require hysterectomy.

Operative procedure.—Once the decision has been taken to terminate the third stage and all preparations, as outlined above, are to hand, the procedure is in the first place to ensure a well-contracted uterus, if necessary by massage, and then to employ the Brandt-Andrews' manoeuvre and failing that, not more than one attempt at Credé's expression. This is done initially without an anaesthetic and after catheterisation of the bladder. If this fails, anaesthesia is induced and Credé's expression is again attempted, which, if unsuccessful, must be immediately followed by manual removal of the placenta.

There is often some difference of opinion about the repair of a perineal laceration or an episiotomy during the waiting period of an abnormally prolonged third stage, but one should have no hesitation in proceeding with it, for not only will it save time, but it will also save blood. The patient is bound to continue to lose a certain quantity of blood from any sizeable laceration and even more so from an episiotomy. Not only is this more humane to the patient, but does not in any way interfere with the completion of the third stage.

Secondary Postpartum Haemorrhage

This is bleeding which occurs after an interval of 24 hours or more following the birth of the child and is most often due to the fact that something abnormal is retained within the uterus, usually a portion of placenta, occasionally a large blood clot or a submucous fibroid. In a series of 97 cases from Sheffield,[7] labelled as secondary postpartum haemorrhage, there was found no satisfactory cause for the bleeding in over half those requiring surgical exploration and in less than a third of them was the retention of placental tissue confirmed histologically. In others, only organising clot, fragments of decidua and uterine muscle were found, yet the results of evacuation of the uterus were good whether placental tissue was found or not. Unfortunately in no less than 3 cases the uterus was perforated by instrumentation for which laparotomy and suture was indicated.

Oestrogens for suppressing lactation are a fairly common cause and bleeding follows usually within a fortnight of their withdrawal.

Retained chorion seldom causes secondary postpartum haemorrhage, and chorion epithelioma, an unlikely possibility, does not cause bleeding before at least three or four weeks after delivery.

Most secondary postpartum haemorrhages reveal themselves within the first week or nine days of the puerperium, but sometimes much later, and often supply advance warning in the form of increased red lochial loss and a low-grade puerperal pyrexia. The condition is potentially very dangerous, and one cannot afford to ignore even a small secondary postpartum haemorrhage because it is almost certain that a very much larger and possibly fatal haemorrhage will follow. I have seen some very alarming haemorrhages of this type. Sonar is of great help in confirming the need for exploration.

It is essential to explore the uterine cavity without undue delay and to be certain that a supply of cross-matched blood is available, because the operation may be by no means bloodless.

If a portion of placenta has been retained for any length of time it tends to become organised and rather densely adherent to the uterine wall, so that not only is its removal difficult but its presence within the uterus may escape detection. I well remember one such case in which the uterus was explored twice and no placental tissue found, yet the patient continued to have alarming haemorrhages and had to be repeatedly transfused. At hysterectomy, which was undertaken eventually as an emergency measure, a large portion of placenta was found densely adherent to the uterine wall in the region of the fundus.

REFERENCES

1. Andrews, C. J. (1940). *Sth. Med. Surg.*, **102,** 605.
2. Bonnar, J., McNicol, G. P. and Douglas, A. S. (1969). In: *Modern Trends in Obstetrics*, **4**. Ed. R. J. Kellar, pp. 162–196. London: Butterworths.
3. Bonnar, J., McNicol, G. P. and Douglas, A. S. (1969). *J. Obstet. Gynaec, Brit. Cwlth*, **76,** 799.
4. Bonnar, J., McNicol, G. P. and Douglas, A. S. (1969). *Brit. med. J.*, **3,** 387.
5. Brandt, M. L. (1933). *Amer. J. Obstet. Gynec.*, **25,** 662.
6. Department of Health and Social Security, Scottish Home & Health Department and Welsh Office (1973). *Notes on Transfusion.* Revised 1973.
7. Dewhurst, C. J. (1966). *J. Obstet. Gynaec. Brit. Cwlth*, **73,** 53.

8. Dewhurst, C. J. and Dutton, W. A. W. (1957). *Lancet*, **2,** 764.
9. Dickins, Aileen M. and Michael, C. A. (1966). *J. Obstet. Gynaec. Brit. Cwlth*, **73,** 460.
10. Embrey, M. P. (1961). *Brit. med. J.*, **1,** 1737.
11. Embrey, M. P., Barbor, D. T. C. and Scudamore, J. H. (1963). *Brit. med. J.*, **1,** 1387.
12. Embrey, M. P. and Garrett, W. J. (1958). *Brit. med. J.*, **2,** 138.
13. Friborg, S. R. C., Rothman, L. A. and Rovinsky, J. S. (1973). *Obstet. and Gynec.*, **41,** 876.
14. Kimbell, N. (1954). *Brit. med. J.*, **2,** 130.
15. Kimbell, N. (1958). *Brit. med. J.*, **1,** 203.
16. MacGregor, W. G. and Tovey, A. D. (1957). *Brit. med. J.*, **2,** 855.
17. Millar, W. G. (1959). *J. Obstet. Gynaec. Brit. Emp.*, **66,** 353.
18. Ministry of Health (1958). *Notes on Transfusion issued for the National Blood Transfusion Service*, London: H.M.S.O.
19. Moir, J. C. (1944). *J. Obstet. Gynaec. Brit. Emp.*, **51,** 247.
20. Moir, J. C. (1947). *Brit. med. J.*, **2,** 309.
21. Moodie, J. E. and Moir, D. D. (1976) *Brit. J. Anaesth.*, **48,** 571.
22. Murdoch, R. (1958). *Lancet*, **2,** 731.
23. Notaras, M. J. (1971). *Lancet*, **1,** 214.
24. Robertson, S. (1967). Ob-Gyn. Collected Letters. *Internat. Correspondence Soc. of Ob-Gyn.*, **8,** 103.
25. Scott, J. S. (1955). *Brit. med. J.*, **2,** 290.
26. Spencer, P. M. (1962). *Brit. med. J.*, **1,** 1728.
27. Wallace, G. (1967). *J. Obstet. Gynaec. Brit. Cwlth*, **74,** 64.
28. Wallace, J. (1972). Personal Communication.
29. Willoughby, M. L. N. (1964). Personal Communication.

CHAPTER XXIII

MATERNAL INJURIES

LACERATIONS of the cervix are not included in this chapter, having been dealt with in the chapter on postpartum haemorrhage, but acute inversion will be considered here, for it is in a sense an obstetrical injury.

UTERINE RUPTURE

There are two types of uterine rupture, complete and incomplete, distinguished by whether or not the serous coat of the uterus is involved. In the former the uterine contents, including fetus and occasionally placenta, may be discharged into the peritoneal cavity, and for this reason it would appear to be the more dangerous of the two varieties. This, however, is not necessarily the case, and the terms complete and incomplete are unfortunate in that they give such an impression. The uterus, once empty, is able to retract, so that the amount of blood in the peritoneal cavity is often mercifully limited. On the other hand, most incomplete ruptures start in the lower segment, where retraction is deficient, so that bleeding can continue briskly both *per vaginam*, between the layers of the broad ligament, and retroperitoneally.

Incomplete rupture with resulting broad-ligament haematoma is commoner than recognised, but fortunately only a proportion of the cases develop to an alarming extent.

When the cervix tears in labour, the lateral rent easily extends into the lower segment, where large veins may be torn and may bleed furiously. In milder cases there may be no more than a troublesome puerperal pyrexia to show for it.

Not all cases of lower segment rupture are incomplete, and in obstructed labour or in difficult and traumatic instrumental deliveries a rent, usually oblique, may occur through all the layers, including the visceral peritoneum. As a general rule, rupture occurring during labour occurs in the lower segment, whereas in pregnancy it is usually in the upper segment, and in this case the onset is often fairly silent and insidious, particularly when a previous classical Caesarean scar gives way.

Ruptures often extend to involve both the cervix and the vaginal vault as well, an accident which not only increases bleeding but often makes any conservative surgical procedure impracticable.

Causes of uterine rupture.—The incidence of uterine rupture is about 1 in 2500 cases and is not becoming so very much rarer nowadays because of an extended aetiology. Between the years 1950 and 1964 there were 143 reported cases in Dublin of which forty-three followed previous Caesarean section. The incidence of scar rupture was 1·4 per cent following lower segment section and 6·4 per cent after the classical operation.

The remainder were traumatic, including 13 due to oxytocin infusion of which eight were in grand multiparae.

The maternal mortality from traumatic rupture was as high as fifteen per cent.[8]

During pregnancy the commonest cause is a previous Caesarean section scar, chiefly the classical variety. Any history of genital-tract infection during the puerperium following such an operation raises serious doubts about the integrity of the scar, and if, as is not unlikely, the placenta in the present pregnancy happens to be sited over the scar, the burrowing action of the villi into what is often an imperfect decidua and the increased vascularity of the area weaken the uterine wall.

Myomectomy scars in the uterus are often quoted as causes of rupture, especially when the uterine cavity has been opened at the previous operation, but this disaster is very rare. Personally I have never met it, and Bonney, a great protagonist of myomectomy, never encountered it in his very large series. The difference here lies in the fact that the uterus after myomectomy is not undergoing involution with the rhythmical contractions which follow Caesarean section, and the tissues, because they are at rest, heal better.

Direct trauma to the uterus is another recognised cause but is extremely uncommon, and it is surprising how much violence the pregnant uterus will withstand.

The uterine wall may be weakened by previous wounds, for example, after manual removal of a morbidly adherent placenta or curettage, with or without perforation, for retained products of conception following abortion. The later in a previous pregnancy that abortion followed by curettage has occurred the greater the risk of perforation at that time, often undiagnosed, and of uterine rupture in a subsequent pregnancy. One of the worst of such cases I have personally encountered was that of a woman admitted so ill that it was difficult to make a diagnosis at all—as is often the case in really desperate emergencies. She was in acute pain and very shocked. The uterus, corresponding in size to thirty-four weeks' gestation, was not hard enough to encourage a diagnosis of abruptio placentae. The fetal heart was absent and the urine was normal. In spite of transfusion her condition rapidly deteriorated. A provisional diagnosis of haemoperitoneum was made though its source was not expected to be uterine in view of her past obstetrical history which was negative, apart from a previous abortion at six months followed by curettage. Laparotomy revealed an enormous quantity of free blood in the peritoneal cavity coming from a small hole in the fundus uteri through which a portion of placenta was presenting. She collapsed on the table in the course of Caesarean hysterectomy and was pulseless for over an hour, but following massive transfusion of eight units of blood she made an uninterrupted recovery.

Concealed antepartum haemorrhage is very occasionally associated with uterine rupture, which adds to the great gravity of the condition, but this too is fortunately a rare complication.

Nowadays no gynaecologist worthy of the name performs the operation of ventrifixation, especially in any woman likely to become pregnant again, for in this case the uterus can only enlarge by the mechanism of sacculation, if abortion does not first occur.

Lastly, pregnancy in a rudimentary horn or an angular pregnancy may result in uterine rupture. Notwithstanding all this, however, there are a number of cases in whom no cause whatsoever can be found, particularly in grand multiparity.

After labour has started, additional causes come into the field, and it is now particularly that a uterus, weakened by rapid and repeated childbearing, may be unequal to the strain.

The use of oxytocic drugs in labour may be dangerous from the point of view of rupture, and for this reason alone they are only employed with full precautions and supervision before the end of the second stage.

Grand multiparity is a contra-indication of their use because of this hazard. The response of the uterus may be unpredictably violent and in a case of my own, a para 9, the first few ml of a dilute oxytocin infusion proved lethal. In spite of supervision and the immediate shutting off of the drip, the uterus "stood on its head" and burst. Caesarean hysterectomy was a matter of minutes but she died ultimately of uncontrollable renal failure.

Version in labour, especially internal version, is a very common cause, and the more advanced the labour the greater does this risk become. Even the gentlest handling provides no guarantee against it. I have myself caused a very extensive rupture of the uterine wall, extending from the round ligament to the cervix and vaginal vault, in performing an internal version in a case of transverse lie with hyperextension of the fetus, although I was surprised at the time by the very great ease and lack of force with which the operation was completed.

Any instrumental delivery, especially if the cervix is not fully dilated, may cause rupture of the uterus, except in cases of low forceps extraction, but with careful application this accident should not occur in experienced hands. Cranioclasm, however, may result in tearing of the uterus, and vaginal walls as well, if great care is not taken in extracting the exposed portions of bone.

Forceful stretching of the cervix which, after all, is no more than a variety of *accouchement forcé*, may cause a tear of the cervix which extends upwards into the lower segment to an uncontrollable degree and is a practice now generally condemned.

The uterus may be ruptured during the course of manual removal of the placenta, but this risk is lessened by keeping the fingers of the hand close together and by avoiding any temptation to claw at the placenta. The steadying influence of the outside hand on the abdominal wall also helps to reduce this risk, which is in any case surprisingly small.

By far the majority of cases of uterine rupture occur either as a result of a previous Caesarean section scar giving way or of obstructed labour. The latter comes into a class of its own. The risk of rupture of a uterus bearing a scar is apparently increased by each pregnancy thereafter, by each succeeding vaginal delivery, by high parity, twins, large fetus and hydramnios.[3]

Labour may be obstructed as a result of disproportion, malpresentation, pelvic tumours and strictures of the cervix which are the result of previous cauterisation, amputation, trachelorrhaphy or, very rarely, some congenital defect. In these cases either the uterus or the cervix must tear, and occasionally an annular separation of the cervix may occur (Fig. 1). In disproportion causing obstructed labour the uterine rupture is sometimes favoured by ischaemia, due to the pressure of the presenting part. The tear in the uterus then spreads from this area.

Threatened rupture and prophylaxis.—Ocasionally a uterine scar that is about to give way may give some advance warning in the form of pain and tenderness localised to the region of the scar.

In obstructed labour with an intact uterus, the lower uterine segment becomes progressively thinned while the upper segment, as a result of retraction, becomes thicker, so that the junction between the two (Bandl's ring) can often be both seen and felt through the abdominal wall. This visible ridge rises progressively in level and is usually oblique. At the same time the intervals between the contractions shorten, until the condition of tonic contraction or tetanic spasm of the uterus is fully developed. Rupture is now imminent. The combination of a Bandl's ring rising appreciably within 20 minutes or so, together with the threat of tonic contraction, indicates the immediate need for delivering the patient by the simplest and therefore safest possible method before rupture actually occurs. Under these circumstances internal version is nothing less than disastrous and, in the case of a shoulder presentation, decapitation is not only simpler but more expeditious. If the child is still alive, Caesarean section is the only reasonable treatment, but when, as is usually the case, the fetus is already dead, craniotomy in a cephalic presentation and other destructive operations as appropriate still have a place. Few obstetricians in civilised communities nowadays have much experience in these operations, because with proper supervision the situation does not arise.

Consequences of rupture.—As a rule, rupture in labour is far more dramatic than that occurring in pregnancy and is more dangerous because shock is greater and infection is almost inevitable. Haemorrhage and shock are the two most immediate risks and may be rapidly fatal.

Prolapse of the bowel is also likely to occur and is also assuredly fatal unless dealt with. Hypofibrinogenaemia may complicate uterine rupture and add defective coagulation to a situation already sufficiently disastrous. It is suggested that amniotic fluid may be forced into the circulation through vessels exposed by incomplete lower segment rupture, commonly in multiparous patients with precipitate delivery.[5] The resulting microcoagulation throughout the vascular tree, especially pulmonary, defibrinates the blood and, besides haemorrhage, the patient suffers collapse with cyanosis and respiratory distress. Finally, sepsis may carry off a patient who manages to survive the other catastrophes. Many cases of incomplete rupture, however, settle down spontaneously, and the haematoma in the broad ligament is ultimately absorbed.

The outlook for the next pregnancy is seriously prejudiced, and to allow a woman subsequently to deliver herself *per vaginam* is very questionable, however carefully and skilfully the rent has been sutured and however successful the antibiotics have been in controlling infection. It is usually wisest to perform elective Caesarean section in the next pregnancy about ten days before term, and in those cases where it is decided to take the risk of vaginal delivery, the forceps should be ready at full dilatation. This eliminates the increased dangers of the second stage.

Symptoms of uterine rupture.—Classically the patient experiences a severe bursting pain, although in a few cases of insidious rupture she may complain of no more than severe discomfort. Fainting is common, and usually there is some external bleeding, although this is variable. Silent rupture is more likely with a lower-segment scar and may be accompanied by no more than a rise in pulse rate. This sign is highly significant in a woman who is now labouring following a previous lower-segment Caesarean section.

Diagnosis of uterine rupture.—In the acute case the diagnosis is not usually difficult because labour comes to an abrupt stop to the accompaniment of great pain and ensuing shock.

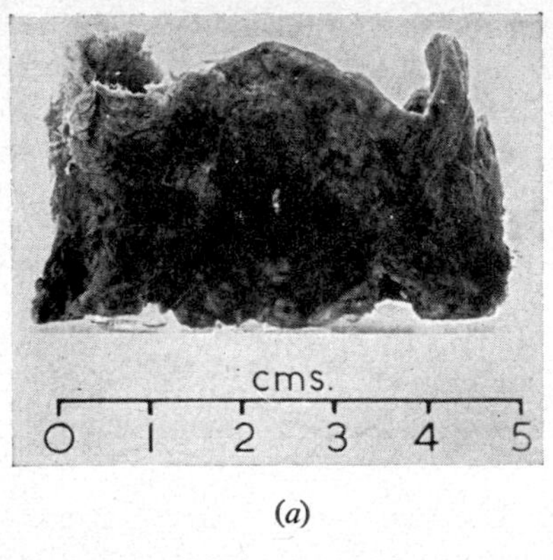

(*a*)

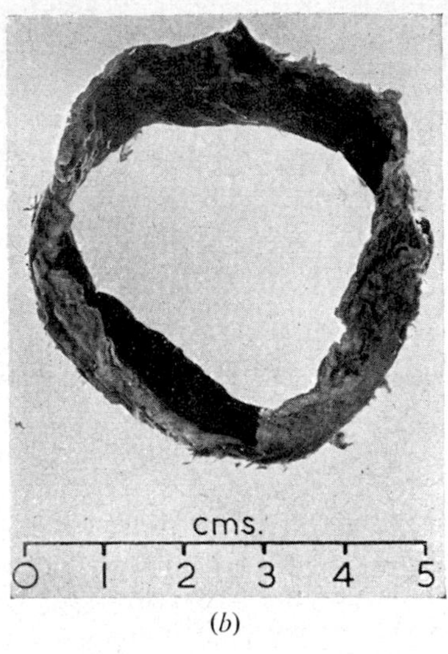

(*b*)

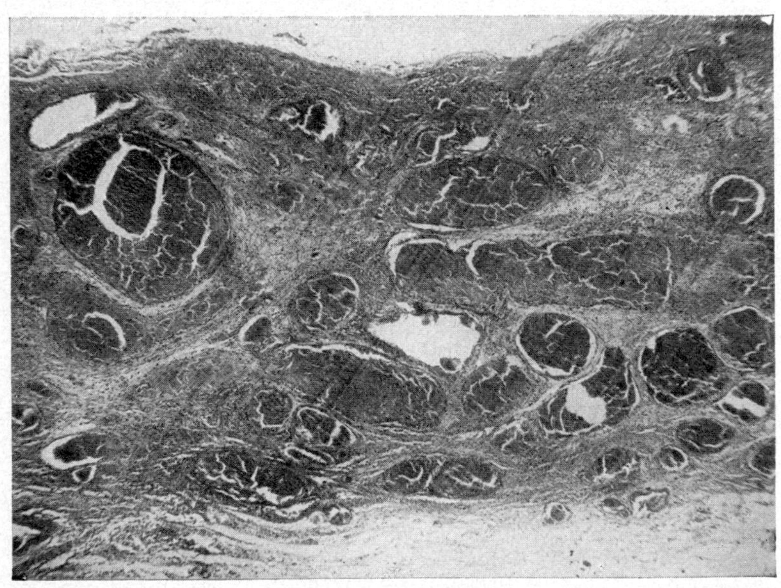

(*c*)

23/FIG. 1.—(*See opposite*.)

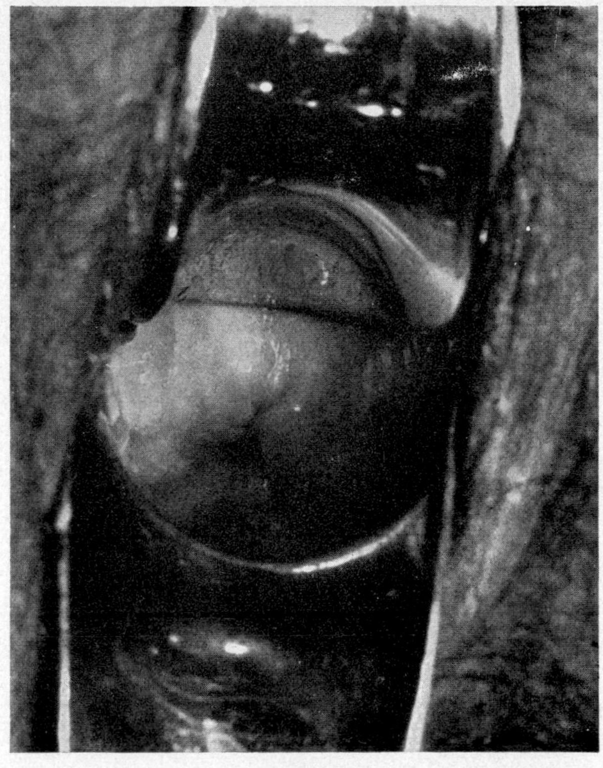

(*d*)

23/Fig. 1.

(*a*) and (*b*). Annular detachment of cervix.
(*c*) Photomicrograph of section of detached cervix showing intense engorgement of the blood vessels, advanced necrosis of all tissues and areas of haemorrhage.
(*d*) Remaining stump of cervix three months after delivery.
(By courtesy of Dr J. P. Erskine and the R.C.O.G. Museum).

Where, however, the onset is insidious, these signs are very much less marked. Nevertheless, contractions cease. The patient is not always shocked at first, and occasionally her condition may remain reasonably good for up to half an hour.

A characteristic sign is the loss of the presenting part from its former position within the pelvis. Indeed, as the fetus is extruded into the abdominal cavity, the fetal parts become easily palpable through the abdominal wall, especially if the patient is thin. The child usually dies, the fetal heart ceasing shortly after rupture.

In cases of complete rupture the now empty and retracted uterus forms a firm swelling to one side of the fetus, while in cases of incomplete rupture the bulge of a retroperitoneal haematoma in the broad ligament can often be felt to one side of the uterus and it may extend into the pelvis down one side of the vagina, bulging into its lumen.

Occasionally rupture occurs at the very end of the second stage of labour, so that vaginal delivery of the fetus is successfully completed. There now follows a very characteristic sign, namely shortening of the cord. This is practically pathognomonic of uterine rupture, with extrusion of the placenta into the abdominal cavity, and I have seen such a case in which this was the first and only obvious clue, since the patient's condition remained, for the time being, very good. The diagnosis was finally confirmed when an attempt was made to remove the placenta manually. On this occasion I well remember the firm, rounded, slippery swelling of the posterior wall of the uterus in front of my hand and the coils of intestine at the back of my fingers as I followed the cord into the peritoneum. The actual rent in the uterus was not noticeable to the examining hand at first.

Sometimes the diagnosis of uterine rupture will only be made after the completion of the third stage, and I recall another case in which collapse occurred during the third stage with the placenta still *in situ* and with only a moderate degree of external bleeding. I removed the placenta manually from the posterior wall of the uterus and did not observe the rupture of a previous classical Caesarean scar in the anterior wall. In the hours which followed, the patient's condition seemed to be far more anaemic than warranted, considering the six units of blood which had already been transfused. Her blood pressure was satisfactory, but, on removing the hot blankets, her flanks were noted to be bulging with blood from an extensive haemoperitoneum. She made an uninterrupted recovery following hysterectomy.

After delivery any case exhibiting a severe degree of shock which is unexpected or unexplained calls for exploration of the uterus forthwith, since many cases of maternal death occur from unsuspected uterine rupture and lacerations of the genital tract.

In Feeney and Barry's series of 45 cases of uterine rupture and perforation there were seven maternal deaths of which six were regarded as avoidable. Three of these deaths were due to failure, within hospital, to diagnose the condition in time.

All cases of previous Caesarean section who have just completed a subsequent vaginal delivery should be examined to assess the state of the old scar in the uterus. This can be done immediately after delivery without an anaesthetic by passing two fingers through the cervix and exploring the lower part of the uterine cavity. Pushing the uterus downwards over the fingers by pressing on the fundus facilitates the examination.

When bleeding continues in spite of a well-retracted uterus, for example after a forceps delivery or breech extraction, it is as well to remember that a laceration of the cervix, if present, may have extended far up into the uterus, and it is necessary to identify the apex. Sometimes, however, the cervix is intact and the bleeding may be coming from a rupture of the vaginal vault. This may not be easy to determine unless the cervix is first grasped with ring forceps and retracted to one side so that the vault can be inspected.

The differential diagnosis is concerned with the other causes of acute abdominal catastrophe, chief among which, in obstetrics, is abruptio placentae in which pain, shock, absence of uterine contractions and the disappearance of the fetal heart sounds likewise occur. Usually, too, there is vaginal bleeding. The uterus, however, in this case is regular in outline, and no swelling either of broad-ligament haematoma or extruded fetal parts can be felt to the side of it. The history of the case may be of some help; nevertheless, it is easy to be mistaken.

Shoulder presentation with the head in the iliac fossa may feel remarkably like a uterus pushed to one side by a fetus extruded through a uterine rent, but in this case rhythmical contraction and relaxation of the uterus will be observed.

After delivery the differential diagnosis is concerned with the other causes of postpartum collapse which have been dealt with in the chapter on that subject, but it behoves one especially to bear in mind the possibility of acute inversion. If in doubt, a vaginal examination should be made, because this is a condition which does not lightly forgive procrastination.

Treatment.—In full-blown complete uterine rupture, laparotomy should be undertaken as soon as possible after a blood transfusion has been started. Having opened the abdomen, three courses of action can be considered, namely hysterectomy, repair of the rupture, and repair and sterilisation of the patient. Of these, hysterectomy is undoubtedly the safest course, for a uterus which has once ruptured may well do so again, and removal of the dangerous and infected organ gives the best prospects for a smooth convalescence. However, especially in a young woman, there may be strong reasons for taking the risk of preserving the uterus and the nature of the rent itself will largely influence the decision.

Undoubtedly the advent of the antibiotics has made the repair and conservation of the uterus a less hazardous procedure, and I have delivered a young woman of two normal babies by the vaginal route, following a previous uterine rupture in which the bowel prolapsed into the vagina. Needless to say, the case caused considerable anxiety, but she was particularly anxious to increase her family and continually threatens to repeat the procedure yet again. It is not desired to give the impression that this line of treatment is favoured, but the patient in question, though well aware of the risks, was insistent. In the majority of cases there can be no doubt that, in a subsequent pregnancy, the safest course is to perform elective Caesarean section just before term.

The third alternative treatment, namely repair and sterilisation, has rather less to recommend it than the other two, because it takes every bit as long as hysterectomy to perform. The only advantage is that the patient is left with the questionable blessing of continued menstruation.

In repairing a uterine rupture it is customary to freshen up the edges of the wound by dissection, but too much time should not be wasted on this. The uterus should be repaired with interrupted sutures in layers, starting with one traction suture at the upper end of the rent and then working from the bottom upwards. In this way it is possible to examine the lowest and therefore the most difficult parts of the repair with the finger passed inside the uterus through the rent before it is finally closed. Great care must be taken not to include the ureter in any of the stitches, especially when the rupture extends to the sides of the lower segment. Prophylactic chemotherapy is of course obligatory.

Before proceeding to hysterectomy, however, one should be fully satisfied that the main source of haemorrhage is not a vaginal vault laceration if a tragic and irrelevant mistake is to be avoided.

In the lesser degrees of incomplete rupture in which the patient's condition remains satisfactory and the parametrial haematoma does not continue to enlarge, it is often possible to adopt a more conservative line, and these cases can be treated by plugging. The haematoma should be cleared out *per vaginam* and the space firmly packed with gauze impregnated with sulphonamide and penicillin. It is important at the same time to exert counter-pressure by means of a pad and abdominal binder, as otherwise blood may collect beyond the pack and behind the peritoneum. Uterine retraction should be maintained with ergot, and full anti-shock treatment should be continued, as appropriate. The pack is removed after 48 hours, the patient being well morphinised and several hours being spent over its gentle withdrawal. In less severe cases, in which the patient's general condition warrants it, morphine, blood transfusion and cat-like observation may suffice.

INVERSION OF THE UTERUS

This is one of the most serious complications in all midwifery. Fortunately it is very rare, although it is impossible to obtain reliable

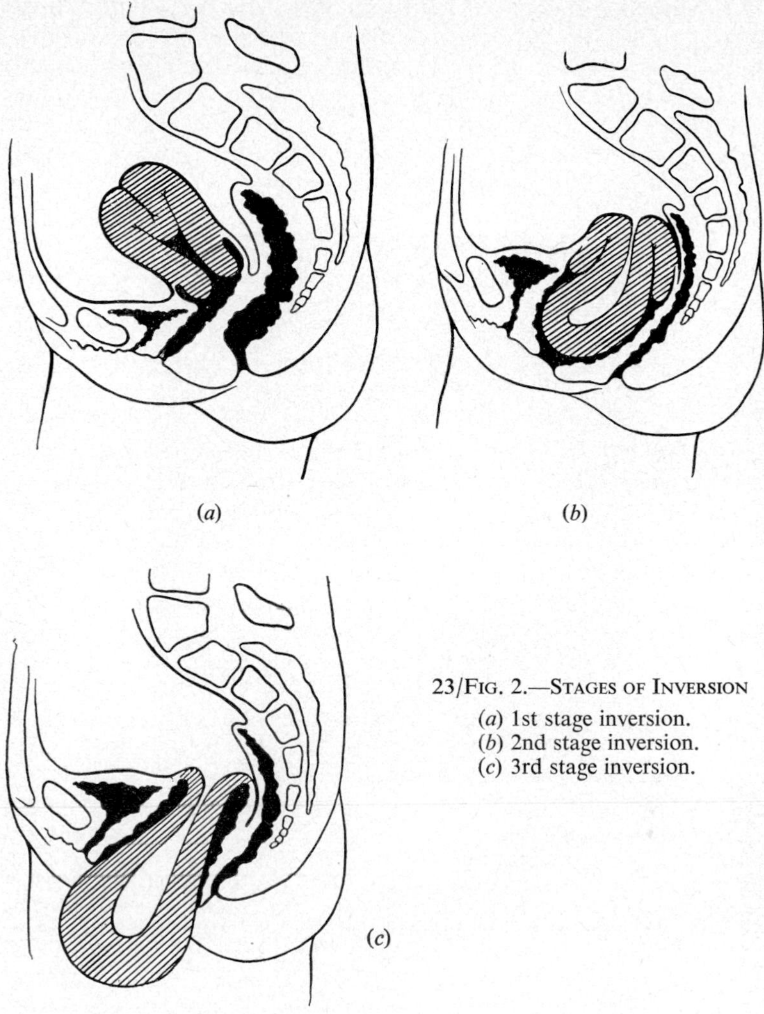

23/Fig. 2.—Stages of Inversion

(*a*) 1st stage inversion.
(*b*) 2nd stage inversion.
(*c*) 3rd stage inversion.

figures of incidence. Reports in the literature estimate it variously as between 1 in 17,000 and 1 in 200,000 deliveries. Most well-run obstetrical services supply reports of their work, and in these inversion is naturally extremely rare. It is in parts of the world where obstetrics is less enlightened that inversion is more common, and it is from these very regions that reports are not as a rule available.

There are three degrees of uterine inversion (Fig. 2). The first degree, which is likely to be missed, is that in which the fundus, in turning itself inside out, does not, however, herniate through the level of the internal os. In the second degree the fundus passes through the cervix and lies within the vagina, and in the third degree, which is very uncommon, the entire uterus is turned inside out and hangs outside the vulva, taking much of the vagina with it (Fig. 3). In other words, in all but the third and rarest degree the inverted uterus does not present to external view and consequently the diagnosis may not be as obvious as would appear.

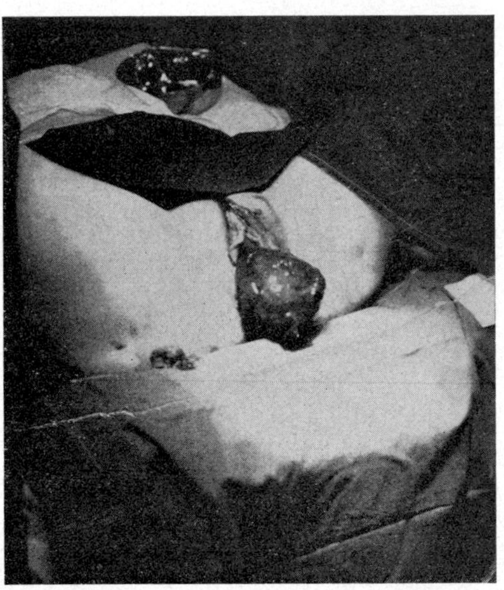

23/Fig. 3.—Acute spontaneous inversion of uterus. Photograph taken within a few minutes of its occurrence with a Polaroid camera, while anaesthetist and colleague made preparations for reducing it. (In my haste the photograph was badly torn.) Cardiac arrest occurred a few minutes later during anaesthesia. Thoracotomy was repeated four times in course of the next 36 hours because of recurrent cardiac arrest. Patient ultimately died without regaining consciousness.

Causes of inversion.—In about four-fifths of the cases some error of management is responsible, although the existence of spontaneous inversion cannot be denied. A fundal insertion of the placenta would appear to be a necessary prerequisite, and has been established in 75 per cent of spontaneous inversions.[2] A second prerequisite at the time of inversion is atony of the uterus. In other words, the hard and well-retracted uterus cannot be inverted.

The association of fundal placental insertion and uterine atony allows a number of more immediate causes to operate. Firstly, pulling on the cord under these circumstances will clearly provoke inversion, and the strongest argument against this practice is that one cannot be certain at the time that the placenta is not inserted at the fundus, although it is the least common position for it to occupy. It takes very little traction to pull such a uterus inside out, and I have demonstrated it to students at Caesarean section, an experiment not to be recommended, because in this case the drop in the patient's blood pressure was quite remarkable and I had some difficulty in replacing the inversion as the remainder of the uterus began to retract behind it.

Again, pressure upon the fundus of the soft uterus in order to expel blood clot or placenta may easily provoke inversion. Thirdly, a short cord may start a spontaneous inversion during the second stage of labour, although more commonly the placenta itself becomes detached. Sometimes, although the cord is not unduly short, it may be wound several times around the baby's neck, and this will produce the same effect.

Precipitate delivery, especially in the erect position, is more likely to provoke inversion than when the patient is lying down.

It has been postulated that occasionally there may be a localised area of uterine atony in the region of the placental site and that a sharp rise in intra-abdominal pressure, for example from violent bearing-down efforts or severe coughing, may initiate the process. In fact, inversion may be due to traction from within via the cord, or pressure from without. In the former case, some degree of abnormal adhesion of the placenta is probably necessary to invert the uterus.

Fibroids at the fundus are possible causes of inversion, but more commonly they only produce the chronic variety in cases wherein a submucous fibroid develops a pedicle and becomes a fibroid polyp. This is a state of affairs which is not met in obstetrics, although it is fairly common in gynaecology.

The rôle of Credé's expression of the placenta in producing inversion must be mentioned. Properly performed with a firm retracted uterus, the danger is practically non-existent, but any such attempt without first ensuring a uterine contraction is, of course, asking for trouble.

There is no specific prophylaxis against inversion except the avoidance of pulling on the cord or of pressing on the fundus of the uterus while it is soft. The patient should not be instructed to change her position, for example from the left lateral to the dorsal position, in the third stage without first ensuring that the uterus is firm, because the rise in abdominal pressure which the effort of movement entails might, in rare instances, initiate inversion.

Risks of inversion.—The immediate effect upon the patient is one of shock, often extremely profound, which comes on even faster than that associated with acute uterine rupture. It should be one of the first diagnostic possibilities to be considered in any patient developing postpartum collapse. Haemorrhage is variable but may be quite severe, especially when the placenta is already detached. The patient who weathers these two risks is still exposed to the likelihood of puerperal sepsis, which the various therapeutic measures adopted to reduce the inversion are likely to aggravate. As in all conditions producing severe shock, anuria and Sheehan's syndrome are possible sequelae. The untreated case is likely to die, but in a few instances spontaneous reduction occurs. In those in which it does not, the inverted uterus becomes infected and proceeds to slough.

Diagnosis.—The patient is usually too shocked to register much in the way of symptoms which, if recorded, consist mainly of severe lower abdominal pain with a strong bearing-down sensation.

The first step in arriving at a diagnosis is to find the whereabouts of the uterine fundus and to note any cupping, dimpling or irregularity of its upper surface. In severe cases the body of the uterus cannot be found at all on abdominal palpation, since it has turned itself inside out into the vagina. Abdominal palpation alone is not enough, and Spain (1946) described two cases in which, although the patients were thin, the abdominal signs of cupping of the fundus could not be demonstrated although they were deliberately looked for. One of the patients died ten days later. In both, the diagnosis was only made on vaginal examination. Any possibility, therefore, that the uterus may be inverted demands vaginal examination. The differential diagnosis is concerned with other causes of postpartum collapse dealt with in another chapter.

Treatment.—The best person to treat uterine inversion is the attendant present at the time of its occurrence. If it can be reduced within a few seconds of its development, the very factors which produce shock will be removed. The treatment is immediate replacement without attempting to remove the placenta from the inverted fundus. As a general rule it is preferable to reduce the inversion with the placenta still attached and to deal with its delivery later. In many of these cases the placenta is morbidly adherent and, in any event, removal exposes the maternal sinuses, which are intensely engorged, to infection. Moreover, bleeding is likely to be very severe and will aggravate the already developing shock. There is another very real risk in removing the placenta from the inverted uterus, namely that the uterine wall can be easily torn and perforated.

There are only two indications for removing the placenta before replacement of the uterus. The first is the necessity to reduce the bulk of the inverted mass in order to get it through a narrowing cervical ring, and the second is when all but a portion of the placenta is already separated. If immediate replacement is not feasible, shock supervenes so quickly that further attempts are no longer safe until the shock is first treated. Within a very few minutes even vaginal examination, unless very gentle, can precipitate or aggravate shock.

Unfortunately, in a number of cases acute inversion occurs in the absence of skilled assistants, so that when first seen the patient is already too shocked for replacement there and then. In these circumstances, or where it is not possible to replace the inversion straightway, the first thing to be done is to convert a third-degree inversion into one of the second degree and to raise the foot of the bed to maintain the inverted mass within the vagina instead of hanging outside. This reduces shock to some extent and, to a lesser extent, the inevitability of infection. Attempts at replacement in the presence of shock may easily prove fatal and should only be made either before shock has come on or after it has been treated.

Having replaced the inverted mass into the vagina, the patient should be given morphia 15–20 mg, and a plasma or saline drip should be set up pending the arrival of cross-matched blood for transfusion.

In domiciliary practice the patient should be treated adequately for shock before submitting her to an ambulance journey into hospital, and the assistance of a flying squad, if available, is invaluable. While awaiting help the patient should be kept warm, and on no account should ergot or oxytocin be given, as these will only aggravate matters and make reduction or replacement virtually impossible for the time being. The vulva is meanwhile kept covered with a sterile pad.

Replacement of the inversion.—The longer this is deferred the more difficult is it likely to be because of the tightening of the cervical ring. A fairly deep anaesthetic should be given, and following the usual antiseptic ritual, an attempt may be made by manual and digital pressure to reduce the inverted mass. If possible an attempt should be made to reduce that part of the uterus which has inverted last, in other words, the part nearest the cervix, rather than dimpling the inverted fundus and trying to push extra thicknesses of uterine wall through the cervical ring. While carrying out this manipulation the other hand should be placed over the abdomen to supply counter support, otherwise the still inverted uterus may be pushed high up into the abdomen with the vagina on the stretch. This increases shock. If this manoeuvre is successful in replacing the uterus, the hand should be kept within its cavity until ergometrine has been given and taken effect. This will reduce the likelihood of a recurrence. Titus, in his book *Management of Obstetrical Difficulties*, recommended packing the uterus to prevent the inversion recurring, but opinion in this country is much less inclined to favour packing of the uterus at any time.

O'Sullivan in 1945 published a simple and very effective method of dealing with inversion by applying intravaginal hydraulic pressure. He himself told me that he came on this method of treatment purely by accident. He was about to reduce an inversion by the traditional methods and, preparatory to doing so, gave the patient a warm antiseptic vaginal douche, in the course of which his forearm blocked the vulval outlet. To his astonishment the inversion disappeared and the uterus returned to its normal position. He has since used this method in at least two dozen further cases deliberately. He passes a douche nozzle towards the posterior fornix and, with the douche can raised no more the one metre above the level of the vagina, he runs in a copious, warm antiseptic solution. An assistant gathers the labia around his forearm so as to block the vulva, and in practically every case the treatment is dramatically successful. This method would appear to be a real advance and is certainly less likely to cause further shock to a patient than manipulation and taxis. I once had a case in which acute inversion of the third degree had occurred four hours previously in domiciliary practice. The mass was pushed into the vagina and covered with a sterile pad and the patient admitted to hospital. Profound shock supervened following vaginal examination which transfusion could not correct. Under deep anaesthesia replacement was undertaken but I found the cervical ring so tight that in spite of combining O'Sullivan's hydraulic method and direct manipulation I could at first prevail nothing. The whole mass felt like a doughy pudding. Presently the ring appeared to move upwards towards the fundus and the last half of the inversion suddenly and miraculously disappeared under the hydraulic pressure of the douche. The patient's recovery was immediate and dramatic.

If all the above methods fail, it is usually because the cervical ring has become too tight and its forcible dilatation will only make matters worse. In long-standing cases Aveling's repositor may be tried, coupled with repeated hot douches but, as a rule, provided the patient's condition can stand the surgical procedure, it is better to resort to operation, of which there are several types. Of these the best known is that of Spinelli in which, using the vaginal approach, the bladder is dissected upwards and pushed out of the way. The ring and the lower part of the inverted uterus, i.e. that part of it nearest the cervix, is divided anteriorly, and the inversion is then replaced, following which the incision is closed with interrupted sutures. An alternative method is that of Küstner, in which the cervical ring is divided posteriorly.

Operation by the abdominal route is another alternative, and an attempt may be made to drag back the inversion from above by the use of Allis forceps. The recently delivered uterus, however, is very liable to tear, in which case reposition may be more easily achieved by incising the ring posteriorly from above according to the method of Haultain. Full anti-shock treatment must be maintained until the patient is out of immediate danger. Bacteriological cultures should be taken from the cervix at the time of replacement, so that appropriate antibiotic treatment may be started with the minimum of delay and as early as possible in a puerperium which is almost bound to be stormy.

PERINEAL AND VAGINAL TEARS

The adoption of the erect posture has endowed humanity with certain well-known penalties. One of these is the fact that the pelvic floor literally lives up to its name at the bottom of the pelvic cavity and is subjected to stresses which in no way apply to quadrupeds. As a result the shape of the birth canal becomes that of a right-angled pipe, the far wall of which is formed by the muscles of the pelvic floor. As the perineum constitutes the common point of insertion for most of these, it comes in for the brunt of the burden in vaginal delivery.

The casual view that the perineum was ordained by nature to tear in childbirth cannot be upheld, for it is a structure of considerable functional importance. A damaged perineum means an ineffective pelvic floor, and the condensations of pelvic fascia, which maintain the pelvic viscera in their normal anatomical positions, cannot afford indefinitely to do without the active muscular support of the levatores ani. Thus, after a latent period of many years, the supports of the uterus, bladder and bladder-neck yield, often in the process of menopausal atrophy, and the patient all too often becomes the victim of prolapse, stress incontinence or both. In this respect a stretched perineum may be almost as bad as a torn perineum, for both lose some of their functional capacity. Furthermore, a torn perineum is a wound in a none-too-sterile part of the body at a time when unnecessary infection cannot be countenanced, and it is only the great vascularity of the part and its local resistance to infection which prevent it from becoming a dangerous portal of entry for sepsis.

TYPES OF PERINEAL TEAR

There are three main degrees of perineal laceration; the first degree involves the hymen, or what is left of it, and fourchette, together with a small distance of vaginal and perineal skin, but the perineal body itself is undamaged. In second-degree laceration the perineal body is ruptured, together with a variable length of posterior vaginal wall. In severe forms the external anal sphincter may be damaged, but provided the lumen of the anal canal is not opened, the case should properly be included in the second degree. The third-degree laceration is obviously the most serious because the anal canal is opened up; in fact, the tear may extend to include the rectum. The patient is incontinent of faeces and the whole wound is inevitably infected from the bowel. This type of injury is a major obstetrical disaster, and unless effectively dealt with may wreck the patient's whole future and make a social outcast of her.

There are a few minor subdivisions of less importance, such as the so-called central tear of the perineum in which an anterior bridge remains intact, the baby being delivered as the term would suggest. The existence of the anterior bridge of unruptured tissue is of no importance and in any case it must be divided before repairing the tear.

Labial lacerations are seldom of any structural significance and do not often call for any reparative procedure. They are, however, very tender, and can be quite a nuisance during the puerperium when they are particularly liable to produce reflex retention of urine.

The causes of perineal tearing are not necessarily the fault of the medical attendant, although the extent thereof may to some extent be a measure of clumsiness. In the past much harm has been done by sister tutors of midwifery who have regarded the torn perineum as a matter for disciplinary admonition of the midwife, with the result that a policy of saving the perineum at all costs tends to be adopted. This is highly undesirable, because an overstretched and devitalised perineum ends up far worse off than a perineum which has been torn and properly sutured. If the perineum is kept on the stretch for a long time by the baby's head, it transmits great pressure to the back of the symphysis pubis and to the region of the bladder neck, so that its supports become permanently weakened, and stress incontinence, even without prolapse, may result. In the reports of most well-run maternity units the episiotomy rate exceeds the perineal tear rate.

Very rapid delivery, on the other hand, is not only unnecessarily damaging to the perineum but is bad for the baby's head. The head may be crowned without causing damage, but the perineum may be needlessly torn in the course of delivering the face. If possible this should be achieved between uterine contractions. The delivery of the posterior shoulder frequently causes damage which the patient has hitherto escaped, and in training students and midwives more emphasis should be placed on skilful handling at this stage than in the delivery of the head itself, because the majority of lacerations caused by the posterior shoulder are unnecessary and largely due to clumsiness.

The narrower the subpubic arch, the more acute the subpubic angle, and the more android in type the pelvis, the farther back will the head have to pass to emerge from under the symphysis pubis. This will certainly increase the extent of perineal damage.

Face-to-pubis delivery, because of the larger fetal diameters concerned, does more damage than delivery with the occiput anterior, and the worst degrees of tear, frequently involving the rectum, are those caused by the unwitting forceps extraction of a head in the unreduced persistent occipitoposterior position.

Breech delivery has a high perineal tear rate, because there is less opportunity for the perineum to stretch adequately, and in primigravidae it is most undesirable that the perineum should hold up the delivery of an aftercoming head, so that episiotomy is more or less standard practice.

Prevention of perineal tears.—It is not intended to give the impression that the perineum should just be allowed to rip, in fact, a conscientious attempt should be made to limit the extent of tearing. Timely episiotomy (under local infiltration anaesthesia) will often forestall a ragged tear. It is certainly impossible to guard the perineum with the fingers, as is so frequently taught, for the force so applied is misdirected and misapplied. Much can be done by allowing completion of the delivery of the head only between pains and by care with delivery of the posterior shoulder. It seems probable that the use of the left lateral position in normal labour is less likely to favour tears than the dorsal position, although the latter has so many other advantages that its use is becoming increasingly general in this country.

Method of repair.—This should be done soon after delivery, and the practice of accumulating the night's tears in hospital until they can all be liquidated the following morning is to be deplored. For one thing, freshly damaged tissues can be more satisfactorily sutured, for another, less time is allowed for the introduction of sepsis, and lastly, the patient deserves to be tidied up after labour and left in peace without the anticipation of stitching in hours to come. There is much to be said for proceeding with the repair while awaiting delivery of the placenta, especially if the tear is not extensive. The only argument against getting to work straightway is in the case of the extensive tear when a good view must be obtained, and it may be very inconvenient to deal with the arrival of the placenta before at least the vaginal skin is properly sewn up.

A good light is essential to work by and a relatively bloodless field is a great help, otherwise the apex of the rent in the vagina will be missed. It is a good plan to cut a vulval pad in two and to push the half pad up into the vaginal vault to absorb any trickle of blood from above. Very adequate anaesthesia can be obtained by the injection of 1 per cent lignocaine infiltrated directly round the region of the tear. Twenty millilitres should be perfectly adequate for the purpose.

The apex of the vaginal tear is now identified, and the vagina is first sutured with continuous catgut so as to produce a good blood-tight joint. This prevents the seepage of lochia into the depths of the perineal wound, which will assuredly occur if the posterior vaginal wall is not properly closed. Failure to observe this precaution results in many repairs breaking down. The perineal body is then stitched, usually with about three or four interrupted No. 1 catgut sutures. While inserting them, the index finger of one hand should press the rectum backwards out of harm's way. These stitches should not be tied tightly; this is a common mistake and discourages rather than facilitates healing. There remains now only the perineal skin. My own preference is for interrupted fine catgut sutures inserted with the knot buried inwards. Some prefer a running subcuticular stitch, but any continuous suture in the event of sepsis tends to prevent drainage. Interrupted nylon or silkworm gut is still very popular in units still accustomed to barbarity and the use of black silk has a touch of black magic about it. Apart from being a natural tissue irritant it involves the patient in the miserable puerperal ritual of stitch removal.

I have never had any trouble from burying under the skin the knots of interrupted fine catgut and the patient is always very comfortable.

The old-fashioned method was to take silkworm gut on large harpoon needles and go through all layers, taking up enormous bites of tissue. This is a very unsatisfactory method, and while the end result may look all very well from the outside, it often leaves no more than a "dashboard" perineum with relatively little substance deep to the skin. My students have attributed to me the remark that women do not micturate on barbed-wire fences. I cannot remember making it but at least they got the message. It might be feared that the delivery of the placenta would break down one's repair, but this is not so, for the placenta is very soft, and any suturing which could not withstand its passage has not been properly done. The possibility of having to undertake manual removal of the placenta may also discourage one from embarking on perineal suture during the third stage, but this should not deter one. The deep sutures need not be tied until after the arrival of the placenta.

It is a common mistake to sew up too tightly, with the result that the patient is considerably embarrassed subsequently by dyspareunia. The tissues of the vulva and vagina shrink during the process of involution, and it should be a rule to ensure that three fingers can be easily inserted simultaneously into the vagina at the end of the operation.

Third-degree Tear

There is no place for local anaesthesia in repairing a third-degree tear. The job has to be done very thoroughly in a proper theatre and a general anaesthetic should be given. The first step is to repair the anus and rectum. Interrupted catgut sutures are used, starting from above and working downwards. They should be inserted in such a way that the knots come to lie within the rectal lumen (Fig. 4). An alternative

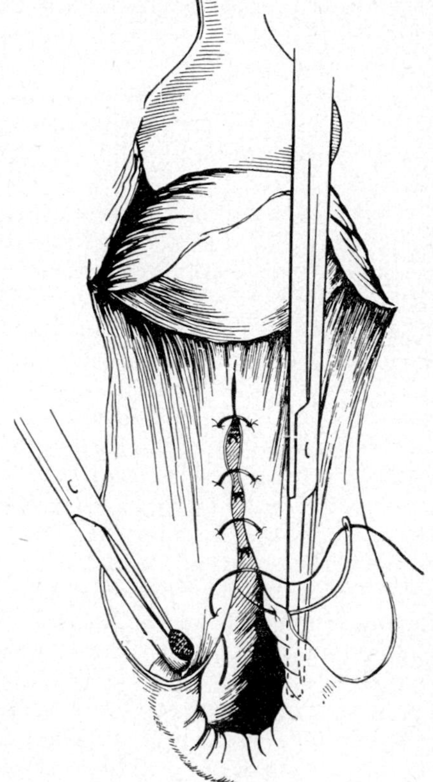

23/FIG. 4.—Repair of the rectum in third-degree tear.

and more fussy method is to insert Lembert sutures which necessitate the tying of knots on the perineal aspect and no advantage is to be gained thereby.

Having repaired the anal canal, the torn ends of the anal sphincter must be found. One side nearly always retracts out of view and must be deliberately sought, whereupon two or three fine mattress sutures are used to produce satisfactory end-to-end apposition of the sphincter. If the tear has been very deep, it may be found to have extended beyond the upper apex of the perineum, in which case the vaginal and rectal rents will correspond, so that it is difficult to repair the rectum as a separate layer. This step is essential nevertheless, and in order to achieve it the rectum should be dissected upwards from the vagina for a distance of a centimetre or two. This is a common region for a residual rectovaginal fistula, not only from failure to observe this precaution, but because there is no appreciable thickness of tissue which can be brought between.

The third-degree tear has now been converted into one of the second degree and the steps of the operation are continued as described above.

The after-treatment is important, and the patient should be kept on a low-residue diet for the next week. Liquid paraffin by mouth is commonly recommended from the second day onwards, but paraffin is extraordinary stuff for finding out leaks and will seep through any available crevices in the surgical repair, thus encouraging non-union, and the patient may be left with a fistula. It is necessary to leave the bowels strictly alone for at least five or six days; thereupon a gentle instillation of a few ounces of olive oil with a soft rubber catheter twice a day should suffice to soften down any faecal masses, so that when the patient has a bowel action at about the end of a week it is a soft, atraumatic one.

In spite of the most careful technique, it not infrequently happens that the repair of a third-degree tear breaks down. There are two reasons for this: either the repair was imperfectly carried out or it breaks down because of sepsis. The patient is now left with a very real disability in the form of some degree of rectal incontinence and will not be comfortable until the trouble is dealt with. Nevertheless, it is not safe to attempt further repair until all signs of local sepsis have cleared up. Usually one prefers to wait for about four months for involution to complete itself, in the hope thereby of operating upon more satisfactory tissues, but in favourable circumstances secondary suture may be undertaken earlier. Every failed attempt prejudices the outlook for subsequent operations.

It is worth noting here, in passing, that patients with unhealed third-degree tears very seldom develop prolapse, in spite of the perineal damage. This is because of the constant effort which the patient unconsciously makes, with what is left of her pelvic floor, to maintain some degree of rectal continence.

A patient who has had a successfully repaired third-degree tear must be carefully managed in any subsequent delivery. If there has been much previous difficulty in curing her, there is much to be said for elective Caesarean section but, if vaginal delivery is decided upon, a generous episiotomy is obligatory. On no account should the scar of the previous repair be subjected to the stresses of labour.

VAULT RUPTURE

This is more common than is usually recognised, and is one of the causes of continued trickling of blood after the completion of the third stage. The lateral margin of the cervix is often involved as well, and if large vessels at the base of the broad ligament are opened up, haemorrhage can be very profuse. In lesser degrees quite a large paravaginal haematoma may form and give rise to a pyrexial puerperium. Attempts to repair a rent in the vaginal vault are fraught with the danger of damaging a ureter, and on the whole these injuries are safest left to themselves to heal. However, if any appreciable degree of bleeding continues, the rent and the space in the cellular tissue beyond it should be packed with gauze, and to prevent the development of a parametrial haematoma, a firm abdominal pad and binder should be applied to exert counter-pressure. The bleeding point is often on the torn vaginal edge and careful suturing deals with it. Nevertheless, if the rent is a large one, it is worth partially suturing, at the same time inserting a drain into the haematoma cavity. These measures will nearly always suffice, but where the haemorrhage is really torrential and cannot be controlled by packing from below, it may be necessary to resort to laparotomy and in very rare instances to hysterectomy, or as an alternative, ligation of the anterior division of the internal iliac artery on the affected side.

EPISIOTOMY

The importance of this little operation is out of all proportion to its simplicity. Nevertheless, it is frequently abused.

An episiotomy is infinitely preferable to an overstretched and devitalised perineum, with its parallel weakening of the supports of the bladder neck. Timely episiotomy can prevent a great deal of damage in this respect and is regarded as an important factor in the prevention of subsequent prolapse. An episiotomy, moreover, will save what might otherwise have been a perineal tear extending to the third degree, because it deflects the direction of tearing to one side of the anus.

The chief virtue of episiotomy lies in the saving of unnecessary wear and tear upon the fetal skull. This is particularly important in cases of prematurity.

A second stage prolonged because of rigidity of the perineum can often be completed satisfactorily without the need for forceps, and the patient may be saved a great deal of unnecessary misery. Lastly, the uterus may be spared some exhaustion, and this will reduce the likelihood of postpartum haemorrhage.

In forceps deliveries, episiotomy is becoming increasingly general, because delivery can be completed with less traumatic force to mother and baby, since it relieves the fetal head of the undesirable rôle of acting as a battering ram on the maternal pelvic floor.

Flew's episiotomy rate in primigravidae was over 50 per cent, yet only 12 per cent were combined with the forceps operation, suggesting, in other words, that episiotomy dispensed with the need for forceps in many cases.

To withhold episiotomy when indicated would be wanton; nevertheless, it constitutes a mutilation, although mild, and if ruthlessly abused without good reason, it will leave a number of women exposed to the likelihood of further perineal troubles in subsequent deliveries, often necessitating repeated episiotomy. This is a minor objection, but it has to be remembered that occasionally a painful and unsatisfactory scar may give rise to dyspareunia. It is as well to repeat episiotomy, when indicated, on the same side as before. It heals just as well and causes less ultimate scarring and possible dyspareunia.

Indications

There are many indications, and the following is a list of most of them:

1. All cases of fetal distress in the second stage demand episiotomy to spare the child further delay, damage and asphyxia in labour.
2. All cases of prematurity for reasons given above.
3. All cases of primigravid breech delivery. It is too late to start thinking about an episiotomy when one runs into trouble with the after-coming head or with extended arms.
4. All cases of face-to-pubis forceps delivery.
5. After previous colpoperineorraphy and after any operation for the cure of stress incontinence in which a vaginal delivery has been decided upon.

The above are absolute indications. To these many would add all cases of forceps delivery in primigravidae.

There follows a list of relative indications:

1. When the subpubic arch is narrow, and the head, because of its consequent posterior displacement, has difficulty in emerging.
2. Failure to advance because of perineal rigidity.
3. When the presenting part has been on the pelvic floor for more than half an hour.
4. Most cases of face presentation, excluding anencephaly.
5. When the perineal skin starts to split and a sizeable tear appears to be a certainty.

A very ragged vaginal tear is an unsatisfactory thing to sew up and this can often be avoided by episiotomy. If an episiotomy is inadequate for the demands made upon it, it will split further, but very seldom indeed into the rectum, whereas tearing of the perineum may easily extend uncontrollably.

Technique

The usual practice is to direct the cut to one side of the midline. A so-called midline episiotomy or perineotomy has little to recommend it, as any extension of the wound will be directed towards the rectum. The time to perform the episiotomy is when the perineum is unquestionably bulging. The length of incision required is then easier to determine, and to do it earlier may result in an unnecessary amount of blood loss which normally the pressure of the presenting part tends to control. On the other hand, to perform episiotomy too late, when the damage from stretching is already done, is also a mistake.

It is sometimes taught that an anaesthetic is not necessary on the argument that the patient is feeling such excruciating pain at this stage of labour that she is unlikely to notice any addition to it. This is nothing less than horrifying brutality, and it is inexcusable not to infiltrate the area of the incision with a few millilitres of lignocaine, 1 per cent, a simple procedure taking a few seconds.

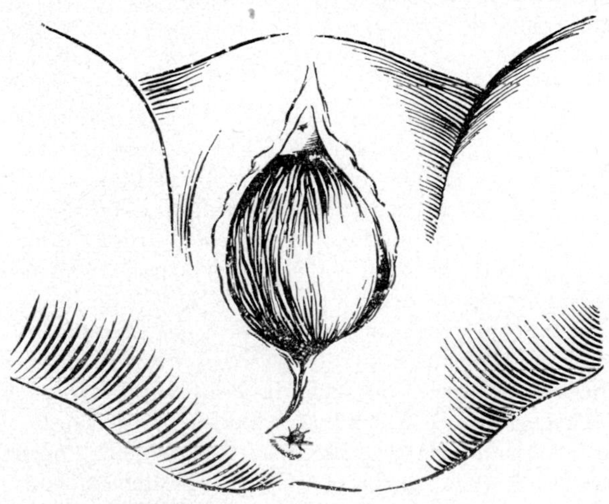

23/Fig. 5.—Line of episiotomy.

The best instrument to use is a strong pair of curved scissors, and the incision should start anteriorly from the midpoint of the fourchette (Fig. 5). It is a common mistake to make an oblique cut starting too far from the midline, for not only may this defeat satisfactory suture but a more vascular area is opened up and bleeding may be excessive. The best procedure is to cut directly backwards for the first part of the incision and then to use the curve of the scissors to direct the incision laterally in the shape of the letter "J" so that it runs to one side of the anal margin. By keeping 2–3 cm away from the latter one can be certain of avoiding damage to the anal sphincter. Personally, I prefer to map out the incision with an unmounted scalpel blade held in the left hand using the scissors only for cutting the vaginal wall.

A finger should be inserted into the vagina as a guard and the whole depth of tissue should be convincingly divided, if possible in one determined cut rather than in a series of nibbles. If brisk bleeding occurs, it is probable that the episiotomy has been done too early, but in any case a powerful bleeding point ought to be picked up with a haemostat, for a patient can lose a surprising quantity of blood from an episiotomy wound in quite a short space of time.

The repair of an episiotomy follows exactly the same lines as for a second-degree tear, but the inner side of the wound tends to retract more than the lateral margin and care must be taken to secure satisfactory alignment.

The practice of performing bilateral episiotomy has now been almost universally abandoned because, although it provides an enormous exposure and the anal canal tends to hinge backwards out of the way like a trap-door, there is a strong likelihood of sloughing, since the blood supply has been interrupted from both sides. For this reason it is better to do a wide single episiotomy than two small bilateral cuts.

There are very few dangers in episiotomy, the chief being blood loss which can always be controlled. Sepsis occurs occasionally and the wound breaks down, but secondary suture as soon as the sepsis has been cleared up is a perfectly satisfactory procecure.

On rare occasions Bartholin's duct is damaged, and some time later a Bartholin's cyst develops. This should never occur if the incision has been started correctly in the midline and only results from recklessly wide lateral cuts.

If deepening shock occurs, as occasionally it may, following episiotomy repair, it is worth including a large paravaginal haematoma among the diagnostic possibilities. Vaginal examination will at once reveal the characteristic lateral bulge. In such a case the repair must be undone, the clot evacuated and proper haemostatic suturing undertaken. Only rarely should packing be necessary.

INJURIES TO THE URINARY SYSTEM

It is not surprising that the urinary tract occasionally suffers some degree of wear and tear considering its unfortunate anatomical proximity to the field of obstetrical battle. All manner of urinary disabilities therefore, ranging from the mild to the severe may be encountered.

Stress Incontinence

During early and late pregnancy some degree of this is common enough to be almost physiological, but the stresses of labour may so weaken the fascial supports of the bladder neck that a permanent disability results, if not forthwith, at least in years to come, particularly at about the time of menopausal involution.

The bladder neck in difficult labour becomes the nut between the crackers, being compressed and devitalised between the back of the symphysis pubis and the advancing fetal head.

Sometimes the anterior vaginal wall is pushed down in front of the presenting part, and it is important to press it up and out of the way during the second stage. Often a perineal tear is carefully avoided at the cost of diminished urinary control, and it is far preferable to perform episiotomy than to leave the head a long time on the perineum. The expeditious use of the low forceps operation, or ventouse, will also cut short prolonged stress upon the bladder neck supports, but forceps applied before full dilatation of the cervix is a potent cause of stress incontinence.

After delivery, postnatal exercises are of great value in forestalling the development of this miserable condition, and it is important that they should be continued after return home when urinary control is inadequate or cystocele threatens. Physiotherapy, here, can perform a very useful function.

If the condition persists at the time of postnatal examination, the temporary support afforded by a suitable pessary until involution is complete may render subsequent operation unnecessary.

If, however, stress incontinence is still troublesome six months after delivery, operative repair by colporrhaphy should be performed regardless of the patient's age or the prospects of further childbearing. The need for this, however, is usually the result of the patient's failure to co-operate in her postnatal exercises and physiotherapy. Stress incontinence is a preventable condition.

Having successfully cured the case surgically, labour must, in later instances, be conducted with due regard to the operative result. Episiotomy at the very least is emphatically indicated, and often Caesarean section may be advisable.

Ureteric Fistula

This is fortunately a very rare complication of vaginal delivery and only the most extreme forms of misdirected trauma are likely to inflict it.

Vesicovaginal Fistula

This is uncommon in enlightened obstetrics, but was a common result of neglected disproportion, particularly in cases of flat pelvis. It may arise either as the result of pressure necrosis of the bladder neck, in which case the fistula develops about a week after delivery when the slough separates, or it may be directly caused by laceration with instruments or, in the operation of cranioclasm, by the jagged ends of skull bones. After symphysiotomy, too, the bladder, no longer fully supported by the pubic framework, may suffer damage. Howsoever caused, the invariable symptom is total urinary incontinence regardless of posture or activity.

The diagnosis is not difficult. The larger fistulae can either be seen, or felt with the finger but the instillation of methylene blue into the bladder may help to reveal very small lesions.

The fistula is usually situated on the anterior vaginal wall, but occasionally it may open into the anterior fornix or even into the cervix or uterus. At lower-segment Caesarean section failure to displace the bladder downwards and out of harm's way before incising the uterus, or careless suturing later, may damage the bladder wall and cause a vesico-uterine fistula. Damage to the bladder at the time of the operation is usually demonstrated by bloodstained urine which is easily tested for by pinching the catheter before withdrawing it and then emptying the urine within over a white towel or swab.

Treatment should be immediate and never deferred even until next day if there is to be any hope of obtaining spontaneous closure. A catheter should be passed into the bladder and anchored with sutures; continuous gentle suction drainage should be maintained for two, or preferably three weeks, keeping the bladder absolutely empty and at rest. I have seen very unpleasant fistulae close spontaneously without more elaborate treatment, but success depends entirely upon instituting drainage before the fistulous track has a chance to epithelialise.

If this treatment fails to close the fistula, operative repair must be undertaken, and there is no need to prolong the patient's wretchedness by waiting for more than three months, since it can safely be assumed that if it has not closed before then nothing short of surgical repair will succeed in effecting a cure.

OBSTETRICAL PALSIES

Although the literature has paid rather scant attention to this subject, palsies as a result of pregnancy and labour are by no means rare, and they constitute a fairly important source of postnatal disability. The commonest form is the appearance of foot-drop, usually unilateral, shortly after delivery or during the first day or so.

The muscles most frequently affected are the dorsiflexors of the foot and toes, though occasionally the glutei, hamstrings, quadriceps and adductors of the thigh may be severally involved.

The lesion is of the lower motor neurone type with flaccidity and wasting. Sensory loss or disturbance is less prominent but is often present. Strenuous vaginal delivery, usually terminating in a forceps operation, is an accepted predisposing condition, but the complication can occur after easy, rapid and normal delivery with a roomy pelvis.

The old explanation that the lesions was caused by direct pressure, either by the fetal head or the forceps blades upon the lumbosacral cord or sacral plexus, is not accepted nowadays, because it does not explain the onset of symptoms many hours after labour, nor the appearance of damage of femoral nerve distribution, and if direct intrapelvic pressure could so operate, one would expect vesical and rectal injury even more often.

Backward rotation of the sacrum in labour has also been thought to result in stretching of the lumbosacral cord and may account for some cases of postnatal sciatica, but the most likely explanation lies in the theory of intervertebral disc protrusion. O'Connell (1944), in giving details of four cases, discussed the likelihood of this factor very clearly, and he considered that the prolapsed disc theory can account for all cases, excluding of course those of peroneal palsy due to misuse of lithotomy poles and stirrups. This explanation is not accepted for all cases however; Chalmers (1949) traced 142 cases in the literature and added another four of which only one was attributed to disc protrusion, the other three being due to compression (two cases) and sacral rotation (one case) and he concluded that different mechanisms could produce the condition. Now, as is well known, the joints of the pelvis increase their mobility in pregnancy, and in pathological degree this may give rise to symptoms of pelvic arthropathy. The effect is believed to be due to "relaxin" or progesterone and can be reproduced in experimental animals. Since it is unlikely that an endocrine effect would select only the pelvic joints, it is reasonable to assume that the vertebral column, too, takes part in the general loosening-up process. In pregnancy, furthermore, lordosis of the lumbar spine may be exaggerated, so that the intervertebral discs become vulnerable to the stress of labour and may herniate. The type of neurological lesion and whether or not it is bilateral will then depend only upon the extent and direction of the disc protrusion. The disc most commonly involved is that between the fifth lumbar and first sacral vertebral body.

On this basis treatment is formulated. Firstly, rest in bed is necessary, sometimes for six weeks in cases which do not readily clear up and where pain persists. A hard board should be placed under the mattress and over the bed-springs to prevent sagging of the back while the patient is relaxed in sleep. Secondly, splinting is applied to prevent damage by unopposed overstretching of the paralysed muscles. Massage and electrical stimulation to the muscles are started fairly early, and active exercise is encouraged with the return of function.

The prognosis is usually favourable and many cases clear up within a few weeks, though it may be necessary to prescribe a spring to raise the front of the shoe in the early stages of ambulation. In severe and resistant cases, in which disability or pain and backache persist, operation upon the prolapsed disc may be required. Nevin (1951) has suggested that cases who develop disc lesions in pregnancy should be delivered by Caesarean section unless a straightforward and easy labour can be confidently anticipated.

REFERENCES

1. Chalmers, J. A. (1949). *J. Obstet. Gynaec. Brit. Emp.*, **56,** 205.
2. Das, P. (1940). *J. Obstet. Gynaec. Brit. Emp.*, **47,** 525.
3. Feeney, K. and Barry, A. (1956). *Brit. med. J.*, **1,** 65.
4. Flew, J. D. S. (1944). *Brit. med. J.*, **2,** 620.
5. Josey, W. E. (1966). *Amer. J. Obstet. Gynec.*, **94,** 29.
6. Nevin, S. (1951). In: *Medical Disorders in Pregnancy*, S. G. Clayton and S. Oram, eds., London: Churchill.
7. O'Connell, J. E. A. (1944). *Surg. Gynec. Obstet.*, **79,** 374.
8. O'Driscoll, K. (1966). *Proc. roy. Soc. Med.*, **59,** 65.
9. O'Sullivan, J. V. (1945). *Brit. med. J.*, **2,** 282.
10. Spain, A. W. (1946). *J. Obstet. Gynaec. Brit. Emp.*, **53,** 219.

CHAPTER XXIV

CAESAREAN SECTION

CAESAREAN section is now performed with increasing impunity, thanks largely to antibiotics, improved anaesthesia and the availability of blood transfusion. It is natural, therefore, that the indications for this operation are being continually extended; nevertheless, there is no excuse for resorting to it because one lacks the obstetrical skill of a previous generation, and it would be a great mistake to regard it as a means of finding a happy issue out of all our obstetrical afflictions. "Caesarean Section—a lethal operation?" was chosen, in fact, as the title of Sir Andrew Claye's William Hunter Memorial Lecture in Glasgow in 1960, in which he reviewed disasters precipitated by ill-chosen indications, unsatisfactory operating conditions, indifferent or inexperienced technique and bad timing.

In these days of small families the baby's right to survival is increasingly recognised, and consequently many of the indications for the operation are now solely concerned with the interests of the infant.

Indications.—The following is a list of indications more or less in order of importance, which, singly or in combination, may sway the obstetrician's decision in favour of abdominal delivery (vaginal by-pass):

1. Fetal distress in the first stage of labour. This indication accounts largely for the rising incidence of Caesarean section in hospital practice. Often the vigorous condition of the baby at birth, in spite of being coated with thick meconium, causes one to wonder how genuine was the distress. The growing use of fetal blood sampling by the Saling method as described in the chapter on labour may help however to reduce the incidence of unnecessary Caesarean section for this indication.
2. More than minor degrees of disproportion.
3. Where previous Caesarean section has been carried out following a failed trial of labour for disproportion.
4. Certain cases of failure to progress, especially with the membranes ruptured for a long time. In these cases the fetal prognosis worsens as labour becomes more and more prolonged.
5. The bad obstetric history. This subject is dealt with more fully elsewhere.
6. Severe degrees of placenta praevia or any case of severe revealed antepartum haemorrhage, when the patient is not in labour and primigravid and the baby still alive.

7. Failed surgical induction. As discussed in the chapter on induced labour, the indications for embarking on induction must be sufficient to make one ready to proceed even farther in order to secure a patient's delivery, should induction fail.
8. Certain cases of fulminating pre-eclamptic toxaemia, in which surgical induction will not terminate the pregnancy quickly enough.
9. Certain classes of malpresentation, usually in association with other abnormalities.
10. Prolapse of the cord with the child still alive and the patient still short of full dilatation of the cervix.
11. A previous repair operation in which symptoms of urinary or rectal incontinence have, with difficulty, been cured. This of course applies also to a history of repair of vesicovaginal fistula.
12. The presence of an established constriction ring in the course of labour with the child still alive and labour prolonged.
13. Many cases of diabetes mellitus.
14. Ovarian tumours complicating pregnancy at term if they cannot be pushed from in front of the presenting part.
15. Cases of fibroids which occupy the pelvis and persist in their threat to obstruct the advance of the presenting part.
16. Elderly primigravidae, in association with other abnormalities. Caesarean section is no guarantee of live birth of the child but, especially after a prolonged period of infertility, subsidiary indications for Caesarean section will, in this case, carry more weight.
17. Certain cases of cardiac disease, in which a perfectly straightforward labour cannot be confidently anticipated as a result of associated abnormalities, major or minor. The use of Caesarean section to provide a means of carrying out sterilisation at the same time is not a valid indication.
18. Cases of carcinoma of the cervix discovered late in pregnancy.
19. Structural abnormalities of the vagina which cannot be expected to stretch adequately or safely to allow the passage of the fetal head. These abnormalities may be either congenital or the result of previous plastic operations on the vagina.
20. History of two previous Caesarean sections.

The case for the lower-segment operation.—For nearly all practical purposes there is only one type of Caesarean section today, namely the lower-segment operation. Its almost universal adoption has contributed a great deal to the safety of Caesarean section. Although the approach is still transperitoneal, there are many reasons for preferring it to the older, classical upper-segment operation. For one thing, it is usually possible to perform the operation with relatively much less blood loss. For another, it takes very little longer to perform; but one of its chief virtues lies in the reduced chances of infection of the general peritoneal cavity because of the low position of the operation area which is less vulnerable. The scar in the uterus lies deep in the pelvis and behind the bladder during the puerperium and the spread of infection tends thereby to be limited. Its greatest advantage, however, lies in the fact that the uterine scar is placed in an area of the uterus which is at rest during the puerperium; this allows far more satisfactory healing. The classical scar in the upper segment is undermined by the rhythmical uterine contractions which follow delivery and loosen the sutures, often causing them to cut out so that only the serous coat of the uterus holds that organ more or less together. Any uterine infection still further interferes with sound healing, and the chances of uterine rupture in a subsequent pregnancy are too high to be countenanced. The classical scar, moreover, is very liable to ooze blood at the end of the operation. This not only encourages infection, but invites the formation of bowel adhesions which rarely complicate the lower-segment operation. In the course of the latter, coils of intestine should not even come within view, and this fact must contribute, to some extent, to the diminished incidence of postoperative ileus. Finally the classical scars which give way in subsequent pregnancy are usually those underlying the placenta. This is almost as likely to happen on the anterior upper-segment wall as the posterior. Implantation of the placenta over an old scar undoubtedly weakens it and in our view it is important to know the position of the placenta in all cases of previous Caesarean section.

Lower-segment Section and Placenta Praevia

There is still a tendency in some quarters to prefer the classical operation for cases of placenta praevia, and for some years the author held this mistaken view, largely out of fear that he might run into uncontrollable bleeding in incising the lower segment. It was not until he started doing the lower-segment operation for placenta praevia that he came to believe what others had already told him. It is true that the front of the lower segment may be very vascular, but with a good technique this should not be troublesome, and certainly the upper segment is, as a rule, more likely to bleed whether the placenta is situated beneath the incision or not.

Another objection advanced is that one may encounter the placenta praevia anteriorly. This should not deter one, for it is only the matter of a second to brush it aside or, if necessary, to rip straight through it. Perhaps the most serious objection is that with an anteriorly placed placenta the uterine wall in the lower segment may be more friable and, therefore, uncontrollable tears may occur, making suture difficult and threatening satisfactory union. There is the further danger that the fetus may bleed from the placenta if the latter has to be incised instead of being pushed aside. Butler and Martin (1954) reported 5 cases of neonatal anaemia as a result of this and Neligan and Russell (1954) likewise encountered the placenta on incising the lower segment in 20 out of 45 cases of placenta praevia. It is recommended, therefore, that the umbilical cord should be clamped as soon as possible if the placenta has been damaged, in order to reduce the fetal blood loss, and a careful watch, by repeated haemoglobin estimates, should be maintained in any baby in which this complication is thought possible. Blood transfusion should be given if the baby's haemoglobin level falls to 90 per cent.

It is unlikely that the scar in the lower segment will again be the site of placenta praevia in future pregnancies. This is an important consideration for reasons already stated.

Classical Caesarean Section

Unfortunately, this cannot be dismissed without some discussion, for it is still too commonly practised. As already hinted, the indications for it must be very few indeed. The following are the only indications which would appear to be valid:

1. The mother is already dead, and one is performing post-mortem Caesarean section in the hopes of securing a live child.
2. When the patient is already so moribund from antepartum haemorrhage due to placenta praevia that every second in delivery may count.
3. When hysterectomy is contemplated at the same time.
4. When some relevant structural abnormality of the uterus exists which makes approach to the lower segment technically impossible.
5. Occasionally in cases of transverse lie no proper lower uterine segment can be identified.
6. In cases of gross kyphosis in which the distance between sternum and pubis is so reduced that the belly is pendulous and the lie transverse. I have only once encountered such a case and it was as much as I could do to avoid placing the incision in the uterine fundus.

Extraperitoneal Caesarean Section

This operation might have had a great future but for the discovery of antibiotics. However it has now fallen into total disuse, along with all manner of types of peritoneal cavity exclusion operation such as I myself tried many years ago. They are difficult, time-consuming and fare no better in convalescence than the standard lower-segment technique. More often traumatic holes made in the bladder require painstaking suture.

Porro Caesarean Section

American authorities are inclined to use this term to cover cases of Caesarean subtotal hysterectomy, but this use of the name Porro is incorrect. As performed in 1877 by Porro, it involved amputation of the uterus at the internal os together with the adnexa and the fixation of the cervical stump in the lower end of the abdominal wound. It is no longer used.

History

The operation of Caesarean section dates of course from antiquity, and was usually employed in the hope of obtaining a living child when the mother was dead or so near to death that maternal survival was not a practical consideration. While the mother was still alive, even so-called primitive peoples employed, as a rule, some form of narcosis, usually alcoholic. The introduction of anaesthetics, however, in the last century brought the operation into more serious consideration.

In 1870 the death-rate from Caesarean section was still in the region of 75 per cent. In 1878 Murdoch Cameron in Glasgow achieved the feat of performing a series of eight Caesarean sections without a maternal death. One of the cases lived to the ripe age of 75. She had an illegitimate pregnancy and a true conjugate of 1½ inches (3·75 cm)—not a good combination in the Scotland of those Victorian days. A meeting of the senior obstetricians of the city debated her fate and Caesarean section was finally agreed, one of the disputants insisting that a minority view be minuted since he regarded the case as borderline!

Quite apart from shock and sepsis, the main reason for maternal death was haemorrhage, because it was the practice, up to that date, to return the uterus to the abdomen unsutured. The success of uterine-wound suture revived interest in the classical type of operation during the last thirty years of the nineteenth century.

All these operations were of the classical variety, and the Porro operation at once produced an enormous improvement in mortality figures for, by suturing the cervical stump into the lower end of the abdominal wound, there was no opportunity for continued intraperitoneal bleeding. Moreover, the main focus of sepsis, namely the body of the uterus, was removed by amputation, and drainage of what was left was of course complete.

The history of lower-segment Caesarean section is older than one would expect, for in 1805 Osiander performed an operation of this type, and in 1821 a disastrous attempt at extraperitoneal Caesarean section was made by Ritgen, in which the patient died although the child was born alive.

At the beginning of this century Frank developed a type of exclusion operation in which he sutured the upper edge of the parietal peritoneum to the visceral peritoneum and incised the uterus transversely through the lower segment, and by 1910 Sellheim was doing an operation which was not very dissimilar from the lower-segment operation of today. The operation, however, appears to have taken a long time to come into vogue, and it was Munro Kerr who did most of all in this country to popularise it.

It is strange to think that the general adoption of the lower-segment operation has taken place only in the last forty years or so. The maternal mortality figures speak for themselves, and the improvement cannot be attributed to antibiotics or to blood banks, neither of which made their appearance until the Second World War, and to this operation alone must go the major credit for the increased safety of Caesarean section.

Incidence of Caesarean Section

This varies very widely in different centres. Hospital statistics give no true picture of how commonly the operation is in fact performed amongst the population as a whole, because the more abnormal cases gravitate there. The figure varies between 1 per cent and 8 per cent according to the nature of the hospital and also according to geographical conditions; for instance, in areas where contracted pelvis, due to rickets, is still relatively common, the incidence of Caesarean section is higher. Our own figure varies between 8 and 10 per cent annually.

Safety of Caesarean Section

The operative mortality had fallen from the level of 75 per cent during the middle of the last century to less than 10 per cent at the beginning of this one, although the classical operation was almost universally performed during this period.

The reasons for which the operation is performed have very often more to do with the death-rate than has the operation itself, and cardiac disease, diabetes mellitus, placenta praevia and abruptio placentae are noteworthy examples.

At present the overall maternal mortality in England and Wales in cases delivered by Caesarean section is 3·5 per thousand and in spite of recent improvements in facilities and techniques the figure remains seven times as high as after delivery by the vaginal route.

The risk of pulmonary embolism, as with all pelvic abdominal operations, still remains with us, but this is very largely a preventable condition. It is not wholly fair to compare the operative mortality of Caesarean section with the mortality of vaginal delivery. Such a comparison, to be valid, should take into account the indications.

Preparation of the Patient

Of all measures, undoubtedly the most important is to exclude any anaemia or to treat it if present. Where blood loss prior to operation has been acute, it should be replaced quantitatively as far as possible before operating. Where chronic anaemia exists, the blood condition ought to be restored at least to a haemoglobin level of 80 per cent pre-operatively. Needless to say, the patient's blood group must be known, and some serum should have been taken already for cross-matching and a supply of a compatible blood should be assured. It would be sheer pessimism to anticipate the need for routine blood transfusion in all one's cases but, when needed, circumstances may brook no delay. The patient who is anaemic is ill-equipped to withstand further haemorrhage at operation, and the effects of bleeding will be magnified. But this is not all, for anaemia not only aggravates the effects of shock but also predisposes the patient to puerperal thrombosis; also resistance to infection may be so lowered by anaemia that her chances of recovery may be prejudiced. It is now our practice in all cases to have a saline drip set up and running slowly before starting the operation. Any intravenous injection or blood transfusion can then be given without delay if necessary.

Another wise precaution is to take a straight X-ray of the abdomen, where time permits, in order to exclude the presence of a fetal abnormality in so far as this is possible. There are two main absolute indications for Caesarean section even when fetal abnormality is radiologically demonstrable. These are, cases of central placenta praevia, and secondly, gross pelvic contraction. In most other cases, however, where a fetal abnormality exists, every attempt should be made to secure vaginal delivery.

In all cases in which the possibility of infection is suspected, it is a wise plan to take a specimen from the vault of the vagina for bacterial culture before operating. The report on the culture will then be available so much the earlier, so that appropriate chemotherapy can be readily instituted. Where there has been no opportunity to take this pre-operative specimen, a swab should be taken from the uterine cavity at operation.

The advisability of operating under what is now referred to as a "chemotherapeutic umbrella" in suspect cases is a debatable matter. Undoubtedly the practice is abused, and antibiotics are given to all sorts of cases quite empirically, with the result that accurate diagnosis of a puerperal infection may be prejudiced and the patient's recovery, far from being accelerated, may actually be delayed. The "umbrella", however, is certainly indicated in cardiac cases in whom the risk of heart-valve vegetations is too serious to countenance.

The stomach should be empty. Unfortunately, especially in those cases who have been some time in labour and have throughout this period been encouraged to drink as much as possible, the stomach is likely to contain large quantities of fluid, and this fact provides one of the greatest risks in the induction of anaesthesia. It is safer to pass a stomach tube and to administer by mouth 14 ml of magnesium trisilicate mixture (BPC) to neutralise any remaining gastric acid.

The abdominal wall and vulva of the patient are shaved and some suitable antiseptic paint is applied. A pre-operative soap-and-water enema is commonly given, provided there is no antepartum bleeding, although we have now abandoned this as a routine practice. A catheter is passed before the patient leaves the ward. The catheter is left *in situ* throughout the operation unspigoted and draining, so that the bladder at all times is unquestionably empty. Premedication is usually restricted to atropine 0·6 mg to dry up secretions, and narcotic drugs are not usually given at the same time because of the possible effect they may have upon the baby's readiness to breathe.

Failure to ensure that the catheter remains well in the bladder throughout the operation can provide a nasty situation in which the full, undrained bladder bulges up following incision of the abdominal parietes and hinders proper exposure of the lower uterine segment. When, as has happened to me, this has occurred at a repeat Caesarean section (in fact the patient's fourth) the necessary dissection was not easy in spite of attempts to squeeze the bladder empty from above. Aspiration with a large syringe would have taken longer than the emergency conditions allowed at the time but the real trouble came after delivery of the baby. The bladder instantly filled up, as so often happens in the third stage of labour, and I was thankful for the stay suture in the lower edge of the uterine incision which I always put in, in order to be able to keep that suture line safely in view and in the interests of bladder safety.

Anaesthesia

The greatest danger period is during the induction of anaesthesia, when vomiting from a full stomach is particularly liable to occur and may result in dangerous degrees of aspiration. Maternal asphyxia is even more dangerous to the baby than it is to the mother herself, and because of the very slow and sluggish circulation of the uterus it may be anything up to a quarter of an hour before the uterus becomes well oxygenated again following acute asphyxia. During this period the baby, even if it does not die, is liable to undertake premature inspiratory movements.

The fairly general improvement in anaesthetic standards is progressively eliminating the once common preference of many obstetricians for spinal and local anaesthesia, often administered by the obstetrician himself.

Epidural anaesthesia, introduced by the lumbar route has largely replaced spinal anaesthesia, especially in cases of prolonged incoordinate labour where it might have been instituted earlier on.

The advantages which apply to both epidural and spinal anaesthesia are that haemorrhage is reduced because uterine tone is not affected. The effect, moreover, on liver and kidneys is negligible, while during the postoperative period there is very little vomiting or intestinal ileus. The child suffers no effects whatsoever from the anaesthetic. Nevertheless, there are certain grave disadvantages. A severe fall in blood pressure may occur in the course of the operation and may be very hard to correct. It is not a safe form of anaesthetic in patients who are severely shocked or suffering from hypotension from any cause. Cases with heart disease are liable to collapse and severe degrees of anaemia make this type of anaesthetic unsuitable. Highly excitable patients are not likely to co-operate well, and in them the technique may be almost impossible to carry out. Hypotensive episodes are of course very much more likely to occur if the patient is left in the supine position and, when on her back, she should be titlted by at least 15 degrees to the left by the insertion of mattress wedges, or by an operating table capable of lateral tilt, in order to take the weight of the gravid uterus off the inferior vena cava (Ansari *et al.*, 1970).

Local anaesthesia still has a useful place in situations where general anaesthetic service is inadequate. Shock is reduced to a minimum and pulmonary complications are very rare. Again, the liver and kidneys suffer no toxic damage and cardiac muscle is not in any way affected. Uterine tone is good throughout, and this also diminishes haemorrhage. Cases of heart disease are regarded as usually suitable.

Unfortunately, there are certain drawbacks to local anaesthesia which prevent its more general adoption. It takes time to secure adequate anaesthesia and often one fails to achieve it completely so that the patient, already frightened, finds that she has to suffer also a certain amount of pain. It is usually impossible by local infiltration methods to make extraction of the head, especially when deep in the pelvis, a painless procedure, and very often the local anaesthetic has to be reinforced at this time with some short-acting general anaesthetic such as thiopentone. Remembering the patient has usually had no narcotic premedication, there can be no doubt that the experience, even if it is not particularly painful, must be psychologically traumatic. The surgeon is often handicapped by the fear of hurting the patient, and this will tend to limit his exposure. The peritoneal cavity will, for the same reason, be less efficiently packed off and the removal of all traces of blood and liquor at the end of the operation is likely to be less thorough. On the whole the Caesarean section carried out under local anaesthesia is often an unpleasant experience for both surgeon and patient, and general anaesthesia is more widely preferred.

Of the inhalation anaesthetics, chloroform has to be mentioned, although its use is dying out. It has the one great advantage that induction is usually smooth, but this feature is more than cancelled by its great dangers, not the least of which is the liability to produce uterine atony and therefore postpartum haemorrhage. In this respect, because chloroform is such a powerful uterine relaxant, it is the worst anaesthetic to use.

Ether is much safer, of course, but the dangers of uterine atony are almost as great. Both ether and chloroform are liable to interfere with the baby's respiratory centre and they are definitely contra-indicated in prematurity and in cases of established fetal distress. Induction of anaesthesia involving the use of ether takes very much longer, and during this time the patient is in considerable danger of vomiting and induction asphyxia. Following ether the postoperative course is likely to be much less pleasant for the patient because of air swallowing, vomiting and ileus.

Halothane, though satisfactory from this point of view, relaxes the uterus dangerously in a manner which ergometrine will not counter, although oxytocin may be more effective. It is therefore not recommended.

Trichloroethylene anaesthesia, although very safe, unfortunately is not usually adequate by itself for the performance of the operation, and there is no inhalation anaesthetic which is entirely satisfactory. I prefer cyclopropane, because induction is smooth and quick, the patient remains well oxygenated and the uterus loses very little retractile power. Nitrous oxide is fraught with more perils than is generally realised, mainly because of the high risk of vomiting.

The introduction of the relaxant drugs of the curare class has made possible the use of very much smaller quantities of inhalation anaesthetic agents with, therefore, a great increase in their safety. The short-acting relaxants are particularly useful and they do not interfere with uterine tone.

A dose not exceeding 250 mg of thiopentone may be given beginning of induction provided the trachea can be intubated forthwith, otherwise this drug cannot be considered as safe in Caesarean section. The majority of our anaesthetics now consist of brief thiopentone induction followed immediately by a short-acting muscle relaxant and immediate tracheal intubation. Any anaesthetist worthy of the name is skilful at passing endotracheal tubes. Those who are not should be discouraged from undertaking obstetric anaesthesia. Anaesthesia is thereafter maintained with nitrous oxide and oxygen and sufficient relaxant to facilitate exposure and wound suture. The patient should regain some measure of consciousness and certainly her cough reflex within a few minutes of the end of the operation.

The choice of the best anaesthetic is a thorny subject on which very few obstetricians and still fewer anaesthetists agree. It shows that no ideal method yet exists. One thing, however, is certain: this type of anaesthesia is not for the occasional anaesthetist, for there are too many pitfalls and dangers, not merely to one life but to two.

Technique of Lower-segment Caesarean Section

The position of the patient during the operation should be dorsal, with a left-lateral tilt of 10–15 degrees; the use of the Trendelenburg position is not only unnecessary but may be harmful. Under certain circumstances, however, it may be necessary to tip the patient in the head-downwards position, especially if the anaesthetist gets into difficulties with induction vomiting, and very occasionally the use of the Trendelenburg position may facilitate delivery of the head when it is deep in the pelvis. Shoulder rests are very dangerous things, and brachial palsies seem to be particularly easily produced in pregnant women at term, especially after the use of relaxants which abolish all muscle protection to the brachial plexus. If one of the arms has to be abducted for the purpose of giving an intravenous injection during the operation, the likelihood of the risk is greatly magnified. Corrugated mattresses prevent this risk entirely.

The catheter is left *in situ* and drains into some loose wool between the patient's legs. The fetal heart should be checked.

After painting and towelling the patient, the operator should examine the abdomen and satisfy himself about the position of the child. In the case of a transverse lie it is better, if possible, to correct this before starting the operation than to rely upon internal version through the incision in the lower segment. In vertex presentation it is worth noting on which side the occiput lies, because, in delivering the head, the occiput should be rotated so that it presents through the uterine wound first.

Incision

We now mostly use a transverse incision of the Pfannenstiel type about two fingersbreadth above the symphysis pubis. The rectus sheath is then divided transversely and peeled off the underlying rectus abdominis muscles, cutting with blunt-pointed scissors to free it deep to the linea alba in the midline and sparing, as far as possible, vessels and nerves laterally. It is desirable to leave the pyramidalis muscles attached to the lower aponeurotic flap and to dissect bluntly behind them as far down as the top of the symphysis pubis. The more practice one has at making this incision the fewer the number of bleeding points that have to be picked up as a rule. The rectus muscles are separated in a vertical direction.

This incision, because it has a better blood supply than the vertical varieties, heals better (Willocks and Gebbie, 1963) and, as in thyroidectomy scars in the neck, the skin edges lie more naturally together and a more cosmetic scar results. A further advantage of this incision is that the fundus of the uterus can be more easily palpated during the first few postoperative hours.

At the last time of taking account at the Queen Mother's Hospital, in the total of 1300 Caesarean sections undertaken at that time there had been only six wound dehiscences and all occurred in midline incisions. We now tend to ignore previous vertical incisions, however awful and unsightly, and make a fresh Pfannenstiel incision. A previous vertical incision with a residual hernia is not an adequate reason for repeating the offence, nor is the time suitable for repair of hernia, as puerperal morbidity is thereby greatly increased. Repeat Pfannenstiel incisions are perfectly feasible and seldom even require excision of the previous scar. Today the only valid indication for using a vertical incision would be the need to remove at the same time a very large ovarian cyst, an unlikely situation as most cysts would have been dealt with earlier and one small enough to escape prior detection could still be delivered through a Pfannenstiel incision.

The peritoneum is now picked up and incised in the upper third of the incision. It is important not to open the peritoneum any lower than this because, during labour and also in late pregnancy, the bladder may be a lot higher than expected and may be accidentally opened. Should this mistake be made, the bladder should at once be repaired in two layers with fine catgut. In enlarging the incision in the peritoneum the upper edge of the bladder should be both felt and looked for. Often a little ooze of blood from the margins of this incision will give warning that one is getting close to the edge of the bladder. Occasionally, because the bladder is so high, it may be felt that an inadequate exposure is being obtained. In these circumstances the incision in the peritoneum can be skirted to one side or the other round the bladder margin. A Doyen's retractor is now inserted, although I now often dispense even with this in order to reduce trauma to the abdominal parietes which may discourage mobility and deep breathing during the recovery phase.

It is better to use a small Doyen retractor than a wide one. Paradoxically a better exposure is obtained thereby, because the assistant can swing a small Doyen retractor to either side of the wound in order to improve the surgeon's access to any particular corner of it. The anterior surface of the uterus is now in view, and it should be noted whether or not there is a serious degree of dextrorotation, which is by no means uncommon, and brings the very vascular left lateral border of the uterus too closely into the field of operation. If large veins present themselves to view on the surface of the uterus, one should suspect such uterine rotation and confirm it by passing a hand in and feeling for the round ligaments and correcting it. It is not always possible to centralise the uterus satisfactorily, but it is as well to be aware of this anatomical variation so that eventually the incision may be started farther on the right side and consequently nearer the uterine midline.

The remainder of the peritoneal cavity is now packed off with roll gauze six inches wide. The left side should be well packed first, because this will help to correct dextrorotation of the uterus, and the pack should extend well down in front of the broad ligament so that spill will not occur. The packing is now continued beneath the margins of the upper part of the incision in the abdominal wall and then well down in front of the right broad ligament. Packing is an important step in the operation, and one's aim should be to prevent any blood or liquor from reaching the general peritoneal cavity. Dry gauze is more efficient than gauze wrung out in warm saline, as it is more absorbent.

Identification of the Lower Segment

This is not difficult. The level at which the serous coat of the anterior wall of the uterus ceases to be intimately applied to the uterine wall and can be slid over the underlying muscle (because of its very loose attachment to it) marks the upper margin of the lower segment. In labour this limit is considerably raised, and often a slight groove marks the junction with the upper segment. In the absence of labour contractions, in prematurity, in cases of transverse lie and in cases of placenta praevia the length of the lower segment is much reduced in comparison, and it is very easy to incise the uterus far too high, perhaps even into the upper segment, which is most undesirable.

The upper edge of the bladder is applied to the front of the lower segment, and is seldom less than 5 cm below this demarcation line, which can usually be seen as a definite groove. The peritoneum of the uterovesical fold is now picked up in the midline with forceps and a stay suture may be inserted, the ends of which are cut 2·5 cm long. This is a useful identification mark in suturing the visceral peritoneum later. The peritoneum is now cut with scissors in the midline above the marker suture and the closed scissors are inserted beneath it both to the left and to the right to open up the space of areolar tissue behind it and to satisfy oneself that there is no danger of injuring the bladder (Fig. 1).

The visceral peritoneum is incised transversely in a curved direction convexity downwards, almost as far laterally as the round ligaments on each side, taking care not to injure the uterine veins. A layer of thin cellular tissue will be found deep to this incision, and it should be picked up with forceps and incised likewise. There may be some venous bleeding at this stage, but for the time being it should be ignored. The lower flap of peritoneum, together with the bladder, is now sponged down behind the symphysis pubis in order to expose a reasonable area of lower segment and to enable the uterine incision to be made as low as possible.

Incision of Uterus

The Doyen retractor is now adjusted so as to include the bladder behind its lip and to keep it out of harm's way during the next stages. Occasionally some large veins may be seen coursing over the uterus, and they should be avoided in making the initial incision. A suitable point is selected roughly in the midline and as low down as possible and a stay suture is here inserted whose ends are left long and held in a clamp. Traction on this suture elevates the uterine wall away from the underlying fetal head and a small transverse incision is made just above it, not more than 2 cm wide (Fig. 2). By restricting the size of the initial incision and by carefully selecting its site it should be possible to proceed without undue haemorrhage, which in any case can usually be controlled temporarily by pressing with the second and third fingers of the left hand on either side of it. The incision is deepened, and between strokes with the knife its depth is palpated with a finger of the left hand. In this way it is often possible to complete the incision without opening the amniotic sac.

One of the possibly ugly moments in Caesarean section is encountered when incising a very thick and vascular lower segment. Failure to reach the uterine cavity may be accompanied by profuse bleeding which defies swabbing and denies a proper view so that blind cutting becomes necessary before too much blood has been allowed to fill up the wound. Poking with the fingers will not achieve entry and deeper cutting is necessary, feeling with the finger tip between each cut for the moment of entry into the uterus, whether the membranes have obliged by protruding through the incision or not. Reckless cutting may injure the underlying baby. This is no time, however, for dilatoriness which will often cost the patient quite serious loss of blood.

Very occasionally one's view may be obscured by fairly brisk venous bleeding from a varicocele of the uterovesical fold or from large veins in the bed of the bladder, but an assistant working a suc-

24/FIG. 1.—Incising the visceral peritoneum.

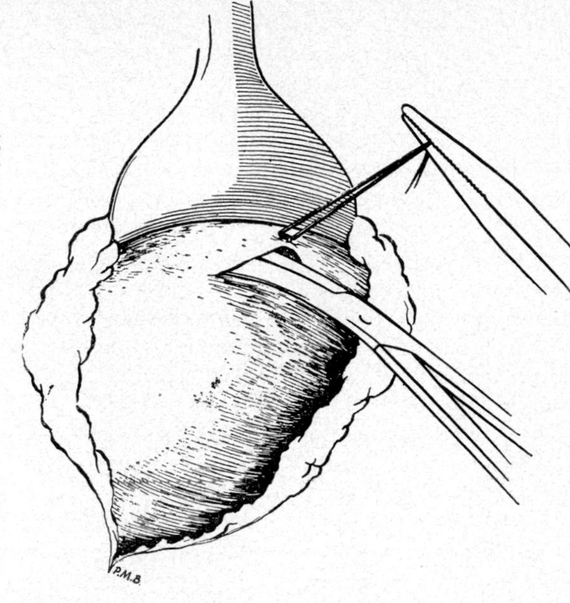

24/FIG. 2.—First incision of uterus.

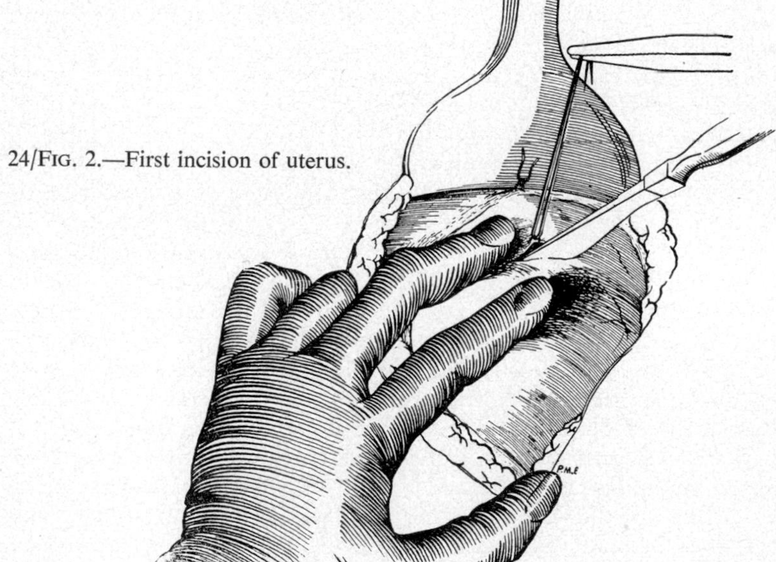

tion apparatus should be able to keep the field sufficiently clear at least to complete the initial incision by touch if not completely by sight.

As soon as the thickness of the uterine wall has been penetrated, first one finger and then two of the left hand are inserted through it and between the membranes and the lower segment itself. These fingers raise up the uterine wall and protect the underlying fetus and the incision is extended laterally in each direction with curved scissors, concavity directed upwards (Fig. 3). It is best always to enlarge the incision to the right before the left, because of the prevalence of some degree of dextrorotation of the uterus which exposes the vessels on the left side to greater risk of injury. Having thus enlarged the incision by 5 cm, the index fingers of both hands are now inserted into its lateral angles and it is stretched open sufficiently to allow the head to be delivered (Fig. 4).

By using the hook of the finger to extend the incision, one is far less likely to damage the great vessels at the sides of the uterus. It is a common mistake not to extend the incision sufficiently far, a mistake which is aggravated by now using the scissors.

By adopting the above precautions one should seldom encounter severe haemorrhage from the lateral angles or an incision which has gone too far outwards. Only on rare occasions is it necessary to deal with large, abnormal vessels on the surface of the uterus by preliminary ligation. Some surgeons having made an initial opening in the uterus, rely entirely upon digital traction to extend it, but by using scissors in the first place as described, the direction of extension is somewhat determined in advance and laceration of the lower uterine flap, especially downwards, is largely prevented. Uncontrolled tears of the lower segment have to be very carefully identified afterwards and sutured.

In this country the transverse uterine incision, as described above, is generally preferred, but across the Atlantic a vertical incision is still popular, so it might be as well to review the arguments in favour of each. The case for the vertical incision is firstly that haemorrhage is likely to be less from the edges of the wound which, being midline, is less vascular. Secondly, in sewing up a vertical incision there is no disparity between the thicknesses of the two edges of the incision, whereas in the transverse incision the upper edge is much thicker than the lower and it is therefore not possible to make such a tidy scar. Thirdly, if the wound becomes infected, it is said by some that thrombosis is less likely to involve the veins at the side of the uterus and encourage embolism, and moreover the lowest end of the vertical incision is lower than the transverse and this may facilitate drainage.

It might appear from the mechanics of labour that a transverse

24/Figs. 3 and 4.—Enlarging uterine incision.

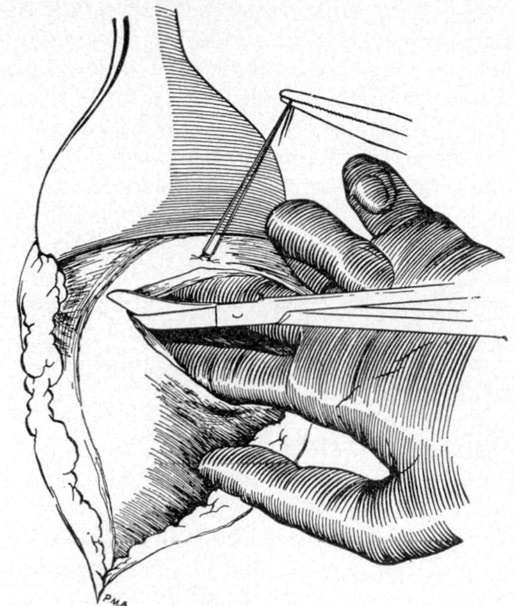

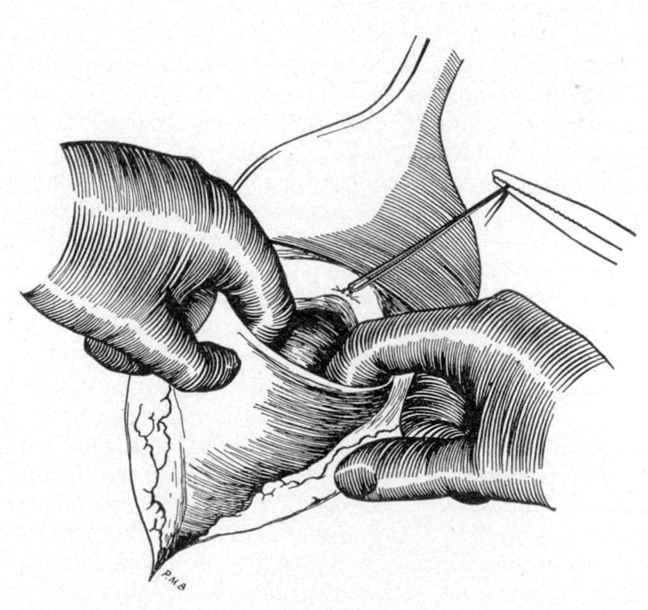

scar in subsequent delivery might prove weaker than a vertical one. This has not been borne out by the experiences of uterine rupture.

The case for the transverse scar, on the other hand, is if anything stronger. A great proportion of the muscle fibres low down in the lower segment are arranged in a circular fashion so that a transverse scar is more suitable anatomically. It is also easier to control the extent of a transverse incision, whereas a vertical one may accidentally be extended too far downwards behind the bladder, and it is often difficult to make a large enough opening without encroaching in an upward direction on the upper uterine segment, thereby defeating the whole purpose of the lower segment operation. In any case, from the point of view of infection, the transverse incision, being lower than the highest part of the vertical incision, is less dangerous. Lastly, the bladder is less likely to be damaged with the transverse incision if the technique described above is carefully followed.

Delivery of the Head

Having opened the uterus, the Doyen retractor is removed in order to make room for the surgeon's hand, which is carefully insinuated so that the fingers can be passed below the head (Fig. 5). Either hand may be used for this manoeuvre, and in the case of a deeply engaged vertex I find it easier to use my left hand in the first place in order to secure disengagement, as I stand on the patient's right. One may be dismayed at first to find that there is not apparently enough room to pass the hand down between symphysis and baby's head, but it is always possible to worm the half-hand between them, especially on the side on which the baby's face lies. No force should be used and gentle persistence will succeed. It may help if the baby's anterior shoulder is pushed upwards by the other hand. A common mistake is to try to lever the head out of the pelvis before the fingers have been passed right round the corner below the baby's head. The difficulty in disengaging it is as much due to vacuum as to tightness of fit, so that it sometimes pays to spread the fingers slightly to facilitate the release of this negative pressure. This is the crucial stage of the operation, and occasionally in difficult cases the use of the Trendelenburg position, already referred to, may help.

As soon as some air manages to get below the head it will be found that the vertex can be quite easily raised to the level of the pelvic brim. It should not be lifted beyond this point. The right hand, if it has not hitherto been used, should now be inserted in place of the left hand so as to act as a scoop in directing the head out through the uterine incision (Fig. 6). It is important to encourage as great a degree of flexion of the head as possible, to bring smaller diameters through the incision and, remembering on which side the occiput

CAESAREAN SECTION

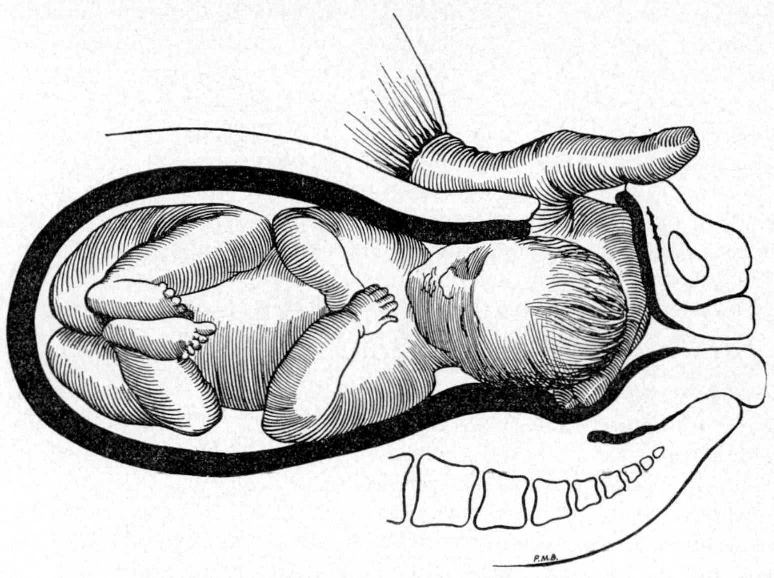

24/FIG. 5.—Action of left hand in delivery of head.

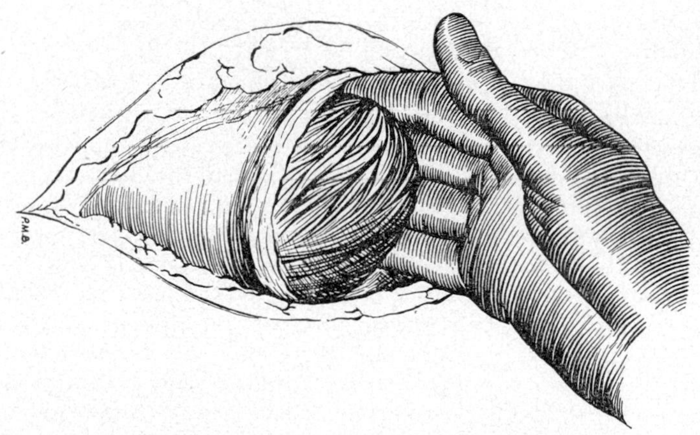

24/FIG. 6.—Right-hand delivery of head.

lies, slight rotation should be imparted to the head to encourage the lambda to present through the wound first, instead of delivering it broadside on and thereby involving the large occipitofrontal diameter. The head is then allowed to be born very slowly.

Difficulties in Delivering the Head

Firstly, there may be some difficulty in reaching below the head with the fingers, and rough handling may provoke accidental tears of the lower segment. Secondly, the head may be found to be so tightly wedged that nothing will move it. This impression is usually false, and more often than not is due to a faulty technique, since if the head has managed to get that far, retreat must surely be possible. As a last resort some recommend thrusting the hand into the vagina and pushing the head up from below, with all its attendant risks of sepsis. An alternative measure is to incise the uterus vertically in the midline so that the original incision becomes an inverted T. This will of course involve the upper segment, but the child can now be delivered by the breech and the head extracted from the depths of the pelvis by traction. Inverted T incisions are more likely to rupture subsequently at the vertical component area and three such cases have been reported in recent years in the annual reports of the Simpson Memorial Maternity Pavilion in Edinburgh. In like manner classical abdominal hysterotomy scars for previous mid-trimester abortion are also less trustworthy.

As already mentioned, the head should not be pushed up above the level of the pelvic brim, for it may easily bob out of reach, in which event the uterine incision tends to shrink, and it can be quite difficult to steer the vertex through it.

Alternative Methods of Delivering the Head

Many surgeons use a pair of obstetric forceps as a routine. It is felt, however, that more damage is likely to be done by cold steel than by the soft hand, and the use of the forceps is either unnecessary, dangerous, or both. The blades are applied with the concavity of the pelvic curve directed towards the patient's feet. It is clearly undesirable to apply them over the anteroposterior diameters of the head which is likely to occur unless the head is first rotated. Now, if the head occupies the pelvis with a loose enough fit to make this rotation possible, it is surely loose enough to allow the passage of a hand. The correct procedure is to rotate the head so that the mouth faces upwards, and then, having applied forceps, to deliver the face first. This at least is a more certain and scientific way of doing it than merely putting on the forceps and hoping that the occiput will emerge first. If there is difficulty in extracting the head from the pelvis with the hand, the brute force which a metal instrument can bring to bear is contra-indicated.

Lately I have gone back more and more to using a single blade of an obstetric forceps as a vectis. It should not be used as a lever to disimpact the head from the pelvis as the bladder may suffer compression injury against the symphysis pubis, nor should the blade be inserted until the head has first been raised level with the top of the symphysis pubis so that care can be taken to make sure that the tip of the blade does not pass through the cervix into the posterior fornix. Lacerations so caused may tax a surgeon's skill to the uttermost in subsequent repair. Some care must be taken to see that the baby's head does not swivel on the blade and get out of control. The advantage however is that the head can be safely extracted through a correspondingly smaller incision in the lower segment since both operator's hand and the baby's head do not have to be simultaneously accommodated in it.

Delivery of the Child's Body and the Prevention of Postpartum Haemorrhage

As soon as the head is delivered the anaesthetist gives an intravenous injection of 0·25 mg ergometrine or Syntometrine. This is an important step and enormously reduces the amount of blood lost. Ampoules usually hold 0·5 mg of ergometrine, and the second half of this dose can be kept in reserve should further intravenous injection be necessary. Given intravenously, the effect is both certain and rapid, and the intramuscular route cannot compare with it in efficacy. A further advantage is that ergometrine produces quite a sharp rise in central venous blood pressure, even in the presence of quite brisk blood loss.

There are many who adopt the fatuous procedure of injecting ergometrine directly into the uterine muscle. Now this is only an intramuscular injection and, as in the case of all such injections, the drug must first find its way into the circulation before it can exert its full effect upon the uterus, with the result that there may be anything up to a few minutes delay before any effect is apparent. Moreover, of all the muscles to choose, the uterine muscle is probably the least suitable, because any spontaneous retraction which it may have undergone after delivery of the head will restrict circulation and, to some extent, delay absorption. It may be thought that the local effect of the drug at the site of injection in the uterus will quickly spread over the whole surface of that organ, but this is unlikely.

Within a few seconds of injecting ergometrine intravenously the uterus contracts well and should be allowed to assist the expulsion of the child's body so that by the time it is completely delivered the uterus has already shrunk considerably. It is then reassuringly firm and placental separation has usually started.

While the intravenous injection is being given immediately after delivery of the head, the child's mouth, pharynx and nostrils are cleared of mucus and blood, etc., with a mechanical suction apparatus. Frequently the baby will now take its first breath. In delivering the shoulders it is usually best to raise the head and allow the posterior shoulder to appear first. There is no need whatever to hurry, and rough handling is only likely to tear the lower segment. The rest of the child's body is now slowly and gently extracted or expelled by the uterine contraction.

The Third Stage

If the above steps have been carefully followed, there should be very little bleeding, and one can profitably wait a minute or two to allow the placenta to separate spontaneously. There is still some debate about how soon the cord should be clamped and divided. Certainly the traditional practice of hurriedly holding the child by the heels high above the uterus while separating it has nothing to recommend it, because fetal blood will siphon back into the placenta from this position. If the need for resuscitation is all that urgent this unnatural type of "venesection" is unlikely to improve matters.

Alternatively the baby may be held below the level of its placenta until pulsation stops, although this is a clumsy manoeuvre without proven value. Our own practice is to allow the baby to lie on the mother's thighs, on its side, at the same level therefore as the placenta, while pharynx and nostrils are aspirated by mechanical suction. Usually the baby will cry by this time and make further resuscitation assaults unnecessary, although it is hard to stop nurses from annoying it thereafter with oxygen funnels.

If pulsation in the cord ceases, or is slowed in cases of fetal asphyxia, the cord is clamped and divided as no further placental transfusion is likely in such instances.

Gunther (1957) showed, by weighing, that babies acquired about 80 ml of blood from the placenta after normal vaginal delivery if cord clamping was delayed. Uterine activity squeezes the placenta and is partly responsible for this physiological type of transfusion.

After dividing the umbilical cord, the stay suture originally placed in the lower flap of the uterine wall is picked up and the Doyen's retractor is replaced. The uterine incision can now be carefully inspected and the lateral corners can be marked by applying Littlewood clamps.

Occasionally one or two vessels on the edge of the incision may be bleeding rather briskly, and these can be controlled by applying Green-Armytage clamps to the wound edge, but they are seldom necessary and can be rather a nuisance by flopping about and getting in the way.

By now the placenta will probably have separated, and firm pressure on the fundus through the abdominal wall will deliver it. Some surgeons make a habit of inserting the right hand and removing the placenta manually. This, however, is only very rarely necessary and likely to provoke more bleeding than allowing the placenta to separate unaided. Cord traction should be "controlled" as described in the previous chapter. I once unwittingly inverted the uterus through the lower segment incision by pulling on the cord, and the effect on the patient's blood pressure was striking. In any case, the cord should not be pulled upon unless the fundus is well contracted and hard. The membranes are often very adherent to the uterine wall and should be delivered very carefully and gently to prevent tearing and leaving large shreds behind. It is often surprising how relatively bloodless the third stage can be by the careful adoption of these procedures.

Drainage of Lochia

If a patient was already in labour at the time of operation, one may not be concerned about uterine drainage, since the cervix will already be partially open, but in elective Caesarean section the closed cervix may prevent discharge of blood. It is most unusual for the cervix not to open sufficiently by the end of the operation to allow blood to drain, but a portion of chorion may, for a time, overlie the internal os and prevent drainage. It is a wise practice to pass the finger down to the internal os from inside the uterus and to satisfy oneself that drainage is possible. In the very rare instances in which the internal os is tightly closed, a Hegar's dilator may be passed through it from above and removed from the vagina at the end of the operation.

Constriction Ring

About 90 per cent of these occur at the junction of the upper and lower uterine segments and, on the rare occasions when present, may prevent delivery of the shoulders. Steady traction will usually succeed in delivering the body of the child, but occasionally it may be necessary to incise the ring vertically. Much more commonly a constriction ring may cause retention of the placenta, in which case the placenta will have to be removed manually.

Suture of the Uterine Wound

The lower flap stay suture now demonstrates its usefulness and prevents a very common and dangerous mistake which I have seen committed twice by surgeons far senior to myself. The posterior wall of the lower segment often bulges into the wound after the delivery of the placenta and the lower flap, if not marked by a stay suture, is liable to drop down into the depths of the pelvis, out of sight in a pool of blood, with the result that one can easily suture the upper edge of the incision to the posterior uterine wall. The mistake is almost certain to be recognised later, but it will mean undoing the stitches.

Blood may well up into the operative field fairly copiously at this stage, and it is necessary to waste as little time as possible in inserting the first layer of sutures. To preserve one's landmarks in the face of this bleeding it is a good plan to mark the centre of the upper edge of the wound with an Allis clamp and to cross this clamp and the stay suture already mentioned, across the palmar surface of the

CAESAREAN SECTION

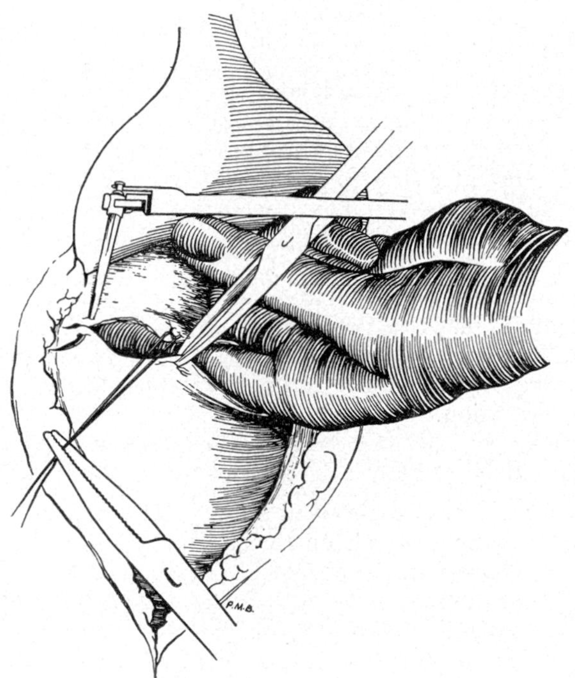

24/Fig. 7.—Closing uterine incision.

index finger of the left hand, thus approximating the edges of the incision in the midline. The index finger is now pointing into the left corner of the incision and, using an eyeless needle with the right hand, it is possible to start the suture line with great accuracy, beginning at the left corner, and thus being certain that no gaps are being left by checking the suture line from inside the uterus with the finger (Fig. 7). With competent assistants one can work very fast with a Reverdin needle, but it is a fairly crude instrument however deftly handled and nowadays we normally use continuous sutures mounted on atraumatic needles.

The whole thickness of the uterine wall, excepting the decidua, is included in a continuous suture of chromicised catgut, and the fact that one is often sewing a thin edge to a fat one should make no difference. On the whole it is undesirable to penetrate the decidual layer as there is the hypothetical possibility that a track may thus be formed for infection to ooze outside the uterus. Accurate suture, excluding the decidua but no more, is reckoned to improve the healing result and the strength of the scar in subsequent labours (Poidevin 1965).

The majority of surgeons prefer to undertake suture of the uterine wound with the uterus lying *in situ* within the abdomen, but an increasing number nowadays choose to eventrate the uterus, dragging the whole organ out into the open through the abdominal incision. This is a subject on which I have an entirely open mind and use either method according to the accessibility of the operating area but if haemorrhage is really troublesome eventrating the uterus may make it easier to suture the uterine incision with less loss of blood. The only nuisance about this is that it may be difficult to return the uterus to the abdominal cavity especially if the Pfannenstiel incision is insufficiently large. Rather than involving oneself in a traumatic struggle with the uterus the task may be made easier by swinging the Doyen retractor round to the upper end of the wound after which the fundus will slip into the peritoneal cavity more easily.

Having inserted the first continuous suture, the situation, so far as haemorrhage is concerned, should be well under control and the field of operation can now be mopped out. A second continuous chromicised catgut suture is now inserted to reinforce the first and should include the layer of pelvic fascia which was originally displaced in exposing the lower uterine segment. This will usually complete haemostasis of the uterine wound, but, if necessary, isolated bleeding points can be underrun with interrupted mattress or "over-and-over" sutures.

Haematomata may occasionally occur, especially at the lateral corners of the incision, as a result of puncturing veins with the needle. These should be controlled from spreading by mattress sutures. All blood is now mopped out of the field and the stay suture originally placed in the lower flap of the uterovesical peritoneum will be seen in the depths of the pelvis and is picked up. The visceral peritoneum is now closed with a continuous catgut suture which will automatically replace the bladder over the wound in the uterus. The resulting scar in the peritoneum of the uterovesical fold will be no more than 3–5 cm long.

All traces of blood are now removed and the roll gauze packing is withdrawn. If the packing has been properly inserted, there should be hardly any visible trace of blood or liquor in the peritoneal cavity.

Closure of the Abdominal Wall

This is closed in layers in the usual manner. Deep tension sutures in the case of vertical incisions produce an unsightly scar. It is better to reinforce the rectus sheath continuous suture line with three further interrupted catgut sutures. The skin is closed with Michel clips, or better still with subcuticular stitching. I have not used dressings, apart from a Nobecutane "varnish" spray, for many years.

One is not infrequently confronted with the case that already has a ventral hernia from previous Caesarean sections which have employed vertical instead of Pfannenstiel incisions and it is tempting to use the occasion of repeat section to repair it. It is far preferable, however, not to attempt formal repair of a hernia amounting to more than simple divarication of the rectus abdominis muscles at the same time as Caesarean section because of the increased shock which is likely and the danger of post-operative distension. The use of the Pfannenstiel incision is still preferable to the vertical even where the latter has been used before, unless it is intended to excise a very unsightly scar. Dressings simply prevent ready inspection of the wound and are uncomfortable to remove. The idea that gauze, no matter how many layers, with its coarse mesh, can keep out bacteria is simply Crimean nonsense. The best dressing of all is Nature's coagulum.

I seldom forbid anything in my unit except unthinking traditionalism and stupidity. The application of a many-tailed bandage, or a "cuirass" of adhesive strapping is one of them. Their only function is to restrict deep breathing during recovery and thus to encourage thromboembolism.

Before leaving the theatre the surgeon should satisfy himself that the uterus is well retracted and any clots which may have collected within its cavity should be squeezed out while the patient is still under an anaesthetic and in no condition to protest. Failure to take this simple precaution may result in a brisk loss of blood when the patient arrives back in the ward.

The catheter is pinched between the finger and thumb and withdrawn, and then any urine within it is released and inspected for the presence of blood. The absence of any naked-eye appearance of blood in the urine is a fairly reliable reassurance that the bladder has not been damaged. If bladder damage is suspected or there is more than a faint degree of haematuria, the patient should be put on continous catheter drainage for at least a week.

Germ-free Caesarean Section

This is nowadays technically feasible and is indicated in cases where there is reason to suspect that the baby may be suffering from hypogammaglobulinaemia. Such a baby is obviously very vulnerable to infections even of the most trivial sort. This immune deficiency syndrome is genetic in origin and a previous history of neonatal death from the disorder in siblings in the mother's history may alert one to the hazard and to the need of delivering by germ-free Caesarean section in the hope of allowing time to transplant tissue-matched bone marrow or possibly thymus.

The technique which we have used at the Queen Mother's Hospital is to use a double laminar airflow system providing a complete screen from bacteria outside, and which includes the operators and the operation area of the patient's abdomen only. Contiguous to this is a second double laminar airflow system at a slightly greater pressure into which the baby is passed after delivery, against the air pressure within the second compartment. This method is much less cumbersome than that described in London using the polyvinyl chloride surgical isolator overlying the patient and through the windows of which the surgeon's hands operated.[2] I have only done such an operation twice. The first was a dress rehearsal for the real case which followed a week later of a woman who had already had two neonatal deaths and no living children, both babies having died from agammaglobulinaemia. It says much for the technique that in this case the meconium of the baby was sterile even at eight days of age, since the full laminar airflow sterile technique was maintained until the baby's immunological status could be ascertained.

After-care

If no blood appears at the vulva at the end of the operation even after squeezing the uterus, it is probable that the cervix is too tightly closed to allow its escape or it may be covered by a sheet of chorion. Nearly always, however, the cervix will open sufficiently within the next hour, but if no blood appears by then, ergometrine 0·5 mg should be injected intramuscularly. If, after a further hour, blood still fails to appear, it may be necessary to dilate the cervix from below with a pair of artery forceps, for the retention *in utero* of lochial discharges is almost certain to produce a stormy convalescence.

For the first few days it is very difficult to be certain that the patient is emptying her bladder completely, unless she has a Pfannenstiel incision which will often permit palpation of a distended bladder and a consequently raised uterine fundus. Retention is unlikely with early ambulation and allowing the patient out of bed to micturate. Our patients, provided their general condition is satisfactory, are encouraged to get out of bed as soon as they want to pass water and certainly within the first 24 hours. The use of bed pans is steadily diminishing.

It is during the early post-operative phase that the services of the physiotherapist are particularly useful. Deep breathing should be firmly encouraged from the first. This, by improving the venous return from the extremities to the heart, does more than anything else to stave off thrombosis in the deep vessels of the calf, etc., and is more important than early ambulation in preventing pulmonary embolism. I have heard of a hospital on the Continent in which the incidence of pulmonary embolism was, for a time, unduly high, so a notice was put up in one of its surgical wards which read, "Breathe hard, cough hard, spit hard", which well illustrates the principle. Leg and ankle movements, if necessary with the encouragement of a physiotherapist in attendance, should be persisted in from the very first. However, to turn an unwilling patient out of bed and sit her in a chair is simply a travesty of the principle of early ambulation. Huddled in a chair and with her legs dependent, nothing could be more calculated to discourage a healthy venous return from the legs and she would be far better off doing her exercises and deep breathing in bed.

The Caesarean section patient has not had her pelvic floor and pelvic ligaments stretched in the process of vaginal delivery, so that the hypothetical risk of prolapse as a result of getting up too soon does not apply. On the second post-operative day there is often a certain amount of gaseous distension of the bowel and the patient may be much troubled by flatulence. As soon as good peristaltic movements can be auscultated, an enema should be given, following which the intestinal tract will rapidly deflate. It is a mistake to give the enema before reasonable peristalsis has returned to the gut because, in that case, the enema is likely to be retained. As a general rule the enema can be given towards the end of the first 48 hours. A Dulcolax or a glycerine suppository may be used instead and we are now giving fewer enemata.

Whether or not the patient lost a large quantity of blood at the time of the operation, the haemoglobin level should always be estimated on the third day, for these patients are often found to be more anaemic than expected. Appropriate treatment will greatly hasten full convalescence. The quantity of blood lost at Caesarean section is always more than most surgeons will admit to, as though their surgical skill is being questioned. The average loss as measured by Wallace using the Perdometer technique was found in fact to be not far short of a litre, and far higher than in most forceps deliveries. Surgeons should recognise that Caesarean section is a "bloody operation" and should be more ready to acknowledge the benefits which transfusion may contribute to speedy post-operative recovery.

Breast feeding can be started on the second day and managed as in normal cases. If convalescence is uneventful the patient can be discharged home safely within ten or twelve days. Earlier dismissal is not a mark of slicker surgery and if embolism is going to occur (as occasionally it will in spite of all precautions) the patient has a better chance of surviving it in hospital.

Complications of Caesarean Section

The first and most important of these is, of course, primary haemorrhage and, as already stated, blood of a suitable group should always be available and unhesitatingly given as indicated. Shock is not usually a common complication unless associated with haemorrhage. It is recognised and treated on the usual lines.

Sepsis, frequently mild, occasionally severe, still remains one of the commonest complications. Many of the cases who have been in labour for some while at the time of the operation are infected and a swab taken at this point will reveal the responsible organism far earlier and make possible the prompt institution of appropriate chemotherapy. Operating under an antibiotic umbrella has the serious drawback that the causal organism may be partially suppressed for the time being and therefore not recognised later. Troublesome resistant strains may be bred. This is particularly true of *Staph. pyogenes*, which is one of the commonest and most serious of the infecting organisms complicating Caesarean section. In spite of modern technique, about a quarter of the cases have to be classified as puerperally morbid. Unfortunately, when serious infection does occur, the peritoneal cavity is inevitably involved and the patient will be more dangerously ill than if she had received the same infection in the course of vaginal delivery.

When Caesarean section has perforce to be undertaken in the presence of already recognisable sepsis, it is as well to anticipate peritonitis and ileus and to pass a nasoduodenal tube at the end of the operation and maintain "suck-and-drip" therapy from the very beginning of the post-operative phase until the bowel regains peristaltic activity. The suction must be continuous and not intermittent and should be limited to about 10 cm water negative pressure to prevent blocking the tube by forcibly sucking gastro-intestinal mucous membrane into its openings. This can be achieved by a very simple device (Fig. 8) which, when connected in series between pump and collecting bottle, safely and effectively limits suction.

The purpose of continuous suction is to remove swallowed air at once and before it has a chance to distend the gastro-intestinal tract for want of peristalsis to pass it on. Intermittent suction fails in this respect and it is the unseen gas which is removed rather than the brown fluid which matters. We now believe that distension causes ileus rather than vice versa.

During the period of continuous aspiration the patient is losing electrolytes, particularly chlorides, and twice-daily biochemical electrolyte balance studies should be undertaken in order to control the drip infusion therapy which is mandatory at the same time. It is the biochemical imbalance of paralytic ileus which is the final killer in peritonitis. Antibiotics may trample down her infection but will not of themselves restore her biochemistry.

It is indeed impressive to watch the convalescence of such a case, whose death from peritonitis would have seemed a certainty a few years ago. With a flat, undistended abdomen, a clean, moist tongue, well hydrated, free from vomiting and passing urine of normal specific gravity she soon masters her infection and emerges from the valley of the shadow of death. I recall the hideous post-operative distension of bygone years, the metallic tinkle on auscultation of otherwise silent intestines, the acute mental awareness of the patient, her rising and weakening pulse and her copious brown vomits, often too large for the standard bedside bowl. How readily prevented and treated today when maternal deaths from peritonitis are almost culpable!

Chest complications are also much commoner after abdominal delivery and account for a number of cases of puerperal pyrexia. These are directly related to the incidence of smoking. Years of propaganda against this filthy habit do not appear to have had much effect. By contrast, post-operative chest complications in the non-smoker are very unusual nowadays.

The formation of a retrovesical haematoma is fairly common after the lower-segment operation, and although the condition usually resolves without much trouble, it probably causes many of the apparently inexplicable post-operative temperatures. The importance, therefore, of haemostasis in producing a smooth puerperium cannot be overstressed.

Some degree of haematuria may occur for the first day or two after operation and may suggest some damage to the bladder. Most commonly it results from the pressure of an unsuitable Doyen retractor and the ministrations of a rough assistant manipulating it. If there is any doubt, however, about the integrity of the bladder, continuous catheter drainage should be instituted.

All temperatures, even though not notifiable, call for full investigation, and in every case a high vaginal or cervical swab should be taken for culture together with a midstream specimen of urine. It is both lazy and foolish to wait until the next day in the hope that the temperature will have subsided, and it should be an absolute rule

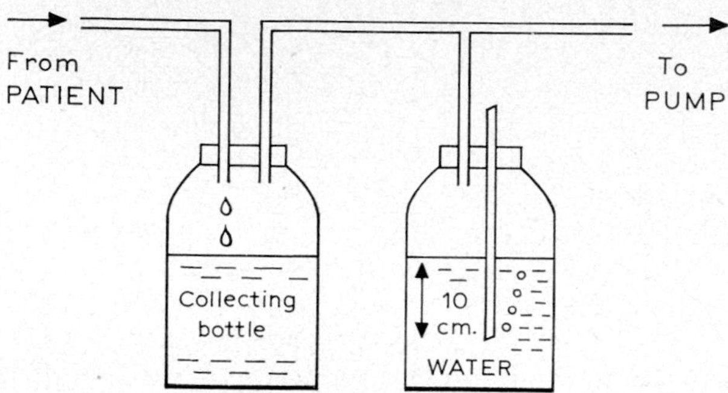

24/Fig. 8.—Limited-suction drainage.

never to start empirical chemotherapy before unadulterated specimens have been taken. A high post-operative pulse and a niggling temperature frequently signify the onset of venous thrombosis or the development of a haematoma which may not be fully apparent for some days. Pulmonary embolism, unfortunately, still remains one of the great risks, although it is very largely a preventable accident. This subject is dealt with more fully in the next chapter.

Repeat Caesarean Section

It used to be said "once a Caesarean always a Caesarean" partly because the operation was done mainly for disproportion, and for this condition the old saying is largely true provided the original diagnosis was genuine. Subsequent babies tend to be larger for the same period of gestation, and if a patient was previously incapable of delivering herself with an intact uterus it would hardly appear reasonable to expect a uterus with a scar in it to perform better. Many primigravid trials of labour, however, fail because of uterine inertia or because of the complicating factor of a persistent occipito-posterior position, and the need for the previous section may have been more due to these than to actual bony disproportion. Under favourable circumstances, therefore, a repeat Casarean section may not be necessary. Nevertheless, a previous Caesarean section casts "a shadow over any future pregnancy" (Jackson, 1961). Today a more up-to-date version of the old saying would be "twice a Caesarean, always a Caesarean".

The main fear, of course, in subsequent pregnancy and labour after Caesarean section is that the scar will rupture. Holland in 1921 reported an incidence of over 4 per cent of scar rupture after previous Caesarean section, but this referred to the classical operation.

Rupture of the lower-segment scar is much less common. It may appear treacherously thin at operation, yet is still unruptured for all that, and it is by no means true to judge that rupture would have occurred just from appearances alone. Poidevin (1959) found that on opening all uteri which have previously been subjected to lower-segment Caesarean section a larger or smaller depressed scar will always be seen. The deformity usually takes the form of a wedge depression but provided it is not more than 5 mm deep the scar can be relied upon not to give way. But when the deformity is deep or irregular the scar should be suspect. These deformities of the uterine wall can only be demonstrated by radiohysterography between pregnancies. Usually, however, one is presented with the problem in a patient already pregnant and has to fall back on the usual gamble on probabilities.

Three factors are mainly responsible for subsequent scar rupture. Firstly, infection of the scar during recovery from the previous section. A history of genital-tract infection should always make one suspicious of the scar's integrity. Many of these cases of supposed scar infection complicating recovery would be found, if examined by sonar, to be due in fact to post-operative haematoma in the operative region.[5, 6] Secondly, implantation of the placenta over the site of the old scar is a common way in which it becomes undermined. This implantation is far less likely to occur over a lower-segment scar than over one in the upper segment. Thirdly, lack of immobility of the healing tissues interferes with sound healing, and this is one of the great reasons why the classical scar so often comes to grief. After delivery the lower segment remains at rest, but the upper segment is undergoing constant and rhythmic activity in the form of "after pains" during the early days of the puerperium, with the result that the stitches tend to cut out or work loose and only the serous coat, which heals very rapidly indeed, may be left intact.

Repeat Caesarean section, then, is chiefly indicated in cases of established disproportion and more commonly after a classical operation, especially if the puerperium was complicated by sepsis. The fact that a patient had a classical operation before is no excuse for inflicting this surgical insult a second time.

The technique of repeat Caesarean section does not differ, except in a few details, from the standard lower-segment operation. The peritoneum ought to be opened as high as possible and with great care, because the bladder may be displaced upwards and intestine may be adherent to the original wound. Adhesions are often surprisingly few, but the uterovesical pouch is usually much shallower than in the fresh case. Some extra care should be taken in sponging down the bladder off the lower segment, because it may be rather more adherent than usual and may thus suffer damage.

It is often quite difficult to identify the exact site of the previous scar in the uterine wall. The number of Caesarean sections to which a patient can be subjected has never been determined, the greatest number in one patient which I have personally encountered being six, though I myself have only performed the last of a series of four and did not on this occasion see fit to sterilise the patient.

Subsequent Vaginal Delivery

It is usual practice to admit to hospital, a fortnight before term, all cases who have had a Caesarean section in any previous pregnancy, of whatever variety, as a precaution against scar rupture. If, however, the history is one of uncomplicated lower-segment section it is permissible to leave the patient at liberty in her own home until labour or just before term. Rupture of such a scar is likely to be slow and insidious before the onset of actual labour.

In any case in whom vaginal delivery is now contemplated, the adequacy of the pelvis should be beyond all question.

It is important, of course, to know whether the placenta is situated in the region of the previous uterine scar in recurrent pregnancy, and this is standard practice in units having a sonar service.

When a lower-segment scar gives way only a little suprapubic pain and tenderness may declare it. Often the first sign may be no more than a persistent unexplained tachycardia. If the diagnosis of rupture is no more even than probable, repeat Caesarean section is safer than a wait-and-see policy.

One is naturally more alert if there is a history of difficulty at the previous operation. When there is no progress in the course of labour the integrity of the scar becomes doubly suspect. It is said that Caesarean section scars can be assessed digitally during labour with the additional help of caudal analgesia but I cannot say that I have ever found it possible to reassure myself by such means.[9] The use of oxytocin in cases under an epidural anaesthetic is debatable in cases of previous Caesarean section. It is however common practice with us, but monitoring must be meticulously maintained in such cases.

After the completion of the third stage in a case who successfully delivers herself *per vaginam*, a digital examination should be made of the inside of the lower segment to determine the integrity of the old scar. The exploration can be done simply with two fingers and a full anaesthetic should not be necessary.

Sterilisation

There are some who offer the patient sterilisation at the time of the second Caesarean section and a certain number of patients will gladly avail themselves of this. In any event the consent of both husband and patient should be obtained in writing and it is unwise to press the patient to consent. The technique of sterilisation is simple, and can be performed without eventrating the uterus. The uterus is displaced to one side and the tube is identified. It is cut between clamps about 3–4 cm from the cornu, and both the cut ends are ligated, the proximal end being ligated preferably with silk or linen thread which diminishes the chances of recanalisation. Further security against another conception is obtained by separating the two ends of the cut tube from each other by a wall of peritoneum. This is best achieved by burying the proximal linen-tied stump of tube with a purse-string suture, picking up the anterior and posterior leaves of the broad ligament from the round ligament to the ovarian ligament. The blind end of the distal part of the tube is now tucked forward under the round ligament with a stitch. This method combines the virtues of simplicity with almost complete reliability. Simple ligation fails too often and is not recommended. Excision of the tubes and cornuectomy is unnecessarily involved and may cause troublesome bleeding.

Puerperal Sterilisation

As a general principle puerperal sterilisation in a woman who has delivered herself *per vaginam* is to be deplored. It is far better to consider the operation in three months time, employing laparoscopy. Not only will the results be more certain following complete involution but in a few cases the patients change their minds meanwhile. This is a right which every woman has and which should be respected. Often the argument is produced that the husband and wife had agreed to sterilisation in the course of the recent pregnancy. This is not a suitable setting for reaching a decision of this sort since the pregnancy may have been unwelcome at the time. The Family Planning argument that the patient might "escape" and fail to report for postnatal sterilisation is nothing less than a blatant denial of a patient's basic human rights. The decision about sterilisation should be made very deliberately between pregnancies. If the fear of another pregnancy supervening in the course of the next few postnatal weeks is medically genuine, the period can be safely covered by the injection of 150–200 mg of medroxyprogesterone (Depo-Provera).

Caesarean Hysterectomy

Apart from malignant disease of the cervix, which will not be discussed here, the indications for hysterectomy following Caesarean section are few indeed (Fig. 9). One may be tempted to consider this procedure because the patient is elderly and the uterus contains a number of fibroids, but the fact that she has managed to conceive and carry her pregnancy to maturity suggests that there is insufficient pathology in the uterus to warrant its removal. As a treatment of concealed accidental haemorrhage, Gibberd's famous statement: "If she is well enough to stand it she is not ill enough to need it" still holds good.

Unless dissection is both thorough and careful, however, one may be shocked, at postnatal examination, to find how much cervix has

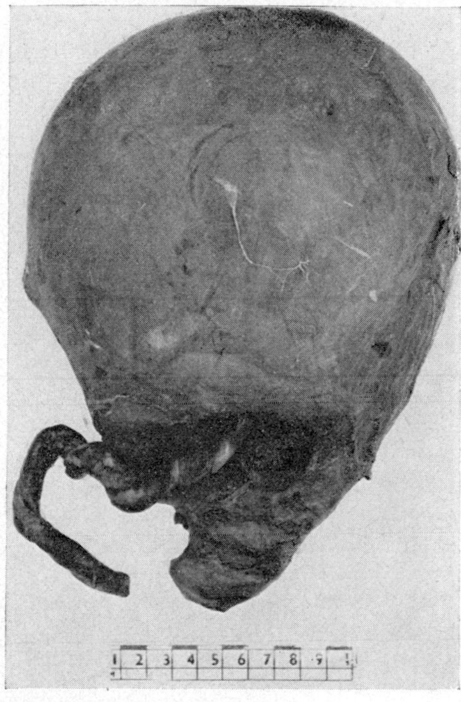

24/FIG. 9.—Caesarean hysterectomy in a multiparous patient with an unsound lower segment scar from previous Caesarean section.

been left behind, so that the hysterectomy may appear to have been more subtotal than total.

One may be very tempted to perform myomectomy at the same time as Caesarean section, but only the more fortunate patients will escape the dire consequences of such surgical folly; quite apart from the fact that in many cases the myomectomy is not even necessary, the great risk lies in the difficulty of securing reliable haemostasis in the bed from which the fibroid has been excised. The tissues of the gravid uterus hold haemostatic sutures badly and they are liable to cut out, and even though they may appear to be holding at the time of the operation they cannot be trusted to continue to do so during the next few post-operative hours. Even the subserous fibroid is no exception to this risk, unless its pedicle is so thin that one ligature will suffice to control it. In addition to the possible loss of excessive quantities of blood at the time of the operation, the puerperium is very likely to be complicated by haemoperitoneum or peritonitis or both. Caesarean myomectomy is not an operation. It is a surgical crime.

Fetal Risks in Caesarean Section

The risks to the baby of the operation itself are largely those of anaesthesia and asphyxia, and it is more often the anaesthetist than the obstetrician who kills the baby at Caesarean section. Maternal asphyxia means inevitably uterine asphyxia and the latter will long outlive the former because of the sluggishness of uterine circulation. I have more than once seen a uterus remain a dusky purple many minutes after a healthy well-oxygenated colour had been restored to the mother, and in each case the condition of the baby was consequently precarious.

The neonatal death rate is influenced by prematurity, since the operation may have had to be undertaken some time before term for obstetrical reasons. In assessing the fetal loss, correction should be made for prematurity, malformations and erythroblastosis. Nevertheless, the fetal death rate is undoubtedly higher than after normal delivery. Respiratory difficulties at birth are certainly more frequently encountered after Caesarean section especially in diabetic mothers, hence our preference for at least an attempt at vaginal delivery after surgical induction. This matter has been dealt with more fully in the chapter on resuscitation of the newborn.

REFERENCES

1. Ansari, I., Wallace, G., Clemetson, C. A. B., Mallikarjuneswoar, V. R. and Clemetson, C. D. M. (1970). *J. Obstet. Gynaec. Brit. Cwlth*, **77**, 713.
2. Barnes, R. D., Fairweather, D. V. I., Reynolds, E. O. R., Tuffrey, M. and Halliday, J. (1968). *J. Obstet. Gynaec. Brit. Cwlth*, **75**, 689.
3. Butler, N. R. and Martin, J. D. (1954). *Brit. med. J.*, **2**, 1455.
4. Claye, A. (1961). *J. Obstet. Gynaec. Brit. Cwlth*, **68**, 577.
5. Donald, I. (1971). *Proc. roy. Soc. Med.*, **64**, 991.
6. Donald, I. (1974). *Amer. J. Obstet. Gynec.*, **118**, 299.
7. Gunther, M. (1957). *Lancet*, **1**, 1277.
8. Jackson, I. (1961). *Practitioner*, **186**, 570.
9. Meehan, F. P., Moolgaoker, A. S. and Stallworthy, J. (1972). *Brit. med. J.*, **2**, 740.

10. Neligan, G. A. and Russell, J. K. (1954). *J. Obstet. Gynaec. Brit. Emp.*, **61,** 206.
11. Poidevin, L. O. S. (1959). *Brit. med. J.*, **2,** 1058.
12. Poidevin, L. O. S. (1965). *Caesarean Section Scars.* Springfield, Ill.: Charles C. Thomas.
13. Wallace, G. (1967). *J. Obstet. Gynaec. Brit. Cwlth*, **74,** 64.
14. Willocks, J. and Gebbie, D. A. M. (1963). *J. Obstet. Gynaec. Brit. Cwlth*, **70,** 284.

CHAPTER XXV

PUERPERAL MANAGEMENT AND COMPLICATIONS

THE puerperium, that period of recovery and involution from pregnancy and childbirth, usually regarded as lasting for six weeks, is rapidly losing medical interest and importance, perhaps dangerously so, because of our modern preoccupation with antenatal care. The lying-in period in maternity hospitals is getting progressively shorter under a variety of stimuli, not the least of them being a shortage of maternity hospital beds, and, one by one, standard nursing procedures which were hitherto regarded as more or less sacrosanct are being thrown overboard. The days of the peasant woman who produced her baby in the fields and then continued with her work now do not seem quite so far away.

Consultants themselves are much to blame for the neglect of this period in a woman's life since so many of them tend to spend only a very small fraction of their time visiting their lying-in wards as compared with the trouble they take over their antenatal cases. The present decline in breast feeding has tended further to rob this period of medical interest and the problems of the baby are coming more and more into the sphere of activity of the paediatrician. It is small wonder, therefore, that patients, once safely delivered, feel that it is all over "bar the shouting" and are anxious to get home.

This tendency to shorten the lying-in period in hospital has received further impetus from the acknowledged risk of the baby acquiring a hospital staphylococcal infection the longer it stays in hospital, but, above all, the medical profession are to blame for this trend by their intellectual neglect of lying-in care now that maternal puerperal sepsis has ceased to be the problem of bygone times.

When I was a student patients lay in bed for over a week until they felt thoroughly weakened by the experience and then were got up and given some hurried lessons in baby bathing and sent home on the tenth day, debilitated by bed rest, still frightened strangers to their babies whom they had had little opportunity to get to know and were told to report again for postnatal examination in six weeks' time. To them the intervening period must have seemed like a very rough sea somehow to be crossed. The institution of Health Visiting on arrival at home provided opportunities for helping a woman at this difficult period in her life and many hospitals, including my own, run a splendid "after-sales service" in the form of mothercraft advice, largely thanks to the initiative of a devoted nursing staff.

Nowadays the increasing practice of early ambulation and rooming-in at least ensure that when a patient does leave hospital after an abbreviated lying-in period she receives less of a psychological and physical jolt.

At present, in Glasgow, the puerpera hardly expects to stay in hospital more than six days and, however many more hospital beds are provided, it is unlikely that the working-class women of this city will come to accept a longer period in hospital as desirable. At the extreme end of the scale we have what is popularly known as the Bradford Experiment in which, in order to secure a greater number of hospital deliveries and the safety thereby provided, a large number of women who are safely delivered and fit are discharged home on the second day.[43] Now it should be pointed out first of all that it was not the primary objective of this so-called experiment simply to increase the number of hospital deliveries on the "sausage machine" principle, but it came about because of an urgent need to increase the number of antenatal beds which could only be got at the expense of the lying-in wards and in so far as this objective is considered the results were highly rewarding. Furthermore a very satisfactory liaison was established with the general practitioners, the local authorities and the domiciliary midwives, which, alone, could make such a scheme satisfactory and workable. Hellman *et al.* (1962) have also described the results of this very early discharge principle in action, usually about the third or fourth day, in Brooklyn, and it is clear that unless the babies, as well as the mothers, are carefully followed up as they would have been had a longer period been spent in hospital, important findings such as neonatal jaundice might escape notice. One cannot help feeling, however, that this is a sorry doctrine of expediency rather like "bowing down and worshipping the devil" and may readily encourage Planning Authorities to curtail their maternity hospital building programmes in the interest of economy and to overwork their hospital staffs at no extra cost to the exchequer. Such a trend could only end in disaster with a rising rate of hospital sepsis the inevitable result. At a time when there is so much talk about personal relations in obstetrics nothing could be more calculated to undermine the happy and fruitful relationship established between most patients and those in hospital who look after them than this sordid and mechanistic view of delivery and its aftermath.

It would not come amiss at this point to consider the Registrars, Housemen and midwives whom such an abuse can easily expose to overwork. They shoulder the heat and burden of the day, and the night as well, and they deserve to be treated as human beings every bit as much as their patients.

Two reasons are often given for the 48-hour dismissal scheme, or even lesser periods. The first is so-called pressure on beds. There is only one honest answer to that problem and that is to provide more beds. If this can be achieved in Glasgow it can be achieved anywhere else and the administrators must be suitably stimulated. The second reason commonly given, particularly from general practice, is that patients dislike hospitals in the same way that many children dislike boarding school. The answer to the second problem is to have better and nicer hospitals. Alas, many British maternity units are structurally quite nasty places, outdated, dingy and depressing, with a rigid discipline, indifferent food and general dreariness, but within the years since the second world war nearly all of them have had a face-lift. What matters more than paint and flowers is the attitude of the staff, particularly the nursing staff.

The decision to allow small children to visit their mothers and the new baby brother or sister was a difficult one to reach. I had always preached in the past that small children were walking test tubes of infection, but this is probably untrue and anyway the patient will be returning to such a milieu with her new baby within a very few days. The children are only supposed to visit their own new baby and not the others. This matter is discussed more fully in Chapter I.

The mothers are thus looked after and relieved of the household responsibilities from which they certainly deserve a rest in the early days of the puerperium, without any of the usual heartache, and it is as well to consider how much better off such a mother is than one sent home very often to conditions which no amount of general practitioner or Health Visitor supervision can ameliorate; in fact as Garrey and his colleagues from the Royal Maternity Hospital, Rottenrow, on the other side of the town, have pointed out, there is often a background of social deprivation and the care or supervision possible at home simply cannot equal that which a modern hospital can provide. There are still far too many homes in the poorer cities without bathrooms, or even indoor sanitation, and the more multiparous the patient, the more does she appreciate the benefit from a period of tender, loving care in a hospital which manages to eschew the traditional types of discipline.

A woman emerging from the months of pregnancy and the hazards of delivery, however normal, deserves a period of tranquillity in which to establish a satisfactory psychological "rapport" with the most important member of the house in a relationship which is most adequately expressed in breast feeding. Nothing is to be gained by the present practice of letting patients home at the end of the first week, or somewhat earlier at a time if lactation is neither safely established nor satisfactorily suppressed.

The simplification of lying-in care has already been mentioned. Over the years in our unit to a large extent we have abolished juggings, swabbings, enemas, catheterisations, removable perineal sutures and in Caesarean section dressings, adhesive strapping, many-tailed bandages and as much as we can condemn as nursing mumbo-jumbo. A similar attitude applies to the newborn. On the other hand we attach considerable importance to good feeding, fresh air and adequate periods of rest both at night and in the afternoon, free of visitations from doctors, students or relatives. Physiotherapists have a particularly important role in training the patient in deep breathing, perineal exercises and leg exercises designed to improve circulation. Women should be encouraged to take an interest in regaining their figures, advised on their diet and brainwashed in a positive attitude towards good health. Unfortunately this cannot be achieved in six lying-in days and to practise gynaecology even in this day and age is to force on one the realisation of how commonly a patient's disabilities such as backache, discharge, poor urinary control, dyspareunia, varicose veins, swollen ankles, obesity and a host of psychosomatic ailments date, from childbirth; surely an indictment of postnatal care. The following is our present schedule of lying-in care.

Schedule of Lying-in Care

(*a*) *Mothers*

1. They are allowed out of bed to go to the lavatory within the first twenty-four hours.
2. They are given a bath on the next day.
3. They wash their own breasts and those who are not yet ambulant are supplied with a basin for the purpose.
4. If the nipples are badly crusted on arrival in the lying-in ward the nurses assist the mothers to bathe the crusts off and, in severe cases, apply olive oil.
5. The mothers apply their own nipple dressings consisting of a mixture of lanolin, gentian violet and tinct. benzoini co. or Massé cream on small squares of lint.
6. Where the breasts are hard, but not obviously engorged, manual expression is carried out, with the assistance of the nurses since the patients are often unpractised in the art. Breast expression is not carried out in more than the mildest cases of engorgement. Instead, reliance is placed upon the use of frusemide (40 mg) or, if available, on an Engel pump.
7. Nurses assist the mothers in the early stages in fixing the baby on the breast.
8. Bedpans and vulval toilet are practically non-existent, except for patients confined to bed for medical reasons.
9. Since the method of suturing the perineum is by using catgut throughout, the Crimean ritual of suture removal on the sixth day is dispensed with.

10. Uncomplicated cases of Caesarean section are treated more or less in the same manner.
11. The use of bidets with running water sprays has made a wonderful difference to perineal comfort and healing.

(*b*) *Babies*

1. The baby is bathed when it is a few hours old in order to remove vernix, meconium and blood. We have considered abolishing this procedure on the ground that vernix is probably a very good skin dressing, but some of these babies are in a very offensive condition after birth and it is feared that the mothers might take it upon themselves to scour the offending material off the babies, to their consequent detriment. The first bathing is done, of course, by the nursing staff, but thereafter the baby receives no further bathing until the day before discharge when the mother undertakes it herself. Hexachlorophane cream removes vernix effectively.
2. At the same time as this initial bathing the cord is cut short and clamped, and spirit is applied, without a dressing, again by the nursing staff.
3. The cord thereafter is treated by the mother on napkin-changing, by the application of spirit.
4. Baby-powders are no longer used.
5. The baby is "topped and tailed" once a day by the mother.
6. The mother does all the nappy changing and obtains the nappies from a wheeled trolley. At each changing of the nappies the mother cleans up the baby's bottom herself.
7. The baby goes to the breast at the age of six hours and thereafter four-hourly, for three minutes on each side. A boiled water feed is given first.
8. The baby stays as much as possible with the mother, including at night, and if it cries during the night the mother is free to feed it herself, provided that not more than one interruption occurs in her sleep. The baby who is restless and won't settle down and is likely to disturb the mother's sleep and that of the other patients is taken outside, but the babies are moved out of the lying-in ward as little as possible. Allowing the babies into bed with the mothers, as at the Coombe Hospital in Dublin, has been considered, but we feel that the occasional accident, even though rare, cannot be chanced, nor could it be defended in the eyes of the public.
9. Bottle-fed babies are fed by nurses only at night, if they require it.

EXAMINATION OF THE NEWBORN BABY

General.—Firstly, check the identity of the baby and that its name tapes are correctly positioned.

In a warm room and in a good light the baby is now examined from head to toe. Caput, any cephalhaematoma and moulding should be noted as this information may be useful in subsequent labours. Cleft palate must be looked for in a good light or it will be missed. Make sure that the arms are fully movable and that there is neither dislocation nor paralysis. Count the fingers.

Always take the first temperature per rectum in order to exclude imperforate anus, unless meconium has been passed already.

There should be full movement of the feet. A calcaneovalgus deformity is usually self-correcting within the next few months, but equinovarus is much more sinister and should be brought to the notice of an orthopaedic specialist.

The spine should be examined with the fingers to exclude spina bifida. If there has been hydramnios, a stomach tube should be passed as soon as possible after birth to exclude oesophageal atresia. In any event the first feed at 6 hours should be one of boiled water, before milk is given or the baby put to the breast, in case there is a tracheo-oesophageal fistula, the effects of boiled water being so much less disastrous.

Look behind the ears for accessory auricles.

The baby's mouth is easily opened by pressing on the lower jaw.

Look behind the anus for any sinus.

The cord clamp or ligature should be secure.

The anteroposterior diameter of the chest should be about the same as the transverse diameter and the heart should be examined for coarse murmurs. The liver is normally about $2\frac{1}{2}$ cm below the right costal margin and the spleen too may be palpable without signifying anything pathological.

Even at birth the testicles are usually in the scrotum. It is futile to try and pull back the prepuce. This cannot be done at this age. The only medical indication for circumcision is ballooning of the prepuce when the child attempts to micturate.

The central nervous system can be readily examined by observing the Moro reflex (startle reflex). It can be evoked by banging the side of the cot or making a loud noise, or even putting a cold hand on the baby's skin, or allowing the head to drop unexpectedly a few inches from one hand to the other. The baby responds by throwing out its arms and then immediately adducting them. The fingers are usually thrown open as well. Absence of this reflex suggests cerebral damage or depression. Sucking reflex is present at birth and the rooting reflex can be demonstrated by touching the corner of the baby's mouth with a teat or the mother's nipple when the baby will immediately search in order to get a hold with its lips. The grasp reflex is demonstrated by stroking the back of the fingers whereupon they extend and the baby will then close them over the examiner's finger.

An attempt at walking with giant strides is made if the baby is held upwards with hands round the thorax as though encouraging it to walk.

Vomiting.—"Possetting" is the term used for the regurgitation of mouthfuls following feeds and is physiological, but excessive vomiting with mucus may require gastric lavage. A case in which the vomiting appears bile-stained should be regarded as due to intestinal obstruction until proved otherwise, and requires urgent investigation.

Jaundice.—Although jaundice is common in the first week of life one must not lose sight of the possible differential diagnosis. If it appears within 24 hours it is certainly not physiological and requires urgent paediatric investigation. Jaundice appearing later, if more than very mild, calls for the estimation of serum bilirubin levels from heel-prick blood. Jaundice may in fact be the presenting feature in cases of ABO incompatibility, infection of the urinary tract, hypothyroidism, septicaemia and galactosaemia. The association of raised levels of bilirubin following induction with oxytocin has been discussed in the chapter on Induction of Labour.

Neonatal hepatitis has been found to be associated with the presence of alphafetoprotein in the baby's serum, levels of 4 mg per 100 ml or more being regarded as significant. This is said to be due to the renewal by the liver of alphafetoprotein synthesis. This compensatory mechanism is lacking in response to the other deadly differential diagnosis, namely, biliary atresia.[51] The diagnosis therefore of physiological jaundice can only be sustained by the exclusion of other possibilities, its mildness and its rapid disappearance. Even so it may be associated with sleepy behaviour on the part of the baby.

Twitching.—During the first 48 hours twitching is most likely to be due to hypoglycaemia and should be urgently checked by dextrostix testing of heel-prick blood. At the same time the possibility of intracranial pressure should be borne in mind and any tension of the anterior fontanelle should be noted.

After the fifth day twitching is almost certainly likely to be due to hypocalcaemic tetany which is more likely to occur with artificially fed babies, due to inadequate calcium levels. It requires treatment with calcium chloride 300 mg in 5 ml given orally three times a day for three days.

Snodgrass *et al.* in 1973 observed that although there was no significant difference between plasma levels of calcium and phosphate and inorganic phosphorus in artificially fed babies, the calcium levels were nevertheless definitely higher and the phosphorus levels lower in breast-fed babies as compared with a number of artificial cows' milk formulae. This possible relationship between phosphate and calcium tetany is being followed up in our hospital at present.[27]

Blood on the napkin.—In female infants this is not uncommon and is a type of pseudomenstruation, presumably due to the withdrawal of blood oestrogen levels following delivery, but staining could be due to the excretion of urates which are pink. It is important however to keep the matter under observation rather than merely to shrug it off in the case of an anxious midwife or mother.

Congenital dislocation of the hip.—This must be sought for in all babies before they leave the obstetrician's care. Failure to carry out this simple examination in the neonatal period may mean that the missed case will not be diagnosed until it fails to walk a year or two later and may then be permanently crippled. It is possible that this failure to examine properly within the first few days of birth may expose the doctor to an action for damages, because the condition is so easily curable if picked up within the first week or two of life. The incidence of congenital dislocation of hip is by no means negligible at about 1·5 per 1,000 and the diagnosis depends upon demonstrating instability in the hip joint. The test for what is commonly referred to as Ortolani's sign only takes a few seconds. To carry it out, the baby is placed on its back with the legs pointing towards the examiner, with the knees fully flexed and the hips flexed to a right angle. The thighs of the baby are grasped in both hands with the middle finger of each placed over the greater trochanter on the outside and with the thumb placed on the inner side. The thighs are then abducted and the middle fingers of the examining bands press forward on the greater trochanters (Fig. 1 *a*, *b*, *c* and *d*). In congenital dislocation of the hip the femoral head suddenly slips forward into the acetabulum with a distinctly palpable "clunk". If pressure is now applied with the thumbs outwards and backwards on the inner side of the thigh, the femoral head again slips out over the posterior lip of the acetabulum.

If the femoral head slips back into the acetabulum again when the pressure is released it is merely unstable, rather than dislocated. Further confirmation in doubtful cases can be obtained by using one hand to grasp the pelvis firmly between a thumb on the pubis and fingers placed behind the sacrum and the other hand can repeat the test on one hip joint at a time.

This test is important because the treatment in early neonatal life is so simple and efficient, and consists simply in maintaining the hips in full abduction and at least 90° flexion with malleable metal splints, which can produce permanent cure by the age of three or four months if applied at once. On the other hand failure to nip in the bud this disabling condition will expose the child to a whole

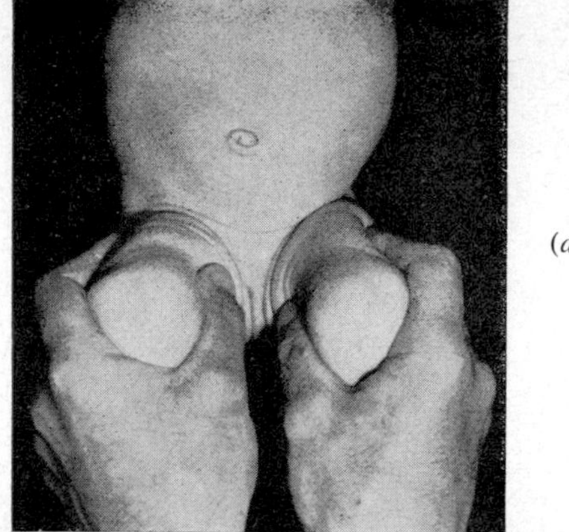

(*a*)

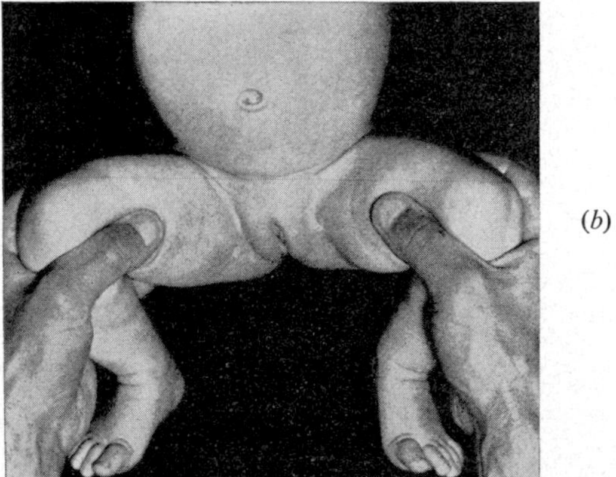

(*b*)

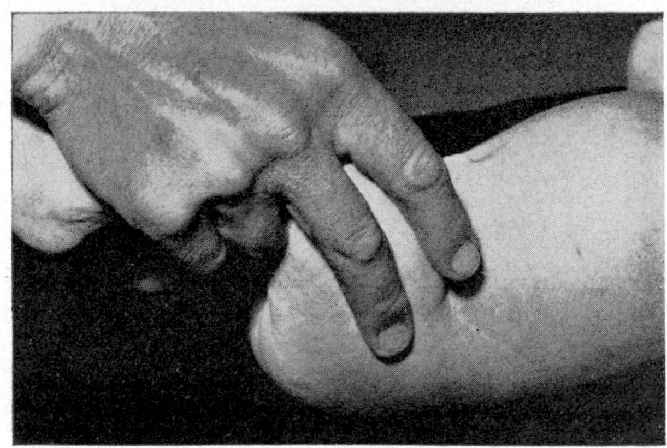

(*c*)

25/Fig. 1

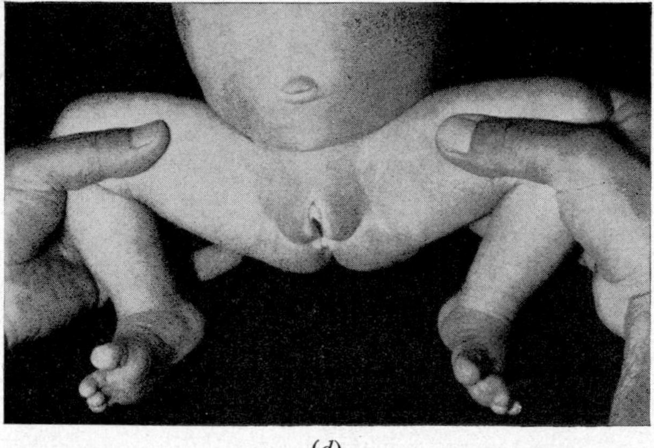

(*d*)

25/FIG. 1 (*see opposite*).—Ortolani's sign. (*a*) Grasping a child's knees and thighs. (*b*) Abducting the hips and pressing forward with the middle fingers of the examining hands. (*c*) Lateral view of the above manoeuvre. (*d*) The heads of the femora have slipped into the acetabulum with the characteristic "clunk".

series of difficult operations in later life, with a high failure rate and a strong chance of osteo-arthritis developing at an early age, to say nothing of the likely permanent crippling which it will suffer.

In spite of all these precautions, nevertheless an occasional case will slip through the net and cases still present later on with congenital dislocation of the hip. It has been postulated that in these occasional cases one is dealing with a type of joint which though clinically normal at birth becomes unstable during the ensuing months, developing signs of dislocation or dysplasia. This possibility makes it desirable to examine the hips of babies routinely at any opportunity which presents itself in later months, even up to the age of two years.[44]

Hydrocephalus and spina bifida.—The quicker these cases can be brought to a paediatric surgeon the less terrible may be the disability in the event of the child's survival, which is nowadays quite likely. It is now reckoned that if operation can be undertaken within the first 24 hours of life, 75 per cent of cases of spina bifida will survive, one-third of them with minimal disability. Even those cases of open meningomyelocele are not beyond salvage. The essential thing here is to prevent drying of the exposed neural canal. A sterile swab soaked in saline should be immediately applied and the child transferred to a paediatric centre without even an hour's delay if there is to be much hope of salvaging neurological function below the waist, including sphincters. With early closure and proper management of hydrocephalus, practically all cases of pure meningocele and

20 per cent of those with meningomyelocele may be spared lower-limb paralysis, and in only 20 per cent of the latter is paralysis likely to be complete or severe. Associated lower-limb deformities may also need correction. Effective surgical treatment of hydrocephalus gives a fair chance that the child will be educationally normal and the condition tends to be self-limiting after the first few years of life. The important thing is to preserve the brain tissue between the ventricles and the inner skull. Sometimes, however, this tissue amounts to no more than a rind.

Neonatal hypoglycaemia.—Normally the blood sugar drops to about 50 mg per 100 ml within the first few hours in babies born at term. It falls even lower in premature babies and adult levels are only slowly regained during the first month, with premature babies again taking longer. The respiratory distress syndrome and exposure to cold greatly increase the tendency to hypoglycaemia.[40] Other aetiological factors, besides prematurity, are dysmaturity or the small-for-dates baby, diabetes, hypoxia, intracranial haemorrhage and infection. The condition may be asymptomatic or symptomatic and when clinical signs appear they most often do so between the ages of 2 and 3 days when the blood sugar may be found to be lower than 20 mg per cent. Unless treated promptly the brain may suffer irreversible damage or the child may die. The symptoms and signs consist of apnoeic attacks, reluctance to feed, jittery movements and a depressed Moro reflex. Convulsions and coma may supervene. The differential diagnosis is that of tetany, meningitis and intracranial haemorrhage. Diagnosis and therapy can be combined by the immediate injection of 1 to 3 g of glucose intravenously—the child's immediate recovery confirming the diagnosis. Asymptomatic hypoglycaemia is thought unlikely to damage the brain,[40] but cerebral damage and mental retardation are more likely if clinical signs are manifested.

Since February, 1965, it was decided in Glasgow to perform a dextrostix test on every infant admitted to the special care nursery at the Queen Mother's Hospital, and the test was repeated six hours later in all those in whom feeding had not yet started. The test was also applied to all infants who had apnoeic attacks or demonstrated other abnormal behaviour. The dextrostix enzyme strip was found very suitable for screening for possible hypoglycaemia and certainly did not fail in any case where the true blood sugar was confirmed as being below 20 mg per 100 ml (1.11 mmol/1). In the first 1,000 consecutive cases so tested no less than 31 cases of hypoglycaemia were picked up.[8] Ten of these cases were asymptomatic and only six were associated with other severe disorders, the remaining 15 being cases of what were called idiopathic symptomatic hypoglycaemia. Of these so-called idiopathic cases, five were dysmature and one premature, most of them had twitchings or convulsions and in about half of them there was cyanosis, apnoea or lethargy. Troublesome vomiting was reported as an almost invariable symptom. This tended to undo the benefits of oral glucose and the most satisfactory treatment has been found to be the intravenous injection of 5 to 10 ml of 50 per cent glucose, followed by a scalp-vein 10 per cent glucose drip at the rate of 60 ml/kg per 24 hours. The crisis is rapidly mastered on this treatment and oral feeding with the addition of glucose 2·5 to 5 g added to the feeds is established as soon as possible.

In the asymptomatic cases of hypoglycaemia 8 out of 10 cases had had some degree of asphyxia at birth and it is suggested that all babies at risk to hypoglycaemia should have dextrostix screening, six-hourly by heel prick during the first 48 hours, whether or not feeding has been started, in order to reduce the later complications of mental retardation. It is thus the practice in our hospital not to wait for signs and symptoms to appear.

Cold injury.—The very great dangers of chilling of the newborn were pointed out from Brighton,[31, 33] although by no means the coldest part of the United Kingdom. The danger would appear to be particularly great in the case of coal-fire heated rooms when, in the small hours of the morning, the fire dies out and the parents continue asleep and unaware of their baby's peril. The hazard is not confined to the homes of the poor. During the two winters from 1961 to 1963, no less than 110 hypothermic babies were admitted to the three major admitting units in Glasgow.[1] The criterion of severe hypothermia was a rectal temperature of 90° F (32° C) or lower, with the thermometer left *in situ* for not less than a minute. The seriousness of such a condition, whether the baby is premature or not, is revealed by the fact that in this series over 40 per cent died. Birth asphyxia and prematurity increase the hazards of this condition and the drowsy, anorexic baby with red cheeks should put the physician on guard. Apart from red skin, the baby feels very cold to the touch and there may be oedema and sclerema, and the limbs may even be frostbitten. The diagnosis is immediately confirmed by the use of a low-reading thermometer. It is noteworthy that of the 110 babies described in this series the diagnosis of severe hypothermia was made in only seven before admission.

Very careful rewarming over a prolonged period of up to two or three days in a properly equipped paediatric unit provides the best chance of recovery.

It is amazing, in fact, what babies will stand in the way not only of asphyxia, but of exposure to cold, and Mann (1963) described the case of a baby which was buried alive in a garden and survived after being dug up by the family dog.

Inborn Errors of Metabolism

So far about 80 of these have been recognised and they are commonly due to a primary enzyme abnormality which is genetically determined. Two of the most important are phenylketonuria and galactosaemia.

Phenylketonuria.—This is an autosomal recessive trait in babies who are homozygous with a deficiency in the enzyme phenylalanine hydroxylase. Normally phenylalanine, which is an amino acid derived from milk, is converted by this enzyme into tyrosine in the liver. In the absence of this change phenylalanine collects in the blood and results in later mental retardation, possibly because of tyrosine deprivation. It appears in the urine as phenylpyruvic acid which can be detected by adding 5 to 10 per cent aqueous ferric chloride drops that produce a green colour. This is the basis of the Phenistix test paper which is applied to the wet nappies, provided the child is already ingesting milk and is old enough (i.e. a few days old) to demonstrate the rising level of unconverted phenylalanine. Unfortunately this simple test may miss some cases or may wrongly diagnose others.[38] This is an important matter in both directions because the missed case may later present as one of mental retardation whereas the wrongly diagnosed case, not properly confirmed biochemically, may be subjected for a long time to an unnatural diet, which has to be low in phenylalanine content causing unnecessary distress to the child and to those looking after it. Therefore the Guthrie test is more favoured.[20]

The Guthrie test depends upon a method of bacterial inhibition assay. The growth of a certain strain of *Bacillus subtilis* is inhibited by beta-2-thienylalanine but this inhibition can be specifically prevented by the presence of phenylalanine and phenylpyruvic acid. A drop of blood is collected by heel prick from the baby, at the age of about a week, onto a piece of rather thick type filter paper. This is autoclaved in order to fix the blood pigments and a small disc of the blood-impregnated filter paper is placed on the surface of a medium containing spores of this bacillus and inhibitory beta-2-thienylalanine. In the presence of phenylalanine, growth of the bacillus will not be inhibited and the diameter of the growth halo is more or less in direct proportion to the amount of phenylalanine in the original blood drop.[42] The same test method can be used to detect maple syrup urine disease or histidinaemia by substituting 2-beta-leucine or 8-azaserine for the inhibitory agent beta-2-thienylalanine. Phenylketonuria, commonly referred to as PKU, is believed to have an incidence of at least 1 : 10,000 of all births. Alas, the mental retardation due to the accumulation of phenylalanine in the blood is only apparent when it is too late to correct, namely, some time after six months, and in Massachusetts already, for example, all newborn infants are required by law to be tested for PKU.

The treatment of this disease consists of a diet free of phenylalanine.

The ideal time for screening tests is towards the end of the first week, and this is one of the disorders which could easily be missed as a result of the policy of early dismissal of mother and baby from hospital, unless a proper organisation exists outside.

Galactosaemia.—This is another autosomal recessive genetic defect in which an enzyme deficiency prevents the conversion of galactose to glucose in the liver and red cells, causing a rise of galactose particularly in the red cells. The galactose is derived from the metabolism of lactose in milk, which is split into glucose and galactose. The results of accumulating galactose levels are mental retardation, cirrhosis of the liver and cataract in those that survive. The mental retardation is irreversible even if a lactose- and galactose-free diet is belatedly started. The enzyme deficiency is that of uridyl transferase and it has been found that a mutant strain of *E. coli* is sensitive to galactose and lacks this enzyme. Growth of the organism is therefore inhibited in the presence of galactose which diffuses through the bacterial cell wall. Again, blood-impregnated filter paper is cut into discs and placed on a medium containing the mutant coliform organism and incubated overnight. A positive test shows bacterial inhibition.[42]

It is thus possible to test for all three types of metabolic error, namely, PKU, maple-syrup urine disease and galactosaemia by taking blood from the baby by heel prick and collecting three or four separate drops of it on thick absorbent filter paper and posting to a central laboratory.

Mongolism

This tragically common form of congenital imbecility is usually due to an extra chromosome, namely, trisomy 21, although in younger women, certain translocations may be responsible. What is particularly noteworthy is that the condition is commoner by far in babies born to mothers towards the end of their reproductive life. There has been much speculation but little proof as to the cause of this. One suggestion is that the older woman has coitus less frequently and consequently an ovum may be fertilised later than might have been the case had the intervals between coitus been shorter.

To the experienced eye mongolism is fairly obvious immediately after birth because of the general appearance of the child. The eyes are the most notable feature, slanting upwards and outwards with marked epicanthic folds confined to the inner angles. The tongue, which later may appear fissured, protrudes from a small mouth, the ears are of a simple shape and both the bridge of the nose and the occiput tend to be flattened. The hands are broad and stubby with short fingers and there is commonly a single deep palmar crease. The little finger curves inwards. A large gap separates the great toe and the second toe. Straight hair and generalised hypotonia complete the clinical picture. Further information may be obtained from an X-ray of the pelvis.[24] This shows a flattened roof to the acetabulum, more horizontal than in the normal case, large flared ilia and elongated tapering ischia. The various angles from the horizontal of the acetabular roof and the iliac flaring are used by radiologists as criteria of mongolism.[2] Such findings are applicable to about 80 per cent of mongols.

PUERPERAL INFECTION

It is not so many years since puerperal sepsis ranked, with haemorrhage and eclampsia as one of the three prime killers in obstetrics. Although the subject has, at any rate for the time being, lost its grimness, it still retains its importance as a source of puerperal disability, and the present lull, which is due to the antibiotics, may not continue indefinitely if the race between the bacterial development of resistance and the production of newer antibiotics ever goes in favour of the former. Nowadays one can get away with all manner of procedures under antecedent circumstances which would have horrified the obstetricians of a generation ago; for example, Caesarean section after a failed attempt at forceps delivery and manual removal of the placenta carried out almost with abandon and sangfroid. We cannot ignore the possibility that the days of dirty surgery and dirty obstetrics may come again if encouraged by years of unpunished, slovenly aseptic technique.

The need for full precautions against sepsis is just as great as ever, although the penalties for neglect are less retributive. It is just over a hundred years since Semmelweis, in 1861, drew attention to the appalling death-rate in the Vienna maternity clinic from puerperal fever, more than 10 per cent of the mothers dying from this hideous cause in some of the wards. Other large maternity units were no better off but Semmelweis managed to reduce the death-rate to about 3 per cent by stricter attention to hygiene and antiseptic ritual.

The introduction by Domagk of prontosil (the first of the sulphonamides) in 1935 for the treatment of streptoccocal infections and its application to obstetrics (Colebrook and Kenny, 1936) has proved one of the greatest advances of the century in this branch of medicine although the mortality from puerperal sepsis was already being slowly reduced even before the advent of this drug and its many successors. Colebrook, writing in 1936, reckoned that in England and Wales 1,200 to 1,500 women died of puerperal sepsis and that 6,000 or 7,000 were desperately ill every year. During my own period of internship, before the Second World War, epidemics were common and necessitated the closing down of maternity departments, so that we were quite used to being rung up by colleagues at other hospitals asking us if we could take on their cases for delivery as they were closed for sepsis, and a sort of give-and-take arrangement was in force throughout the town.

Since deaths from sepsis have been almost eliminated, our attention is now focused on maternal morbidity, as distinct from mortality. Moreover, the problem of neonatal infection has not only become relatively more important but is developing as a menace in its own right absolutely.

Notification

The State still retains its interest in puerperal morbidity and the notification of puerperal pyrexia is legally compulsory. The standards of notification have been altered, as it appeared that the net was not being cast widely enough and it is now necessary to notify any temperature (as before, whether genital in origin or not) reaching 38° C on any one occasion within the 14 days following delivery, whereas formerly this temperature had to be maintained or to recur within a period of 24 hours during the first three weeks. (The former regulation still applies in Scotland and, under Central Midwives Board regulations, midwives must notify to a doctor any pyrexia during the lying-in period of 14 days and must notify the Local Health Authority of any temperature of 38° C occurring within 21 days after childbirth or miscarriage.) Apart from the bureaucratic welter so caused, there is no harm, but I think that a far better index of the surgical cleanliness of an obstetric unit would be provided by the incidence of "sticky eyes" in the newborn.

Sources of Pyrexia

In order of numerical importance, urinary-tract and genital-tract infections come foremost, followed by breast infections. A small remainder is made up of thrombosis, respiratory-tract infection and other non-obstetric causes. The significant point to observe is the large number of cases in whom no pathology is ever found, and this should serve as a reminder against the wanton and indiscriminate use of antibiotics without established indications.

Aetiology of Genital Infection

The responsible bacteria and sources of infection are either endogenous, for example in the case of *E. coli*, anaerobic streptococci and usually *Cl. welchii*, or exogenous as in the Lancefield group A haemolytic streptococcus and *Staph. pyogenes*. In the former some alteration in environment or the lowering of resistance as a result of trauma or the presence of debris endows a common inhabitant of the lower genital tract with pathogenicity. In the latter the infection is introduced by an external agency.

Colebrook's lessons of several years ago were taken well to heart when he pointed out the great dangers of contact with cases of scarlet fever, tonsillitis, otitis media, erysipelas, sinusitis, burns, paronychia, whitlow and impetigo, and he also drew attention to the silent carrier rate of Group A haemolytic streptococci in the throats of healthy attendants. The exclusion of carriers of this type of infection from maternity departments has been achieved with moderate success for years, but this has proved impracticable with carriers of pathogenic staphylococci, and Mary Barber *et al.* (1949) found a 60 per cent carrier rate among the nursing and medical staff in a large obstetric hospital in London. Her findings will be discussed later.

Infected dust constitutes another source of cross-infection, and since the total exclusion of carriers of pathogens is not feasible without closing down every department in the world, a thorough aseptic and antiseptic technique constitutes the second main line of defence. More than half the cases of genital infection have had some type of obstetrical interference, which operates aetiologically either as a means whereby infection is introduced or by which endogenous latent infection may gain a foothold on devitalised tissues.

Bacteriology

The denizens of the past, namely the haemolytic streptococci, Groups A, B, C and G, have become much less important numerically, particularly the first-mentioned, and the anaerobic streptococcus now heads the list. In the Calman and Gibson series[7] the organisms responsible were listed as follows in 141 cases of genital infection:

Anaerobic streptococcus, 34 per cent
Staph. pyogenes, 23 per cent
Non-haemolytic streptococci, 19 per cent
Strep. viridans, 11 per cent
E. coli, 8 per cent

There were no cases due to the Group A haemolytic streptococcus in this series, although Gibson subsequently had a crop of them. The "also-rans" include the *Cl. welchii*, the *Strep. faecalis*, pneumococci and gonococci.

The most ugly feature, however, in the changing bacteriology of our time is the rapid emergence of antibiotic-resistant bacteria, the chief offender at present being the staphylococcus, although other species are beginning to follow suit. This is a man-made problem entirely and is due to the injudicious use of powerful antibiotics. To quote an American witticism, "Fewer bugs are nowadays sensitive to penicillin and there are fewer patients that aren't!" Staphylococcal infection in hospital which is penicillin-resistant (as is likely) is almost certainly a cross-infection, whereas 95 per cent of staphylococci in the world outside are sensitive.

The situation is likely to deteriorate steadily in spite of teaching and propaganda in medical schools, and junior medical officers in hospitals are as remiss as general practitioners in prescribing the wrong antibiotic in inappropriate dosage to the patient who could have recovered without it anyway.

The pathogenicity of staphylococci is initially determined by finding out whether or not they can produce the enzyme coagulase which is responsible for the formation of protective fibrin round the infecting bacteria. The term "staphylococcus pyogenes" refers to coagulase-positive staphylococci.

In tracking down the source of staphylococcal epidemic, phage-typing is undertaken. Bacteriophages, of which over 20 are used in the classification of staphylococci, are in fact viruses which cause lysis of bacteria. By the use of different phages it is possible to identify characteristic lysis patterns and thus to track down the common source of infection. Phage-type 80/81 is a particularly troublesome strain in causing staphylococcal epidemics in maternity hospitals and the most recent epidemic in Glasgow was due to this cause.

Streptococcal typing first of all depends upon demonstrating the capacity to haemolyse blood. Where this is complete, the colonies show clear zones surrounding them on blood agar plates. This is called beta-haemolysis. A less complete type of haemolysis (alpha-haemolysis) applies to the *Streptococcus viridans*. Only some of the beta-haemolytic streptococci, however, are virulent and these have to be further grouped and typed. Lancefield grouping, of which Group A is by far the most important and virulent, is undertaken by using precipitation tests with anti-sera prepared against the different carbohydrate surface antigens which each streptococcal groups possesses. There are thus 13 Lancefield groups of haemolytic streptococci from A to O, missing out I and J. Although B, C and G may be pathogenic, Group A is the important one. In each Lancefield group the streptococci can be further typed which again is important in tracking down the source of an infection.

The two most important anaerobic organisms in obstetrics are the anaerobic streptococcus and *Cl. welchii.* Growth of these is inhibited in the presence of oxygen. Culture must therefore be undertaken in truly anaerobic conditions and in requesting a bacteriological report in cases of suspected genital-tract infection it is important to ask for anaerobic as well as aerobic culture.

If an infection cannot be stamped out at once with the initial loading dose, the less susceptible mutants, which are liable to appear at random at any time, may survive and with continuing inadequate dosage resistant strains will develop by selective breeding. This is called multiple-step resistance and inadequate dosage is largely to blame. Certain species of organism, however, can develop high resistance to streptomycin in a single step, for example, *Mycobacterium tuberculosis* in which mutants with natural high resistance already exist in considerable numbers. This is why it is necessary to treat tuberculous infection with not less than two antibiotics because, statistically, one is much less likely to encounter organisms with double resistance.

Staphylococci are less dependent than most organisms upon random mutation to produce penicillin-resistant strains, and the resistant population is thus very easily produced even with large doses of penicillin. Such staphylococci produce the enzyme penicillinase which destroys the penicillin molecule. The importance of the newer types of penicillin lies in their ability to avoid destruction by penicillinase, for example, methicillin (Celbenin), cloxacillin (Orbenin), or cephaloridine (Ceporin). The following Table lists the usual antibiotic sensitivities of some of the commonly encountered pathogens in obstetric practice.

When dealing with very severe infection, for example septicaemia, one may have initially to work on what McAllister calls the "best guess" principle, certainly in the first instance. As in recent years the likelihood that the offending organism has been either an *E. coli* or a *Staph. aureus,* he recommends either an aminoglycoside such as gentamicin or tobramycin, to both of which coliforms as well as *Staph. aureus* are 100 per cent sensitive, or alternatively he recommends a cephalosporin such as cephaloridine, cephalothin, cephradine or cephazolin, plus a lincomycin or metronidazole for the Bacteroides species. Of the cephalosporins only cephalexin and cephradine are suitable for oral administration. Even the intelligent use of available antibiotics in no wise minimises the need for the full supportive therapy such as steroids, central venous pressure monitoring, the use of mannitol to encourage urinary output, oxygen, bicarbonate and some such drug as chlorpromazine.[28]

The sensitivity of a given organism to various antibiotics is determined by exposing the organism to concentrations of the antibiotic

25/TABLE 1

ANTIBIOTIC SENSITIVITIES OF THE COMMON PATHOGENS

	Penicillin	Erythromycin	Fusidic Acid	{Methicillin {Cloxacillin	Ampicillin	Cephaloridine	Chloramphenicol	Tetracyclines	Nitrofurantoin	Neomycin	Streptomycin	Kanamycin	Polymyxins
Staph. pyogenes	v	v	+	+	v	+	v	v		v	v	v	
Str. pyogenes	+	+			+	+	+	+			h	h	
Str. faecalis	vh	+			+	v	+	+	+		h	h	
Haemophilus	h	+			+	v	+	+			+	+	+
Coliforms	h				+	+	+	+	+	+	+	+	+
Proteus	h				v	+	+	h	+	+	+	+	
Pseudomonas							h	h		+	+		+
Cl. welchii	+				+	+	+	+					
Neisseria gonorrhoeae	v	+	+		+	+	+	+			+		

+ sensitive; h sensitive to high concentrations; v variably sensitive

(With acknowledgments to W.H.O. Technical Report No. 210)

such as would be found in the tissues in the treated patient and observing whether or not growth is effectively inhibited. This can be done either by using standard dilutions, commonly made up in broth to which the organism is added, or quite a number of antibiotics can be tested out at the same time on a single culture plate impregnated with a series of discs which will produce zones of inhibition of bacterial growth depending on the degree of sensitivity. A large number of sensitivity results may be produced at one time but it is essential to use pure cultures of the organism, which means that other bacteria in the case of mixed flora must first be got rid of. This alone takes about 36 hours, so that a full sensitivity report, unless one is dealing with a single organism, cannot be obtained in under a couple of days. As a result antibiotic therapy cannot be truly definitive, except in clear-cut and obvious cases at the very start of an infection, the severity of which, however, may demand immediate action. The initial choice of antibiotic must therefore be a wise one, depending upon the likely type of infection and the efficacy of the antibiotic used, bearing in mind the danger of breeding resistance or encouraging the growth of other organisms so that the last state of the patient is worse than the first, and there should be no delay in delivering the specimen at the earliest possible moment to the bacteriologist in order to facilitate his task of obtaining pure cultures for sensitivity testing.

Penicillin is destroyed by gastric acid and therefore can only be given by mouth if in an acid-resistant form such as phenoxymethyl penicillin (penicillin V). Otherwise it must be given by injection. The penicillinase-resistant penicillins such as methicillin and cloxacillin have already been mentioned. The latter is reasonably acid-resistant and can be given by mouth one hour before meals in 500 mg doses, six-hourly. Cloxacillin can also be given by intramuscular injection, 250 mg up to 1 g four- to six-hourly. The broad-spectrum penicillin, ampicillin (Penbritin), is particularly useful because it resists gastric acid, can be efficient given by mouth, and concentrates highly in the urine. Unfortunately its resistance to penicillinase is less marked.

Streptomycin although having a broad spectrum has the double drawback of being useless by mouth and relatively toxic, particularly towards the eighth cranial nerve. I once had a case of bilateral wrist drop which was attributed to this drug. It should not be used for the treatment of coliform infections, for example, when other safer drugs are available. Kanamycin is also ototoxic and, like streptomycin. may accumulate in the bloodstream if there is renal impairment, The ability of any antibiotic to be excreted in the urine must be taken into account in both the choice and dosage of drug. Kanamycin has to be given by injection (0·5 to 1 mega-unit daily in divided doses for not more than six days) whereas neomycin must be given orally. Neomycin is also useful topically and for "sterilising" the gut from which it is not absorbed. It has therefore a limited place in obstetrics quite apart from its discouraging toxicity which contra-indicates parenteral administration.

The tetracyclines should never be used in pregnancy because of the evil effects of discoloration which they produce on a baby's teeth. They may also interfere with fetal bone growth. Their use should be restricted entirely to women who are puerperae and who are not breast-feeding their babies. There is thus seldom an indication to use tetracyclines in obstetrics. The damage to the fetus is not related to the dose nor the duration of administration.

Chloramphenicol would be one of the most useful of all antibiotics because of its wide range of activity and ease of administration, usually by the oral route, were it not for the very real danger of agranulocytosis which practically contra-indicates its use in obstetrics where other antibiotics can be used instead.

Nitrofurantoin (Furadantin) is mainly useful against organisms infecting the urinary tract including *E. coli*, *Proteus* and *Str. faecalis*. It is given in tablet form four times a day after meals, commonly 100 mg each dose.

Co-trimoxazole (Bactrim, Septrin) is a mixture of the sulphonamide sulphamethoxazole and trimethoprim. This last interferes with bacterial folic acid metabolism. The combination is bactericidal and acts both against Gram-positive and Gram-negative organisms. The usual dose is two tablets (80 mg of trimethoprim and 400 mg of sulphamethoxazole) twice daily. It is more effective than the sulphonamides alone to which so many coliforms are nowadays resistant.

The erythromycin group (macrolides) is mainly useful in reserve against penicillin-resistant staphylococci. Most other Gram-positive organisms are sensitive as well. Because of low solubility the drugs are usually given by mouth in enteric-coated capsules, 1–2 g daily, in divided doses. If given parenterally a larger volume has to be administered in order to dissolve the drug than when given intravenously.

There is more to the choice of an antibiotic than a knowledge of sensitivity which may have to be awaited over the course of a couple of days. If the art of prescribing is not to degenerate into mere witchcraft, it is as well to take some note of how these drugs are believed to act.

Sulphonamides compete with para-aminobenzoic acid which is structurally similar and which certain bacteria require in the course of folic acid metabolism. In other words they producd a metabolic pathway block. If, however, the bacteria do not require para-aminobenzoic acid they demonstrate sulphonamide resistance and even in the case of sensitive organisms the presence of pus will supply the metabolites which would otherwise have been blocked; therefore sulphonamides become ineffective where there is frank suppuration.

The penicillins, on the other hand, interfere with the formation of tough bacterial cell envelopes which alone protect them from lysis due to osmotic pressure. The polymyxins, however, alter the function of the cell membrane so that important substances leak out of the cell causing its death.

The tetracyclines and chloramphenicol interfere with protein synthesis, thus discouraging growth.

It will now be seen that there are two types of effect. Either the antibiotic kills the cell by its effect upon the cell membrane or the envelope, as in the case of the penicillins and polymyxins, or the metabolism necessary for the survival of the cell is interfered with as in the case of the sulphonamides and tetracyclines. The bactericidal drugs, as their name implies, can kill the bacteria outright, whereas the bacteriostatic merely inhibit their development and growth, preferably until such time as the host has had time to build up his own defences, but withdrawal of the drug too soon will allow the original bacterial population to go ahead unchecked. The following drugs for example are bactericidal:

Penicillins
Streptomycin
Polymyxins
Erythromycin in high concentration
Fusidic acid

The following drugs are bacteriostatic:

Sulphonamides
Tetracyclines
Chloramphenicol
Erythromycin in low concentration

Bearing these points in mind and taking account of the likely infecting organism from the clinical condition of the patient, an intelligent choice of antibiotic drug can be made while still awaiting confirmatory sensitivity reports. Therefore, if possible in the early stages of an infection, a bactericidal drug, which will kill the organism outright, is preferable to a bacteriostatic drug which will merely hold the infection in abeyance during the course of treatment. It is infinitely preferable to start with a narrow-spectrum antibiotic rather than to shoot one's bolt with a broad-spectrum drug which may presently confront one with resistant organisms of a most intractable kind, unless the patient's condition is so serious as to warrant the risk.

Pseudomonas infections are a particularly ugly reward for using broad-spectrum antibiotics ill-advisedly. This organism can produce serious enteropathic infections in the vulnerable, particularly premature, baby. Here the choice of antibiotics is very much limited and colistin and carbenicillin are the most effective. A less serious secondary infection following antibiotic therapy is infection with *Candida albicans*, which, if it becomes established in the intestinal tract can be very troublesome for a long time. I, myself, have personal experience of this very unpleasant complication of antibiotic therapy.

In many respects it is better to use combined therapy with more than one antibiotic rather than one very broad-spectrum drug and as a general guide the bactericidal drugs are usually synergistic and do not antagonise each other, for example, penicillin and streptomycin, whereas antagonism is usual between bactericidal and bacteriostatic drugs.

When confronted with an acute infection one's immediate choice, if appropriate, is penicillin because of its low toxicity and its potent bactericidal effect. Unfortunately some patients are allergic to the penicillins and this extends as a rule to the newer drugs of this class. One must bear in mind the ease with which resistant strains can be easily selected out with the chosen drug especially in hospital practice and for this reason drugs like streptomycin and erythromycin should not be used alone. The presence of pus will render the sulphonamides useless and in considering the treatment of urinary infections one wants to choose a drug which is excreted in high concentration and active form in the urine, but must at the same time ensure that there is no renal excretory impairment, otherwise dangerously high blood concentrations of the drug may develop. This danger is particularly true of streptomycin and kanamycin. The general condition of the patient and whether vomiting is persistent or not may determine the route of dosage, for example intravenous or oral.

As a general rule one should not use a steam roller where a sledge hammer will do. On the other hand the intention is to give the bacteria a proper clout, not just a gentle stroke. Underdosage therefore is dangerous.

In our unit in Glasgow no antibiotic may be prescribed without the specific sanction of the consultant in charge of the case and never before the necessary swabs have been taken for culture. In New Zealand, antibiotic prescribing seemed to go "haywire". In 1955, for example, the antibiotics bill, in a population of only 2 million, exceeded £400,000 and this figure excluded penicillin and streptomycin; nor did it include those drugs used in hospitals. (*Lancet* Editorial, August 11th, 1956.)

Morbid Anatomy

The nature and extent of the pathology in puerperal sepsis depends upon certain factors. Firstly, the patient's general resistance to infection is of paramount importance because it influences both the efficacy and the speed of operation of the general defence mechanisms of the body. It depends upon the state of the blood, the absence of anaemia, particularly anaemia recently acquired as a result of exsanguination, and the state of general health which it is one of the objects of good antenatal care to promote. Next comes the initial state of the tissues locally at the beginning of the puerperium, the effects of trauma being obviously adverse. Thirdly, the nature of the pathology depends on the one hand upon the organism responsible and its virulence, and on the other upon the nature of the inflammatory response and its ability to localise the infection at its site.

It matters less whether a patient has pelvic peritonitis or parametritis than whether her infection is due to the anaerobic streptococcus or the *E. coli*, and the gross manifestations of the disease, upon which the clinical signs are based are profoundly influenced by the type of organism responsible and the characteristic type of response. For example, in the case of the haemolytic streptococcus, the local response is not gross; abscesses, if present at all, tend to be small and the barrier erected to the spread of the infection is often ineffective. The clinical signs of inflammation are the result of the struggle between attack and defence, and since in this instance the defence is more mobile than static, the body as a whole is readily overrun with the infection and septicaemia may quickly develop. The rise in pulse rate is often far more characteristic than the rise in temperature, and where the inflammatory response is minimal, as in the most serious cases, the temperature may be subnormal. The small vessels draining the uterus contain infected thrombi which liberate the bacteria into the blood stream in showers. Likewise the infection may sail through the wall of the uterus, hardly bothering it enough to interfere with involution, and may infect the peritoneal cavity which, too, may put up a very half-hearted protest. This is the picture in the cases coming to a fatal issue. A more efficient inflammatory response locally will save the patient's life, often with the formation of an abscess.

The above is in marked contrast to infections due to *E. coli*, in which the local response is far more vigorous and large abscesses are readily formed.

The *Staph. pyogenes*, characteristically, causes the formation of multiple small abscesses. Although a satisfactory response to infection more readily occurs, septicaemia and metastatic infection are common. The *Strep. viridans* is important because of its property of causing vegetations to grow on heart valves previously deformed either as a result of rheumatic disease or through congenital anomaly.

The anaerobic streptococcus, now numerically so important, is associated with a history of trauma, particularly lacerations of the cervix opening up the tissues of the parametrium, and the presence of retained products of conception. The inflammatory response is considerable, resulting in offensive lochia and often a type of induration of the pelvic cellular tissues which has been likened to plaster of Paris. The veins draining the pelvic organs become the seat of gross thrombophlebitis, from which little chunks of infected clot are liable to break away, producing pyaemic abscesses in the lungs. These cases run a prolonged course with intermittent fever and rigors.

The *Cl. welchii* is often present in a healthy vagina, but it becomes invasive in the presence of traumatised and devitalised tissue. A dead fetus retained *in utero* also provides such a culture medium, and for this reason surgical induction of labour should not be practised in cases of intra-uterine death. The two outstanding features in infection from this organism are haemolysis and the formation of gas which, in fatal cases, not only produces marked tissue emphysema, but also what is known as the "foamy liver".

Investigation

Any case of pyrexia in the puerperium should be regarded as due to a genital tract infection until the contrary is proved, because of the great risks at stake. It is a wise rule, therefore, to take vaginal and cervical swabs, as well as a clean specimen of urine, for culture forthwith and not to await developments. This rule should be followed even though the physical signs unequivocally suggest an extra-genital infection. The temperature and the bacteriology are far more important nowadays than physical signs in the abdomen and pelvis. Until recently a high vaginal swab was considered adequate, but we no longer think so. It is true that in the case of an infection of the uterine cavity with the haemolytic streptococcus, culture from the vagina is just as likely to demonstrate an overwhelming predominance in the growth of this organism as a swab taken from the cervical canal, but high vaginal swabs can be misleading in less outspoken cases, in that they may, in the absence of an overriding intra-uterine infection, yield cultures of normal vaginal inhabitants which are not necessarily pathogenic.

What is almost as important as the collection of the bacteriological specimen is its method of despatch. The late afternoon on a Friday is about the worst possible moment because it may not reach the laboratory in time for proper culture to be set up, so that all manner of irrelevant bacteria may falsify the picture. Even urine is a first-class culture medium and it is increasingly the practice now to send specimens to the laboratory as soon as they are obtained without even waiting for the end of a round or a clinic. If working, however, at a distance from a bacteriological department it is worth preparing a Gram-stained film on the spot. In the case of urine, some of the specimen should be examined forthwith after spinning down and looking for pus cells and bacteria in a wet specimen under a cover slip. There are still antisocial individuals who have not the common decency to cover a wet specimen with a cover slip and simply soil the objective lens of the microscope, much as day-trippers soil the countryside with their litter. The mentality is roughly the same.

Large numbers of vaginal squames and very few pus cells in a urine specimen will almost certainly indicate a badly taken and contaminated specimen (Fig. 2).

If sending specimens by post, sometimes a transport medium such as Stuart's may be used, in which case the best plan is to dip the swab with which the specimen was taken into the little bottle of medium and break off the stick inside the bottle before applying the screw cap.

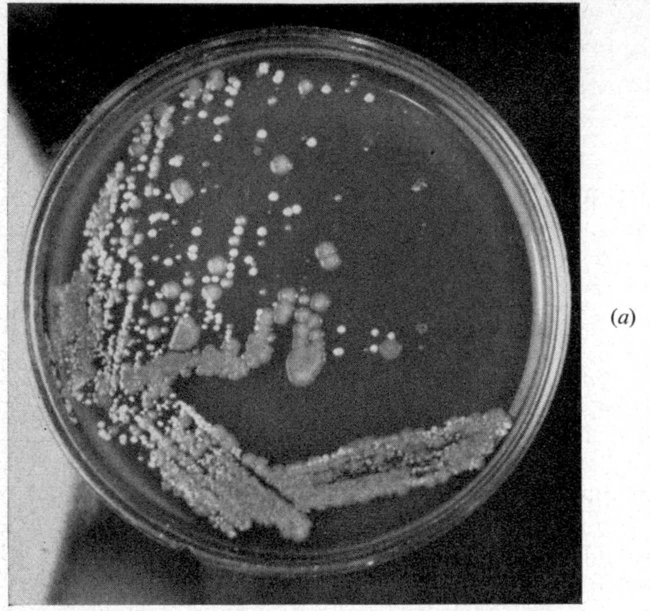

(*a*)

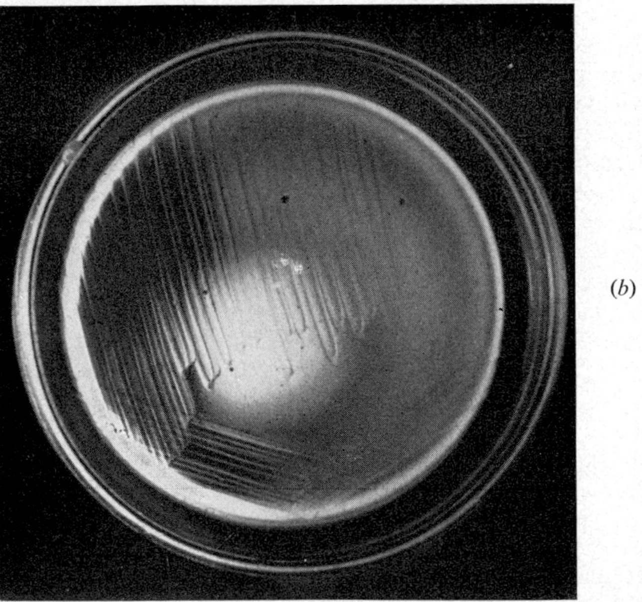

(*b*)

25/Fig. 2.—Culture plates showing (*a*) the heavy contamination of a casually taken MSU, compared with a catheter specimen (*b*) taken 2 hours later from the same patient.

In setting up one's own cultures it is best to use blood agar plates both aerobically and anaerobically for pus, and for urine a MacConkey medium is likely to be best for coliforms and enterococci (Fig. 2).

The next best thing to immediate delivery to the bacteriologist is refrigeration until the specimen can be collected. The report from a badly handled or mishandled specimen is worse than no report at all.

It goes without saying that these specimens should be taken before any chemotherapy or antibiotics are prescribed. Among the many evils of prophylactic chemotherapy is the partial suppression of relevant bacteriological evidence without suppression of the disease process. As soon as the specimens have been taken, antibiotics may now be given empirically at first while awaiting the bacteriologist's report and later corrected or modified in accordance with these findings. Anaerobic culture is just as important as aerobic and should never be omitted. Whenever there is a spiking temperature, or rigors, blood culture should be undertaken as well. Even in the absence of concrete bacteriological evidence, any case exhibiting a temperature which has defied the usual treatments for more than 10 days should be regarded as possibly due to the anaerobic streptococcus.

Lastly, and I say lastly advisedly, a proper clinical examination of the patient must be carried out. The reason for putting matters in this order is that the possibility of a genital infection is so often discounted by the absence of local physical signs; but as has been said before, these signs depend upon the nature and the extent of the inflammatory response and, if present, represent a willingness on the part of the tissues to resist the infection. This examination will not only include the urine, a sample of which should always be examined on the spot with a microscope before waiting for the pathologist to announce the presence or absence of pus cells, but the breasts should be scrutinised, the chest gone over and the legs searched for signs of puerperal thrombosis. The perineum should be inspected for infection of any wounds sustained, in which case the removal of some of the sutures may be necessary and a rectal examination will detect a pelvic inflammatory collection. A point to remember is that puerperal pyelitis, apart from pyrexia, is usually symptomatically silent with neither loin pain nor tenderness.

General Treatment

The patient is nursed in isolation and all the usual details of general nursing care apply, as in any acute febrile illness. An adequate fluid intake must be maintained and sufficient rest must be ensured by the administration of analgesics or sedatives. Any serious degree of anaemia must be combated by blood transfusion in order to give the patient a fighting chance to resist her infection. All the antibiotics in the world will avail little if the patient is exsanguinated.

Local treatments, intra-uterine glycerine (except for certain saprophytic types of case) and the application of local heat have all gone by the board, and the specific treatment of today is now concentrated in the judicious use of the appropriate antibiotic, hence the importance of the bacteriologist.

The general hazards of antibiotics.—The ills which may affect the patient treated with sulphonamides or the antibiotics have been categorised under five main headings:[26] 1. Allergic and anaphylactic reactions. 2. Gastro-intestinal disorders. 3. Renal lesions. 4. Neurological disorders. 5. Blood dyscrasias.

The first group, due to hypersensitivity, comprises angioneurotic oedema, asthma, sweating, collapse and sudden death. Emergency treatment consists in the immediate subcutaneous injection of 0·1 ml of a 1 in 1,000 solution of adrenaline hydrochloride, repeated and repeated as necessary, keeping the syringe needle *in situ* until a total of 1 ml has been given. The more chronic types of allergic response, mainly urticarial, can be treated by antihistamines given orally.

The tetracycline group are particularly liable to cause diarrhoea and gastro-intestinal upsets, often due to a resistant staphylococcal enteritis and occasionally to infection with *Candida albicans*.

The dangers of crystalluria and anuria from sulphonamides are well known, but, with the main exception of penicillin, the antibiotics also are occasionally capable of causing albuminuria and lower nephron nephrosis.

The chief neurotoxic effects are vertigo and deafness due to damage to the vestibular and auditory divisions respectively of the eighth nerve.

Of the blood dyscrasias, leucopenia and agranulocytosis are the commonest and expose the patient to the risk of fulminating streptococcal infection without the natural powers of resistance. Penicillin, which is guiltless in this matter, may be urgently necessary to combat such an infection in a patient half-killed by other antibiotics. The production of white cells may, in fortunate instances, be stimulated by intramuscular injection of nucleotide (BPC) 40 ml per day, and the oral administration of pyridoxine hydrochloride 50 mg t.i.d. and folic acid 20 mg daily.

Bone-marrow aplasia occasionally occurs, especially after sulphonamides and chloramphenicol, and may necessitate repeated transfusion with whole fresh blood.

PROPHYLAXIS

It goes almost without saying that good midwifery comes foremost. Throughout the chapters of this book reference is constantly made to the adverse effect in respect of maternal morbidity which follows so many of the complications described. Many of these cannot be prevented, but the skill exhibited in meeting them with the maximum regard for the maternal tissues is reflected in straightforward puerperal convalescence. The saving of blood at all times and in all places is not only one of the first objectives of sound obstetric practice, it is vital to the patient's speedy recovery, and no amount of prophylactic chemotherapy can justify or mitigate a disregard for this principle. Notwithstanding all the care in the world, however, puerperal sepsis will continue to occur sporadically, but epidemics surely demonstrate serious loopholes in technique.

Although the sting has been removed from the haemolytic streptococcus, epidemic staphylococcal infection has to some extent taken its place. The investigation of a high rate of staphylococcal infection in infants (which, as stated before, gives a good indication of surgical cleanliness or the lack of it) occurring in a large institution in London in 1949, as described by Barber, Hayhoe and Whitehead, is a model of bacteriological detective work, and many similar reports have followed since then. The findings of these workers are worth quoting. Firstly, infections encountered were predominantly penicillin-resistant, from which the inference can be drawn that they were due to hospital cross-infection, since resistant strains of staphylococci in the population at large are in a distinct minority. The investigation was continued throughout the better part of the year, and it was found that between 60 and 70 per cent of the nursing and medical staff were at some time nasal carriers of *Staph. pyogenes* and that the strains were penicillin-resistant in over 80 per cent. The heaviest growths were obtained from the members of the permanent staff, and the proportion of nurses and pupil midwives carrying these resistant strains rose with the duration of their stay at the hospital, rising from about 20 per cent on their first enrolment on the staff to 66 per cent after three months there. A control series was taken from a London store, from which 62 of the employees were examined, and although half of them were carriers of *Staph. pyogenes*, there were no penicillin-resistant cases among them. There was also noted a seasonal variation in the incidence of infection among the babies, which reached its peak in February at 22 per cent and fell to 8 per cent in August, but in most of the other months was fairly constant between 11 and 14 per cent. It would appear, therefore, that there is inevitably a reservoir of infection in the noses of a high percentage of workers in hospital from which bedding, hands, clothes, instruments and utensils may become infected. Hospitals, too, breed their own varieties of pathogenic coliforms, particularly in gynaecological wards, which put up the risks of catheterisation for example. Every time a bed is made the air becomes filled with dust, impregnated with organisms from the bedding, so that it is remarkable that the infection rate is not higher than it is.

From the above, the lessons to be drawn are obvious. Clearly the institution so investigated is no isolated instance. Every hospital in the land is seeking to curtail staphylococcal cross-infection. Since

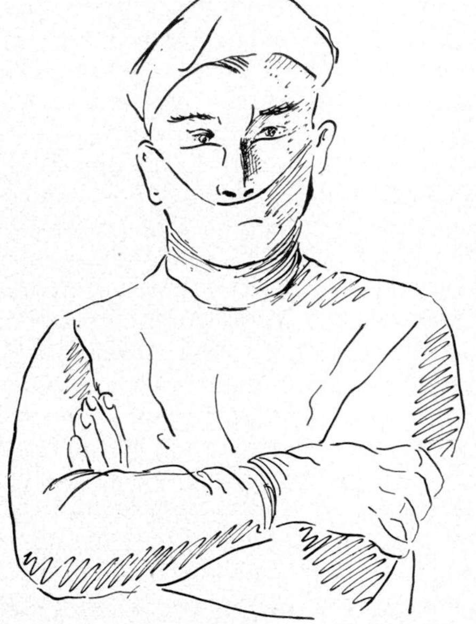

25/FIG. 3—Bad mask-wearing. A travesty of aseptic technique. Note also the left hand! The axilla, even after gowning, is not a sterile area.

it is not practicable to send two-thirds of the staff of hospitals off duty, one has to fall back upon the rigid observance of a first-class aseptic and antiseptic technique. The following steps are therefore recommended:

1. **Mask-wearing.**—Colebrook's recommendations have lost none of their force, yet how seldom does one meet a proper technique. The masks should be supplied sterile and, once put on, should not be touched by the hands and certainly not pulled down under the chin. A very deplorable practice must be mentioned here in order to condemn it, namely the wearing of the mask over the mouth *but under the nose!* (Fig. 3).

Unfortunately there are many who are guilty of this serious breach of technique and, worn in this fashion, a mask is worse than useless, as it just rubs staphylococci off the lower end of the nasal septum and scatters them at large.

2. **Gowns.**—Freshly laundered gowns or coats should be kept at the entrance to each lying-in ward and donned on entry. Clothes are dirty things, and it is only prudent to avoid, by a change of outer

clothing, the carrying of infection from one ward to another. This practice is far from usual, unfortunately.

3. **Gloves.**—Dry sterile gloves should be used for all vaginal examinations and operative work, after a conscientious scrub-up. Putting on non-sterile gloves and then rinsing them in antiseptics or rubbing them over with antiseptic cream is not satisfactory, and the attitude should be that what is good enough for general surgeons (who would not dream of operating without dry sterile gloves) should be *almost* good enough for obstetricians!

4. **Isolation facilities.**—These must be adequate, and the accommodation for septic cases should be provided, preferably in another building or at least in another part of the block, and the staff concerned should not do duty in both clean and unclean wards. Barrier nursing constitutes no more than a dangerous pretence at taking adequate precautions. Maternity departments in general hospitals should be in buildings separated from the general wards. Unfortunately, in many hospitals of the older type this is not feasible.

5. **Infection among personnel.**—Members of the staff suffering from sore throats, colds, boils, whitlows, paronychia and other such ailments, even though mild, should be swabbed and immediately suspended from duty, and whenever infection occurs that is anything more than sporadic, a search should be made for the source.

6. **Septic babies.**—These should be sent, together with their mothers, to the isolation ward. They are a potent source of epidemic infection.

7. **Antiseptics.**—These, though indispensable, should be regarded as a subsidiary line of defence. Creams should be coloured with some dye to indicate the areas of application. Our present preference is for hexachlorophane. Chlorhexidine (Hibitane) is a magnificent antiseptic but it is expensive. Savlon is cheaper and very satisfactory.

8. **Control of dust.**—Dust is an important source of cross-infection, always worse after bedmaking. The oiling of blankets and floors has been tried out. The first has certain laundering difficulties and the second has a depressing effect upon the appearance of the floor. Colebrook found that staphylococci can remain viable in blankets for many weeks. Boiling blankets shrinks them and autoclaving turns them into felt. Soaking them in antiseptics or oils has the further disadvantages of being likely to induce sensitivity reactions in some patients. The ultimate answer is to provide Terylene blankets in hospitals. These can be safely sterilised.

All dry-sweeping and the use of brooms should be replaced by vacuum cleaning.

9. **Bed-pans.**—These should be sterilised with steam as soon as used. On no account should cloth bed-pan covers ever be used. Disposable bed-pan linings have now replaced the traditional bed-pan with us, thus eliminating yet another source of cross-infection.

10. **Disposal of vulval pads.**—These should be placed at once in a bin with a fly-proof, automatically closing lid and should be collected twice a day and burnt. Strong paper container-bags are very useful for lining the bins. Disposal lifts are ideal. They are safer than chutes which have been found to "funnel" bacteria from one floor to another.

The Problem of Neonatal Sepsis

During the 1950s this problem in maternity units had become so acute as to question, once more, the desirability of institutional confinement in completely normal cases. Within twelve months no less than four maternity departments in the West of Scotland, for example, had epidemic outbreaks necessitating the temporary closure of two of them, including the whole of our own maternity hospital. The trouble is endemic in all units and those who say they have none are usually those with the poorest facilities for bacteriological investigation, the lowest standards of observation and the least clinical honesty.

We now recognise that no septic lesion in a newborn baby is trivial, however superficial or minor it may appear to be. Even a small septic skin spot may apparently heal rapidly in hospital yet provide a latent focus of infection which, some weeks later, breaks out as a fixation abscess, for example in lung, or as osteomyelitis, meningitis or septicaemia. The connection of this major illness with the earlier transient lesion is often missed and the maternity unit remains blissfully ignorant of its part in the subsequent disaster.

In an allegedly "clean" maternity department Barber and Burston reported that 65 per cent of all babies went home with penicillin-resistant strains of staphylococci, and Hutchison and Bowman in Newcastle-on-Tyne found that colonisation of the infant nose and umbilical stump by *Staph. pyogenes* occurred in exactly two-thirds of all babies in one or other site within 24 hours of birth. Cross-infection appeared to be from infant to infant. They too found that some of the hospital strains of staphylococci carried home persisted and spread within the family for up to six months. It would appear that babies in hospital cannot avoid being colonised with staphylococci. What really matters is what sort of staphylococci. The umbilical stump is now increasingly recognised as a primary site of multiplication of these organisms and source of spread. Open exposure of the umbilicus to the air is favoured in most units as a means of accelerating mummification of the umbilical stump and the usual modern practice is either to clamp or ligate the stump very close to the umbilicus and remove the distal tissue. Occlusive dressings are distrusted by most of us on the grounds that it is hard to believe that bacteria cannot penetrate them, and because they encourage moisture and interfere with inspection.

The anterior nares of the babies also become quickly infected with staphylococci and so great is the problem that Williams (1958) observed that 15 per cent of babies developed at least some staphylococcal lesion, even though trivial. In an interesting experiment involving the positioning of babies in nurseries in relation to an index baby carrying a recognisable strain of staphylococcus, Wolinsky *et al.* (1960) found that the spread of infection was predominantly by organisms carried by the nurses and not by the index babies and that even after one sole exposure over 50 per cent of the babies could acquire the strain from the appropriate nurses as determined by umbilical and nasal cultures. From this work it is clear that a baby is in more peril from being handled by a nurse than by lying in a cot next to an infected baby. The magnitude of the problem has been particularly well recognised in Australia where as many as 41 per cent of babies have been found to have developed clinical evidence of staphylococcal infection and 100 per cent of them at five days old carried staphylococci. Plueckhahn (1961) blamed the busy life which the babies suffered at the hands of the nursing staff, ranging from full bathing to weighing, eye toilet four-hourly, cot-making and being changed, to the accompaniment of much coming and going of the staff and dirty linen being sorted within the same atmosphere. As a result of these disturbing figures the nursing management of these babies was drastically overhauled and produced a most astonishing decrease in minor staphylococcal disease from 41 per cent in 1956 to 4·7 per cent in 1960, achieved by restricting these routine nursing procedures, by employing rooming-in and dry-washing the babies with hexachlorophane. The institution of these more up-to-date techniques was also rewarded by a reduction in subsequent admissions of babies to hospital for staphylococcal disease and a considerable fall in the incidence of breast abscess in the mothers. Since babies must acquire staphylococci they are more likely to acquire epidemic varieties of virulent and antibiotic-resistant strains in hospital than if born at home and certainly Elias-Jones *et al.* (1961) found this rate to be more than double in the case of the former. Nevertheless, as Williams (1961) has pointed out in a survey of North-West London, there was also an appreciable incidence of nasal carriage of *Staph. aureus* in babies born at home, in fact little different from those born in hospital, and one cannot assume that domiciliary delivery protects the baby altogether from what has now become a modern widespread problem. The possibilities of competitive colonisation by harmless staphylococci as an alternative to high-powered methods of protection from exposure has yet to be worked out.

Unfortunately not only the staphylococcus but now the *E. coli* is providing new problems in cross-infection. The latter is now identifiable by serotyping and it would appear that many of these infections are transmitted from the mother's own bowel. Often, however, hospital strains of *E. coli* are the source of trouble.

The epidemic strains of staphylococcus are all penicillin-resistant and already resistant to many or most of the commonly used antibiotics. This situation is likely to get worse with the present indiscriminate misuse of all and every drug unless some potent antibiotic, e.g. erythromycin, is kept strictly up one's sleeve and used only to save life in certain segregated instances.

Staphylococci of phage-type 80/81 are common offenders—as in our own epidemic in Glasgow, and also in Australia, New Zealand, Canada and the United States. Phage-typing, however, gives little indication of virulence but serves to track down a possible source of infection.

What then can one do in the face of so widespread a problem? The most rigid enforcement of the rules of surgical asepsis must come first. Domiciliary delivery might get over the difficulty but would expose the patient and her child to too many other hazards, except in cases "carefully selected" for their expected normality. Early dismissal from hospital is a compromise solution but is hardly fair on the type of patient most in need of rest and attention. The increased use of rooming-in and entrusting the mother with as much as possible of the handling of her baby certainly cuts down cross-infection between babies and constitutes yet another reason for early ambulation in the fit puerperal mother.

Additional Steps to Control or Curtail Infection among Babies

1. Any case of neonatal sepsis, however minor, must be isolated.
2. Overcrowding in the nurseries is dangerous and should be avoided.
3. Baby bathing is a fatuous, unnecessary and sentimental ritual which is largely overdone and provides opportunities for the spread of infection. The babies should be cleaned in their cots, sterile wool should be used and their towels should be separate.
4. Masks should always be worn by the staff whenever handling babies.
5. The number of nurses handling any individual baby throughout its stay in hospital should be limited as far as possible.
6. There should be no communal changing tables.
7. In addition to wearing gowns, the hands should be properly washed and dried on paper towels. Hospital hand towels are dangerous and should be abolished.
8. All feeding utensils should be boiled after use if not disposable.

Teats which were re-used were responsible for an outbreak a few years ago of a *Pseudomonas aeruginosa* epidemic in one of the other paediatric units in Glasgow and it would appear that the common practice of sterilising teats by immersion in Milton hypochlorite (1:80) solution, as is the usual practice, was not always adequate. This technique was replaced by gas sterilisation with ethylene oxide with a dramatic drop in the positive percentage on rectal swabbing of babies in the unit.[30]

9. The cot bedding should be of Terylene. An alternative although less efficient method is to enclose the blankets in small cotton bags.

10. The babies should be removed from the lying-in wards while floor-sweeping or bed-making is in progress. The commonest type of neonatal infection is the sticky eye. The use of prophylactic eye-drops, once so important in the prevention of gonococcal ophthalmia, has now been abandoned in many institutions. It does nothing to cut down the incidence of sticky eye and, in fact, it may provoke its increase. It is, nevertheless, important to take swabs at once from any eye showing conjunctival infection, after which eye-drops such as Albucid or penicillin may be started straightaway pending the bacteriologist's report, and the baby and its mother with it must be isolated.

BREAST INFECTIONS

There can be no doubt about the advantages of breast feeding for both mother and child and yet, except in the more intelligent strata of the community, breast feeding is unquestionably on the decline. Newson and Newson (1962) have disposed of the popularly held belief that it was the desire of the mother to get back to gainful employment which made her anxious to give up breast feeding at the earliest possible moment. They showed in their survey in Nottingham, an area of high level of employment of women, that even by the time the baby was twelve months old fewer than 2 per cent of the mothers were back at their full-time work and less than 8 per cent had even part-time jobs; they observed that over and over again the physical reasons at first given for failure to breast feed were cover for underlying attitudes of mind ranging from a vague sense of inconvenience to a deep-seated revulsion. Fifty-five per cent of those interviewed admitted that they had not wanted to breast feed and would not have continued anyway, 28 per cent said they would have liked to breast feed and the remainder were in the "don't know" class. Only about 1 in 10 of the mothers had continued to feed for as long as six months. So much for the success of medical and nursing propaganda. The position in Glasgow is exceptionally discouraging. Many of the older multiparae do their best to discourage the young primigravida and take the line that it is an awful nuisance and a terrible tie. This attitude is most marked amongst those living in the worst and most overcrowded housing conditions, where lack of peace and privacy militate against breast feeding, but one often feels that family doctors find it easier and less trouble to put a baby on the bottle than to encourage the falterer with all the determination which it sometimes requires. It is no use trying to encourage a favourable attitude towards breast feeding in the few hectic days which the Glasgow working-class woman is prepared to stay in hospital after delivery. The brainwashing can only succeed, if at all, in the course of antenatal care. We ascertain, earlier in pregnancy, the patient's wishes in regard to breast feeding and prepare accordingly. Breast milk is every baby's birthright. Failure to breast feed is a source of very real disappointment to many women, and in the large majority of cases is due to neglect on the part of the patient's nurses and doctors.

The psychological aspects and importance of breast feeding are incalculable but, on the more physical plane, human breast milk is the ideal diet for the neonate which no substitute, however ingenious its composition, can wholly replace. The statement, so often made to mothers who are having difficulties with lactation, that their milk is disagreeing with the baby is in every instance a flagrant travesty of the truth, and it would be far more accurate to diagnose that the nurse was disagreeing with the mother. The following is a brief summary of the advantages of breast feeding:

1. Human breast milk, by having a relatively higher content of lactalbumin as compared with cows' milk, which has relatively more caseinogen, is more easily digested.
2. It is safe.
3. The chances of gastro-enteritis are much reduced.
4. It is far simpler than the conscientious preparing of feeds.
5. It is cheap.
6. Overfeeding at the breast is practically impossible after the first fortnight.
7. Uterine involution is unquestionably assisted. Suckling provides powerful sensory stimuli in the highly innervated nipple. These reach the innervation of the posterior pituitary and stimulate the production of oxytocic hormone. This not only provokes the milk-ejection reflex by its action on the myo-epithelial elements surrounding the mammary alveoli but acts, of course, directly upon the uterus as well.
8. Subsequent breast carcinoma is less common after a series of successful periods of lactation.

Feeding bottles are hardly necessary for the woman who succeeds in breast feeding her child, because she will manage to lactate until the child is old enough to drink directly from a cup at about eight or nine months, which is about the correct time for weaning, although from the age of six months or from the time when the child has reached a weight of 6–7 kg, whichever is the sooner, additional food in the form of groats, Farex or simple broths will have been given.

The seeds of failure to breast feed are often sown during the patient's stay in hospital and, paradoxically, it is often those patients who during this period seemed to have a super-abundance of milk who dry up so often shortly after their return home. The cause of the trouble nearly always lies in an uncorrected overdistension of the breasts occurring during the first puerperal week. A rise of milk pressure within the breast alveoli discourages secretion by flattening the alveolar columnar cells and occluding the surrounding capillaries. The baby, confronted with a breast surface almost as hard as a brick wall, cannot properly apply its jaws behind the lacteal sinuses in the nipples as it should and, instead of drawing the nipple into its throat, simply champs to no purpose on the nipple itself, abrading it, making it vulnerable to infection and wholly failing to relieve the fullness of the breasts. Small wonder, then, that it loses interest and the breasts, too, take the hint and start to dry up. Waller's results (1946) in Woolwich were so remarkable that his case stands proven up to the hilt. He managed to obtain a successful lactation rate at 6 months of 83 per cent in primigravidae and Blaikley *et al.* (1953), following Waller's principles, managed to double the 6-month success rate at Guy's Hospital to 51 per cent as against only 26 per cent in a control series. Anyone who visited the British Hospital for Mothers and Babies, Woolwich, in Waller's day will have appreciated at once the reasons for his enormous success, which was due, not only to his own intensive personal supervision, but also to the whole-hearted and enthusiastic support which his nursing staff supplied.

This shows what can be done when doctors, nurses and patients are all determined—an unusual combination. A review of the reasons for abandoning breast feeding within the first three months has been made by Hytten *et al.* (1958) who studied a sample of primiparae in Aberdeen numbering 106. Seventy-four had given up by three months and all but two experienced one or more difficulties in breast feeding. The commonest complaints were of excessive crying by the baby, maternal fatigue, breast and nipple troubles and inadequate milk.

It is neither dignified nor profitable for the staff to engage in a battle of wills with a patient who, in her heart of hearts, has no desire or intention of breast feeding. The difficulty is to spot the losers before any conflict is about to arise and this requires a more thorough knowledge of the patient's temperament than most harassed clinicians possess in hospital practice. Bearing in mind that many cases are likely to suffer some initial discouragement in getting the baby to take an interest in what they have to provide (and some babies are insultingly sleepy when first put to the breast), one's best hope is to forestall these difficulties before they ever assume any size. It is as well to warn the mother about "fourth day puerperal blues". This is where Waller's principles, summarised later, of establishing a ready flow of milk before delivery itself and avoiding any trace of engorgement in the breast, give lactation the chance of a flying start. Where the likelihood of failure is reinforced by an unsatisfactory psychological attitude it is better to suppress lactation from the very start.

Lactation can be suppressed by a variety of methods ranging from nothing at all to most elaborate hormone combinations. The breasts are so often literally crying out to exercise their natural function that it sometimes takes a lot of wanton effort to suppress it and the placebo technique has something punitive about it. A series of untreated cases has been compared with those receiving a homeopathic dose of 5 mg of stilboestrol twice a day, with an average stay in hospital of only 4·76 days after delivery.[29] This can hardly be called stilboestrol suppression. We ourselves used to go in for a massive dosage scheme of stilboestrol, namely 15 mg thrice daily, followed by 10 mg likewise, then 5 mg and tapering off thereafter, and our experience accords with that of Hodge in 1967, who found a 12 per cent failure rate with stilboestrol as against a 65 per cent failure rate without it. We then carried out a number of alternative suppression schemes involving diuretics and stilboestrol in each of our main wings, including intramuscular injections of 2 ml of Mixogen which contain both oestradiol and testosterone. As a result of all this we came to agree a final policy which consists of simply binding the breasts and giving frusemide 40 mg as required.[39] One dose was found often to be sufficient if started early enough and no patient required more than eight doses. Mammary discomfort was dealt with by adequate analgesia provided by paracetamol, dihydrocodeine (DF118), if necessary intramuscularly, or pentazocine. Distalgesic was found to have the additional virtue of not constipating the patient. The advantages of giving up oestrogens including stilboestrol were soon apparent. In the first place there was less "rebound filling" of the breasts after dismissal home[9] and perhaps most important of all the incidence of oestrogen-withdrawal bleeding was considerably reduced. Finally the chances of the patient developing deep venous thrombosis were lessened. A note is sent with the patient advising her general practitioner that we have purposely withheld oestrogens and this policy seems to be working well particularly in the women in the older age groups who are more prone to thrombosis.

Where there has been a history of antenatal venous thrombosis it would certainly be unwise to use oestrogens in suppressing lactation in the puerperium.[14]

A tenfold increase in the incidence of puerperal thrombo-embolism has been reported in women whose lactation was suppressed with oestrogens as compared with those who were breast feeding.[13]

Aetiology of Breast Infections

Breast abscesses are a preventable condition. Waller had only 4 such in 10,000 cases in 9 years at Woolwich, and the usual incidence which most institutions suffer does little credit to their management of lactation. The essence of the matter lies in the state of the nipples and the prevention of overdistension of the breasts. Staphylococcal cross-infection does the rest. Overdistension exposes even good nipples to traumatic suckling, but poor nipples themselves are often associated with ducts choked with colostrum. Engorgement, with its surrounding oedema, still further prevents the proper drainage of milk. The stage is now set for the access of pathogenic organisms via nipple cracks and abrasions, so that engorgement turns to mastitis and mastitis to abscess formation.

Prophylaxis in pregnancy.—Since breast infections are preventable by the satisfactory establishment and maintenance of lactation, prophylactic measures should be undertaken in pregnancy. These consist firstly in teaching the patient the art of manual expression of the breasts. This not only establishes the flow of milk and clears the ducts of colostrum blockage, but endows the patient with a skill in advance in combating overdistension in the early days of the puerperium. It also means that lactation is smoothly established at the outset of the puerperium without the usual hectic course of milk coming in with a rush on the third day. This manual expression and clearance of colostrum should be kept up from the 36th week onwards. The hypothetical value of colostrum to the baby as a source of maternal antibody is insignificant in comparison with its nuisance value in causing duct blockage. Secondly, the nipples should be rendered fit for lactation. This will depend not only upon the texture of skin but more upon the property of *protraction.* In order to determine the presence of protraction or retraction it is not merely enough to tug on the nipples. They should be properly tested by pinching the areola between finger and thumb and observing whether the nipple comes forward or tends to buckle inward. Where protraction by this simple test appears to be inadequate, the wearing of Waller glass shells during the later part of pregnancy will make a very beneficial difference. Apart from ordinary washing with soap and water, the skin of the nipples does not require any of the more traditional methods of hardening it up, for example, the use of spirit which simply encourages the later appearance of cracks and fissures.

Prophylaxis in the puerperium.—Every effort is directed to the prevention of engorgement and distension, because in this event spontaneous leakage of milk from the breast stops, and the organ becomes tense and oedematous to the danger of the nipple. Breast feeding should, therefore, be stopped as soon as the breasts become tight, and manual expression should be started as soon as an outflow of milk can be obtained, shortly after which the oedema will subside and breast feeding can be resumed. Oxytocin nasal sprays have been found helpful by some by stimulating the ducts to eject milk. In breasts which tend to get rather tight, it is a good plan to perform manual expression before the feed in order that the baby has a softer breast to deal with, and residual milk at the end of the feed should be expressed likewise. When suckling and expression are insufficient to relieve engorgement or the threat of it, stilboestrol should be prescribed without hesitation, and if the breasts remain tight in spite of suckling and expression, the need for this drug is urgent. Five mg stilboestrol should be given at once in early cases, but the dose should be adjusted at each feed time to suit individual need. One can safely give up to 20 mg in one dose without fear of suppressing lactation, provided suckling can be quickly resumed, in which case the mechanical stimulus thereof will more than counter the inhibitory effects of the drug. The effect of stilboestrol on the breasts lasts up to about 8 hours, so that repeated dosage may be necessary, but the effect is dramatic and the success of the treatment depends upon the promptitude with which it is instituted.

Summary of Waller Procedures

1. Teach the art of manual expression before delivery. This may make it unnecessary afterwards.
2. Encourage protraction, if necessary with the help of shells.
3. At the threat of engorgement give stilboestrol 5 mg four-hourly.
4. Where engorgement is rapid and severe, give up to three doses of 20 mg of stilboestrol four-hourly and then reduce the dose rapidly.
5. Institute manual expression of the breasts as soon as the swelling and oedema start to subside.

Waller found that stilboestrol was needed in about 5 per cent of his cases to control milk retention.

Non-surgical Treatment of Mastitis

The antibiotics have not proved an unmixed blessing in breast infections and their indiscriminate use may mask the cardinal signs of inflammation and cause delay in surgical intervention, which is as important as ever, though the extent of operation has to some extent been modified lately. The antibiotics are admirable for aborting an infection if given early enough, but after the disease has become firmly established, they fail to secure full resolution, so that a chronic induration of the breast may be induced which may even mimic a lactation carcinoma. Ultimately in these cases one makes a belated incision, ploughing through a vascular density of inflamed tissue which bleeds furiously and only a small quantity of pus may reward one's efforts. The patient ends up with a much more persistent disability than she would have had if antibiotics had not, in the first place, delayed the decision to operate.

It is often difficult to decide whether pus is likely to be found before operating. To wait for signs of fluctuation is to wait too long, since this will only be found in neglected cases. Aspiration with a wide-bore needle is not very rewarding, and it is a good rule to diagnose the presence of pus simply on the grounds of suspicion.

The baby should not be put to the breast while the infection is active and as long as pathogens can be isolated from the milk, or while the nipple is cracked. Both nipple and breast should be rested with the help of stilboestrol and gentle manual expression, provided it is not painful. If the condition cannot be fairly smartly aborted it is better to suppress lactation outright.

Surgical Drainage

From the above it is clear that surgical drainage is just as important as formerly and that procrastination with antibiotics interferes with its ultimate efficacy. Any breast in which inflammation does not rapidly resolve with stilboestrol, the antibiotics and the immediate cessation of breast feeding, should be suspected of having formed pus, and the presence of a brawny oedema over the skin makes the diagnosis almost a certainty. Under a general anaesthetic a radial incision is made over the affected area and a finger is introduced into the wound to open up and drain all loculated areas. If the incision has to be placed in the upper quadrants of the breast, counter drainage through a lower incision is often necessary. The quicker pus is evacuated, the less will be the disorganisation of the breast tissue and the shorter the course of the illness. Neglected cases can run a very tedious course.

Ancillary lines of treatment should not be omitted in dealing with breast abscess. All breast feeding should be stopped at once because, even though the other breast is normal, continued suckling therefrom produces cross-stimulation of the inflamed breast. Stilboestrol should be vigorously prescribed. In a great many of these cases, even though healing is very rapid, it is not possible thereafter to re-establish lactation. This takes us back to the paramount importance of the prophylactic measures outlined earlier.

Bottle Feeding

Within the last few years sterile pre-packed feeds have been introduced into maternity and children's hospitals both in this country and the United States. These feeds are available in full- and half-cream varieties in 100-ml volumes, made up in disposable bottles, marked in 20-ml increments. The teat is of the screw-type, made of latex and likewise disposable but this considerably increases the cost, so that many units keep a separate teat for each baby in his own hypochlorite solution which seems to be a sound economic compromise.[17]

Amounts as large as 100 ml would naturally be largely wasted by premature babies and those on tube feeding, for whom 25-ml feeds would be more appropriate. The cost of such a scheme is to a large extent offset by the economy in staff and in not having to provide a special milk-preparation department and its staff. The milk which the baby receives is identical in composition with what he will receive on returning home from properly made up dried-milk powder of the same manufacture. The mother therefore will be faced with no additional difficulty.

Clearly such a scheme is not universally available.

From the mother's point of view evaporated milks are simpler to prepare than dried milks. The former are reconstituted by adding two parts of milk to three parts of water.

Babies weighing less than 2,500 g require special care in feeding and the help of a specialist paediatric unit. Those between 2,500 g and 3,000 g are likely to require feeds approximately 3-hourly, while those above 3,000 g may be fed normally.

If there has been any history of polyhydramnios, the passage of a soft rubber tube into the stomach is mandatory to exclude a diagnosis of oesophageal atresia and in any case a first feed should always be of boiled water or 5 per cent dextrose. The first feed is given within six hours of birth, or earlier in the case of the smallest babies, but the average baby should certainly be fed within eight hours of birth. If the baby shows no interest whatsoever in feeding by the end of 24 hours the possibility of cerebral birth injury or damage from hypothermia may have to be considered. Our own normal practice is to encourage feeding on demand if breast feeding.

The normal baby born at term will take at least 15 ml/kg birth weight per day, working up to at least 120 ml/kg by the end of the first week. Many take more, for example, 40 ml/kg building up to 150 ml/kg and some even up to 200 ml/kg.[46]

A good fluid intake reduces plasma bilirubin, which is highly desirable especially in the jaundiced. Unfortunately these are just the babies who are often sleepy and disinclined to feed. It is better to tube-feed than allow a baby to become dehydrated from inadequate fluid intake.

All normal babies should have regained their birth weight by the end of the first week and thereafter gain steadily.

Not many units have ethylene oxide gas sterilisers and immersion in Milton hypochlorite solution for both bottles and teats after preliminary washing normally suffices. Naturally mothers managing at home have to be taught a proper hygienic drill with regard to feeding utensils. This is one of the fields where the increased safety of breast feeding is obvious among the less privileged classes.

Water that has been boiled should be used for making up the feed. The instructions on the tin of a given powder must be faithfully followed. A common mistake is to use a heaped scoop instead of a level scoop of mixture and it is far better to give a feed which is too dilute than one which is too concentrated.

Compared with human milk, cows' milk contains very much more protein and very much less lactose. Most dried-milk formulae consist of cows' milk to which iron and vitamins have been added. Vitamin D has usually been added to partially evaporated tinned milks.

Because of the higher content of minerals in cows' milk, the baby is likely to have a higher concentration of phosphates in the blood and lower concentrations of calcium than in the breast-fed case, and as a result have an increased risk of tetany convulsions; also a larger amount of urea and minerals have to be excreted by the kidneys, which may encourage dehydration. The addition of sugar, usually sucrose, may be necessary to bring the ratio of protein to carbohydrate more into line with that of human milk.

THROMBOSIS

Thrombosis rears its ugly head just as much in midwifery as in general surgery, although, apart from cases delivered by Caesarean section, the more dramatic end result, namely embolism, is relatively uncommon; nevertheless, a potent source of maternal disability lies here, and many a case of venous misery in later life owes its origin to thrombosis occurring after childbirth. The events of the puerperium rank with a family history of ulceration and the association of obesity in the aetiology of this serious disability of middle age.

There are two main varieties of thrombosis:

Ileofemoral thrombosis.—This is segmental in nature, and may extend from the internal iliac vein as far down as the profunda femoris, or upwards into the common iliac vein. It is due to the proximity of an inflammatory process within the pelvis and it produces the acute variety of white leg. It is a true inflammatory thrombophlebitis.

Phlebothrombosis of calf.—This is the more common variety. Clotting occurs in the venous sinuses within the soleus muscle. These sinuses are without valves, and the thrombosis may spread along the veins draining into the posterior tibial vein, whereupon oedema of the ankles appears. From here the thrombosis may spread to involve the popliteal vein, resulting in considerable swelling and pain, and, finally, the femoral vein may become involved to the accompaniment of the full-blown clinical picture of white leg. Although the origin of white leg in this instance is different from the first, the condition is now hard to distinguish from that due to ileofemoral thrombophlebitis. Thus it will be seen how the condition of white leg can arise, either as a result of inflammatory thrombophlebitis or non-inflammatory phlebothrombosis. In thrombophlebitis the infection reaches the vein along the perivenous lymphatic channels and, as a result of inflammation, the endothelium in the threatened vein is destroyed, so that thrombosis occurs. In phlebothrombosis, on the other hand, the venous endothelium is intact.

Aetiology of Phlebothrombosis

Stasis is the most important single factor, and this of course is favoured by immobility, shock and a poor venous return to the heart because of shallow postoperative respiration. Pre-operative or antepartum anaemia is also an important aetiological factor, and stasis may be caused locally by the careless use of lithotomy poles and operating table straps. There are also other contributory causes to venous stasis in the legs, namely prolonged labour, haemorrhage, manipulations, dehydration, prolonged anaesthesia (particularly with chilling while under its influence), and the use of binders after delivery which interfere with respiration. After surgical operation, and in our case particularly after Caesarean section, there is a marked alteration in the coagulability of the blood, the fibrinogen is increased, platelets are more numerous and they clump together more readily. The relative increase in thrombosis after Caesarean section is therefore explained.

Ochsner and De Bakey (1940) considered that the mechanical blockage resulting from an intravascular clot or the lymphatic obstruction caused by perivenous inflammation is not enough to explain the full syndrome of white leg, and they suggested arterial vasospasm as being responsible for the full clinical picture, pointing out that ligation alone of a main vein is not followed by oedema or white leg. They considered that the arterial spasm is reflexly induced from the thrombosed segment of vein, and were able to reproduce this spasm by causing an experimental endophlebitis with chemicals. They showed, furthermore, that this reflex arc could be blocked by interruption of the sympathetics. As a result of the spasm, pressure within the capillaries is raised, and the endothelium, as a result of anoxia, leaks fluid into the tissues; in addition, they held that the arteriolar spasm results in a decrease in the rate of flow of lymph, causing a rise of osmotic pressure and the establishment of a vicious circle with more oedema.

The diagnosis of clinically obvious cases, swollen, blue or white, is not difficult, but less florid cases may require more sophisticated methods of identification such as phlebography and radioiodine.[125] Alternatively, Doppler ultrasound may be used, applying the transducer over the femoral vein in the groin with the patient semi-reclining and with the thigh or calf squeezed by a pressure cuff. The venous blood flow is reduced in cases of recent occlusion.[16] I have only occasionally tried this technique and cannot claim enough experience of it to be convinced of its value.

The Objectives of Treatment

There are several facets to consider:

1. The prevention of further clot propagation. In the case of embolism this is vitally necessary.
2. The alleviation of symptoms, which may be very severe.
3. The prevention of pulmonary embolism.
4. The prevention of residual disability and sequelae.

In the case of ileofemoral thrombophlebitis, the ultimate prognosis, as regards function, is often better than in severe types of phlebothrombosis starting in the calf. Recanalisation commonly occurs in the former, but when it occurs in the latter the patient is left with an incompetent venous system, so that, usually about two years later, she may be greatly troubled with pain in the legs on standing, oedema and later ulceration. It has to be noted that the inflammatory reaction in the leg which may be apparent in association with phlebothrombosis is a result and not a cause of clotting in a calf vein, which may have been previously normal.

Obstetricians tend to lose sight of the late effects of this complication of pregnancy.

Methods of Treatment

Thrombosis after delivery or operation is largely a preventable condition. Anaemia and rough handling of tissues at the time can to some extent be avoided, and haemo-concentration can be countered by an adequate fluid intake during the early days of the puerperium. Venous stasis should be discouraged by the active use of the muscles of the extremities in bed, which is more effective than early ambulation, and by exercises in deep breathing which increase the rate of the venous return to the heart.

Non-specific methods.—When thrombosis threatens or appears, the affected leg, or preferably both, should be raised above the level of the heart. This can be achieved by putting the foot of the bed up on blocks. Bicycle-type exercises should be encouraged as soon as the reduction in pain will permit their use, and massage can be instituted usually within two days. These methods alone are often all that is necessary without resorting to more elaborate lines of treatment and are effective in quickly reducing oedema and cutting short the disability. Elevating the legs by raising the foot of the bed alone will quadruple the rate of venous flow and is the most important single measure, but elevation as frequently practised by raising the leg on pillows and sandbags, by thus immobilising it, destroys half the point of the treatment. Mobility must not be restricted.

Heparin.—This is the most important, the safest and the most certain of the anticoagulant drugs. It is prepared from mammalian lung and liver. It is one of the strongest organic acids produced within the body, bears a strongly negative electrical charge and is able to combine with various basic compounds in the blood. It acts in several ways, chiefly by preventing the action of thrombin on fibrinogen. It also acts as an antiprothrombin and reduces the conglutination of the platelets and the consequent liberation of blood-clotting enzymes. Its effect, therefore, is to prolong clotting time. Heparin should be given by intravenous injection. It should not be given intramuscularly or subcutaneously, even with the addition of hyaluronidase and 2 per cent procaine, because a haematoma may develop at the injection site, the extent of which may be difficult to control, and great pain will be produced. The usual dose is between 8,000 and 10,000 international units administered four-hourly, although in serious emergencies, such as massive pulmonary embolism, 25,000 international units may be injected forthwith (1 mg equals 100 units). The effect is fully reached within about 60 seconds of administration and tails off within the next four hours, hence the need to repeat the injection. One's objective in treatment should be to increase the patient's clotting time threefold, and one should not be satisfied with a clotting time of less than twelve minutes. Subsequent doses are regulated according to the clotting time achieved. Heparin has the great advantage that the further propagation of clot is immediately suppressed and the case can be brought under control at once, so that, within 48 hours, massage can often be instituted and the patient can be got out of bed as soon as oedema and tenderness show signs of settling.

For some reason clinicians are often reluctant to use this drug, not only because of the inconvenience of giving intravenous injections, but because of the fear that a dramatic haemorrhage may result. Fortunately a ready antidote to heparin exists in the form of a 1 per cent solution of protamine sulphate which may be given intravenously in doses of 5–10 ml. Payling Wright reckoned that 1 ml of this solution is equivalent in antidote effect to 1,000 international units of heparin. This antidote, which should always be available when a case is being treated by heparin, acts by neutralising the negative charge on the heparin molecule. A transfusion of fresh blood should be given in addition, and any available or necessary methods adopted of arresting haemorrhage locally. Overdosage with protamine sulphate may produce a paradoxical anticoagulant effect. It is clearly not desirable to abolish the anticoagulant effect of the heparin completely and as a rough-and-ready guide bleeding can be brought under adequate control by giving sufficient protamine sulphate to counteract about half the last quantity of heparin given.

Dicoumarol and allied substances.—Dicoumarol and its allies, e.g. phenindione (Dindevan) and warfarin sodium (Marevan), act upon the clotting powers of the blood by preventing the liver from synthesising prothrombin from vitamin K. They also prevent the formation of Factor VII. They are not destroyed in the stomach and can therefore be given by mouth, but their effect is somewhat indirect and delayed because at the time of first administration active prothrombin already in circulation will continue to operate for many hours.

These synthetic anticoagulants are closely related chemically to vitamin K and they probably act by competitive inhibition usurping the place of this vitamin as well as its function in the synthesis particularly of prothrombin. Dicoumarol has now given place to the more easily managed Dindevan and Marevan, the latter being more recent and having advantages of more prolonged action and more easily stabilised control in long-term treatment.

It will be appreciated that these drugs do not affect the clotting time directly and the control of dosage is carried out by estimating the prothrombin time usually by the Quick one-stage method, or the prothrombin and proconvertin (P. & P.) method of Owren, and more recently the thrombotest (Owren, 1959).

Quick's method uses oxalated venous blood from which the plasma is separated. To the latter a standard thromboplastin solution is added and then calcium chloride. The time taken for coagulation is recorded and either expressed as a multiple of the clotting time of a normal control plasma, e.g. $2\frac{1}{2}$ times, or as a percentage of normal prothrombin activity which is calculated by a formula:

Prothrombin activity (percentage of normal) $= \frac{K}{PT - A}$ when PT is prothrombin time in seconds, and K and A are constants of 303 and 8·7 respectively.

In Owren's P. & P. method the plasma is diluted to increase sensitivity and bovine plasma, lacking in certain thromboplastin factors but a good source of fibrinogen and Factor V (proaccelerin) is added. Calcium chloride is then added to complete the reaction and the coagulation time is noted. A graph is plotted of the prothrombin time of normal pooled plasma in a series of dilutions to express the range of times from 100 per cent to one per cent prothrombin. The result of the coagulation time of the sample under test is compared with the same time on this graph, from which can then be read off corresponding prothrombin percentage concentration. The therapeutically desired result is in the range of about 10–14 per cent of normal prothrombin concentration.

The thrombotest is designed to evaluate all four factors which these oral anticoagulants may suppress, namely Factor II (prothrombin), Factor VII (proconvertin), Factor IX (Christmas factor) and Factor X (Stuart-Prower factor). This is achieved by an all-in-one reagent (thrombotest) containing crude cephalin, thromboplastin from ox or horse brain, adsorbed bovine plasma freed from the four factors concerned but containing the other clotting factors not affected by the anticoagulants and finally calcium chloride. This reagent is reconstituted with distilled water and can be used for testing capillary blood or venous samples.[36]

Results are obtainable with little technical equipment or skill in 2–3 minutes and are expressed as a percentage of normal. Anticoagulant therapy should aim at about 10 per cent (range 6–15 per cent). I have lived thus myself for ten years!

These anticoagulants and the present methods of control are now regarded as safe, but certain factors should be borne in mind which may seriously modify the patient's response. Aspirin, and in fact salicylates generally, exaggerate the increase in prothrombin time and should be avoided. They also reduce platelet adhesiveness. Their even greater danger is that of an uncontrollable haematemesis. Broad-spectrum antibiotics, by influencing the intestinal flora and thus interfering with the synthesis of vitamin K may, apparently, potentiate the anticoagulant effect. Chlorpromazine and phenylbutazone also exaggerate these effects and may have been inadvertently prescribed to control the patient's symptoms. Secondary infection, debilitating conditions and renal failure favour over-reaction, while diarrhoea and liquid paraffin may interfere with absorption and reduce the effect. Haematuria is usually the first sign of overdosage, and a haemorrhagic tendency is not usually exhibited until the prothrombin falls to 10 per cent of normal.

Usually the effect of phenindione is in full swing with adequate dosage within 18 hours. Following the withdrawal of the drug, the effects persist for several days. Dosage is usually 200 mg by mouth initially, followed by a daily dose of 100 mg, more or less, according to the results of prothrombin estimations which should be repeatedly made as long as the patient continues on this treatment. The dose for warfarin sodium is much lower, 40–50 mg, followed by a maintenance daily dose of 3–20 mg according to prothrombin tests. Overswings take longer to correct and stabilise.

The antidotes to overdosage are the transfusion of fresh blood and the injection of vitamin K. Vitamin K_1 (phytomenadione) is more efficient than vitamin K and, injected intravenously (5 mg) or given orally (15 mg), can restore a normal prothrombin level within a few hours. Severe bleeding may require up to 20 mg Konakion intravenously given very slowly. Fresh blood transfusion is more rapidly effective and counteracts the drug at once, but further transfusion may be necessary later as the drug already absorbed continues to operate.

The medical treatment of deep venous thrombosis has been fully discussed by Kakkar (1971) and our own experience too has found very little place for surgery, especially as limb viability in obstetrics is rarely, if ever, in question.[25]

Venous ligation.—This operation is favoured by certain general surgeons and is designed to prevent pulmonary embolism, but it has little place in obstetrics and further thrombosis and embolism may arise proximal to the ligature. Recurrent embolism in spite of anticoagulant therapy may, however, necessitate it, but I would first suspect the determination with which the treatment had been pushed. I have yet to meet the case in which I was convinced of the necessity for the operation. Ligation can be performed with impunity up to the lower inferior vena cava, although later disability in the affected leg may be serious in years to come. If ligating a femoral vein, it is usually preferable, where applicable, to tie off the vein distal to the profunda femoris. However, the prompt treatment of embolism, or the threat thereof, with heparin should render this operation unnecessary.

Outline of Treatment in Specific Instances

There is no set line of treatment for thrombosis as a whole, but the following are some remarks applicable to the different varieties.

Mild cases of deep thrombosis and cases of superficial thrombosis.—The treatment recommended is to raise the foot of the bed on blocks and to encourage muscle activity as soon as possible in order to defeat venous stasis and to prevent the persistence of oedema. The risk of pulmonary embolism in superficial thrombophlebitis is small in obstetrics and in our view does not justify the use of anticoagulants, except in postoperative cases, for example after Caesarean section, or if the process appears to be spreading.

Severe cases of thrombosis and puerperal white leg.—In this condition the patient is in considerable pain at first and exercises cannot, therefore, be prescribed initially. The legs, as before, should be elevated by raising the foot of the bed and a short course of heparin is given, as outlined earlier, to prevent propagation of the clot *in situ* and the development of additional thrombosis elsewhere. Meanwhile a more prolonged course of treatment with phenindione or warfarin is got under way. Because these drugs appear in breast milk, lactation should be suppressed. After 48 hours, with the subsidence of pain, massage and gentle movements can be started. Still keeping the legs elevated, full movements and active exercises should be in full swing after about 7 days. An no time should the legs be immobilised with sandbags and roller towels, as was so often practised in the past. The legs are kept raised until the oedema has almost disappeared, usually within about 12 days of this treatment, after which the patient may be allowed up provided a really e*fficient* elastic support, to include the whole foot, heel and leg, is applied before rising. This support should be used unfailingly whenever the patient is out of bed for a further six months. It is important to treat these cases very strictly, as only thereby can residual disability be prevented.

It remains now to discuss the duration of anticoagulant therapy. The general mistake is to stop too soon. Anything less than three weeks is inadequate and patients so treated and recovering would probably have done quite well without it. Treatment should be maintained for long enough to allow the clot to undergo fibrinolysis or to become thoroughly fibrosed and firmly attached to the vein wall. If pulmonary embolism has occurred the treatment should be continued for several months in order to prevent subsequent pulmonary hypertension and congestive cardiac failure.

Pulmonary embolism.—This is nowadays second only to pregnancy toxaemia as a cause of maternal death. Although it is much more common relatively after Caesarean section than after vaginal delivery, nevertheless the Ministry of Health Confidential Enquiry Reports on Maternal Deaths (1955–57) indicated that 114 out of 157 cases of fatal embolism followed vaginal delivery and in half of them warning had been given in the form of signs of deep thrombosis or previous small emboli. The greater the physical signs in the leg the less is the risk of pulmonary embolism, and when one leg is severely affected and the patient develops an embolus, it is probable that the source is in the apparently unaffected leg. The traditional story of the patient who sits up in bed, asks for the bed pan and drops dead from pulmonary embolism is misleading in the likely sequence of events. It is more probable that the effort associated with defaecation, by distending the veins with raised intravenous pressure, is responsible for the detachment of the clot.

Seventy per cent of emboli come from the calf or the profunda system and 30 per cent from the internal iliac veins. A large embolus produces such shock and vagal inhibition that the patient dies at once. In more than half the cases, however, the immediate effects are not fatal at first, but there occurs a secondary post-embolic thrombosis within the pulmonary arteries which increases the degree of lung infarction. Treatment must be very prompt, not only to counter the patient's immediate shock, but also to prevent this secondary thrombosis and a recurrence of fresh embolism. Clinically the patient may have a mild fever suggesting thrombosis which, sometimes after settling for a few days, is followed by a brisk rise in pulse rate and then further fever signifying minor embolism. The immediate symptoms of embolism are related mainly to hypotension, namely faintness, breathlessness and tachycardia. Pleural pain and haemoptysis are often not present and diagnosis may be difficult, although portable chest radiography may help by demonstrating a rise in the level of the diaphragm and clouding of the costophrenic angle from partial lung collapse.[5]

Emergency treatment consists in the immediate intravenous injection of morphia 15 mg and a massive intravenous injection of heparin (25,000 international units). There is now believed to be a further beneficial effect of heparin, since it has been found that it inhibits the vasoconstrictor action of 5-hydroxytryptamine (serotonin) which is released in the early stages of clot propagation by the lysis of blood platelets.

Since the clinical signs in pulmonary embolism are out of proportion to the size of the clot or the volume of infarcted lung, and are due to the liberation of such a humoral agent, it can be seen that heparin's action transcends the prevention of further clot propagation and has the additional rôle of first-aid countering of the systemic effects of the catastrophe. Oxygen is supplied by mask. Noradrenaline may be necessary to maintain an adequate blood pressure and tachycardia is countered with digitalis. During the next 48 hours heparin is given four-hourly to maintain a clotting time of over 12 minutes. This will prevent the propagation of further clotting, and at the end of 48 hours the risk of detachment of clot already formed will have largely disappeared as a result of organisation. The feet are kept up by elevation of the foot of the bed as mentioned before and movements are encouraged as early as possible. The effect of dicoumarol is too late to make it anything more than an "also ran", and it is on heparin that we must rely for getting the case immediately under control during the first critical 48 hours. Nevertheless, warfarin treatment is instituted as soon as possible to cover the longer-term treatment.

If the patient lives more than two hours after the first attack, and this is true in more than half the cases, prompt treatment along these lines will provide an excellent chance of recovery.

POSTNATAL ADVICE

There is little point in sending a patient away with instructions to return in six weeks time unless she is given advice on how to manage meanwhile. She should be encouraged to seek official advice rather than that of her alleged friends should her breasts give trouble or should she be in doubt about baby feeding. Postnatal exercises which can be done as a matter of habit without interfering with housework should be prescribed as follows:

Postnatal Exercises

These exercises should be done each day for at least six weeks. Do exercises 1–4 six times and work up to twelve times. They can be done while working round the house. Exercises (1) and (2) are very important.

(1) Standing peeling potatoes or standing at bus stop (with legs crossed at ankles or one heel in hollow of opposite foot—ballet stance)—press thighs together, pull up between legs, pull in abdomen and tighten seat muscles. Hold it all tight while you count four then let it all relax slowly. (This is the movement you would do if you were trying to prevent the passage of water or a bowel movement.)

(2) Standing with back against wall—pull in abdominal wall, tighten seat muscles—(imagine you are tucking your tail between your legs) and try to get lower part of back to touch the wall. This exercise can also be done in sitting position with back against chair or lying on bed with knees bent up and pressing back into bed.

(3) Standing—pull one leg up at the hip so that one leg is shorter than the other. Keep your knee straight; foot should be right off the ground. Repeat with other leg.

(4) Standing—feet together, knees together, thighs pressed together. Move along the floor for a short distance as if "twisting".

(5) Pull in abdomen before bending down to pick up anything. Always pull in abdomen before doing any housework which involves bending.

(6) Do not attempt to lift anything which is very heavy. When lifting an object of moderate weight—bend knees and keep back straight.

(7) Pram pushing. Do not crouch over pram. Keep upright and keep pram close to you. Hold the handle lightly, with elbows easy. Shoulders neither braced nor raised nor depressed but level. When pushing pram uphill lean slightly forward from the hips and bend knees slightly, but don't crouch. See that you are breathing easily.

A problem which is likely to be uppermost in the patient's mind, although one to which she may feel too reticent to confess, is the question of resumption of marital relations and how, for the meantime, to avoid further pregnancies. After the first month there need be no restriction with regard to the former although the patient is unlikely to be much interested and young husbands should be particularly warned that this is no unnatural phenomenon. The fear of conceiving straight away is very real. It is usual to prescribe the contraceptive pill only after the first period has re-established itself, but in the exceptionally fertile woman there is no reason why it should not be prescribed from the very first. Intra-uterine contraceptive devices have a high drop-out rate if inserted before eight weeks at least or preferably twelve.

Postpartum sterilisation, easy enough surgically during the first days of the puerperium, while the fundus of the uterus is still easily accessible through a very small incision, is an operation which I have never really liked. For one thing it is not a very suitable time for a woman to make such an irrevocable decision and for another the baby's hold on life may still be precarious. The failure rate is also higher due to recanalisation and I now much prefer to carry out the operation through a laparoscope, which makes it a very minor procedure, after three months.

Pending these measures the patient's husband should be advised to use condom contraception, or a depot progesterone injection may be given intramuscularly, e.g. Depo-Provera 150–250 mg.

Immunisation Procedures

BCG vaccination against tuberculosis should be carried out within the first few days of birth. The baby should receive its first injection for diphtheria, whooping cough and tetanus at the age of three to four months followed by second and third injections at intervals of a month each. Poliomyelitis vaccine by mouth can be given at four to six months of age followed by second and third doses at intervals of four to six weeks. A booster injection for diphtheria, whooping cough and tetanus should be given at the age of eighteen months and smallpox vaccination carried out during the second year.

REFERENCES

1. Arneil, G. C. and Kerr, Margaret M. (1963). *Lancet*, **2,** 756.
2. Astley, R. (1963). *Brit. J. Radiol.*, **36,** 2.
3. Barber, M., Hayhoe, F. G. J. and Whitehead, J. E. M. (1949). *Lancet*, **2,** 1120.
4. Barber, M. and Burston, J. (1955). *Lancet*, **2,** 578.
5. Barritt, D. W. and Jordan, S. C. (1961). *Lancet*, **1,** 729.
6. Blaikley, J. B., Clarke, S., Mackeith, R. and Ogden, K. M. (1953). *J. Obstet. Gynaec. Brit. Emp.*, **60,** 657.
7. Calman, R. M. and Gibson, J. (1953). *Lancet*, **2,** 649.
8. Campbell, Marie, A., Ferguson, Isobel, C., Hutchison, J. H. and Kerr, Margaret M. (1967). *Arch. Dis. Childh.*, **42,** 353.
9. Cole, B. W. and Pitts, N. E. (1966). *Practitioner*, **196,** 139.
10. Colebrook, L. (1936). *J. Obstet. Gynaec. Brit. Emp.*, **43,** 691.
11. Colebrook, L. (1955). *Lancet*, **2,** 885.
12. Colebrook, L. and Kenny, M. (1936). *Lancet*, **1,** 1279.
13. Daniel, D. G., Campbell, H. and Turnbull, A. C. (1967). *Lancet*, **2,** 287.
14. Duncan, I. D., Coyle, M. G. and Walker, J. (1971). *J. Obstet. Gynaec. Brit. Cwlth*, **78,** 904.
15. Elias-Jones, T. F., Gordon, I. and Whittaker, L. (1961). *Lancet*, **1,** 571.
16. Evans, D. S. and Cockett, F. B. (1969). *Brit. med. J.*, **2,** 802.
17. Francis, P. E. M. and Thompson, M. (1971). *Nursing Times*, 24th June.
18. Garrey, M. M., Paterson, M. M. and Evans, J. M. (1964). *Lancet*, **2,** 1057.
19. Gillespie, W. A., Simpson, K., and Tozer, R. C. (1958). *Lancet*, **2,** 1075.
20. Guthrie, R. and Whitney, S. (1964). *Phenylketonuria.* Children's Bureau Publication No. 419. Washington, D.C.: U.S. Dept. of Health, Education and Welfare.
21. Hellman, L. M., Kohl, S. G. and Palmer, J. (1962). *Lancet*, **1,** 227.
22. Hodge, C. (1967). *Lancet*, **2,** 286.

23. Hutchison, J. G. P. and Bowman, W. D. (1957). *Acta paedia (Uppsala)*, **46,** 125.
24. Hytten, F. E., Yorston, J. C. and Thomson, A. M. (1958). *Brit. med. J.*, **1,** 310.
25. Kakkar, V. V. (1971). *Brit. J. hosp. Med.*, **6,** 741.
26. Kekwick, A. (1956). *Brit. med. J.*, **1,** 796.
27. Kerr, M. M. (1976). Personal communication.
28. McAllister, T. A. (1975). *Scot. med. J.*, **20,** 85.
29. MacDonald, D. and O'Driscoll, K. (1965). *Lancet*, **2,** 623.
30. Maclaurin, J. C. (1969). Report on Outbreak of *Pseudomonas aeruginosa* in a pediatric unit. Glasgow: Glasgow Royal Maternity Hospital.
31. Mann, T. P. (1955). *Lancet*, **1,** 613.
32. Mann, T. P. (1963). *Nursing Times*, **59,** 15.
33. Mann, T. P. and Elliott, R. K. (1957). *Lancet*, **1,** 229.
34. Newson, L. J. and Newson, E. (1962). *Brit. med. J.*, **2,** 1744.
35. Ochsner, A. and De Bakey, M. (1940). *J. Amer. med. Ass.*, **114,** 117.
36. Owren, P. A. (1959). *Lancet*, **2,** 754.
37. Plueckhahn, V. D. (1961). *Brit. med. J.*, **2,** 779.
38. Population screening by Guthrie test for phenylketonuria in S.E. Scotland. Report by Consulting Paediatricians and Medical Officers of Health (1968). *Brit. med. J.*, **1,** 674.
39. Russell, T. V. N. (1974). Personal communication.
40. Shelley, Heather J. and Neligan, G. A. (1966). *Brit. med. Bull.*, **22,** 34.
41. Snodgrass, G. J. A. I., Stimmler, L., Went, J., Abrams, M. E. and Will, E. J. (1973). *Arch. Dis. Childh.*, **48,** 279.
42. Stevenson, J. S. and Scott, J. (1967). *Hlth Bull. (Edinb.)*, **25,** 47.
43. Theobald, G. W. (1959). *Brit. med. J.*, **2,** 1364.
44. Walker, G. (1971). *Brit. med. J.*, **3,** 147.
45. Waller, H. (1946). *Arch. Dis. Childh.*, **21,** 1.
46. Wharton, B. and Berger, H. M. (1976). *Brit. med. J.*, **1,** 1326.
47. Williams, R. E. O. (1958). *Publ. Hlth. Rep. (Wash.)*, **73,** 961.
48. Williams, R. E. O. (1961). *Lancet*, **2,** 173.
49. Wolinsky, E., Lipsitz, P. J., Mortimer, E. A. and Rammelkamp, C. H. (1960). *Lancet*, **2,** 620.
50. Wright, H. P. (1953). *Brit. med. J.*, **1,** 987.
51. Zeltzer, P. M., Foukalsrud, E. W., Neerhout, R. C. and Stieham, E. K. (1974). *Lancet*, **1,** 373.

CHAPTER XXVI

POSTMATURITY AND DYSMATURITY

To the practising obstetrician the problem of postmaturity constantly recurs and it is surprising how little guidance most of the textbooks supply. How far is it a clinical entity in its own right? How much does it matter? How can one be sure that the case is postmature? What are the risks and what steps should be taken to counter them?

The difficulties arise from the absence of any fixed criteria. Size of infant alone is not enough, for the postmature baby is not always unduly large and, conversely, very large and apparently postmature babies may be born before the 40th week of pregnancy.

If postmaturity is abnormal, there should be some evidence of abnormality either in mother, child or in the process of labour, and a diagnosis by dates alone is all too often not supported by any such concrete and abnormal findings. The expected date of delivery, as reckoned by Naegele's rule, can only be calculated from the beginning of the last menstrual period and, except in rare instances, it cannot be known precisely when conception occurred.

The average duration of pregnancy so calculated is 280 days, and if this period is exceeded by 14 days or more it is reasonable to believe pregnancy to be prolonged, but this is not the same thing as saying that it is abnormal without other evidence. As Wrigley (1958) said, there can no more be an "exact" time for gestation than an "exact" height or an "exact" weight for everyone.

Before diagnosing postmaturity with confidence, more than one criterion should be satisfied.

Finn Bøe used three standards:

1. Pregnancy had exceeded 290 days;
2. Fetal length exceeded 54 cm;
3. Fetal weight exceeded 4,000 g (approx. 8¾ lb).

All three conditions were satisfied in 2 per cent of cases which were thus classified as postmature, but only the first is ascertainable with any accuracy before the actual delivery.

The incidence of postmaturity, then, will clearly vary widely according to the arbitrary standards employed.

In Aberdeen, for example, McKiddie found that 24·6 per cent of 6,803 pregnant women went more than seven days beyond their expected date, while Rathbun in America found that 13·2 per cent (approximately half the above percentage) had overrun their dates by more than a fortnight.

McKiddie noted no significant difference in the age groups of patients becoming "postmature". Where the provisional diagnosis of postmaturity is confirmed retrospectively by taking into account the baby's size, as regards both length and weight, the true incidence of postmaturity is certainly more in the region of 2 per cent. The babies of multiparae tend to be heavier at birth than their elder siblings were, but their length is not increased in the same ratio, so that if both factors are reckoned, postmaturity is no more likely to be confirmed.

It is probable that the incidence of true postmaturity satisfying two or more criteria would be more common were it not for the prevalence of induction of labour as a therapeutic measure to forestall it.

Aetiology

Not much is yet known about the causes of postmaturity. The earliest beginnings of pregnancy are unlikely to provide an explanation, for it is generally agreed that the ovum can be fertilised only within the first twenty-four hours of ovulation. Coitus may, however, provoke ovulation outside the normal time limits, and although embedding of the fertilised ovum does not occur for a further five to eight days, nevertheless, it must occur at least two days before the menstrual flow would have been due or menstruation will follow; thus it will be seen that provoked ovulation later in the cycle would, at the most, account for no more than a week of apparent postmaturity.

Pregnancy can be artificially prolonged in lower animals, such as rabbits, by administering large doses of progesterone, and it is very likely that in humans endocrine influences play a large part, but progesterone in the human species has not been found capable of producing this effect.

As poor nutrition and bad social conditions can cause prematurity, so, conversely, an improved standard of living might be expected to encourage pregnancy to be prolonged, but there is nothing to suggest that it occurs to any abnormal extent. Finn Bøe noted that since 1900 there had been a tendency for the duration of pregnancy and the size of babies to be increased on average, though only to a slight degree, particularly where pregnancy mainly coincided with the summer months; but during the privations of the German occupation of Norway, pregnancy was not appreciably shortened, although birth weights tended to fall, presumably as a first result of malnutrition.

Hereditary factors are of the most certain importance and postmaturity tends to recur in successive pregnancies in the same woman, which is a point of some prognostic significance. The condition often runs in families.

Lastly, the diabetic patient and the diabetic-prone or "prediabetic" woman tend to produce oversize and "postmature" infants.

Legal Aspects

These can be very vexing. The plaintiff is usually the supposed father who is disputing paternity on the grounds that he has had no opportunity to cohabit with his wife within the usually accepted limits of pregnancy's duration. These are not pleasant cases in which to give evidence and all the possible signs of postmaturity will have to be carefully weighed. No official upper limit has been fixed by the courts, and since the onus of proof lies with the plaintiff, the mother is likely to be given the benefit of any doubts, and doubts there will nearly always be. It is quite certain that no judicial decision will ever alter the husband's attitude and, whatever the result of the action, the child is bound to suffer in either case.

To state categorically that a pregnancy of, for example, 330 days is impossible in a given case is often beyond the competence of a medical witness to decide in the present state of our knowledge, and the courts are likely to seek subsidiary evidence of chastity, or the reverse, in the mother, in trying to reach a decision, and the case will not simply be dismissed on precedent alone.

The famous case, many years ago, of Gaskill *v.* Gaskill was dismissed in the mother's favour, there being no corroborative evidence whatever of lack of chastity; in this instance pregnancy was stated to have lasted for 331 days, and, if one were to be guided by precedent it would appear that any period of gestation within that figure would in subsequent actions, be upheld. Furthermore, advances on this figure might come to be accepted without any foreseeable limit. More recently, however, the case of Preston Jones *v.* Preston Jones went in the opposite direction and the stated duration of pregnancy was 360 days.

Pathology

If postmaturity is an abnormal condition it must, of course, have its own pathology.

Firstly, the fetus is increased in size, to the possible detriment of labour. Secondly, ossification proceeds apace and results in a head which is not only larger but definitely harder and therefore less able to mould in labour. Thirdly, oxygen saturation is diminished, and though to some extent compensated for by fetal polycythaemia, the postmature infant is liable to approach the verge of intra-uterine asphyxia.

Barcroft and Young, taking samples of blood from the anterior fontanelles of rabbit fetuses while still *in utero* found a progressively diminished oxygen saturation level from term onwards until death occurred from asphyxia due to postmaturity. A similar mechanism has been demonstrated in humans (Walker and Turnbull, 1953; Walker, 1954).

Walker found that there was a progressive fall in the percentage level of oxygen saturation in umbilical vein blood during the second half of pregnancy from 70 per cent at about the 30th week, 60 per cent just before term and deteriorating rapidly to 30 per cent by the 43rd week—a level at which meconium-staining of the liquor, as a consequence of asphyxia, was inevitable. Furthermore, Walker and Turnbull found that this adverse trend was accelerated in cases of pre-eclamptic toxaemia or where there had been bleeding earlier in pregnancy.

From a study of the clearance rates of radiosodium from the myometrium, Moore and Myerscough (1957) inferred that the rate of uterine blood flow was reduced in normal primigravidae past term and that pre-eclampsia reduced the clearance rates still further. They admitted, however, a wide range of rates in normal subjects, which limits the value of the method in trying to decide which case is outliving its placental efficiency.

The influence of increasing maternal age was also reckoned by Baird (1957) to reduce placental sufficiency so that the Aberdeen school favours routine induction of labour in all primigravidae over the age of 25 whose pregnancy runs beyond the 41st week.

An entirely opposite view stemmed from Belfast where Bancroft-Livingston and Neill (1957), from a careful study likewise of umbilical venous blood, showed no correlation whatever between the oxygen level thereof and either fetal or maternal age.

Their finding would certainly indicate that the association of postmaturity and intra-uterine hypoxia has been overstressed and most authorities nowadays take an intermediate view between these rival schools of thought.

Fetal haemoglobin has a greater affinity for oxygen than adult haemoglobin, and the ratio of the fetal to the adult variety falls progressively in later pregnancy, and presumably still more in protracted pregnancy, so that even if placental efficiency did not lessen, this of itself would contribute to anoxia.

The placenta is an ageing organ, though to what extent its functional capacity is lowered is not fully known. Although its weight is increased, much of its substance is infarcted and therefore useless. The structural evidences of ageing, however, are not fully matched by loss of efficiency, and the rate of transfer, for example, of radio-sodium per gram of placental weight is known to increase at least right up to term.

Microscopic examination does not help as yet in recognising placental ageing.

Calcification of the placenta is negligible in prematurity, but is more evident when the case has become postmature, whether assessed by radiography, chemistry or histological examination; nevertheless, its presence is not reliably related to adverse effects on the fetus.

The postmature fetus, besides being more exposed to anoxia, has also to live in a restricted environment of a progressively diminishing volume of liquor amnii, which may handicap the processes of labour. From the 37th week onwards the volume of liquor gets rapidly less (Elliott and Inman, 1961) from an average amount of about 1,200 ml until by the 43rd week it may be no more than 100 ml in all, a clinical point which may be noticeable to the same observer supervising the case.

Clinical Signs and Diagnosis

Mistaken dates account for more errors in diagnosing post-maturity than any other factor and should be very carefully scrutinised. As recounted earlier, women candidates at examinations commonly assure me that less than half of all women are cast-iron sure about the date of their last period. The patient may, however, give accurate information, but conception may have occurred during a cycle which happened to be prolonged.

Normally ovulation occurs approximately fourteen days before menstruation and fertilisation of the ovum is unlikely to take place more than a day or two after it. If the menstrual cycle is one, for example, of seven weeks, this would introduce a positive error of three weeks in calculating the expected date of delivery from the onset of the last menstrual flow. It is therefore necessary to know the history of the menstrual rhythm. Where it has previously been as regular as clockwork, errors are less likely to be made, but even these cases are subject to unpredictable arrhythmia occasionally, and it is always possible that ovulation might have been delayed in any given instance. Since ovulation can be provoked, out of turn, by coitus, another source of error becomes apparent. Where a reliable history of isolated acts of intercourse can be obtained, some guidance may be forthcoming, since the ability of spermatozoa to fertilise the ovum does not usually outlive thirty-six to forty-eight hours, although living spermatozoa can sometimes be found in the cervix after as long as a week.

During antenatal supervision a record should always be made of the time of quickening, which will pin down the duration of pregnancy at that time to at least sixteen weeks. Records of the size of the uterus are far more valuable in the earlier months of pregnancy than in the later and careful notes at the time may prevent many subsequent doubts.

Normally the maternal weight stops increasing at about term and begins to fall. This is a useful sign that the case is at least mature but Browne (1962) attached even greater importance to this sign and regarded it as evidence of placental insufficiency so commonly associated with prolonged pregnancy. On examining the abdomen of the postmature case, the relative quantity of liquor to the size of the baby may appear palpably reduced. The child has increased muscle tone, giving an impression of ramrod rigidity, but this impression is largely due to the diminished amount of liquor. The value of this observation is enhanced if it is made by the same pair of hands at each visit (Wrigley, 1946).

Vaginal examination is sometimes helpful. A deeply engaged head, well applied to a thinned lower uterine segment and a ripe cervix, will suggest that the child is at least mature.

Attempts at fetal mensuration by clinical means, although of slight help in assessing prematurity, are unlikely to assist much in estimating postmaturity. The length of the fetus in a well-flexed attitude (and herein lies the mischief) is usually double the direct distance of breech to vertex, which at term is not less than 50 cm.

Radiology may provide some help, by a study of ossification centres, though errors of up to four weeks are possible here.

The ossification centre of the cuboid usually appears at term and its appearance denotes probable maturity. The centre at the upper end of the tibia appears at about the same time but is less reliable, while the lower end of the femur usually begins to ossify somewhat earlier. Even twins, however, may show differing evidences of maturity on the basis of ossification centres (Cope and Murdoch, 1958).

Cephalometry by X-rays is often disappointing largely because it is difficult to be sufficiently certain of the distance of the fetal head from the X-ray tube and errors are magnified on the film, and when one is dealing in significant fractions of a centimetre, it is easy to see how small errors of technique can spoil results.

The biparietal diameter, on average, increases by 0·17 cm or more each week in the last few weeks of pregnancy. Our own technique of employing sonar for measuring the biparietal diameter *in utero* has been described on numerous occasions.[17, 18, 19, 47, 48] In our opinion the biparietal diameter is more closely related to maturity than it is to actual birth weight and this is a very useful point. A biparietal diameter of 9·8 cm, for example, indicates maturity at the very least and one of 10·1 cm or over strongly suggests that the case is postmature even though the weight itself may not exceed 3·2 kg (7 lb). In our practice, decisions as to maturity and postmaturity are more readily made by sonar than by resorting to radiography.

Campbell's modification of our ultrasonic method of biparietal cephalometry has now stood the test of time. Carried out between the 20th and 30th week of gestation it can, in competent hands, correctly assess the maturity to within plus or minus 9 days in 95 per cent of cases.[12] Unfortunately the accuracy falls off markedly as term approaches.

The earlier in pregnancy that a patient is examined the better, and single readings are not enough. The importance of serial readings cannot be questioned in cases of doubt. Not only will inaccuracies of measurement be ironed out thereby but departures from normal growth rates can be reliably recognised.[48] When these rates fall below the 5th percentile 82 per cent of babies studied at Queen Charlotte's Hospital have been found to be below the 10th percentile of weight for gestation and 68 per cent were below the 5th percentile. Even more noteworthy was the finding that retarded ultrasonic growth rates were associated significantly with more low Apgar scores at birth, gross fetal abnormalities and perinatal deaths.[13] Other workers have abundantly confirmed these observations.[24] More refinement still can be expected from simultaneously measuring transthoracic and transabdominal diameters and areas which promise to define and chart intra-uterine growth with even more precision. As it is, cephalometry by sonar is already more reliable than radiology and studies of liquor amnii.[41]

In units lacking ultrasonic facilities the liquor amnii provides useful information, particularly regarding lecithin : sphingomyelin ratios which at least indicate pulmonary maturity though not fetal maturity itself when exceeding 2·5:1. Likewise creatinine levels reflect fetal renal maturity, levels of 1·6 mg/100 ml roughly indicating 36 weeks gestation and 2 mg/100 ml being likely at term.[33] What used to be postulated under the hypothetical name of "surfactant" is now recognised as dipalmitoyl lecithin which is believed to be synthesised from the increase in free fatty acids to be found in fetal lungs near term.[36] All tests on liquor amnii are really only tests of maturity for certain organs and not the fetus as a whole, and therefore are only indirect indices of overall fetal growth *in utero*, unlike what can be provided by sophisticated sonar. Doubtless I am prejudiced!

Diagnosis after delivery should be confirmed if only to guide one in future pregnancies, because postmaturity is often recurrent and the course of the present labour may provide very helpful information in years to come. The two most definite postpartum signs are a birth weight of over 4,500 g (10 lb) and a fetal length of more than 54 cm. The closure of the posterior fontanelle is too variable a sign to be trusted.

There is one important sequence of events which is worth mentioning in regard to postmaturity: occasionally a patient at or about term appears to go into labour and then, before getting properly under way, all signs of labour cease and pregnancy drags on for perhaps a week or more; hormonal influences are probably at work in discouraging true labour from establishing itself. When this happens one should be warned that maturity has been reached and overstepped and there is a strong case for not withholding induction for more than a few days because of the possibility of intra-uterine fetal death. If maternal weight is dropping at the same time, there should be even less hesitation in regarding the case as postmature.

Occasionally there arises the problem of the case which is unquestionably mature, or postmature, in whom the cervix is as unripe as the spout of a tea-pot. Calder and his colleagues[11] have found an effective method of ripening the cervix by administering prostaglandin extra-amniotically by the "single shot" technique, employing a xylose gel vehicle, three to six ml, containing 240–480 μg prostaglandin E_2 through a Foley catheter introduced through the cervix with a 20-ml balloon. This is both simple and effective in hastening the onset of induced labour.

Attempts at assessing biological maturity by cytological study of cervical and vaginal smears have been made at a number of centres, but reports are conflicting. So much depends upon the quality of the cytology.

More definite is a study of the cells within the liquor amnii, but this entails either deliberate amniocentesis or artificial rupture of the membranes if they have not already ruptured spontaneously. The investigation is therefore not as useful as often as its simplicity would otherwise indicate. It was noted by Brosens and Gordon that a 0·1 per cent aqueous solution of Nile Blue sulphate stained mature fetal squamous cells orange. The Nile Blue test was first introduced to confirm or refute the diagnosis of premature rupture of the membranes, but it was observed that the proportion and intensity of orange-stained cells increased with the maturity. In fact between the 38th and 40th week of pregnancy there is a very sharp rise in the percentage of such cells to over 50 per cent, whereas the percentage is less than 10 per cent at 36 weeks. Sharp, however, found that with this test no orange-stained cells could be found in hydramnios.

The study of pregnanediol and oestriol excretion rates (particularly the latter) may also declare diminishing placental function, but unless serial records have been made over a long time and diurnal variations can be studied in sufficient detail to discount them, the evidence is not likely to be of much help to the clinician faced with a given problem.

Effects and Hazards of Postmaturity

In the genuine case the risks are very real. Already short of oxygen the baby will not tolerate further hypoxia well in labour, and may die of intrapartum asphyxia. This risk is by no means uncommon and the stillbirth rate in postmaturity, 5–6 per cent (Rathbun), is not far short of twice that of babies born at term, largely due to this factor. In the past so much attention has been focused on the increased weight and size of the baby that this most important aspect of physiology has been sometimes overlooked.

It is true that the head is larger, and this may make labour more difficult, especially as it does not readily mould, but there is some compensation in the fact that the head is harder and therefore protects the brain better from mechanical injury. Certainly these babies stand difficult forceps deliveries rather better than most, and there should be no hesitation in applying the forceps as soon as fetal distress (which is asphyxial) appears in the second stage of labour. Signs of fetal distress are much commoner than usual both before and during labour.

Fortunately the neonatal death rate is not significantly altered once the postmature baby has been safely born.

Labour itself is likely to be slightly prolonged and is often associated with a deflexed fetal attitude and a high incidence of occipito-posterior position.

Uterine inertia of one variety or another may complicate these labours. It is difficult here to distinguish cause and effect and post-maturity may even be a manifestation of uterine dysfunction as well as a cause of it.

It is not surprising, therefore, that the operative delivery rate is enormously increased and, which is noteworthy, this particularly applies to the more serious procedures, high mid-cavity forceps applications, difficult rotations and Caesarean section. Finn Bøe quoted an operative rate of 29 per cent (44 per cent in primigravidae), of which 19 per cent were Caesarean sections and 6 per cent craniotomies, a figure which would hardly obtain today. The postpartum haemorrhage rate is also increased and is worse in the primigravida. These factors, together with the possibility of maternal intrapartum pyrexia, adversely affect puerperal morbidity.

Even after safe delivery of the head, delay may occur with the shoulders in the case of a large baby and not a few are lost through this complication.

Although intracranial haemorrhage accounts for some fetal deaths, the percentage of unexplained stillbirths increases with the degree of postmaturity.

The fetus that is suffering from hypoxia in labour, and is therefore distressed, not only passes meconium because of sphincter relaxation but is likely to inhale it in the course of its hypoxic gasps, giving rise to the meconium-aspiration syndrome. This is not uncommon in the postmature and because of the great respiratory efforts which may be made, pulmonary alveoli may rupture or be ruptured by attempts at resuscitation, giving rise to neonatal pneumothorax.

Another fetal complication of postmature labour accompanied by hypoxia is the consumption of blood clotting factors by diffuse intravascular coagulation.[14] It has been suggested that this may damage the liver and other vital organs. The damage is due to hypoxia rather than to postmaturity *per se*.

Malpresentations are commoner, especially breech presentation, and because the baby is larger the effects are likely to be more serious.

When labour is inert, which is often the case, especially when the head is too large to "bed down" well in the pelvis and so stimulate contractions, the risks of intrapartum asphyxia are greatly magnified, so that the need for operative delivery becomes more clamant; the relatively diminished quantity of liquor also contributes to dystocia, and the fact that the head may be well engaged and there are no signs of disproportion does not justify a complacent attitude.

In enumerating this formidable list of complications resulting from postmaturity, it may seem that the dangers have been overstressed, since the majority of cases deliver themselves satisfactorily. But a majority result is not good enough, and to foresee a risk is to go half-way towards circumventing it.

MANAGEMENT

There would be no problem if all inductions worked safely and infallibly and if prematurity never resulted by mistake. We cannot afford to lose sight of the possibility that, in postmaturity, artificial rupture of the membranes may carry with it even greater risks to the baby than those which it is hoped to prevent by such interference. Even a failed medical induction is not without its adverse effects upon the patient and the inertia in labour which may follow induction is closely bound up with demoralisation of the patient, or her obstetrician (Gibberd, 1958).

All are nowadays agreed that the combination of postmaturity with pre-eclampsia, hypertension or any history of bleeding earlier in this pregnancy carries risks of intra-uterine fetal anoxia, and possibly death, which far exceed those of even unsuccessful induction.

All cases therefore of hypertensive disease or of pre-eclampsia or where abortion has threatened earlier or where there has been accidental haemorrhage, however slight, should not be allowed to overrun their dates and become postmature, but labour should be induced with determination.

The use of the Saling amnioscope[35] provides a view of the forewaters and the liquor beyond and if the liquor appears clear with flakes of clean vernix within it one is encouraged to assume that the case can safely be allowed to continue undelivered for another half week at least; in this way one's hand may be stayed from carrying out injudicious induction in the false belief that the patient was postmature. We occasionally carry out this procedure more often to reinforce a decision already taken not to induce than for any other valid reason, though, of course, amniotomy can easily be undertaken under direct vision at the same time if amnioscopy is included in the technique of induction.

If at induction the liquor is found to be stained with meconium the possibility of having to undertake Caesarean section should be carefully considered. In such cases the fetal heart must be very vigilantly watched and if labour is not very expeditious Caesarean section may indeed be indicated, although here again the decision may be reinforced or modified by fetal scalp blood sampling by the Saling technique.[4] The fetal heart may not give much warning of imminent fetal death during labour.

The use of an oxytocin drip undoubtedly raises the percentage of successful inductions of labour, but if the liquor is scanty and stained with meconium it may increase fetal asphyxia.

Uterine irritability, as an index of the imminence of labour or of the likelihood of success following induction, can be assessed by some such test as that devised by Eddie (1963) in which minimal but increasing dosage of oxytocin, 0·01 to 0·1 units, are administered by dilute intravenous injection and the threshold of uterine response observed.

Caesarean section should be very readily considered in all cases in which labour, following induction, persistently hangs fire or whenever signs of fetal distress appear. One cannot escape the impression that uterine inertia and postmaturity are sometimes linked to a common disorder of uterine function and the combination should be taken seriously.

A special warning must be made about the dangers of postmaturity in the presence of a fetal monster, including anencephaly. Many years ago Munro Kerr drew attention to the fact that about half the cases complicated by anencephaly, if left to their own devices, went postmature. In such circumstances a very dangerous situation may arise in which, when the patient ultimately goes into labour (and I had one such case who went to 46 weeks) the small "head" slips through the partially dilated cervix and comes to press on the pelvic floor and stimulate very powerful uterine contractions, so that the patient endeavours to deliver herself by bearing down before full dilation and before the shoulders can be accommodated by the undilated cervix. In the case referred to above the patient ruptured her lower uterine segment, developed an amniotic embolus and cardiac arrest, a desperate combination of circumstances, which after many hours of cardiac massage had all the unhappy ritual of death on the table and finally defeated all our efforts.

No plea is made for routine induction at 42 weeks or some such arbitrary standard, for far more mistakes are likely to be made through errors in diagnosing or assessing postmaturity than disasters are likely to be avoided thereby. It would be better stated that when a case has overrun her dates by 14 days one ought to have concrete indications for not inducing labour.

No baby is the better for weighing more than 4 kg (approximately 9 lb) at birth and the mother may ultimately be much the worse for it.

It would be as well to reiterate two rules:

1. Beware of fetal distress.
2. Beware of delay with large shoulders.

OBSTRUCTED SHOULDERS

This problem is only likely to occur in postmaturity when delivering a very large baby, in fact it may prove the worst part of it. My sorriest experience of it concerned an elderly primigravida with a 14 lb (6·36 kg) baby. (Her husband had weighed 15 lb (almost 7 kg) at birth—an important point to note in postmaturity and one which I overlooked in this case.) After rotating and delivering the head with Kielland's forceps I then ran into trouble with impaction of the anterior shoulder and wasted too much time trying to free it and before using the whole hand to bring down the posterior arm. In that hectic fifteen minutes of brute force, of which one could only be ashamed, the baby died. It is a nightmarish situation and one should be ready for it as soon as it is clear that the anterior shoulder is going to impact.

If not in the lithotomy position the patient must be immediately put there, or failing that, the left lateral position. The dorsal position is worse than useless as it is impossible to pull the head far enough back to free the point of the anterior shoulder. The lithotomy position allows the use of fundal pressure from above which the left lateral position does not, and is to be preferred.

The head is drawn backwards rather than pulled, remembering that the brachial plexus is vulnerable to overstretching, determined fundal pressure is applied from above and an attempt is made with the fingers to encourage rotation of the anterior shoulder under the symphysis. This usually does the trick and as soon as the point of the anterior shoulder is free the head can be lifted forwards and the posterior shoulder delivered. If this fails, general anaestheia should be induced at once, an attempt meanwhile being made to rotate and push the shoulders round "*à la* Løvset", so that the posterior shoulder now becomes anterior, using a hand on the abdomen to assist rotation and trying to avoid dislodging the shoulders upwards. Too much time should not be wasted on this manoeuvre which is likely to fail if the baby is really huge and tightly wedged. An alternative method is described by Holman (1963). In this method the primary attention is focused on the posterior shoulder, and the head, instead of being drawn backwards, is drawn downwards and forwards in the axis of the pelvis and, preferably with the help of a second pair of hands, the anterior shoulder is pressed caudally in relation to the fetus in order to reduce the transverse diameter across the shoulders. Fundal pressure is at the same time maintained.

Needless to say an episiotomy is an important adjunct to any such technique. By now, general anaesthesia should have been induced and the hand, if necessary the whole hand, is introduced to bring out the posterior shoulder or even to deliver the posterior arm. This procedure is very damaging to the maternal pelvic floor.

Sometimes, on introducing the whole hand the reason for the delay may be revealed in the form of an unsuspected gross fetal abnormality, such as fetal ascites, etc., and embryotomy may be required.

If the baby is already dead cleidotomy makes possible an easy delivery of impacted shoulders. Strong scissors which will not buckle are required and the most accessible clavicle, usually the anterior, is felt for and brought as far as possible within reach by traction of the head backwards. I have never performed cleidotomy in the living fetus nor seen it done. For one thing the decision to undertake it on a living child would not be made until all other attempts at delivery had failed, by which time the baby would be dead and the immediate relation of the subclavian vessels below the clavicles is enough to discourage one.

Likewise the decision to use a hook is never made at the time as such instruments of a bygone age are never available when the emergency arises. That they would damage the brachial plexus and fracture or separate an epiphysis of the humerus is more than likely and up to the very last experience encourages one that a more normal delivery of the shoulders will yet be achieved, as is usually the case. Nevertheless, disasters from obstructed shoulders still occur and in retrospect provide some of the most mortifying recollections in obstetrics.

DYSMATURITY

This is an important subject and goes by a variety of names, including "the small-for-dates baby", "placental insufficiency", "intra-uterine growth retardation" (hideously, "IUGR") and so-called "postmaturity syndrome", but "dysmaturity" is both brief and descriptive.

By international agreement all babies with birth weights below 2,500 g ($5\frac{1}{2}$ lb) are classified as premature but, as the 1958 Perinatal Mortality Survey carried out in the United Kingdom indicated, one out of three of these babies is not premature at all, but, in fact, dysmature. Dysmaturity has a totally different pathology from prematurity and a different prognosis too and taking the long view in those that survive, the premature baby, weight for weight, is likely to fare far better, both physically and intellectually, than its dysmature counterpart, that is to say provided it survives the immediate neonatal period. In babies with birth weights below the tenth percentile the mortality is very much higher in the case of the premature than the dysmature by a factor of about five, and survival depends more upon gestational age than on weight itself. For one thing the incidence of respiratory disease syndrome (RDS), that killer of the premature in spite of improved management, is much less common in the dysmature. Against this has to be set the well-known risk of sudden attacks of hypoglycaemia in the first few days of neonatal life in dysmaturity, presumably due to the antecedent run-down in glycogen reserves associated with hypoxia. Meconium aspiration for the same reason may complicate birth and call for immediate aspiration under direct laryngoscopic vision.

Another serious feature which may occur within the first day or two of life in the dysmature is the consumption of clotting factors due to microcoagulation and consequent coagulation deficiencies during the first day of life. Low thrombotest (Owren) results have been noted in low-birth-weight infants with signs of cerebral damage, as compared with matched controls not so damaged, and it has been suggested that the brain damage in the low-thrombotest group of those that survived is due to cerebral haemorrhage associated with fibrin depletion from disseminated intravascular coagulation.[10] High haematocrit levels may be connected with the phenomenon of microcoagulation and the appearance of purpura.

Oedema can be more easily provoked by fluids in the dysmature but feeding at the level of 90 ml/kg body weight instead of 65 ml is favoured by paediatricians.

It is a tragic fact that dysmaturity may be a recurrent condition in some women, by no means those confined to the poorer social classes. Postmaturity and fetal abnormality may both be associated with dysmaturity but there are certain general conditions well known to be associated with intra-uterine malnutrition and hence dysmaturity, such as pre-eclamptic toxaemia, all hypertensive conditions, recurrent antepartum haemorrhage chronic renal disease and many cases of heart disease. Diabetes also produces its own type of dysmaturity.

We define nowadays as dysmature any baby whose birth weight is below the tenth percentile of weight for gestation according to the Lubchenko Tables.[30, 47] These tables, based upon Caucasian types of women, were drawn up in Colorado where there are residential areas at high altitudes and the figures may be slightly less than for other parts of the Western world, but they serve to indicate dysmaturity where the gestation period is clearly known. A further distinction between dysmaturity and prematurity can be made by employing the Nile Blue sulphate stain on the cells of the liquor amnii, as it has been observed[39] that the percentage of orange-stained cells is not affected by dysmaturity and corresponds to the known gestational age.

Commonly, the dysmature infant is scraggy with poor subcutaneous fat and has a poor resistance to cold. The liver reserves of glycogen are poor and these babies are particularly liable to dangerous attacks of hypoglycaemia which, if not treated promptly, may result in permanent mental damage. The brain is normally developed in accordance with the gestational age, as are the lungs, which however, are liable to the effects of meconium inhalation because fetal distress *in utero* is common.

Ischaemia of the placental site would appear to be a factor common to most cases,[45] because experimental ischaemia of one horn of a gravid rat uterus has been shown in the second half of pregnancy to produce stunting of the fetuses contained within it. This observation would support what is known about reduced placental blood flow in hypertensive states, for example. The placenta is not just a filter for the passage of oxygen or glucose or small molecules. In actual fact work is done by the placenta in transferring even these substances across the so-called barrier, so that placental insufficiency results not only in chronic hypoxia but also in chronic subnutrition. Normally the placenta weighs about a sixth of the weight of the infant, but in dysmaturity it may weigh appreciably less and the villous surface area is said to be much reduced.

If we could accurately assess placental function during pregnancy we would have solved one of the biggest classes of unresolved obstetrical problems today. Attention is therefore being focused upon hormone excretion levels in the maternal urine. Of all the forms of urinary hormone assay the measure of oestrogens gives more information about the growth and development of the fetus than any other form.[32] The ratio of the usual oestrogens, namely oestriol, oestrone and oestradiol, is usually given as 3:3:1 in the non-pregnant woman but in pregnancy the ratio goes up tenfold in the case of oestriol; in other words an enormous increase in oestriol is secreted by the placenta and gives the best biochemical index of placental function and is generally preferred to pregnanediol excretion curves. Of the steroids in rapid transit between the fetoplacental unit and the mother, oestriol sulphate is the main component and measuring it is more likely to provide useful clinical information than any other compound.[29]

Pregnanediol levels less closely indicate blood levels of progesterone than do urinary levels of oestrogen as indices of plasma oestrogen levels. Chorionic gonadotrophin levels are even less reliable in regard to placental function. Oestriol secretion by the placenta depends upon the activity of the fetal adrenal cortex and this, in its turn, depends upon ACTH from a functioning fetal pituitary. The anencephalic pregnancy therefore produces very low oestriol levels.

Oestriol excretion levels as isolated tests are of very little use and proper curves should be drawn from repeated assay. Even so, low levels do not always indicate placental insufficiency and the scatter is wide. As Klopper (1965) has remarked, "It is difficult to represent the changing picture of retarded fetal growth without producing a bewildering web of crisscross lines," and falls in oestriol output may be "reflections of an underlying disease process affecting the feto-placental unit."

There are indeed many pitfalls in getting accurate and worthwhile oestriol results even accepting the fairly wide variation in day-to-day excretion levels, which necessitate averaging at least two or three consecutive 24-hour collections of urine. Often, bad results are due to bad specimen collection and it is usual practice to check that a urinary specimen is indeed a 24-hour collection by estimating creatinine content in the whole sample. Normally this is fairly stable within about 20 per cent per person every day; somewhere about 900 mg a day according to the patient's weight. Any specimen which suddenly shows, for example, 500 mg can certainly be discarded as an incomplete 24-hour collection.

Only a minority of hospitals can undertake this volume of biochemical work which is by no means easy and even we, with our extravagant facilities, have to restrict our oestriol studies to the following groups:

History of dysmaturity in previous pregnancies;
Cases where the uterus is small for known dates;
Maternal diabetes, or hypertensive conditions;
Chronic renal disease;

Recurrent antepartum haemorrhage;
Certain cases of cardiac disease.

In addition, dysmaturity is suspected where there has been a loss of maternal weight in pregnancy or a gain of only a very few pounds. Scanty liquor is also sometimes a sign of dysmaturity.

It seems to us that growth retardation can be even more accurately and directly estimated by actually measuring fetal growth and, as already mentioned, the use of sonar to measure the growth rate of the biparietal diameter is now increasingly employed by us.[40, 46, 47] At least with this technique the answers are immediate and any fall-off in growth rate as compared with a standard chart is regarded as ominous. It is now our practice to combine biparietal diameter growth curves with oestriol excretion curves on the same chart (Fig. 1). Both techniques may reinforce unequivocally a clinical impression that intra-uterine growth is retarded and may indicate the need for elective delivery of the fetus before it is too late. Here at least is a concentrated attack on the problem of macerated stillbirth.

What then of the survivors? As Coyle and her colleagues in Dundee have warned, a 24-hour excretion of less than 3 mg of oestriol indicates the likelihood of intra-uterine fetal death in the near future, although this is not invariable. In their follow-up study of 14 babies whose mothers had a low oestriol excretion rate during pregnancy Wallace and Michie (1966) found that only 8 were completely normal, 2 were seriously handicapped neurologically and were mentally retarded, a third had a hemiplegia, another had retarded speech and subnormal behaviour, another was retarded and "over-active", and one had a minor neurological abnormality. These are daunting observations. Furthermore there is an increased incidence of intracranial haemorrhage because many of these babies had thrombotest levels less than 10 per cent of normal, which even vitamin K_1 may not correct soon enough.[26] Dysmature babies therefore should be tested for clotting defects, particularly of prothrombin, and treated if there is any suspicion of intracranial haemorrhage by fresh-frozen plasma or fresh blood while waiting for vitamin K_1 to take effect. Another serious complication of dysmaturity, as already mentioned, is neonatal hypoglycaemia which has been described in the previous chapter. This must be tested for routinely and treated urgently with intravenous glucose.

It is naturally a matter of increasing concern to follow up babies who have shown signs of intra-uterine growth retardation and dysmaturity and even to relate the long-term findings to the period during pregnancy when growth was observed to have lagged behind normal. For instance in a study of such cases with a mean age of four years it has been noted that in cases with retarded ultrasonic cephalo-

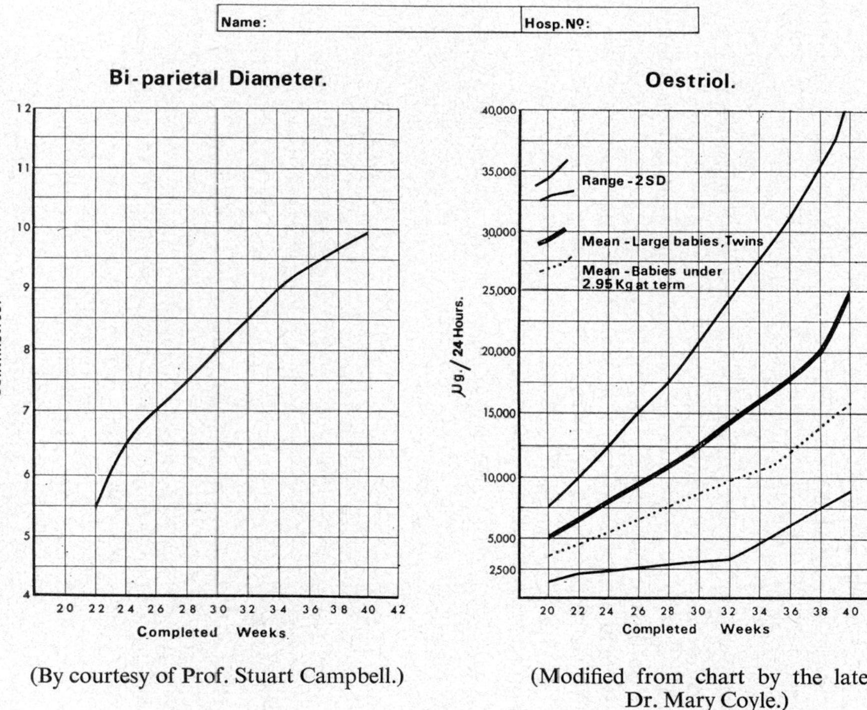

(By courtesy of Prof. Stuart Campbell.)

(Modified from chart by the late Dr. Mary Coyle.)

26/Fig. 1

metry curves, recognised before 34 weeks gestation, both height and weight were below the tenth percentile. The situation, including school performance, was noted to be even worse when the growth lag occurred even earlier in pregnancy.[23] More modern methods of care for these potentially handicapped children would appear to be capable of mitigating their unfavourable prognosis from a depressing former figure of 33–70 per cent, including mental handicap, to about 14 per cent.[38] Much of the damage is due to hypoxia, hypoglycaemia and hyperbilirubinaemia which are, to an increasing extent, treatable. Drillien attributes the earlier poor results in the 1950s to the practice then of delayed feeding.[20] She classifies low-birth-weight infants under three headings:

1. Those prematurely delivered and with developmental abnormalities. A poor prognosis here.
2. Those where the growth is retarded from hypoxia or malnutrition during the third trimester. These may have minor degrees of mental retardation and neurological abnormality.
3. Those prematurely delivered with weights appropriate to the period of gestation. The prognosis in these is quite good with proper modern premature-baby care.

It is all very well for the obstetrician to recognise dysmaturity *in utero* and to deliver the baby into a more congenial environment at the optimum moment, but if the baby is to have a real chance of being spared the possible hideous sequelae of dysmaturity in later life he must be transferred urgently to the care of a paediatric special department. Therefore cases of suspected dysmaturity in pregnancy should be delivered only in a highly equipped hospital with these facilities.

REFERENCES

1. Baird, D. (1957). *Brit. med. J.*, **1,** 1061.
2. Bancroft-Livingston, G. and Neill, D. W. (1957). *J. Obstet. Gynaec. Brit. Emp.*, **64,** 498.
3. Barcroft, J. and Young, I. M. (1945). *J. exp. Biol.*, **21,** 70.
4. Beard, R. W. and Morris, E. D. (1965). *J. Obstet. Gynaec. Brit. Cwlth*, **72,** 496.
5. Bøe, Finn (1950). *Acta obstet. gynec. scand.*, **30,** Suppl. 1.
6. Bøe, Finn (1951). *Acta obstet. gynec. scand.*, **30,** 247.
7. Brosens, I. and Gordon, H. (1965). *J. Obstet. Gynaec. Brit. Cwlth*, **72,** 342.
8. Brosens, I. and Gordon, H. (1966). *J. Obstet. Gynaec. Brit. Cwlth*, **73,** 88.
9. Browne, J. C. M. (1962). *Brit. med. J.*, **2,** 1080.
10. Bryant, G. M., Gray, O. P., Fraser, A. J. and Ackerman, A. (1970). *Brit. med. J.*, **4,** 707.

11. Calder, A. A., Embrey, M. P. and Tait, T. (1976). Personal communication.
12. Campbell, S. (1969). *J. Obstet. Gynaec. Brit. Cwlth*, **7**, 603.
13. Campbell, S. and Dewhurst, C. J. (1971). *Lancet*, **2**, 1002.
14. Chadd, M. A., Elwood, P. C., Gray, O. P. and Muxworthy, S. M. (1971). *Brit. med. J.*, **4**, 516.
15. Cope, I. and Murdoch, J. D. (1958). *J. Obstet. Gynaec. Brit. Emp.*, **65**, 56.
16. Coyle, Mary G., Greig, M. and Walker, J. (1962). *Lancet*, **2**, 275.
17. Donald, I. (1968). *Brit. med. Bull.*, **24**, 71.
18. Donald, I. and Brown, T. G. (1961). *Brit. J. Radiol.*, **34**, 539.
19. Donald, I. and Abdulla, U. (1967). *Brit. J. Radiol.*, **40**, 604.
20. Drillien, C. M. (1971). *Lancet*, **2**, 697.
21. Eddie, D. A. S. (1963). *Brit. med. J.*, **1**, 73.
22. Elliott, P. M. and Inman, W. H. W. (1961). *Lancet*, **2**, 835.
23. Fancourt, R., Campbell, S., Harvey, D. and Norman, A. P. (1976). *Brit. med. J.*, **2**, 1435.
24. Flamme, P. (1972). *Brit. med. J.*, **3**, 384.
25. Gibberd, G. F. (1958). *Lancet*, **1**, 64.
26. Gray, O. P., Ackerman, Ann and Fraser, Anne J. (1968). *Lancet*, **1**, 545.
27. Holman, M. S. (1963). *S. Afr. med. J.*, **37**, 247.
28. Klopper, A. (1965). Research on Steroids. *Trans. 2nd Meeting International Study Group for Steroid Hormones*, pp. 63–83.
29. Klopper, A. (1970). *Ann. clin. Res.*, **2**, 289.
30. Lubchenko, Lula D., Hansman, Charlotte, Dressler, Maria and Boyd, Edith (1963). *Pediatrics*, **32**, 793.
31. McKiddie, J. M. (1949). *J. Obstet. Gynaec. Brit. Emp.*, **56**, 386.
32. Macnaughton, M. C. (1967). *Amer. J. Obstet. Gynec.*, **97**, 998.
33. MacVicar, J., Logan, R. W. and Barnard, W. P. (1973). *Scot. med. J.*, **18**, 84.
34. Moore, P. T. and Myerscough, P. R. (1957). *J. Obstet. Gynaec. Brit. Emp.*, **64**, 207.
35. Morris, E. D. and Beard, R. W. (1965). *J. Obstet. Gynaec. Brit. Cwlth*, **72**, 489.
36. Possmayer, F. (1973). Paper read to Gynaecological Society of Canada, Vancouver.
37. Rathbun, L. S. (1943). *Amer. J. Obstet. Gynec.*, **46**, 278.
38. Rawlings, G., Reynolds, E. O., Stewart, A. and Strang, L. D. (1971). *Lancet*, **1**, 516.
39. Sharp, F. (1968). *J. Obstet. Gynaec. Brit. Cwlth*, **75**, 812.
40. Thomson, H. E., Holmes, J. H., Gottesfeld, K. R. and Taylor, E. S. (1965). *Amer. J. Obstet. Gynec.*, **92**, 44.
41. Underhill, R. A., Beazley, J. M. and Campbell, S (1971). *Brit. med. J.*, **3**, 736.
42. Wallace, Sheila J. and Michie, Eileen A. (1966). *Lancet*, **2**, 560.
43. Walker, J. (1954). *J. Obstet. Gynaec. Brit. Emp.*, **61**, 162.
44. Walker, J. and Turnbull, E. P. N. (1953). *Lancet*, **2**, 312.
45. Wigglesworth, J. S. (1966). *Brit. med. Bull.*, **22**, 13.

46. Willocks, J., Donald, I., Duggan, T. C. and Day, N. S. (1964). *J. Obstet. Gynaec. Brit. Cwlth*, **71,** 11.
47. Willocks, J., Donald, I., Campbell, S. and Dunsmore, I. R. (1967). *J. Obstet. Gynaec. Brit. Cwlth*, **74,** 639.
48. Willocks, J. and Dunsmore, I. R. (1971). *J. Obstet. Gynaec. Brit. Cwlth*, **78,** 804.
49. Wrigley, A. J. (1946). *Proc. roy. Soc. Med.*, **39,** 569.
50. Wrigley, A. J. (1958). *Lancet*. **1,** 1167.

CHAPTER XXVII

PREMATURITY

"The Obstetrician delivers the baby from the Mother;
the Paediatrician delivers the baby from the Obstetrician!"
—*Ex-Glasgow Colleague.*

Any attempt greatly to reduce the present wastage of fetal life calls for a successful attack upon the problems of prematurity, for no single obstetrical misfortune is more extravagant in this respect, and half of all neonatal deaths occur in premature infants. There are three facets to consider, namely, the prevention of premature labour, its management when it becomes inevitable and the rearing of the infant so born. Such a child's initial handicaps are easy to appreciate when one reflects that an infant born at thirty-two weeks has lost one-fifth of the normal span of intra-uterine life, and it is surprising, therefore, that even greater degrees of prematurity than this are still compatible with full and normal subsequent development.

The responsibility for the first two sides of the problem lies with the obstetrician, but the third is now increasingly the paediatrician's concern in any sizeable and up-to-date maternity unit, and good team work between the two services is essential.

Definition

There is no satisfactory definition of prematurity, which really means birth before the thirty-seventh week, and for want of a better standard, birth weights of 2,500 g ($5\frac{1}{2}$ lb) and under have been arbitrarily accepted for the purpose of classifying births as premature. Unfortunately this definition takes no account of babies that are in fact dysmature. In other words they are small for dates, and at whatever gestational age birth occurs their weights are considerably below average levels. This subject was dealt with in the previous chapter, but it also overlaps into the differential diagnosis of prematurity and there is much to suggest a different sort of prognosis too. Walker (1967) holds that babies below the 25th percentile up to 37 complete weeks of pregnancy should be classed as cases of poor intra-uterine growth. Whatever standards are used, however, there can be no doubt that dysmaturity is a syndrome in its own right and differs from prematurity, and there seems to be general unanimity with the opinion expressed by Drillien (1964) that babies born with a very low birth weight because of a shortened gestation period develop relatively better subsequently than babies born with the same low birth weight which cannot be accounted for by prematurity.

The Perinatal Mortality Survey (Butler and Bonham, 1963) showed that just over one-third of low-birth-weight babies in fact are not prematurely born. The condition is likely to be recurrent and in Walker's Dundee series of 215 mothers with babies weighting 2,500 g or less at 39 weeks or more, 10 per cent had had several small-for-dates babies and a quarter of them had had at least one other child similarly dysmature. Many of these women showed a poor weight gain in pregnancy after 30 weeks.

There are certain characteristic pathological features in the dysmature baby which help to distinguish it from the premature, for example, Wigglesworth (1967) stated that histological examination of the pulmonary alveoli and renal glomeruli showed structures corresponding to the gestational age which may be of course at term or later in spite of the baby's small size. Also there is a much raised ratio of brain to liver weight from the normal figure of about 3:1 to 6:1 in these cases.[21] Their livers are not only relatively smaller but deficient in glycogen[64] and this may be the reason why they are vulnerable to hypoglycaemia.[65] This last complication may have something to do with mental retardation, and blood sugar levels below 20 mg/100 ml (less than 1·1 mmol/l) are regarded as critical and worth prompt correction whether symptoms and signs are clinically present or not.

At least the accepted standard of weight is easy to apply and cannot be argued about. Admittedly there are racial differences in mean birth weight for given maturity, and in the case of males this is reputedly 100 g greater than that of females, but these differences are not large; the greatest source of possible wrong classification is in twins who naturally tend to be underweight for their period of gestation, and this leads to the classifying of nearly half of all twins as "premature".

Incidence.—This varies between 4 and 10 per cent, and depends more upon the social and economic status of the mother than upon anything else, or rather, as Drillien (1957) has shown, more upon the social and economic circumstances of the mother's childhood upbringing than on her state after marriage. In other words, the social grade of the baby's maternal grandfather has more influence upon its chances of being prematurely born than has the grading of its own father. Previous abortion, including so-called "therapeutic abortion," increases the incidence of prematurity to over 14 per cent, as has been found in Hungary.

Over England and Wales, as a whole, the incidence of prematurity has remained stationary at 7 per cent and the post-war rise in the general standard of living has not yet had a chance to affect it. The figure is, of course, influenced by the fact that over a third of all stillbirths are prematurely born; the incidence of live-born prematures is thus lower (e.g. 5 per cent in Scotland). In other words, although prematurity can be a cause of stillbirth, even more often is stillbirth a factor in producing a higher prematurity rate, although in this case premature labour is merely incidental to previous intra-uterine fetal death. The Sub-Committee of the Central Health Services Council reporting on the prevention of prematurity and the care of premature infants (1961), regarded the problem as sufficiently large in the United Kingdom to justify the provision of at least six cots for premature infants or ill, newborn infants for every 1,000 live births. This need in any sizeable maternity unit should preferably be met by the provision of separate nurseries for premature babies born inside the Maternity Hospital and those born in domiciliary practice, because of a possible different bacteriological status.

Survival chances.—In any large series it can be seen that the chances of survival are directly proportional to the maturity. This can only be a rough guide in assessing the prognosis in a given case, of course, and one would do better to take more note of the child's actual vigour, which is a far more reliable guide. A birth weight of under 900 g gives a chance of about 1 in 30 only, whereas at 1,350 g the chances are nearly 10 times as good at 1 in 3 or even better. At 1,800 g these odds are reversed in favour of survival, and at $2\frac{1}{4}$ kg one should be able to save most of the cases.

The same Sub-Committee reported that 46 out of every 100 live premature infants weighting 1,500 g or less (3 lb 4 oz) died within the first 24 hours in 1959 and that only 34 were alive at the end of the fourth week, whereas an additional 500 g in birth weight up to 2,000 g (4 lb 6 oz) more than quartered the death rate within the first twenty-four hours and more than doubled the survival rate in the first month.

It is interesting to note that of those who die, nearly half do so within the first 24 hours and a further 15 per cent die within the second, so that about two-thirds of the deaths occur in under 48 hours, that is, within a period profoundly influenced by the obstetrician's management of the case in labour, since minor injuries at delivery and minor infections contracted are often sufficient to kill a premature infant.

Causes of Prematurity

As all the factors which initiate labour are not yet known nor understood, it is often not possible to state why a particular labour should be premature, and in fact over half the cases remain unexplained. This naturally handicaps prophylaxis.

Of these complicating conditions, pre-eclamptic toxaemia is the chief offender (36 per cent), followed by hypertension 17 per cent and placenta praevia 12 per cent. With the first two a few precious extra weeks can sometimes be gained by early recognition and careful treatment, and in the case of placenta praevia there is nowadays an improvement in both prematurity rate and fetal salvage, thanks largely to Macafee's influence on the management of this condition more than 30 years ago.

It is to be noted that pre-eclamptic toxaemia is a cause of prematurity more through the need to terminate pregnancy than through its own direct effects on the woman, although, less often, it may kill the baby *in utero*, thus causing the premature stillbirth of a macerated fetus.

Beyond these three chief causes listed above there are a large number of conditions each of which makes a small contribution to the prematurity rate. Hydramnios, by distending the uterus beyond what it will tolerate; abruptio placentae, which may be either a manifestation of toxaemia or may be simply the expression of the mechanism of abortion, though on a grander scale. Fetal abnormalities, often a cause of miscarriage in earlier weeks, may occasionally cause a spontaneous interruption of pregnancy or, if diagnosed, may call for induction. They also are frequently associated with hydramnios. Syphilis, always quoted as a cause, particularly of premature stillbirth, is less commonly so nowadays, in fact, in far less than 1 per cent of cases, thanks mainly to routine diagnosis in early pregnancy and modern treatment. Genetic factors are also clearly responsible in certain women who seem, often repeatedly, unable to go through to term. Cervical incompetence, or rather an undue readiness of the cervix to dilate may be a factor and justify the insertion of a Shirodkar type of stitch (see Chapter II).

Severe cardiac lesions predispose to premature labour and conversely postmaturity is not common in cardiac disease. Fibroids are often unpredictable in their effect on pregnancy, but inasmuch as they may provoke abortion, so too they may provoke premature labour. The effect, however, can only be regarded as mechanical when the mass of fibroids is exceptionally large, and in the average case endocrine factors are probably at work. Erythroblastosis, mainly through the changes produced in the placental villi, may terminate pregnancy early and disastrously. Trauma is responsible for a few cases, not the least common being that of external version, and for this reason, if an anaesthetic is necessary, such an operation is best postponed to within four weeks of term. Psychological shocks can bring on labour at any time in patients whose hold on pregnancy is none too secure. Chronic nephritis is now recognised as a fairly rare complication but is certainly a cause, either of itself, or through the need to terminate pregnancy.

Any serious illness, especially those producing very high temperatures, e.g. pyelitis and pneumonia, can also bring on labour, and it is important to control hyperpyrexia for this as well as for other reasons.

Of all the abdominal operations likely to be followed by premature labour, appendicectomy in a severe case associated with gross peritonitis is the most important, the peritonitis rather than the operation, of course, being the real cause. Myomectomy could be equally disastrous to continued pregnancy but few gynaecologists today are rash enough to undertake it.

Listeriosis (infection with *L. monocytogenes*) is recognised as a cause of premature stillbirth. Seeliger's monograph (1961) gave a full account of the condition. It was first noticed, about 1926, as an infection occurring in rabbits and guinea-pigs, although it can also occur in sheep, goats and rodents. If a baby is born alive having contracted such infection *in utero* it may demonstrate a confusing clinical picture of otherwise unexplained encephalitis, meningitis, septicaemia, pneumonia and conjunctivitis. The pregnant woman is believed to be very susceptible to this condition. The organism, which resembles coryza bacteria, can be cultured from meconium, conjunctival sacs, cerebrospinal fluid and throat swabs of affected babies and the infection can also be identified serologically. It is sensitive to a wide range of antibiotics although streptomycin produces resistant strains readily. An infected mother may yield Listeria in blood, urine or cerebrospinal fluid. If the baby is born alive there may be pyrexia, jaundice, cyanosis, dyspnoea, signs of cerebral irritation and, at necropsy, lesions may be found in the central nervous system and foci of necrosis in lung and spleen. The placenta contains granulomatous lesions, and there may be similar lesions in the adrenals. There may be a gap of two or three months between the contraction of the infection by the mother and the delivery of an affected infant, often stillborn or frequently premature and dying in the neonatal period. Accounts of this condition from West Germany have not been matched in this country and I personally cannot recall a case in my own experience. Only two cases in five years have been found in Glasgow but there was an epidemic in New Zealand in 1970.[7]

Premature, spontaneous rupture of the membranes is usually followed by premature labour within the next ten days, but the cause of the membrane rupture is usually obscure.

There remain malnutrition and overwork, not exactly diseases in themselves, but probably more important than all in the above subsidiary list put together.

It has already been said that the prematurity rate is an index of social and economic well-being. Baird, for example, showed a rate of 9·18 per cent in hospital cases, whereas the rate was only 5 per cent among those who could afford nursing-home confinements and only 3·9 per cent in those rich enough to engage the services of a specialist. There is no suggestion that the latter two groups had treatment superior to that of the hospital cases, and the differences must be due either to the food they eat or to the easefulness of their lives in pregnancy, and there is no doubt that the poorer woman is usually overworked, either through the need to keep herself in employment, or through the lack of help in household duties. Maternal diet, according to Thomson (1951), has to be very poor indeed for it to have much effect upon birth weight.

In Holland there was acute famine from November 1944 to May 1945 due to war conditions, and the women who were in mid-pregnancy during this period gave birth to babies subsequently of markedly reduced birth weight.[54]

What is known as the Oslo Experiment is worth noting. During the years 1931–38 a home for unmarried pregnant girls, in which the inmates were cared for throughout pregnancy, showed the very low prematurity rate of 2·2 per cent, whereas the rate was 16 per cent in the case of emergency admissions of such girls not so supervised.

In spite of the war the standard of living in this country and in the U.S.A. has unquestionably risen in the poorer classes, and this factor, coupled with the development of the modern paediatric service, has approximately halved the premature neonatal death-rate since 1926.

Effects of Prematurity—Pathology

These are very variable, and the apparent degree of hypoxia at birth and in the first few hours of life is not necessarily paralleled by later evidences of permanent damage, so that one would be wrong to despair even in the face of repeated cyanotic attacks. Nevertheless, no one would believe frequent or prolonged hypoxia to be anything but harmful and some mental and intellectual defects can be attributed to this cause. More than five such attacks, however, signify a very bad prognosis.[26]

Cerebral haemorrhage is very common and is likely to be present in over 10 per cent of premature infants however delivered, including cases born by Caesarean section. There are many obvious reasons for this: the softness of the skull provides poor protection, allows rapid and dangerous degrees of moulding, and, even without a tentorial tear being sustained, back pressure in the vein of Galen is easily induced by the stress disturbances of intracranial anatomy. Secondly, the smaller veins and capillaries are more fragile than normal and do not withstand well the engorgement of even minor degrees of asphyxia. Of the latter, massive intraventricular haemorrhage (Figs. 1 *a* and *b*) is the most characteristic lesion and is usually due to the hypoxic engorgement and rupture of a vessel in the floor of one of the lateral ventricles. The blood may then track through to the subarachnoid space. This type of lesion is found in the more severe degrees of prematurity and in the ultra-premature and is entirely asphyxial in origin, having nothing whatever to do with trauma, unlike subdural bleeding.[15]

The possibility that this type of bleeding may be associated with hypoprothrombinaemia should not be overlooked. This is commoner than generally recognised.[75] If this is indeed found to be present correction is achieved most rapidly by transfusion with fresh-frozen plasma. Injections of vitamin K_1 are far more effective and safer than vitamin K analogues, but take longer than fresh blood or plasma to reverse the defect.

Throughout the body there are fewer blood vessels, a fact which favours tissue anoxia and the ready development of oedema.

Because of poor muscle development, venous return to the heart is poor. This is particularly noticeable in the relatively stagnant circulation of the extremities.

Heart failure is readily superimposed on asphyxia and pulmonary oedema develops rapidly, still further increasing hypoxia and congestion. Such a baby can literally drown in its own pulmonary oedema fluids.

The fragility of the capillary vessels can be demonstrated by applying suction to an area of skin which will show haemorrhages at about half the negative pressures necessary to provoke the same effect in the mature infant. Particularly common effects of asphyxia are subserosal haemorrhages, especially in heart, lungs and liver, also haemorrhages in the pia-arachnoid in addition to the cerebral ventricles.

Disorders of pulmonary aeration, including atelectasis, are the commonest of all the causes of neonatal death. Asphyxial deaths thus accounted for 66 per cent of the series published by us in 1958; any successful method of overcoming this would, of itself, make a tremendous difference to chances of survival.

It is believed that the respiratory centre is so immature that it only responds to degrees of hypercarbia which in themselves may be nearly lethal, and as a result of this the centre becomes even less sensitive—another instance of the vicious circle.

We have studied pulmonary expansion after birth in both mature and premature babies by a variety of techniques involving spirometry, electromanometry of intrathoracic pressures, and by radiography (Donald, 1954, 1957; Donald and Steiner, 1953; Donald *et al.*,

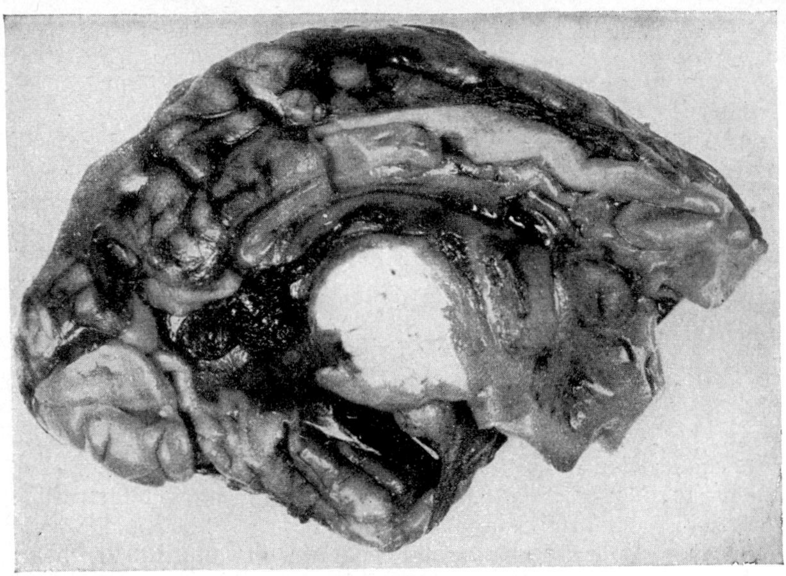

27/FIG. 1 (*a*)—Intraventricular haemorrhage.
(By courtesy of Dr. A. E. Claireaux.)

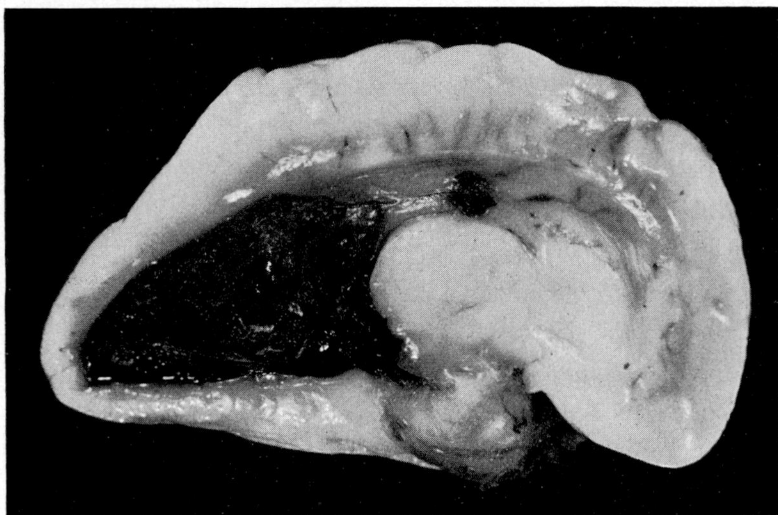

27/FIG. 1 (*b*)—The area of subependymal bleeding which eventually ruptured into the ventricle is shown anterior to the clot. It is situated on the floor of the body of the lateral ventricle and the clot has been partially removed in this part of the ventricle to expose the bleeding point.
(By courtesy of Dr. Jean Scott.)

1958), and we believe that aeration of the lungs is very rapid indeed, occurring within a few minutes of the onset of vigorous crying,[60] although it was formerly thought that expansion was not complete for many days. Vigour at birth, however, is essential and in the case of the premature baby is more important than birth weight. For the premature infant who lacks the strength to overcome the moist cohesion of the alveolar walls and the resistances of the lung tissue itself to expansion, atelectasis may persist for several days and during this critical period infection is all too liable to develop in areas of lung thus particularly predisposed, so that the case easily and often slides into one of full-blown bronchopneumonia. Poor protective coughing reflexes, furthermore, fail to deal with aspirated foreign material. Apart from pneumonia, the child is prone to all forms of sepsis, especially intestinal and skin infections, and is poorly equipped to cope with them. Much of this is preventable.

Passive immunity acquired from the mother increases steadily towards term. The readiness of the tissues generally and of the infected tissues in particular to become oedematous restricts circulation in the affected part and so handicaps the fight against infection and magnifies its local effects.

Anaemia is common, largely because the main stores of iron are only laid down in the last few weeks of pregnancy. The haemoglobin level should, therefore, be carefully watched in the neonatal period and thereafter.

Fetal shock in the course of delivery may easily occur, but is even more liable to appear as a result of handling and disturbance during the first day or two.

Jaundice comes on early and is often very deep because the liver is unable to remove bile constituents from the blood sufficiently readily; these babies are often, as a result, more than usually sleepy and reluctant to feed. The kernicterus of prematurity is independent of haemolytic disease (see later) and may develop if the serum bilirubin is allowed to rise above 20 mg per 100 ml (340 μmol/l). Even lower levels than this in the vulnerable tissues of the premature baby's brain may be responsible for the lowering of the mean intelligence quotient later on in the smallest premature babies and the recognised risk of neurological sequelae. This is due to low albumin levels and consequent reduction in the bilirubin-binding capacity.

In the matter of metabolism generally the processes are defective in degree rather than lacking altogether, for example, the synthesis of prothrombin and of the haemoglobin molecule is slow. To this factor is attributed the tendency to haemorrhagic disease.

Because of feeding difficulties and an immature digestive metabolism, signs of malnutrition may easily develop and the premature infant is more than usually prone to rickets in later months.

Hernia, of various sorts, is more common in prematurity, for which poor muscle development is mainly responsible.

The kidneys, by reason of immaturity, are less able to excrete urine differing widely in osmotic pressure from that of blood, their concentrating power is poor and they are less able to alter water and salt excretion rates in response to the needs of the moment. It is not uncommon for no urine to be passed at all for the first day or two. The more mature the kidney the more numerous the nephron units. Developing nephrons complete their development after birth, but no new units are formed, so that there may be a nephron deficiency.[57]

Deficiencies in heat regulation.—The smaller the creature the greater must be the ratio of surface area, from which heat is lost, to volume and therefore the metabolic needs are correspondingly greater; for instance, a mouse will consume its own weight in food in about four days. Add to this the fact that the premature infant has very little subcutaneous fat to insulate it and the discrepancy is even more pronounced. This, however, is not all, for it is impossible, often for some weeks, for the child's digestive apparatus to cope with a quantity of food sufficient to produce the necessary number of calories. Even so, metabolism is defective to some degree, so that the fully available amount of heat is not produced, and, furthermore, the muscles whose activity is normally a very important source of heat generation are, in this case, poorly developed.

One should aim to nurse the baby in an environment which maintains a difference between rectal and skin temperature of less than 0·5° C. This indicates a satisfactory level of heat conservation.

It will be seen therefore that heat is poorly generated and rapidly dissipated, rather like a budget which cannot be balanced. This simile is even more apt than at first sight, because the control mechanism is also immature and incapable of checking wild swings in temperature, which the baby's relative inability to sweat does little to stabilise. One cannot work long with premature infants without being struck with the fantastic ranges of rectal temperature which may be demonstrated within a few hours.

Signs and Features of Prematurity

1. *Weight.* As stated before, a maturity of less than 37 weeks is the only satisfactory criterion.

2. *Length.* This is usually less than 47 cm.

3. Very little subcutaneous fat is present, a fact which gives the infant its characteristically scraggy appearance and makes the toes and fingers at first glance appear unusually long.

4. The skin, as a result of this, has a brick-reddish colour, feels very thin and wrinkles easily.

5. Lanugo, a fine downy hair, is plentiful.

6. Vernix caseosa is very scanty or absent. Vernix is composed of sebaceous material, and the glands in the skin which produce it are still immature.

7. The skull bones are very thin. This sign is hardly of much clinical help, but is one of the most serious features of prematurity in the course of labour. It is usually said that in premature labour excessive moulding occurs to the detriment of the cranial contents, but this is not quite accurate, for when moulding occurs in mature labour the vault of the skull gradually alters its shape and maintains this alteration for some hours, and, of course, does not alter appreciably between uterine contractions. With the premature infant, however, the soft skull tends to be squeezed into a different shape with each contraction and has not the rigidity necessary fully to maintain the change in shape between each onslaught. This denies the brain and intracranial ligaments the chance to adapt themselves progressively.

On the release of pressure after delivery of the head, which may be very sudden, the damaging effects are particularly exaggerated. In the case of a breech birth, all the advantages of a small after coming head may be cancelled by the rapid alterations in skull shape which can occur.

8. The size of head relative to body is greater than at term; this increases the hazards of breech delivery.

9. The testicles are undescended.

10. The labia minora are exposed and apparently project because the labia majora are poorly developed, mainly through being deficient in fat.

11. Urine secreted is scanty and in fact none may be passed for up to 3 days after birth.

12. Jaundice is liable to come on early and is deep because of the slow clearance of bile pigments.

13. There is a marked tendency to hernia of various types because of poor muscle development.

14. The ears are very soft and flabby because what little cartilage they contain is particularly soft.

15. The nails are often stated not to have grown as far as the finger-tips. While long nails do not occur, this reputed shortness is, in fact, seldom seen.

16. Radiology may fail to show the ossification centres generally reputed to appear at or near term, e.g. lower end of femur and cuboid, but there is quite a wide range of variability here, often of several weeks.

The diagnosis of prematurity is therefore not difficult; what is more uncertain is to be able to assess its degree.

Dubowitz scoring.—This is a good system from Sheffield which takes full clinical account of 10 neurological and 11 "external" criteria for assessing gestational age in a baby, and can be applied by doctor or nurse with practice in ten minutes, using only clinical observation and no fancy apparatus.

There is also good correlation with birth weight although boys have slightly higher levels than girls. It can be applied reliably up to the age of five days.

Its great virtue lies in its objectivity and the emphasis it places upon good clinical examination.

A descriptive leaflet is issued by Messrs Cow and Gate.

Scores of from 0 up to 4 are given for each of the 21 clinical features giving an absolute maximum of 70. In fact the likely scores at 34 weeks gestation are about 35, at 36 weeks over 40, at 38 weeks just short of 50 and almost 60 at 40 weeks in normally developed children.

Prior to delivery, when we have to rely on ultrasonic mensuration of the fetus, it is our view that the biparietal diameter alone is more nearly related to maturity than is actual weight, and others too have found it to provide a better index than urinary oestriol excretion rates or human placental lactogen.[62] Sonar can do better still if lower transthoracic diameters are measured too. Hansmann noted that the ratio of head to thorax diameter decreases to unity as term approaches and thereafter falls still further, and a similar alteration in ratio in the case of abdominal circumference at the level of the ductus venosus occurs after the thirty-sixth week.[13] In cases of intra-uterine growth retardation the ratio remains well above one.

Long-term Effects of Prematurity

It is said that Sir Isaac Newton, at his birth, could have been pushed into a two-pint pot, and none would deny his intelligence; nevertheless, the chances of mental deficiency have to be carefully considered. As the treatment of prematurity continues to improve, one may well speculate upon the likelihood of burdening society with beings so handicapped mentally or physically that it might have been better if Nature had been allowed to take her ruthless course, but so far as modern success has gone to date this is by no means necessarily the case. If, however, the fetus which today is regarded as previable is ever, as a matter of course, reared to full maturity and beyond, more discouraging factors may well come to light.

Surveys such as that of Knoblock *et al.* (1956) indicated an overall likelihood of neurological abnormality of approximately 8 per cent, as against 1·6 per cent in mature controls matched by social grading, birth order and race, but the mental deficiency rate was only strikingly higher (8·8 per cent) in the smaller birth-weight groups of 1,500 g

(3·3 lb) or less. These handicaps have been abundantly confirmed by Drillien (1959), who has shown that in babies weighing less than 3 lb at birth there is not only retardation in weight and to a lesser extent in growth but, what is much worse, 14 per cent of her series in this group had an estimated I.Q. less than 70 and would be in need of special schooling, and nearly half were considered very dull. Where the birth weight was over 2 kg there was no difference in subsequent mental development, but below that figure the intellectual capacity of the babies would appear to be more or less inversely proportional to birth weight. Douglas (1960) likewise made a controlled study (in so far as it is possible to control such a study) of the later school records of all children born during the first week of March, 1946, which provided 706 babies weighing less than 2,500 g at birth, each child being matched with a control weighing more than this, but otherwise selected on the basis of sex, position in the family, the mother's age, her social grouping and home social conditions. The subsequent school records of the prematures were consistently lower than those of the controls and, what is more, the handicap became more marked as the age increased; for example, from eight years to eleven, only 9·7 per cent of the premature babies gained places in Grammar Schools as compared with 22 per cent of the controls, but it was pointed out that the complex social causes of prematurity are undoubtedly a very major factor in the handicaps of these babies, rather than low birth weight *per se*.

Now, a prematurely born child may owe some of its small birth weight to one of three classes of cause. First, because of its parent's stature, it may be small for genetic reasons. Secondly, pregnancy may have been interrupted therapeutically for some obstetrical indication. Thirdly, something may have interfered with intra-uterine development. The dangers of mental retardation would appear to be mainly confined to the last group and the analysis by Douglas (1956) which was carried out on eight-year-old children by means of reading, vocabulary and intelligence testing, indicates that although premature children scored less than their controls, most markedly so in reading, the worst group were those in whom no obstetric nor genetic explanation could be found for their low birth weight. In other words, as might be expected, intra-uterine handicaps to development are more important than actual birth weight, which may be the result of extraneous interference, for example, induction of labour. So far, however, it can be said that the premature infant has a very good chance of catching up in its development by the third or fourth year with four provisos:

(1) No gross or oft-repeated anoxia must be allowed to occur and so damage the central nervous system;

(2) There must be no damage to immature tissue;
(3) There must be no unfavourable genetic factors;
(4) The social grading of the parents does not fall within the lowest groups.

More recent reports give a more cheerful view of the development prospects of the low-birth-weight infant, especially if born since 1960, thanks to the great strides which have been taken since then in paediatric care, especially as regards hypoglycaemia, hyperbilirubinaemia, hypoxia and early nutrition.[18] The normal level of neonatal blood glucose is 30–60 mg/100 ml (1·66–3·33 mmol/l). Levels below 20 mg/100 ml (1·11 mmol/l) are abnormal and dangerous to the central nervous system.

The ratio of brain weight to liver is normally 3:1 whereas in cases of intra-uterine malnutrition the ratio may be as high as 7:1 because of reduced liver size.[2] Delayed feeding, as used to be practised, aggravates the situation and may be rewarded with mental retardation and cerebral palsy.

Obstetrical complications, *per se*, such as pre-eclamptic toxaemia, malpresentation, respiratory distress syndrome, even jaundice, convulsions and signs of cerebral irritation, are not incompatible with a subsequent reasonable intelligence quotient, provided cases of gross neurological or sensory damage are excluded.[53] In other words apparently normal children would seem to have a chance of normal intellectual development.

The problem of atelectasis remains paramount.

Respiratory Distress Syndrome
(Pulmonary Syndrome and Hyaline Membrane)

The four conditions, pulmonary syndrome of the newborn, intraventricular haemorrhage (already described), pneumonia and birth trauma were found by Bound *et al.* (1956) to account for two-thirds of all neonatal deaths in their survey of neonatal mortality and they too noted, as I, too, had in 1954, that these conditions are not distinguishable during life by ordinary clinical, as distinct from radiological, methods and the baby behaves in a remarkably similar way in each.

The term "pulmonary syndrome of the newborn" is a very useful one and was introduced by Bound and his colleagues at University College Hospital to describe cases of secondary resorption atelectasis together with one of the following: hyaline membrane, intraalveolar haemorrhage or pulmonary oedema. The term Respiratory Distress Syndrome (RDS) is now more fashionable.

Hyaline membrane consists of an eosinophilic membrane of patchy distribution which is plastered against the walls of the air passages, especially the alveolar ducts, and which obstructs aeration (Figs. 2 and 3). Distal to these points of obstruction the alveoli collapse and become filled with fluid.[57]

The general belief is that deep aspiration is necessary to set the stage for the development of this membrane, for it is not to be found in the lungs of stillborn infants. The sequence of events would appear to be firstly the development of severe fetal anoxia before or at birth resulting in the deep inspiration of liquor which is not, of itself, sufficient to obstruct subsequent breathing. If the child is delivered by Caesarean section without the compression of its thoracic cage by the normal processes of labour, this membrane is even more likely to develop. Amniotic fluid, as is well known, contains thromboplastic material. This reacts with fibrinogen which is diffused from the pulmonary circulation into the alveoli and alveolar ducts where it is converted to fibrin, which has been identified as the main constituent of hyaline membrane along with other elements such as lipid and squamous remnants from the liquor amnii.[36]

In 1959 Avery and Mead described a lipoprotein, named pulmonary surfactant, which normally lines the alveoli and which may have something to do with preventing pulmonary collapse. Others, for example, Pattle *et al.* (1962) confirmed their finding that this lining substance is not present in infants dying of the respiratory distress syndrome. Prematurity is the main cause of a deficiency of surfactant. Asphyxia is also said to be a cause, either by damaging the cells in the alveoli which synthesise it or because in asphyxia there may be an exudation of fibrinogen which inactivates it. This substance, formerly called surfactant, is now known to be lecithin. Gluck and colleagues[37] in a series of over 300 amniocenteses noted that the phospholipid concentration in liquor increased rapidly after 35 weeks gestation and heralded pulmonary maturity. On thin-layer chromatography the size of the lecithin spot can be compared with that of sphingomyelin and a ratio between them observed. The lecithin : sphingomyelin (or L:S) ratio rises from 1:1 at 35 weeks to sometimes as high as 7:1. Figures above 2:1 indicate fetal pulmonary maturity, since these phospholipids not only originate in increasing quantity as the lungs mature but the lecithin element more markedly so than sphingomyelin.[37] Lecithin levels of 3·5 mg/100 ml would appear to be critical[9] but it is simpler and quicker to examine the L:S ratio which, if satisfactory, practically ensures that the baby will not suffer from RDS.

The action of the lecithin is to reduce the surface tension and hence the moist cohesion of the alveolar walls and so permit their expansion with the onset of respiratory effort.

The maturation of the L:S ratio has been found not to occur in

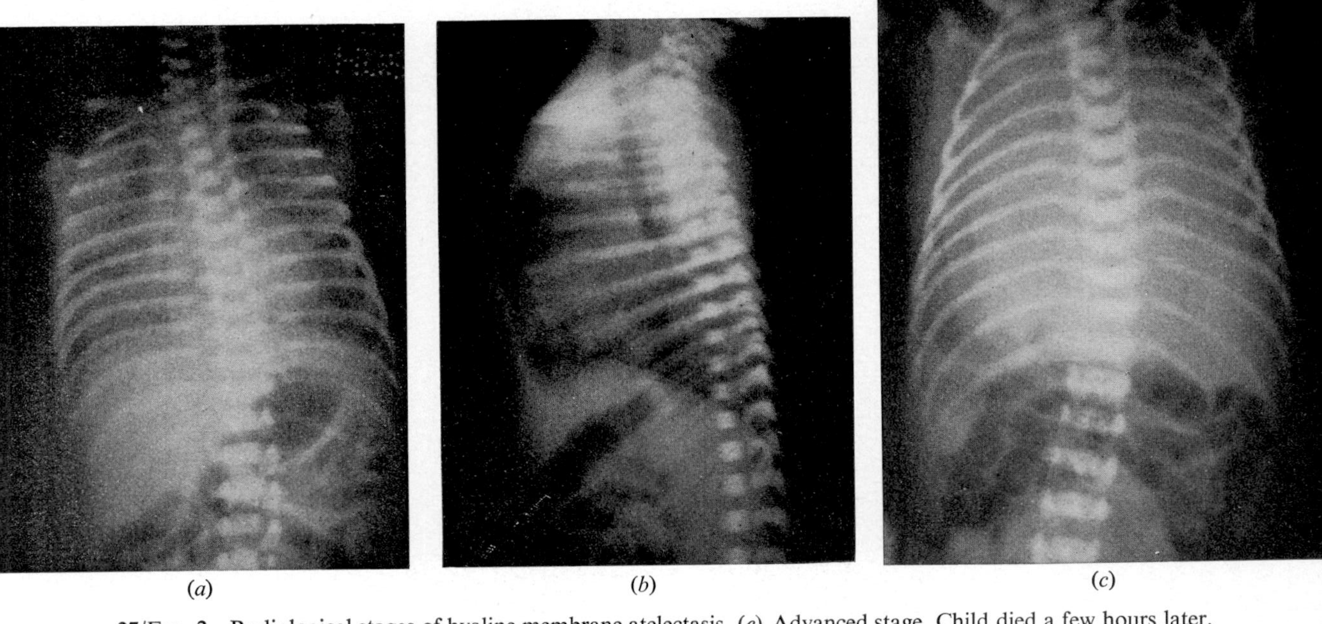

(a) (b) (c)

27/FIG. 2—Radiological stages of hyaline membrane atelectasis. (c) Advanced stage. Child died a few hours later. (By courtesy of Prof. R. E. Steiner.)

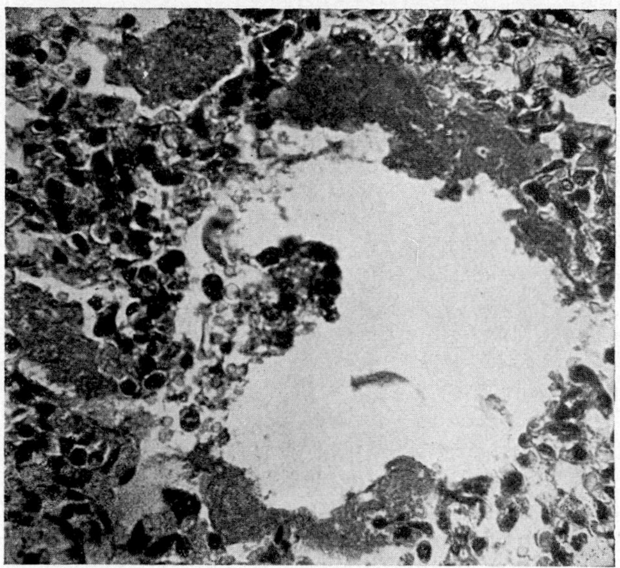

27/Fig. 3—Hyaline membrane in alveolar duct.
(By courtesy of Dr. A. E. Claireaux.)

some cases of pregnancy complicated by diabetes or severe Rh-haemolytic disease.[73]

As an alternative to shallow chromatography a simple "shake test" has been devised.[17] This depends on the ability of the surfactant substance in the liquor to generate stable foam bubbles in the presence of ethanol, which eliminates other substances such as proteins, bile salts and fatty acids which could otherwise also foam on shaking and give false positive results. The test is simple to perform although the details are exacting and would be beyond my own patience, requiring the admixture of varying amounts of liquor amnii made up in known concentrations in 0·9 per cent saline to which is added an equal amount of 95 per cent ethanol. The tubes are then shaken vigorously for all of fifteen minutes and then stood vertically and examined fifteen minutes later for a stable ring of bubbles at the meniscus. We do not use it.

The distribution of the membrane, plastered around the walls of the alveolar ducts, is due to the passage of air caused by the baby's respiratory efforts. The membrane, consequently, is not found in cases of stillbirth.

It is very likely that the persistence of the membrane within the lungs is due to a deficient pulmonary circulation, because the vascular bed within the lungs has not been adequately opened up for one reason or another, usually inadequate respiratory activity. Thus the membrane, or its precursor substance, is neither absorbed nor got rid of, except in babies capable of exhibiting the necessary respiratory vigour. It is the commonest cause of secondary atelectasis.

The fact that premature infants are more than usually susceptible may be further explained by their very weak powers of eliminating foreign matter from their lungs and of opening up their pulmonary circulation quickly.

As explained in the chapter on resuscitation of the newborn in the section describing the first breaths of life, the exercise of negative intrathoracic pressure by the baby in its attempts to inspire air also encourages the flow of blood into the lungs. The blood then returning from the lungs raises the left atrial pressure within the heart and closes the foramen ovale. In addition to this, it has been shown by Dawes *et al.* (1953–56) that there is initially a reversed flow from left to right through the ductus arteriosus which does not close functionally for the first few hours until the percentage oxygen saturation of the blood has risen from about 60 per cent at birth to over 90 per cent. In this way, blood returning from the lungs to the left atrium and ventricle is partly shunted back through the still patent ductus arteriosus into the pulmonary circulation for a second helping of oxygen—an ingenious mechanism while the lungs are still relatively inefficient from persistent atelectasis (Born *et al.*, 1954).

It has, moreover, been shown by Lind and Wegelius (1954) that the ductus, after closure, may reopen early in the neonatal period if provoked by neonatal anoxia. In this case, if through inadequate respiratory activity the pulmonary circulation has not been sufficiently opened up, the original high resistance in the pulmonary circuit persists and blood is thereby encouraged to bypass the lungs by going from right to left through the reopened ductus. As a result, less blood returns from the lungs to the left atrium so that a pressure gradient develops between right and left atria, and the foramen ovale reopens. In other words, reversion to the fetal type of circulation has taken place and a full cyanotic attack results.

The chain of events described above explains the clinical picture in the pulmonary syndrome. The respiratory rate shortly after birth is around 70 per minute, but if this does not fall below 50 by the end of the second hour the possibility that the baby is developing the respiratory distress syndrome should be considered and a chest X-ray obtained. Acute left heart failure may be revealed. An important alternative diagnosis may also be made by an X-ray taken at this age, namely, that of diaphragmatic hernia. In such a case transfer to a paediatric unit with full surgical facilities is immediately necessary and oxygenation should be maintained with an endotracheal tube throughout the journey; otherwise the intestines may simply fill up, especially if oxygen is given by a mask, and the baby may become dangerously embarrassed from mediastinal displacement.

The course which is run is fairly characteristic; the baby is usually premature, practically never postmature, and appears well at birth, and may even for a time maintain a healthy colour. Crying, however, is not well sustained and within a few hours, sometimes within twenty minutes, the first signs of respiratory distress develop. These consist of whimpering and expiratory grunting and movement of the alae nasi. Presently signs of inspiratory recession of the chest wall appear, especially in the subcostal regions and also, to a less obvious extent, in the intercostal spaces and suprasternal area. In very severe cases the whole sternum is dragged inwards by the child's inspiratory efforts.

Clearly the child is now literally fighting for its breath and Karlberg *et al.* (1954) reckoned that in such respiratory distress the effort of breathing is between two to five times as great as normal. Our own researches encourage us in a similar view.

Radiographs taken at this time show the developing changes which we have described as a fine miliary mottling, proceeding to coalescent areas of non-aeration and leading finally to total lung radio-opacity with only the bronchial tree outlined because of the air within it (Donald and Steiner, 1953).

After a variable number of hours the baby gives up the unequal struggle in the face of such difficulty and stops breathing. A cyanotic, or grey, attack follows. This may be the first of a series which finally ends in death, usually within two or three days, and often within twelve hours, but never in less than two hours.

We believe that milder cases of the pulmonary syndrome may survive if possessed of sufficient respiratory vigour to overcome it, and provided acidosis can be meanwhile corrected and biochemical homeostasis in all respects achieved.

Such membrane is cleared only with very great and prolonged difficulty, and only those babies sufficiently vigorous to be able to manage on unaffected lung portions are likely to survive. So far, the one hope is to maintain life until respiratory compensation occurs. Even neonatal babies can generate their own surfactant after birth.

Prophylaxis and Premature Birth

Since premature birth is often deliberately brought on because of some maternal condition which either jeopardises the mother's health or carries with it the threat of intra-uterine fetal death, e.g. pre-eclamptic toxaemia, the only prophylactic measures that can be employed here are tied up with the early recognition of the disorder and, as far as possible, the control of its severity in order to justify prolonging pregnancy for a few more weeks. But there are many conditions which in themselves endanger neither mother nor unborn child through the continuation of pregnancy, but which carry a high prematurity rate.

Important instances in the latter group are cases of multiple pregnancy, hydramnios without demonstrable fetal abnormality, a large mass of fibroids, severe cardiac lesions (in which induction of labour is not indicated), malnutrition and profound debility, and that group of patients who recurrently and for no apparent reason go into premature labour.

In such cases as these, notice must be taken of the liability to start labour, and an extra few weeks may be gained by keeping the patient in bed. Unless she has had a previous series of obstetrical disappointments, a healthy woman with twins is unlikely to be willing to go to bed for the last few weeks of her pregnancy on the off-chance that her children might not be prematurely born, but cases of triplets should be strongly urged to co-operate in this precaution.

Once the threat of premature labour has revealed itself by the onset of labour pains or by the rupture of membranes or a show, the patient should of course be put to bed and kept there. Even the leakage of liquor is not inevitably followed straight away by labour, although it is more than probable, and with strict care the leak may seal itself, at least temporarily, and a futher ten days or more may be gained. There may be some doubt about whether the fluid draining is liquor amnii or urine from incontinence. The smell may be characteristic, but a useful method of distinguishing the two is to give methylene blue by mouth which discolours urine only. Another method to distinguish between the seepage of liquor and urine is to allow a drop of fluid to dry on an ordinary microscope slide and to look at it under low power. Aborisation crystals may be seen in the case of liquor but not in urine. Another test described by Fell (1960) is to take the soiled pad and fold it over an Albustix protein detector, and squeeze. Because of the protein in liquor amnii a positive reaction will be obtained. Unfortunately this is also true of vaginal discharges and we have found the method yields too many false positive results. We commonly employ the Nile Blue sulphate test using a 0·1 per cent aqueous solution (see previous chapter) which can be very quickly undertaken as a side-room procedure. Fetal cells present in the liquor show up as anucleate orange-stained cells, often in clusters. Unfortunately the more premature the case the less reliable is the test and, annoyingly enough, the more premature the case, the more serious the matter of premature membrane rupture. Undoubtedly the best of all methods is to use one's nose, a method denied to the many nicotine addicts within our profession.

If it is established that the membranes have indeed ruptured, the seriousness of the case will depend upon the degree of prematurity and the baby's chances of survival on that ground alone. Meanwhile the risks of amnionitis rise with the passing of each day so that the baby may die *in utero* from infection or shortly thereafter. If the pregnancy has reached 35 weeks and the fetus appears reasonably grown it is safer to encourage labour, if necessary with oxytocin infusion, since one is sitting on a time-bomb.

If premature labour threatens with membranes ruptured at 30–32 weeks one would hope to stave off labour and in doing so avoid the contraction of infection by all possible means including the use of antibiotics.

There must be no local interference apart from vaginal bacteriological swab-taking. An ultraconservative policy on these lines can be very rewarding and I kept one pregnancy going for a futher month in spite of continuous seepage of liquor and the child is now a brilliant medical student.

Caesarean section at 31 weeks in fetal interests is a cowardly way out and simply transfers mortality from the stillbirth table to the neonatal death table of figures, the patient being unjustifiably grateful for the surgical assault on her uterus in the misguided belief that everything possible has been done.

If labour threatens with contractions occurring regularly every ten minutes or less, the decision to treat the threat with energetic medication is a clear one. Immediate removal to hospital with full paediatric facilities is, of course, essential since no incubator for transport is better than the mother's own womb.

During this period of trying to prolong pregnancy, the bowels should be left severely alone and adequate sedatives given. Undoubtedly, morphia is efficient but, in the event of labour proceeding, it carries the risk that delivery may occur while the fetus is still within the range of its effects. The barbiturates will, therefore, be found to be more generally serviceable, e.g. Sodium Amytal 200 mg repeated up to three times within 24 hours, or Seconal in similar dosage.

In hospital more sophisticated therapy is available. Intravenous ethyl alcohol has had a long innings but is no more than seventy per cent effective in postponing labour. The diuretic effect of alcohol is known to be due to its power to inhibit the release of antidiuretic hormone from the neurohypophysis and its effect on oxytocin release is similar. It is given in 9·5 per cent concentration in a 5 per cent dextrose/water solution.[34] The loading dose is 15 ml/kg body weight in the first hour or two. This is then cut back to a maintenance dose of one tenth, i.e. 1·5 mg per hour. The dosage is maintained for several hours after the threat has worn off and the blood levels of alcohol will be a little below the Breathalyser limit, usually between

0·09–0·16 per cent. It must be remembered that the baby will be inebriated to the same extent.

Success can only be claimed if labour is postponed by three days or more and failure is certain if the membranes are already ruptured.

We never had much convincing success with isoxsuprine and more recently we have adopted salbutamol as giving better results than alcohol. Salbutamol is a beta-adrenoceptor stimulant and significantly reduces uterine activity. Our practice to date has been to add 5 mg (5 ml) to 500 ml of 5 per cent dextrose solution which gives a concentration of 10 μg per ml, equivalent to 15 drops from a normal giving set, intravenously. The infusion is started at 10 drops per minute and increased by a further 10 drops every five to ten minutes until contractions cease or an infusion rate of 50 drops (33 μg) per minute is reached. This can be stepped up every twenty minutes until a maximum rate of 80 drops is reached if uterine contractions have not ceased before.

The treatment is abandoned if the cervix dilates after six hours of treatment or if maternal tachycardia above 140/min occurs.

If contractions are suppressed the infusion at the appropriate rate is maintained for a further hour and then halved for six hours and still further progressively reduced during the next six hours when the patient can be maintained on oral tablets (4 mg salbutamol) six-hourly for a week.

Apart from tachycardia, tremor and palpitations may necessitate reducing the dosage and, as with the other drugs of this class, cardiac disease and antepartum bleeding are contra-indications and alcohol is to be preferred.

Orciprenaline and ritodrine act similarly but I have no personal experience of them. The management and effects are similar. A large multi-centre study of 91 patients in premature labour has been reported from Belgium[72] indicating an 80 per cent success rate with ritodrine.

Naturally, since premature birth has such a high risk of being followed by the respiratory distress syndrome which may be lethal and is due to pulmonary immaturity, considerable interest is being shown in any crash programme which can accelerate lung maturation before delivery.

The human placenta is permeable to glucocorticoid substances which are believed to accelerate the development of pulmonary surfactant, and will improve the L:S ratio already referred to. Liggins and Howie[47] by the use of betamethasone before actual delivery were able to demonstrate a marked reduction of neonatal death rate from hyaline membrane disease and incidentally also from intraventricular haemorrhage in the very small babies which is, itself, the result of asphyxia.

The beneficial effect is maximal 48 hours after such medication during which period delivery should be staved off. The theoretical objection that the baby's resistance to infection would be thereby reduced has not materialised, but the treatment is useless if given only after birth. In our own practice we have combined treatment with salbutamol with intramuscular injections of 1 ml (4 mg) betamethasone 21-phosphate every eight hours up to a total of six doses and have not employed routine antibiotic therapy even though the membranes are already ruptured, unless there is a bacteriological indication for it.

That the L:S ratio can be improved by such glucocorticoid therapy, given time, there can be little doubt but we still feel it is a "once and for all" type of treatment, not to be repeated.

Conduct of Premature Labour

When it is clear from the dilatation of the cervix that labour will inevitably proceed, an enema should be given, for nothing will now be gained by uterine inertia. Analgesic drugs should be used as sparingly as possible. Morphia and its derivatives, as already hinted, are poison to the premature infant, and even 10 mg of morphia will depress respiration in a premature infant born as much as six or seven hours later. Pethidine is preferable, although chloral and paraldehyde are safest. Premixed gas and oxygen analgesia, 50/50, for example by the Entonox apparatus is useful and perfectly safe. If labour hangs fire because of inertia we begin to fear the possibility of intra-uterine infection to which the premature fetus is very vulnerable and we therefore give cephaloridine by intramuscular injection, 500 mg twice daily.

The use of oxytocin to accelerate labour is seldom necessary. I have already referred scathingly to the use of Caesarean section in very premature labour.

Throughout labour the patient should be kept in bed, because delivery is often precipitate and unexpected.

Because of the excessively rapid and dangerous moulding which the fetal head may undergo, its egress should be facilitated by an adequate episiotomy whenever it appears that the perineum is causing more than a moderate resistance to delivery. This can be done quite simply and quickly following local infiltration with about 8–10 ml of 2 per cent lignocaine when the head is on the perineum. This is more than ever important with a breech delivery, and in all such cases the head should be very slowly and gently delivered, steadying the vault of the skull with the wide palm of the hand rather than with the fingers. The protective value of forceps such as

Wrigley's is commended. The ventouse should not be used on the soft premature head.

When the child has been born, its pharynx should be sucked out with a rubber-ended mucus-extractor at once and before dividing the cord. Swabbing out the inside of the mouth with gauze is very damaging to the lining of the cavity and should not be practised. The common types of mucus-extractor are inefficient, dirty and dangerous, because the midwife has to blow down them to clear them. A pump-driven sucker is far more satisfactory. (See chapter on Resuscitation of the Newborn.)

The cord is not divided until pulsation in it ceases, as thereby a few extra millilitres of blood are not lost to the baby. This hardly matters in a mature infant which is born with polycythaemia, but anaemia in the premature infant has to be remembered.

The child is now placed, preferably uncovered, in a warm atmosphere of oxygen in an incubator and is left alone. It is surprising how quickly a combination of warmth and oxygen will revive such an infant.

The breathing is at first so shallow that it may be imperceptible, but provided the colour remains a healthy pink there is no cause for immediate concern. The cases which go grey and toneless at this stage have a bad prognosis, and many of these are the victims of intracranial bleeding. Even so, more harm results from so-called resuscitative measures than from relying solely on oxygen and warmth. Tracheal intubation is often practised, and oxygen under positive pressures of up to 30 cm of water can be administered, but the present general view does not favour this line of treatment, except in emergency, because of the disturbance to the child which it entails, the risk of introducing infection, and damage which may be caused to the lining of the air passages.

The main indication for intubation in these desperate cases is prolonged apnoea which is even more damaging. Considering how fatal the handicaps of atelectasis may prove within the next forty-eight hours, it is possible that in expert hands intubation and some form of assisted respiration may come to be more widely used in the future. We have practised such a technique, using nylon catheters, in ultrapremature cases with some success in pulmonary aeration (Donald *et al.*, 1958), employing one of the writer's electronically controlled patient-cycled respirators. Intubation tends, after all, to be reserved for the more moribund cases and therefore the frequency of disappointment is bound to be high.

There are many indications that interest in artificial respiration in severe cases of the respiratory distress syndrome is being revived in some quarters. For example, in a small but controlled trial in Aberdeen[61] the difference in survival in cases treated by intermittent positive-pressure ventilation over many hours was striking. Our own work along these lines, using augmented respiration so as to assist a baby's own spontaneous efforts and relieve it of some of its appalling physical load in attempting to aerate atelectatic lungs, may even presently have a second innings, long after our work on the subject in the early 1950s has been forgotten.[22–26] This, of course, is no new phenomenon. It is only simple forms of treatment, after all, that manage to jump the ditch at the first attempt, and trying to maintain artificial respiration in a tiny, cyanotic and grossly atelectatic baby is hard and discouraging work. The present vogue is for continuous positive airways pressure (CPAP), to be described later.

MANAGEMENT OF THE PREMATURE INFANT

There are four cardinal features in the treatment and rearing of the premature infant, and their importance runs in the following order:

(1) Maintenance of body temperature;
(2) Prevention of infection;
(3) Treatment of pulmonary atelectasis;
(4) Nutrition.

In addition, there are the more general aspects of nursing care.

Maintenance of Body Temperature

The importance of this is often not sufficiently stressed. These babies chill off very quickly and can be seen to develop a condition of irreversible peripheral circulatory failure, the so-called grey attack, for which either pulmonary atelectasis or an inadequate supply of oxygen may be blamed, a mistake which the available but incidental evidences at autopsy tend to support. Such attacks are very liable to follow even short periods of exposure or handling and attempts to feed. Rectal temperatures are, of course, taken as infrequently as possible in order to reduce disturbance of the child, but such information is invaluable. The surrounding cot or atmosphere temperature should be so adjusted that the baby's rectal temperature is maintained at about 35·5° C, which is often a difficult matter. As a general guide, if the baby is clothed the cot temperature should in the first instance be 30° C near the baby's body and 25° C in the rest of the cot. If, on the other hand, the baby is being nursed naked in an incubator, the temperature inside it should be 35° C. Adjustments can then be made according to the baby's temperature reactions. The dangers of overheating and burning are very great in the absence of thermostatically controlled safety cut-out switches.

Rectal temperatures are taken with special thermometers reading down to 25° C.

If the whole room can be heated to an even temperature of up to 30° C so much the better.

The term "thermo-ventral environment" is the catch phrase to indicate conditions involving minimal oxygen consumption. This is recognised as satisfactory if the skin temperature dose not differ by more than half a degree from the rectal.

The atmosphere must have a humidity of at least 75 per cent. All incubators have special humidifiers incorporated, and in hospital units the air is automatically conditioned and humidified. In the home, however, a steam kettle should be used.

Oxygen supplied to the baby should be bubbled through warmed water, since dry, neat oxygen may act as a pulmonary irritant.

Babies, on their reception into a premature unit, are often found to have very low temperatures which must be restored carefully before irreversible changes set in. In the Glasgow series,[3] two babies with temperatures actually below 77° F (24° C) survived—surely a record!

Prevention of Infection

There is almost no measure which can be taken to minimise this risk which could be called far-fetched, and no precaution can be safely omitted. From this point of view a premature infant is better off nursed in a good private house than in an inadequately equipped hospital. The development of premature baby units in the larger hospitals is no fanciful fad, and staffing of such units has to be on a lavish scale to make the nursing ritual possible or even tolerable for those who run it, and the nursing staff should not work elsewhere. Every member should have nose and throat swabs taken on enrolment, whenever they return to duty following any infectious illness, including the common cold for which absence from work is obligatory, and routinely every four weeks. The taking of the full holiday allowances is likewise important.

No visitors other than the baby's father should be allowed to enter, and of all possible visitors it must be remembered that young children are far the most dangerous.

Psychological deprivation has to be balanced against the calculated risk of infection.

All entrants to the unit, including doctors, should put on freshly laundered coats or gowns which belong specially to the unit, because all day-to-day clothing is dirtier than one would imagine. These coats or gowns should be frequently replaced and sent to the laundry and should hang on pegs or racks not used by ordinary clothing.

Hands must be washed between handling each child, preferably with hexachlorophane soap.

The unit should be divided into a series of small rooms in which all the infants below 1,800 g (4 lb), or those not securely thriving, are strictly isolated, and each of these isolation rooms is entered through an air lock of double doors, only one of which is opened at a time. The doors should be of the swing type on springs and without handles. Each of these small rooms is centrally heated and air-conditioned to the right humidity and optimal temperature. In temperatures below 29° C the babies must be clothed.

The larger and older premature infants may be nursed in one room together, as it is seldom practicable to have enough isolation rooms, and the larger nursery, which is less heated, is a stepping-stone to the world outside.

Each room has it own washing and baby bathing facilities, and a separate gown is donned by the nurse for each child that she has to handle. All floors may be treated regularly with spindle oil to reduce dust-borne infection.

Milk and feeding utensils are prepared in the unit's own kitchen or pre-packaged, and feeds are prepared before and not after nappy changing.

Infants admitted from outside the hospital are particularly suspect, and should be separately nursed. For infants born following a long labour with early rupture of the membranes, cephaloridine, 12 mg/kg body weight, or kanamycin, 10–15 mg/kg body weight are given over 24 hours intravenously at first and later by mouth. The three main types of infection encountered are broncho pneumonia, skin and conjunctival infections and gastro-enteritis. Meningeal infections should be a very rare disaster, but may follow aspiration of *E. coli* infected liquor.

No inflammatory lesion can safely be regarded as too trivial for energetic treatment, and *Staph. pyogenes,* often penicillin-resistant, can light up an epidemic overnight.

Nowadays Gram-negative organisms are proving particularly troublesome. *Pseudomonas aeruginosa* and *Aerobacter aerogenes* appear readily in intensive care units with their high humidity, and Group B non-haemolytic Streptococci from the vagina can become pathogenic.[50]

Treatment of Pulmonary Atelectasis

A child's first breath remains a marvel, the mechanism of which has not yet been fully explained, but very great effort (40–90 cm H_2O) is clearly necessary to open up the alveoli, and this may prove beyond the child's power (Donald, 1957). Crying produces a sharp rise in pressure in the air passages against the resistance of the partially closed glottis, but premature infants are often too weak to cry, and under such circumstances it may take four days for full lung expansion to occur. It is remarkable at autopsy how small an amount of aerated lung can manage to support life, at any rate for a few hours, but the clinical picture during life is fairly characteristic. Breathing is both shallow and rapid, in fact, respiratory rates of over 60 a minute are common, and this is mechanically inefficient and exhausting to the baby and may not be maintained. The clinical features of atelectasis and the pulmonary syndrome have already been described. Hyaline membrane accounts for very many of these cases, but is not always demonstrable.

Clearly the aspiration of meconium and mucus at birth invites atelectasis, and the first step is to remove it from the mouth and pharynx before this can occur. What is noticeable, however, is how unusual it is to find a bronchial tree blocked with mucus at autopsy in cases dying with pulmonary atelectasis; this finding weakens the case for treatment by bronchoscopic suction, which should be reserved only for the very occasional case of clinically unilateral atelectasis. This manoeuvre demands the skill of one who is highly practised in it because of the disturbance and handling involved, and can only be appropriate when the blockage is high enough in the bronchus to be accessible. The natural riddance of mucus depends mainly upon an intact ciliated epithelium in the bronchial tree, and traumatic procedures, besides their general harm, can only increase reactionary oedema and produce yet more mucus. It may well be that much of the exudate blamed for non-aeration is a product rather than a cause of asphyxia.

Laryngeal spasm may at times prevent air entry, for which a small bead of mucus may be responsible.

During the first hours, the baby will often drool from its mouth large quantities of mucus, but this has probably been produced recently by the baby itself and has nothing to do the aspirated material; much of it probably comes directly from the stomach, in which organ it is very readily secreted, and for this reason and for the possible risk of subsequent aspiration, it is more logical to suck out the stomach contents; this is a routine procedure on first receiving the baby into the unit.

The differential diagnosis of neonatal pulmonary atelectasis is often open to error. Bronchopneumonia has already been mentioned, and often the diagnosis cannot be made before the child is beyond chemotherapeutic aid, but an equally common error is to diagnose the case as suffering from intracranial haemorrhage. In fact, the behaviour of the baby in these conditions can be very similar, and in addition to this all three conditions may co-exist. An X-ray is vital.

In recognising the reluctance of premature babies' lungs to expand, it has occurred to many workers to try to achieve adequate oxygenation by other means, though most of these methods are used chiefly for resuscitation at birth rather than during the course of the critical first three days.

One method popular for some years was to supply oxygen via the intestinal tract as described by Akerren and Furstenberg or by Yllpo's method, but it is now discredited. The writer's method of augmenting respiratory effort by patient-triggered respirators encouraged us, but required unremitting supervision on a technical as well as medical level and one's principal stand-by has hitherto remained the supply of humidified oxygen in a suitable incubator. If central cyanosis persists in spite of 35 per cent oxygen concentrations, Po_2 monitoring is necessary. Higher concentrations are regarded as dangerous for prolonged periods. Oxygen is supplied in the hope that the child will oblige by breathing it, but although you can take a horse to water you cannot make it drink!

In spite of a growing amount of experimental work, theorising, talking and writing, in all of which I, too, have participated, the subject of the respiratory distress syndrome seemed to be heading for a stalemate until a fresh approach to the subject, largely under the stimulus of Usher (1961) in Montreal, altered the direction of attack, namely, an attempt to control the biochemistry of the mixed metabolic and respiratory acidosis which are lethal features of the condition. Until I heard an address by Usher to the Neonatal Society in London, I had regarded the ultimate deaths of these babies as primarily due to cardiac and peripheral circulatory failure, brought about by hypoxia and exhaustion from the mechanical difficulties of achieving and maintaining aeration of lungs whose alveolar walls, because of prematurity, were reluctant to expand and whose circulatory filling was not sufficiently encouraged by adequate respiratory effort; hence my concentration upon the technique of augmented respiration. This may be an important side of the problem but is only part of the truth. The biochemical derangement associated with the condition is profound. In both types of acidosis the pH of arterial blood may be very low, often below 7, even as low as 6·5, and in fact most cases with a pH of less than 7 are doomed. In addition there is a low bicarbonate reserve and increased base deficit. In respiratory acidosis, the Pco_2 is very high. The normal range is between 30 and 40 mm Hg and the case is serious if the level rises above 70 mm Hg and hopeless if over 150 mm Hg. Metabolic acidosis is always present and to it may be added respiratory acidosis, but there is never respiratory acidosis alone. Much of the former is probably renal in origin. Bircarbonate levels are low, for example 15 to 20 as against a normal 22 mEq/l. The additional respiratory acidosis which complicates hyaline membrane disease, for example, may show P_{CO_2} levels in excess of 100 mm of mercury although the baby for a time is pink. These measurements can be made with the micro-Astrup apparatus which is capable of measuring pH, P_{CO_2} and plasma bicarbonate in milliequivalents per litre. Usher's recommended technique was to correct this acidosis by dripping glucose and sodium bicarbonate through an anterior scalp vein. My own paediatric colleagues, Professor Hutchison and Dr Margaret Kerr, have modified the technique and employed it very extensively with the most encouraging results (Hutchison *et al.*, 1962, 1964). Usher in fact opened the way to modern biochemical homeostasis.

In their first series of 100 cases they included only severe cases with the following criteria common to all:

1. Expiratory grunting;
2. Tachypnoea (over 60 per minute);
3. Inspiratory recession of the chest wall;
4. Cyanosis without oxygen;
5. Characteristic radiographic changes.

As well as this, all the infants showed some degree of oedema and most of them developed icterus. On clinical grounds alone therefore these babies were at very high risk.

Using heparinised samples of blood obtained by heel prick the degree of metabolic acidosis, as well as respiratory acidosis, is determined by means of the micro-Astrup apparatus. The former is correctable by intravenous sodium bicarbonate and this was given by a polythene catheter in the umbilical vein in a dose depending on the base excess and with the practical assumption that the extracellular space in the baby could be presumed to be about 35 per cent of the body weight. Using a solution, therefore, of 8·4 per cent sodium bicarbonate, as 1 mEq is equal to 1 ml of this mixture, the dose was calculated on the formula of:

Base excess in mEq/litre × 0·35 × the body weight in kilograms.

The more modern preference is to reduce the strength of the sodium bicarbonate solution to a sixth of the former concentration, namely to 15 mEq/100 ml because the injection of grossly hyperosmolar solutions dehydrates the intracellular fluid content.

In other words a sort of *in vivo* titration of the baby with sodium bicarbonate. Further micro-Astrup estimations are carried out 30 minutes later and more sodium bicarbonate given as indicated, the aim being to raise the pH to between 7·35 and 7·4. Thereafter the acid-base equilibrium is monitored more or less hourly and the dose of sodium bicarbonate prescribed accordingly. The total daily fluid intake is adjusted to 60 ml/kg with 15 per cent glucose instead of fructose since the latter lowers the pH.

An incidental beneficial effect is a likely diuresis and this is particularly helpful in the "waterlogged" baby of a diabetic mother. Very early on, hyperbaric oxygen up to 3 atmospheres absolute pressure was found to be of no benefit.

Unfortunately the sodium bicarbonate treatment does not relieve the high P_{CO_2} values which indicate severe respiratory acidosis, and attempts have been made to raise the pH with buffer substances such as THAM or TRIS (tris-hydroxymethylaminomethane). The results in this respect, however, are disappointing and it still remains to be seen whether the addition of augmented respiration will improve the prognosis in these desperate cases with rising P_{CO_2} levels in spite of treatment. Nevertheless the biochemical correction alone of the metabolic acidosis by the above technique has resulted in a striking improvement in mortality rates from otherwise uncomplicated cases of respiratory distress syndrome, from about 45 per cent to 11·5 per cent[42, 43] and already such results have had the effect of modifying obstetrical treatment. We are now less hesitant to undertake Caesarean section, for example, in prematurity and in conditions such as antepartum haemorrhage and diabetes known to predispose the baby to this dreaded complication, especially if a satisfactory L:S ratio is obtainable on amniocentesis.

Formerly one would have expected at least half the cases, or more, to die. What is even more encouraging is that follow-up, although necessarily short so far, has shown few complications although umbilical vein phlebitis and pyaemia may occur. It is now more usual to cannulate an umbilical artery, which has the additional advantage that arterial samples can easily be obtained through the same catheter.

Even a normal baby at term is born with a mild acidosis, both metabolic and respiratory, of which the respiratory element (the raised P_{CO_2}) is eliminated presently after birth by efficient pulmonary ventilation, but the metabolic acidosis takes longer to correct and pulmonary function is the principal method by which the infant maintains its acid-base balance. When, for any reason, respiratory function fails, the derangement of metabolism becomes profound and is associated with hyperkalaemia to a lethal degree. This brings us back to where we started and the baby that breathes and cries well gets out of its acidosis and stays out of it.

In addition to therapeutic homeostasis the period 1965–1970 witnessed the heyday of ventilators, which were not without their dangers. Now grunting is one of the clinical features of the respiratory distress syndrome, and Chu[14] and Harrison and colleagues[41] recognised this as a modified Valsalva manoeuvre. They noted that grunting of course ceased on intubating the baby but as the intrapleural pressures fell so the arterial oxygen levels fell too. They recognised that grunting was a protective mechanism in order to raise the arterial oxygen. This mechanism also illustrates the benefits of crying.

These observations led to the development of continuous positive airways pressure (CPAP) treatment. This involves pressure therapy via an endotracheal tube, or a box or bag using a neck seal.[6, 39] A similar mechanism could be invoked by applying negative pressure (CNAP) to the thorax, again using a neck seal, but this has obvious disadvantages.

Using pressures of 12 mm Hg or less, a great improvement in arterial oxygen levels can be obtained, and this removes the need to supply oxygen concentrations of more than 35 per cent.

Boxes, bags, neck seals and prolonged use of endotracheal tubes all have their drawbacks and the favoured method of administering CPAP is by nasopharyngeal tubes fitting snugly through both nostrils but not tightly enough to cause necrosis.

If an oral gastric tube is passed into the stomach first, aspiration can be carried out without interfering with the treatment.[58]

Since the introduction of CPAP in 1971 babies with even severe respiratory distress syndrome, if weighing more than 1,500 g have a very good chance of survival.

Nutrition

A baby large and strong enough to suck should be put to the breast, six-hourly after the first day and three-hourly on the third and subsequent days until its weight has reached 3 kg when four-hourly feeding can be instituted. A large proportion of premature infants, however, are not sufficiently vigorous, and there remains a choice of the following methods of feeding:

(1) Tube feeding;
(2) Bottle feeding;
(3) Nasojejunal feeding for the very ill or premature;
(4) Intravenous hyperalimentation.

The accent is now on maintaining homeostasis so there is an increasing tendency to start fluids within 3 hours, orally or intravenously.

In such an infant, each feed may be fraught with danger. In the first place the swallowing reflexes may be functionally inadequate to prevent aspiration of milk into the trachea; secondly, vomiting and regurgitation, especially common in association with cerebral irritation, may cause aspiration; and thirdly, "grey attacks" may follow the feed even without foreign matter being aspirated; this last mishap is largely provoked by the disturbance and handling entailed, but possibly reflex factors from the stomach operate as well. Because of the aspiration risk, nasogastric feeding is generally preferred to the other methods in the very weak and ultrapremature, and can certainly be more expeditious. The utensils should of course be boiled before use and the nurse should wash her hands as in all handling manoeuvres. A fine polythene catheter is simply passed via the nose down to the lower end of the oesophagus, the length of tube being equal to the distance from the bridge of the nose to xiphisternum + 5 cm. The feed is slowly run in from a funnel or syringe. The tube should be pinched firmly on withdrawal so as to prevent any leakage of milk from its tip while passing the epiglottis. An experienced nurse can gauge well whether the baby is satisfied with the amount given.

The dangers of neonatal hypoglycaemia are now fully recognised. Following a small feed of 2–5 ml of boiled water, full-strength breast milk is given; this should be pasteurised rather than boiled since boiling destroys the protective immunological properties of the milk. The breast milk is obtained by manual expression from the mother's breast or from a bank supply.

In a racily written communication by Smallpeice and Davies (1964), immediate feeding with full-strength breast milk is recommended even in those babies not interested in sucking at breast or bottle, in which case a polythene tube is passed through a nostril well down into the stomach. The tubes can be kept for as long as a week but bottle or breast feeding is encouraged as soon as the tube can be dispensed with. Under this scheme feeds are started within two hours of birth and rapidly stepped up from a total of 60 ml/kg of body weight (1 oz/lb body weight) on the first day, to 150 ml/kg body weight ($2\frac{1}{2}$ oz/lb body weight) on the seventh day. This quantity, divided into small frequent amounts, is put into the stomach often hourly at first in the very precarious babies, up to three-hourly, as soon as possible. The advantages claimed for this early type of feeding are that it almost eradicates symptomatic hypoglycaemia and lowers the serum bilirubin. Furthermore it shortens the period taken for the baby to regain its birth weight and it is even suggested that the incidence of neurological sequalae of prematurity may be diminished. This trial was conducted on babies weighing between 1 and 2 kg at birth and therefore presented quite a challenge, but the authors drove home the thrust, presumably referring to delayed feeding, that, "many well-meant advances in the care of the premature baby over the last 20 years have been disastrous."

The premature baby is born with an iron deficit that cannot be made good by natural feeding, so that after six weeks, by which time its digestion should be able to cope, it is advisable to give oral iron, e.g. ferrous gluconate or sodium iron edetate (Systron); additionally in babies of less than 1,800 g, folic acid, 100 μg twice weekly from the age of two weeks, combats the anaemia of prematurity.

General Nursing Details

In addition to the principles already enumerated, the following points are observed:

The baby is nursed in a cot or incubator and is not bathed; in fact cleaning is reduced to the minimum and is done with hexachlorophane cream, avoiding broken skin and removing immediately to prevent possibly toxic absorption. There is no need whatever, nor is it desirable, to clean off all the vernix. The routine oiling of the baby has now been abandoned.

Nappies or pieces of gauze tissue are placed under the buttocks and not round the baby, so that they can be replaced with the minimum of disturbance.

No cord dressing is applied. Such ritual, besides being useless, prevents proper inspection. No bath is given until the cord has separated and not even then unless the baby's condition warrants it. Until the first bath the baby is simply "top and tailed" with plain water when necessary.

Weighing should be daily and temperature taking *per rectum* is, if possible, kept down to three-hourly for the first twenty-four hours and then twice daily.

No routine treatment is given to eyes, ears or nostrils unless the development of some local infection calls for it. The routine use of eye-drops as a prophylaxis against infection probably does more to encourage the sticky eye than to prevent it, and the scouring out of nostrils and ears with cotton-wool is both mischievous and meddlesome.

There is probably no branch of nursing which is quite so exacting and certainly none more important than the care of the premature infant, but it is also one of the most rewarding.

The average stay in the unit is between six and seven weeks, but it is doubtful if any similar period at any other time in the child's life will have been better spent (Fig. 4).

KERNICTERUS

This is a lethal condition which is common in both haemolytic disease and prematurity. It refers to any type of cerebral jaundice in which the basal nuclei of the brain become heavily stained with bile pigments and suffer degenerative changes. The distribution and the nature of the lesion are similar, whether associated with prematurity or haemolytic disease. As a factor in neonatal death it is of considerable importance, and Claireaux[16] found it responsible for 33 out of 376 deaths in infants within the neonatal period, giving an incidence of 8·8 per cent.

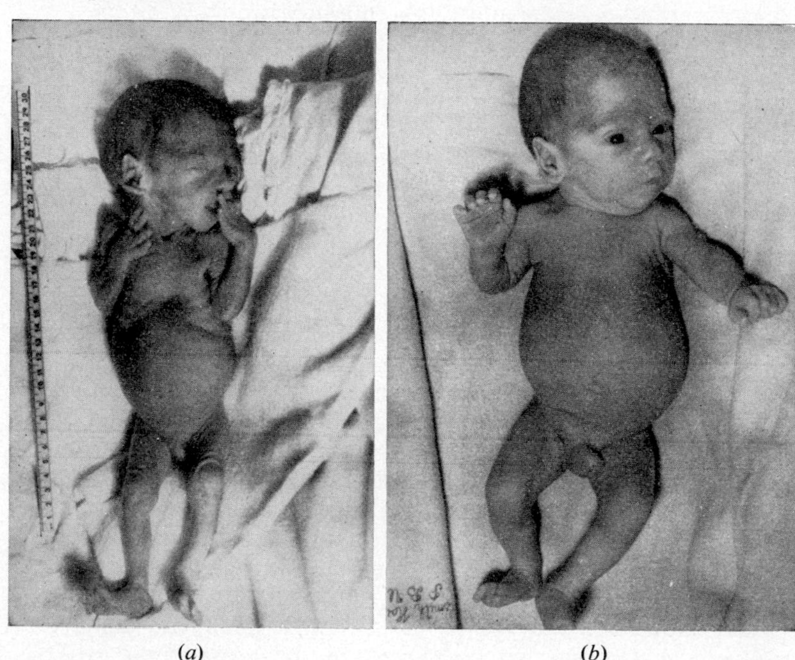

(*a*) (*b*)

27/FIG. 4.—Gross prematurity. (*a*) Birth weight 1 lb 14 oz (618 g). Note persistence of subcostal inspiratory recession in a very premature infant at 17 days. (*b*) Same infant 6 weeks later.

Kernicterus cannot occur without hyperbilirubinaemia and hyperbilirubinaemia cannot occur without jaundice. The mechanism by which this type of central nervous damage is incurred is very different in the two major conditions producing it, namely, haemolytic disease and prematurity, but now that the metabolism of bilirubin is better understood the mechanism is clearer. The subject has been well reviewed by Claireaux (1960). Bilirubin is a natural product of red cell haemolysis. In its unconjugated form it is highly toxic, particularly to cells within the central nervous system which for one reason or another, such as hypoxia, may be rendered vulnerable. Unfortunately bilirubin, though soluble in alcohol and fat, is not so in water, and until this solubility can be achieved it cannot be excreted in the bile. Conjugation, however, with glucuronic acid within the liver under the influence of the enzyme glucuronyl transferase converts it to bilirubin glucuronide which is soluble, non-toxic and readily excreted in the bile. Each gram of haemoglobin can produce as much as 35 mg of bilirubin on haemolysis. Normally, large quantities are therefore not produced (except in haemolysing conditions) and are rapidly converted to the soluble and non-toxic form.

Hyperbilirubinaemia can therefore readily occur when the conversion mechanism is swamped by haemolytic conditions or it may occur if there is some interference with this enzyme transformation. Unfortunately the latter is the case in neonates to some extent, but even more so in prematurity. The mechanism is also defective in rare conditions such as congenital non-haemolytic jaundice (Crigler-Najjar syndrome).

Barbiturates, although on the way out in general medicine, have still a useful role in obstetrics, not only as good sedatives in threatened premature labour but because they actually improve the baby's liver enzyme capacity for conjugating bilirubin and therefore helping to cope with neonatal jaundice in the premature.

On the other hand, when jaundice is obstructive in type, the bilirubin has already been converted to the harmless and soluble glucuronide before it is dammed back in the circulation and therefore kernicterus does not occur. Bilirubin is thus the responsible agent and may operate by being produced in excess as in haemolytic disease due, for example, to the Rhesus factor, or to congenital spherocytosis (abnormal red cell fragility) or it may not be conjugated sufficiently readily, as in functional immaturity of the liver in the premature and in congenital familial non-haemolytic jaundice.

Unconjugated bilirubin can be reduced by exchange transfusion, phenobarbitone and, interestingly, by phototherapy. Lund and Jacobsen in 1974 noticed that more bilirubin in unconjugated form was excreted as a result of 24 hours' phototherapy, especially by the blue part of the visible spectrum. Phototherapy degrades bilirubin by photo-oxidation so that the concentration of unconjugated bilirubin excreted in bile is approximately doubled and less bilirubin in the conjugated state is excreted. These photo-oxidation products are water-soluble and therefore more readily excreted. Ultraviolet light should however be screened out by filters and the baby's eyes should be protected with goggles during treatment.

Diazepam, so widely used in obstetrics, has as its vehicle sodium benzoate, which can cause kernicterus by competitive albumin binding, leaving free lipid-soluble unconjugated bilirubin to damage the basal ganglia. We have had such a case in a young unsupervised unmarried eclamptic girl who was treated with diazepam and Heminevrin. The baby, which was very premature and weighed only

0·84 kg, lived for six days but died from kernicterus. Fetal interests would appear to be not well served by diazepam in the face of severe jaundice with prematurity or in haemolytic disease.

In congenital bile-duct atresia one is dealing with the more harmless obstructive variety. In galactosaemia the liver is damaged by the toxic action of one of the metabolites of galactose, because of the lack of a specific enzyme necessary for the proper breakdown of this sugar. As a result of the periportal fibrosis and cirrhosis which can thus be caused, the bile canaliculi contain plugs of inspissated bile and an obstructive type of jaundice results. Although mental defects may occur they do so for a different reason than from kernicterus.

When hyperbilirubinaemia is due to infection such as, for example, umbilical sepsis, or viral infections, both bilirubin and bilirubin glucuronide levels may be raised, the danger of kernicterus again coming from the former. Finally a very disturbing type of kernicterus can be due to iatrogenic hyperbilirubinaemia either because a drug increases haemolysis directly or acts as a metabolic competitor. The analogues of vitamin K have been incriminated on both counts. Vitamin K_1, for example phytomenadione (Konakion), is both safer and more effective. This vitamin is essential for the formation within the body of prothrombin, factor VII and factor X. Vitamin K_1 is reputed to be harmless in fact and, as mentioned in the section on the ventouse, it is our practice to carry out a thrombotest examination of the premature newborn baby's blood and because hypoprothrombinaemia is much commoner than formerly recognised. We have no hesitation in giving 1 mg intramuscular injection repeated as necessary according to results.

It is known that bilirubin is readily bound to plasma albumin, which makes it less liable to affect the cells within the central nervous system. In prematurity the level of this albumin is low. Therefore there may be an increase in the amount of dissociated bilirubin in the blood stream. Furthermore, salicylates and sulphonamides may compete with bilirubin for attachment to this albumin and may therefore enable toxic amounts of unconjugated and non-protein-bound bilirubin to reach the central nervous system. Some such mechanism as this probably accounts for the fact that kernicterus may occur at different levels of serum bilirubin and that there is no critical level above which kernicterus is inevitable nor below which this dreadful complication is unlikely to occur. Nevertheless, in general principle, the higher the level of bilirubin the greater the hazard. The more premature the infant, the lower the bilibrubin level necessary to produce kernicterus, and the more damaged the brain cells by hypoxia, the more readily are they predisposed to this type of damage. In such cases Govan and Scott considered that pigmentation was a secondary factor, as they had found similar lesions in the brains of premature infants dying in the first few days of life before jaundice had made its appearance. It may well be that the cells of the nuclei have first to be damaged to make them susceptible to pigmentation, and of all the predisposing causes anoxia and prematurity operating together would appear to be the most likely.

The clinical features of the two classes of kernicterus differ mainly in the age of onset. Whereas in haemolytic disease the jaundice usually comes on very rapidly after birth, in prematurity the jaundice appears about the third or fourth day, death occurring at about the end of the first week. In the case of haemolytic disease, anaemia is progressive, but in the premature infant so afflicted there is often a history of asphyxia at birth or soon after; it is liable to recurrent attacks of cyanosis, is feeble and frequently oedematous. Signs of cerebral irritation are often manifest, but, serious though the condition is, premature babies often recover from severe degrees of jaundice. There remains considerable anxiety about the cerebral damage which may have been sustained, and about the chances of intellectual impairment.

Since the risk of kernicterus is to some extent proportional to the serum bilirubin level and begins to operate when this level exceeds 15 mg per cent (250 μmol/l), becomes highly probable at 25 mg (416 μmol/l) per cent and a cast-iron certainty at 40 mg per cent (680 μmol/l), a rising level is now accepted as an outright indication for exchange transfusion regardless of the aetiology since, at all costs, the mental damage associated with kernicterus is to be avoided. The transfusion removes the albumin/bilirubin complex. However, the exchange has to be carried further than in haemolytic disease because this albumin/bilirubin complex is contained not only within the vascular compartment of the body, but in the extravascular fluid as well and diffusion back into the circulation may produce a sort of rebound phenomenon. The transfusion may therefore have to be repeated. In spite of the risks of exchange transfusion, particularly in the weak and premature, bilirubin levels over 20 mg per 100 ml (340 μmol/l) are regarded by most workers as a full indication for the procedure.

A survey of the Society of Medical Officers of Health has been reported by McDonald (1962) which deals with the neurological and ophthalmic disorders in children with birth weights of 4 lb (1,800 g) or less. Of those who had already died more than half had had some neurological disorder and of those still alive nearly a quarter were found to have either a neurological or an ophthalmic disorder. How much of the former was due to kernicterus remains to be worked out by further prospective study. Of the ophthalmic disorders, myopia is common, and retrolental fibroplasia, an even more terrible consequence of prematurity, now believed to be mainly iatrogenic in origin.

RETROLENTAL FIBROPLASIA

This condition became at one time a serious factor in congenital blindness. It occurs only in premature infants whose birth weight is less than 5 lb ($2\frac{1}{4}$ kg) and was first described by Terry in 1942. The end point of the disease is blindness with searching nystagmus, due to the presence of bilateral vascularised opaque membranes behind the lens, together with retinal detachment.

The findings of the Medical Research Council investigation have supported the popular view that the disease is caused by the too liberal use of oxygen in prematurity.

The Medical Research Council investigators noted that the chances of spontaneous regression without treatment were 44 per cent and they doubted the real value of corticotrophin or returning the child to its former high-oxygen environment, although the number so treated was too small for firm conclusions. The likelihood of developing retrolental fibroplasia increases with the duration of oxygen therapy, but only a few hours of oxygen toxicity suffice to induce retrolental fibroplasia, the danger level of Po_2 in arterial blood being in the region of 160 mm Hg.[69] Certainly concentrations of oxygen above 35 per cent for longer than a few hours are both dangerous and unnecessary.

Supervision should be maintained up to the sixth month of life at least, but if signs have not appeared by then they will not do so subsequently.

With the progressive elimination of gonococcal ophthalmia from our maternity departments, retrolental fibroplasia now constitutes the biggest single cause of blindness in children.

REFERENCES

1. Akerren, Y. and Furstenberg, N. (1960). *J. Obstet. Gynaec. Brit. Emp.*, **57,** 705.
2. Anderson, J. M., Milner, R. D. G. and Strich, S. J. (1966). *Lancet*, **2,** 372.
3. Arneil, G. A. and Kerr, M. M. (1963). *Lancet*, **2,** 756.
4. Avery, M. E. and Mead, J. (1959). *Amer. J. Dis. Child.*, **97,** 517.
5. Baird, D. (1945). *J. Obstet. Gynaec. Brit. Emp.*, **52,** 217.
6. Barrie, H. (1972). *Lancet*, **1,** 776.
7. Becroft, D. M. O., Farmer, K., Seddon, R. J., Sowden, R., Stewart, J. H., Vines, A. and Wattie, D. A. (1971). *Brit. med. J.*, **2,** 747.
8. Bembridge, B. A., Coxon, M., Moulton, A. C. L., Jackson, C. R. S. and Smallpiece, V. (1952). *Brit. med. J.*, **1,** 675.
9. Bhagwanani, S. G., Fahmy, D. and Turnbull, A. C. (1972). *Lancet*, **1,** 159.
10. Born, G. V. R., Dawes, G. S., Mott, J. C. and Widdicombe, J. G. (1954). *Cold Spr. Harb. Symp. Quant. Biol.*, **19,** 102.

11. Bound, J. P., Butler, N. R. and Spector, W. G. (1956). *Brit. med. J.*, **2,** 1260.
12. Butler, N. R. and Bonham, D. G. (1963). *Perinatal Mortality*, p. 142. Edinburgh: Livingstone.
13. Campvell, S. and Wilkin, D. (1975). *Brit. J. Obstet. Gynaec.*, **82,** 689.
14. Chu, J. *et al.* (1967). *Pediatrics*, **40,** 709.
15. Claireaux, A. E. (1958). In: *Modern Trends in Paediatrics*, 2nd series. London: Butterworth.
16. Claireaux, A. E. (1960). *Brit. med. J.*, **1,** 1528.
17. Clements, J. A., Platzker, A. C. G., Tierney, D. F., Hobel, C. J., Creasey, R. K., Margolis, A. J., Thibeault, D. W., Tooley, W. H. and Oh, W. (1972). *New Engl. J. Med.*, **286,** 1077.
18. Davies, P. A. and Stewart, A. L. (1975). *Brit. med. Bull.*, **31,** 85.
19. Dawes, G. S., Mott, J. C., Widdicombe, J. G. and Wyatt, D. G. (1953). *J. Physiol. (Lond.)*, **121,** 141.
20. Dawes, G. S., Mott, J. C. and Widdicombe, J. G. (1954). *J. Physiol. (Lond.)*, **126,** 523.
21. Dawkins, M. J. R. (1964). *Proc. roy. Soc. Med.*, **57,** 1063.
22. Donald, I. (1954). *J. Obstet. Gynaec. Brit. Emp.*, **61,** 725.
23. Donald, I. (1957). *Brit. J. Anaesth.*, **29,** 553.
24. Donald, I. and Lord, J. (1953). *Lancet*, **1,** 9.
25. Donald, I. and Steiner, R. E. (1953). *Lancet*, **2,** 846.
26. Donald, I., Kerr, M. M. and MacDonald, I. R. (1958). *Scot. med. J.*, **3,** 151.
27. Douglas, J. W. B. (1956). *Brit. med. J.*, **1,** 1210.
28. Douglas, J. W. B. (1960). *Brit. med. J.*, **1,** 1008.
29. Drillien, C. M. (1957). *J. Obstet. Gynaec. Brit. Emp.*, **64,** 161.
30. Drillien, C. M. (1959). *J. Obstet. Gynaec. Brit. Emp.*, **66,** 721.
31. Drillien, C. M. (1964). *The Growth and Development of the Prematurely Born Infant*, p. 77. Edinburgh: Livingstone.
32. Dubowitz, L. M. S., Dubowitz, V. and Goldberg, C. (1970). *J. Pediat.*, **77,** 1.
33. Fell, M. R. (1960). *Lancet*, **1,** 1295.
34. Fuchs, F., Fuchs, A. R., Poblete, V. F. and Risk, A. (1967). *Amer. J. Obstet. Gynec.*, **99,** 627.
35. Gaisford, W. and Schofield, S. (1950). *Brit. med. J.*, **1,** 1404.
36. Gitlin, D. and Craig, J. M. (1956). *Pediatrics*, **17,** 64.
37. Gluck, L., Kulovich, M. V., Borer, R. C., Bremner, P. H., Anderson, G. G. and Spellacy, W. N. (1971). *Amer. J. Obstet. Gynec.*, **109,** 440.
38. Govan, A. D. T. and Scott, J. M. (1953). *Lancet*, **1,** 611.
39. Gregory, G. A., Kitterman, J. A., Phibbs, R. H., Tooley, W. H. and Hamilton, W. K. (1971). *New Engl. J. Med.*, **284,** 1333.
40. Hansmann, M. (1974). *Gynäkologe*, **7,** 26.
41. Harrison, V. C., Heese, H. de V. and Klein, M. (1968). *Pediatrics*, **41,** 549.
42. Hutchison, J. H., Kerr, M. M., McPhail, M. F. M., Douglas, T. A., Smith, G., Norman, J. N. and Bates, E. H. (1962). *Lancet*, **2,** 465.

43. Hutchison, J. H., Kerr, M. M., Douglas, T. A., Inall, J. A. and Crosbie, J. C. (1964). *Pediatrics*, **33,** 956.
44. Karlberg, P., Cook, C. D., O'Brien, D., Cherry, R. B. and Smith, C. A. (1954). *Acta paediat.* (*Uppsala*), **43,** Suppl. 100.
45. Knoblock, H., Rider, R., Harper, P. and Pasamanick, B. (1956). *J. Amer. med. Ass.*, **161,** 581.
46. Lancet. Editorial. 1974. **2,** 1056.
47. Liggins, G. C. and Howie, R. N. (1972). *Pediatrics*, **50,** 515.
48. Lind, J. and Wegelius, C. (1954). *Cold Spr. Harb. Symp. quant. Biol.*, **19,** 109.
49. Lund, H. T. and Jacobsen, J. (1974). *J. Pediat.*, **85,** 262.
50. McAllister, T. A. (1976). Personal Communication.
51. McCormick, C. O. (1947). *Textbook on Pathology of Labor, the Puerperium and the Newborn*, 2nd edit. St Louis: C. V. Mosby Co.
52. McDonald, A. D. (1962). *Brit. med. J.*, **1,** 895.
53. McDonald, A. D. (1964). *Brit. J. prev. soc. Med.*, **18,** 59.
54. McLaurin, J. (1977). Personal Communication.
55. Medical Research Council (1955). Report of Conference on Retrolental Fibroplasia. *Brit. med. J.*, **2,** 78.
56. Ministry of Health, Central Service Council (1961). *Report of Sub-Committee on the Prevention of Prematurity and the Care of Premature Infants.* London: H.M.S.O.
57. Morison, J. E. (1962). *Foetal and Neonatal Pathology.* London: Butterworth & Co.
58. Novogroder, M., MacKuanying, N., Eidelman, A. I. and Gartner, L. M. (1973. *J. Pediat.*, **82,** 1059.
59. Pattle, R. E., Claireaux, A. E., Davies, P. A. and Cameron, A. H. (1962). *Lancet*, **2,** 469.
60. Potter, E. L. (1952). *Pathology of the Fetus and the Newborn.* Chicago: Year Book Publishers.
61. Reid, D. M. S., Tunstall, M. E. and Mitchell, R. G. (1967). *Lancet*, **1,** 532.
62. Robinson, H. P., Chatfield, W. R., Logan, R. W. and Hall, F. (1974). *Ann. clin. Biochem.*, **11,** 15.
63. Seeliger, H. P. R. (1961). *Listeriosis.* Basel: S. Karger.
64. Shelley, H. J. (1964). *Brit. med. J.*, **1,** 273.
65. Shelley, H. J. and Neligan, G. A. (1966). *Brit. med. Bull.*, **22,** 34.
66. Smallpeice, V. and Davies, P. A. (1964). *Lancet*, **2,** 1349.
67. Terry, T. L. (1942). *Amer. J. Ophthal.*, **25,** 203, 1409.
68. Thomson, A. M. (1951). *Brit. J. Nutr.*, **5,** 158.
69. Tizard, J. P. M. (1971). *Proc. roy. Soc. Med.*, **64,** 771.
70. Usher, R. (1961). *Pediat. Clin. N. Amer.*, **8,** 525.
71. Walker, J. (1967). *Proc. roy. Soc. Med.*, **60,** 877.
72. Wesselius-de Casparis, A., Thiery, M., Yo Le Sian, A., Baumgarten, K., Brosens, I., Gamissans, O., Stolk, J. G. and Vivier, W. (1971). *Brit. med. J.*, **3,** 144.
73. Whitfield, C. R., Chan, W. H., Sproule, W. B. and Stewart, A. D. (1972). *Brit. med. J.*, **2,** 85.
74. Wigglesworth, J. S. (1967). *Proc. roy. Soc. Med.*, **60,** 879.
75. Willoughby, M. L. N. (1967). Personal Communication.
76. Yllpo, A. (1935). *Acta paediat.* (*Uppsala*), **17,** Suppl. 1, 122.

CHAPTER XXVIII

Rh FACTOR

THE term haemolytic disease of the newborn has now largely supplanted the more clumsy and less euphonic name "erythroblastosis fetalis". The essential underlying pathology is an active haemolysis of the fetal red cells before, at, or shortly after birth, and the three conditions, hydrops fetalis, icterus gravis neonatorum, and haemolytic anaemia in the newborn, are now recognised to differ only in degree and to be related to the one disease process. The discovery of the Rh factor, the recognition of its clinical importance and the practical applications of this knowledge in therapy constitute one of the great romances of modern research where theory, observation and practice have, in the space of a very few years, pieced themselves together to form a coherent picture.

In 1939 Levine and Stetson discovered an atypical immune agglutinin in a woman who had been delivered of a stillborn fetus. In the next year Landsteiner and Wiener discovered the Rh antigen. These workers started preparing immune sera in animals by giving injections of blood from another animal, and they came thus to immunise rabbits with blood from the rhesus monkey and found that the resulting immune serum agglutinated the majority of human bloods, but by no means all. In other words, in the majority of humans there is a factor which was common to the rhesus monkey. This factor is known as the Rh factor, and those who possess it are classed as Rh-positive and those whose bloods are not agglutinated by the immune rabbit serum are called Rh-negative.

Landsteiner and Wiener in 1940 detected an Rh antibody in the serum of an Rh-negative woman who had experienced haemolytic reactions after a transfusion with Rh-positive blood. In 1941 Levine observed the relationship between the presence of an Rh antibody in Rh-negative women whose pregnancies resulted in haemolytic disease of the baby or in certain cases of stillbirth. From this point progress was very rapid both in the United States of America and in Great Britain, and it was soon found that there was more than one Rh factor until at last, in 1944, Fisher's CDE classification made sense out of a growing and bewildering confusion.

Iso-immunisation

Iso-immunisation has been defined as the process whereby immune antibodies are produced in one individual in response to the injection of antigen from another individual of the same species (hence the prefix *iso*), this last individual possessing antigens which the first lacks. It follows, therefore, that there are three possible methods by which iso-immunisation can occur. The first and most obvious method is by the transfusion of unsuitable blood. In the case of the ABO groups, reactions are immediate, as immunity to the appropriate factors is inherent in the individual's make-up, although recent interest has been aroused in the possibility of anti-A reactions, but in the case of the Rh groups this immunity is actively acquired. Reaction is therefore not immediate, but immunity develops later, occasionally within a week, and repeated transfusions of unsuitable blood in respect of the Rh factor heighten the response. A second and less common method of iso-immunisation is by the intramuscular injection of unsuitable whole blood. This, in the past, has featured in the treatment of a variety of conditions, but is not numerically important. The third and most interesting method is the result of pregnancy, whereby an Rh-negative woman, pregnant with an Rh-positive child, manages by one means or another to receive into her own circulation some of her child's Rh-positive red cells which act as antigens. Any interruption, however minute, in the placental barrier between circulations of mother and child will allow the antigenic fetal red cells to enter the maternal circulation.

The obvious time for fetal cells to leak through into the maternal circulation, of course, is with the delivery of the placenta where damage to this organ, in the course of its separation and expulsion, may liberate cells into maternal venous sinuses sufficiently open to receive them. It is possible that the routine use of ergometrine at the beginning of the third stage may be responsible for the increase of iso-immunisation by squeezing fetal blood cells into the maternal circulation, but this has not yet been proven. Other forms of placental accident, even minor, in the course of pregnancy, such as placental separation from any cause may likewise cause iso-immunisation even in the first pregnancy. There is now a growing weight of evidence that fetal cells enter the circulation in small numbers even in quite normal pregnancies, since they can be recognised by their content of fetal haemoglobin. In many cases the ABO group of the baby is incompatible with that of the mother and the fetal cells are immediately destroyed. Finn *et al.* (1961) found that these feto-maternal microtransfusions were much less likely to occur in the case of women who were bearing an ABO incompatible baby. Fraser and Raper (1962) have, however, identified these ABO incompatible fetal cells early in the puerperium, but their life in the maternal circulation is a short one. This may explain the fact that Rh iso-immunisation is less likely to occur where ABO incompatibility exists between mother and child. What is surprising is that iso-immunisation does not occur in every case in which an Rh-negative woman bears an Rh-positive child, but the phenomenon is doubtless dependent upon the size, quantity or repetition of the antigenic stimulus. Once the mother has become immunised, her serum will contain antibodies for most of the rest, if not all, of her life. These antibodies pass with little hindrance across the placenta in subsequent pregnancies and work havoc on the red cells of any fetus whose blood is Rh-positive and therefore susceptible to their action. It follows, therefore, that if iso-immunisation has occurred as a result of pregnancy, the results are most likely to appear, not in that pregnancy, but in subsequent ones, although this is not always so, and any solution in placental continuity, for example from a threat to miscarry or an antepartum haemorrhage, can provoke sensitisation in susceptible individuals. Nevertheless, it is most unlikely that a patient can become sensitised in the course of a given pregnancy before the 5th month. If, therefore, antibodies are found to be present as early as, for example, three months, previous sensitisation is indicated, and even a previous abortion occurring as early as 12 weeks may have been responsible.

The relative importance of unsuitable transfusion in iso-immunising a patient is now lessening with the more general adoption of precautions in respect of the Rh factor when transfusing women of childbearing age, so that whereas in 1950 about a third of our Rh cases with children affected with haemolytic disease gave a history of such a transfusion in the past, the figure is now very low indeed.

The chances of iso-immunisation occurring are very much greater from unsuitable transfusion than from bearing Rh-positive children and it has been found that a transfusion of volunteers with two spaced intravenous injections of $\frac{1}{4}$ ml of Rh-positive blood sensitised 40 per cent of them, but that if such injections were repeated often, the figure could be raised to 90 per cent. By contrast the Rh-negative woman who has two Rh-positive babies has still only a 1 in 12 chance of being iso-immunised.

The proportion of people who are Rh-negative varies according to race. For example, in China it is most uncommon, and it might be suggested that the older civilisation of the Chinese has, by a process of natural selection, bred out an undesirable gene, but in England 16·8 per cent or 17 per cent of people are in this category. Of this 17 per cent of Rh-negative women three, on average, are likely to marry Rh-negative men, so that their chances of having infants affected with haemolytic disease are nil. Of the remaining 14, six are likely to marry homozygous Rh-positive husbands with a 1 in 12 chance of their second child being affected, and eight are likely to marry heterozygous Rh-positive husbands with a consequently reduced chance, at 1 in 15, of having an affected second child. The more pregnancies that a woman has, who is unsuitably mated in respect of the Rh factor, the more likely is she to have, sooner or later, an affected child, and haemolytic disease tends to be more severe with each repetition. For example, the first child to be affected has a 90 per cent chance of spontaneous survival. If the patient was not sensitised before a given pregnancy, she is practically certain not to produce a child stillborn because of haemolytic disease, but if she has been previously sensitised, the stillbirth rate is about 30 per cent and if, having a homozygous Rh-positive husband, she has already had one stillbirth, the chances of a repetition of this disaster are as high as 80 per cent.[38] After two Rh stillbirths the outlook indeed becomes poor.

The majority of cases of haemolytic disease of the newborn are due to Rh incompatibilities, but there are other blood group systems which are independent of ABO or Rh grouping and which may in rare instances produce iso-immunisation. These include the MNS, P, Lutheran, Kell, Lewis, Duffy and Kidd blood group systems. When haemolytic disease occurs within the ABO incompatibility group it is nearly always in the case of Group O mothers with Group A babies and very occasionally Group B,[44] but all these are rare phenomena compared with the Rh group of iso-immunisation. According to Walker (1959) the incidence of haemolytic disease of the newborn due to Rh incompatibility was about six out of every thousand babies in England and Wales and until now fifteen were stillborn out of every hundred affected babies. The problem is therefore a large one.

Subgroups

The division of all humanity into the two classes, Rh-positive and Rh-negative, is an over-simplification of the facts, although in general it serves well enough. Wiener started the ball rolling by finding a serum which reacted in only 70 per cent out of the 85 per cent of known Rh-positive people, the remaining 15 per cent being unaffected. This led to the acknowledgment of at least two components of the Rh-positive group which were called Rh_1 and Rh_2, and it was not long before the study of atypical reactions led to the discovery of further subgroups such as Rh′, Rh″, Rh_y, etc. Fisher's CDE classification is now more generally accepted, as it is far easier to understand, its only disadvantage being that it is inconvenient to use in speech. The CDE classification is based upon the theory that each Rh gene is made up of three components selected from three allelomorphic pairs, namely C or *c*, D or *d*, E or *e*, giving for example a gene such as C*d*E. Mathematically the possible combinations of these elements would supply us with eight Rh types of gene, but since every individual inherits genes from both parents, the full genotype must always contain a double set of *cde* letters, for example CD*e*/*cde*. The identification of each of these six possible letters is done by means of antisera which are specific. The commonly available antisera are anti-C, anti-D, anti-E and anti-*c*. The antisera *e* and *d* are rare or not available. The accompanying table shows the relationship of the various types to each other and the more obsolete Rh_1 and Rh_2 sort of classification.

In general, the distinction between Rh-positive and Rh-negative patients is made with anti-D serum, which is the most important of the series. It will be seen that the recessive so-called Rh-negative gene has to be regarded as a definite entity possessing antigenic properties of its own, and cases have been cited in which an Rh-positive serum agglutinated all Rh-negative cells encountered by it. Such a serum might be expected to contain anti-*d*, but this is a rare phenomenon. It now appears, therefore, that when an individual lacks any one of the many Rh components, iso-immunisation may occur if this component is introduced artificially. The matter is important because, unfortunately, reactions can occur within the Rh group itself.

Other subdivisions, even of this subgrouping, continue to emerge, for example, on the C–*c* locus of the Rh gene a third alternative has been identified, namely C^w. This often exists in combination with plain C. Of the four above-mentioned antisera which are fairly widely available, the anti-C is usually in the form of anti-C + C^w. Pure anti-C and pure anti-C^w are rarer.

In reproduction each parent hands on the first or the second half of his or her full genotype so that, for example, a case of group CD*e*/*cde* hands on either CD*e* or *cde* to the offspring. In any instance where there is a possibility of handing down a choice of either D or *d*, the case is regarded as heterozygous, and will pass on to the next generation either an Rh-positive or an Rh-negative gene, but where there is a big D in both halves of the genotype, the parent is homozygous and can only pass on an Rh-positive gene. Likewise, where there is a little *d* in both halves, the parent must breed true to type as Rh-negative. All so-called Rh-negative people must, by definition, have a little *d* in each half of the genotype and are therefore homozygous. Heterozygous persons, though in reality half Rh-positive and half Rh-negative, will always be classified as Rh-positive because D is dominant to *d*.

The practical importance in obstetrics is that the heterozygous fathers have an even chance of passing on an Rh-negative gene, so that the child of an Rh-negative mother has an even chance of being itself Rh-negative and therefore most unlikely to be the victim of haemolytic disease. Only iso-immunisation to the less usual factors can prevent this rule from being an absolute certainty.

Showing Reactions using Standard Sera in Typing

Cells of Subgroup	*Fisher Classification*	*Anti-C (anti-Rh₁)*	*Anti-D (Standard anti-Rh)*	*Anti-E (anti-Rh₂)*	*Anti-c*
Rh_1	CD*e*	+	+	−	−
Rh_2	*c*DE	−	+	+	+
Rh′	C*de*	+	−	−	−
Rh″	*cd*E	−	−	+	+
Rh_y	C*d*E	+	−	+	−
Rh_o	*c*D*e*	−	+	−	+
Rh_z	CDE	+	+	+	−
Rh (rh)	*cde*	−	−	−	+

N.B.—Anti-D (standard anti-Rh) reacts with 85 per cent (normal Rh of population), but misses Rh′, Rh″, and Rh_y Anti-C reacts with 70 per cent of population and distinguishes Rh_2 (15 per cent of population).

Antibodies

Antibodies can be detected in the sera of iso-immunised individuals in varying titre. Now, as it happens, anti-D is not only the commonest but also the most serious, and it has been found that there are two types of anti-D, one of which agglutinates D cells suspended in saline and the other which fails to do so but renders them incapable of being subsequently agglutinated by the first-mentioned antibody, also known as the complete or saline anti-D. In other words, the second type has a blocking action. This blocking antibody, however, will agglutinate D cells if they are suspended in 20 per cent albumin. Alternative names for the blocking antibody are albumin or incomplete antibody. It has been found in experimental iso-immunisation of volunteers with injections spaced every three months that the titre of saline antibody rises at first and then subsequently falls, whereas the titre of albumin antibody rises steadily throughout, and it is thought that the albumin antibody probably represents a later development of the process of iso-immunisation- and therefore indicates a more advanced degree. This explains a well recognised clinical fact that the presence of albumin antibody in maternal serum indicates a far worse prognosis than in the case of saline antibody only and saline titre predominance usually signifies a better prognosis for the child. Albumin antibody is known to pass the placenta, but the saline variety probably does not, so that the former is the main factor in haemolytic disease.

It is more important to recognise the preponderance of one or other types of antibody than the actual level of titre. As is well known, the titre gives little indication of the severity of disease which may be expected in the child, and it may even rise somewhat in a pregnancy with an Rh-negative fetus which is not exposed to risk.

Clinical Picture

Clinically haemolytic disease takes the form of hydrops fetalis, icterus gravis neonatorum, of which kernicterus is often a sequel, and lastly congenital haemolytic anaemia.

Hydrops fetalis is almost invariably fatal and the child is usually stillborn. Mollison reckoned that somewhere between 5 and 10 per cent of all still births were due to haemolytic disease.[33, 34] The fetus usually dies *in utero*, characteristically about six weeks before term, although it may be much earlier. It is often pale and very oedematous, but occasionally may be macerated and show no sign of oedema. The oedema is commonly so severe as to influence the attitude which the baby adopts *in utero*. This is likened to the Buddha position (Fig. 1) and is of considerable diagnostic significance radiologically. In cases of hydrops there may also be seen, on X-ray, a halo round the scalp,

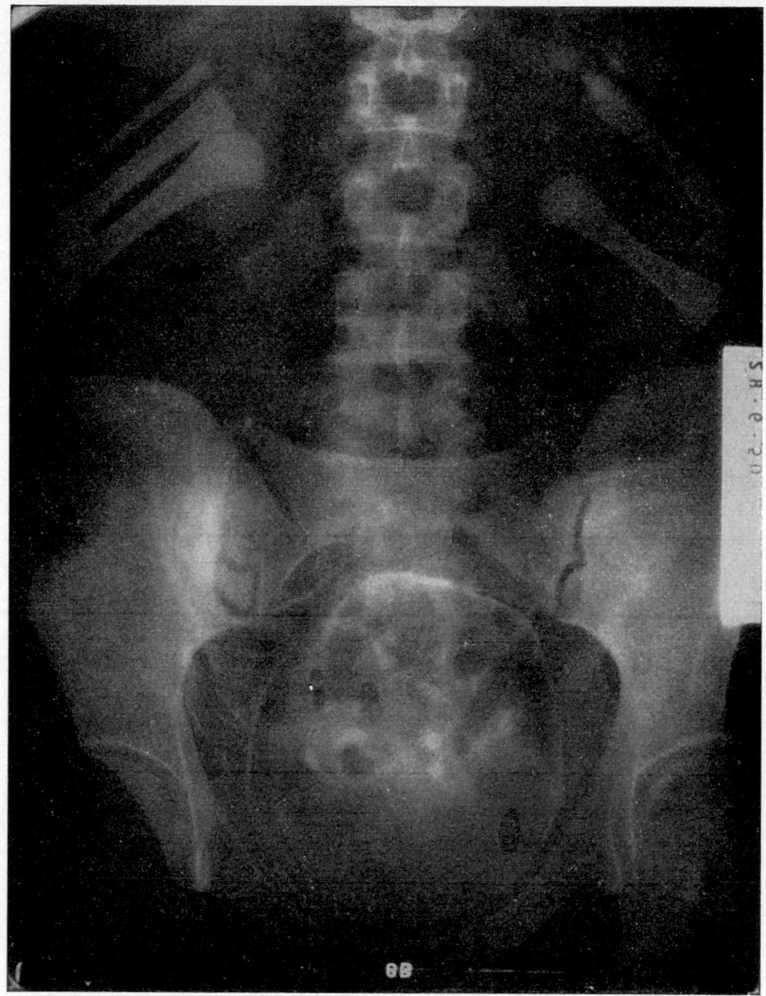

28/Fig. 1.—Hydrops. Inverted Buddha position.
(By courtesy of Prof. R. E. Steiner.)

but it is only significant if this halo is actually displaced from the skull, in which case it indicates intra-uterine death rather than hydrops (Barnett, personal communication).

Apart from the gross oedema which is usual, the liver and spleen are greatly enlarged as is the placenta which is pale and oedematous with swollen villi.

Premature labour is common, and even those cases born alive seldom live without treatment for more than a few hours. Haemolytic disease is not the only cause of fetal oedema at birth, but is certainly the commonest. Congenital syphilis and severe congenital heart disease may produce the same effect, and if in doubt the underlying diagnosis should be established serologically.

Icterus gravis neonatorum, the commonest variety, usually affects the babies born at term who, though initially apparently well, may become jaundiced within the hour or nearly always within the first twenty-four hours after birth. Progressive anaemia is also associated with the condition, but may be masked clinically by jaundice. The spleen and liver are usually enlarged.

This type of jaundice has to be distinguished from the physiological jaundice of neonatal life which is never so intense and comes on after the second day, is only transient and is not associated with anaemia.

The jaundice of prematurity has been fully described in the previous chapter. Although haemolytic in nature, the basis of this jaundice in the premature infant lies in its inability, because of immaturity, to deal with the products of physiological haemolysis. The mature liver of a baby born at term readily conjugates bilirubin with glucuronic acid, thus rendering it innocuous, but in prematurity the liver is less capable of dealing rapidly with free circulating bilirubin. Confusion with the jaundice of haemolytic disease may be encouraged by the early appearance of neurological signs, but serological tests should distinguish the two.

Congenital bile-duct atresia causes an obstructive type of jaundice which, however, does not make its appearance until after the first week of life. Again blood serology is negative.

Severe congenital syphilis may also cause jaundice, but other stigmata of syphilis are present, especially radiological evidences of osteochondritis, and the Wassermann reaction is positive.

Kernicterus.—After the first few days, the child suffering from icterus gravis neonatorum may develop signs of cerebral irritation with head retraction, twitchings and spasticity. Death occurs about the end of the first week, and at necropsy the basal ganglia of the brain are found to be stained with bilirubin. Some of the cases survive, but may later show signs of cerebral damage, choreo-athetosis, deafness and mental backwardness. The chances of kernicterus developing are largely proportional to the bilirubin concentration in the blood for, whereas in the normal child the serum bilirubin at birth is about 30 μmol/l, in icterus gravis the figure is 50–100 μmol/l at first, rising steeply thereafter to danger levels of over 275 μmol/l. The subject of hyperbilirubinaemia in the newborn is also fully described in the previous chapter.

Congenital haemolytic anaemia.—This is the mildest form of the disease, and haemolysis is sufficiently slow to prevent signs of jaundice appearing. The destruction of a child's Rh-positive cells can continue up to six weeks at a rate which, at any time, is unpredictable, but most of the damage is likely to occur within the first fortnight.

The blood shows a characteristically large number of nucleated red cells, seldom less than 10 for every 100 white cells present and occasionally as high as 200,000 per mm^3. The reticulocyte count may be as high as 10 per cent. These cases actually have the best prognosis, as they do not develop kernicterus and only the anaemia has to be treated; this presently burns itself out with the gradual elimination of maternal antibody.

Rh antibodies have been identified in the maternal milk, and for this reason the wisdom of allowing breast feeding has been questioned, but the general opinion nowadays is that the child is not likely to be harmed in this manner.

Rh TESTING

The determination of the Rh group of all pregnant patients should be made at the first antenatal visit and a test for the presence of antibodies should be done in the case of all who are Rh-negative, whatever their parity. It is now the practice of most modern units to screen all patients for antibodies regardless of their Rhesus group, as occasionally other antibodies will be discovered.[45] These rarer types of antibodies can themselves cause haemolytic disease and would otherwise be missed. The scheme in use is to screen all patients using a sensitive enzyme-treated cell test. This screening is repeated in Rh-negative women at the 28th week and 34th to 36th week of gestation as well, but if in any patient an antibody is detected, the antibody titre is estimated at least every month from the time of its discovery onwards and the husband's blood is also obtained for grouping and genotyping. It is on the basis of this type of screening that the programme for amniocentesis is worked out. If the antibody test at the 34th week is positive following a negative test at booking, it suggests that immunisation has occurred in the course of this pregnancy. This is a definite but uncommon risk. The antibody titre is only loosely related to the degree of haemolytic disease in the child, but any preponderance of albumin antibodies, whatever the titre, is more ominous. The acquisition of this information at about the 34th week of pregnancy allows plenty of time for arrangements for delivery to be made in an institution.

For testing maternal blood for the presence of antibodies about 5 ml should be collected in a clean bottle without oxalate or any anti-clotting substance.

AMNIOCENTESIS

This is indicated whenever the antibody Coombs' titre rises to more than 1:8, or when there is a history of a previously severely affected baby that was either stillborn or required exchange transfusion. The amniocentesis is first carried out at any time between the 25th and the 32nd week of gestation depending upon history or titre. The purpose of amniocentesis is to determine the level of bilirubin and bilirubinoid substances within the liquor, whose concentration exactly reflects the degree to which the baby is affected with haemolytic disease. Using a full aseptic technique a lumbar puncture needle of gauge 18 is inserted through the abdominal wall into the amniotic cavity. Too fine a needle becomes too easily blocked by vernix caseosa. A local infiltration with 1 per cent lignocaine provides all the anaesthetic that is necessary and the main difficulty in the operation is finding a free pool of liquor amnii from which 10 ml can be withdrawn. This can be difficult especially in later pregnancy when the liquor is more scanty, but mainly in cases of occipito-posterior postition, frank breech presentation and in the very obese patient.

When the placenta is on the anterior uterine wall there may be difficulty in avoiding it, so that instead of liquor blood is withdrawn and I have seen a case of fatal fetal intra-amniotic haemorrhage from this sort of accident. It is our invariable practice now always to locate the placenta by sonar, not just in a general sort of way but to establish its precise margins, before ever undertaking amniocentesis. Traversing the placenta may indeed cause a leak of fetal red cells into the maternal circulation and this is reputed to increase the degree of iso-immunisation and to worsen the subsequent prognosis in later pregnancies, although it is unlikely to have much immediate effect on the present pregnancy because it takes some weeks for further degrees of iso-immunisation to occur. However reports from Newcastle,[12, 13] reviewing a fairly large number of cases of amniocentesis, states that there is no real evidence that amniocentesis increases the severity of haemolytic disease in the current or subsequent pregnancy, nor directly alters the maternal antibody titre. Most of us would, however, regard any possible feto-maternal transfusion as undesirable and would avoid it if we could, hence the desirability of accurate localisation of the placenta first.

It is as well to take note of the position and attitude of the fetus and with arms and legs flexed a gap can definitely be palpated between the upper and lower limbs in an area in which diminished resistance can also be palpated.[40] In this region the needle is inserted at right angles to the skin. This point will usually be found on the side opposite to the baby's back and below the umbilicus, except in breech presentation when it may be higher. In over 1,000 such cases in Manchester there were no complications such as premature labour or placental abruption and the operation was successful in 95 per cent of cases. Where the specimen of liquor amnii is bloodstained it may still be serviceable if immediately centrifuged and filtered.

An alternative approach is the space behind the fetal neck, but this too can be unrewarding.

If the presenting part can be satisfactorily displaced upwards, well out of the pelvis, a transisthmic approach below it in the midline may prove less traumatic, but the bladder must be assuredly empty.[1] Specimens of urine sent by mistake seldom evoke charitable comments from one's laboratory colleagues!

The sample of liquor may have been contaminated from previous bloody taps but the discoloration is more brown or red-brown and cloudy than in the case of massive intrafetal haemolysis.[9]

It is no longer safe to regard the depth of golden coloration of the liquor as a reliable index of the severity of the disease as even fairly pale specimens may, on proper analysis, indicate quite high levels of bilirubin. Specimens should therefore be subjected to spectrophotometric analysis.

It is important to protect the specimen from strong light and therefore it should be collected and sent to the laboratory in a dark glass bottle. If there is any likely delay in testing the specimen it should be refrigerated.

Immediately after amniocentesis a specimen of maternal blood should be taken by venepuncture and tested for the presence of fetal cells as an index of feto-maternal transfusion, which is particularly likely if the placenta has been pierced. Since taking the precaution of localising the placenta by sonar and avoiding it, the incidence of demonstrable feto-maternal bleeding has been strikingly reduced.[45]

If in an Rh-negative woman the tap is bloodstained she should be given 50–100 μg of anti-D immunoglobulin there and then (see later). This precaution will not harm the fetus.

The specimen is centrifuged to remove vernix and is now examined for its bilirubin content and associated bilirubinoid substances. For this purpose spectrophotometry is quicker and more accurate than biochemical methods of estimation. Liley (1963) reported there were at least seven bilirubinoid pigments which contributed to the optical density absorption peak at 450 mμ.

The optical density of the liquor is plotted on semi-logarithmic paper against a range of wavelengths ranging from 350 mμ to 700 mμ. Interest is concentrated at the 450 mμ range, but it is worthless to take a reading of optical density there without taking into account the curve as a whole, as it is the deviation from the normal curve at 450 mμ which matters, and bilirubinoid pigment is quantitated by the optical density deviation from the normal curve at this wavelength. This precaution is necessary because a number of factors affect the range of optical density of the liquor amnii as a whole. Plotting the optical densities at each wavelength on the ordinate logarithmically and the actual wavelengths on the abscissa axis, the absorption curve of normal liquor will be seen to be more or less a straight line within the range of 365 to 600 mμ, but where there is a concentration of bilirubin-like pigments there is a deviation from this more or less straight line at approximately 450 mμ with a slightly less consistent peak at 415 mμ (Liley, 1961). A baseline is therefore drawn tangentially to the curve at approximately 365 mμ to the 550 mμ level and the height of the bulge or deviation at 450 mμ in terms of difference of optical density gives the quantity of pigment present (Fig. 2).

Normally the pigmentation of liquor amnii as a whole diminishes with increasing maturity which therefore has the effect of accentuating the significance of the "deviation bulge" in later weeks (Fig. 3). It is thus important to know the maturity. Therefore, for any given period of gestation the height of the spectrophotometric bulge at 450 mμ falls within one of the three well-known Liley zones. In Zone 1 (the lowest), the baby is either unaffected or only mildly so and can probably safely be allowed to go to term. In the intermediate Zone 2, which is a somewhat unreliable zone on which to base a prognosis, the baby can probably be allowed to develop *in utero* beyond the 34th week, but is likely to require premature delivery. In Zone 3, the highest zone, the baby is very severely affected and intra-uterine death is either imminent or hydrops fetalis already likely. If this state of affairs exists after the 34th week immediate delivery should be undertaken and, if before the 34th week, when the degree of prematurity would wreck any chances of survival, only intra-uterine transfusion may be able to stave off disaster and may, especially if repeated, allow a little more time for further development *in utero* in order to achieve a degree of viability some time after the 34th week. Nevertheless Liley (1963) in a study of 400 cases warned that there were possible errors in assessing the severity of haemolytic disease, often from examining the wrong fluid, of which the commonest is probably fetal urine from puncture of the bladder, or fetal ascitic fluid, or the liquor of a twin sac or from aspirating an undiagnosed ovarian cyst.

This last improbable accident has happened in my own unit and when the patient complained of the cessation of movements after amniocentesis it was assumed that intra-uterine death had occurred. Unfortunately the antibody titre also appeared to rise and intra-uterine death seemed certain. This provided yet another instance of attempts to induce labour with repeated oxytocin drips in what was an ovarian cyst in a

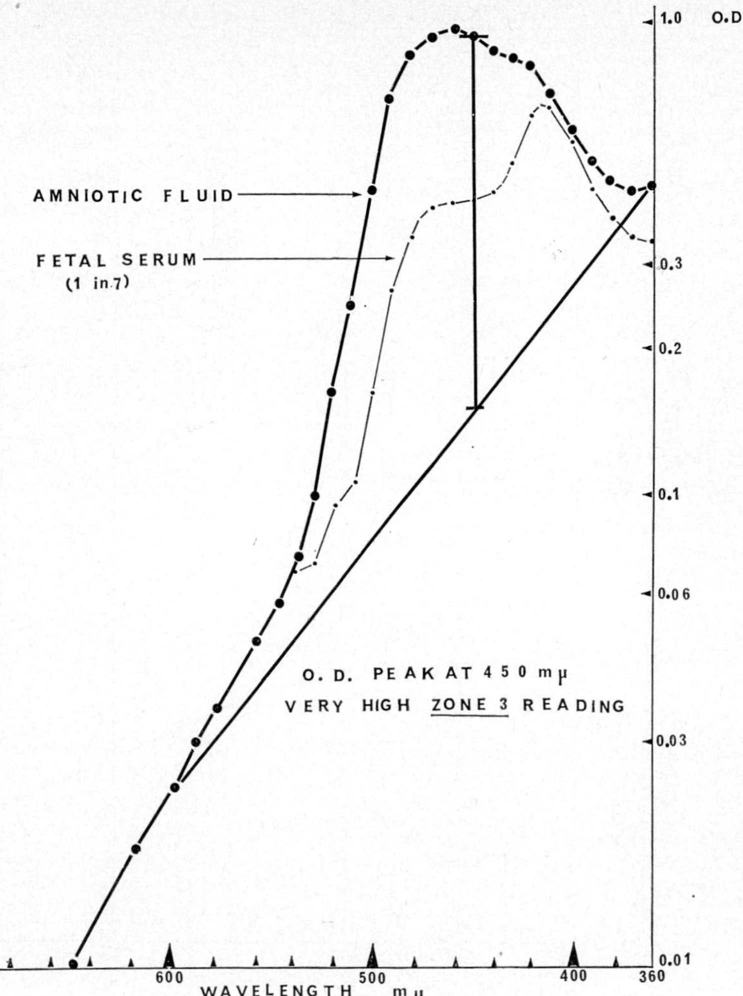

28/FIG. 2.—Shows the "bulge" at 450 mμ demonstrating the deviation from a normal optical density curve. The fetal serum levels of bilirubin mirror those of liquor amnii.

(By courtesy of Dr. M. L. N. Willoughby.)

patient who was not pregnant at all. There were many other unfortunate aspects to this case, inasmuch as the patient had had an illegitimate pregnancy before marriage, about which her husband was in ignorance, had iso-immunised in that pregnancy and had had a series of disasters thereafter, so that there was a large psychological guilt factor, and the husband's reaction was mainly one of fury at the suggestion that his

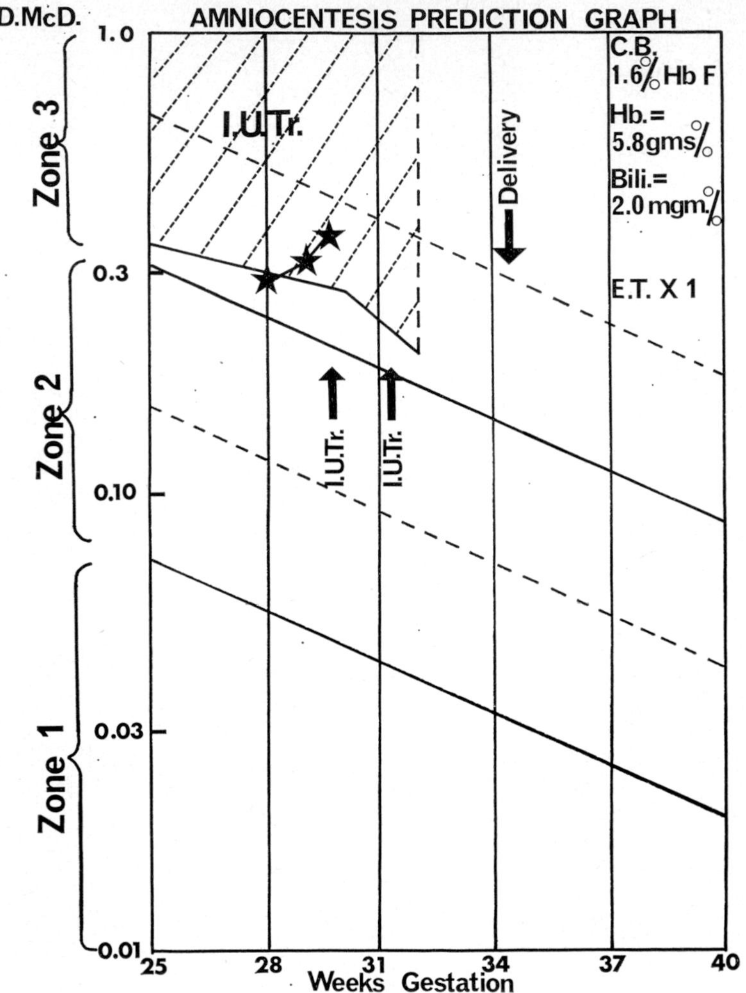

28/Fig. 3.—Successful case, brought to reasonable maturity by intra-uterine transfusion on basis of zoning prognostication and requiring exchange transfusion (E.T.) after delivery.

(By courtesy of Dr. M. L. N. Willoughby.)

wife hadn't even been pregnant, as though this were a matter for personal reflection on himself.

The other source of error which Liley pointed out was the estimation of the wrong pigment due to contamination with blood or serum, meconium and in cases of duodenal atresia, and he strongly recommended what is now the common practice of repeated testing, especially in Zone 2 cases, to indicate in which direction the prognostic trend is developing.

The value, therefore, of repeated amniocentesis and spectrophotometric analysis in relation to the Liley zones is that they not only indicate when heroic measures such as intra-uterine transfusion are necessary in order to prevent intra-uterine death before the 34th week, but also (and this is perhaps even more valuable numerically) they prevent many a case from being induced unnecessarily early and must by now have avoided many deaths from unwarranted prematurity (Fig. 3).

Testing the Baby at Birth

As soon as the baby is born, 10 ml of cord blood should be collected in a heparinised tube for haemoglobin estimation and Coombs' testing. The blood can be collected from the placental end of the severed cord but, to avoid contamination with Wharton's jelly, it should not be squeezed out. If the cord is not clamped early the haemoglobin level rises. Therefore, in order to get a true picture, a sample should be taken at once. An affected baby is bound to have a positive Coombs' test so that an answer should be very readily available. A blood smear is also made for the detection of immature red cells.

The haemoglobin level at birth is an important part of the investigation, as it gives a quantitative as well as qualitative index of the severity of the disease, since the length of survival without treatment is more or less proportional to the haemoglobin concentration. Lastly the serum bilirubin is estimated.

Coombs' Anti-human Globulin Test

Since the antibodies whose presence we are seeking are contained in the globulin fraction of human serum, the test is made with rabbit serum which has been sensitised to human globulin. An Rh-positive child (who is therefore at risk) has cells which have been exposed to Rh antibody and will therefore have adsorbed antibody on to the cell surfaces. As a result of this, rabbit anti-human globulin serum will agglutinate them, but it is first necessary to remove all the remaining human globulin present in the specimen of the child's serum. This is done by washing the cells with saline.

The method is to take about ½ ml of cord blood to which is added at least 10 ml of normal saline and mix by repeatedly inverting the tube. The mixture is now spun down for two minutes and the supernatant saline is removed with a pipette and replaced with more fresh saline. This washing in saline is repeated two or three times and removes any antibody which is not fixed to the red cells and which might neutralise the anti-globulin in the rabbit serum. A 10 per cent suspension is now made of these washed red cells in saline, and one drop of the suspension is placed on a clean tile with one drop of diluted anti-human globulin serum. Control tests are set up with normal saline instead of the rabbit serum and, as additional safeguards, cells which are known to be sensitised and cells known to be unsensitised are also set up against the testing serum. The tile is gently rocked in a warm atmosphere for up to seven minutes and agglutination denotes a direct positive Coombs' test. Since the fetal red cells may be affected as early as the 5th month of pregnancy, the Coombs' test may be positive from that time onwards.

The Place of Induction of Premature Labour

Although antibodies can cross the placenta to the fetus from the end of the first half of pregnancy, the worst damage appears to be done in the last four weeks of pregnancy. A balance has therefore to be struck between increasing damage from haemolytic disease due to continued existence *in utero*, and the dangers of prematurity which the baby so affected stands badly. Amniocentesis, however, has taken the guesswork out of the management and it is far better to deliver a baby prematurely and carry out exchange transfusion than to encourage undue haemolysis by hanging on too long. Only the mildest cases, therefore, should be allowed to go as far as term and postmaturity has nothing whatever to be said for it as an additional complication. The premature induction of labour therefore has the largest single place in the obstetrical management. The purpose of induction is to secure delivery and if the induction hangs fire delivery should be secured by vaginal bypass if necessary and without hesitation. Needless to say expert paediatric services must be immediately on hand.

Where a previous stillborn is definitely attributable to haemolytic disease and the father is homozygous, the chances of recurrent stillbirth are so high (90 per cent) if spontaneous labour is awaited, that premature delivery either by induction or by Caesarean section is called for.[39]

It is unfortunate that estimation of the lecithin:sphingomyelin ratio of the liquor amnii is less than usually reliable in assessing fetal maturity from the point of view of neonatal respiratory distress, for, as with maternal diabetes, the progressive rise towards term of this ratio may not occur.[42] It is therefore difficult to choose the optimum moment for delivery, and one may wait too long, with a resultant intra-uterine death.

Intra-uterine Transfusion

Delivery before the 34th week is so readily rewarded by a neonatal death that every attempt should be made to secure this degree of maturity at least, but the most severely affected babies are liable to die *in utero* often long before this time. In order to stave off intra-uterine death, intra-uterine transfusion, introduced by Liley in 1963, provides hope of salvage in these desperate cases. Success greeted him in the fourth case in which the operation was performed. In the first two cases the fetus was already hydropic and death followed within 24 hours of the transfusion and in the third previous case a mildly hydropic fetus died *in utero* after the second transfusion undertaken at 33 weeks.

This procedure has captured the imagination of the whole obstetrical world, because it represents the first successful attempt at directly correcting a fetal disorder before birth. Using local anaesthesia and an 8-cm Tuohy needle of gauge 16, Liley found that the layers of the uterine wall and abdominal wall of the fetus could be identified especially by observing the resistance encountered to saline injection.

The principle of intra-uterine transfusion is based upon the fact that the fetus very readily absorbs blood directly from the peritoneal cavity, far more readily so in fact than an adult, and on examination of a case successfully transfused and badly in need of it, a high preponderance of donor cells instead of the fetal cells belonging to the baby is found. Having entered the peritoneal cavity with the Tuohy needle, a Portex epidural catheter is fed down the needle which is then withdrawn, and confirmation that the catheter is, in fact, in the peritoneal cavity is confirmed by observing the biconcave shadows radiologically of a radio-opaque dye, such as 3 ml of Urografin, lying between loops of bowel and under the diaphragm. Warmed, packed cells, Rhesus-negative of course, are now slowly injected over about 20 minutes into the peritoneal cavity in amounts ranging, according to the size and maturity of the baby, up to about 110 ml. This success was quickly followed up in Lewisham, London.[19, 20] A rough guide as to the quantity of blood to be transfused is to calculate the number of weeks gestation over 20 and to multiply by ten, e.g. at 30 weeks 100 ml would be an appropriate amount. Fortnightly intra-uterine transfusions are usual as all donor cells are likely to have been absorbed by then. In fact, there is post-mortem evidence that the blood is completely absorbed within ten days of the intraperitoneal transfusion and that the process may even occur earlier.[20] Fetal movements already begin to improve by then. The X-ray dosages involved in the procedure may be considerable, and figures as high as 35 rads to the maternal skin and about 3 rads to the fetus have been suggested, though not as yet confirmed.[3] To reduce the irradiation dosage, an image intensifier is recommended and is particularly useful in the earlier weeks of pregnancy in helping to identify the position of the fetal intestines. This is achieved by injecting 15 ml of Urografin about a day before the proposed intra-uterine transfusion. The fetus swallows the dye and thus shows up its own intestines.

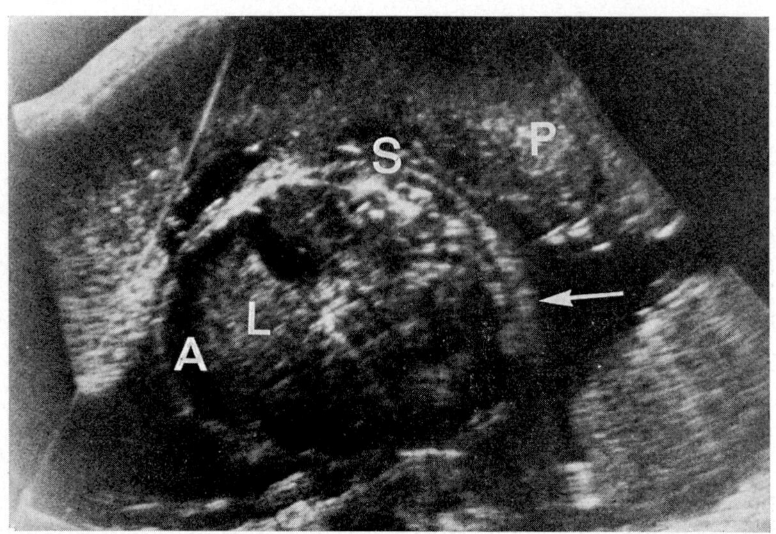

28/Fig. 4.—Fetal ascites displayed by sonar. Note ascites (A), liver (L), fetal spine (S), and hydropic placenta (P). Arrow marks the oedematous abdominal wall. Transverse section through fetal trunk. Diasonograph grey-scale picture.
(By courtesy, Dr Roger Wild, Western General Hospital, Edinburgh.)

If straight radiography demonstrates hydrops fetalis, failure is almost certain, but minor degrees may not be beyond help. Radiological assessment may show a small increase in the thickness of the scalp or the subcutaneous tissues over spine and ribs following the injection of contrast medium into the amniotic cavity.[5] The scapula may likewise be displaced away from the ribs because of the thickening of the soft tissues of the shoulder, but scalp thickness probably represents the best index of severity of hydrops.

Sometimes a severe degree of fetal ascites can be demonstrated by sonar (Fig. 4). To pump blood into a peritoneal cavity already distended with fluid is to invite cardiac failure in the fetus and this accounts for some of the mortality attending the operation. It is highly desirable to remove as much fluid as possible (in our experience over 50 to 100 ml) before injecting the blood.

The operation sounds very much more easy than in fact it is, because the area of abdominal wall through which access to the peritoneal cavity is sought with a needle is often very limited and all sorts of structures may be inadvertently pierced, such as lung, liver and particularly fetal bladder, which is often distended with about 50 ml of urine. Injection of the test dye into the bladder shows a torpedo-shaped shadow rather than the biconcave shadows surrounding loops of bowel. If the tip of the needle is in some inappropriate part of the baby, such as muscle for example, there will be resistance to saline injection, and if the needle is not inside the fetus at all, any dye injected will be so immediately diluted as not to be properly visible.[5] As accurate an image as possible must be in the operator's mind of the exact position and attitude of the fetus, and this will depend as much upon palpation as upon radiography, although the application of skin markers to the mother's abdominal wall may help in the identification of landmarks.

Warmed, packed cells are used and the injection is then topped up with 2 g of albumin in 10 ml to combat hypoproteinaemia in the fetus. It is usually recommended, too, that blood be stored for a brief period not exceeding a day or two in order to kill off the lymphocytes. Regional Transfusion Centres have, with the object of removing donor lymphocytes, adjusting the haemoglobin content, and facilitating administration, traditionally supplied washed cells. But in our region in recent years there have been two disasters from infection which these premature and moribund babies have had little ability to withstand. The practice has now given way to that of supplying unwashed cells, since the hypothetical danger of colonising the fetus with donor lymphocytes is less than that of infection.[41]

In assessing the success of intra-uterine transfusion, account should be taken of the maturity at which it is performed, because the later in pregnancy the better will be the apparent results,[13] particularly if some unnecessary operations are included. It may well indeed be that the indications for intra-uterine transfusion will be extended in the future as a result of present enthusiasm, but Liley has reminded us that "what is necessary is more important than what is possible and extreme measures are best reserved for extreme situations".

Maternal Plasmaphaeresis

From Canada in 1968 came a report of the attempt to remove maternal antibodies by repeated and intensive plasmaphaeresis, i.e. separating the mother's red cells from her plasma and returning them to her suspended in plasma from healthy Rh-negative donors. [4]The authors certainly demonstrated the speed with which the antibodies are re-formed within a very few days, and doubted the efficacy of the treatment. Nevertheless, after removing 46 litres of plasma over a nine-week period, the fetus survived in spite of a neglible reduction in Rh antibody titre.

We, too, have had some success with this very drastic treatment, undertaken twice or thrice weekly in desperate cases. It was certainly a psychological ordeal for the mother, especially, as so often happened, the baby died during later intra-uterine transfusion, or shortly thereafter. The policy was therefore changed in favour of continuing plasmaphaeresis and avoiding intra-uterine transfusion until the baby could be safely delivered.[46] Under this regime two out of three babies survived, the third dying from the respiratory distress syndrome.

Since then a much larger combined series has come from Liverpool and Bristol.[17] From these reports it would appear that maternal plasmaphaeresis has a very real contribution to make, although elimination of intra-uterine transfusion is unlikely, in spite of its hazards for the baby.

Exchange Transfusion

This operation has made an enormous difference to the chances of affected babies who survive delivery. It is greatly superior to "topping up" or simple transfusion, and it has the further advantage that a great deal of the excess bilirubin is at the same time removed from the baby's circulation, thus reducing the chances of kernicterus developing. Mollison introduced the technique to this country and convinced us in an early series by losing only 8 out of 62 cases so treated, whereas 36 out of 54 treated by simple transfusion succumbed. Other advantages of exchange transfusion are that the child is put right as a rule in one go and the antibodies passively acquired from the mother are also to a large extent quantitatively eliminated, whereas with simple transfusion the antibodies remain as a hangover and the process may have to be repeated many times.

Although most exchange transfusions will be undertaken within the first 24 hours of the baby's life it is nevertheless necessary to repeat the operation, sometimes more than once, especially with high serum bilirubin levels, in the course of the first week. Attempts to maintain the serviceability of the umbilical stump by saline dressings usually fail because the base of the cord stump dries in spite of the dressings. It is far better to cut right down to the root of the umbilicus and it is then usually possible to catheterise the umbilical vein up to the sixth day. If there is any difficulty in identifying the vein in the umbilical stump, Yong (1965) recommended applying a small artery forceps on either side of the umbilical rim and turning the forceps outwards, thus everting the umbilicus, when the vein will be revealed. On rare instances where the umbilical bed is deep he suggested making two small incisions in the umbilical rim above and below, in order to facilitate the eversion of the umbilicus by further rotating the artery forceps outwards.

Indications for Exchange Transfusion at Birth

1. A haemoglobin less than 105 per cent (15·5 g);
2. Cases of prematurity with a positive Coombs' test regardless of the haemoglobin level, because of the increased liability to kernicterus;
3. All cases of very rapidly developing jaundice in which the serum bilirubin exceeds 5 mg per cent;
4. All cases in which there is a history of previous severely affected infants, provided the Coombs' test is, in this instance, positive.

Requirements for Exchange Transfusion

Rh-negative blood, of the same ABO group as the baby's, must be used, in order to avoid the effects of the possible presence of anti-A or anti-B agglutinins. Nowadays one is usually aware in advance of the possible need for an exchange transfusion before the baby is even born and blood should be obtained in advance and cross-matched with the mother's own serum. The former practice of packing the red cells has now been abandoned and, in fact, the less the blood is interfered with before transfusion the better. The blood should not be more than five days old and the amount required is about 80–100 ml per half kg of body weight. With larger children, therefore, a litre of blood should be available for the operation in order to provide sufficient cells.

The following instruments are required:

Two 20-ml syringes;
Two three-way cocks connected in series;
Umbilical vein catheters, No. 6 or No. 9;
Heparin saline solution 1 ml (1,000 Toronto units) in 100 ml normal saline;
Saline manometer.

Technique of Exchange Transfusion

Death may occur with cardiac failure and a high venous pressure. The operation should always start, therefore, with the withdrawal of 40 to 50 ml of blood as a form of venesection before pumping in any of the Rh-negative blood, so that the operation is conducted throughout at a discount.

The baby is placed on an electric blanket and full aseptic ritual is observed. A mucus extractor, preferably a mechanical type of sucker, should be available for immediate use. The cord is sliced to a length of about 1 cm and profuse bleeding indicates a high venous pressure.

The arteries seldom bleed. The vein is identified and seized with very fine forceps and the polyvinyl catheter is introduced. Usually some obstruction is encountered at the level of the abdominal wall, and it can be negotiated more easily by pulling the cord downwards towards the child's pubis in order to straighten out the vein. Occasionally the cord itself is not negotiable, in which case it is advisable to shorten it. About 7 cm length of catheter is inserted and the saline manometer is connected. A refinement is to read the manometer with the help of a ruler and a spirit level led from the front of the infant's chest to the manometer scale in order to get an accurate zero reading. Normally the venous pressure is between 2 and 4 cm of saline and higher pressures make preliminary venesection of about 50 ml obligatory, before proceeding to the exchange transfusion. All the apparatus should be flushed from time to time with heparinised saline and a nurse should be at hand to maintain a pumping score.

On no account should the operation be hurried, and a minimum time of 1½ hours should be allowed. Twenty ml of the child's blood are sucked out and 20 ml of donor blood are given back in return. The individual exchange amounts should not exceed 20 ml at a time, and in small, premature infants the amounts should be less. About two and a half minutes should be allowed for the introduction of each 20 ml, and the rate of giving should be both slow and consistently even. The venous pressure should be estimated with a manometer from time to time and a careful watch kept against overloading. The operation is not without its immediate mortality, and these babies are very liable to collapse suddenly, so that one cannot be too careful.

Donor blood preserved in acid-citrate-dextrose has a pH as low as 6·5 and there is indeed danger of aggravating a metabolic acidosis already present in the newborn.[2, 30] This adds to the hazards of exchange transfusion and it is recommended that one milli-equivalent of sodium bicarbonate be given for every 100 ml of blood transfused and in fact it is desirable to carry out acid-base estimations both before transfusion and during it.

Because of the risk of tetany from the use of citrated blood, 2 ml of calcium gluconate in 10 per cent solution can be given every 20 minutes throughout the procedure, or 1 ml of this solution for every 100 ml of blood given.

By this means an 80–90 per cent replacement of the baby's blood is achieved. A repeat exchange transfusion is often necessary in order to get rid of excess circulating bilirubin and thereby to prevent kernicterus, and it is obligatory to estimate the serum bilirubin every day for the first few days. If the level exceeds 20 mg per cent, the exchange transfusion should be repeated. This should be done very slowly, possibly in two parts, to allow tissue bilirubin to be got rid of. The continued serviceability of the umbilical vein is best maintained over a few days by the insertion of a marker—a sort of polythene spigot.

Even the most severe cases with haemoglobin levels below 50 per cent may be salved by this dramatic procedure, but in these cases the need for patience and slow replacement is even greater.

Adjuvant therapy, such as phototherapy, should of course be maintained (see chapter on Prematurity). Phenobarbitone is also useful because of its ability to increase glucuronyltransferase enzyme activity in the fetal and neonatal liver, concerned with bilirubin clearance from the plasma. The recommended dose of phenobarbitone is 2 mg/kg of body weight, administered 6–8-hourly.[31]

Late Prognosis

Considering how ill and how premature these babies often are it is surprising that the long-term results are as good as they are.[36] Mental subnormality, and hearing defects have to be watched for, but it is difficult at present to distribute blame amongst the various factors of prematurity, hyperbilirubinaemia, and hypoxia. These are cases where salvage can be particularly rewarding.

Future Pregnancies

Once a woman has had one affected child the outlook for further children is likely to be no better, but much will depend upon whether the husband is homozygous or heterozygous. Unfortunately, about three-quarters of the fathers of affected children are in fact homozygous, in which case the outlook is bleak for the particular marriage in this respect, because there is a tendency for the disease to be more severe in each successive instance. However impressive intra-uterine transfusion, how much better to prevent iso-immunisation in the first place!

The work of Finn *et al.* (1961) started off the experimental studies on prevention of Rh haemolytic disease. This team in Liverpool[6] have used a modification of the Kleihauer method of detecting fetal blood cells in the maternal blood by using a citric-phosphate buffer, and on blood smear the adult cells appear as ghosts but the fetal red cells as dark, refractile bodies. Alternative staining techniques with Biebrich scarlet and aniline blue have been claimed to give fewer false positive results than the traditional Kleihauer test.[10] They have thus investigated the incidence of transplacental fetal bleeding, its relation to Rh antibodies and the time at which this type of bleeding occurs in pregnancy.[6, 7, 8, 11] It would appear that the placental barrier normally protects five out of six women at risk from iso-immunisation, at least until damage to the placental barrier is inflicted at labour. These workers then tried to prevent iso-immunisation in male Rh-negative volunteers by injecting anti-D serum shortly after a sensitising dose of Rh-positive cells tagged with radiochromium. The anti-serum coated a lot of the Rh-positive cells and caused the disappearance of more than half of them within two days. This led to the suggestion that Rh-negative women might be given an injection of blocking anti-D serum immediately after labour to protect them from sensitisation by destroying the Rh-positive cells, which at this time are particularly likely to invade the maternal bloodstream. Clearly, however, this prophylaxis would achieve nothing in those who were already immunised by fetal red cells before labour.

Where the fetal blood, however, is incompatible with the mother's the fetal cells are at once destroyed. It will be seen therefore that ABO incompatibility between fetus and mother provides almost complete protection against Rh iso-immunisation. This early work has since come to ample fruition and it is interesting to note that Professor Clarke described in his Lumleian Lecture to the Royal College of Physicians in London in 1967 that his interest in these genetic studies in Rh-haemolytic disease was fostered by his study of the evolution of mimicry in certain types of butterfly. The research was carried a stage further by roughly the same Liverpool team headed by Clarke (1963). A combined study was then undertaken in a number of centres in England and in Baltimore, the English groups including Liverpool, Sheffield, Leeds and Bradford. The final results have fully confirmed that a high degree of protection can thus be obtained.[35]

These workers, using groups of Rh-negative male volunteers (who in Liverpool were blood donors, but in Baltimore were inmates of the Maryland State Penitentiary), sought to coat the antigenic Rh-positive erythrocytes with incomplete anti-D, since this prevents antibody formation when subsequent injections of Rh-positive cells are made into Rh-negative circulations, thus demonstrating the blocking action of incomplete antibody. By this means they found that it was possible to give three or four stimuli in the form of Rh-positive cells without the development of immune antibodies in three out of twenty-one people previously treated with plasma containing predominantly incomplete antibodies. These workers believe that it is necessary to clear about 95 per cent of injected cells finding their way into the circulation within 24 hours of entry if the antibody production is to be prevented. It looks as though this can, in fact, be achieved with anti-D antibody which is without saline activity but with a high incomplete titre. To overcome the risks of hepatitis a concentrated gamma-globulin preparation containing incomplete anti-D antibodies only is desirable.

The evidence would now appear to be overwhelming that a very large majority of cases at risk of sensitisation to the D-antigen can be protected by a timely injection of anti-D gamma globulin which, if it is to be effective, must be given within the first 36 hours following delivery, as it is during labour that the greatest feto-maternal bleeds may occur. This does not deny the existence of possible leaks of fetal cells into the maternal circulation during pregnancy, which could produce immunisation before delivery itself, and for this reason the Winnipeg workers have favoured the giving of small antenatal doses of anti-D gamma globulin, not in themselves sufficient to harm the fetus, in order to clear the maternal circulation of these cells during pregnancy.[18]

Supplies of anti-D immunoglobulin are at last adequate. This requires the immunisation of male volunteers, and post-menopausal women volunteers, prepared to be deliberately immunised and to make regular donations of their serum. Plasmaphaeresis, the process of removing erythrocytes from the patient's serum and then returning them to him, will help to improve supplies, and it is estimated that 15 donors each providing a litre of plasma per month could serve a population of one million.

It is now possible to implement the following recommendations:

A standard dose of 100 μg anti-D immunoglobulin should be given to all Rh-negative women having Rh(D)-positive babies, within 60 hours of delivery and preferably less, regardless of parity or ABO compatibility.

For Rh-negative women having a pregnancy terminated or aborting spontaneously before the 20th week of gestation the standard dose is 50 μg.

All such cases requiring anti-D immunoglobulin should also be screened by some test such as the Kleihauer, to detect large feto-maternal haemorrhages (e.g. more than 2 fetal cells per low-power field), in which case a larger dose may have to be given, or repeated, at once, and further screening carried out until they are free of all fetal cells.

Rh-negative women having procedures or episodes which might damage the placenta should also have the benefit of prophylaxis and screening. Such events as amniocentesis, antepartum bleeding and external version under anaesthesia should be so regarded. The smaller 50 μg dose should suffice for pregnancy of less than 20 weeks gestation but otherwise the dose is 100 μg, and screening is desirable as well.

For screening, a 10 ml venous sample should be taken, of which 2 ml are placed in a citrate tube. At delivery the same amount of cord blood should be taken. The specimens are then tested for Rh and ABO grouping and the presence or absence of Rh antibodies. Where indicated, Kleihauer testing should be carried out.

At the same time the baby's blood can be Coombs tested and the levels of bilirubin and haemoglobin estimated.

The object of the Kleihauer test is to detect major feto-maternal bleeds. It is too insensitive to eliminate the need for prophylactic treatment of eligible cases in general.

100 μg of anti-D immunoglobulin can neutralise 4 ml of fetal cells, which latter should disappear from the maternal blood within about six hours. This constitutes a form of therapeutic titration.

This vigorous policy should, within a generation reduce the Rh problem to about a tenth of its present size but it can never eliminate it altogether.

Women will rightfully come to demand the protection of their children from Rh haemolytic disease.

The question of therapeutic abortion and sterilisation may arise, but there is no legal or ethical sanction for taking such a drastic step, and it has to be remembered that the patient might one day remarry, possibly an Rh-negative second husband. Even a history of repeated stillbirths due to haemolytic disease does not rule out the possibility of a subsequent survivor.

REFERENCES

1. Amy, J. J. (1973). *Europ. J. Obstet. reprod. Biol.*, **3/5,** 167.
2. Barrie, H. (1965). *Lancet*, **2,** 712.
3. Blackwell, R. J. (1934). Personal communication.
4. Bouman, J. M., Peddle, L. J. and Anderson, C. (1968). *Vox Sang. (Basel)*, **15,** 272.
5. Campbell, B. L. (1966). *Brit. J. Radiol.*, **39,** 81.
6. Clarke, C. A., Donohoe, W. T. A., McConnell, R. B., Woodrow, J. C., Finn, R., Krevans, J. R., Kulke, W., Lehane, D. and Sheppard, P. M. (1963). *Brit. med. J.*, **1,** 979.
7. Clarke, C. A. (1967). *Brit. med. J.*, **2,** 7.
8. Clarke, C. A. (1967). *Brit. med. J.*, **4,** 7.
9. Clayton, E. M., Waller, D. H. and Foster, E. B. (1969). *Obstet. and Gynec.*, **34,** 641.
10. Clayton, E. M., Foster, E. B. and Clayton, E. P. (1970). *Obstet. and Gynec.*, **35,** 642.
11. Clayton, E. M., Waller, D. H., Foster, E. B. and Dudley, R. B. (1970). *Amer. J. Obstet. Gynec.*, **107,** 704.
12. Fairweather, D. V. I., Murray, S., Parkin, D. and Walker, W. (1963). *Lancet*, **2,** 1190.
13. Fairweather, D. V. I., Tacchi, D., Coxon, A., Hughes, M. I., Murray, S. and Walker, W. (1967). *Brit. med. J.*, **2,** 189.
14. Finn, R. (1970). *Brit. med. J.*, **2,** 219.

15. Finn, R., Clarke, C. A., Donohoe, W. T. A., McConnell, R. B., Sheppard, P. M., Lehane, D. and Kulke, W. (1961). *Brit. med. J.*, **1,** 1486.
16. Fraser, I. D. and Raper, A. B. (1962). *Brit. med. J.*, **2,** 303.
17. Fraser, I. D., Bothamley, J. E., Bennett, M. O., Airth, G. R., Lehane, D., McCarthy, M. and Roberts, F. M. (1976). *Lancet*, **1,** 6.
18. Friesen, R. F., Bouman, J. M., Barnes, P. H., Grewar, D., McInnis, C. and Bouman, W. D. (1967). *Amer. J. Obstet. Gynec.*, **97,** 343.
19. Holamn, C. A. and Karnicki, J. (1964). *Brit. med. J.*, **2,** 594.
20. Karnicki, J. (1966). *Proc. royl Soc. Med.*, **59,** 83.
21. Landsteiner, K. and Wiener, A. S. (1940). *Proc. Soc. exp. Biol. (N.Y.)*, **43,** 223.
22. Landsteiner, K. and Wiener, A. S. (1941). *J. exp. Med.*, **74,** 309.
23. Levine, P., Burnham, L., Katzin, E. M. and Vogel, P. (1941). *Amer. J. Onstet. Gynec.*, **42,** 925.
24. Levine, P., Katzin, E. M. and Burnham, L. (1941). *J. Amer. med. Ass.*, **116,** 825.
25. Liley, A. W. (1961). *Amer. J. Obstet. Gynec.*, **82,** 1359.
26. Liley, A. W. (1963). *Amer. J. Obstet. Gynec.*, **86,** 485.
27. Liley, A. W. (1963). *Brit. med. J.*, **2,** 1107.
28. Liley, A. W. (1963). *Pediatrics*, **35,** 831.
29. Liley, A. W. (1963). *Pediatrics*, **35,** 836.
30. Macrae, D. J. (1965). *Lancet*, **2,** 950.
31. McMullin, G. P., Hayes, M. F. and Arora, S. C. (1970). *Lancet*, **2,** 949.
32. Mollison, P. L. (1951). *Blood Transfusion in Clinical Medicine.* Oxford: Blackwell Scientific Publications.
33. Mollison, P. L. (1953). Personal communication.
34. Mollison, P. L., Mourant, A. E. and Race, R. R. (1952). *Medical Research Council Memorandum, No. 27.* London: H.M.S.O.
35. Multiple Authors: Prevention of Rh-Haemolytic Disease: Final Results of the "High-Risk" Clinical Trial. Combined Study from Centres in England and Baltimore. (1971). *Brit. med. J.*, **2,** 607.
36. Richings, J. (1973). *Lancet*, **1,** 1220.
37. Walker, W. (1959). *Brit. med. Bull.*, **15,** 123.
38. Walker, W. and Murray, S. (1956). *Brit. med. J.*, **1,** 187.
39. Walker, W., Murray, S. and Russell, J. K. (1957). *Lancet*, **1,** 348.
40. Walker, A. H. C. (1966). *Proc. roy. Soc. Med.*, **59,** 82.
41. Wallace, J. (1971). Personal communication.
42. Whitfield, C. R. and Sproule, W. B. (1972). *Lancet*, **1,** 382.
43. Wiener, A. S. (1941). *Amer. J. clin. Path.*, **14,** 52.
44. Wiener, A. S., Freda, V. J., Wexler, I. B. and Brancato, G. J. (1960). *Amer. J. Obstet. Gynec.*, **79,** 567.
45. Willoughby, M. L. N. (1967). Personal communication.
46. Willoughby, M. L. N. (1976). Personal communication.
47. Yong, C. K. (1965). *Brit. med. J.*, **2,** 1125.

CHAPTER XXIX

ULTRASONICS IN OBSTETRICS (SONAR)*

THE term "sonar" is used to cover this subject in order to distinguish it from high-power ultrasound, which is employed in a number of destructive processes in industry and as a therapeutic source of heat generation at depth within the tissues in therapeutics. Sonar employs energies so low that it is difficult even to measure them.

The breakthrough, if such it can be called, came most easily in gynaecology and obstetrics[25, 34] because in the former, tumour masses come readily to laparotomy, often within a matter of days, and a diagnosis can be quickly confirmed or revised. Medical disorders such as, for example, hepatomegaly and splenomegaly are less immediately explored surgically and by the time the case comes to necropsy the whole picture may have altered from the time at which the original sonar investigation was made. In pregnancy the outcome of the case is likely to be known within a matter of weeks and again there is a ready feedback of information. In this way it was possible for those of us who work in this field to develop an extensive experience very rapidly over the space of a few years and our mistakes have been every bit as instructive as our successes.

Definition

Sonar stands for "sound, navigation and ranging" and is akin to "radar". This technique was developed by Professor Langevin for the French and British Admiralties during the First World War to combat the growing U-boat menace.[49] Later, in time of peace, it was used for oceanographic exploration. The term therefore acknowledges its historical maritime origins.

The reason for using ultrasound instead of ordinary sound is that energy generated as ultrasound is emitted in beam form of predictable velocity with very little divergence. The precise point of origin of an echo therefore can be determined, and when dealing with a multiplicity of echoes such as occurs within the human body, their

* Much of the material in this chapter was published in the Silver Jubilee number of the *Journal of Obstetrics and Gynaecology of India* (Volume xxv, pp. 70–84), and the author wishes to make his acknowledgments to the editors.

positions can be mapped out and displayed by cathode ray oscillography.

Differences between Sonar and X-rays

Both Sonar and X-rays can penetrate tissues far more efficiently than light or heat, which lose energy more extensively from the surface inwards. Both ultrasonic and X-ray energies are transmitted in wave form but thereafter all points of similarity cease. In the case of X-rays the energy belongs to the electromagnetic spectrum, in which the higher the frequency (and therefore the shorter and more refined the wavelength) the more effective is the penetration of bodily tissue. Ultrasound on the other hand is simply sound of such a high frequency (and therefore short wavelength) that it is inaudible to animal hearing, which in the case of the human seldom exceeds a frequency of 20,000 vibrations a second (20 KHz). In medical diagnosis, sonar uses frequencies in the megahertz, i.e. million per second, range, but unlike X-rays the higher the frequency the *less* readily does the ultrasonic beam penetrate tissues. Penetration must therefore be secured by a sufficiently low frequency, with a concomitant sacrifice of resolution. At a commonly employed frequency of $2\frac{1}{2}$ million vibrations a second ($2\frac{1}{2}$ MHz) the wavelength in tissue is of the order of 0·7 mm and is too coarse for histological purposes. Therein lies an inherent limitation. The diagnosis of malignancy, for example, can be no more than suggested on inferential grounds, and still rests upon histological study.

A radiograph is essentially a shadow picture with the patient situated between the source of X-rays and a screen or photographic plate on the far side. Shadows depend partly upon the densities of the tissues traversed and to an even more important extent upon their mineral content, particularly that of calcium. Ultrasonic pictures on the other hand are "reflection maps". Numerous attempts have been made to produce shadow pictures as in the case of X-rays, but there is no method comparable to the photographic film for recording ultrasonic shadows by a through-transmission technique, which for sonar requires a mosaic diaphragm of some quartz-type of material with piezo-electric qualities (see later) which has to be maintained under vacuum and scanned by an electron beam. The need for the vacuum on one side of the material limits the size that can be used to about 10 cm at most and, compared with photographic film, the resolution of any picture is very low.

From the above it will be seen that X-rays of a fetus *in utero* are useless until the fetal skeleton at least has enough mineral content to give a shadow, whereas in the case of sonar the fetus in its surrounding liquor is not so very different from a submarine in the ocean and the echo phenomenon can be utilised.

Generation of Ultrasonic Energy and Processing of Signals

This requires a transducer, i.e. something which transforms one type of energy into another and vice-versa, in this case electrical energy into mechanical and mechanical energy into electrical (as in a gramophone pick-up). This is achieved by the piezo-electric effect, direct and converse. Only certain materials, initially quartz but nowadays more usually barium titanate or lead zirconate, have these piezo-electric qualities when cut as crystals along certain given axes. Wafers of these crystalline material, when struck by a controlled electrical discharge, respond by mechanical distortion at right angles to that discharge (the converse piezo-electric effect). The crystals are damped so that each electrical "blow" causes a brief mechanical oscillation lasting about 1½ microseconds. These electrical blows are distributed at a predetermined pulse repetition frequency (PFR) and the frequency with which the crystal rings, expressed in megahertz, depends upon the material, its thickness and dimensions. The commonly employed pulse repetition frequencies range from 25 up to 1,000 per second. We use a PFR of 600. It will be seen therefore that between each pulse there is a relatively long silent period during which the transducer is capable of receiving returning echoes. Each echo arrives back in turn, according to the depths from which it is received, in the form of mechanical energy which on striking the crystal face is converted by the piezo-electric effect into an electrical signal and this, after very extensive amplification and processing, can be applied to the deflection plates, cathode or grid of a cathode ray oscilloscope for visual display, or for any other display method of choice (Fig. 1).

Commonly in obstetrics and gynaecology one crystal is used both to transmit and to receive ultrasonic energy, except in the case of continuous ultrasonic machines employing the Doppler principle (see later), which employ two transducers, one transmitting and one receiving.

Echoes are generated whenever an ultrasonic beam in its passage through the body encounters a boundary, or interface as it is now known, between two different types of tissue. Every tissue in the body has its own specific acoustic impedance which is a product of the speed of the sound wave passing through it (c) and the density of that tissue (ρ). Both of these factors are known.

The specific acoustic impedance of any given tissue is therefore "ρc". The amount of energy reflected (E_r) at an interface between two differing substances or tisues (1 and 2) as compared with the impingent energy (E_i) is expressed in Rayleigh's law:

$$E_r = E_i \left(\frac{\rho_1 c_1 - \rho_2 c_2}{\rho_1 c_1 + \rho_2 c_2}\right)^2$$

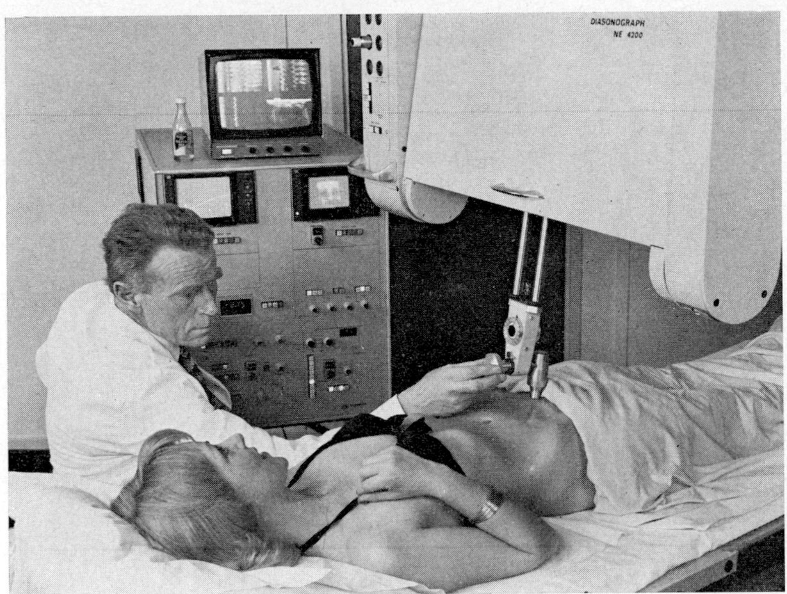

29/FIG. 1.—Diasonograph apparatus (EMI/Nuclear Enterprises Ltd) being operated by the author. All ultrasonograms throughout this book have been taken with this type of apparatus.

Expressed in direct language, this fraction of energy reflected can be calculated as the square of the quotient derived from the difference in the acoustic impedances divided by their sum.

The greater the difference in acoustic impedance of the tissues on either side of an interface, the stronger therefore will be the echo. Where the difference in acoustic impedance is very large, for example at a gas interface between the wall of intestine and the flatus contained within its lumen, more than 99 per cent of the energy is reflected. This limits the usefulness of sonar in gastro-intestinal diagnosis. More commonly only some of the energy is reflected, a little may be absorbed in the form of heat too small to be measured and the rest, in somewhat attenuated form, passes onwards into the rest of the body until it meets the next tissue interface and so on.

It is a pity that the ultrasonic characteristics of blood, pus, cerebrospinal fluid, urine, ascites and all other biological fluids are not distinguishable since they do not themselves contain sufficient reflecting properties. Haemoperitoneum therefore is not diagnosable as such but only as "echo-free fluid".

Ultimately the echoes may become so weak and the ultrasonic beams so attentuated that no information at depth can be obtained. To some extent this disadvantage can be countered by increasing the sensitivity of the amplifier, particularly to echoes emanating from a great depth, by a compensating electronic system of "time-varied gain"; that is to say, the longer it takes an echo to return, and therefore the greater its depth, the more is it automatically magnified. In this way the echo from the far parietal bone of the fetal head can be magnified to match that of the proximal parietal bone and likewise a posteriorly situated placenta can be visualised from the anterior aspect of the patient.

Where there are few interfaces, little energy will be reflected or absorbed, nor will there be much attenuation. In no instance is this more obvious than in the case of fluid-containing structures such as cysts. One of our earliest observations[34] was therefore that cysts demonstrated their far walls with great clarity, whereas a fibromyoma tended to attenuate the ultrasonic beam until it was progressively harder to make out its dimensions and depth. The bladder, too, transmits ultrasound equally well when full of urine, since it behaves like an ovarian cyst.

These early observations led to a ready ability to distinguish between solid and cystic masses and our first interest was in differentiating massive ascites from massive ovarian cysts.[27] In the case of cysts the contours could be readily mapped, whereas in ascites the intervention of bowel floating amongst the fluid produced a mass of echoes whose distribution might help to indicate the nature of the ascites, for example that due to peritoneal carcinomatosis. An ovarian cyst containing many echo-reflecting components might suggest by its very complexity that it might be malignant although, as already stated, the diagnosis of malignancy must rest on histological examination.

It has already been mentioned that the penetration which can be achieved by the ultrasonic beam is inversely proportional to the frequency. This provides a measure of the transparency of a given tumour mass to ultrasound. We now refer to its "transonicity". A fluid-filled cyst is transonic at a high frequency, for example of 5 MHz as easily as $2\frac{1}{2}$ MHz, whereas a fibromyoma might be easily transonic at $1\frac{1}{2}$ MHz, be poorly so at $2\frac{1}{2}$ MHz, and not transonic at all at 5 MHz. However the vascularity of a tumour mass influences its transonic properties and in pregnancy fibromyomata are more transonic than they would be in the non-pregnant, or particularly in the postmenopausal state. Areas of degeneration produce echoes within the substance of the fibroid since they may interrupt the steady attenuation of the beam as it passes through them.

When making a diagnosis therefore, whether it be of tumour mass, placental tissue or pelvic viscera in general, these physical factors have to be taken into account, namely, the frequencies employed, the power and amplification settings expressed as a ratio in terms of decibels, the time-varied gain used, also expressed in decibels, and the resulting character of the echoes.

The Two Types of Diagnostic Ultrasound

In medical practice two main varieties of ultrasound are used. The least complicated is that which employs the Doppler effect.[4, 41] Here a continuous beam of ultrasound is aimed at a moving, reflecting interface such as the fetal heart. The movement towards and away from the transducer shortens or lengthens respectively the time taken for that echo to return to it and hence the apparent frequency is noticably changed. This alteration can be processed as either an auditory or a visual signal. With such apparatus the fetal heart can be picked up, often from the 11th week of pregnancy onwards. The use of the Doppler principle is also applied to circulation blood flow studies but, it will be noted, this simple information depends on the existence of moving structures.

The other main class of ultrasonic echo sounding depends upon the pulse/echo principle. This allows echoes to be spatially separated in time and thus to be mapped. It is therefore used in differential

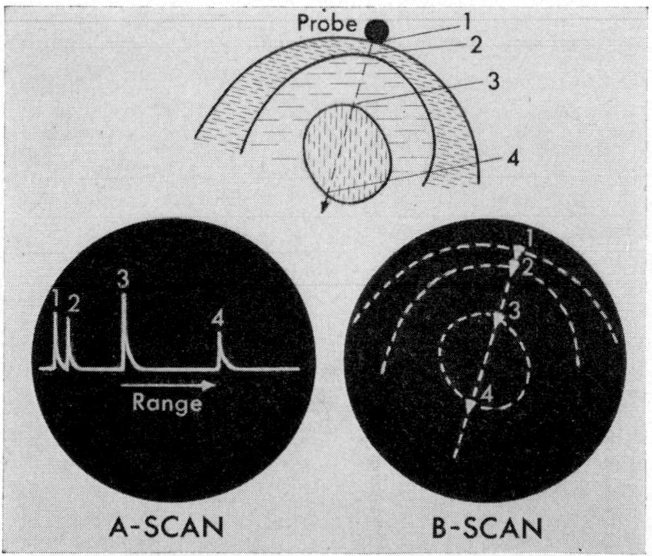

29/FIG. 2.—Diagram representing the differences between A-scan and B-scan (see text). The upper picture represents a hypothetical body with the probe placed upon the surface and directing the beam obliquely inwards, encountering three underlying interfaces; these are represented on the left of the figure as vertical blips (A-scan) and on the right in B-scan as light dots whose position corresponds to the position of each echoing interface within the body.

diagnosis since the appearances, often characteristic, are increasingly recognised. The two methods can be used in conjunction.

METHODS OF PRESENTATION OR DISPLAY

A-Scan

The simplest form, A-scan, is unidimensional. In this the echoes are superimposed as vertical deflections or "blips" on the time-base sweep of a cathode ray tube, the signal being applied to the appropriate deflector plate (Fig. 2). The distance from left to right on this time-base sweep represents the depth of origin of the reflecting interface and the height of the blip represents the strength of that echo, which in its turn depends on the difference in acoustic impedance on either side of the interface. In the case of the fetal skull these differences in acoustic impedance, compared with liquor and surrounding uterine muscle, are considerable, and the echoes are readily recognised. Time-varied gain compensation can bring the far echo from the posterior parietal bone up to parity with the near one. The midline structures, mainly the falx, produce weaker echoes midway between the two (Fig. 3). Biparietal cephalometry provides the most frequent indication for the use of A-scan.[26]

A-scan is applicable in the measurement of the distances between structures whose position is known. In ultrasonic echo sounding, as in the case of light physics, the laws of reflection and refraction apply and good echoes can only be received if the ultrasonic beam strikes the reflecting interface at perpendicular or what is called "normal incidence", otherwise the reflected beam is diverted away from the receiving transducer, and if the angle of incidence exceeds the critical angle, refraction, too, will occur, with consequent misleading distortion.

Biparietal Cephalometry

Biparietal cephalometry is only accurate and useful in so far as the true diameter can be identified.[33] By mapping the head first by a two-dimensional technique (see later) and calculating the angles of its attitude correctly a proper A-scan measurement can be made.[8] This technique requires practice and precision but we aim for errors of less than 1 mm (Figs 3 and 4).

Biparietal cephalometry supplies about two-thirds of the workload of most ultrasonic departments in obstetric units. It is the only measurement of the head which can be made independently of the presentation or the degree of flexion or deflexion attitudes. Fortunately it is also the easiest to reach, particularly in vertex presentations, since the head commonly engages in the occipitolateral position, and the anterior parietal eminence is fairly accessible provided the head

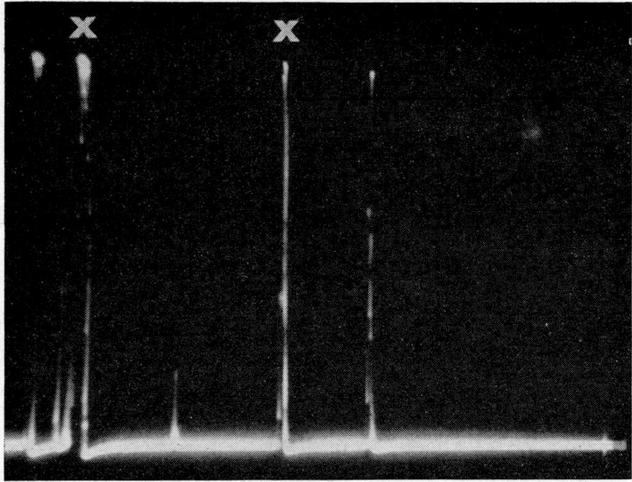

29/Fig. 3.—Fetal biparietal cephalometry by A-scan. The distance between the two large blips (X—X) is proportional to the biparietal distance. Note the smaller midline echo.

is not too deeply engaged. (In this event the examination can be facilitated by allowing the patient's bladder to fill and lowering the head of the examination couch in order to disengage the head sufficiently.)

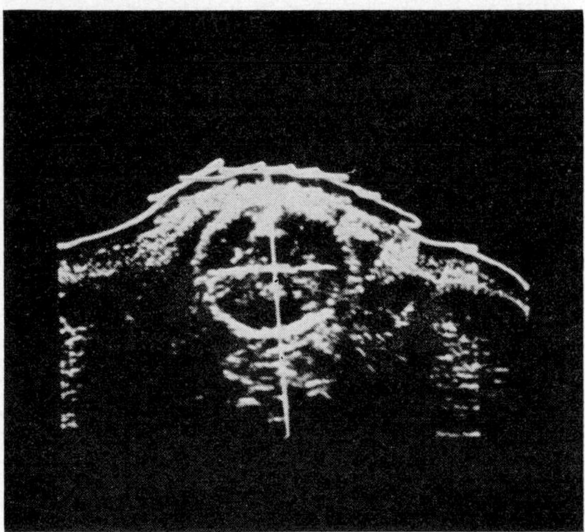

29/Fig. 4.—Demonstration of the position of the biparietal diameter on B-scan. The measurement of the biparietal diameter cannot be made so accurately here as by measuring the position of the leading left edges of the appropriate blips on A-scan.

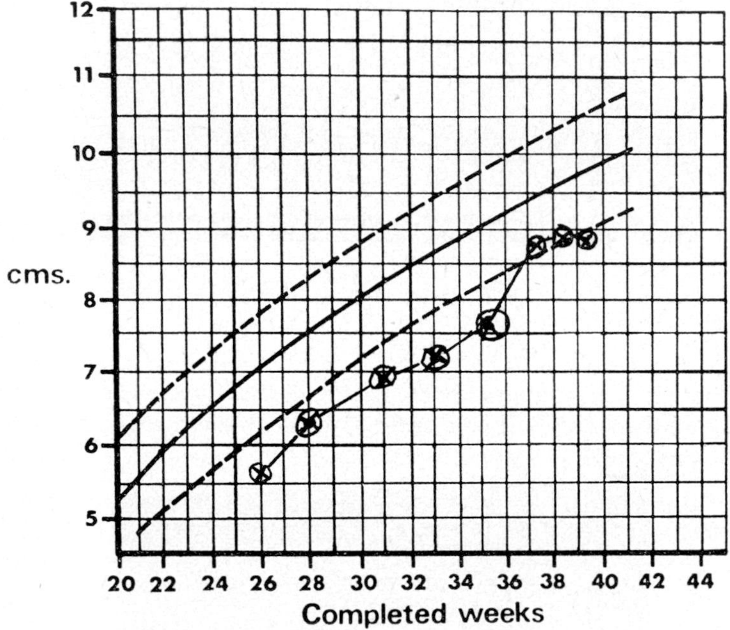

29/Fig. 5.—Intra-uterine growth retardation showing biparietal diameter "lag curve" in a dysmature baby. Delivery by Caesarean section at term because of apparent cessation of growth and bad obstetric history. Oestriol excretion amounts throughout the last 10 weeks of pregnancy were less than 55 μmoles per 24 hours. Birth weight was 2·08 kg.

(By courtesy of Appleton-Century-Crofts, New York. *Obstetrics and Gynaecology Annual, 1977*, edited by Ralph Wynn, M.D.)

Numerous studies have shown that there is greater correlation between the biparietal diameter of the fetal head and the maturity of the fetus than between the actual weight and maturity.[19, 64, 65] If the thoracic measurements are combined with biparietal measurements a better estimate of fetal weight can be made.[2, 39, 61] The sequential study of biparietal diameters provides an index of intra-uterine growth rate and therefore of fetal well-being, and it is standard

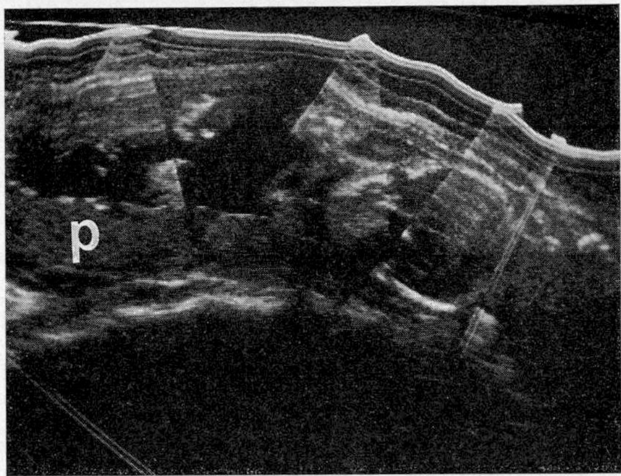

29/FIG. 6(*a*).—Longitudinal scan, cephalad to left, of normally growing pregnancy in a woman with three previous mid-trimester abortions. Fetal head is to right. Maturity 25 weeks. Note placenta posteriorly situated (p) and maternal aorta behind. (Grey-scale picture.)

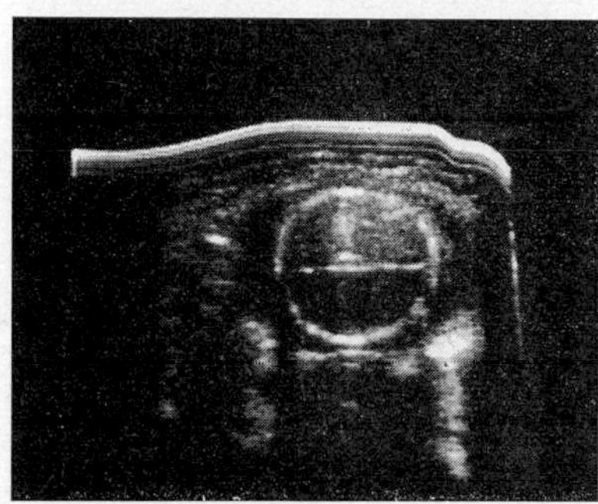

29/FIG. 6(*b*).—Same head of fetus as in 6(*a*) in transverse view in almost perfect biparietal plane. Note circular shape of head at this stage.

practice with us and many other units to use this technique at repeated intervals and to plot the growth curve in conjunction with oestriol excretion rates in the hope thereby of recognising the fetus which is showing intra-uterine growth retardation (Fig. 5). In this instance the slope of the curve becomes more horizontal than the norm. We use the curve established by Campbell while working in our department.[8] In contrast, mistaken dates will show a growth slope which, although not coinciding with the accepted curve, runs more or less parallel to it.

This technique serves to monitor intra-uterine fetal health on the basis of the argument that a fetus outrunning its placental nutritional reserve fails to grow adequately. This also helps to reduce mistakes in estimating maturity, especially when induction is being contemplated. Lastly it may indicate a degree of disproportion, due to an overgrown head, likely to complicate labour. X-ray cephalometry is, by comparison, notoriously unreliable, since any errors in estimating the distance of the fetal head from the X-ray tube or screen are thereby magnified.

The best estimates of maturity can be made before the thirtieth week, up to which time the head is so circular that its diameter is easily measured (Fig. 6). From the thirtieth week onwards the head acquires a more oval shape with a longer occipitofrontal than biparietal diameter, and therefore the technique becomes not only more difficult but also more open to error. Readings therefore early in pregnancy are of great value.

Two-dimensional B-Scan Presentation

In this system the signal from the returning echo to the transducer is applied to the cathode or grid of a cathode ray tube, thereby increasing or reducing the electron emission from the cathode gun. This alters the brightness of the dot of light created by the impinging electron beam on the tube phosphor. The brightness is thus to some extent intensity-modulated according to echo strength. Furthermore the direction of the ultrasonic beam is taken into account in the positioning of this dot of light upon the cathode ray screen, so that it geometrically represents its position of origin within the body. In this way a whole succession of dots can build up a continuous contour (Fig. 2). Bearing in mind the need for an ultrasonic beam to strike an interface at normal incidence, B-scanning may miss a great deal of available information unless it is compounded by a system of transducer-rocking so that as many interfaces as possible are identified, if not from one direction then from another.[20, 33, 34] Thereby more echo information may be obtained but always at the expense of some resolution. Even so, echoing interfaces which are not orientated at normal incidence in all three dimensions may deflect echo information and the structure may only be properly visualised if the whole probe system is tilted into a more appropriate plane. A search technique is therefore always necessary. In the case of fetal cephalometry we commonly search for the head first of all in longitudinal section to find its angle of asynclitism if any, and we then scan transversely at the predetermined point with the whole scanning head tilted to this angle.[8] The measurements should match, whether the biparietal dimensions are measured in longitudinal or transverse section. Failure to carry out this technique in full is bound to lead to bad results.

Time-motion Display

This is used to depict graphically the movement pattern of a structure, such as for example the fetal heart. While the Doppler technique is successful for simply detecting its presence and its rate, it indicates nothing of the pattern of movement itself. Robinson in this department has developed time-motion scanning for the earliest detection of the fetal heart within the first few weeks of pregnancy.[53] First of all the fetus is identified within its sac by compound B-scanning. Simultaneously the A-mode is applied to a second screen and pulsation is watched for in the form of vertical blips being displaced at an appropriate rate, around 160 beats per

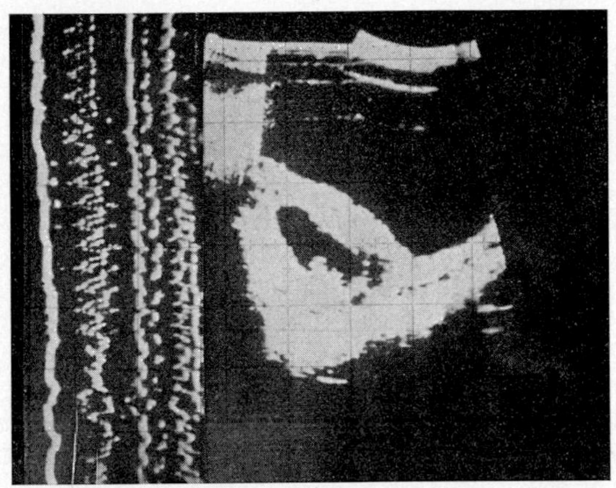

29/FIG. 7.—Nine-week fetus (menstrual age) lying at the bottom of early gestation sac in anteverted uterus viewed through full maternal bladder. Time-motion display of fetal heart superimposed to left of picture.

second, from left to right and vice-versa, on the A-scan trace. Having therefore determined which point of the fetal mass on B-scan contains the pulsating structure, the third method of display is now brought into play in which the time-base sweep is spread at a known rate across the face of the tube from below upwards. The echoes, instead of being represented as blips are converted to intensity-modulated light dots and with the movement progressively of the time-base sweep these light dots trace a movement pattern across the face of the tube (Fig. 7). The fetal heart can thus be detected far more early than by the Doppler technique, even by the 6th week after the onset of the last menstrual period. Proof positive is thus obtained, even at this early stage, of continuing intra-uterine fetal life. This movement pattern can also be sought in any structure which might be thought to be the second head of a twin when in fact one might be looking at the thorax and heart of a single fetus. The pulsating structure prevents one from making such a mistaken diagnosis of twins.[24]

PATIENT MANAGEMENT

For a diagnostic technique to be acceptable it must not involve the patient in pain, indignity or hazard. Sonar meets these requirements admirably. The patient lies simply upon an examination couch and normally the examination is made through the anterior abdominal wall. Since an air interface reflects over 99 per cent of ultrasonic energy, good contact has to be made with the patient's skin. Here two techniques are available. The earliest methods involved immersing the patient naked in a tank of water. This is clearly not acceptable particularly in the sick or the pregnant. Another alternative is to apply a flexible tank of water to the abdominal wall, coupled with some air-excluding jelly. This method is still used but for the patient who is supine it increases the likelihood of hypotensive phenomena. It is cumbersome, uncomfortable and restricting. Furthermore the interface between tank and skin reflects very powerfully and the depth of water has to exceed that of any subsequent echo thereafter, otherwise a series of false reverberations will be set up which interfere with the resulting picture.

The Australian technique of having a patient on a more or less vertical frame gets rid at least of the supine, hypotensive difficulties.[44] Our own preference has always been for direct-contact scanning, applying the transducer probe directly to the abdominal wall. Coupling is achieved by liberally smearing the abdominal wall with an air-excluding lubricant; warmed olive oil is easily the least objectionable. Poor quality pictures are commonly obtained from an insufficiently liberal use of air-excluding oil.

The technique is quick and this is important as sometimes patients begin to feel faint after lying in the dorsal position on a hard examination couch, due to the supine hypotensive syndrome. In this case the examination must either be halted and the patient turned on to her side, or the need for this may be temporarily postponed by raising her feet up in the air on the shoulders of an assistant and also by lowering the head end of the couch.

When the direct-contact method is used, as is our practice, the patient experiences no discomfort nor does she feel any sensation, and even a very sick patient can be examined without being moved from her bed.

USES AND INDICATIONS FOR SONAR

The current scale of usage is shown in Table 1.

29/TABLE 1

ULTRASONIC EXAMINATIONS AT QUEEN MOTHER'S HOSPITAL, 1975

Class of examination	*Number*
Biparietal cephalometry	2057
First trimester	911
Placental localisation	737
Non-pregnant	112
Kidneys and liver	203
Neonatal ventriculography	18
Retained products	137
Total	4175

The following is a list of the main indications for investigations by sonar.

29/TABLE 2

INDICATIONS FOR SONAR INVESTIGATIONS IN PREGNANCY

Early pregnancy	*Middle and late pregnancy*	*Puerperium*
Early gestation sac	Fetal growth rate	Retained products
Implantation site	Maturity	Involution
Growth rate	Twins	Caesarean scars
Blighted ovum	Associated tumours	Haematoma
Placental differentiation	Hydramnios	Associated tumours
Maturity	Placentography	Urinary retention
Early diagnosis of twins	Placental development	Renography
Abortion—all varieties	Rh placental changes	Puerperal pyrexia
Retained products	Caesarean section scar integrity	
Hydatidiform mole	Renal complications	
Associated pelvic tumours		

EARLY PREGNANCY

Until we came to use the full bladder as a method of gaining ultrasonic access to the depths of the pelvis,[15] our examination of the gravid uterus was restricted to cases where the uterus was already palpable over the symphysis pubis. However, to an increasing extent since 1963 we have been able to examine the pregnant uterus from the very early stages of gestation,[16, 22]

The full bladder displaces bowel which would otherwise interfere with the examination, and provides an extremely efficient sounding tank with practically no intermediate absorption of ultrasonic energy.[38] The uterus which is not even enlarged can be examined equally well whether retroverted or anteverted.

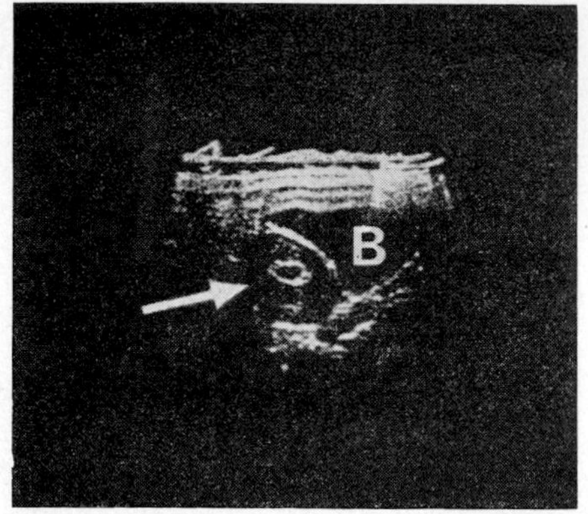

29/FIG. 8.—Very early intra-uterine pregnancy. The gestation sac (arrow) is nidated at a reasonably high level within the uterine corpus which is partially outlined behind a semi-full bladder (B). Period of gestation: six weeks plus 5 days' amenorrhoea in a normal cycle.

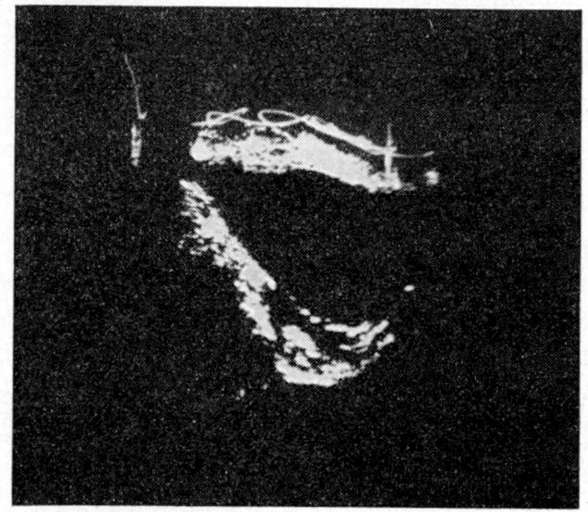

29/FIG. 9.—A very early pregnancy after between six and seven weeks' amenorrhoea with a low implantation, in which pregnancy proceeded no further than very early abortion.

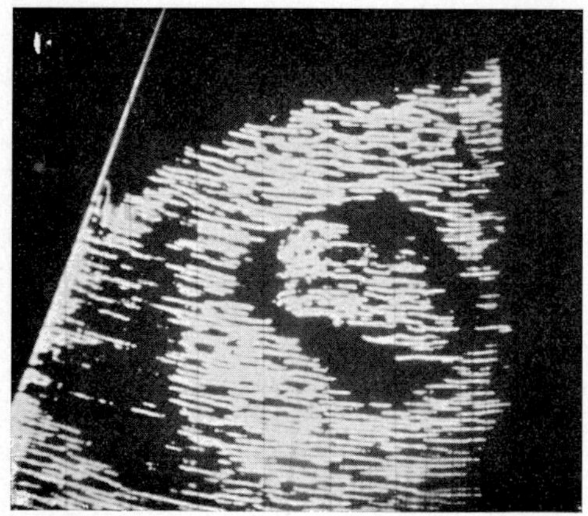

29/FIG. 10.—Early ten-week fetus in enlarged view showing early development of ? cerebral vesicles to left.

(By courtesy, Dr Judy Caines.)

A gestation sac first appears as a fine, white ring, often before the sixth week of gestation (menstrual age) (Fig. 8). The level of nidation can also be observed. In favourable circumstances this should be in the upper segment. A low level of the gestation sac may indicate the imminence or the start of the abortion process (Fig. 9).

By the seventh week of amenorrhoea it is usually possible to identify the fetal pole within the gestation sac with certainty (Fig. 7), and even to measure its crown/rump length (Fig. 10).[54] This fixes maturity very reliably to within about half a week.

Using the time-motion display method the fetal heart can be picked up from the sixth week of amenorrhoea onward (Fig. 7),[53] and if it cannot be found by the end of the seventh week it signifies the possibility that intra-uterine fetal death has already occurred and that the ovum is blighted.

Blighted Ovum

The phenomenon of blighted ovum is now recognised as very common, often recurrently so in the woman with a bad history. Some of these cases are due to genetic abnormalities[12] and chromosome karyotyping is always undertaken whenever we can obtain the tissue ultimately passed. Frequently the patient may not even be aware of her conception and may simply think her "period" was delayed. Several signs indicate the diagnosis of blighted ovum in addition to the absence of a demonstrable fetal heart.[35] These are: a poorly formed ring with speckling, or a gestation sac ring which is incomplete; in other cases the ring is consistently empty and no fetal pole can be found in it (anembryonic blighting); and finally, all signs of further growth are absent over the course of a week or more (Fig. 11*a* and *b*).

If the patient has been examined because of a history of bleeding and a provisional diagnosis made of threatened abortion, the discovery of ovum blighting spares her much unnecessary treatment aimed at conserving the pregnancy and the inevitable disappointment later.

Abortion

It is in the study of abortion in all its varieties that sonar has much to offer since, by examination through a full bladder, it is easy to determine whether the uterus is empty or not, or whether it contains an intact pregnancy or retained products of conception from an incomplete abortion.[20] So great is the reliance which we have now come to place upon this, that, provided a patient is not actually bleeding heavily, we do not subject cases of abortion to routine curettage unless the presence of retained products indicates it (Fig. 12*a* and *b*). This has made a very marked difference to our bed usage.

Maturity

So accurate is the estimate of maturity now in early pregnancy that the information may be vital later on towards its end.[22, 54]

The rate of fetal growth *in utero* is now clearly well recognised and greatly influences the prognosis.

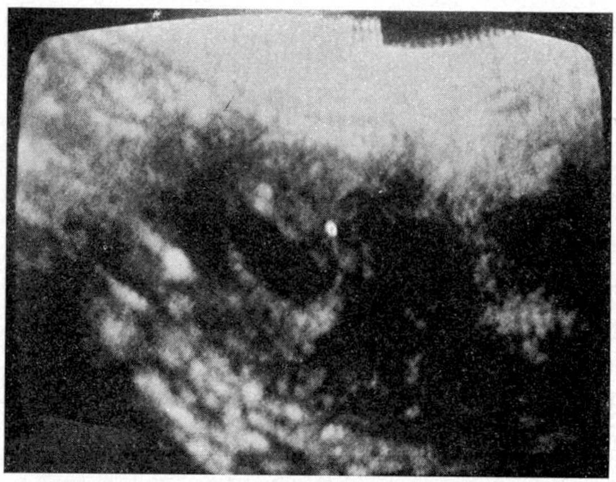

29/Fig. 11(*a*)—Blighted ovum with minimal signs of fetal echoes in gestation sac in spite of enlargement. Eight days later aborted a $2\frac{1}{2}$ cm diameter sac while flying over mid-Atlantic. Specimen retrieved.

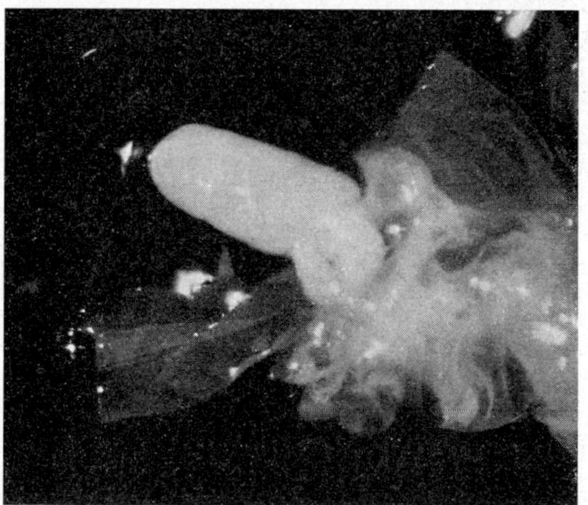

29/Fig. 11(*b*).—Retrieved specimen of blighted ovum. On tissue culture it proved be have an abnormal karyotype.

(By kind permission of the mother, herself a gynaecologist.)

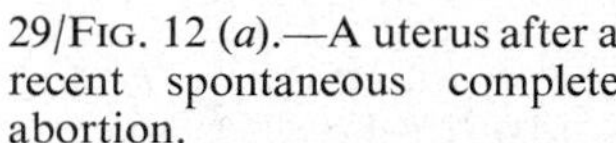

29/Fig. 12 (*a*).—A uterus after a recent spontaneous complete abortion.

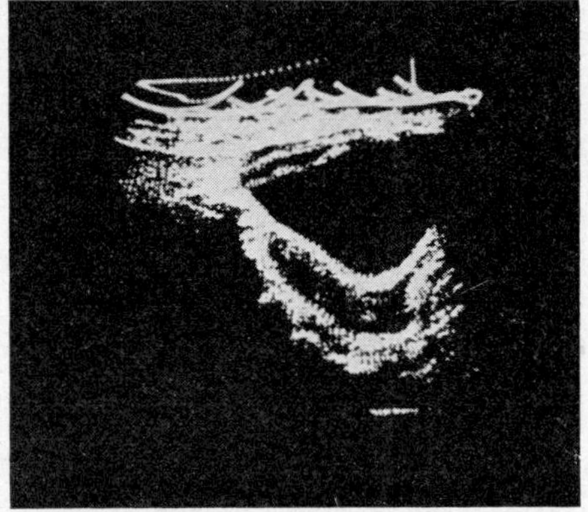

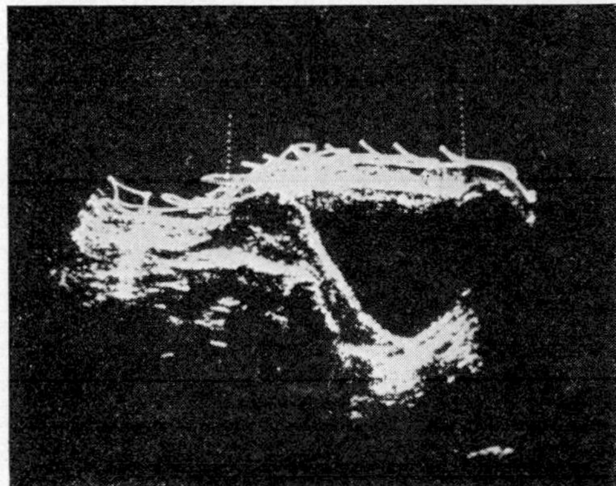

29/Fig. 12 (*b*).—A recent incomplete abortion with retained products of conception in the upper segment and a curious "waisting", often seen in cases of recent abortion. Length of uterine cavity was found to be four inches (10.16 cm), and retained products of conception were later removed.

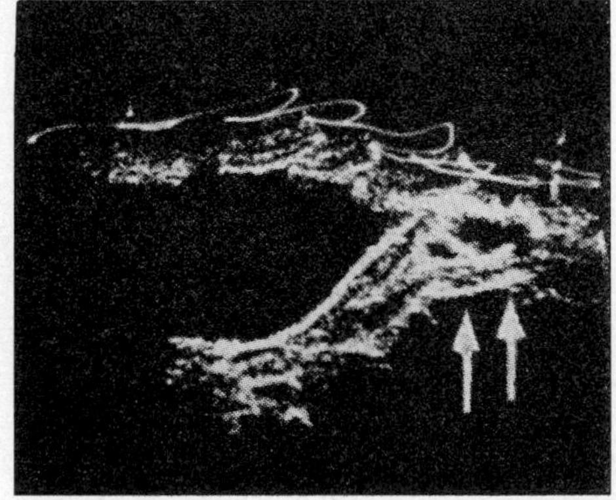

29/Fig. 13.—Twin gestation sacs (two arrows) in a uterus displaced upwards and behind a very full bladder. Period of amenorrhoea: 7½ weeks. Investigated for threatened abortion. Twin pregnancy continued. In this picture the fundus of the uterus is to the right.

Twins

A diagnosis of twin pregnancy can be made often well before the end of the first trimester (Fig. 13) and the feat of diagnosing quintuplets by sonar at the ninth week, at Queen Charlotte's Hospital in London, is now famous.[9]

Occasionally by the eleventh week and more often by the twelfth week of amenorrhoea the fetal head may be identified on B-scanning. From then onwards the fetal head provides the best index of maturity, since the growth is rapid at this stage of pregnancy.

Ectopic Pregnancy

Our biggest disappointments have been in the diagnosis of ectopic pregnancy. In so far as the gestation sac may be seen within the uterus one may be assured that the case is not one of ectopic pregnancy. Otherwise the ultrasonic findings differ every bit as much as the clinical, physical signs, and depend upon which stage of disease is encountered ranging from the unruptured tubal pregnancy to tubal abortion with peritubal and pelvic haematocele, and frank rupture with acute haemoperitoneum. There may in fact be considerable difficulty in distinguishing between a pelvic abscess and pelvic haematocele and even haemorrhage from a corpus luteum.[18] The best that can be said is that sonar may provide an indication for examining the patient by laparoscopy so that in our department mistaken laparotomies for possible tubal pregnancy are now very rare.

"Large for Dates"

A common request for sonar examination in early pregnancy is made because the patient appears clinically "large for dates". This may be simply a question of mistaken maturity, easily settled by sonar,[10] but even more important is the diagnosis of a complicating pelvic tumour and the ability to distinguish between that due to a fibromyoma, for which the treatment is conservative, and that due to an ovarian tumour, which demands laparotomy in its own right (Fig. 14).[21]

Hydatidiform Mole

Bleeding in early pregnancy may provide problems in differential diagnosis which sonar does much to resolve. The varieties of abortion have already been mentioned, but striking success can be achieved in the diagnosis of hydatidiform mole long before other evidences, such as the passage of vesicles, warn the physician of the patient's very great danger.[52] The appearances of hydatidiform mole are those of a clearly transonic speckled mass within the uterus (Figs

15 and 16) which remains transonic with the posterior wall of the uterus still visible on reducing the gain settings of the apparatus by 15 decibels, even though the speckles themselves may be suppressed by this manoeuvre. Furthermore the diagnosis can be confirmed at the very high frequency of 5 MHz, a precaution which should always be undertaken if one is to avoid the mistake which we have made in the past of confusing myxomatous degeneration of a fibromyoma with hydatidiform mole.[17]

The diagnosis of fetal abnormality within the first half of pregnancy is only possible in a limited number of instances. For example the inability to find the fetal head raises seriously the possibility of anencephaly. Spina bifida is hard to diagnose using two-dimensional scanning, and requires a particularly lucky sectional view of the vertebral column (Fig. 17). Occasionally kidneys can be seen and also urine within the bladder. Hydramnios gives very characteristic appearances of large quantities of fluid with blob-like echoes floating within, presumably due to fetal limbs (Fig. 18).[58] The fetal thorax with the pulsating heart within it can be found and distinguished from a fetal head.

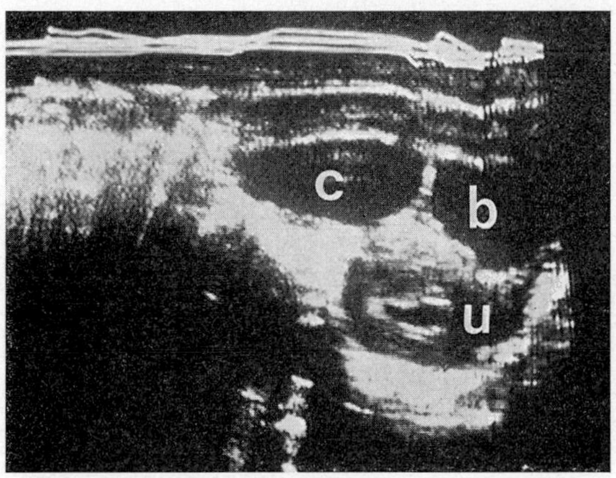

29/FIG. 14.—Ovarian cyst (c) above uterus (u) containing an anembryonic blighted ovum. Partially full bladder (b). Patient had had nine weeks' amenorrhoea after ceasing to take the contraceptive pill. Pregnosticon test positive.

When dealing with the possibility of abnormality in early pregnancy the role of sonar is chiefly in its ability to localise the placenta and indicate a safe site for amniocentesis. Placental differentiation can be observed progressively from the tenth week of pregnancy onwards and by the time at which amniocentesis is normally carried out, namely between the 14th and 16th weeks of pregnancy, localisation can be very efficiently determined.[3] This has enormously

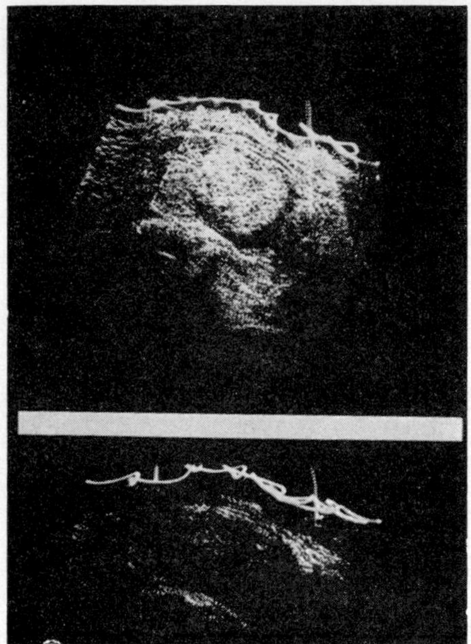

29/Fig. 15.—Hydatidiform mole visible in upper picture, at high-gain amplification, as a mass of "speckles" which become almost invisible at low gain (lower picture).

increased the safety of amniocentesis and reduced the risks of fetomaternal transfusion. Maturity can also be determined at the same time and is necessary for the interpretation of alphafetoprotein levels.

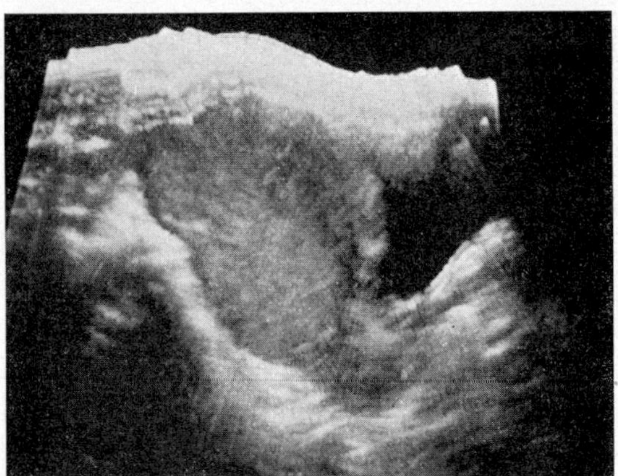

29/Fig. 16.—Grey-scale ultrasonogram of a recurrent hydatidiform mole, for the second time in the same patient.

(By coutresy, Mr A. D. Christie, Perth.)

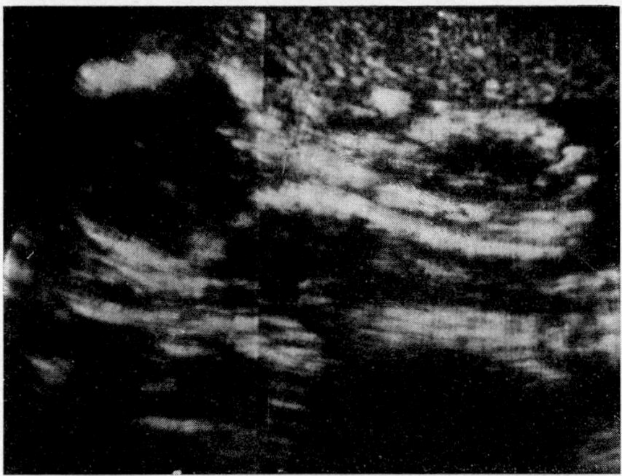

29/Fig. 17.—Fetal spine and head in enlarged view. Normal 17-weeks gestation in a case whose last pregnancy was anencephalic. The "tram-line" appearance of the spine is characteristic.

LATER PREGNANCY

The presentation of the fetus, even in the very obese patient, is not difficult since the head can be so easily found. It is recognised by its sharp contour and by the existence of a "mid-equatorial line", believed to be due to the falx (Fig. 4). Furthermore it contains no pulsating structures, unlike the thorax.

Growth and Maturity

Biparietal cephalometry represents the greatest single use of sonar in obstetrics. Not only is it immensely useful in determining maturity

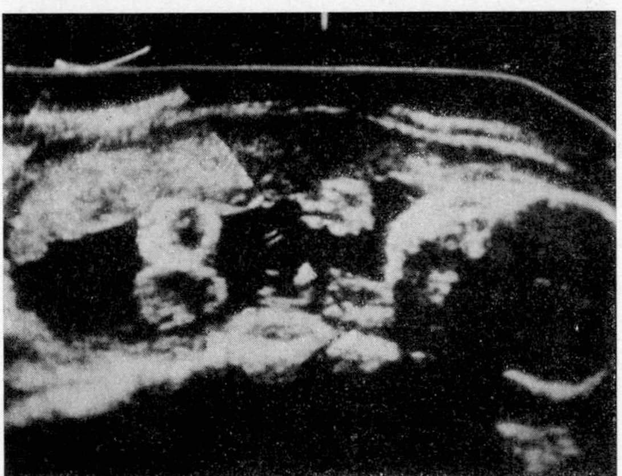

29/Fig. 18.—Hydramnios demonstrated by blob-like limb echoes in abundant liquor amnii. Fetal head to right, and upper anteriorly-situated placenta on left of picture.

but even more so in studying fetal growth rate. Except for sudden accidents in pregnancy, it is believed that the fetus which dies from placental subnutrition or insufficiency may give earlier warning of growth retardation.[1, 26] Combined with oestriol curves, which we undertake simultaneously, it is possible, by sonar, to recognise life-threatening dysmaturity and to interrupt the pregnancy before intra-uterine death occurs. This method of screening fetal growth is applied in all conditions known to interfere with it, such as, for example, hypertensive disease, renal disease, diabetes, and in all cases of a bad obstetric history (Fig. 5).

Ultrasonic measurements can be combined with transthoracic and transabdominal mensuration at the level of the ductus venosus, which is fairly easily identified on transverse sectional scanning, and a better forecast can then be made of fetal weight, which is less important.[11] But the technique may also help to distinguish between microcephaly and immaturity since the ratio of these measurements does not normally fall to unity under 36 weeks gestation.

Placental Location

Placentography is another common reason for employing sonar in obstetrics, and sonar is generally recognised as providing the method of choice since it is apparently safe, is easily repeated, and can be undertaken at any stage of pregnancy (Fig. 19); in fact, the earlier the easier.[32, 37, 45] It is indicated in all cases of antepartum haemorrhage and is singularly successful in identifying placenta praevia (Fig. 20). It is also employed in all cases of unstable lie, and always before amniocentesis.

With regard to the diagnosis of placenta praevia it is interesting to observe that the placenta in earlier pregnancy may appear to encroach upon the lower uterine segment and even to cover the os but in some cases, presumably with the taking up of the lower segment, the situation may improve and the placenta towards the end of pregnancy may appear to have "migrated" away from the praevia position.[42] The converse fortunately does not occur and a placenta identified earlier in pregnancy as safely within the upper segment does not later appear as one of placenta praevia.

With a properly positioned scan it should be possible to identify the fetal surface of the placenta by the very definite white line first observed by Kobayashi (Fig. 19).[43]

Our interest is now much concerned with studying the actual structure of the placenta particularly with regard to Rh haemolytic disease, diabetes and any condition likely to influence placental structure, size and growth.[24] The Rhesus placenta is certainly very large and thick and ultrasonically more opaque, but in making these estimates maturity has to be taken seriuosly into account since the

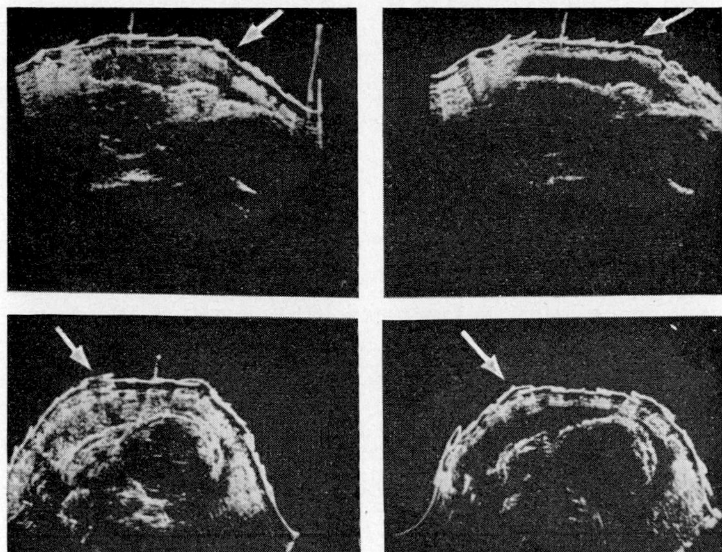

29/FIG. 19.—Upper anterior placenta. The two top pictures are in longitudinal section at high-gain and low-gain amplification respectively. The two lower pictures are of the same case scanned in transverse section at umbilical level, showing the placenta situated anteriorly and somewhat to one side.

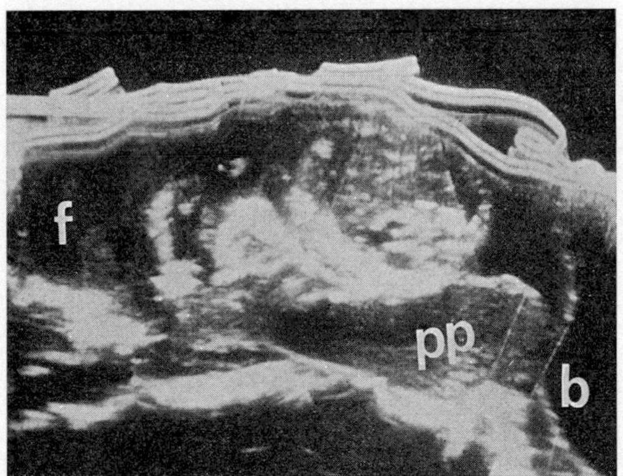

29/FIG. 20.—Major degree of posterior placenta praevia (pp) overlying cervical os, whose site is revealed by partially filled bladder (b). Fundal fibroid (f) to left of picture. 28 weeks gestation treated by conservative rest in hospital until emergency Caesarean section, necessary at 38 weeks for haemorrhage.

relative size of the placenta to the conceptus as a whole is greater in earlier pregnancy than at term.

A practical point worth remembering in placentography is to examine when the bladder is moderately full. This helps to indicate the position of the lower segment and facilitates the diagnosis of placenta praevia (Fig. 20).

"Large for Dates"—Differential Diagnosis

The diagnosis of twins depends in later pregnancy on the identification of two separate fetal heads (Fig. 21). It is also useful to determine which of the two heads is the larger, that of the first or that of the second-coming twin, since the hazards to the second twin are greatly magnified if it is the larger of the two. The diagnosis of triplets is not so easy because it is difficult to depict all three heads in one two-dimensional plane.

Hydramnios, as Sunden (1964) has demonstrated, is revealed by clear areas of fluid in which are curious, blob-like echo complexes, probably due to limbs floating in plentiful liquor amnii. This appearance is pathognomonic (Fig. 18).

Inability to demonstrate the fetal head at any level indicates anencephaly. Hydrocephaly is easy to recognise (Fig. 22).

Pelvic tumours associated with pregnancy are a particularly important field of ultrasonic investigation, since the presence of a large uterus in the second half of pregnancy may conceal a tumour, particularly in the very obese subject.

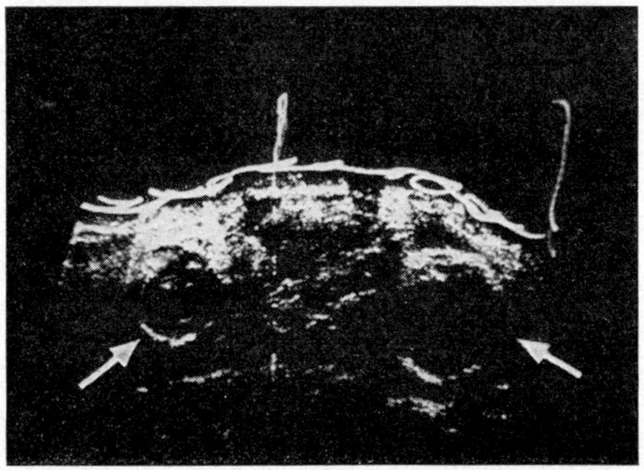

29/Fig. 21.—Twin heads at 29 weeks; the fundus of the uterus is on the left of the figure. Note that the second-coming head is the smaller of the two.

Previous Caesarean Section

In cases who have undergone Caesarean section in a previous pregnancy, examination of the scar, using the full-bladder technique, is worthwhile.[24] This requires very careful scanning from side to side across the whole length of the scar, and one is particularly alerted if the posterior surface of the bladder appears to be irregular or puckered.

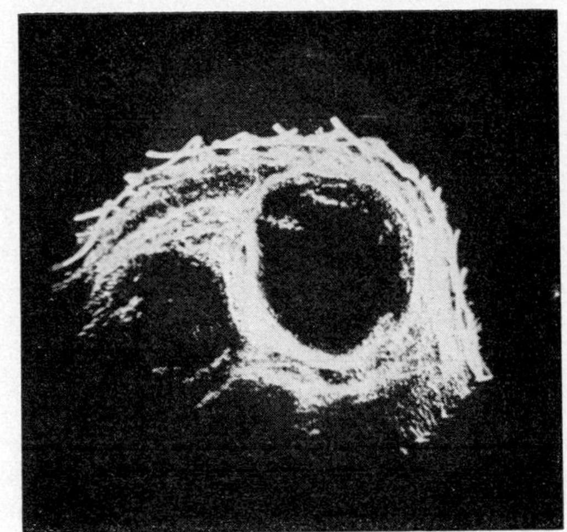

29/FIG. 22.—Hydrocephalus. The biparietal diameter, 13.75 cm, was measured by sonar. A tongue of placenta is indicated (top left of the figure). Two litres of fluid were removed by tapping the head by the abdominal route, avoiding the placenta (top right of the figure).

Fetal Abnormalities

Fetal abnormalities can usually only be detected in the case of the fetal head, for example, anencephaly, hydrocephalus and microcephaly (Fig. 22). As technique improves, spina bifida and cardiac and renal abnormalities will be more readily recognised but so far, sonar may at best do no more than indicate the need for radiography.

Puerperium

Cases of secondary postpartum haemorrhage have frequently to be examined by sonar to determine whether or not there are retained secundines. Subinvolution can likewise be differentiated. Often it is very obvious that the apparent failure of the uterus to involute is due to retention of urine, which is easily demonstrated without incurring the risks of catheterisation.

In a few instances we have picked up pelvic tumours in the puerperium which had previously escaped detection during the pregnancy. Cases of Caesarean section undergoing a stormy convalescence are worth examining. It may be found that a large haematoma is associated with the lower segment scar.[23] This can be differentiated by sonar from the bladder in front and the involuting uterus behind and may be seen to track at different levels towards the abdominal wall.

GREY SCALING

Until recently all echo information was provided on an "all-or-none" basis. That is to say that either a white echo dot was visible or it was not. This was partly because of the need to cut off irrelevant electronic "grass" and partly because of the limited range of echoes that could be handled.

The purpose of grey scaling is really to study tissue texture, and this is likely to be most useful in examining the placenta and also in examining the internal structure of the liver. In such an examination there should be no sacrifice in anatomical detail.

Our appreciation of tissue texture as distinct from anatomical structure was largely limited until recently by the dynamic range of standard cathode ray tubes which is restricted to about 16 decibels. Previously, therefore, attempts had to be made to compress the range of echo strengths logarithmically in order to include the maximum amount of information without at the same time introducing artefacts.[46, 47]

This hurdle has recently been overcome by the principle of "scan conversion". This was first developed in radio communication due to the need to convert American television, with its 525-line system, to the standard European 625-line system.[28, 29]

Ordinarily, cathode ray tubes convert electric signals into light when the electron beam on which they are carried, strikes an incandescent phosphor on the cathode ray tube face. In scan conversion the cathode ray beam emitted from the electron gun, modified in accordance with received echoes, strikes a silicon storage target, as in the Lithicon storage tube, which is coated with a fine mosaic of silicon oxide and silicon whose particles form a multiple array of capacitors capable of accepting a momentary charge. Their size is smaller even than the width of the impingent beam from the electron gun, which can itself be focused, but whose size is now the limiting factor in resolution.

The silicon oxide/silicon target does not itself emit visible light, but is raster-scanned by an electron beam which "reads" it. The information so picked up is then fed on to a standard television display unit (Fig. 23).

At least ten shades of grey can thus be presented without sacrifice of anatomical detail (see Frontispiece and Figs. 24–27). Resolution, too, is thus enormously improved since the light dot or "spot size" as it is called, on an ordinary phosphor screen or worse still, that induced from a storage mesh behind it in the case of a storage oscilloscope is, by comparison, of very coarse size.

The Lithicon storage scan-concertor tube has the additional advantage of what is called a "peak-value" memory which means that, within limits, it cannot be overloaded by inexperienced scanning and overwriting.

Our own apparatus incorporates not only scan conversion but also variable storage facilities with zoom magnification in addition to standard A-scan, B-scan and time-motion display systems.

The limit has almost been reached of what can be done with single transducer systems and the time has come to graduate from the "pin-hole camera" stage to "movie type cinematography". This brings us to real-time scanning.

REAL-TIME SCANNING

Here lies the direction of future development.[31] Real-time scanning involves the very rapid acquisition of two-dimensional pictures as in cinephotography, fast enough to be free of flicker, which means a frame rate of over 20 per second at least, and preferably more.

This is not easy to achieve with single-transducer systems because such rapid movement at the skin surface would be intolerable to the

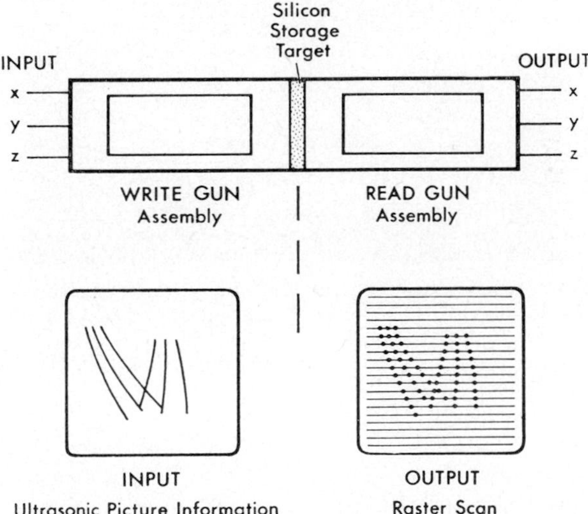

29/Fig. 23.—Diagram of principle of scan conversion. The echo information is written on to the silicon target (centre of diagram) using x, y, and z co-ordinates and this is then read in raster form and displayed on a standard television tube. It offers a more flexible format for processing and storage.

(By courtesy of Editor, *British Journal of Radiology*.)

29/FIGS. 24–27.—The following figures illustrate what can be achieved in grey-scaling with scan conversion.

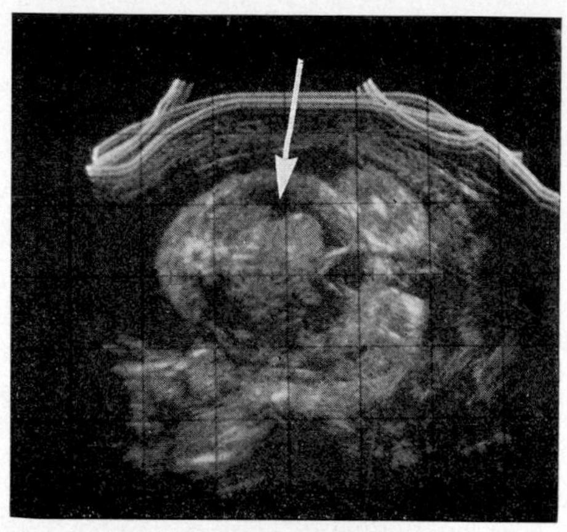

29/FIG. 24 (*a*).—Hydrops fetalis. Transverse section through lower trunk. Note spinal canal to left (white circle), ascitic fluid (arrow) and fetal bladder between thighs in Budda position.

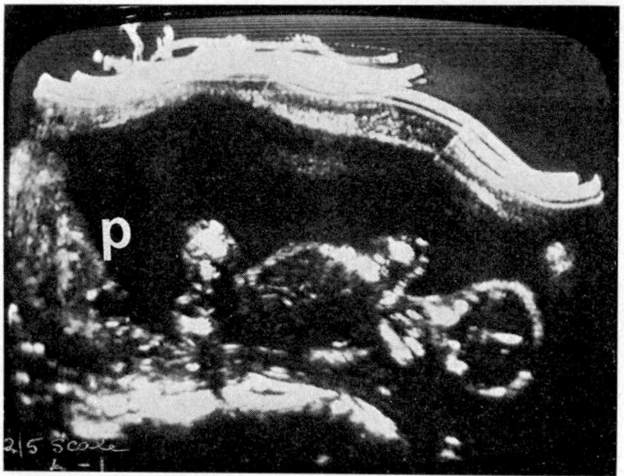

29/FIG. 24 (*b*).—Same case in longitudinal section. Breech presents. Gestation 31 weeks. Note Rh placenta (p). Successful intra-uterine transfusion after removal of 200 ml ascitic fluid. Baby ultimately succumbed three weeks later following premature delivery at 34 weeks as a "living hydrops" in spite of maternal plasmaphaeresis meanwhile.

(By courtesy, Dr Mary Pont.)

patient, and a stand-off tank system, as in the long-established Vidoson, is necessary. In this a single or, more recently, triple, transducer is mounted on a rotating cylindrical arm resembling that in a modern dish-washing machine inside a water filled tank. A parabolic mirror behind the rotating arm reflects a series of parallel beam lines projected through a plastic window fixed, with some air-excluding medium, to the patient's abdominal wall. As with all tank

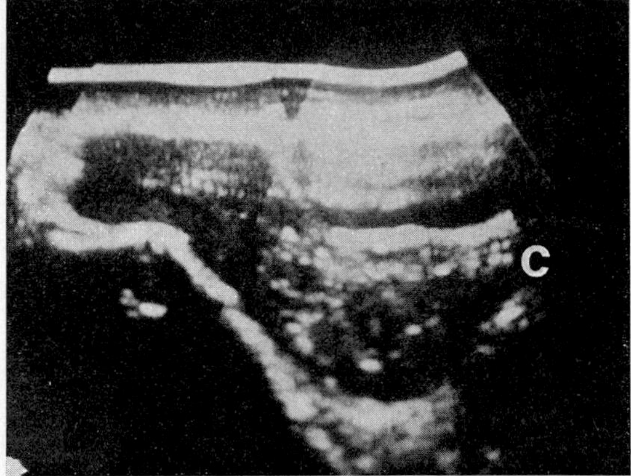

29/Fig. 25.—Inevitable abortion in progress. Dead 14-week fetus in lower part of uterus, and cervix (c) already dilating. Upper segment to left is already empty. Patient aborted one hour later.

systems, the length of the water column must exceed the depth of the structure within the body which it is hoped to examine, otherwise a series of reverberations corresponding to the depth of the water tank would spoil the picture. This adds greatly to the bulk of the scanning head. There are also limitations to resolution, and to the speed of frame presentation in order not to "trip over" preceding pictures.

The more modern approach is the use of multi-element transducer heads, sequentially fired in linear array, e.g. 1,2,3,4/2,3,4,5/3,4,5,6 and so on. With an array of 64 transducers, as for example in the

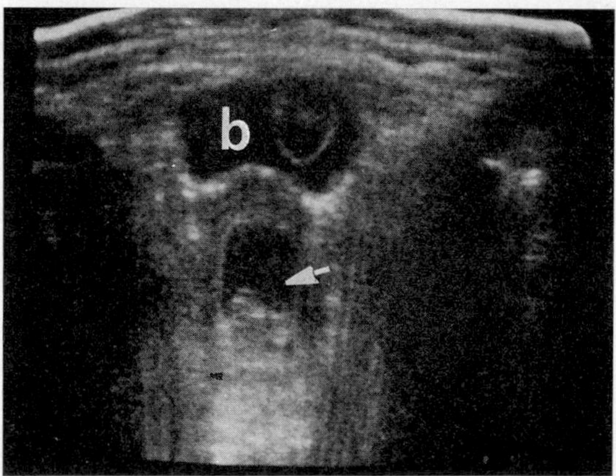

29/Fig. 26.—Incarcerated retroverted gravid uterus containing 13-week fetus (arrow). Note Foley catheter in bladder (b).

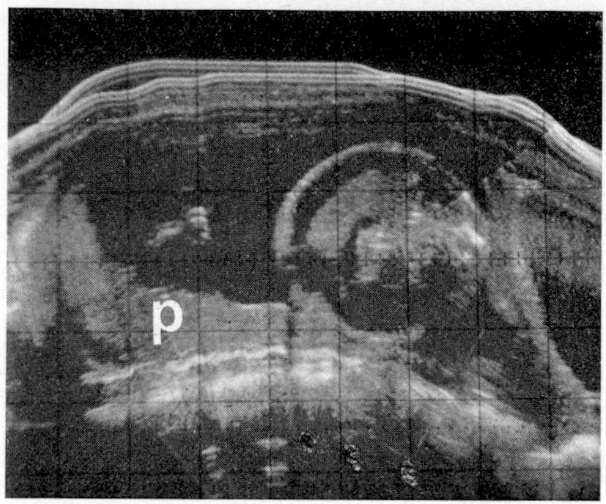

29/FIG. 27.—Mid-trimester fetus, head to right, with hydramnios. Chorio-angiomatous appearance of placenta (p).

(By courtesy, Dr Beresford Buttery, Melbourne, Australia.)

A.D.R. machine, 61 lines of discrete echoes are produced in sufficiently rapid succession to produce real-time pictures which can be recorded on videotape. Alternative new systems involve a phased array of fewer transducers within a highly mobile probe head in which, from a single viewpoint on the surface of the patient, an electronic sector-sweep scan is made wherever the operator wishes to look. This is achieved by firing each crystal in the probe head a minute fraction of time after its predecessor so that the ultrasonic wave front can be rapidly "steered" in a whole series of directions within the sector being examined.

I have had some experience of both systems. As yet they cannot match the pictorial quality of static single-transducer systems in current use; and cost, of course, is a factor to take into account; but in handling such probe systems one has the impression of extending the clinical range of one's palpating hands—altogether an exciting experience! To watch a baby in the middle trimester put its hand to its face as if to suck its thumb, or to observe its breathing movements[5] is truly amazing.

SAFETY

It remains to consider the question of the safety of this new diagnostic technique, particularly in pregnancy where it might be expected that rapidly growing fetal tissues were most vulnerable to the onslaught of any type of energy.

The hazards of X-radiology are already well known,[57] and by analogy there is a very natural fear that the same may apply to sonar, but the latter employs a mechanical as distinct from an ionising type of energy and the biological effects are different. High-power ultrasound can indeed produce heating and cavitation but this is not the case with diagnostic sonar. A great deal of work has already been done and the literature has become very extensive on the question of safety, but surprisingly little in the way of adverse results has so far been demonstrated. Teratogenesis and interference with normal development have not so far been found in spite of extensive search,[40] and much experimental work has been done on rodents, for example, right through to the second generation, in a search for mutagenic effects.[14, 56, 66]

The preliminary reports of chromosome defects, emanating from Cape Town,[50] turned out to be completely without foundation when the work was repeated at a number of other centres including our own.[1, 6, 7, 13, 51, 62, 63] Even placental enzyme changes have not been found.[55] High energies can produce damage occasionally in chick embryos at very early stages of gestation before the 13-somite stage, with exposure at point-blank range.[59, 60] Chick embryo capillaries lying parallel to a beam of standing ultrasonic rays demonstrate concentration and stasis of red cells at nodal points and possibly some endothelial damage,[36] but these experimental situations are far removed from clinical usage. The subject of the biological effects of ultrasound as used in diagnosis has been very fully reviewed by the writer in another volume,[30] and so far, experimental work has yielded reassuringly negative results. One of the problems is to know in which direction to look.

It has to be admitted that so far the whole subject of safety has been far more taken up with conjecture than with concrete experimental fact. Present-day ultrasonic diagnostic machines use such small levels of energy that they would appear to be safe, but the possibility must never be lost sight of that there may be safety threshold levels possibly different for different tissues, and that with the development of more powerful and sophisticated apparatus these may yet be transgressed.[30, 48] In the meantime the scope and usefulness of sonar, particularly in obstetrics and gynaecology, is gathering increasing momentum and ever-widening acceptance.

REFERENCES

1. Abdulla, U., Campbell, S., Dewhurst, C. J. and Talbert, D. (1971). *Lancet*, **3,** 829.
2. Anderson, G. V. and Niswonger, J. W. (1965). *Amer. J. Obstet. Gynec.*, **91,** 563.
3. Bang, J. and Northeved, A. (1972). *Amer. J. Obstet. Gynec.*, **114,** 599.
4. Bishop, E. H. (1966). *Amer. J. Obstet. Gynec.*, **96,** 863.

5. Boddy, K. and Dawes, E. S. (1975). *Brit. med. Bull.*, **31,** 3.
6. Boyd, E., Abdulla, U., Donald, I., Fleming, J. E. E., Hall, A. H. and Ferguson-Smith, M. A. (1971). *Brit. med. J.*, **2,** 501.
7. Buckton, K. E. and Baker, M. V. (1972). *Brit. J. Radiol.*, **45,** 340.
8. Campbell, S. (1968). *J. Obstet. Gynaec. Brit. Cwlth*, **75,** 568.
9. Campbell, S. and Dewhurst, C. J. (1970). *Lancet*, **1,** 101.
10. Campbell, S. and Newman, G. B. (1971). *J. Obstet. Gynaec. Brit. Cwlth*, **78,** 513.
11. Campbell, S. and Wilkin, D. (1975). *Brit. J. Obstet. Gynaec.*, **82,** 689.
12. Carr, D. H. (1965). *Amer. J. Obstet. Gynec.*, **97,** 283.
13. Coakley, W. T., Slade, J. S. and Breeman, J. M. (1972). *Brit. J. Radiol.*, **45,** 328.
14. Connolly, C. and Pond, J. B. (1967). *J. biomed. Engng.*, **2,** 112.
15. Donald, I. (1963). *Brit. med. J.*, **2,** 1154.
16. Donald, I. (1965). *Amer. J. Obstet. Gynec.*, **93,** 935.
17. Donald, I. (1965). *J. Obstet. Gynaec. Brit. Cwlth*, **72,** 907.
18. Donald, I. (1967). In: *Fifth World Congress of Gynaecology and Obstetrics*. Ed. C. Wood. p. 530. Australia: Butterworth.
19. Donald, I. (1967). *Brit. J. Radiol.*, **40,** 604.
20. Donald, I. (1968). *Brit. med. Bull.*, **24,** 71.
21. Donald, I. (1969). *Amer. J. Obstet. Gynec.*, **103,** 609.
22. Donald, I. (1969). *J. Pediat.*, **75,** 326.
23. Donald, I. (1971). *Proc. roy. Soc. Med.*, **64,** 991.
24. Donald, I. (1974). *Amer. J. Obstet. Gynec.*, **118,** 299.
25. Donald, I. (1974). *Ann. roy. Coll. Surg. Engl.*, **54,** 132.
26. Donald, I. (1974). *Scot. med. J.*, **19,** 203.
27. Donald, I. (1974). *Ultrasound in Med. and Biol.*, **1,** 109.
28. Donald, I. (1975). *Scot. med. J.*, **20,** 177.
29. Donald, I. (1976). *Brit. J. Radiol.*, **49,** 306.
30. Donald, I. (1976). The biological effects of ultrasound. In: *Present and Future of Diagnostic Ultrasound.* Eds I. Donald and S. Levi. pp. 20–32. Rotterdam: Kooyker Scientific Publications.
31. Donald I. (1976). *J. clin. Ultrasound*, **4,** 323.
32. Donald, I. and Abdulla, U. (1968). *J. Obstet. Gynaec. Brit. Cwlth*, **75,** 993.
33. Donald, I. and Brown, T. G. (1961). *Brit. J. Radiol.*, **40,** 604.
34. Donald, I., MacVicar, J. and Brown, T. G. (1958). *Lancet*, **1,** 1188.
35. Donald, I., Morley, P. and Barnett, E. J. (1972). *J. Obstet. Gynaec. Brit. Cwlth*, **79,** 304.
36. Dyson, M., Woodward, B. and Pond, J. B. (1971). *Nature*, **232,** 572.
37. Gottesfeld, K. R., Thompson, H. E., Holmes, J. H. and Taylor, E. S. (1966). *Amer. J. Obstet. Gynec.*, **96,** 538.
38. Hall, A. H. (1972). Second world congress on ultrasonics in medicine. *Excerpta med.* (*Amst.*), **277,** 271.
39. Hansmann, M. (1974). *Gynäkologe*, **7,** 26.
40. Hellamn, L. M., Duffus, G. M., Donald, I. and Sunden, B. (1970). *Lancet*, **1,** 1133.
41. Johnson, W. L., Stegall, H. F., Lein, J. W. and Rushmer, R. F. (1965). *Onstet. and Gynec.*, **26,** 305.

42. King, D. L. (1973). *J. clin. Ultrasound*, **1**, 21.
43. Kobayashi, M. (1968). Personal communication.
44. Kossoff, G., Garrett, W. J. and Robinson, D. E. (1965). In: *Ultrasonic Energy: Biological Investigations and Medical Applications*. Ed. E. Kelly. p. 365. Urbana: Univ. of Illinois Press.
45. Kossoff, G. and Garrett, W. J. (1972). *Aust. N.Z. J. Obstet. Gynaec.*, **12**, 117.
46. Kossoff, G. and Garrett, W. J. (1972). *Obstet. and Gynec.*, **40**, 299.
47. Kossoff, G., Garrett, W. J. and Radovanovich, G. (1974). *Aust. J. Radiol.*, **18**, 62.
48. Lancet Editorial (1970). **1**, 1158.
49. Langevin, M. P. (1928). *Revue Général de l'électricité*, **23**, 626.
50. MacIntosh, I. J. C. and Davey, D. A. (1970). *Brit. med. J.*, **3**, 92.
51. MacIntosh, I. J. C., Brown, R. C. and Coakley, W. T. (1975). *Brit. J. Radiol.*, **48**, 230.
52. MacVicar, J. and Donald, I. (1963). *J. Obstet. Gynaec. Brit. Cwlth*, **70**, 387.
53. Robinson, H. P. (1972). *Brit. med. J.*, **4**, 466.
54. Robinson, H. P. (1973). *Brit. med. J.*, **4**, 28.
55. Robinson, H. P., Sharp, F., Donald, I., Young, H. and Hall, A. H. (1972). *J. Obstet. Gynaecc. Brit. Cwlth*, **79**, 821.
56. Smyth, M. G. (1966). In: *Diagnostic Ultrasound*. Eds C. C. Grossman, J. H. Holmes, C. Joyner and E. W. Parnell. pp. 296–299. New York: Plenum Press.
57. Stewart, A., Webb, J., Giles, D. and Hewitt, D. (1956). *Lancet*, **2**, 447.
58. Sunden, B. (1964). *Acta obstet. gynec. scand.*, **42**, Suppl. 6.
59. Taylor, K. J. W. and Dyson, M. (1972). *Brit. J. hosp. Med.*, **8**, 571.
60. Taylor, K. J. W. and Pond, J. B. (1972). *Brit. J. Radiol.*, **45**, 343.
61. Thompson, H. E., Holmes, J. H., Gottesfled, K. R. and Taylor, E. S. (1965). *Amer. J. Obstet. Gynec.*, **92**, 44.
62. Watts, P. L., Hall, A. H. and Fleming, J. E. E. (1972). *Brit. J. Radiol.*, **45**, 335.
63. Watts, P. L. and Stewart, C. R. (1972). *J. Obstet. Gynaec. Brit. Cwlth*, **79**, 715.
64. Willocks, J., Donald, I., Duggan, T. C. and Day, N. (1964). *J. Obstet. Gynaec. Brit. Cwlth*, **71**, 11.
65. Willocks, J., Donald, I., Campbell, S. and Dunsmore, I. R. (1967). *J. Obstet. Gynaec. Brit. Cwlth*, **74**, 639.
66. Woodward, B., Pond, J. B. and Warwick, R. (1970). *Brit. J. Radiol.*, **43**, 719.

APPENDIX A

"The Midder Bag"

A. Midwifery case with detachable and washable lining
Portable steriliser
Obstetric forceps to taste, e.g. Milne Murray, Kielland, Wrigely
3 Sponge forceps (ratchet-handled)
Ovum forceps
2 Large artery forceps
4 Small artery forceps
Vulsellum
Drew Smythe catheter
Scissors, large straight Mayo
Scissors, dressing
Scissors, strong curved
Dissecting forceps
Sims speculum, large
Bivalve speculum
Bard-Parker scalpel handle
Bard-Parker scalpel blades
Needle holder
Needles, various
Catgut No. 1 and No. 0 chromicised
Hegar's dilators (including large)
Spoon-flushing curette
Mouth gag
Tongue forceps
Guedel's airway (adult and child size)
Endotracheal tube
Laryngoscope with adult and infant blade
Aneurysm needle (small)
Circumcision shield
Mucus catheters
Trilene inhaler, e.g. Cyprane
Catheters, soft rubber
Torch light
Obstetric "helper"

Drugs:
- Prilocaine hydrochloride ½ per cent (Citanest)
- Entonox
- Pethidine
- Morphia
- Sparine. Omnopon
- Ergometrine
- Pitocin or Syntocinon
- Hyoscine
- Atropine
- Nikethamide
- Amyl nitrite
- Paraldehyde (for intramuscular injection).
- Largactil ampoules 50 mg, 100 mg

B. Gladstone-type bag with detachable and washable lining
2 kidney dishes
Sphygmomanometer
Stethoscope
Rubber or polythene sheeting
Rubber apron
Gloves (sterile)
Finger stalls.
Trilene
Albustix or Multistix
Clinitest
Acetest
Gauze dressing and roll
Sterile distilled water
Transfusion-giving set
Dried plasma
Saline for intravenous use
pHiso-Med antiseptic cream.

C. Portable foot operated suction pump.

APPENDIX B

Eclampsia

Equipment to be kept in readiness:

Mouth gag and prop
Lint-covered wooden spoon
Oxygen cylinder (full!)
Mask for oxygen
Guedel's airways
Tongue forceps
Hand lamp
Intravenous giving sets
Heminevrin 0·8 per cent (500 ml) 3 bottles
Apresoline (hydrallazine) 20 mg ampoules
Diazoxide 300 mg in 20 ml
Morphine 15 mg
Valium (diazepam) 10 mg ampoules
Epidural anaesthesia (if available).

APPENDIX C

Resuscitation of Newborn

Equipment to be kept in readiness in labour room:

Reception tray for infant
Mucus suction catheters (MacRae type—disposable)
No. 4 French catheters with square-cut ends for aspiration
Nasal catheters
Syringes (10 ml and 20 ml)
Adapters to suit
Oxygen cylinder (full) and key
Humidifying Woulfe bottle
Plastic funnel and/or mask for supplying oxygen
Baby airway
Infant laryngoscope
Battery (functioning!)
Endotracheal catheters and adapters (Warne)
Gauze swabs
Syringe (1 ml), with small needles for intravenous injection into cord
Narcan Neonatal (counteracts Fortral)
Veritain ampoules (0·02 g/1 ml)
Ampoule files
Heated towels and blankets
Sterile cord ligatures or disposable clamps
Sodium bicarbonate 8·4 per cent (1 mEq/ml)
Aquamephyton (vitamin K_1) 5 mg ampoules
Silver Swaddler (Henley's Medical Supplies) for transport of baby to hospital.

APPENDIX D

Flying Squad Equipment

(Doctor and midwife accompany)

A. *Tray of box*:

Sphygmomanometer
Stethoscope
Fetal stethoscope
Poly bag containing:
  1 Gown
  1 Underpad
  1 Plastic draw sheet
  1 Bin sac
  6 Sanitary towels
4 Packets gauze swabs
2 Packets cotton-wool balls
2 Sterile hand towels
3 Grey, 3 Green } Medicuts
2 Syringes (30 ml)
2 Syringes (20 ml)
2 Syringes (10 ml)
2 Syringes (5 ml)
2 Syringes (2 ml)
1 Insulin syringe
2 Extension sets with final filter

1 Bottle Dextrostix and lancets
6 Green, 6 Yellow } Gillette needles
6 Blood bottles
Ampoule Syntometrine
Pr scissors
Thermometer
2 Bottle-holders
Blood-giving set
Arm splint
2 Catheters and spigots
2 Cut-down cannulae
Roll Elastoplast
Airstrip dressings
Tacky labels
2 Mediswabs
Mouth wedge
Drugs:
  2 Ampoules pethidine 100 mg
  2 Ampoules morphine 15 mg
  1 Ampoule papaveretum 20 mg
  (These drugs are kept in the Controlled Drugs cupboard.)

B. *Base of box*:

Delivery box with Iowa needle
Pelvic examination box
Set of delivery instruments in bowl
Sterile gown and hand towel
Packet of green towels
Cut-down set
Recording material
Poly bag containing:
  Placenta bag
  Razors: bin sac

Sodium Amytal
Syntometrine
Syntocinon

(2) Calcium gluconate
Hydrocortisone
Lanoxin
Largactil
Sparine
Phenobrabitone

Swabs
Hand towel
2 Blood administration sets
Portable drip stand
Hunter lamp
2 Boxes of drugs: (*see* Chapter on Labour)
(1) Adrenaline 1 mg
Aminophylline
Ergometrine
Insulin
Lasix
Diazepam
Water for injection
2 Blankets
Intravenous fluids:
2 Plasma
2 Water for injection
1 Ringer lactate
1 Normal saline
1 Dextrose 5 per cent
10 Pairs sterile gloves.

APPENDIX E

Baby Born Outside

(Senior midwife accompanies)

A. *Delivery pack contents*:
Table cover
Under-buttock drape
Abdomen drape
Disposal bag
Cord clamp
Gallipot
3 Waxed bowls
24 Cotton-wool balls
2 Maternity pads
2 Swabs
2 Anal pads
2 Paper towels
1 Baby wrap
1 Large tray (placenta bowl).

B. *Case contents*:
Eezi-scrub brushes
Silver Swaddler
Waxed bag (for placenta)
CSSD packet containing:
  2 Small Spencer Wells forceps
  1 Pair of scissors
CSSD packet containing:
  2 Large Spencer Wells forceps
  1 large pair of scissors
Plastic drawsheet
1 Nurse's white gown
2 Mucus extractors
2 Ampoules of Syntometrine
1 Ampoule of ergometrine
Bottle of sodium chloride
2 Savlon sachets
Cord clamp
Bottle of methylated spirit
2 Thermometers—low reading and normal
Pair of gloves—sterile
Sphygmomanometer and stethoscope
2 Razors
Syringe (20 ml) and Jacques catheter
Syringe (2 ml) and needles
Delivery summary sheet (for recording purposes)
Set of procedure instructions
Hibitane obstetric cream
K.Y. jelly
4 Maternity pads
2 Incontinence pads
Change for telephone
Blease resuscitator
Sparklet O_2 cylinder
Nightgown
Packet of 10 Raytex swabs.

APPENDIX F

Ultrasonic Measurements

(Queen Mother's Hospital)

Biparietal Diameters (after Campbell)

Weeks	Cm	Weeks	Cm
13	2·25	28	7·56
14	2·84	29	7·82
15	3·32	30	8·13
16	3·69	31	8·29
17	4·01	32	8·54
18	4·39	33	8·80
19	4·72	34	8·98
20	5·04	35	9·22
21	5·36	36	9·30
22	5·66	37	9·49
23	6·12	38	9·62
24	6·42	39	9·75
25	6·73	40	9·85
26	6·94	41	9·91
27	7·31		

Crown/Rump Length (after Robinson)

Weeks	Days	Mm
7+	0	10
	2	12
	4	14
8+	0	17
	2	19
	4	22
9+	0	25
	2	27
	4	29
10+	0	33
	2	35
	4	39
11+	0	43
	2	46
	4	50
12+	0	55
	2	59
	4	64
13+	0	68
	2	72
	4	76
14	0	85

APPENDIX G

INFORMATION FOR PATIENTS

Specimen of booklet issued to patients of The Queen Mother's Hospital, Glasgow

General.—This maternity hospital, completed in 1964 under the National Health Service, has been paid for out of your taxes. It is therefore your hospital. Everything has been done to provide the atmosphere of a comfortable hotel rather than of a hospital. Nevertheless in the background is every up-to-date surgical facility and laboratory resource for coping with all types of emergency. We have looked, as far as we can, into the future in order to be able to take the fullest possible advantage of all new research discoveries. We have also to undertake our share of the training of the next generation of doctors and nurses. Above all, our primary objective is to provide a comprehensive maternity service for our patients under the best possible conditions. Consequently the Board and Staff are proud of the Queen Mother's Hospital and hope that you will be too.

We are trying to run this hospital with the minimum of rules for patients in the belief that, once they understand that everything possible is being done for them, they will wish to co-operate in making everyone around them particularly other patients, as happy as possible. So far we have had no reason to regret this policy.

Accommodation.—Apart from the Labour Ward Suite where your baby will be born the hospital is mainly made up of single and four-bedded rooms. There are also a small number of rooms of two and five beds. As far as possible we try to give a patient on admission a choice between a room to herself or a room in the company of others.

There are no private rooms and the cost of all treatment is met by the National Health Service. There is nothing in the way of treatment or care that you or any other patient can buy.

The wards open out on to what we call "Day Spaces" which are furnished with tables and television and radio sets and comfortable chairs specially suited for pregnant women. This is a place where you can meet your visitors and talk to your friends and to each other in comfort.

Telephone.—The telephone number of this hospital is ... The doctors have individual radio page sets which they carry in their coats enabling them to be called at once.

Admission.—In the course of your antenatal preparation you will be taught the signs that labour is starting. When you think that your labour has started and that you should be coming into hospital, get your husband or friend to telephone the hospital at the above number and state that you are coming in presently, giving your full name and, if possible, your hospital registration number. If you have a relative who has a car and can bring you in you are free to come by this means but you may come by ambulance. If you wish an ambulance the hospital will arrange it for you. Please telephone first in either case.

Please bring soft slippers, your toothbrush, a hairbrush, your toilet articles, a nightdress if you wish, a dressing gown if you have one, and Antenatal Appointment Card. It is not essential, however, to bring anything into hospital with you as we can supply all your needs. If possible, get your husband or a friend to come with you so as to take away any clothes or luggage which will not be needed while you are in hospital. If you bring your own nightdresses and underwear you will have to get them washed at home as the hospital laundry does not undertake private laundering.

In labour you will be given a room in the Labour Ward Suite to yourself in which you will spend the time of your confinement. Your husband can visit you there as often, and for as long as he wishes while you are in labour and may be present at the birth of the baby if you both wish. Husbands are welcome and a small sitting room is provided for them where they can relax. All operations both major and minor are undertaken in one of three adjacent operating theatres which are kept at instant readiness. Your husband, of course, cannot reasonably expect to be present in an operating theatre, but, as long as labour is normal you may find him a great comfort. This is a matter for you both to decide between yourselves.

Your Baby.—After your baby is born, you and your baby, provided he is fit and well, will be together in each other's company in the same room. This is called "rooming in". During this period you will be taught how to manage your baby in all respects and will get to know him thoroughly so that he is no stranger to you when you return home. Some women are keen to breast feed and others are equally anxious not to. We wish to make it clear that there is no compulsion in either direction and the choice is yours entirely. Your wish is usually ascertained well before labour. If you state that you do not wish to feed your baby nothing further will be said; your breasts will be dried up and your baby will be started on the bottle. Many women are anxious and keen to breast feed their baby and we certainly agree with them that this is the best way to bring up a baby. During the lying-in period Sister and the nursing staff will give you all the help you require to get the baby feeding well on the breast. You will find the results very rewarding for there is no better way for a baby to start its young life and no better or more natural food for it. Quite apart from this, in breast feeding a mother and her baby develop an understanding between each other which nothing will ever replace. Doctors think that breast feeding is every baby's birthright, but, by no hint or suggestion will we force this point of view on you if you wish otherwise. It is your baby after all and our job is to help you.

In order to make absolutely certain of your baby's identity he is double-labelled at birth. The name bracelets must not be tampered with or disturbed.

Lying-in Period.—This is the time spent in hospital after the birth of your baby and it has two main purposes; firstly, to get you as fit as possible after your labour, so that you can return home confident and able to cope with your new life; and secondly, to ensure that your baby has a safe start in life, that all his early feeding problems have been overcome and that you know how to manage him. We prefer not to make a set routine period of time for this important part of maternity care but to judge each case upon its needs and merits. You will however observe certain features. Adequate periods of rest are interspersed with properly graduated activity. The old days of keeping a normal case in bed for many days after having a baby have now gone and you will be encouraged to be up and active as soon as the doctors feel it is safe for you to do so. Under medical and nursing advice you will find that you have a choice of baths, showers and bidets for personal hygiene. Bidets are extremely helpful and are well worth learning how to use. Physiotherapists will also instruct you in methods of recovering your figure and getting your muscles back into tone.

Shopping.—Newspapers are sold from a trolley which comes round every day. On Mondays, Wednesdays and Fridays a mobile shop with toilet requisites, etc., will be wheeled round the wards by members of the Ladies Auxiliary Committee. Profits from the Ladies Auxiliary shop are used for the benefit of patients.

Meal Times.

8 a.m.	Breakfast
10 a.m.	Milk Drink
12 midday	Dinner
3 p.m.	Afternoon Tea
6 p.m.	Supper
9 p.m.	Hot Drinks

Visiting.—We try to avoid set rules about visiting but the following points may be of guidance and help. Visits are very important in the day-to-day life of a patient in hospital, but they can also tire a patient if overdone. With the exception of her husband it is suggested that *twenty minutes* is long enough for most patients.

There are no fixed visiting hours but the most convenient times from both the patient's point of view and that of the Staff is in the late afternoon after about 3 o'clock. Most patients are ready for bed not long after 8.30 p.m. and should be allowed the opportunity for a good night's rest. Visitors should avoid meal times because we have found that patients do not eat their meals properly if they have visitors present at the same time. Visitors, except husbands, should keep away while patients are feeding their babies because their presence distracts the mother and the baby does not feed so well. There is a rest period after lunch for all patients from 1 p.m. to 2.45 p.m. during which they should not be disturbed.

In the morning the doctors are busy going round and seeing the patients. At any time when doctors or nurses are dealing with the patient visitors will be asked to wait in the Hall until she is ready to be visited.

Visitors should always inquire from Sister or Staff Nurse whether the time is suitable.

The number of visitors is not formally restricted. It is obvious that if every patient had more than two visitors at one and the same time, the Day Spaces and wards would get overcrowded. It is hoped that patients and visitors will use their common sense.

We do not wish to exclude young children from visiting their mothers but they should not be brought into the presence of other patients' babies because of the very real danger that any of them might be incubating whooping-cough or some other such infection which would hardly be fair to another woman's child. Young children, therefore, should only visit their mothers either in the Day Spaces or in a single room—not in the wards.

For obvious reasons visitors are asked not to pick up and disturb babies.

Visitors with sore throats, colds, 'flu, diarrhoea, or any other infectious disease should, of course, stay away, because they are dangerous to patients and babies.

Visits by Clergy.—Your minister, priest or rabbi is welcome to visit you at any time. He is requested simply to announce himself to the Sister or Staff Nurse first. As far as possible privacy for any religious rites will be arranged.

Bus Routes.—Described as appropriate.

Smoking.—There can now be no doubt that smoking shortens life and encourages in years to come a number of extremely unpleasant diseases like bronchitis, heart disorders, breathing troubles and, worst of all, lung cancer. We feel that it is our duty to point out that this is now an accepted medical fact. You will not see any doctor or nurse smoking in your presence anywhere in the hospital. Visitors should not smoke while in the hospital. An exception might be made in the case of the husbands' room. Nevertheless you are free to smoke if you wish, provided that you do not inconvenience other patients. There is no need to smoke secretly in bathrooms and washplaces, making them unpleasant for others. You may smoke whenever you like—but not, please not, in the presence of other women's babies. If you are a smoker, please help us to keep the hospital fresh and unspoiled for the patients who will follow you by using the ash trays in the Day Spaces.

Social Worker.—If you have any personal or family problem connected with your confinement, you should make arrangements to see the Medical Social Worker. She is trained to give specialised help and advice on a variety of problems and she can be seen privately at the Antenatal Clinic. It is also possible to see her by appointment and if you wish to avail yourself of this service you should telephone her Department. If you wish to see her when you are in the ward, Sister will be pleased to arrange this.

Medical Certificates.—Please ask Sister about the Certificates to which you are entitled and she will help you to fill up the necessary forms and advise you what to do with them. As you probably know, money benefits are available to women who are covered by National Insurance and you should not lose the opportunity of claiming them.

Hairdressing.—A hairdressing service is available from Monday to Friday at very modest cost.

Money and Valuables.—It will be useful to have some petty cash but you will not need big sums of money. Please avoid bringing a lot of money or valuables with you. Large sums or valuables should be deposited with Sister for safe keeping and a receipt obtained. The Board of Management cannot accept responsibility for the loss of money or valuables which are not officially deposited with them for safe custody.

Mail and Telegrams.—Please ask your friends to address you by your full name, including your first name, and, where possible, the ward, to ensure prompt delivery of your letters and telegrams.

Telephone.—You may make outgoing telephone calls by means of the mobile public telephone which can be wheeled to your bedside if you are not able to get up and go to the call boxes in the hospital.

On Discharge from Hospital.—When taking your baby home you should have ready the following clothing outfit:

Vest	Mitts
2 Nappies	Bonnet
Gown	Shawl
Matinee Coat	

If your baby is bottle fed, remember to provide a supply of dried milk, bottles and teats at home for him.

Your family doctor will receive straight away a summary of your record while in hospital. A Health Visitor will call and will be able to advise you on a great many points. Please make sure that you know the arrangements for your post-natal examination. Please keep the appointment.

Registration of the Baby's Birth.—By law the birth of your baby must be registered within 21 days. The address of the Registration Office is . . .

Complaints and Comments.—We hope that you will find your stay with us both happy and comfortable. If, however, you have a complaint, please bring it to our notice. Complaints and suggestions should be addressed to the District Administrator. Unless they require urgent action, they will be brought before the medical and nursing staff at their weekly joint meetings when all suggestions for improving the services of our hospital are considered. If we can find a way of doing anything better we are naturally anxious to do so.

ALL GOOD WISHES

INDEX

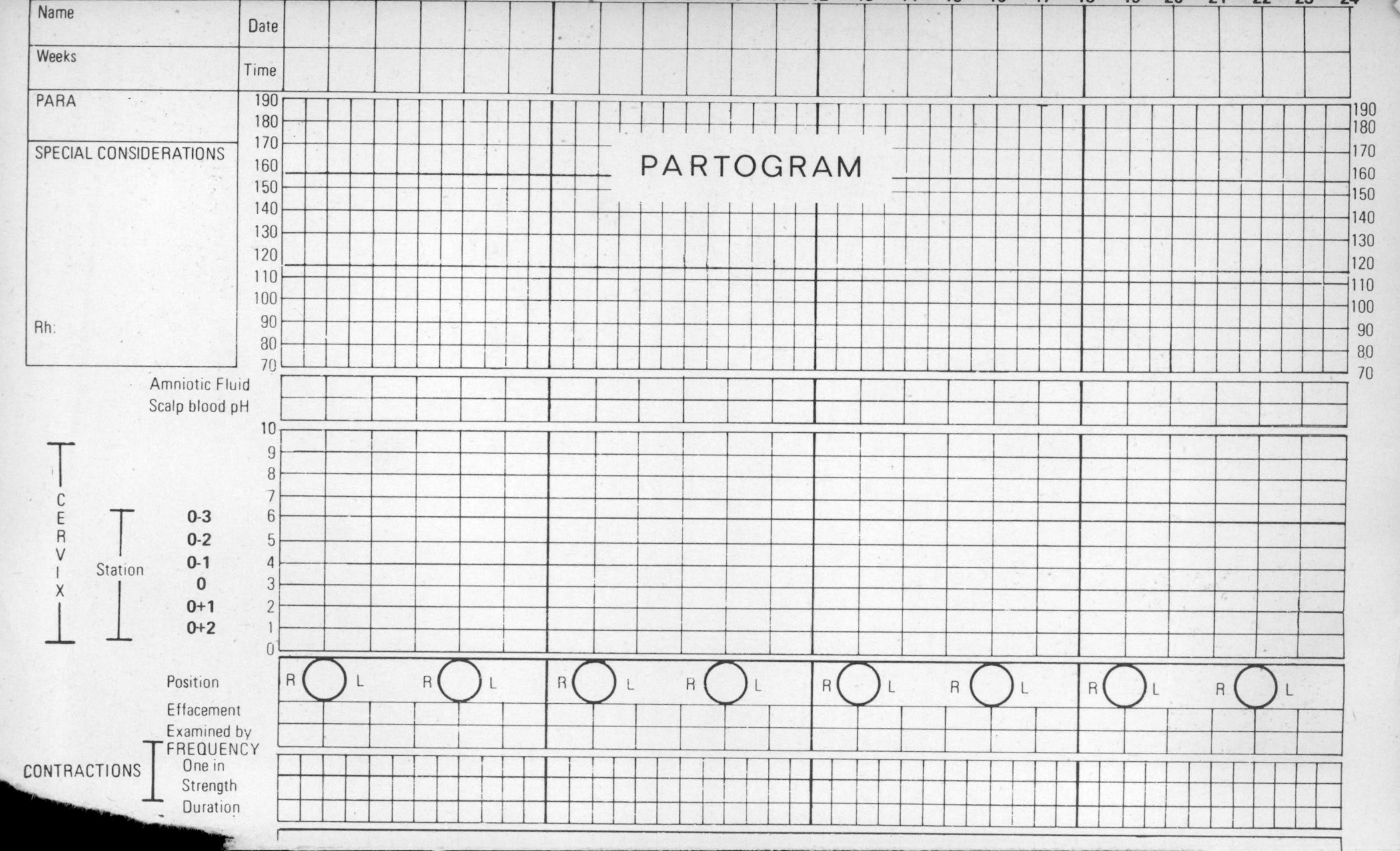
PARTOGRAM
Name
Weeks
Date
Time
PARA
SPECIAL CONSIDERATIONS
Rh:
190 180 170 160 150 140 130 120 110 100 90 80 70
Amniotic Fluid
Scalp blood pH
10 9 8 7 6 5 4 3 2 1 0
CERVIX
Station
0-3
0-2
0-1
0
0+1
0+2
Position
R L
Effacement
Examined by
CONTRACTIONS
FREQUENCY
One in
Strength
Duration
12 13 14 15 16 17 18 19 20 21 22 23 24